# Copeland and Afshari's
# Principles and Practice of
# CORNEA

***System requirement:***

- **Operating System—Windows XP or above**
- **Web Browser—Internet Explorer 8 or above, Mozilla Firefox and Safari**
- **Essential plugins—Java & Flash player**
  - Facing problems in viewing content—it may be your system does not have Java enabled.
  - If Videos don't show up—it may be the system requires Flash player or need to manage flash setting
  - You can test Java and flash by using the links from the troubleshoot section of the CD/DVD.
  - Learn more about flash setting from the link in the troubleshoot section.

***Accompanying CD/DVD Rom is playable only in Computer and not in DVD player.***

CD/DVD has Autorun function—it may take few seconds to load on your computer. If it does not work for you then follow the steps below to access the contents manually:

- Click on my computer
- Select the CD/DVD drive and click open/explore – this will show list of files in the CD/DVD
- Find and double click file—"launch.html"

# DVD CONTENTS

# Copeland and Afshari's
# *Principles and Practice of*
# CORNEA

## Volume 2

*Editors*

**Robert A Copeland Jr** MD
Professor and Chairman
Department of Ophthalmology
Howard University College of Medicine
Howard University Hospital
Washington, District of Columbia, USA

**Natalie A Afshari** MD FACS
Professor of Ophthalmology
Director of Centers of Excellence at Duke Eye Center
Director of Cornea and Refractive Surgery Fellowship
Duke University Eye Center
West Campus Durham, North Carolina, USA

*Foreword*

**Claes H Dohlman** MD PhD

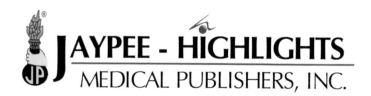

**Jaypee Brothers Medical Publishers (P) Ltd**

**Headquarters**
Jaypee Brothers Medical Publishers (P) Ltd
4838/24, Ansari Road, Daryaganj
New Delhi 110 002, India
Phone: +91-11-43574357
Fax: +91-11-43574314
**Email: jaypee@jaypeebrothers.com**

**Overseas Offices**

J.P. Medical Ltd
83, Victoria Street, London
SW1H 0HW (UK)
Phone: +44-2031708910
Fax: +02-03-0086180
**Email: info@jpmedpub.com**

Jaypee-Highlights Medical Publishers Inc.
City of Knowledge, Bld. 237, Clayton
Panama City, Panama
Phone: +507-301-0496
Fax: +507-301-0499
**Email: cservice@jphmedical.com**

Jaypee Brothers Medical Publishers (P) Ltd
17/1-B Babar Road, Block-B, Shaymali
Mohammadpur, Dhaka-1207
Bangladesh
Mobile: +08801912003485
**Email: jaypeedhaka@gmail.com**

Jaypee Brothers Medical Publishers (P) Ltd
Shorakhute, Kathmandu
Nepal
Phone: +00977-9841528578
**Email: jaypee.nepal@gmail.com**

Website: www.jaypeebrothers.com
Website: www.jaypeedigital.com

**Inquiries for bulk sales may be solicited at:** jaypee@jaypeebrothers.com

This book has been published in good faith that the contents provided by the contributors contained herein are original, and is intended for educational purposes only. While every effort is made to ensure accuracy of information, the publisher and the editors specifically disclaim any damage, liability, or loss incurred, directly or indirectly, from the use or application of any of the contents of this work. If not specifically stated, all figures and tables are courtesy of the editors. Where appropriate, the readers should consult with a specialist or contact the manufacturer of the drug or device.

*Copeland and Afshari's Principles and Practice of Cornea (Volume 2)*

*First Edition:* **2013**

ISBN 978-93-5090-172-4

*Printed at Ajanta Offset & Packagings Ltd., New Delhi.*

## *Dedicated to*

My loving and caring wife Candie and our three wonderful children Kennedie,
Robert III and Lucas. They were the reason why I embarked on this
quest to write and complete this textbook.

**Robert A Copeland Jr**

My parents for their incredible love and support.

**Natalie A Afshari**

# CONTRIBUTORS

**Justin Aaker** MD
Director of Cornea and External Disease
Scott and White Eye Institute
Temple, Texas, USA

**Lamis Abdel-Aziz** MBChB
Department of Ophthalmology
Harrogate District Hospital
North Yorkshire , UK

**Chrysavgi Adamopoulou** MD
Georgetown University Hospital
Washington Hospital Center
Department of Ophthalmology
Washington, District of Columbia, USA

**Natalie A Afshari** MD FACS
Professor of Ophthalmology
Director of Centers of Excellence at
Duke Eye Center
Director of Cornea and
Refractive Surgery Fellowship
Duke University Eye Center
West Campus Durham, North Carolina, USA

**Amar Agarwal** MS FRCS FRCO
Chairman and Managing Director
Dr Agarwal's Group of Eye Hospitals
Chennai, Tamil Nadu, India
Professor of Ophthalmology
Sri Ramachandra Medical College
Chennai, Tamil Nadu, India

**Iqbal Ike K Ahmed** MD FRCSC
Fellowship Director
Glaucoma and Advanced Anterior
Segment Surgery
Assistant Professor
Department of Ophthalmology and
Vision Sciences, University of Toronto
Toronto, Ontario, Canada

**Brian Alder** MD
Department of Ophthalmology
Duke University School of Medicine
Durham, North Carolina, USA

**Eduardo C Alfonso** MD
Director
Bascom Palmer Eye Institute
Kathleen and Stanley J Glaser
Chair in Ophthalmology
University of Miami Miller School of Medicine
Miami, Florida, USA

**Hind M Alkatan** MD
Senior Consultant Ophthalmologist
Chair of Pathology and Laboratory
Medicine Department
King Khaled Eye Specialist Hospital
Riyadh, Saudi Arabia

**Norma Allemann** MD
Professor
Department of Ophthalmology
Federal University of São Paulo-UNIFESP
Brazil
Adjunct Professor
Department of Ophthalmology and
Visual Science
University of Illinois at Chicago-UIC
Chicago, Illinois, USA

**Alfred L Anduze** MD MH
Island Medical Center
Kinghill, US Virgin Islands

**Arundhati Anshu** MMed (Ophth) FRCS (Ed)
Corneal and External Eye Disease
Service Consultant
Singapore National Eye Centre
Singapore, Singapore

**Fahd Anzaar** MD
Forbes Family Medicine
Forbes Regional Hospital
Monroeville, Pennsylvania, USA

**James V Aquavella** MD
Professor of Ophthalmology
University of Rochester
Flaum Eye Institute
Rochester, New York, USA

**Penny A Asbell** MD FACS MBA
Professor of Ophthalmology
Director of Cornea and
Refractive Services
Department of Ophthalmology
Mount Sinai School of
Medicine New York
New York, USA

**Kerry K Assil** MD
Medical Director
The Assil Eye Institute
Beverly Hills, California, USA

**Richard M Awdeh** MD
Assistant Professor of
Ophthalmology and Pathology
Director, Technology Transfer
Bascom Palmer Eye Institute
Miami, Florida, USA

**Dimitri T Azar** MD MBA
Dean, College of Medicine
BA Field Chair of
Ophthalmologic Research
Distinguished Professor
of Ophthalmology
Pharmacology and Bioengineering
University of Illinois at Chicago
Chicago, Illinois, USA

**Adel Barbara** MD MRCOphth
Medical Director of Hadassah Optimal
The Refractive Surgery Unit of Hadassah
Hospital in Haifa
Director of the National Center for the
Treatment of Keratoconus
President of the Refractive Surgery Society
Israel

**Ramez Barbara** MBChB
Department of Opthalmology
Bnei-Zion Medical Center
Technion Haifa, Israel

**Neal P Barney** MD
Professor
Department of Ophthalmology and
Visual Sciences
University of Wisconsin School of
Medicine and Public Health
Madison, Wisconsin, USA

**Mounir Bashour** MD CM PhD FRCSC FACS
Medical Director
LASIK MD
Associate Professor
McGill University
Montreal, Canada

**Sayan Basu** MBBS MS
Ophthalmologist, Biostatistician and
Scientist
Cornea and Anterior Segment Services
Sudhakar and Sreekanth Ravi Stem Cell
Biology Laboratory
Kallam Anji Reddy Campus, L V Prasad
Eye Institute (LVPEI)
Hyderabad, Andhra Pradesh, India

**Carolyn A Bates** PhD
Biomedical Strategic Communications
Tustin, California, USA

**Emily Baum**
San Diego, California, USA

**Michael W Belin** MD
Professor of Ophthalmology and
Vision Science
University of Arizona
Southern Arizona VA Healthcare System
Tucson, Arizona, USA

**John P Berdahl** MD
Vance Thompson Vision
Assistant Professor of Ophthalmology
Sanford University of South Dakota
School of Medicine
Sioux Falls, South Dakota, USA

**Brett Bielory** MD
Clinical Research Fellow, Cornea and
Refractive Surgery
Bascom Palmer Eye Institute (Miami Campus)
University of Miami-Miller
School of Medicine
Miami, Florida, USA

**Felix Bock** PhD
Laboratory Leader
Cornea Lab
Experimental Ophthalmology
LFI Gebäude 13
University Hospital of Cologne
Cologne, Germany

**Charles S Bouchard** MS MD
The John P Mulcahy Professor and
Chairman of Ophthalmology
Department of Ophthalmology
Loyola University Medical Center
Maywood, Illinois, USA

**Frank W Bowden III** MD FACS
Medical Director
Bowden Eye and Associates
Assistant Clinical Professor of
Ophthalmology
University of Florida, Jacksonville
Jacksonville, Florida, USA

**Kraig S Bower** MD
Associate Professor of Ophthalmology
Director of Refractive Surgery
Wilmer Eye Institute
Johns Hopkins University
Baltimore, Maryland, USA

**Kevin M Bowman** MD
Clinical Instructor
Department of Ophthalmology
Cornea Service
University of Minnesota
Minneapolis, Minnesota, USA

**James A Bradley** BS
Research Assistant
Boston Foundation for Sight
Needham, Massachusetts, USA

**Ninita Helen Brown** MD PhD
Department of Ophthalmology
Howard University Hospital
Washington, District of Columbia, USA

**Marieke Bruinsma** PhD
Netherlands Institute for Innovative
Ocular Surgery (NIIOS)
Rotterdam, The Netherlands

**Matthew Brumm** MD
Lecturer
Department of Ophthalmology and
Visual Sciences
University of Michigan
Ann Arbor, Michigan, USA

**Salim I Butrus** MD
Clinical Professor
Department of Ophthalmology
Georgetown University Medical Center
Washington, District of Columbia, USA
Director, Cornea Service
Department of Ophthalmology
Washington Hospital Center
Washington, District of Columbia, USA

**Alan N Carlson** MD
Professor of Ophthalmology
Chief
Corneal and Refractive Surgery
Duke Eye Center
Durham, North Carolina, USA

**John B Cason** MD
Commander, US Navy
Assistant Professor, Uniformed Services
University of the Health Sciences
Naval Medical Center San Diego
San Diego, California, USA

**Lorenzo J Cervantes** MD
OptiCare PC
Waterbury, Connecticut, USA

**Garrick Chak** MD
Gavin Herbert Eye Institute
University of California, Irvine
Irvine, California, USA

**Wallace Chamon** MD
Professor
Department of Ophthalmology
Federal University of
São Paulo-UNIFESP
Sao Paulo, Brazil

**Toby Y B Chan** MD FRCSC
Clinical Fellow
Glaucoma and Advanced Anterior
Segment Surgery
Department of Ophthalmology and
Vision Sciences
University of Toronto
Toronto, Ontario, Canada

**Devron H Char** MD
President, Tumori Foundation
Clinical Professor, Department of
Ophthalmology University of California
San Francisco (UCSF)
Clinical Professor, Department of
Ophthalmology Stanford University
Stanford, California, USA

**Bashira A Charles** PhD
Post-Doctoral Research Fellow
Center for Research on Genomics and
Global Health
National Human Genome Research Institute
National Institutes of Health
Bethesda, Maryland, USA

**James Chodosh** MD MPH
David G Cogan Professor of
Ophthalmology in the Field of Cornea and
External Disease
Massachusetts Eye and Ear Infirmary
Howe Laboratory
Harvard Medical School
Boston, Massachusetts, USA

**Jessica Chow** MD
Clinical Instructor
Bascom Palmer Eye Institute
University of Miami
Miami, Florida, USA

**Janine Austin Clayton** MD
Acting Director, Office of Research on
Women's Health
Office of the Director
National Institutes of Health
Department of Health and Human Services
Bethesda, Maryland, USA

**Tia B Cole** MScPH
Research Associate, Tumori Foundation
The Tumori Foundation
California Pacific Medical Center
Davies Campus
San Francisco, California, USA

**Michael Coleman** MD
Department of Ophthalmology
Kresge Eye Institute/
Detroit Medical Center
Detroit, Michigan, USA

**Robert A Copeland Jr** MD
Professsor and Chairman
Department of Ophthalmology
Howard University College of Medicine
Howard University Hospital
Washington, District of Columbia, USA

**Matthew D Council** MD
Assistant Professor
St Louis University School of Medicine
Department of Ophthalmology
Saint Louis University Eye Institute
St Louis, Missouri, USA

**Claude L Cowan Jr** MD MPH
Clinical Professor of Ophthalmology
Georgetown University Medical Center
Veterans Affairs Medical Center
Washington, District of Columbia, USA

**John W Cowden** MD
Chairman and Roy E Mason
Distinguished Professor
Mason Eye Institute
Department of Ophthalmology
University of Missouri School
of Medicine
One Hospital Drive
Columbia, Missouri, USA

**Andrea Cruzat** MD
Cornea Clinical Research Fellow
Massachusetts Eye and Ear Infirmary
Harvard Medical School
Boston, Massachusetts, USA
Attending Cornea and
Refractive Surgey Specialist
Department of Ophthalmology
Doctor Sotero Del Rio Hospital
Santiago, Chile

**Claus Cursiefen** MD
Professor and Chairman
Department of Ophthalmology
University of Cologne
Köln, Cologne, Germany

**Yassine Daoud** MD
Assistant Professor of Ophthalmology
Cornea, Cataract, and
Refractive Surgery Services
Wilmer Eye Institute
Johns Hopkins Medical Institutions
Baltimore, Maryland, USA

**Isabel Dapena** MD PhD
Netherlands Institute for Innovative
Ocular Surgery (NIIOS)
Rotterdam, The Netherlands

**Sophie X Deng** MD PhD
Assistant Professor of Ophthalmology
Cornea and Uveitis Division
Jules Stein Eye Institute
Los Angeles, California, USA

**John J DeStafeno** MD
Director of Refractive Surgery
Chester County Eye Care Associates
West Chester, Pennsylvania, USA

**Uday Devgan** MD FACS FRCS(Glasg)
Private Clinic
Devgan Eye Surgery
Los Angeles and Beverly Hills,
California, USA
Chief of Ophthalmology
Olive View UCLA Medical Center
Associate Clinical Professor of
Ophthalmology
Jules Stein Eye Institute
UCLA School of Medicine
Los Angeles, California, USA

**Deepinder Kaur Dhaliwal** MD LAc
Associate Professor of Ophthalmology
University of Pittsburgh School of
Medicine
Director, UPMC Eye Center, Monroeville
Director, Cornea Service
Director, Refractive Surgery Service
Director, Cornea Fellowship Program
Director and Founder, Center for
Integrative Eye Care
UPMC Eye Center
Medical Director, UPMC Laser/
Aesthetic Center
Pittsburgh, Pennsylvania, USA

**Martin Dirisamer** MD
Netherlands Institute for Innovative
Ocular Surgery (NIIOS)
Rotterdam, The Netherlands

**Ali Djalilian** MD
Associate Professor of Ophthalmology
University of Illinois Eye and
Ear Infirmary
University of Illinois at Chicago
Chicago, Illinois, USA

**Andrew Doan** MD PhD
Assistant Clinical Professor
Ophthalmology
Loma Linda University
Loma Linda, California, USA

**Terrence J Doherty** MD
Loden Vision Centers
Nashville, Tennessee, USA

**Peter C Donshik** MD
Clinical Professor
University of Connecticut Health Center
Farmington, Connecticut, USA

**Hon Vu Duong** MD
Clinical Instructor of Ophthalmology
Westfield-Nevada Eye & Ear
Las Vegas, Nevada, USA
Senior Lecturer of Neurosciences
Anatomy and Physiology
Nevada State College
Henderson, NV
Las Vegas, Nevada, USA

**Konstantinos Droutsas** MD PhD
Netherlands Institute for Innovative
Ocular Surgery (NIIOS)
Rotterdam, The Netherlands

**Harminder Singh Dua** MBBS DO
    DO(Lond) MS MNAMS FRCS FRCOphth
    FEBO MD PhD
Chairman and Professor of Ophthalmology
University of Nottingham
England, UK
President, The Royal College of
Ophthalmologists, UK
President, European Society of Cornea
and Ocular Disease Specialists (EuCornea)
President, European Association for Vision
and Eye Research Foundation (EVERf)
Editor-in-chief, British Journal of
Ophthalmology
Division of Ophthalmology and
Visual Sciences
B Floor, Eye ENT Centre
Queens Medical Centre
University Hospital
Nottingham, England, UK

**Gawain Dyer** MD
Department of Ophthalmology
Howard University of Ophthalmology
Washington, District of Columbia, USA

**Benyamin Y Ebrahim** MD
Department of Ophthalmology
Georgetown University Medical Center
Washington Hospital Center
Washington, District of Columbia, USA

**William H Ehlers** MD
Associate Professor
University of Connecticut Health Center
Farmington, Connecticut, USA

**Edgar Mauricio Espana** MD
Assistant Professor
Cornea, External Disease and
Refractive Surgery
University of South Florida
Tampa, Florida, USA

**Per Fagerholm** MD PhD
Professor of Ophthalmology
Linkoping University
Linkoping, Sweden

**Daoud S Fahd** MD
Visiting Fellow in Cornea
University of Illinois at Chicago
Chicago, Illinois, USA

**Marjan Farid** MD
Director of Cornea, Refractive and
Cataract Surgery
Co-Director of the Cornea Fellowship
Program
Assistant Professor of Ophthalmology
Gavin Herbert Eye Institute
University of California, Irvine
Irvine, California, USA

**Brad H Feldman** MD
Philadelphia Eye Associates
Philadelphia, Pennsylvania, USA

**Larry Ferdinand Jr** MD
Gulfcoast Eye Center
Ocean Springs, Mississippi, USA

**John Forrester** MD FRCSE FRCSG FRCOphth
Emeritus Cockburn Professor and
Head of Department
University of Aberdeen
Scotland, UK
Professor of Ocular Immunology
University of Western Australia
Perth, Australia

**Mitchell H Friedlaender (Late)** MD
Head
Division of Ophthalmology
Scripps Clinic
Adjunct Professor
Department of Molecular and
Experimental Medicine
The Scripps Research Institute
La Jolla, California, USA

**Thomas A Fuchsluger** FEBO MSc
Consultant, Department of
Ophthalmology
Head, Lions Cornea Bank North
Rhine-Westphalia
Düsseldorf University Hospital
Heinrich-Heine-University
Düsseldorf, Germany

**Anat Galor** MD
Assistant Professor of Clinical
Ophthalmology
Bascom Palmer Eye Institute, University
of Miami Miller School of Medicine
Staff Physician
Miami Veterans Medical Center
Miami, Florida, USA

**Nerea Garagorri GanTxegui** PhD MBA
Senior Researcher of Biomaterials
TECNALIA
Health Division
Mikeletegi pasealekua 2
San Sebastian, Spain

**Prashant Garg** MD
Associate Director Cornea and Anterior
Segment Services
G Chandra Sekhar Distinguished
Chair of Education
LV Prasad Eye Institute
Hyderabad, Andhra Pradesh, India

**Sumit (Sam) Garg** MD
Vice Chair of Clinical Ophthalmology
Medical Director, Gavin Herbert Eye
Institute
Assistant Professor of Ophthalmology
University of California Irvine
Irvine, California, USA

**Harmeet S Gill** MD DABO FRCSC
Oculofacial Plastic and Orbital Surgeon
Lecturer, Department of Ophthalmology
and Vision Sciences
University of Toronto
Toronto, Ontario, Canada

**Kenneth Mark Goins** MD
Professor, Clinical Ophthalmology
Medical Director, Iowa Lions Eye Bank
Cornea and External Diseases
University of Iowa Hospitals and Clinics
Iowa City, Iowa, USA

**May Griffith** PhD MBA
Professor of Regenerative Medicine
Linkoping University
Linkoping, Sweden

**Davinder S Grover** MD MPH
Associate Physician
Glaucoma Associates of Texas
Dallas, Texas
Associate Clinical Instructor
University of Texas, Southwestern
Medical School
Dallas, Texas, USA

**Arun C Gulani** MD MS
Chief Surgeon and Fellowship Director
Gulani Vision Institute
Jacksonville, Florida, USA

**Rebat M Halder** MD
Professor and Chairman
Department of Dermatology
Howard University College of Medicine
Washington, District of Columbia, USA

**Pedram Hamrah** MD
Henry Allen Cornea Scholar, Cornea and
Refractive Surgery Service
Massachusetts Eye and Ear Infirmary
Assistant Professor
Department of Ophthalmology
Harvard Medical School
Boston, Massachusetts, USA

**Mona Harissi-Dagher** MD FRCSC DABO
Assistant Professor of Ophthalmology
Université de Montréal, Montréal
Québec, Canada

**David J Harris Jr** MD FACS
Clinical Associate Professor and Chief
Ophthalmology Section
Department of Surgery
The University of Tennessee Graduate
School of Medicine
Knoxville, Tennessee, USA

**Mike P Holzer** MD FEBO
Associate Professor and Director of
Refractive Surgery
International Vision Correction Research
Centre (IVCRC)
Department of Ophthalmology
University of Heidelberg
Heidelberg, Germany

**Hugo Y Hsu** MD
Associate Professor of Clinical
Ophthalmology
Department of Ophthalmology
Keck School of Medicine of the University
of Southern California
Doheny Eye Institute
Los Angeles, California, USA

**Andrew Huang** MD
Professor of Ophthalmology
Department of Ophthalmology and
Visual Sciences
Washington University
St Louis, Missouri, USA

**Takeshi Ide** MD
Vice Director
Minamiaoyama Eye Clinic
Tokyo, Japan

**Soosan Jacob** MS DNB FRCS
Senior Consultant Ophthalmologist
Dr Agarwal's Group of Eye Hospitals
Chennai, Tamil Nadu, India

**Deborah S Jacobs** MD
Medical Director
Boston Foundation for Sight
Needham, Massachusetts, USA
Assistant Clinical Professor of
Ophthalmology
Harvard Medical School, Boston, MA
Faculty, Cornea Service
Massachusetts Eye and Ear Infirmary
Boston, Massachusetts, USA

**Naima Jacobs-El**
Department of Ophthalmology
Howard University Hospital
Washington, District of Columbia, USA

**Bennie H Jeng** MD
Associate Professor of Ophthalmology
University of California, San Francisco
Co-Director, UCSF Cornea Service
Chief, Department of Ophthalmology
San Francisco General Hospital
San Francisco, California, USA

**R Duncan Johnson** MD
Clinical Instructor of Ophthalmology
Jules Stein Eye Institute
UCLA School of Medicine
Los Angeles, California, USA
Private Clinic, Inland Eye Specialists
Murrieta, California, USA

**Leslie S Jones** MD
Associate Professor, Residency Program
Director, and Director of Glaucoma Services
Howard University
Department of Ophthalmology
Washington, District of Columbia, USA

**John W Josephson** MD
Cornea and Refractive Surgery
Dulles Eye Associates
Lansdowne, Virginia, USA

**Mona A Kaleem** MD
Department of Ophthalmology
Howard University Hospital
Washington, District of Columbia, USA

**Vardhaman Kankariya** MD DNB (SN)
CORNEA (DEC) REFRACTIVE (IVO, Greece)
FICO (UK), FAICO (Ref Surg)
Former Fellow Refractive Surgery-IVO
University of Crete, Greece
LASIK and Refractive Surgeon Cornea
and IOL Implant Surgeon
Sai Surya Eye Care Pvt Ltd
Ahmednagar, Maharashtra, India

**Stephen S Khachikian** MD
Cornea Cataract and Refractive Surgery
Black Hills Regional Eye Institute
Rapid City, South Dakota
University of South Dakota
Vermillion, South Dakota, USA

**Bilal Faiz Khan** MBBS MD
Consultant Ophthalomologist
Associate Dean
United Medical and Dental College
Karachi, Pakistan

**Wei-Boon Khor** MRCSE Mmed
Associate Consultant, Corneal Service
Singapore National Eye Centre
Singapore, Singapore

**Earl Kidwell** MD
Clinical Associate Professor
Director of the Oculoplastic and
Orbit Service
Department of Ophthalmology
Howard University College of Medicine
Washington, District of Columbia, USA

**Peter Kim** BSc(Med), MBBS(Hons), FRANZCO
Sydney Eye Hospital
Macquarie Street Eye Surgeons
Sydney, Australia

**Terry Kim** MD
Professor of Ophthalmology
Duke University School of Medicine
Director of Fellowship Programs
Cornea, Cataract, and Refractive Surgery
Duke University Eye Center
Durham, North Carolina, USA

**Stephen D Klyce** PhD FARVO
Adjunct Professor of Ophthalmology
Mount Sinai School of Medicine
Port Washington, New York, USA

**Jon Konti** MD
Cornea/Refractive Surgeon
Ophthalmic Surgeons and Physicians
Tempe, Arizona, USA

**Ronald R Krueger** MD MSE
Professor of Ophthalmology
Cleveland Clinic Lerner College of
Medicine of Case Western Reserve
University
Medical Director, Department of
 Refractive Surgery
Cole Eye Institute
Cleveland Clinic
Cleveland, Ohio, USA

**Lucia Kuffova** MD PhD
Senior Lecturer, Honorary Consultant
Ophthalmologist
Section of Immunology and Infection
(Ocular Immunology)
Division of Applied Medicine
School of Medicine and Dentistry
University of Aberdeen
Aberdeen, Scotland, UK

**Nikhil L Kumar** BMED GradDipRefractSurg
MPH FRANZCO
Clinical Senior Lecturer
Cornea, Refractive and Cataract Surgery
Australian School of Advanced Medicine
Macquarie University, NSW
Sydney, Australia

**Ruben Kuruvilla** MD
Department of Ophthalmology
Mount Sinai School of Medicine
Department of Ophthalmology New York
New York, USA

**George D Kymionis** MD PhD
Lecturer
Institute of Vision and Optics (IVO)
Ophthalmology Department
Medical University of Crete
Herklion, Greece

**Neil Lagali** PhD
Integrative Regenerative Medicine Centre
Department of Clinical and
Experimental Medicine
Linkoping University
Linkoping, Sweden

**Jonathan H Lass** MD
Charles I Thomas Professor and Chairman
University Hospitals
Department of Ophthalmology and
Visual Sciences
Case Western Reserve University
Medical Director of the Cleveland Eye Bank
Cleveland, Ohio, USA

**Hong-Gam Le** BA
Research Assistant
Boston Foundation for Sight
Needham, Massachusetts, USA

**Erik Letko** MD
Corneal Consultants of Colorado
Littleton, Colorado, USA

**Vasilios S Liarakos** MD
Netherlands Institute for Innovative
Ocular Surgery (NIIOS)
Rotterdam, The Netherlands

**James C Loden** MD
President
Loden Vision Centers
Nashville, Tennessee, USA

**Jay M Lustbader** MD
Chairman, Departments of
Ophthalmology
Georgetown University Hospital and
Washington Hospital Center
Professor of Ophthalmology, Georgetown
University School of Medicine
President, Washington National Eye Center
Washington, District of Columbia, USA

**Francis S Mah** MD
Director, Cornea and External Disease
Co-Director, Refractive Surgery
Scripps Clinic Torrey Pines
La Jolla, California, USA
Consultant
Charles T. Campbell Ocular
Microbiology Laboratory
University of Pittsburgh School of Medicine
Pittsburgh, Pennsylvania, USA

**Mercede Majdi** MD
Research Fellow
University of Illinois Eye and Ear Infirmary
University of Illinois at Chicago
Chicago, Illinois, USA

**Alex Mammen** MD
Cornea, External Disease, and Refractive
Surgery Service
Clinical Assistant Professor of
Ophthalmology
University of Pittsburgh School of Medicine
Pittsburgh , Pennsylvania, USA

**Stephanie Jones Marioneaux** MD
Assistant Professor
Department of Ophthalmology
Eastern Virginia Medical School
Norfolk, Virginia, USA

**William D Mathers** MD
Petti Professor of Ophthalmology
Department of Ophthalmology
Oregon Health and Sciences University
Portland, Oregon, USA

**Zale Mednick** BA MD
Department of Ophthalmology
Queen's School of Medicine Kingston
Ontario, Canada

**Jodhbir S Mehta** Bsc (Hons) MBBS FRCOphth
FRCS (Ed)
Co-Head, Corneal and External Eye Disease
Consultant Refractive Service
Singapore National Eye Centre
Head, Tissue Engineering and
Stem Cells Group
Singapore Eye Research Institute, (SERI)
Associate Professor
Duke-NUS Graduate Medical School
Associate Professor
Department of Ophthalmology
Yong Loo Lin School of Medicine, NUS
Singapore, Singapore

**Mohit Mehtani** MD
Georgetown University Hospital
Washington Hospital Center
Washington, District of Columbia, USA

**Gerrit RJ Melles** MD PhD
Director
Netherlands Institute for Innovative
Ocular Surgery (NIIOS)
Rotterdam, The Netherlands

**Michael Mequio** MD
Ophthalmology United States Air Force
MacDill AFB
Tampa, Florida, USA

**Shahzad I Mian** MD
Terry J Bergstrom Professor
Associate Chair, Education
Associate Professor
Department of Ophthalmology and
Visual Sciences, University of Michigan
Ann Arbor, Michigan, USA

**Behrad Y Milani** MD
Research Fellow
University of Illinois Eye and Ear Infirmary
University of Illinois at Chicago
Chicago, Illinois, USA

**Darlene Miller** DHSC MPH CIC
Research Assistant Professor
Scientific Director-Microbiology Laboratory
Anne Bates Leach Eye Hospital
Bascom Palmer Eye Institute
University of Miami School of Medicine
Miami, Florida, USA

**Ammar Miri** MSc MRCS
University of Nottingham, England, UK
Aleppo University Hospital, Aleppo, Syria
Trust Ophthalmologist
Division of Ophthalmology and
Visual Sciences
B Floor, Eye ENT Centre
Queens Medical Centre
University Hospital, Derby Road
Nottingham, England, UK

**Majid A Moarefi** MD
Research Fellow
University of Illinois Eye and Ear Infirmary
University of Illinois at Chicago
Chicago, Illinois, USA

**Karim Mohamed-Noriega**
International Clinical Fellow
Singapore National Eye Centre (SNEC)
Singapore Eye Research Institute (SERI)
Singapore, Singapore
Professor, Dept of Ophthalmology
Faculty of Medicine and
University Hospital
Autonomous University of Nuevo Leon
(UANL), San Nicolás de los Garza
Nuevo León, Mexico

**Rajiv R Mohan** PhD
Professor of Ophthalmology, Resident
Research Coordinator Mason Eye Institute,
School of Medicine and College of
Veterinary Medicine University of
Missouri-Columbia
Columbia, Missouri, USA

**Jamal M Mohsin** BS
American University of Antigua
School of Medicine
Coolidge, Antigua

**Maryam Mokhtarzadeh** MD
Fellow
Ophthalmic Genetics and Visual Function
Branch, National Eye Institute/National
Institutes of Health
Bethesda, Maryland, USA

**Mikelson MomPremier** MD
Department of Ophthalmology
Howard University Hospital
Washington, District of Columbia, USA

**Kyros Moutsouris** MD
Netherlands Institute for Innovative
Ocular Surgery (NIIOS)
Rotterdam, The Netherlands

**Miguel Naveiras** MD
Netherlands Institute for Innovative
Ocular Surgery (NIIOS)
Rotterdam, The Netherlands

**Vanessa Ngakeng** MD
Cataract and Laser Institute
Mishawaka, Indiana, USA

**Lisa Nijm** MD JD
Warrenville EyeCare and LASIK
Medical Director
Cornea, External Disease and
Refractive Surgery
Warrenville, Illinois, USA
Assistant Clinical Professor of
Ophthalmology
University of Illinois Eye and Ear Infirmary
Department of Ophthalmology and
Visual Sciences
Chicago, Illinois, USA

**Terrence P O'Brien** MD
Professor of Ophthalmology
Charlotte Breyer Rodgers Distinguished
Chair
Ophthalmology Director Refractive Surgery
Bascom Palmer Eye Institute
Department of Ophthalmology
University of Miami Miller
School of Medicine
Palm Beach Gardens, Florida, USA

**Stephen G Odaibo** MD
Department of Ophthalmology
Howard University Hospital
Washington, District of Columbia, USA

**Michael A Page** MD
Assistant Professor
Cornea and External Disease
University of Minnesota Department of
Ophthalmology and Visual Neurosciences
Minneapolis, Minnesota, USA

**Deval R Paranjpe** MD FACS
Assistant Professor of Ophthalmology
Drexel University College of Medicine
Director, Cornea Service
Allegheny General Hospital
Allegheny Ophthalmic and Orbital
Associates
Pittsburgh, Pennsylvania, USA

**Gitane Patel** MD MPH
Associate Ophthalmologist
West Coast Eye Care
San Diego, California, USA

**Yannis M Paulus** MD
Byers Eye Institute at Stanford
Stanford University Medical Center
Palo Alto, California, USA

**Carlos Pavesio** MD
Consultant Ophthalmologist
Director
Medical Retina Service
Moorfields Eye Hospital
London, UK

**Charles J Pavlin** MD FRCS
Professor
Department of Ophthalmology and
Visual Sciences
University of Toronto
Toronto, Ontario, Canada

**Animesh Petkar** MD
Department of Ophthalmology
Howard University Hospital
Washington, District of Columbia, USA

**Roswell R Pfister** MD
Clinical Professor of Ophthalmology
University of Alabama
Birmingham, Alabama, USA
President
The Eye Research Foundation
Birmingham, Alabama, USA

**Roberto Pineda** MD
Associate Professor of Ophthalmology
Harvard Medical School
Director of Refractive Surgery
Massachusetts Eye and Ear Infirmary
Boston, Massachusetts, USA

**Bozorgmehr Pouyeh** MD
Medical Graduate
Tehran University of Medical Sciences
Tehran, Iran

**Christina R Prescott** MD PhD
Assistant Professor of Ophthalmology
Cornea, External Disease and
Refractive Surgery
Wilmer Eye Institute
Johns Hopkins Medicine
Baltimore, Maryland, USA

**Francis W Price Jr** MD
President, Price Vision Group
Indianapolis, Indiana, USA

**Marianne O Price** PhD
Executive Director, Cornea Research
Foundation of America
Indianapolis, Indiana, USA

**Julian A Procope** MD
Horizon Eye Care Group
Harrisburg, Pennsylvania, USA

**Ying Qian** MD PhD
Cornea, Uveitis and External Disease
Department of Ophthalmology
Kaiser Permanente
Oakland, California, USA

**Ruth Quilendrino** MD
Netherlands Institute for Innovative
Ocular Surgery (NIIOS)
Rotterdam, The Netherlands

**Saima M Qureshi** MD
Department of Ophthalmology
Howard University Hospital
Washington, District of Columbia
USA

**Omar N Qutub** MD
Department of Dermatology
Howard University Hospital
Washington, District of Columbia
USA

**Kavita Rao** MD
Consultant Cornea
Cataract and Refractive Surgery
Aditya Jyot Eye Hospital
Mumbai, Maharashtra, India

**John J Requard** BS
108 Acorn Hill Lane
Apex, North Carolina, USA

**Nikisha Q Richards** MD
Department of Ophthalmology
Howard University Hospital
Washington, District of Columbia, USA

**Marie-Claude Robert** BSc MD
Ophthalmology Department
Notre-Dame Hospital
Montréal, Québec, Canada

**Guillermo Rocha** MD FRCSC
Cornea and Refractive Surgery
Ocular Immunology
GRMC Vision Centre
Brandon, Manitoba, Canada

**Jason Rodier** MD
Postdoctoral Fellow
Mason Eye Institute
University of Missouri
Columbia, Missouri, USA

**Gina M Rogers** MD
Attending Physician
Eye Physicians and Surgeons of Chicago
Chicago, Illinois, USA

**David Rootman** MD FRCSC
Professor, University of Toronto
Department of Ophthalmology and
Vision Sciences
Toronto Western Hospital
Toronto, Ontario, Canada

**Noel Rosado-Adames** MD
Cornea Fellow
Duke Eye Center
Durham, North Carolina, USA

**George OD Rosenwasser** MD CEBT
Medical Director, Central Pennsylvania
Eye Institute and Gift of Life Donor
Program Eye Bank
Hershey, Pennsylvania, USA

**Jocelyn A Rowe** MD
Department of Ophthalmology
Mount Sinai Medical Center
Chicago, Illinois, USA

**Roy S Rubinfeld** MD
Clinical Associate Professor of
Ophthalmology
Georgetown University Medical Center
Senior Attending
Washington Hospital Center
Washington, District of Columbia
USA

**Sina J Sabet** MD FACS
Assistant Professor, Departments of
Ophthalmology and Pathology
Georgetown University Medical Center
Washington, District of Columbia
USA

**Dalia Galal Said** MD FRCS
University of Nottingham, England, UK
Research Institute of Ophthalmology
Cairo, Egypt
Consultant Ophthalmologist
Division of Ophthalmology and
Visual Sciences
B Floor, Eye ENT Centre
Queens Medical Centre
University Hospital, Derby Road
Nottingham, England, UK

**Virender S Sangwan** MS
Associate Director
L V Prasad Eye Institute
Head, Cornea and Anterior Segment
Ocular Immunology and Uveitis Service
LV Prasad Eye Institute
Hyderabad, Andhra Pradesh, India

**Naazli M Shaikh** MD
Chief of Ophthalmology
Cornea Specialist
Department of Ophthalmology
Veterans Administration Orlando
Florida, USA
Assistant Professor, Ophthalmology
University of Central Florida
College of Medicine
Assistant Professor, Ophthalmology
Department of Ophthalmology
Howard University Hospital
Washington, District of Columbia
USA

**John D Sheppard** MD MMSc
President, Virginia Eye Consultants
Professor of Ophthalmology
Microbiology and Molecular Biology
Ophthalmology Residency Research
Program Director
Clinical Director, Thomas R Lee Center for
Ocular Pharmacology
Eastern Virginia Medical School
Norfolk, Virginia, USA

**Mark D Sherman** MD
Cornea/External Disease and Uveitis Service
Pacific Eye Surgeons
San Luis Obispo, California
Assistant Clinical Professor
Department of Ophthalmology
Loma Linda University School of Medicine
Loma Linda, California, USA

**Mohamed Abou Shousha** MD
Saint Louis University School of Medicine
Department of Ophthalmology
Saint Louis University Eye Institute
St Louis, Missouri, USA

**Daniel N Skorich** MD
Department of Ophthalmology
Essentia Health-Duluth Clinic
Duluth, Minnesota, USA

**David Smadja** MD
University Hospital of Bordeaux
Ophthalmology Department
Anterior Segment and
Refractive Surgery Unit
Hopital Pellegrin
Place Amelie Raba-Leon
Bordeaux, France

**Janine Smith-Marshall** MD
Assistant Professor of Ophthalmology
Director of Pediatric Ophthalmology and
Strabismus Service
Howard University Hospital
Washington, District of Columbia, USA

**Oluwatosin U Smith** MD
Glaucoma Associates of Texas, Dallas, Texas
Clinical Assistant Professor of Ophthalmology
University of Texas South Western,
Dallas, Texas, USA

**Ronald E Smith** MD
Professor and Chairman
Department of Ophthalmology
Keck School of Medicine of the University
of Southern California
Doheny Eye Institute
Los Angeles,California, USA

**Jason E Stahl** MD
Durrie Vision
Overland Park, Kansas, USA
Assistant Professor of Ophthalmology
Kansas University Medical Center
Prairie Village, Kansas, USA

**Anne Steiner** MD
Director
North Shore-Long Island Jewish
Ocular Surface Center
Assistant Professor of Ophthalmology
Hofstra North Shore—
LIJ School of Medicine
New York, New York, USA

**Roger F Steinert** MD
Irving H Leopold Professor and Chair
Professor of Biomedical Engineering
Director, Gavin Herbert Eye Institute
University of California
Irvine, California, USA

**Stephen C Kaufman** MD PhD
Lyon Professor of Ophthalmology
Director of Cornea and Refractive Surgery
University of Minnesota
Mineapolis, Minnesota, USA

**Christopher N Ta** MD
Professor of Ophthalmology
Byers Eye Institute at Stanford
Stanford University Medical Center
Palo Alto, California, USA

**Khalid F Tabbara** MD ABO FRCOphth (Ed)
Medical Director
The Eye Center and The Eye Foundation
for Research in Ophthalmology
Riyadh, Saudi Arabia
Clinical Professor
Department of Ophthalmology
College of Medicine, King Saud University
Riyadh, Saudi Arabia

Adjunct Professor
The Wilmer Ophthalmological Institute of
The Johns Hopkins University
School of Medicine
Baltimore, Maryland, USA

**Donald Tiang-Hwee Tan** FRCSE FRCSG
FRCOphth FAMS
Medical Director
Singapore National Eye Centre
Professor of Ophthalmology
Yong Loo Lin School of Medicine
National University of Singapore
Singapore, Singapore

**Joseph Tauber** MD
Clinical Professor of Ophthalmology
Kansas University School of Medicine
Tauber Eye Center
Kansas City, Missouri, USA

**David Taylor**
Product Manager
Advanced Diagnostic Devices
Reichert Technologies
New York, New York, USA

**Onsiri Thanathanee** MD
Cornea and Refractive Surgery Service
Department of Ophthalmology
Srinagarind Hospital
Khon Kaen University
Khon Kaen, Thailand

**William Trattler** MD
Director of Cornea
Center For Excellence in Eye Care
Miami, Florida, USA

**Kazuo Tsubota** MD
Professor and Department Chair
Department of Ophthalmology
Keio University School of Medicine
Tokyo, Japan

**Ira J Udell** MD
Arlene and Arthur Levine Professor and
Chairman
Hofstra North Shore-Long Island Jewish
School of Medicine
Chairman, Department of Ophthalmology
North Shore-Long Island
Jewish Health System
Great Neck, New York, USA

**Daniel Vítor Vasconcelos-Santos** MD PhD
Associate Professor of Ophthalmology
Director of Uveitis Service
Universidade Federal de Minas Gerais
Belo Horizonte, Brazil

**David D Verdier** MD
Clinical Professor
Department of Surgery
Ophthalmology Division
Michigan State University College of
Human Medicine
Verdier Eye Center, PLC
Grand Rapids, Michigan, USA

**Ryan Vida** OD
Senior Instructor of Ophthalmology
University of Rochester Medical Center
Clinical Faculty
Flaum Eye Institute
Refractive Surgery Center
Rochester, New York, USA

**Samir Vira** MD
Department of Ophthalmology
Loyola University Medical Center
Maywood, Illinois, USA

**Xiao Chloe Wan** MD
Department of Ophthalmology
University of Chicago
Chicago, Illinois, USA

**Ming Wang** MD PhD
Clinical Associate
Professor of Ophthalmology
University of Tennessee
International President
Shanghai Aier Eye Hospital
Shanghai, China
Director
Wang Vision 3D Cataract and LASIK Center
Nashville, Tennesssee, USA

**George O Waring IV** MD
Assistant Professor of Ophthalmology
Medical University of South Carolina
Director of Refractive Surgery
Storm Eye Institute
Medical Director
Magill Vision Center
Charleston, South Carolina, USA

**Robert S Weinberg** MD
Chairman Ophthalmology
Johns Hopkins Bayview Medical Center
Wilmer Eye Institute at Bayview
Baltimore, Maryland, USA

**Jayne S Weiss** MD
Chairman
LSU Department of Ophthalmology
Herbert E Kaufman MD Endowed Chair
Professor of Ophthalmology, Pathology
and Pharmacology
Director
LSU Eye Center, LSUHSC
New Orleans, Louisiana, USA

**Mark E Whitten** MD
Medical Director
Whitten Laser Eye
Charlotte Hall, Maryland, USA

**Fasika Woreta** MD MPH
Cornea Fellow
Bascom Palmer Eye Institute
University of Miami Health System
Miami, Florida, USA

**Takefumi Yamaguchi**
Research Fellow, Cornea and Refractive
Surgery Service
Massachusetts Eye and Ear Infirmary
Harvard Medical School
Boston, Massachusetts, USA

**Ru-Yin Yeh** MD
Netherlands Institute for Innovative
Ocular Surgery (NIIOS)
Rotterdam, The Netherlands

**Sonia N Yeung** MD PHD FRCSC
Clinical Assistant Professor
University of British Columbia
Department of Ophthalmology
Cornea Service
Vancouver Hospital Eye Care Centre and
St Paul's Hospital
Vancouver, British Columbia, Canada

**Sonia H Yoo** MD
Professor of Ophthalmology
Bascom Palmer Eye Institute
University of Miami
Miami, Florida, USA

**Salman J Yousuf** DO MS
Department of Ophthalmology
Howard University Hospital
Washington, District of Columbia, USA

**Gerald W Zaidman**
Clinical Professor of Ophthalmology and
Vice-Chairman
New York Medical College
Valhalla, NY, Department of
Ophthalmology
Westchester Medical Center
Valhalla, New York, USA

**Siamak Zarei-Ghanavati** MD
Assistant Professor
Cornea Department and Eye Research
Mashhad Center University of
Medical Sciences
Mashhad, Iran

**Wadih Zein** MD
Staff Clinician
Ophthalmic Genetics and Visual function
Branch, National Eye Institute/National
Institutes of Health
Bethesda, Maryland, USA

# FOREWORD

The cornea of the eye is not very impressive in terms of size (11 mm diameter, a half mm thick). Does it deserve the attention of a two volume text written by some of the world's greatest experts in the field? Yes indeed—for obvious reasons: eight to ten million people in the world are blind (20/400 or less, best eye) from corneal disease—sometimes with resulting comorbidities such as glaucoma. These patients are our responsibility and this new treatise can greatly help us to help them. It is a remarkably complete and comprehensive text with accompanying surgical DVDs. It covers the latest thoughts in basic and clinical science, current up-to-date clinical research, worldwide epidemiology of the various corneal diseases, recently developed diagnostic techniques, and cutting edge medical and surgical treatments of the various corneal ailments.

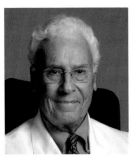

New treatments include antivirals, modern dry eye treatments, collagen crosslinking for keratoconus, scleral lenses for ocular surface disease, immunomodulation, etc. Surgical techniques is getting extensive coverage, particularly for endothelial keratoplasty, deep lamellar grafts, keratoprosthesis, refractive surgery, among others. The surgical DVDs are of crucial importance.

In this text, the editors—both distinguished academic ophthalmologists and famous for their contributions in specialized areas—clearly have had the ambition to create a monumental text, both encompassing and at the same time providing a large number of sharply focused chapters, authored by the ultimate experts. The quality is superb throughout. It should appeal to all trainees and should be a must for practicing ophthalmologists, cornea specialists and medical libraries. The editors should be congratulated for accomplishing a highly academic, readable and overall a very useful guide to a better cornea practice. All in all, this text promises to be around as the last word for a very long time.

**Claes H Dohlman** MD PhD
Professor of Ophthalmology
Harvard Medical School
Massachusetts Eye and Ear Infirmary
Boston, Massachusetts, USA

# PREFACE

In volume one, we delve into the common cornea topics of structure, physiology, anatomy, infectious etiologies, dystrophies, degenerations, tumors, and immunological and metabolic conditions. In addition, volume one explores innovative advances that are reshaping the field, such as corneal biomechanics, prosthetic replacement of the ocular surface ecosystem(PROSE), treatment for ocular surface disease, gene therapy in the cornea, as well as a biosynthetic alternative to human donor tissue. Each chapter is complete with an exhaustive literature review. And, because of the diligence of our contributors, each segment is current, relevant and expertly written.

The second volume is dedicated to corneal surgery. In this book we have tried to give an update on standard corneal procedures, as well as new and emerging techniques like collagen crosslinking, Descemet's stripping endothelial keratoplasty (DSAEK or DSEK), Descemet's membrane endothelial keratoplasty (DMEK), deep anterior lamellar keratoplasty (DALK), intrastromal corneal implants, the use of light adjustable lenses in cataract surgery following corneal refractive surgery, and the various femtosecond laser applications in anterior segment surgery. We have also included two more features—white papers conveying in a stepwise manner how to perform a particular surgery, and a litany of edited surgical DVDs demonstrating actual surgery—that we hope will substantiate this book as a universally credible reference, an effective learning tool, and a utilitarian resource for practicing surgeons.

**Robert A Copeland Jr**
**Natalie A Afshari**

# ACKNOWLEDGMENTS

First and foremost, our hearts go out to patients worldwide, who have suffered through blindness due to corneal disease. We are so very humbled and so very privileged to offer this two-volume comprehensive text to the ophthalmology community, in hopes of building upon our knowledge to better care for you. We are indebted to a team of world-class contributors who have so graciously offered their knowledge, experience, and pedagogy to produce this text. These authors spent days of their valuable time on their chapters and DVDs, and they produced some real classics in scientific writing for which we are truly grateful.

As in every successful endeavor, there are individuals behind the scenes that have helped to bring this major undertaking into fruition. We want to thank our families for allowing us the time to commit to such a project. Our children sat patiently many weekends and evenings next to us while we worked on this task. Their patience was admirable. We are indebted to our residents, fellows, colleagues, administrative assistants, patients and the Jaypee Brothers Medical Publishers, New Delhi, India team for their support with this book. We lost a great friend and colleague with the passing of Mitchell H Friedlaender MD during this project. His numerous contributions to the field of Ophthalmology will be surely missed. Without your hard work and sacrifice this would not have been possible. This is your book.

# CONTENTS

## Volume 1
## Part 1: Fundamentals

### Section 1: Basic Science

## Section 2: Examination and Evaluation Techniques

## Section 6: Ocular Surface Disease

## Section 7: Metabolic and Congenital Disease

## Section 8: Conjunctival Corneal Dysplasia and Malignancy

# Section 9: Trauma

## Section 10: Corneal Dystrophies and Degenerations

## Section 11: Corneal and Conjunctival Manifestations of Dietary Deficiencies

## Section 12: Contact Lenses

## Section 13: Emerging Innovation

# Volume 2

## Section 14: Cornea Surgery

## Section 15: Corneal, Scleral and Conjunctival Surgery: Supportive and Protective

## Section 18: Corneal Instrumentation

## Section 19: Appendix

# SECTION 14

# Cornea Surgery

## CHAPTER

**History of Cornea Surgery**
*Daoud S Fahd, Norma Allemann, Wallace Chamon, Dimitri T Azar*

# CHAPTER 67

# History of Cornea Surgery

*Daoud S Fahd, Norma Allemann, Wallace Chamon, Dimitri T Azar*

## ⋗ INTRODUCTION

Cornea surgery encompasses surgical procedures that aim at replacing all (or part) of the cornea, or altering its curvature to correct for errors of refraction.

Corneal transplantation, aside from blood transfusions, is the most commonly performed, and most successful organ/tissue transplant, due to the avascular nature of the cornea and the advances in donor preservation techniques.

The evolution of cornea surgery, from experiments on animals in the 1700s to the present use of lasers to assist in surgery, went through many advancements and changes.

In this chapter, we will be discussing the timeline of events that lead to keratoplasty and refractive surgery as we know them today. We will present an overview of the succession of techniques in keratoplasty (both penetrating and nonpenetrating), in addition to a review on the different methods employed to correct ocular refractive errors.

## ⋗ HISTORY OF KERATOPLASTY

### Corneal Grafting Envisioners and Initial Studies

Ideas of restoring corneal clarity date back to the first century when the Greek physician Galen (130–200) suggested restoring the clarity of an opaque cornea. More than a century and a half later, Guillaume Pellier de Quengsy envisioned the use of a glass implant in opaque corneas in 1771, and Himly proposed penetrating corneal transplant in 1813.[1,2] Before the 19th century, the lack of proper anesthesia made cornea surgery difficult, and it was not until the mid-nineteenth century that ether and chloroform began to be used. Cornea surgery was then possible;

however, the inexistence of sutures and adequate surgical instruments, as well as postanesthesia coughing, increased postoperative complications.

Many studies and experimentations were done initially. Some did not yield positive results, but all of them helped to form and define the techniques that we use today in transplantation.[1,2]

The first human corneal transplant was from a porcine donor and was done by Kissam in 1844. In 1880s a human donor penetrating keratoplasty (PKP) was performed by Wolfe however it was unsuccessful.[1,2]

### Era of Heteroplasty (1800–1900)

Before the 20th century, donor corneas could not be obtained from human cadavers; therefore, animal heteroplastic donor corneas were used. In 1884, a major breakthrough in cornea surgery came when Koller proposed the use of topical cocaine for corneal anesthesia, with repeated applications of cocaine on the cornea becoming the standard of care.[3]

The modern corneal transplantation is based on the fundamentals of ophthalmic surgery that were laid by von Graefe as well as the first lamellar transplant that was done by von Hippel using his own trephine. Von Hippel reported in 1888 a patient with a 20/200 vision after lamellar keratoplasty (LKP) from a rabbit donor.[4] Fuchs then reported in 1894, on 30 cases of homologous transplants using von Hippel's trephine with 'good results' in 11 eyes, two of which showed improvement in vision.[1,2] The original trephine described by von Hippel in 1888 was composed of a handheld cylinder that was pressed on the cornea to puncture it.[4]

The circular trephines were initially composed of a solid handle on a cylinder with a reusable blade. The blade had to be sharpened continuously; hence the round shape of the trephine was altered with each sharpening. The trephines were not transparent, thus centration was difficult to control resulting in large amounts of postoperative astigmatism, in addition to inadvertent injury to the iris and lens.

## Era of Homoplasty (1900–Present)

The first successful PKP in humans, was performed by Zirm in 1905, in Austria, with long-term survival of the transplanted graft.[5,6] Prior to the 1930s, however, there was limited growth of PKP, since the source of corneas was living individuals with diseased eyes and clear corneas (hence obtaining a cornea was not an easy task). In 1930s, Elschnig published the first series of corneal transplants with a success of approximately 22%.[7]

By the 1930–1940s, retrobulbar anesthesia replaced cocaine anesthesia. An exponential growth of successful PKP followed. The reasons for this growth were multiple: (i) The slit biomicroscope was discovered and this led to better elucidating the corneal anatomy and more detailed description of pathology; (ii) Antibiotics started being used and this led to decreasing postoperative risk of infection, (iii) Anesthesia and aseptic techniques improved, and (iv) Eye banks were established with the ability to successfully use cadaveric eyes for transplants.

### History of the Eye Banks

Filatov proposed the use of cadaveric human donors and established the first eye bank in Odessa, Russia.[8] The first American eye bank was in New York City and was established by R Townley Paton in 1944 and was called the 'Eye Bank for Sight'. The Eye Bank Association of America was later established in 1961 and recorded an amazing number of 2000 transplants that same year.

Advances were being made in the preservation media and this prolonged the viability of donor corneas. After Magitot had discovered, in 1912, an antiseptic preservation medium that could preserve the donor cornea up to 8 days,[9] McCarey and Kaufman, in 1974, developed the M-K medium that preserved corneas up to 2 weeks.[10]

Concurrently with the establishment of eye banks, advances in donor cornea preparation started. In addition to the importance of preservation of tissue, the issue of matching the donor button to the recipient bed plays a very important role.

Before 1973, the recipient cornea was always trephined from the anterior surface to the endothelium. Many factors alter the diameter of the trephined cornea, including the intraocular pressure and the blade sharpness, which resulted in buttons having diameters larger than that of the trephines used.[11]

In 1973,[12] the posterior punch technique with suction-based donor holders was devised. It produced a circular button with a regular and even edge profile.

The use of artificial chambers, popularized in the 1980s,[13] and the storage of donor tissue as corneoscleral buttons instead of whole eyes allowed further sophistications in tissue preparation allowing more precise matching of donor button and recipient bed with smoother interfaces.[14] The artificial chambers provided better preservation of the endothelium, allowing for increased success in posterior lamellar keratoplasties that were later devised.

During the same period, donor corneas underwent extensive screening for specific viruses, such as HIV and Creutzfeldt-Jakob, and previous corneal surgery. This resulted in safer procedures, as well as increased survival and more predictable outcomes of transplanted corneas.[15]

Since the use of desiccated lenticules by Urrets-Zavalia,[16] the desire for a readily available source of prepackaged, uniform thickness donor tissue has been present. Rich[17] used a technique published by Barraquer[18] to produce parallel-faced, smooth surface lamellar corneal donor tissue of a known thickness that could be kept stored in liquid nitrogen until the time of surgery. These cryolenticules gave relatively good results (more than 60% of the eyes had a final vision of 20/40 or better with around 30% getting to 20/20 or better). They showed a delayed visual recovery but no rejection over a period of 10 years; hence their use in areas where there are no eye banks was popularized.[14]

## Later Stages of Homoplasty Era

Following the period of exponential growth in keratoplasty, suturing techniques evolved and materials used became more sophisticated. Prior to 1970s, braided silk was used for cornea suturing. Silk was rapidly degraded and produced significant tissue inflammation, both of which can cause potential problems in wound dehiscence and postoperative failure. In 1970s, nylon was introduced for suturing: it produced very little inflammation, was nonabsorbable, and had a tensile strength that is maintained for around 1 year. 10-0 was chosen since it provided adequate strength while still being easy to handle. Its ability to be stretched to 125% its length provided a leeway for error, a more reproducible suture tension and, therefore, a better way of decreasing induced astigmatism. Other materials had been used such as polypropylene and polyester (Mersilene) and stainless steel.[19]

Suturing techniques included simple interrupted radial sutures and/or continuous sutures. A comparison between continuous 10-0 nylon sutures and interrupted 9-0 silk sutures in 1975 showed equal success in terms of graft clarity but less astigmatism with a continuous nylon suture.[20]

Consequent to the development of finer surgical instruments, sutures and needles, and with the advent of the surgical microscope as well as the knowledge of the endothelial function, results obtained with corneal transplants in the second half of the century were more encouraging. Seminal work by Frederik Stocker[21] on the structure and function of the human endothelium led to better understanding the reasons behind the maintenance of corneal clarity and the dehydrated state.

In the late 1970s, clear-center, disposable trephines were built that circumvent the previously mentioned problems of centration and injury of anterior chamber structures. Some of these trephines used manual advancement of the blade, while others were mechanical. Drews created a cone type of trephine,[22] Donaldson added a handle for stability,[23] Miller designed an open branding-iron configuration,[24] and Doughman created a hollow tube holder that accepted varying size blades.[25]

The single point trephines were later devised: they have a ring that sits on the sclera or on the limbus, thus reducing corneal distortion. Two such trephines include the Lieberman limbal suction-fixation trephine,[26] and the Crock trephine.[27]

Combination trephines, like the Hanna trephine that was popularized by Warring and Hanna in 1989,[28] have a limbal-based suction system that would minimize movement of both the cornea and the trephine allowing maintenance of the centration during the procedure. The trephine is mechanical, can be easily controlled, and has a preset depth, thus limiting its entry into the anterior chamber.

Much progress has been made in the understanding of the factors controlling trephination. Attempts to improve on hand-held instruments have led to suction trephines and motorized devices described above, and more recently, nonmechanical, laser-based, donor and recipient corneal preparation, as will be discussed later.

The most common postoperative complication is astigmatism which may be secondary to donor-recipient mismatch, corneal topographic abnormalities in donor or recipient, suturing techniques or individual healing processes. Initially, the aim of transplantation was restoration of corneal clarity, however with the advent of refined techniques and the improvement in the material available, the emphasis on postoperative astigmatism increased. Since the 1970s, the role of suturing in determining postoperative refractive error and the role of suture removal in their management have been extensively examined. The use of spectacles and contact lenses to correct postoperative astigmatism emerged and surgical techniques began with incisional techniques involving the graft wound, introduced by Troutman as relaxing incisions and wedge resection in 1977.[29] In the 1980s, astigmatic keratotomy, which uses a diamond blade to make transverse incisions at the steep meridian (not in the graft wound) and radial keratotomy (RK) were used to reduce postoperative astigmatism and myopia. With the launching of the excimer laser in the 1990s, surface treatment was applied on postkeratoplasty corneas to correct any residual/induced error.[30]

## Current Evolution in Keratoplasty

By the early 1990s, PKP gained a lot of momentum due to its success and the advancement of the surgical techniques. The idea of removing only the portion of the cornea that is diseased and leaving the recipient's normal anatomic layers intact aimed to do the least amount of resection, with the least amount of risk, for the greatest amount of benefit. Replacing only the anterior stroma in case the stroma is scarred, or replacing the endothelium in case of endothelial failure became the next step in corneal transplantation.

The integrity of the globe in LKP is maintained and the recipient's healthy tissue is kept, minimizing immunologic reactions. In addition, the fact that the PKP wound is transverse across all collagen fibers makes it a weak point, with reports of wound gape after suture removal or globe rupture after mild trauma as high as 7%.[31] Despite the fact that very early transplants were lamellar, PKP were the exclusive keratoplasty procedure performed in the first half of the 20th century. It was not before recent years that the shift to LKP outdid penetrating procedures (Fig. 1).

### Deep Anterior Lamellar Keratoplasty

Lamellar keratoplasty can be subdivided into anterior or posterior LKP. Initially, before the 1950s, anterior LKP was the procedure of choice over PKP. However, this

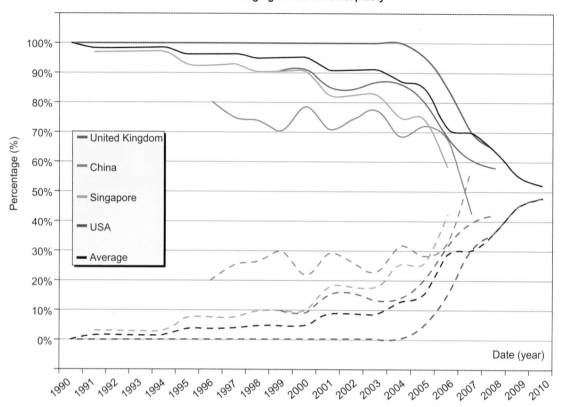

**Fig. 1:** Evolution of lamellar (LKP) and penetrating (PKP) keratoplasties over time. Solid lines represent PKP, dashed lines represent LKP. Colors represent data from the same study. Data pooled from studies done in United Kingdom,[32] China,[33] Singapore[34] and from the Eye Bank Association of America. Part of the data was extrapolated from the published graphs
*Source*: Reprinted with permission from the 2010 Eye Banking Statistical Report by the Eye Bank Association of America. Copyright© 2011EBAA®, Washington, DC; www.restoresight.org. All Rights Reserved

procedure was a tedious, time consuming manual process that left the patients with a best expected visual acuity of 20/30 or worse,[35] PKP was faster and visual results were more promising.[36]

Anterior LKP has always been used for tectonic grafting in cases of recurrent pterygia (in which lamellar grafting would provide a new 'barrier' Bowman's layer), peripheral ulcerative diseases (such as Mooren's ulcer), rheumatoid arthritis, and noninflammatory (Terrien's) degeneration.[14]

In deep lamellar anterior keratoplasty, the objective is to remove all stromal tissue overlying the recipient pupillary zone, leaving just the recipient Descemet's membrane and endothelium, creating the smoothest recipient bed possible. Before 1975, surgical techniques by Malbran[37] and Gasset[38] achieved quite deep keratectomies with transplantation of full thickness corneas with only the donor endothelium removed. Patients had good postoperative visual acuities

(80% had 20/40 or better), however the graft-host bond was weak and this contributed to postoperative pseudo-anterior chamber interface formation.[39] In 1984, Archila[40] described the 'air-bubble technique' of Descemet's membrane separation which was further popularized by Anwar.[41]

### Automated Lamellar Therapeutic Keratoplasty

A main problem with early lamellar surgeries was the irregularities produced at the interface. Smoothening out the surfaces of the donor and recipient allowed for better graft outcomes. Automated and laser-assisted lamellar keratoplasties have been shown to result in optimally-smooth lamellar dissection, and hence better postoperative visual acuity. In automated lamellar therapeutic keratoplasty (ALTK), a microkeratome device is used to cut the donor corneal button while it is on the artificial anterior chamber.[42] The dissection results in a smoother corneal surface that leads to decreased postoperative haze.

## Posterior Lamellar Keratoplasty

Prior to 1999 lamellar endothelial keratoplasty was unsuccessful. Recently, with the advent of instrumentation and the advancement of techniques, its results became more promising. Figures 2A to G show the progression of posterior LKP techniques.

The technique was originally described by Barraquer in 1951.[43] He described a technique in which a superficial rectangular hinged-flap was dissected and a circular opening was trephined in the remaining stroma. Then, a round lenticule of donor posterior cornea tissue containing healthy endothelium was transplanted. The lenticule and the flap were secured in place with sutures. In 1965, Polack repeated Barraquer's proposal, but, due to the postoperative increased astigmatism, the higher rate of endothelial cell loss and the flap problems, the technique was abandoned.[44] In 1993, Ko and colleagues successfully transplanted corneal endothelium in rabbits using a sclerolimbal approach.[42] Jones and Culbertson[45] revived the old Barraquer technique, using a microkeratome to create a thick hinged flap that was then retracted and a 7.0 mm diameter trephine was used to resect the recipient posterior stroma. A posterior lamellar donor button and the flap were then sutured into place. In 1998, Melles and colleagues were the first to present a successful posterior lamellar graft in humans.[46] They had refined the sclerolimbal technique to dissect the posterior part of the stroma and trephine a posterior stromal lamella through a limbal incision, thus keeping the anterior stroma undisturbed. Then, a donor button consisting of posterior stroma and endothelium was injected through the same incision followed by an air bubble in the anterior chamber.[47] The presence of air in the anterior chamber, and the endothelial pump mechanism are thought to promote adherence of the donor to the recipient, thus alleviating the need for sutures.[48]

The surgery was initially termed posterior lamellar keratoplasty (PLK); later, Terry and Ousley refined the technique and the instruments and coined the term deep lamellar endothelial keratoplasty (DLEK).[49] When Descemet's stripping was added to the surgical technique, in 2004, it was renamed Descemet's stripping endothelial keratoplasty (DSEK).[50,51] The later introduced use of automated microkeratomes to prepare donor corneas changed the name of the procedure to Descemet's stripping automated endothelial keratoplasty (DSAEK).[52-54] To improve visual outcome by means of creating a smoother graft interface,[55] refinements in the technique[56]

and development of Descemet's membrane endothelial keratoplasty (DMEK) were described. In DMEK only the endothelium with its attached Descemet's membrane (and no stroma) is replaced.[57] Variations on the technique had been reported by Studeny and by McCauley.[58,59]

In 2003, Seitz and colleagues proposed the use of the femtosecond (FS) laser technology to perform PLK.[60] In this technique the laser firing sequence for the trephination begins in the anterior chamber and moves progressively forward through endothelium, Descemet's membrane and posterior stroma.[60] In 2007, Cheng and colleagues performed the first femtosecond laser-assisted lamellar endothelial keratoplasty (FLEK) in humans.[61]

## Phototherapeutic Keratectomy

Excimer laser phototherapeutic keratectomy (PTK) has been investigated since 1988. Gartry and colleagues started a laboratory investigation in 1988 to study the effect of the excimer laser on the anterior stroma in cadaveric eyes followed by experiments on patients with band keratopathy.[62] Afterwards, different authors reported independently about the use of the excimer laser to ablate the surface of the cornea with high precision and minimal collateral damage to treat surface corneal lesions and irregularities.[63-65] Sher and colleagues reported on a multicenter study using the excimer laser to ablate anterior stromal and superficial scarring from postinfectious and posttraumatic causes, including inactive herpes simplex virus, anterior corneal dystrophies, recurrent erosions, granular dystrophy, and band keratopathy. This led to improvement of the scars and improvement in visual acuity in around half the patients. The authors also noted a hyperopic shift in most of the patients.[65] Stark and colleagues reported in 1992 on the first long follow-up of patients who underwent PTK.[66] Fagerholm and colleagues reported favorable results of 166 patients operated in Sweden and reemphasized the induced hyperopic shift.[67]

The procedure received food and drug administration (FDA) approval in 1995 for the treatment of anterior corneal disorders (affecting less than one-third of the cornea) that significantly degrades visual acuity. It offers an alternative to LKP due to the precise control of amount of tissue ablated, its ease of use, the provision of a smooth base for corneal re-epithelialization, the relatively fast visual recovery and the ability to retreat if need be. Disadvantages of this technique include possible hyperopic shift, scarring, and postoperative discomfort and haze.[68]

CHAPTER 67

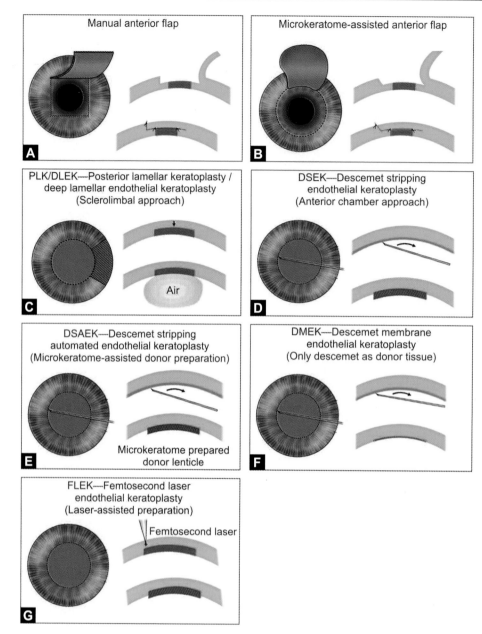

**Figs 2A to G:** Evolution of posterior keratoplasty techniques: The early technique involved fashioning an anterior flap manually as described by Barraquer in 1951 (A), or using a microkeratome as described by Polack in 1965. (B) The anterior flap is lifted and a posterior corneal button trephined. The donor posterior cornea is sutured in place. (C) Posterior Lamellar Keratoplasty, later termed Deep Lamellar Endothelial Keratoplasty using a sclerolimbal approach in which the endothelium is stripped and a donor posterior lamellar graft is inserted and reapposed using air (first described by Ko in 1993 and Melles in 1998). (D) Descemet's Stripping Endothelial Keratoplasty using a modified Sinskey hook through a corneal incision. A thick posterior donor corneal button is apposed using air. Gorovoy, in 2006, proposed using a microkeratome to improve donor tissue preparation and coined the term Descemet's Stripping Automated Endothelial Keratoplasty. (E) Tappin in 2006 reported on transplanting Descemet's membrane only, renaming the procedure Descemet's membrane endothelial keratoplasty. (F) Seitz in 2003 and Cheng in 2007 proposed using the femtosecond laser to prepare donor and recipient; (G) In a procedure called Femtosecond Laser Endothelial Keratoplasty

## Keratoprostheses and Xenotransplants

Despite the fact that PKP is the most successful transplant, the scarcity of donor tissue and some ocular surface pathology might prevent a transplanted cornea from remaining viable. In such cases, the use of a keratoprosthesis, would come into play.

Since 1950s, different approaches for keratoprosthesis have been described based on the ideas of one of the first envisioners of corneal transplant, Pellier de Quengsy.[69] Keratoprostheses are particularly resilient to a hostile environment such as the dry keratinized eye resulting from severe Stevens–Johnson syndrome, ocular cicatricial pemphigoid, trachoma and chemical injury and its rigid optical cylinder permits excellent image quality. Although complications are frequently associated to keratoprostheses, they can effectively restore good visual function in patients considered untreatable by conventional corneal transplantation.

Soon after the second world war some authors realized that polymethylmethacrylate (PMMA) could be used to replace the cornea.[70-73] In the beginning of the 1960s the osteo-odonto-keratoprosthesis was described by Strampelli and colleagues[74] followed by a description by Choyce[75] and then by Dohlman and colleagues.[76] Nowadays several models of keratoprostheses are available, including the Boston keratoprosthesis, the osteo-odonto-keratoprosthesis, the Alphacor, the Chirila keratoprosthesis, the Pintucci Biointegrable keratoprosthesis, Moscow Eye Microsurgery Complex keratoprosthesis (MICOF)[77,78] and the Supra-Descemetic synthetic cornea (that is still being developed).[79,80]

## Laser-assisted Penetrating Keratoplasty

Excimer lasers and FS lasers are both used in cornea surgery. Though their effects complement each other, their mechanism of action differs. Table 1 summarizes some important features specific to the excimer and the FS lasers.

At the end of the 1980s, Lang and colleagues described a novel technique using excimer laser to perform corneal trephination.[81-83] This technique showed a better outcome of PKP.[84]

In 1999, with the advent of the FS laser, the ability of non-mechanical trephination emerged. Clinical applications of laser trephination were pioneered by Naumann in Germany, who has used 193 nm excimer lasers to produce both donor and recipient cuts. In a randomized trial, both myopia and astigmatism were less in laser cut than in mechanically cut eyes.[84]

The donor tissue is prepared using a corneoscleral button mounted in an artificial chamber and cut to match

**Table 1:** Table describing different properties of excimer and femtosecond lasers

| | Excimer | Femtosecond |
|---|---|---|
| Wavelength | 193 nm | 1053 nm |
| Light spectrum | Far UV | Near infrared |
| Tissue effect | Photoablation | Photodisruption |
| Focusing | Collimated beam | Focused beam at any desired depth |
| Suction | Not needed for operation | Needed for proper focusing |
| Tissue clarity | Beam ablates scar-tissue differently | Unaffected by haze |
| Tissue penetration | Absorbed by the first tissue encountered | Penetrates transparent tissue |

UV: Ultraviolet

the recipient tissue. A spiral or raster pattern of FS laser can be used, and the donor corneal button sutured to the recipient residual bed.[60]

In 2008, Yoo et al. reported a case series of FS laser-assisted anterior lamellar keratoplasty (ALK) and introduced the concept of sutureless ALK.[85] They programmed the depth of the FS laser lamellar cuts based on anterior segment optical coherence tomography measurements of the depth of the anterior corneal pathology. They spared the normal posterior corneal tissue, enough to maintain the structural integrity of the cornea.[86]

## Different Trephination Configurations

In 1999, Naumann and colleagues proposed a revolutionary concept of nonmechanical trephination of the cornea using a 193 nm laser.[84]

The laser, known as the FS laser, has a frequency in the order of 10–15 sec, enabling it to deliver high energy to a focused point. It works by photodisrupting tissue: high-power ionizing laser pulses dissociate electrons from their atoms creating a rapidly expanding cloud of free electrons and ionized molecules (plasma). A shock wave is thus created, followed by a cavitation bubble that ultimately results in tissue disruption.[87] The short duration of the laser pulse delivers tens of megawatts of laser energy with a maximum collateral damage of 1 μm.[88] It was approved by the FDA for use in lamellar LKP in 2000. Its use for full thickness keratoplasty was approved in 2005.

The use of the laser for donor and recipient trephination leads to better control over trephining, with the ability to set the depth, diameter, and margin of the corneal buttons.

CHAPTER 67

Early surgical outcomes of laser-assisted PKP show better natural alignment of the donor and host anterior surfaces, improved sealing of the incision, reduced tissue distortion and improved wound tensile strength.[89] All these result in a faster visual recovery with astigmatism comparable to or slightly better than traditional blade trephination PKP.[86]

The use of laser revived a long-forgotten technique of multileveled, stepped and corneal trephination. Patterns such as mushroom shaped, top-hat, zig-zag, Christmas tree and dove-tail became easier to make.[90] These provide better donor-recipient interlocking and less postoperative astigmatism.[87] Table 2 compares indications and outcomes of different forms of keratoplasty.

# ⯈ HISTORY OF REFRACTIVE SURGERY

Today, patients may choose from a large portfolio of refractive surgery, mainly keratorefractive procedures. Keratorefractive surgeries are able to correct low-order optic aberrations (myopia, hyperopia and astigmatism) and higher order aberrations. Presbyopia and treatment of patients with keratoconus have been described but still need to be validated.

All procedures reshape the cornea and induce corneal changes by affecting the corneal stroma. These procedures can be classified as incisional, collagen-altering, keratomileusis, laser-assisted and intrastromal-implant refractive surgeries. Incisions result in wound gape, collagen-altering surgeries use thermal energy to cause focal contraction in collagen architecture, keratomileusis mechanically adds (or subtracts) tissue from the cornea to reshape it, laser-assisted surgeries use excimer or FS lasers to subtract tissue, implants change the corneal shape and/or its refractive index.

## Incisional Corneal Refractive Surgery

The earliest report of using an incision to alter the shape of the human cornea was in 1885, when Schiotz used a limbal relaxing incision in a patient who underwent cataract surgery and observed flattening in the incised meridian.[91] In 1894, Bates noticed that traumatic peripheral corneal scars resulted in flattening along the scar meridian with no effect on the perpendicular meridian.[92] The first description of the astigmatic effect of nonpenetrating incisions placed near the limbus dates back to 1898 and is credited to the Dutch ophthalmologist Lans.[27] In 1939, Sato was the first to publish reports describing his attempts to refine incisional refractive surgery with anterior and posterior corneal incisions.[93] The problem however, was that his incisions compromised the endothelial cells and caused corneal edema. Yenaleyev operated on 426 cases and found that radial incisions in the anterior peripheral cornea could treat up to 4 Diopters (D) of myopia.[94] The Russian ophthalmologist, Fyodorov later developed a systematic process of anterior RK and treated thousands of myopic patients with greater predictability.[95] In the United States, primate and human-cadaveric eye experiments, done in the early 1980s showed flattening of the cornea (of an average between 6 and 11 diopters), with 90% of the effect seen after 8 radial incisions.[96,97] In 1978, Bores performed the first RK in America.[98]

Merlin popularized curved, partial-thickness incisions with a rationale that they remain equidistant from the center of the cornea throughout and pass through cornea of consistent thickness.[99] The technique was termed arcuate keratotomy, and it involved placing 1 or 2 deep, curved corneal incisions perpendicular to the steep meridian of astigmatism. The incisions could either be performed freehand or with the help of an arcitome (Example: Hanna MoriaArcitome).[28] Limbal relaxing incisions (LRI) are a form of arcuate keratotomy in which the incisions are placed closer to the limbus and were described for the first time by Hanna in 1989.[100] They were popularized and described to be done simultaneously with cataract surgery to correct minor astigmatism by Budak in 1998.[101]

**Table 2:** Indications, technique and outcomes of penetrating keratoplasty (PKP), deep anterior lamellar keratoplasty (DALK), Descemet's stripping endothelial keratoplasty (DSEK) and Descemet's membrane endothelial keratoplasty (DMEK)

| | | PKP | DALK | DSEK | DMEK |
|---|---|---|---|---|---|
| **Indications** | Anterior stromal disease | + | + | – | – |
| | Posterior stromal disease | + | + | + | – |
| | Endothelial disease | + | – | + | + |
| **Surgery** | Difficulty | + | ++ | ++ | +++ |
| | Surgery time | + | ++ | + | ++ |
| | Open sky | + | – | – | – |
| | Sutures | + | + | – | – |
| | Astigmatism | ++ | + | – | – |
| **Postoperative** | Time to recovery | +++ | ++ | ++ | + |
| | Graft dislocation | ± | – | + | ++ |
| | Graft survival | + | ++ | ++ | ++ |
| | Postoperative change in topography | +++ | ++ | + | ± |
| | Visual outcome | ++ | + | + | ++ |

In 1981, the United States National Eye Institute (NEI) initiated a multicenter trial for the Prospective Evaluation of Radial Keratotomy (PERK). Patients had 8 radial incisions equidistantly-spaced around a clear central optical zone of 4 mm or less. The study allowed 70% of patients who had 8 radial incisions to correct for a myopic refraction from −2.00 D to −8.00 D with a cylindrical component less than 1.50 D to be spectacle-independent for distance.[102]

The results of incisional surgery were impressive; however they had a large margin of error with results not very predictable in all patients. The longer follow-up of the PERK study demonstrated that more than 40% of eyes presented progressive hyperopia after 10 years of the procedure.[102] This, together with the advent of lasers, led to the procedures being practically abandoned.

## Collagen Alteration Surgery

### Thermokeratoplasty

The biomechanical properties of the cornea are not significantly affected by temperatures less than 50°C; however, between 70°C and 80°C, the stromal collagen lamellae shows significant shrinkage; and intermolecular bonds begin to dissolve, resulting in irreversible necrosis and permanent destruction of the corneal tissue.[103] In 1889, Lans noticed that radial burns in rabbit eyes steepen the cornea.[74] Gasset and Kaufman used the same technique in the 1970s in an attempt to treat keratoconus,[75] and Acquavella used it to treat corneal hydrops.[76] Results were initially good, but long-term complications and regression of its effect ensued.[73] Fyodorov and Newmann were the first to use the technique as a refractive surgery technique and coined the term thermokeratoplasty. In the 1980s, they used a nichrome tip probe to heat the corneal stroma to 600°C in an attempt to correct hyperopia.[104] This altered collagen structure and resulted in refractive changes, but unfortunately, its results were not as predictable as expected and did not last for a long enough time.

### Laser Thermal Keratoplasty

In the early1990s, the first contact probe holmium yttrium-aluminum-garnet (Ho:YAG) laser thermal keratoplasty (LTK) procedure was developed for the treatment of hyperopia.[105] In 2000, investigations in Germany showed success with hyperopia treatment[106] and LTK was then FDA approved in the same year.

Other heating methods for LTK were also tried, including hot copper wires,[107] carbon dioxide lasers,[108] diode lasers,[109] and cobalt: magnesium fluoride lasers.[110]

### Conductive Keratoplasty

Conductive keratoplasty (CK) as an alternative to thermokeratoplasty.[111] Although 1.6 MHz radiofrequency probes had been proposed in the United States since the beginning of the 1980s,[112,113] the use of modern 350 KHz CK probes is credited to Antonio Mendez. He developed in 2002, the procedure was FDA approved for the treatment of mild to moderate (0.75–3.00 D), previously untreated, spherical hyperopia.[107] In 2004, the FDA approved it for the temporary induction of myopia in the nondominant eye of presbyopic hyperopes or emmetropes.[107]

CK uses the electrical conductive properties of the cornea to propagate energy through the stroma and generate heat. In theory, the use of electric energy propagation through the cornea, more than its thermal conductive characteristics, would generate a more homogeneous and cylindrical thermal footprint that may minimize regression over time.[114] The energy is delivered to the corneal midperiphery resulting in central steepening. The source of energy is a high-frequency alternating electric current.

## Keratomileusis

In the late 1940s, Jose Ignacio Barraquer performed freehand lamellar dissection in conjunction with excision of the stroma. In 1964, he termed the technique myopic keratomileusis.[115] The technique involved removal of part of the central stroma leading to flattening of the cornea and improvement in myopia. A corneal cap was removed using a mechanical microkeratome, and the stroma was frozen and processed with a specially designed cryolathe.[116] Results were not very predictable, and complications were not scarce.[117] Krumeich, in an effort to decrease the complications of freezing the cornea during myopic keratomileusis, designed a technique known as nonfreeze keratomileusis. The corneal cap was cut using a mechanical microkeratome, and transferred to a Teflon dish with the epithelium facing down. The cap was maintained in place by suction. The dish had convex and concave concavities that make different parts of the stroma bulge up to correct myopia and hyperopia respectively. A mechanical microkeratome was then used again to cut off any bulging stroma.[115,116,118] Further improvements on the technique were proposed by Ruiz and Rowsey, and named the procedure *In Situ* Keratomileusis. This technique involved removing a corneal cap using a mechanical microkeratome and then cutting a lenticule from the residual stromal bed using the same microkeratome. The cap was then replaced and sutured.[117,119,120] This resulted in flattening of

**CHAPTER 67**

the overall corneal curvature and correction of myopia. Guimarães described for the first time nonsutured myopic keratomileusis under topical anesthesia.[121]

All the above-mentioned procedures had limited predictability of correction and high risk of potential complications. Due to the high amount of postoperative complications and the presence of lasers, a search for a better technique with fewer complications led to the development of Laser *In Situ* Keratomileusis (LASIK).

## Laser Assisted Surgery

### Excimer Laser Assisted

Photorefractive keratectomy (PRK): Initially, refractive surgery involved incisions or burns to alter corneal shape, however with the advent of the laser, the use of the excimer and the FS lasers to ablate and photo disrupt the cornea became the prevalent method of refractive error correction. Nowadays, two laser types are used in cornea surgery, the excimer laser (that ablates tissue) and the FS laser (that photodisrupts tissue).

The excimer (excited dimer) laser principle is related to excitation of gases to release energy. The gases (argon and fluoride) used are stable in their normal low-energy state. When a high-voltage electrical discharge is delivered in a laser cavity containing these gases, these gases combine to form a higher-energy excited-gas state compound. Upon dissociation of this high-energy compound, a photon of energy (proportional to the energy bond between the gas molecules) is released. This wavelength of light energy [193 nm, in the ultraviolet C (UVC) range] is amplified in the laser system and results in the production of a high-energy discrete pulse of laser energy. The 193 nm excimer laser energy is absorbed by the proteins, glycosaminoglycans and nucleic acids that make up the cornea and thus results in breaking of molecular bonds. The corneal molecular fragments are then ejected from the surface of the cornea at supersonic speeds (forming the effluent plume seen during laser treatment). This process is called 'ablative photodecomposition'.

Taboada and Archibald reported the use of the excimer laser on the corneal epithelium in 1981 at the Aerospace Medical Association Meeting.[122] In 1983, Trokel and colleagues showed how the excimer laser could be used to ablate bovine corneal stroma in a manner that was similar to RK.[123] Puliafito defined an excimer laser emission of 193 nm as ideal in terms of leading to a maximum ablation efficiency, and at the same time limiting collateral thermal damage.[124] In 1985, Seiler performed the first excimer laser

treatment in a blind eye. He later was the first to perform excimer laser astigmatic transverse keratectomy.[125] 193 nm excimer laser ablation for correction of astigmatism was first reported in 1991.[126] The first mention of the use of the excimer laser for correction of myopia in a living human eye in the United States was in 1989 by McDonald and colleagues.[127]

*Laser in situ keratomileusis (LASIK)*: Laser *in situ* keratomileusis involves creating a sub-Bowman flap and reflecting it back. This is followed by intrastromal excimer laser ablation after which the flap is repositioned in place.[128] Historically, the foundation for LASIK is largely credited to Barraquer. In 1988, Pallikaris initiated the use of the excimer laser in studies on rabbit eyes.[129] This led to his investigation of the laser in sighted human eyes in 1991. In the early 1990s, two research groups headed by Pallikaris[130] and Buratto[131] independently described a technique that combined two existing technologies: the microkeratome and the excimer laser. Pallikaris coined the term LASIK for this new technique, and Buratto named the technique photokeratomileusis (PKM). Buratto's technique involved removing a keratomileusis cap and performing laser on it,[132] while Pallikaris' technique involved the treatment of the stromal bed.[130] In 1991, Pallikaris and colleagues described the basis of the technique that is used nowadays, lifting a hinged flap and applying laser energy to the residual stromal bed.[129]

### Femtosecond Laser Assisted

The femtosecond (FS) laser creates a resection plane for lamellar cuts using a 1040 nm wavelength beam with a spot size less than 1 mm, and a pulse repetition rate in the MHz range. It can perform horizontal and vertical cuts in the cornea with very minimal collateral damage, thus it can be successfully used to promote corneal trephination and LASIK flaps.

*Flap creation*: The advents of FS laser over microkeratomes include better control over flap creation in which customization of the diameter, hinge and depth of the flap is more precise and independent of the corneal shape and curvature, with less flap-related complications. The IntraLase was FDA approved for LASIK flap creation in 2001.[133] The first report on its efficiency in LASIK flap creation was published in 2003.[134]

*Femtosecond Lenticule EXtraction FLEX®*: Femtosecond Lenticule EXtraction (FLEX), initially developed by Carl Zeiss Meditec[135] and popularized in their FS laser VisuMax, uses solely the FS laser for refractive procedures.

It involves making two cuts in the cornea that intersect in the periphery, creating a lenticule, which is ultimately removed, thus altering the curvature of the cornea.[136] Initial reports in non-seeing eyes, highly myopic eyes, and amblyopic eyes were first published in 1998.[137,138] Sekundo and colleagues published about the feasibility and efficacy of FLEX to correct myopia.[136]

*Intracor®*: INTRACOR was developed by Technolas Perfect Vision.[139] It is designed to correct presbyopia in emmetropic patients. The FS laser is used to create a series of concentric circular cuts intrastromally, centered around the visual axis without reaching the surface. This leads to a biomechanical change in the center of the cornea, causing it to shift slightly anteriorly, thus becoming hyperprolate and enhancing near vision. The corneal epithelium, Bowman's layer, and anterior stromal fibers are preserved during this process.[140]

## Intrastromal Implants

### Rings

Reynolds, in 1993, proposed altering the corneal surface by placing intrastromal corneal rings.[141,142] Initially, the implants were PMMA rings inserted through a peripheral single corneal incision into a circumferential corneal channel. The rings were then refashioned into rings segments thus making their implantation easier. Two main types of intracorneal ring segments (ICRS) received CE approval in 1996 and FDA approval in 1999.[143] In 2000, Colin reported the first clinical results of ICRS use in keratoconus.[144] The ICRS have various cross-sectional designs, diameters, thicknesses and arc-lengths. Initially, Intacs and Ferrara rings were developed, but KeraRings®, Bisantis® segmented perioptic implants, and Myorings® were later introduced with all of them still present on the market today.[143]

## CORNEAL COLLAGEN CROSSLINKING

Collagen crosslinking (CXL) involves the use of ultraviolet light to increase interlamellar collagen linkages. The idea to use this approach to treat keratoconus was conceived in Germany in the 1990s by a research group at Dresden Technical University[145] and initial clinical results were published by Seiler and collaborators in 2003.[146] It involves using ultraviolet A (UVA, 370 nm) light and 0.1% riboflavin-5-phosphate (vitamin B) at a radiance of $3\,mW/cm^2$ to crosslink the central cornea. This results in

stiffening of the cornea, up to 300%.[147] A newer proprietary technique,[148] FlashLinking® Crosslinking, was evaluated by Rocha et al. in 2008. It involves the use of a fast curing crosslinking material that induces corneal collagen stiffening after a 30 second exposure to UVA irradiation.[149] In 2011, AvedroInc®, another proprietary technique received FDA orphan-drug status to perform corneal crosslinking in the treatment of keratoconus (www.clinicaltrials.gov, NCT01344187).

## APPENDIX

Summary of important landmarks in keratoplasty

| Author | Year | Contribution |
|--------|------|--------------|
| Galen | 130–200 | Idea of restoring transparency of an opaque cornea |
| Darwin | 1760 | Idea of removal of an opaque cornea by trephination |
| Quengsy | 1771 | Idea of implanting a clear glass instead of the opaque cornea |
| | 1796 | First circular cutting of the cornea |
| | 1800s | Discovery of anesthesia and antiseptic measures |
| Himly | 1813 | Idea of replacing opaque cornea with clear cornea in animals |
| Reisinger | 1824 | Penetrating transplants in rabbits |
| Bigger | 1837 | First successful transplant in animals |
| Königshofer | 1839 | Squared lamellar transplants |
| Mühlbauer | 1840 | Triangular lamellar transplants |
| Steiner | 1843 | First use of trephines in animals |
| Kissam | 1844 | Penetrating transplant with porcine corneas |
| Sellerbeck | 1878 | Unsuccessful keratoplasty with fetal corneas |
| Wolfe | 1880 | Penetrating transplant in bridge with temporary success |
| Koller | 1884 | Topical cocaine for corneal anesthesia |
| Von Hippel | 1886 | First trephine |

*Contd...*

CHAPTER 67

| Author | Year | Contribution |
| --- | --- | --- |
| Von Hippel | 1888 | Heterologous lamellar transplant with success in one patient |
| Fuchs | 1894 | Homologous lamellar transplant in 30 patients |
| Zirm | 1905 | Penetrating transplant with permanent success |
| Löhlein | 1910 | Lamellar transplants in bridge in animals |
| Magitot | 1911 | Cornea preservation for 8 days |
| Forster | 1923 | Triangular rotational penetrating grafts studies |
| Thomas | 1930 | Crossed contention sutures studies in animals |
| Elschnig | 1930 | Contention sutures in humans |
| Castroviejo | 1931 | Contention sutures with conjunctival flaps |
| Filatov | 1935 | First eye bank (Odessa, Russia) |
| Paton | 1945 | First US eye bank (New York) |
| | 1930 | Development of the slit biomicroscope |
| Maumanee | 1941 | Graft rejection recognized as a clinical entity |
| Stocker | 1953 | Description of structure and function of human endothelium |
| | 1961 | Eye Bank Association of America |
| Urrets-Zavalia | 1966 | Use of desiccated lenticules for LKP |
| | 1970 | Use of 10-0 nylon sutures for cornea surgery |
| | 1970 | Introduction of specular microscope for corneal examination |
| | 1974 | McCarey-Kaufmann donor preservation medium |
| | 1980s | Astigmatic and radial keratectomies |
| Archila | 1985 | Air-bubble technique for anterior LKP |
| | 1989 | Hanna semi-automated trephine |
| | 1992 | Optisol donor preservation medium |
| | 1989 | First idea of use of laser for trephination |

*Contd...*

| Author | Year | Contribution |
| --- | --- | --- |
| Juhasz | 1990 | Prototype of first ophthalmic surgical femtosecond laser |
| | 1990s | Topical and subconjunctival anesthesia |
| Jones | 1998 | Endothelial lamellar keratoplasty |
| Naumann | 1999 | Laser trephination |
| | 2000 | FDA approval for femtosecond use for lamellar keratoplasty |
| Terry | 2001 | Deep lamellar endothelial keratoplasty |
| Anwar | 2002 | Big-bubble technique of DALK |
| Busin | 2003 | Stepped grafts (reverse mushroom) using femtosecond laser |
| Melles | 2004 | Posterior lamellar keratoplasty |
| Ignatio | 2004 | First results of use of laser in PKP published |
| | 2005 | FDA approval for IntraLase use for PKP |
| | 2005 | First human full thickness femtosecond transplant |
| Price | 2005 | Descemet's stripping endothelial keratoplasty |
| Buratto | 2007 | First case series of femtosecond PKP |
| Yoo | 2008 | Sutureless femtosecond ALK |

LKP: Lamellar keratoplasty; FDA: Food and Drug Administration; DALK: Deep anterior lamellar keratoplasty; PKP: Penetrating keratoplasty; ALK: Anterior lamellar keratoplasty

## ▶ ACKNOWLEDGMENT

MIDWEST Eye-Bank Association.

## ▶ REFERENCES

1. Olson RJ. Corneal transplantation techniques, in the cornea. In: Kauffmann HE, McDonald MB, Barron BA, Waltman SR (Eds). Churchill Livingstone: New York; 1988. pp. 743-85.
2. Paton RT. History of corneal grafting in Keratoplasty. In: Paton RT (Ed). McGraw-Hill: New York. 1955. pp. 4-35.
3. Liljestrand G. Carl Koller and the development of local anesthesia. Acta Physiol Scand Suppl. 1967;299:1-30.
4. Von Hippel A. Eine neue methode der Hornhauttransplantation. Arch Ophthalmol. 1888;34:105-30.

5.  Zirm EK. Eineerfolgreichetotale keratoplastik. Graefes. Arch Clin Exp Ophthalmol. 1906;64:580-93.

6.  Zirm, EK. Eineerfolgreichetotale keratoplastik (a successful total keratoplasty). Refract Corneal Surg. 1989;5(4):258-61.

7.  Elschnig A. Keratoplasty .Arch Ophthalmol. 1930;4:165-73.

8.  Filatov V. Transplantation of the cornea. Arch Ophthal. 1935;13:321-47.

9.  Magitot A. Recherchesexpérimentalessur la surviepossiblie de la cornéeconservée en dehours de l'organismeetsur la kérato-plastiedifférée. Ann d'Ocul. 1911;146:1-34.

10. McCarey BE, Kaufman HE. Improved corneal storage. Invest Ophthalmol. 1974;13(3):165-73.

11. Van Rij G, Waring GO 3rd. Configuration of corneal trephine opening using five different trephines in human donor eyes. Arch Ophthal. 1988;106:1228-33.

12. Brightbill FS, Polack FM, Slappey T. A comparison of two methods for cutting donor corneal buttons. Am J Ophthalmol.1973;75(3):500-6.

13. Maguen E, Villaseñor RA, Ward DE, et al. A modified artificial anterior chamber for use in refractive keratoplasty. Am J Ophthalmol. 1980;89:742-44.

14. Terry MA. The evolution of lamellar grafting techniques over twenty-five years. Cornea. 2000;19(5):611-6.

15. McDonnell PJ, Falcon MG. The lamellar corneal graft for optical indications. Eye (Lond). 1988;2:390-4.

16. Urrets-Zavalia AJ. Lamellar keratoplasty with homologous material preserved by spontaneous desiccation. Int Ophthalmol Clin. 1966;6(1):79-98.

17. Rich L. A technique for preparing corneal lamellar donor tissue using simplified keratomileusis. Ophthalmic Surg. 1980;11:606-8.

18. Barraquer J. Basis of refractive keratoplasty. Arch Soc Am Ophthal Optom. 1967;6:21-68.

19. Jongebloed WL, Rijneveld WJ, Cuperus PL, et al. Stainless steel as suturing material in human and rabbit corneas: A SEM-study. Doc Ophthalmol. 1988;70:145-54.

20. Boruchoff SA, Jensen AD, Dohlman CH. Comparison of suturing techniques in keratoplasty for keratoconus. Ann Ophthalmol. 1975;7:433-6.

21. Stocker, Georgiade NA. The endothelium of the cornea and its clinical implications. Trans Am Acad Ophthalmol Otolaryngol. 1953;51:669-786.

22. Drews RC. Corneal trephine. Trans Am Acad Ophthalmol Otolaryngol. 1974;78(2):OP223-4.

23. Donaldson WB, Haining WM. A new corneal trephine. Trans Ophthalmol Soc U K. 1978;98(1):14-5.

24. Miller D. A new microsurgical corneal trephine. Ophthalmic Surg. 1979;10(7):55-8.

25. Doughman DJ. Corneal trephine holder. Ophthalmology. 1978;85(8):875-6.

26. Lieberman DM. A new corneal trephine. Am J Ophthalmol. 1976;81(5):684-5.

27. Crock GW, Pericic L, Chapman-Smith JS, et al. A new system of microsurgery for human and experimental corneal graftin. I. The contact lens corneal cutter, stereotaxic eye holder, donor disc chuck, and frame. Br J Ophthalmol. 1978;62(2):74-80.

28. Waring GO 3rd, Hanna KD. The Hanna suction punch block and trephine system for penetrating keratoplasty. Arch Ophthalmol. 1989;107(10):1536-9.

29. Troutman RC. Microsurgery of the anterior segment of the eye. In: Troutman RC (Ed). St Louis: CV Mosby. Volume 2. 1977.

30. John ME, Martines E, Cvintal T, et al. Photorefractive keratectomy following penetrating keratoplasty. J Refract Corneal Surg. 1994;10(2 Suppl):S206-10.

31. Abou-Jaoude ES, Brooks M, Katz DG, et al. Spontaneous wound dehiscence after removal of single continuous penetrating keratoplasty suture. Ophthalmology. 2002;109(7):1291-6.

32. Keenan TD, Carley F, Yeates D, et al. Trends in corneal graft surgery in the UK. Br J Ophthalmol. 2011;95(4):468-72.

33. Xie L, Qi F, Gao H, et al. Major shifts in corneal transplantation procedures in north China: 5316 eyes over 12 years. Br J Ophthalmol. 2009;93(10):1291-5.

34. Tan DT, Mehta JS. Future directions in lamellar corneal transplantation. Cornea. 2007;26(9 Suppl 1):S21-8.

35. Anwar M. Dissection techniques in lamellar keratoplasty. Br J Ophthalmol. 1972;56(9):711-13.

36. Richard JM, Paton D, Gasset AR. A comparison of penetrating keratoplasty and lamellar keratoplasty in the surgical management of keratoconus. Am J Ophthalmol. 1978;86(6):807-11.

37. Malbran E, Stefani C. Lamellar keratoplasty in corneal ectasias. Ophthalmologica. 1972;164(1):59-70.

38. Gasset AR. Lamellar keratoplasty in the treatment of keratoconus: conectomy. Ophthalmic Surg. 1979;10:26-33.

39. Morrison JC, Swan KC. Full thickness lamellar keratoplasty: a histologic study in human eyes. Ophthalmology. 1982;89:715-9.

40. Archila EA. Deep lamellar keratoplasty dissection of host tissue with intrastromal air injection. Cornea. 1984;3(3):217-8.

41. Anwar M, Teichmann KD. Big-bubble technique to bare Descemet's membrane in anterior lamellar keratoplasty. J Cataract Refract Surg. 2002;28(3):398-403.

42. Behrens A, Dolorico AM, Kara DT, et al. Precision and accuracy of an artificial anterior chamber system in obtaining corneal lenticules for lamellar keratoplasty. J Cataract Refract Surg. 2001;27(10):1679-87.

43. Barraquer J. Queratoplastia: Problemasqueplantea la fijacion del injerto. in 16th Concilium Ophthalmologicum Acta. London: British Medical Association. 1951

44. Polack FM. Queratoplastia lamelar posterior. Rev Peru Oftalmol. 1965;2:62-4.

45. Jones DT, Culbertson WW. Endothelial lamellar keratoplasty (ELK). Invest Ophthalmol Vis Sci. 1998;39:S76.

46. Melles GR, Lander F, Beekhuis WH, et al. Posterior lamellar keratoplasty for a case of pseudophakic bullous keratopathy. Am J Ophthalmol. 1999;127(3):340-1.

47. Melles GR, Eggink FA, Lander F, et al. A surgical technique for posterior lamellar keratoplasty. Cornea. 1998;17(6):618-26.

48. Terry MA, Ousley PJ. Replacing the endothelium without corneal surface incisions or sutures: the first United States clinical series using the deep lamellar endothelial keratoplasty procedure. Ophthalmology. 2003;110(4):755-64.

49. Terry MA, Ousley PJ. Endothelial replacement without surface corneal incisions or sutures: topography of the deep lamellar endothelial keratoplasty procedure. Cornea. 2001;20(1):14-8.

CHAPTER 67

50. Price FW, Price MO. Descemet's stripping with endothelial keratoplasty in 50 eyes: a refractive neutral corneal transplant. J Refract Surg. 2005;21(4):339-45.

51. Melles GR, Wijdh RH, Nieuwendaal CP. A technique to excise the descemet membrane from a recipient cornea (descemetorhexis).Cornea. 2004;23(3):286-8.

52. Gorovoy MS. Descemet-stripping automated endothelial keratoplasty. Cornea. 2006;25(8):886-9.

53. Price FW, Price MO. Descemet's stripping with endothelial keratoplasty in 200 eyes: Early challenges and techniques to enhance donor adherence. J Cataract Refract Surg. 2006; 32(3):411-8.

54. Price MO, Price FW. Descemet's stripping with endothelial keratoplasty: comparative outcomes with microkeratome-dissected and manually dissected donor tissue. Ophthalmology. 2006;113(11):1936-42.

55. Price MO, Price FW. Endothelial keratoplasty—a review. Clin Experiment Ophthalmol. 2010;38(2):128-40.

56. Tappin M. A method for true endothelial cell (Tencell) transplantation using a custom-made cannula for the treatment of endothelial cell failure. Eye (Lond). 2007;21(6):775-9.

57. Melles GR, Ong TS, Ververs B, et al. Descemet membrane endothelial keratoplasty (DMEK).Cornea. 2006;25(8):987-90.

58. McCauley MB, Price FW, Price MO. Descemet membrane automated endothelial keratoplasty: hybrid technique combining DSAEK stability with DMEK visual results. J Cataract Refract Surg. 2009;35(10):1659-64.

59. Studeny P, Farkas A, Vokrojova M, et al. Descemet membrane endothelial keratoplasty with a stromal rim (DMEK-S). Br J Ophthalmol. 2010;94(7):909-14.

60. Seitz, B, Langenbucher A, Hofmann-Rummelt C, et al. Nonmechanical posterior lamellar keratoplasty using the femtosecond laser (femto-plak) for corneal endothelial decompensation. Am J Ophthalmol. 2003;136(4):769-72.

61. Cheng YY, Pels E, Nuijts RM. Femtosecond-laser-assisted Descemet's stripping endothelial keratoplasty. J Cataract Refract Surg. 2007;33(1):152-5.

62. Gartry D, Kerr Muir M, Marshall J. Excimer laser treatment of corneal surface pathology: a laboratory and clinical study. Br J Ophthalmol. 1991.75(5):258-69.

63. Seiler T. The Excimer laser. An instrument for corneal surgery. Ophthalmologe. 1992;89(2):128-33.

64. Dausch D, Schroder E. Treatment of corneal and scleral diseases with the excimer laser. A preliminary report of experiences. Fortschr Ophthalmol. 1990;87(2):115-20.

65. Sher NA, Bowers RA, Zabel RW, et al. Clinical use of the 193-nm excimer laser in the treatment of corneal scars. Arch Ophthalmol. 1991;109(4):491-8.

66. Stark WJ, Chamon W, Kamp MT, et al. Clinical follow-up of 193-nm ArF excimer laser photokeratectomy. Ophthalmology. 1992;99(5):805-12.

67. Fagerholm P, Fitzsimmons TD, Orndahl M, et al. Phototherapeutic keratectomy: long-term results in 166 eyes. Refract Corneal Surg. 1993;9(2 Suppl):S76-81.

68. McCally RL, Connolly PJ, Stark WJ, et al. Identical excimer laser PTK treatments in rabbits result in two distinct haze responses. Invest Ophthalmol Vis Sci. 2006; 47(10):4288-94.

69. Chirila TV, Hicks CR. The origins of the artificial cornea: Pellier de Quengsy and his contribution to the modern concept of keratoprosthesis. Gesnerus. 1999;56(1-2):96-106.

70. Stone W, Herbert E. Experimental study of plastic material as replacement for the cornea; a preliminary report. Am J Ophthalmol. 1953;36(6:2):168-73.

71. Stone W. Alloplasty in surgery of the eye. N Engl J Med. 1958;258(12):596-602.

72. Gyorffy I. Acrylic corneal implant in keratoplasty. Am J Ophthalmol. 1951.34(5:1):757-8.

73. Macpherson DG, Anderson MJ. Keratoplasty with acrylic implant. Br Med J (Clin Res Ed). 1953;1:330-53.

74. Strampelli B, Valvo A, Tusa E. Osteo-odonto-keratoprosthesis in a case treated for anchylobepharon and total simbleraphon. Ann Ottalmol Clin Ocul. 1965;91:462-79.

75. Choyce P. Management of endothelial corneal dystrophy with acrylic corneal inlays. Br J Ophthalmol. 1965;49(8):432-40.

76. Dohlman CH, Brown SI. Treatment of corneal edema with a buried implant. Trans Am Acad Ophthalmol Otolaryngol. 1966;70(2):267-80.

77. Huang Y, Dong Y, Wang L, et al. Long-term outcomes of MICOF keratoprosthesis in the end stage of autoimmune dry eyes: an experience in China. Br J Ophthalmol. 2012;96(1): 28-33.

78. Huang Y, Yu J, Liu L, et al. Moscow eye microsurgery complex in Russia keratoprosthesis in Beijing. Ophthalmology. 2011;118(1):41-6.

79. Gomaa A, Comyn O, Liu C. Keratoprostheses in clinical practice—a review. Clin Experiment Ophthalmol. 2010;38(2):211-24.

80. Hicks C, Crawford G, Chirila T, et al. Development and clinical assessment of an artificial cornea. Prog Retin Eye Res. 2000;19(2):149-70.

81. Lang GK, Koch JW, Schröder E, et al. Configuration of corneal incisions with the excimer laser: an experimental study. Fortschr Ophthalmol, 1989;86(5):437-42.

82. Lang GK, Schroeder E, Koch JW, et al. Excimer laser keratoplasty. Part 2: Elliptical keratoplasty. Ophthalmic Surg. 1989; 20(5):342-6.

83. Lang GK, Schroeder E, Koch JW, et al. Excimer laser keratoplasty. Part 1: Basic concepts. Ophthalmic Surg. 1989;20(4):262-7.

84. Seitz B, Langenbucher A, Kus MM, et al. Nonmechanical corneal trephination with the excimer laser improves outcome after penetrating keratoplasty. Ophthalmology. 1999;106(6): 1156-64.

85. Yoo SH, Kymionis GD, Koreishi A, et al. Femtosecond laser-assisted sutureless anterior lamellar keratoplasty. Ophthalmology. 2008;115(8):1303-7.

86. Bahar I, Kaiserman I, Srinivasan S, et al. Comparison of three different techniques of corneal transplantation for keratoconus. Am J Ophthalmol. 2008;146(6):905-12.

87. Shousha MA, Yoo SH. New therapeutic modalities in femtosecond laser-assisted corneal surgery. Int Ophthalmol Clin. 2010; 50(3):149-60.

88. Kurtz RM, Horvath C, Liu HH, et al. Lamellar refractive surgery with scanned intrastromal picosecond and femtosecond laser pulses in animal eyes. J Refract Surg. 1998;14(5):541-8.

89. Farid M, Kim M, Steinert RF. Results of penetrating keratoplasty performed with a femtosecond laser zigzag incision initial report. Ophthalmology. 2007;114(12):2208-12.

90. Lee J, Winokur J, Hallak J, et al. Femtosecond dovetail penetrating keratoplasty: surgical technique and case report. Br J Ophthalmol. 2009;93(7):861-3.

91. Schiotz HA. Ein fall von hochgradige hornhautastigmatismus nachstar extraction: besserung auf operativen Wege. Archiv für Augenheilkunde. 1885;15:179-81.

92. Bates WH. A suggestion of an operation to correct astigmatism.1894. Refract Corneal Surg. 1989;5(1):58-9.

93. Sato T. Crosswise incisions of Descemet's membrane for the treatment of advanced keratoconus. Acta Soc Ophthalmol (Jpn). 1942;46:469-70.

94. Yenaleyev FS. Experience of surgical treatment of myopia. Ann Ophthalmol USSR. 1979;3:52-5.

95. Durnevv VV. Characteristics of surgical correcion of myopia after 16 and 32 peripheral anterior radial non-perforating incisions, in Surgery of anomalies in ocular refraction. In: SN Fyodorov (Ed). The Moscow Research Institute of Ocular Microsurgery: Moscow; 1981. pp.33-5.

96. Steel D, Jester JV, Salz J, et al. Modification of corneal curvature following radial keratotomy in primates. Ophthalmology. 1981;88(8):747-54.

97. Salz J, Lee JS, Jester JV, et al. Radial keratotomy in fresh human cadaver eyes. Ophthalmology. 1981;88(8):742-6.

98. Bores LD, Myers W, Cowden J. Radial keratotomy: an analysis of the American experience. Ann Ophthalmol. 1981;13(8):941-8.

99. Binder PS, Waring GO III. Keratotomy for astigmatism, in Refractive Keratotomy for Myopia and Astigmatism. In: Waring GO III (Ed). Mosby Year Book: St Louis, MO. pp. 1085-1198.

100. Hanna KD, Jouve FE, Waring GO, et al. Computer simulation of arcuate and radial incisions involving the corneoscleral limbus. Eye (Lond). 1989;3( Pt 2):227-39.

101. Budak K, Friedman NJ, Koch DD. Limbal relaxing incisions with cataract surgery. J Cataract Refract Surg. 1998;24(4):503-8.

102. Waring GO, Lynn MJ, McDonnell PJ. Results of the prospective evaluation of radial keratotomy (PERK) study 10 years after surgery. Arch Ophthalmol. 1994;112(10):1298-308.

103. Sporl E, Genth U, Schmalfuss K, et al. Thermomechanical behavior of the cornea. Ger J Ophthalmol. 1996;5(6):322-7.

104. Neumann AC, Fyodorov S, Sanders DR. Radial thermokeratoplasty for the correction of hyperopia. Refract Corneal Surg. 1990;6(6):404-12.

105. Seiler T, Matallana M, Bende T. Laser thermokeratoplasty by means of a pulsed holmium: YAG laser for hyperopic correction. Refract Corneal Surg. 1990;6(5):335-9.

106. Gudmundsdottir E, Jonasson F, Jonsson V, et al. "With the rule" astigmatism is not the rule in the elderly. Reykjavik Eye Study: a population based study of refraction and visual acuity in citizens of Reykjavik 50 years and older. Iceland-Japan Co-Working Study Groups. Acta Ophthalmol Scand. 2000;78(6):642-6.

107. Ismail MM, Alio JL, Perez-Santonja JJ. Noncontact thermokeratoplasty to correct hyperopia induced by laser in situ keratomileusis. J Cataract Refract Surg. 1998;24(9):1191-4.

108. Peyman GA, Larson B, Raichand M, et al. Modification of rabbit corneal curvature with use of carbon dioxide laser burns. Ophthalmic Surg. 1980;11(5):325-9.

109. Thompson VM, Seiler T, Durrie DS, et al. Holmium: YAG laser thermokeratoplasty for hyperopia and astigmatism: an overview. Refract Corneal Surg. 1993;9(2 Suppl):S134-7.

110. Horn G, Spears KG, Lopez O, et al. New refractive method for laser thermal keratoplasty with the Co: MgF2 laser. J Cataract Refract Surg. 1990;16(5):611-6.

111. Mendez G, Mendez A. Noble, Conductive keratoplasty for the correction of hyperopia, in surgery for Hyperopia and Presbyopia. In: Sher N (Ed). Williams & Wilkins: Baltimore; 1997. pp. 163-71.

112. Rowsey JJ, Doss JD. Preliminary report of Los Alamos Keratoplasty Techniques. Ophthalmology. 1981;88(8):755-60.

113. Rowsey JJ. Los Alamos keratoplasty techniques. Eye and Contact Lens. 1980;6(1):1-12.

114. Haw WW, Manche EE. Conductive keratoplasty and laser thermal keratoplasty. Int Ophthalmol Clin. 2002;42(4):99-106.

115. Swinger C, Krumeich J, Cassiday D. A new device for viable refractive keratoplasty. Invest Ophthalmol Vis Sci. 1985; 26(Sup):51.

116. Rama PCW, Genesi C, Azar D. Excimer laser intrastromal keratomileusis (LASIK), in Refractive Surgery. In: Azar DT (Ed). Appleton & Lange: Stamford, Connecticut. 1997. pp. 455-69.

117. Hagen KB, Kim EK, Waring GO. Comparison of excimer laser and microkeratome myopic keratomileusis in human cadaver eyes. Refract Corneal Surg. 1993;9(1):36-41.

118. Krumeich JH, Knuelle A. Non-freeze epikeratophakia (live epikeratophakia). Fortschr Ophthalmol. 1990;87(1):20-4.

119. Bas AM, Nano HD. In situ myopic keratomileusis results in 30 eyes at 15 months. Refract Corneal Surg. 1991;7(3):223-31.

120. Ruiz LA, Rosey J. In situ keratomileusis. Invest Ophthalmol Vis Sci. 1988;29(sup):392.

121. Barraquer JI. The history and evolution of keratomileusis. Int Ophthalmol Clin. 1996;36(4):1-7.

122. Taboada J, Archibald CJ. An Extreme Sensitivity in the Corneal Epithelium to Far UV ArF Excimer Laser Pulses. In Preprints Aerospace Medical Association Meeting. San Antonio, TX. May 4, 1981.

123. Trokel SL, Srinivasan R, Braren B. Excimer laser surgery of the cornea. Am J Ophthalmol. 1983;96(6):710-5.

124. Puliafito CA, Steinert RF, Deutsch TF, et al. Excimer laser ablation of the cornea and lens. Experimental studies. Ophthalmology. 1985;92(6):741-8.

125. Seiler T, Bende T, Wollensak J. Correction of astigmatism with the Excimer laser. Klin Monbl Augenheilkd. 1987;191(3):179-83.

126. McDonnell PJ, Moreira H, Clapham TN, et al. Photorefractive keratectomy for astigmatism. Initial clinical results. Arch Ophthalmol. 1991;109(10):1370-3.

127. McDonald MB, Kaufman HE, Frantz JM, et al. Excimer laser ablation in a human eye. Case report. Arch Ophthalmol. 1989;107(5):641-2.

128. Seiler T, Bende T, Winckler K, et al. Side effects in excimer corneal surgery. DNA damage as a result of 193 nm excimer laser radiation. Graefes Arch Clin Exp Ophthalmol. 1988;226(3):273-6.

CHAPTER 67

129. Pallikaris IG, Papatzanaki ME, Siganos DS, et al. A corneal flap technique for laser in situ keratomileusis. Human studies. Arch Ophthalmol. 1991;109(12):1699-702.

130. Pallikaris IG, Papatzanaki ME, Stathi EZ, et al. Laser in situ keratomileusis. Lasers Surg Med. 1990;10(5):463-8.

131. Buratto L, Ferrari M, Genisi C. Keratomileusis for myopia with the excimer laser (Buratto technique): short-term results. Refract Corneal Surg. 1993;9(2 Suppl):S130-3.

132. Buratto L, Ferrari M, Rama P. Excimer laser intrastromal keratomileusis. Am J Ophthalmol. 1992;113(3):291-5.

133. Ratkay-Traub I, Juhasz T, Horvath C, et al. Ultra-short pulse (femtosecond) laser surgery: initial use in LASIK flap creation. Ophthalmol Clin North Am. 2001;14(2):347-55.

134. Nordan LT, Slade SG, Baker RN, et al. Femtosecond laser flap creation for laser in situ keratomileusis: six-month follow-up of initial U.S. clinical series. J Refract Surg. 2003;19(1):8-14.

135. Bendett M. Apparatus and method for ophthalmic surgical procedures using a femtosecond fiber laser. Carl Zeiss Meditec AG. IMRA America Inc. 2003.

136. Sekundo W, Kunert K, Russmann C, et al., First efficacy and safety study of femtosecond lenticule extraction for the correction of myopia: six-month results. J Cataract Refract Surg. 2008;34(9):1513-20.

137. Krueger RR, Juhasz T, Gualano A, et al. The picosecond laser for nonmechanical laser in situ keratomileusis. J Refract Surg. 1998;14(4):467-9.

138. Ratkay—Traub I, Ferincz IE, Juhasz T, et al. First clinical results with the femtosecond neodynium-glass laser in refractive surgery. J Refract Surg. 2003;19(2):94-103.

139. Koziol J. Method for producing a multifocal corneal surface using intracorneal microscopic lenses. 2003.

140. Holzer MP, Mannsfeld A, Ehmer A, et al. Early outcomes of INTRACOR femtosecond laser treatment for presbyopia. J Refract Surg. 2009;25(10):855-61.

141. Burris TE. Intrastromal corneal ring technology: results and indications. Curr Opin Ophthalmol. 1998;9(4):9-14.

142. Burris TE, Baker PC, Ayer CT, et al. Flattening of central corneal curvature with intrastromal corneal rings of increasing thickness: an eye-bank eye study. J Cataract Refract Surg. 1993;19 Suppl:182-7.

143. Pinero DP, Alio JL. Intracorneal ring segments in ectatic corneal disease—a review. Clin Experiment Ophthalmol. 2010; 38(2):154-67.

144. Colin J, Cochener B, Savary G, et al. Correcting keratoconus with intracorneal rings. J Cataract Refract Surg. 2000;26(8):1117-22.

145. Sporl E, Huhle M, Kasper M, et al. Increased rigidity of the cornea caused by intrastromal cross-linking. Ophthalmologe. 1997;94(12):902-6.

146. Wollensak G, Spoerl E, Seiler T. Riboflavin/ultraviolet-a-induced collagen crosslinking for the treatment of keratoconus. Am J Ophthalmol. 2003;135(5):620-7.

147. Wollensak G, Spoerl E, Seiler T. Stress-strain measurements of human and porcine corneas after riboflavin-ultraviolet—A-induced cross-linking. J Cataract Refract Surg. 2003;29(9): 1780-5.

148. Herekar S. Method and material for in situ corneal structural augmentation. PriaVision Inc: USA. 2008.

149. Rocha KM, Ramos-Esteban JC, Qian Y, et al. Comparative study of riboflavin—UVA cross-linking and 'flash-linking' using surface wave elastometry. J Refract Surg. 2008;24(7):S748-51.

# Corneal, Scleral and Conjunctival Surgery: Supportive and Protective

## C H A P T E R S

# CHAPTER 68

# Ophthalmic Applications of Tissue Adhesives in Anterior Segment Surgery

*Brian Alder, Terry Kim*

## ☞ INTRODUCTION

Tissue adhesives have been widely applied in the field of ophthalmology since the 1960s. Traditionally, nonbiodegradable cyanoacrylate-based adhesives have been the primary tissue adhesive applied off-label in a variety of settings, though recently, biodegradable fibrin-based adhesives have been increasingly utilized as well. A variety of novel adhesives are also currently in development. Primarily used for external surface procedures (e.g. conjunctiva, cornea), tissue adhesives have also found applications in retina, glaucoma and oculoplastic procedures. In section I, the authors review cyanoacrylate-based and fibrin-based adhesives and their various applications. Section II provides an overview of multiple novel adhesives currently under investigation.

## ☞ CYANOACRYLATE- AND FIBRIN-BASED ADHESIVES

### Cyanoacrylate-based Adhesive

First discovered in 1942, cyanoacrylates (aka 'super glue') have long been used in ophthalmic surgery.[1-3] The FDA first approved cyanoacrylates as a medical adhesive in 1998, though prior to this date they were commonly used off-label. Chemically, cyanoacrylates are synthetic monomer esters of cyanoacrylic acid with an alkyl side chain (Fig. 1).[4] The side chain can be modified to create bonds with differing properties, including strength and biocompatibility. In general, as the alkyl side chain increases in the number of carbon atoms, it increases

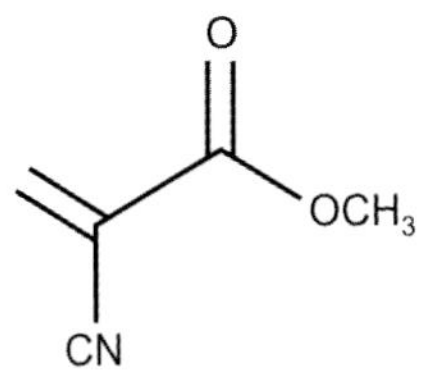

**Fig. 1:** Chemical structure of methyl cyanoacrylate

in biocompatibility, though decreases in shear and compression strength. Earlier cyanoacrylate-based glues contained alkyl side chains with few carbons and were much more toxic to human tissues as their degradation byproducts include cyanoacetate and formaldehyde.

Cyanoacrylate-based glues harden as they polymerize through contact with weak bases (e.g. cells) or water. They can be applied both wet or dry, but tend to have better bond strength in wet conditions.[4]

### Fibrin-based Adhesive

Fibrin-based adhesives, while long in use in abdominal and thoracic surgery, have only recently been widely applied in ophthalmic surgery.[5] A biological-based glue, they are generally more biocompatible than cyanoacrylate-based adhesives and incite a less prominent inflammatory response from the host tissue.[6] Fibrin-based adhesives consist of two components: fibrinogen and thrombin. When mixed, these components engage in the final steps of the coagulation cascade (Fig. 2) to form a bond. While more biocompatible, fibrin-based adhesives carry the disadvantages of increased cost and time to prepare as well as a theoretical risk of viral transmission.

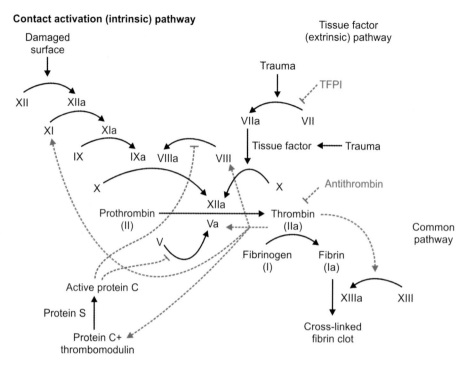

**Fig. 2:** Coagulation cascade

## ✦ OPHTHALMIC USES OF CYANOACRYLATE-AND FIBRIN-BASED TISSUE ADHESIVES

### Pterygium

Fibrin-based adhesives have been gaining popularity for use in pterygium surgery (Figs 3 to 5). In 1993, Cohen et al. reported on the use of fibrin-based adhesive to secure conjunctival autografts during pterygium excision.[7] More recently, Marticorena et al. presented a case series of 20 patients who underwent primary pterygium excision with conjunctival autograft using fibrin-based adhesive.[8] They found that there were no cases of recurrent pterygium, no cases of significant postoperative pain, and only 25% of patients reported mild foreign body sensation. Multiple reports have confirmed these results.[9] Similarly, Jain et al. reported on the successful use of fibrin-based glue for attaching human amniotic membrane graft in primary pterygium surgery, with decreased surgical time and improved patient comfort postoperatively.[10]

Many researchers have compared the use of fibrin-based adhesives and sutures in pterygium surgery. Uy et al. examined the efficacy of fibrin adhesives and suturing in the attachment of conjunctival autograft following pterygium excision. They found that the surgical time for the sutured group was almost twice as long as that of the

adhesive group, and that at 2 months postoperatively, all the autografts were attached in both groups (N=11 in both groups).[11]

Bahar et al. reported both short-term (3 weeks) and long-term (12 months) comparative results of fibrin glue and Vicryl sutures in conjunctival closure following pterygium excision. Surgical time was significantly shorter in the fibrin-based adhesive group. The fibrin glue group had significantly less pain, foreign body sensation, epiphora, and hyperemia both in the short and long term. There were no differences in pterygium recurrence rates at 12 months.[12,13] Karalezli et al. showed similar results when comparing fibrin glue and sutures in the securing of amniotic membrane grafts following pterygium excision.[14,15]

### Cornea

Cyanoacrylate-based adhesives have long been used to treat corneal perforations and impending corneal perforations (Figs 6 and 7). First reported in 1968 by Webster et al.[16] these adhesives have been an effective intervention in the treatment of perforations or impending perforations, with a relatively low complication rate. While effective, cyanoacrylate-based adhesives can cause significant foreign body sensation, conjunctival hyperemia, inflammation, corneal neovascularization, and are not biodegradable (Fig. 8).[17]

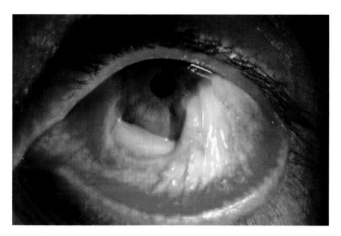

**Fig. 3:** Patient with visually significant pterygium
*Source:* Terry Kim

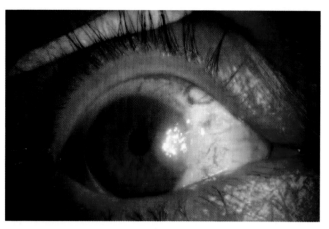

**Fig. 4:** Same patient status post pterygium excision with amniotic membrane graft attachment with fibrin-based adhesive
*Source:* Terry Kim

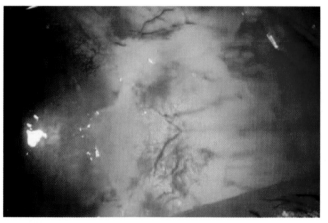

**Fig. 5:** Same patient status post pterygium excision with amniotic membrane graft attachment with fibrin-based adhesive
*Source:* Terry Kim

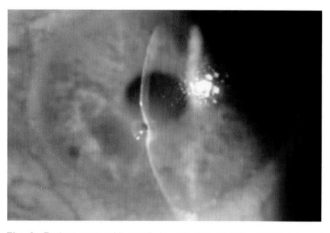

**Fig. 6:** Patient seen with small, less than 3 mm impending corneal perforation
*Source:* Chrisopher J Rapuano

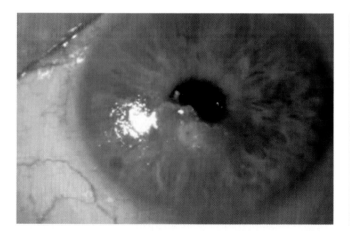

**Fig. 7:** Same patient following treatment with cyanoacrylate-based adhesive
*Source:* Chrisopher J Rapuano

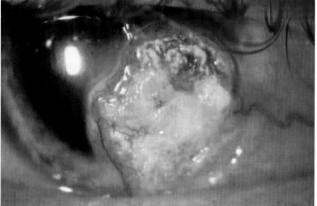

**Fig. 8:** Complications associated with cyanoacrylate-based adhesives including conjunctival hyperemia, increased inflammation, and corneal neovascularization
*Source:* Terry Kim

CHAPTER **68**

More recently, fibrin-based glues have also been used in the treatment of corneal perforations. Sharma et al. compared the efficacy of fibrin-based adhesives and cyanoacrylate-based adhesives in the treatment of small (< 3 mm) perforations.[18] They found that both adhesives were effective in successfully treating small perforations, and noted that while time to healing was greater with fibrin-based glue, there was significantly increased corneal neovascularization and rate of giant papillary conjunctivitis with cyanoacrylate-based glue. The efficacy of fibrin-based glues in the treatment of small corneal perforations was confirmed by Siatiri et al. in 2008.[19]

## Cataract Surgery

Clear corneal incisions have become the most commonly used incision in cataract surgery in the United States, far outpacing the use of scleral tunnel incisions.[20] While clear corneal incisions provide a faster surgical technique, there has been recent scrutiny over the possible increased rate of postoperative endophthalmitis in clear corneal cataract surgery. Cooper et al. found a three-fold increased risk of endophthalmitis in clear corneal incision cataract surgery compared to scleral tunnel incision cataract surgery, while other case reviews have shown that the clear corneal incision is safe, without a significant risk of endophthalmitis.[21,22]

Multiple studies have shown that in the early postoperative period, the clear corneal incision has low integrity with a tendency for early postoperative hypotony.[23-25] This fragility of the incision and hypotony can lead to the ingress of extraocular fluids and other contaminants, theoretically increasing the risk of endophthalmitis (Fig. 9).[26]

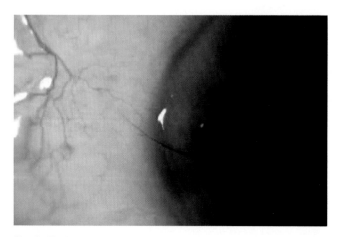

**Fig. 9:** Eyelash migration into clear corneal incision following cataract surgery
*Source:* Terry Kim

Multiple studies have been performed to evaluate the efficacy of various tissue adhesives in the closure of clear corneal incisions during cataract surgery. In 2005, Meskin et al. showed that 1–2 drops of a cyanoacrylate-based adhesive to the clear corneal incision at the end of cataract surgery results in water-tight wounds. In most cases, by the second postoperative visit, no adhesive was noted at the wound, though over half of the patients complained of transient foreign body sensation, and several had diffuse conjunctival hyperemia.[27]

Multiple studies have shown that, when compared to sutureless closure techniques, clear corneal incisions closed with cyanoacrylate-based adhesives have greater wound resistance to leakage, as well as decreased ingress of extraocular fluids (e.g. India ink).[28,29]

Shigemitsu et al. examined the tensile strength of clear corneal incisions in white rabbit eyes following various closure techniques including: sutureless, 10-0 nylon suture, cyanoacrylate-based adhesive, and fibrin-based adhesive. They found that both at 4 days and at 28 days after surgery, incisions closed with both tissue adhesive groups achieved tensile strengths comparable to wounds closed with 10-0 nylon suture.[30]

Histopathologic studies have likewise been performed to compare inflammatory response to clear corneal incisions closed by various methods. Several reports in animal models confirm that incisions closed with fibrin-based adhesives incite a greater inflammatory response than those closed with sutures. On the other hand, cyanoacrylate-based adhesive appears to incite less inflammation than sutures.[31,32]

## Glaucoma

Fibrin-based adhesives have been used in the management of bleb leakage following glaucoma surgery. In 1996, Asrani et al. reported on the successful use of autologous fibrin tissue adhesive in the treatment of bleb leakage in nine of twelve eyes.[33]

Grewing et al. reported two cases of a temporary sclerotomy tamponade achieved with fibrin-based adhesive in cases of post-trabeculectomy hypotony. Both eyes developed postoperative hypotony with large choroidal effusions, but no bleb leakage. Fibrin-based adhesive was applied subconjunctivally in the vicinity of the sclerotomy to achieve tamponade, which resulted in normalization of the intraocular pressure and the development of a functioning bleb at 6 months.[34]

In 2006, Kahook et al. reported on the use of fibrin-based adhesive as a substitute to sutures in several steps during implantation of a glaucoma drainage device. In 14 consecutive patients, glue was used in place of sutures to close the conjunctiva, secure the pericardium patch graft and secure the tube to the sclera. Clinical outcomes were compared to 28 consecutive cases using standard sutured technique. At 3 months, there were no differences in the intraocular pressure (IOP), the rate of glaucoma drop usage, or postoperative complication rate in either group. The surgical time was significantly less in the fibrin-based adhesive group (about half).[35]

## Other

Tissue adhesives have also been applied in the fields of oculoplastics and vitreoretinal surgery. Sonmez et al. reported the use of cyanoacrylate-based adhesive to perform bedside tarsorrhaphy following application of a bandage contact lens in immobilized comatose patients with recalcitrant exposure keratopathy.[36]

Cyanoacrylate glue has been used during retinal detachment repair surgery. Transvitreal application of cyanoacrylate-based adhesives to the retinal breaks during vitrectomy has been shown to achieve stronger chorioretinal adhesions compared to cryopexy, though with possibly greater toxicity to adjacent tissues.[37-39]

## ▶ NOVEL TISSUE ADHESIVES

### Biodendrimer-based Adhesives

Biodendrimers (aka dendritic macromers) are large polymers characterized by highly branched, repeating subunits that can be precisely controlled to form hydrogels of varying chemical composition, structure, and molecular weight (Fig. 10).[40] In addition to their use as tissue adhesives, these hydrogels that have been used for various medical applications, including drug delivery and wound healing.[41]

Biodendrimer-based adhesives have been applied in the setting of corneal wound healing. In 2004, Wathier et al. compared clear corneal wound integrity in enucleated eyes after closure by self-sealing, a single 10-0 nylon suture, and application of a biodendrimer-based adhesive. They found that leaking pressures (i.e. IOP at which leakage is seen from the wound) were 2–3 times higher in adhesive-sealed wounds compared to sutured wounds.[41] Similar results were found by the same group when corneal wound integrity was tested using an artificial anterior chamber to closely control IOP.[42]

Histologic studies carried out *in vivo* in a chicken model show that after about 1 month, there is significantly less corneal scarring in wounds closed with biodendrimer-based adhesives compared to those closed with nylon

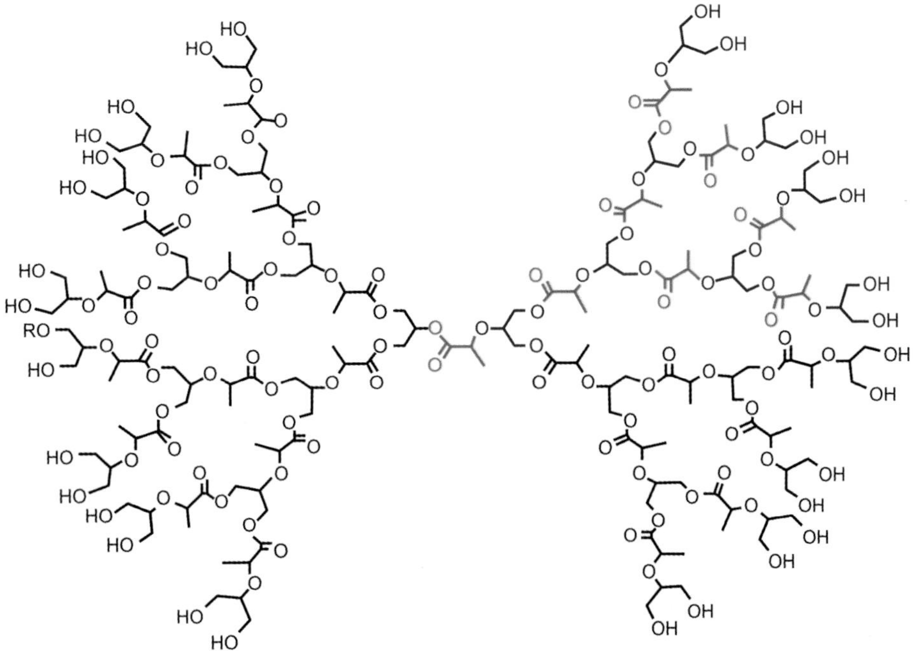

**Fig. 10:** Biodendrimer
*Source*: Velazquez et al., Arch Ophthal 2004, reprinted with permission

CHAPTER

68

sutures.[43] These reports also note about five times shorter closure time with biodendrimer-based adhesives versus sutures.

Biodendrimer-based adhesives have been shown to be effective in the treatment of corneal lacerations (Fig. 11). Velazquez et al. reported on the leakage rates in enucleated eyes with both 4.1 mm central linear and stellate corneal lacerations. They found that wounds closed with adhesive had a significantly higher leakage pressure compared to those wounds closed with 10-0 nylon suture, and that both methods achieved adequate closure (Fig. 12).[44]

Biodendrimer-based adhesives have also been studied in the setting of laser *in situ* keratomileusis (LASIK). They have been shown to effectively secure the corneal flap to the stroma, and are clear, easy to apply, and soft to touch, with possible application in flap dislocation or epithelial ingrowth.[45]

## Polyethylene Glycol-based Adhesives

Polyethylene glycol (PEG)-based adhesives are synthetic polymers that are biocompatible and can be engineered to produce hydrogels of varying flexibility, absorption, and consistency, allowing for multiple potential uses.[46] *In situ* polymerizing PEG-based hydrogels have been approved as duramater sealants, lung sealants, and abdominopelvic adhesions barriers.[47]

Singh et al. showed that PEG-based adhesives effectively prevented the ingress of India ink through 20 gauge and 23 gauge sclerotomies, while there was some ingress through sutured and unsutured wounds.[48] Similarly, Hariprasad et al. reported that leakage pressures for 23 gauge sclerotomies were significantly higher for wounds closed with PEG-based adhesives compared to sutureless wounds.

On review of the current literature, fewer reports on anterior segment uses of PEG-based hydrogels exist, though there are some reports of its use as a sealant of full-thickness corneal wounds.[49]

## Chondroitin Sulfate-based Adhesive

Chondroitin sulfate is a linear polysaccharide comprised of glucuronic acid and C-acetyl-galactosamine, which is found in the extracellular matrix of tissues. Thus, chondroitin sulfate-based adhesives are potentially more biocompatible and less inflammatory than other tissue adhesives. Reyes et al. reported on leakage pressures of clear corneal incisions in enucleated rabbit eyes closed with chondroitin sulfate-based adhesives as well as those closed with one and three 10-0 nylon sutures. There was no difference between the two sutured groups, though the leakage pressure of wounds closed with tissue adhesive was significantly higher.[50]

Recently, a chondroitin sulfate-based adhesive has been cross-linked with PEG to improve biocompatibility and maintain minimal tissue inflammation. This adhesive has been shown to significantly increase leakage pressures of clear corneal incisions compared to sutures.[51]

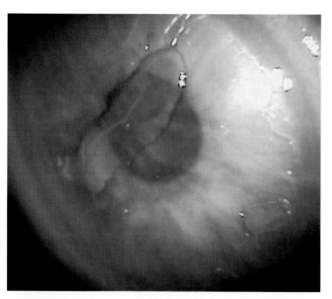

**Fig. 11:** Linear corneal laceration treated with biodendrimer
*Source:* Velazquez et al., Arch Ophthal 2004, reprinted with permission

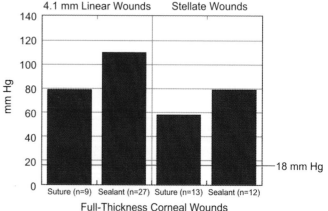

**Fig. 12:** Velazquez et al. found that wounds closed with biodendrimer sealant had higher leaking pressures than those closed with suture
*Source:* Velazquez et al., Arch Ophthal 2004, reprinted with permission

## Acrylic Copolymer-based Adhesives

Another novel tissue adhesive is an acrylic copolymer-based formulation that consists of cyanoacrylate as a copolymer with ethyl maleate. This acrylic copolymer-based adhesive has been shown to be equivalent to sutures in the closure of conjunctiva both in terms of integrity as well as inflammatory response.[52] It has also been shown to produce greater tensile strength in the closure of clear corneal incisions compared to sutures or sutureless closures, but also produces a greater inflammatory response.[53]

## ‣ CONCLUSION

Tissue adhesives have long been used in the field of ophthalmology and are receiving increased awareness and attention. Both traditional cyanoacrylate-based and fibrin-based adhesives, as well as multiple novel adhesives, are finding more and more applications in ophthalmic surgery. Primarily used off-label in corneal and conjunctival wound closure, they also have been applied in multiple other fields. The practicing ophthalmic surgeon must keep informed as the use of tissue adhesives may play a larger role in ophthalmic surgery in the future. Hopefully, further clinical and laboratory research efforts will result in the development of an adhesive specifically designed and utilized for ophthalmic application.

## ‣ REFERENCES

1. Refojo MF, Dohlman CH, Ahmad B, et al. Evaluation of adhesives for corneal surgery. Arch Ophthalmol. 1968;80: 645-56.
2. Trott AT. Cyanoacrylate tissue adhesives. An advance in wound care. JAMA 1997;277:1559-60.
3. Refojo MF. Current status of biomaterials in ophthalmology. Surv Ophthalmol. 1982;26:257-65.
4. Vote BJ, Elder MJ. Cyanoacrylate glue for corneal perforations: a description of a surgical technique and a review of the literature. Clin Experiment Ophthalmol. 2000;28:437-42.
5. Chan SM, Boisjoly H. Advances in the use of adhesives in ophthalmology. Curr Opin Ophthalmol. 2004;15:305-10.
6. Thompson DF, Letassy NA, Thompson GD. Fibrin glue: a review of its preparation, efficacy, and adverse effects as a topical hemostat. Drug Intell Clin Pharm. 1988;22:946-52.
7. Cohen RA, McDonald MB. Fixation of conjunctival autografts with an organic tissue adhesive. Arch Ophthalmol. 1993;111:1167-8.
8. Marticorena J, Rodriguez-Ares MT, Tourino R, et al. Pterygium surgery: conjunctival autograft using a fibrin adhesive. Cornea. 2006;25:34-6.
9. Koranyi G, Seregard S, Kopp ED. Cut and paste: a no suture, small incision approach to pterygium surgery. Br J Ophthalmol. 2004;88:911-4.
10. Jain AK, Bansal R, Sukhija J. Human amniotic membrane transplantation with fibrin glue in management of primary pterygia: a new tuck-in technique. Cornea. 2008;27:94-9.
11. Uy HS, Reyes JM, Flores JD, et al. Comparison of fibrin glue and sutures for attaching conjunctival autografts after pterygium excision. Ophthalmology. 2005;112:667-71.
12. Bahar I, Weinberger D, Dan G, et al. Pterygium surgery: fibrin glue versus Vicryl sutures for conjunctival closure. Cornea. 2006;25:1168-72.
13. Bahar I, Weinberger D, Gaton DD, et al. Fibrin glue versus vicryl sutures for primary conjunctival closure in pterygium surgery: long-term results. Curr Eye Res. 2007;32:399-405.
14. Karalezli A, Kucukerdonmez C, Akova YA, et al. Fibrin glue versus sutures for conjunctival autografting in pterygium surgery: a prospective comparative study. Br J Ophthalmol. 2008;92:1206-10.
15. Kucukerdonmez C, Karalezli A, Akova YA, et al. Amniotic membrane transplantation using fibrin glue in pterygium surgery: a comparative randomised clinical trial. Eye (Lond). 2010;24:558-66.
16. Webster RG, Slansky HH, Refojo MF, et al. The use of adhesive for the closure of corneal perforations. Report of two cases. Arch Ophthalmol. 1968;80:705-9.
17. Kim T, Kharod BV. Tissue adhesives in corneal cataract incisions. Curr Opin Ophthalmol. 2007;18:39-43.
18. Sharma A, Kaur R, Kumar S, et al. Fibrin glue versus N-butyl-2-cyanoacrylate in corneal perforations. Ophthalmology. 2003; 110:291-8.
19. Siatiri H, Moghimi S, Malihi M, et al. Use of sealant (HFG) in corneal perforations. Cornea. 2008;27:988-91.
20. Leaming DV. Practice styles and preferences of ASCRS members—2003 survey. J Cataract Refract Surg. 2004;30: 892-900.
21. Cooper BA, Holekamp NM, Bohigian G, et al. Case-control study of endophthalmitis after cataract surgery comparing scleral tunnel and clear corneal wounds. Am J Ophthalmol. 2003;136:300-5.
22. Monica ML, Long DA. Nine-year safety with self-sealing corneal tunnel incision in clear cornea cataract surgery. Ophthalmology. 2005;112:985-6.
23. Chawdhary S, Anand A. Early post-phacoemulsification hypotony as a risk factor for intraocular contamination: in vivo model. J Cataract Refract Surg. 2006;32:609-13.
24. Taban M, Sarayba MA, Ignacio TS, et al. Ingress of India ink into the anterior chamber through sutureless clear corneal cataract wounds. Arch Ophthalmol. 2005;123:643-8.
25. Aralikatti AK, Needham AD, Lee MW, et al. Entry of antibiotic ointment into the anterior chamber after uneventful phacoemulsification. J Cataract Refract Surg. 2003;29:595-7.
26. Chee SP, Bacsal K. Endophthalmitis after microincision cataract surgery. J Cataract Refract Surg. 2005;31:1834-5.
27. Meskin SW, Ritterband DC, Shapiro DE, et al. Liquid bandage (2-octyl cyanoacrylate) as a temporary wound barrier in clear corneal cataract surgery. Ophthalmology. 2005;112:2015-21.
28. Hermel B. [Studies on the use of tissue adhesives in cataract microsurgery]. Polim Med. 1980;10:3-18.

CHAPTER 68

29. Ritterband DC, Meskin SW, Shapiro DE, et al. Laboratory model of tissue adhesive (2-octyl cyanoacrylate) in sealing clear corneal cataract wounds. Am J Ophthalmol. 2005;140:1039-43.

30. Shigemitsu T, Majima Y. The utilization of a biological adhesive for wound treatment: comparison of suture, self-sealing sutureless and cyanoacrylate closure in the tensile strength test. Int Ophthalmol. 1996;20:323-8.

31. Alvarado Valero MC, Mulets Homs E, et al. [Bioadhesives in ocular surgery]. Arch Soc Esp Oftalmol. 2001;76:559-66.

32. Henrick A, Kalpakian B, Gaster RN, et al. Organic tissue glue in the closure of cataract incisions in rabbit eyes. J Cataract Refract Surg. 1991;17:551-5.

33. Asrani SG, Wilensky JT. Management of bleb leaks after glaucoma filtering surgery. Use of autologous fibrin tissue glue as an alternative. Ophthalmology. 1996;103:294-8.

34. Grewing R, Mester U. Fibrin sealant in the management of complicated hypotony after trabeculectomy. Ophthalmic Surg Lasers. 1997;28:124-7.

35. Kahook MY, Noecker RJ. Fibrin glue-assisted glaucoma drainage device surgery. Br J Ophthalmol. 2006;90:1486-9.

36. Sonmez B, Ozarslan M, Beden U, et al. Bedside glue blepharorrhaphy for recalcitrant exposure keratopathy in immobilized patients. Eur J Ophthalmol. 2008;18:529-31.

37. Hartnett ME, Hirose T. Cyanoacrylate glue in the repair of retinal detachment associated with posterior retinal breaks in infants and children. Retina. 1998;18:125-9.

38. McCuen BW, Hida T, Sheta SM, et al. Experimental transvitreal cyanoacrylate retinopexy. Am J Ophthalmol. 1986;102:199-207.

39. Sheta SM, Hida T, McCuen BW. Experimental transvitreal cyanoacrylate retinopexy through silicone oil. Am J Ophthalmol. 1986;102:717-22.

40. Encyclopedia M-HST. In: McGraw-Hill Encyclopedia of Science and Technology: The McGraw-Hill Companies, Inc; 2005.

41. Wathier M, Jung PJ, Carnahan MA, et al. Dendritic macromers as in situ polymerizing biomaterials for securing cataract incisions. J Am Chem Soc. 2004;126:12744-5.

42. Johnson CS, Wathier M, Grinstaff M, et al. In vitro sealing of clear corneal cataract incisions with a novel biodendrimer adhesive. Arch Ophthalmol. 2009;127:430-4.

43. Berdahl JP, Johnson CS, Proia AD, et al. Comparison of sutures and dendritic polymer adhesives for corneal laceration repair in an in vivo chicken model. Arch Ophthalmol. 2009;127:442-7.

44. Velazquez AJ, Carnahan MA, Kristinsson J, et al. New dendritic adhesives for sutureless ophthalmic surgical procedures: in vitro studies of corneal laceration repair. Arch Ophthalmol. 2004;122:867-70.

45. Kang PC, Carnahan MA, Wathier M, et al. Novel tissue adhesives to secure laser in situ keratomileusis flaps. J Cataract Refract Surg. 2005;31:1208-12.

46. Hariprasad SM, Singh A. Polyethylene glycol hydrogel polymer sealant for vitrectomy surgery: an in vitro study of sutureless vitrectomy incision closure. Arch Ophthalmol. 2011;129:322-5.

47. Cosgrove GR, Delashaw JB, Grotenhuis JA, et al. Safety and efficacy of a novel polyethylene glycol hydrogel sealant for watertight dural repair. J Neurosurg. 2007;106:52-8.

48. Singh A, Hosseini M, Hariprasad SM. Polyethylene glycol hydrogel polymer sealant for closure of sutureless sclerotomies: a histologic study. Am J Ophthalmol. 2010;150:346-51 e2.

49. Kalayci D, Fukuchi T, Edelman PG, et al. Hydrogel tissue adhesive for sealing corneal incisions. Ophthalmic Res. 2003;35:173-6.

50. Reyes JM, Herretes S, Pirouzmanesh A, et al. A modified chondroitin sulfate aldehyde adhesive for sealing corneal incisions. Invest Ophthalmol Vis Sci. 2005;46:1247-50.

51. Strehin I, Ambrose WM, Schein O, et al. Synthesis and characterization of a chondroitin sulfate-polyethylene glycol corneal adhesive. J Cataract Refract Surg. 2009;35:567-76.

52. Alio JL, Gomez J, Mulet E, et al. A new acrylic tissue adhesive for conjunctival surgery: experimental study. Ophthalmic Res. 2003;35:306-12.

53. Alio JL, Mulet ME, Cotlear D, et al. Evaluation of a new bioadhesive copolymer (ADAL) to seal corneal incisions. Cornea. 2004;23:180-9.

SECTION 15

# Conjunctival Flaps

*Anne S Steiner, Ira J Udell*

## ❧ INTRODUCTION

Conjunctival flaps have been employed for the treatment of recalcitrant ocular surface diseases since Scholer first described the technique in 1877.[1] It was Gunderson, however, with his paper published in 1958 who revolutionized the procedure by describing a thin conjunctival flap and made the procedure more successful and therefore more frequently performed.[2,3] With the evolution of the treatment of severe ocular surface diseases the need for the conjunctival flap has decreased over time. When first described, Gunderson's primary indications for performing this procedure were herpes keratitis, recurrent erosions and bullous keratopathy. Fortunately, currently there are more medical options, as well as vision improving procedures available to treat these conditions. However, there are still many situations in which this surgery can be employed to maintain the integrity of the ocular surface, increase patient comfort, decrease the use of chronic medications and provide better cosmesis.[4] In this chapter, we will describe the current indications for conjunctival flaps, as well as the various techniques for this procedure and its possible complications.

## ❧ INDICATIONS

The current indications for a conjunctival flap (Table 1) include providing comfort to a blind and painful eye secondary to an irregular ocular surface, to maintain the integrity of the ocular surface in an eye with a nonhealing epithelial defect, and as a last resort, to supply support to a corneal ulcer unresponsive to standard therapy.

**Table 1:** Indications for conjunctival flap

- Blind and painful eye
- Nonhealing epithelial defects
- Recalcitrant microbial keratitis
- Corneal descemetocele

Conjunctival flaps are generally reserved for eyes with limited visual potential. These flaps may be used as a temporary mechanism to heal the cornea and provide relief to the ocular surface as the flap may be lifted upon stabilization of the cornea and a subsequent penetrating keratoplasty may be performed.[5]

### Blind Painful Eye

In an eye with limited visual potential and surface irregularity causing significant ocular discomfort, a conjunctival flap can provide a regular surface and therefore significant relief from pain. Additionally, it may enable the patient to avoid enucleation as most patients would prefer to keep a non-seeing eye if they could be relieved of discomfort. In the preoperative evaluation, one should place topical anesthetic on the eye to ensure that the pain is in fact surface pain and not pain from a disorganized eye. If the patients' pain is in fact, secondary to surface issues the topical anesthetic should provide significant relief of the patients' discomfort. However, there are cases in which patients have a mixed mechanism for their pain with partial relief of discomfort with the administration of topical anesthetic. In these cases, the decision of what procedure to perform must be decided on an individual basis.

## Nonhealing Epithelial Defect

Nonhealing epithelial defects are seen in patients with neurotrophic corneas, exposure keratopathy, chronic ulcers and chronic limbal stem cell deficiency. The most commonly encountered cause of neurotrophic keratitis is herpes keratitis. When these defects are unresponsive to standard treatments, such as ocular lubrication, bandage contact lens,[6] suture tarsorrhaphy or the prosthetic rehabilitation of the ocular surface ecosystem device (PROSE – Boston Foundation for Sight), conjunctival flap is a reasonable option. In these cases, the conjunctival flap provides metabolic support during the corneal healing process, as well as stability to the ocular surface. There are papers in the literature, however, which advocate conjunctival flap as the preferred surgical treatment over suture tarsorrhaphy for neurotrophic ulcers. The authors advocate this in light of the better cosmetic appearance of a thin conjunctival flap and the more consistent healing of the cornea which they obtained with this procedure.[7]

## Recalcitrant Microbial Keratitis

Fortunately, effective medical options are currently available for the treatment of microbial keratitis leaving this as a less common indication for a conjunctival flap. However, there are multiple reported cases in the literature of microbial keratitis unresponsive to standard medical therapy in which a conjunctival flap was successfully employed as an aid to the healing process. These cases are reported in patients with bacterial, amebic and fungal infections.[8,9] Case reports in which recalcitrant acanthamoeba keratitis was treated with conjunctival flap in combination with deep lamellar keratoplasty or corneal cryotherapy resulted in resolved infection, stabilization of the cornea and eventual successful penetrating keratoplasty. However, the outcomes of conjunctival flap use in the setting of fungal keratitis appear less successful. Sanders et al. reported a case series of nine patients treated with conjunctival flaps for fungal keratitis.[10] In this series, four patients had disease progress to corneal perforation through the flap.

## Corneal Descemetocele and Perforation

Eyes with progressive thinning and poor visual potential not amenable to corneal transplantation may be temporized with a conjunctival flap. In the case of a corneal perforation, however, some authors recommend performing a thick conjunctival flap, leaving tenons capsule adherent to the overlying conjunctiva in order to secure the perforation and prevent fluid from accumulating between the cornea and the flap with associated shallowing of the anterior chamber.[11,12] Thick flaps may be difficult to obtain and may have a higher tendency to retract. Therefore, we do not advocate conjunctival flap alone as the treatment of choice for a corneal perforation. We would combine a tectonic corneal graft with a conjunctival flap to re-establish the ocular integrity.

## ❧ PERIPHERAL CORNEAL DISEASE

Progressive peripheral corneal thinning as seen in Moorens ulcer, peripheral ulcerative keratitis or peripheral ectasia may reach a point where the eye can be compromised. In these cases, a peripheral conjunctival flap is an option, focusing the flap on the area of pathology and leaving the remainder of the cornea untouched. However, in the case of peripheral pathology secondary to autoimmune diseases, it would be recommended to perform a conjunctival resection instead with adjunctive topical and/or systemic therapy as deemed appropriate for the clinical situation.

## ❧ DISADVANTAGES

The main disadvantages to consider when evaluating a patient for a conjunctival flap are inability to accurately monitor intraocular pressure, limited view of the cornea and anterior chamber precluding accurate monitoring of ocular pathology, and decreased visual acuity when the conjunctival flap covers the visual axis (Table 2). In cases of peripheral or partial conjunctival flaps, these disadvantages are eliminated. Patients should also be aware of the change in their ocular appearance which may occur and be considered a cosmetic disadvantage. The cornea may have an opaque white appearance, and the conjunctiva may appear mildly injected on a chronic basis. In general, regression of the conjunctival blood vessels occurs weeks to months after surgery, and the cosmetic appearance improves.[4] However, a conjunctival flap may be performed to enhance the cosmetic appearance if it is performed in preparation for a prosthesis.

| **Table 2:** Disadvantages of conjunctival flap |
|---|
| • Inability to accurately monitor intraocular pressure |
| • Limited view of the cornea and anterior chamber |
| • Decreased visual acuity when the conjunctival flap covers the visual axis |
| • Cosmetic disadvantage |

## ❧ TECHNIQUE

Accurate preoperative evaluation is essential to perform a successful conjunctival flap. All patients should have a thorough slit-lamp evaluation with particular attention paid to the mobility of the superior conjunctiva. The surgical area should be meticulously inspected for any signs of previous surgery, such as glaucoma procedures or previous sclera buckles, which are common in these patients. The area should also be inspected for any evidence of scarring as seen in ocular cicatricial pemphigoid, graft versus host disease, previous radiation, Stevens Johnson syndrome or chemical burns which may be seen in patients with chronic ocular surface disease secondary to loss of limbal stem cells. Additionally, as previously mentioned, if the procedure is being performed for relief of pain, one should ensure that the pain is relieved with topical anesthesia.

The conjunctival flap procedure is generally performed with retrobulbar or peribulbar injection of anesthesia. In cases of a patient who may be uncooperative, general anesthesia can be employed.

### Total Flap

The most commonly performed technique for a total conjunctival flap (Fig. 1) is the technique described by Trygve Gunderson of a thin conjunctival flap.[2] The procedure is described in the order in which it is performed:

- After the performance of a retrobulbar or peribulbar injection, the eye is prepped and draped in the usual sterile ophthalmic fashion.
- A lid speculum is placed into the surgical eye.

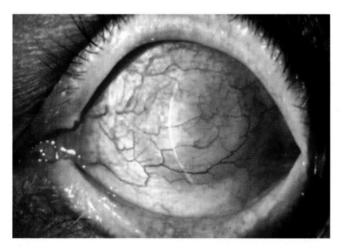

**Fig. 1:** Total conjunctival flap
*Courtesy*: Richard K Forster

- The corneal epithelium is removed in its entirety either with a dry WekCel sponge or #59, #15 or #57 blade. It is important to be meticulous about the epithelial removal in order to prevent the formation of epithelial cysts in the future.
- A 6-0 spatulated double-armed nylon or similar traction suture is placed in the superior cornea or perilimbal sclera at approximately 12 o'clock position, depending on the status of the superior limbal tissue.
- At this point, a 360° peritomy is performed. Others perform the superior dissection described below first and then proceed to complete the peritomy 360°.
- The eye is infraducted to expose the entire superior bulbar conjunctiva. Ideally, one would like to obtain access 16–18 mm posterior to the limbus as the free flap tends to retract especially if partially scarred. It is helpful to use a marking pen to mark the distance from the limbus prior to beginning any dissection.
- Two percent lidocaine with 1:100000 epinephrine is injected in the subconjunctival space posterior to the intended incision taking care not to penetrate the conjunctiva in the area which will be used to create the flap. Others recommend to insert the needle closer to the lateral rectus and using a cotton swab sweep the fluid superiorly in order to create a plane between the conjunctiva and tenon's layer.
- A 2 cm incision 16–18 mm posterior to the limbus concentric with the limbus is made with the aid of a blunt tip scissors and nontoothed anatomical forceps. Situations with less than 14 mm of available tissue generally create tension and retraction of the flap.
- The dissection of the conjunctiva from tenon's capsule is continued anteriorly to the limbus, taking great care not to create a buttonhole in the conjunctiva. When the limbus is reached, the conjunctival tissue is dissected from the limbus.
- At this point, the traction suture is removed and the bipedicle flap is slid over the surface of the cornea. One may find it necessary to perform a further dissection both nasally and temporally in order to free the tissue and decrease tension on the flap when it is slid over the cornea. Additionally, it may be necessary to create relaxing incisions at 4 and 8 o'clock for this purpose.
- The flap is secured to the inferior conjunctiva/episclera and to the superior limbus with interrupted nylon or vicryl sutures.
- The superior tenon's is left bare to re-epithelialize. One should not attempt to close the conjunctival defect superiorly as this may result in ptosis.

## Partial Flap

- A partial conjunctival flap (Fig. 2) is performed to cover a localized corneal lesion. The preferred technique of a partial conjunctival flap depends on the location of the lesion which one desires to cover.
- For central or paracentral corneal pathology, the technique is similar to that of a full conjunctival flap but the width of the conjunctival tissue being transplanted over the cornea is smaller. The size of the corneal lesion is measured with calipers and an area 30% larger is measured and marked on the superior conjunctiva. The corneal epithelium is removed over the area of the cornea which will be covered. The marked conjunctival area is then dissected using the same technique as in the previously described Gunderson flap and is slid over the cornea and secured with interrupted nylon sutures through the cornea.
- For inferior issues, on occasion, an inferior partial conjunctival flap may be performed using this technique applied to the inferior conjunctiva. Additionally, an inferior flap may be performed in situations where there is poor superior conjunctiva, such as from previous glaucoma or retinal surgery.
- For peripheral corneal lesions, a conjunctival advancement flap can be employed. A peritomy is performed of the adjacent conjunctiva, when the conjunctiva is deemed to be freely mobile. It is then advanced to cover the peripheral corneal pathology and secured in place with interrupted nylon sutures. One should note, however, that this particular partial flap has a higher rate of retraction and therefore the area covered needs to be increased to allow for retraction.

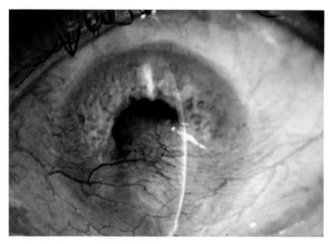

**Fig. 2:** Partial conjunctival flap
*Courtesy:* Richard K Forster

## ▶ POSTOPERATIVE CARE

Generally, the patient is started on topical antibiotic drops, as well as cycloplegics for 1–2 weeks postoperatively. Steroid antibiotic combinations may be suitable in situations where there is no infection or significant thinning. The nylon sutures may be removed as early as 4 weeks postoperatively. The conjunctival flap may thin and become more transparent over the course of a month, and one may be able to examine the anterior segment through the flap at that time.

## ▶ COMPLICATIONS

The vast majority of complications (Table 3) associated with the conjunctival flap procedure can be avoided with meticulous preoperative planning and surgical technique.

### Buttonholes

The formation of a buttonhole in the conjunctival flap is the most common complication of conjunctival flap surgery and can occur from the needle used for the subconjunctival lidocaine injection or simply secondary to conjunctival manipulation with forceps or scissors. Buttonhole formation may also occur from poor visualization during surgery. One should take great care to inject the subconjunctival lidocaine peripheral to the area to be used for the flap. Additionally, one should use nontoothed forceps to handle the conjunctiva as well as blunt tip scissors. One should also be meticulous to control bleeding in order to maintain good visualization of the surgical area. If a conjunctival buttonhole is inadvertently created, one can attempt to suture it closed; however, even with successful intraoperative closure of the buttonhole, there remains a significant risk of this area expanding postoperatively. One may also attempt to slide the flap laterally in order to avoid placing the buttonhole over the cornea.

| **Table 3:** Complications of conjunctival flaps |
| --- |
| • Buttonholes |
| • Flap retraction |
| • Hemorrhage |
| • Epithelial inclusion cyst |
| • Ptosis |

## Flap Retraction

The conjunctival flap may retract; this is more common in a flap that is under traction or has had a buttonhole. It is important to perform a careful peritomy and to separate the conjunctiva from all of its attachments to Tenon's capsule. If flap retraction does occur, one can attempt to resuture the flap to its original location; however, another flap would be difficult to create because of the lack of adequate conjunctiva.

## Hemorrhage

Hemorrhage under the conjunctival flap may occur, but has no long-term sequalae on the quality and effectiveness of the flap; however, it may result in a more opaque flap. One should keep in mind that patients who are taking any form of anticoagulants, i.e. aspirin, plavix or coumadin are at higher risk for hemorrhage with this procedure and if possible, it may be appropriate to discontinue these medications preoperatively. Additionally, patients taking these anticoagulants are at higher risk for intraoperative bleeding. Meticulous cautery and control of bleeding intraoperatively is essential as rarely postoperative bleeding can cause significant blood loss. The authors have encountered a case in which a patient on plavix underwent a conjunctival flap procedure and postoperatively required a blood transfusion secondary to excessive postoperative bleeding and decreased hematocrit.

## Epithelial Inclusion Cyst

These may occur secondary to incomplete removal of the corneal epithelium which creates cysts beneath the flap, most commonly at the limbus. Meticulous removal of the corneal epithelium is preventative. The treatment is surgical excision of the cyst in its entirety if it does not spontaneously regress. However, excision is not necessary if this is purely for cosmesis.

## Ptosis

Postoperative ptosis has been reported and is not uncommon; however, authors agree that many of the patients undergoing conjunctival flap surgery do have pre-existing ptosis and therefore the rate is difficult to report. It is theorized that the ptosis is secondary to inadequate dissection of the conjunctiva from tenon's causing traction at the superior fornix resulting in a mechanical ptosis. Others believe that ptosis results from aggressive dissection high in the superior fornix. Most authors agree that in most clinical scenarios in which conjunctival flap is considered, the benefits which this procedure brings to the patient outweigh the risk of ptosis.

## ⊱ REFERENCES

1. Scholer KW. Jahresberichte uber die Wirksamkeit der Augen-Klinik, in der Jahren 1874-1880. Herlin: H Peters; 1881.
2. Gunderson T. Conjunctival flaps in the treatment of corneal disease with reference to a new technique of application. Arch Ophthalmol. 1958;60:880-7.
3. Gunderson T, Pearlson HR. Conjunctival flaps for corneal disease: their usefulness and complications. Trans Am Ophthalmol Soc. 1969;67:78-95.
4. Alino AM, Perry HD, Kanellopoulos AJ, et al. Conjunctival flaps. Ophthalmology. 1998;105:1120-3.
5. Geria RC, Zarate J, Geria MA. Penetrating keratoplasty in eyes treated with conjunctival flaps. Cornea. 2001;20:345-9.
6. Gassett AR, Kaufman HE. Bandage lens in the treatment of bullous keratopathy. Am J Ophthalmol. 1970;69:252-9.
7. Lugo M, Arensten JJ. Treatment of neurotrophic ulcers with conjunctival flaps. Amer J of Ophthalmol. 1987;103:711-2.
8. Cremona G, Carrasco NA, Tytiun A, et al. Treatment of advanced Acanthamoeba keratitis with deep lamellar keratectomy and conjunctival flap. Cornea. 2002;21:705-8.
9. Mauger TF, Craig E. Combined Acanthamoeba and stenophomonas maltophilia keratitis treated with a conjunctival flap followed by penetrating keratoplasty. Cornea. 2006;25:631-3.
10. Sanders N. Penetrating keratoplasty in the treatment of fungal keratitis. Am J Ophthalmol. 1970;70:24-30.
11. Khoudodust A, Q Quinter AP. Microsurgical approach to the conjunctival flap. Arch Ophthalmol. 2003;121:1189-93.
12. Portnoy SL, Insler MS, Kaufman HE. Surgical management of corneal ulceration and perforation. Surv Ophthalmol. 1989; 34:47-58.

# Scleral Transplantation: Supportive and Protective

*Frank W Bowden III*

## ✦ INTRODUCTION

Scleral transplantation has multiple applications in ophthalmic surgery, which serve to restore functional and structural integrity to the globe and adnexal structures. Scleral grafts have been used primarily as a durable and readily available biologic material in the management of scleral defects and thinning disorders. Scleral transplantation techniques have been used in selected situations in corneal surgery, glaucoma surgery, retinal surgery, oculoplastic surgery, as well as dental surgery.

Scleral disorders which threaten the globe include penetrating trauma, as well as inflammatory conditions which result in collagen destruction. These disorders are encountered in surgical and nonsurgical scleral trauma, infectious scleritis and immune-mediated necrotizing scleritis. Examples of surgical trauma include pterygium surgery and epibulbar tumor resection. Pterygium surgery may result in scleral melt particularly when a bare scleral technique is coupled with adjunctive antimetabolite or radiation therapy. Epibulbar neoplasm resection may result in partial or full thickness scleral defects. Nonsurgical scleral injury may be encountered in penetrating globe trauma and severe chemical burns, which result in ischemic necrosis of the sclera. Infectious scleritis may be encountered as a consequence of scleral extension of peripheral corneal ulcers. It may also result from infectious complications of pterygium surgery, glaucoma surgery and vitreoretinal surgery. Noninfectious necrotizing scleritis may be associated with systemic autoimmune diseases, such as rheumatoid arthritis, polyarteritis nodosa, relapsing polychondritis, and Wegener's granulomatosis. The most recognizable and destructive example of immune-mediated scleritis is scleromalacia perforans.

Collectively, these disorders may potentially result in severe thinning with scleral perforation. Uveal prolapse, choroidal hemorrhage and endophthalmitis may ensue with visual loss. Immune-mediated scleral destruction is particularly problematic due to the risk of recurrent disease following scleral transplantation. Timely recognition of underlying pathophysiologic mechanisms along with prompt medical and tectonic surgical intervention is critical for effective management of scleral melting disorders. Medical therapy in the presence of infectious scleritis involves obtaining appropriate microbiologic evaluation of scrapings or biopsy material. Effective topical and systemic antibiotic therapy are required prior to lamellar or full-thickness scleral grafting to avoid recurrent infection, wound dehiscence and graft sloughing.[1] Medical therapy in the presence of immune-mediated scleral thinning involves a thorough rheumatologic evaluation and serologic testing. Appropriate systemic immunosuppressive therapy to control local inflammation and vasculitis is critical to avoid immune rejection and resorption of a scleral graft.[1]

## ✦ SCLERAL GRAFT

Human sclera possesses several unique characteristics which contribute to its popularity and effectiveness as a connective tissue material suitable for transplantation. It is curved to conform to the shape of the globe in scleral reinforcement procedures. It also adapts well to the shape of the eyelid in oculoplastic procedures. Human sclera has a high tensile strength permitting suture fixation as well as effective tectonic support of the globe. Due to its hypocellular and avascular structure, it evokes little inflammatory reaction with transplantation.

The sclera demonstrates a significant nerve density as evidenced with the severity of pain experienced in patients with scleritis. The density of nerve fibers in the sclera, however, is less than that seen in corneal tissue. Thus, it is felt to impart a reduced risk of prion disease infectivity with scleral tissue compared to cornea, and far less than neural tissue.[2] Limitations of scleral tissue for transplantation include its susceptibility to host pathophysiologic factors and its requirement of mucosal coverage. In specific situations, its availability may as well be limited.

Sclera graft tissue may succumb to the same insults, which have caused inflammatory or ischemic thinning, melting or perforation of the host sclera. As previously noted, local and systemic medical therapy must stabilize the scleral bed prior to transplantation. Donor scleral grafts exposed to mucosal surfaces must be covered with a basement membrane material to avoid desiccation, sloughing, infection and wound dehiscence. Epithelial migration over the scleral surface is generally limited; however, it may be seen with small area scleral patch grafts. Autologous conjunctiva is usually available for scleral graft coverage. It is usually mobilized from an adjacent area of the ocular surface. A popular alternative surface substrate material is amniotic membrane tissue (AMT).[3] This basement membrane with avascular stroma possesses growth factors which promote epithelialization. Despite the presence of an intact conjunctival surface, noninflammatory resorption of scleral tissue has been observed on occasion in the absence of systemic immune factors. This has been encountered in particular with glaucoma surgery wherein sclera and other biologic tissues have been preserved with the tutoplast method.[4]

Preserved scleral tissue is available through the eye bank system, as well as through commercial processing. Eye bank sclera is subjected to standardized donor screening. It may be prepared and distributed as a whole globe or fractional portions of the scleral wall. Eye bank scleral preservation involves either freezing or dehydration. Both methods reduce tissue antigenicity and bacterial contamination.

Frozen scleral tissue may be kept up to 3 months. Scleral preservation by dehydration with alcohol or glycerin permits room temperature storage of sclera with a prolonged shelf life of up to one year. Scleral rehydration and rinse are required prior to transplantation. The scleral tissue pliability and ease of manipulation are restored with rehydration. Though alcohol dehydration offers

antibacterial effect, HIV and Creutzfeld Jakob disease transmission are not completely eliminated. Effective donor screening must be relied upon to minimize the remote risk of viral and prion disease transmission. Host immune factors, low prion tiers in sclera, and a prolonged incubation of Creutzfeld Jakob disease (CJD) contribute to a remote risk of disease transmission in the event that donor sclera was harvested from an individual later found to have CJD.[2] Commercially processed (Tutoplast) scleral tissue is preserved with a proprietary method which renders it biologically inert and dry with a 5-year shelf life. Organic and inorganic solvents are used in the proprietary tutoplast preservation method, which has demonstrated HIV-1 and prion inactivation.[5,6] Surface antigens in the sclera are also destroyed. Dehydration and terminal sterilization by irradiation are performed prior to packaging. This process has an insignificant effect on the integrity of the collagen matrix.

## ▶ ANESTHESIA OPTIONS

The optimal route and choice of anesthesia during scleral transplantation is based on multiple factors. The general health status of the patient must account for the presence of systemic cardiovascular disease, pulmonary disease, renal disease and metabolic disorders. The size and extent of the scleral defect must be considered along with relevant clinicopathologic factors, such as infection and vasculitis. The specific application of the scleral graft will also affect anesthetic selection, particularly in glaucoma, retinal and oculoplastic procedures.

Topical anesthesia with and without subconjunctival anesthetic infiltration involves the least risk to the patient. However, its utility is limited to small anterior scleral defects and corneoscleral thinning disorders, such as a peripheral ulcerative keratitis. It has demonstrated efficacy in tube shunt surgery with scleral graft, as well as with filtering bleb revisions. Retrobulbar and peribulbar regional anesthesia are more desirable in those patients with larger areas of scleral thinning which extend posteriorly. It may be anticipated in this situation that additional globe manipulation for exposure and hemostasis would be required. Particular care must be exercised to evaluate the globe for staphyloma or imminent perforation sites prior to regional anesthesia to avoid excessive orbital volume expansion. This event may lead to elevated intraocular pressure with attendant risk of scleral rupture and extrusion of ocular contents. Regional anesthesia is also particularly well-suited for elderly or debilitated patients with autoimmune disease or significant cardiopulmonary risk for general anesthesia.

General anesthesia may be necessary in those patients with scleral thinning of uncertain dimension or extent. It is also advised in those who may be judged to be poorly cooperative with regional anesthesia. General anesthesia further permits the repair of scleral defects, as well as eyelid reconstruction when a scleral substitute material must be harvested from elsewhere on the patient's body. Optimal preoperative control of systemic diseases, in particular hypertension, diabetes and vasculitis is warranted with general anesthesia to minimize preoperative morbidity.

## SCLERAL GRAFT TECHNIQUES

### Scleral Perforation Repair

In general, scleral transplantation technique requires a customized approach which reflects the location and dimensions of the scleral defect, as well as integrity of surrounding tissues. Split-thickness or full-thickness scleral grafts may be utilized as the situation warrants to maintain a smooth ocular surface. In general, rapidly absorbable sutures are to be avoided in the scleral onlay grafts to avoid dehiscence. Popular suture choices include nylon and vicryl. Perilimbal edges of a scleral graft require a 10-0 nylon or 9-0 nylon suture closure. Posterior edges of the scleral graft warrant a 7-0 or an 8-0 nylon or vicryl suture fixation. In selected situations, bioadhesive materials, such as Tisseel glue may secure the onlay scleral graft to the globe, particularly in the absence of perforation or ectasia. Adjacent sclera must be intact and healthy to permit scleral graft fixation in either case. Lin et al. have demonstrated effectiveness of bioadhesive material in the repair of a large scleral ulcer.[7] Zeppa et al. have also demonstrated a successful sutureless tube shunt surgery technique in 15 eyes.[8]

The tissue integration of homologous scleral grafts has been studied in dogs by Johnson et al.[9] Full thickness and partial thickness scleral grafts were shown to evoke little inflammatory reaction with rapid healing following microscopic evaluation 4–7 months following surgery.

In human scleral transplantation, the basic onlay technique described by Obear and Winter has been effective in managing scleral thinning and perforation (Figs 1A and B).[10] The basic tenets of their method involve adequate exposure of the scleral bed with a limbal or fornix-based conjunctival peritomy. Next, a careful inspection of the scleral defect is followed by debridement of necrotic

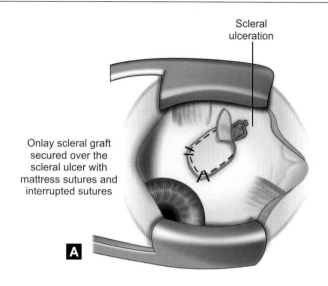

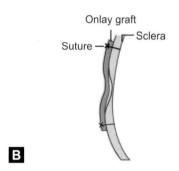

**Figs 1A and B:** Onlay scleral graft technique

or suppurative scleral tissues. Hemostasis with bipolar cautery is usually preferred. Normal or uninvolved scleral margins are indentified to define the dimensions of the scleral defect and to provide the sites for anchor sutures for the scleral graft. A template is created of the scleral defect to permit a customized sclera patch to be fashioned. Obear and Winter recommended an oversized graft by 5–10 mm to allow for sufficient tissue overlap and suture fixation to ensure tectonic success. An interrupted mattress suture closure is recommended with multiple sutures to achieve a secure fixation. In the case of scleral perforation, gentle compression of bulging choroid is feasible with the scleral onlay graft. A variation of this approach has been used with success wherein light cautery to bulging choroid may affect shrinkage prior to the scleral graft placement.[11] A paracentesis may also reduce intraocular pressure to facilitate suture of the scleral patch without tension. When perilimbal thinning and perforation is encountered, the thickness of the scleral graft may be trimmed to conform to the contour of the perilimbal sclera without edge overlap.

10-0 nylon sutures also may extend into the cornea to secure coapted edges of the sclera and cornea. Posterior lesions may require temporary rectus muscle detachment and replacement for complete exposure of healthy adjacent sclera. Finally, Obear and Winter recommended effective closure of conjunctiva over the scleral graft to avoid scleral sloughing. In general, scleral grafts must be covered by a basement membrane material to avoid desiccation and inflammatory necrosis with resorption.[12] When effective conjunctival closure over the scleral graft is not possible due to adjacent conjunctival scarring or surgical resection, pedicle conjunctival flaps, as well as free conjunctival grafts from the same or opposite eye may be employed. Alternatively, amniotic membrane tissue may be applied by suture fixation or bioadhesive glue techniques.

In the specific situation involving a small scleral defect located anteriorly or juxtalimbal, a lamellar sclera autograft technique may be utilized.[13] This option has particular importance when donor scleral tissue is not available. A 'trap door' scleral flap may be created by a dissection of the sclera hinged at the edge of the defect.[14] The flap size should approximate the size of the scleral defect, usually 2–5 mm. The flap is reflected over the defect and secured with interrupted nonabsorbable sutures (Figs 2A and B). Larger

scleral defects may require a free lamellar scleral autograft harvested from either eye.[15] Multiple reports have demonstrated successful management of Mooren's ulcer, perilimbal scleromalacia, and senile scleromalacia with the lamellar autograft techniques.[16] Lamellar sclerokerato plasty has also been effective with corneoscleral ulcerations, such as Terriens degeneration.[17,18]

Several perioperative considerations are important for successful scleral transplantation.[13] Preoperative systemic immunosuppressive therapy must be continued to avoid scleral graft resorption. Preoperative systemic antibiotic therapy must be accompanied by close clinical monitor to ensure effective management of infectious scleritis prior to scleral transplantation. Routine postoperative antibiotic therapy may include topical and systemic medication. To reduce the risk of globe rupture with manipulation, intravenous mannitol may be used along with paracentesis to reduce the intraocular pressure. Optimal exposure may be facilitated with bridle sutures of 6-0 vicryl through the limbus at 6 and 12 o'clock. Following the surgery, a pressure patch and aqueous suppression therapy to control the intraocular pressure are helpful to minimize the risk of operative site hematoma or wound dehiscence. In addition, topical steroid and cycloplegic therapy are included. Close

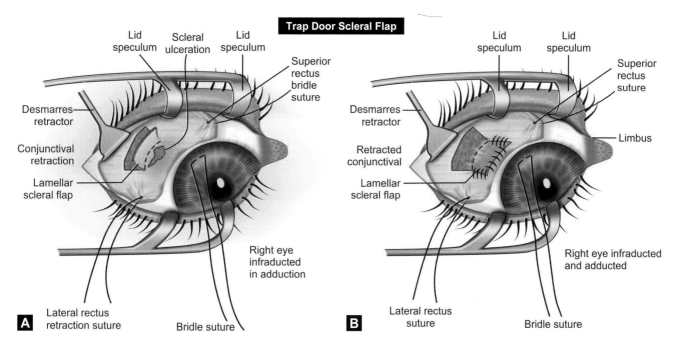

**Figs 2A and B:** (A) Lamellar scleral autograft created adjacent to scleral ulceration; (B) Hinged lamellar scleral autograft secured over adjacent scleral ulceration site

**70 CHAPTER**

monitoring of the ocular surface is necessary to ensure the absence of scleral exposure due to conjunctival retraction or wound dehiscence. Vigorous lubrication and occlusion therapy is necessary to ensure rapid epithelialization of the ocular surface.

## Glaucoma Surgery

Scleral graft techniques involved in glaucoma surgery are modified to manage unique issues related to drainage tubes and dysfunctional filtering blebs. The proximal tube of a drainage device must be covered with a compatible biologic tissue to protect the overlying conjunctiva from mechanical erosion by the plastic tube. The consequence of tube exposure with conjunctival breakdown may include iritis, blebitis, endophthalmitis, and progressive tube shunt extrusion.[19] A homologous scleral patch graft is usually cut to a 4x6 mm dimension for optimal tube shunt and sclerostomy site coverage. The patch graft is usually secured to the sclera with several 8-0 vicryl sutures (Fig. 3). The conjunctiva is usually closed over the scleral graft with a 9-0 vicryl suture with a vascular needle to achieve watertight closure. Aslanides, et al. have described a novel technique with a lamellar scleral autograft, which proved useful when donor sclera was unavailable.[20] Zeppa et al. described the effective use of bioadhesive material to secure the scleral patch in Ahmed valve procedures in 15 patients.[8] No tube erosions or complications were noted in the sutureless technique.

When a tube shunt fails due to contracture of the bleb, loss of intraocular pressure control results. A bleb revision may include a partial pseudocapsule excision. A scleral graft is required to cover the tube shunt plate prior to conjunctival closure. A dysfunctional filtering bleb with hypotony may result from trabeculectomy with adjunctive antimetabolite therapy with overfiltration. In the absence of a bleb leak, hypotony may result from partial flap necrosis with overfiltration. A bleb revision may require a scleral patch or lamellar autograft to cover the sclerostomy site and control aqueous egress.[21,22] Selective compression with the anchoring sutures may effectively reduce fluid outflow and direct aqueous egress posteriorly. Releasable sutures may be used to modulate the intraocular pressure. Mobilization of the adjacent conjunctiva by direct advancement or pedicle rotation may be necessary to cover the scleral graft without wound tension.[23] In the presence of extensive conjunctival scarring, a free autologous conjunctival graft or amniotic tissue may be effective options to cover the scleral graft.

Noninflammatory scleral graft resorption may be encountered on occasion in the presence of an intact overlying conjunctiva following tube shunt surgery.[4] The loss of the scleral graft exposes the eye to the risk of tube erosion through the conjunctiva[24] (Fig. 4). The specific mechanism of resorption is not clear. It occurs without symptoms. It is observed in the absence of systemic vasculitis and without regard to the method of preservation. Patients with implanted tube shunts require careful clinical observation of the tube and scleral graft indefinitely to monitor the ongoing risk of tube exposure. Clinically, patients with tube exposure may often present with minimal irritation symptoms which may progress to foreign body sensation and tearing. Bleb leaks may be encountered with loss of

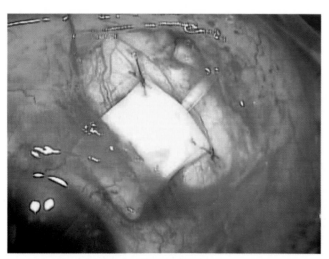

**Fig. 3:** Scleral patch graft coverage of proximal portion of drainage tube

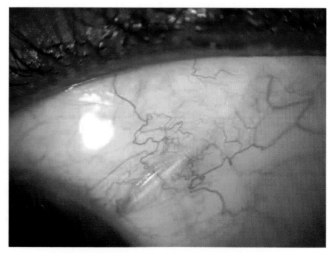

**Fig. 4:** Exposed tube with conjunctival erosion following scleral graft resorption

bleb function and iritis. Management of the conjunctival erosion requires immediate topical broad spectrum antibiotic therapy. The method of surgical intervention will depend on several factors. These include the size of the conjunctival erosion, the extent of tube exposure, the presence of intraocular inflammation and the status of the bleb function. Based on the duration of tube exposure and the size of the conjunctival breakdown, the surgeon must determine whether to retain the tube, to replace the tube with an extender or to replace the shunt device. With significant shunt plate exposure or extrusion, the drainage device must be explanted as the subtenons bleb site becomes lined with conjunctival epithelium. Though a conjunctival closure is not necessary, direct sclerostomy closure with an 8-0 vicryl is warranted to stabilize the anterior chamber. When the tube shunt device is retained, the conjunctival opening is enlarged with sharp dissection. Blunt tipped scissors are used to undermine the adjacent conjunctiva on either side of the tube by 3–4 mm. Care is taken to avoid a conjunctival buttonhole. The scleral allograft tissue is then cut to a 4x6 mm dimension. It is then tucked into the conjunctival pocket opening overlying the tube and secured to the sclera with a bioadhesive material (Tisseel) or an 8-0 vicryl suture. The conjunctiva is then mobilized to cover the graft by direct advancement (Figs 5A and B). A free conjunctival autograft or AMT may also be used to cover the scleral graft when conjunctival scarring prevents direct closure. 9-0 vicryl suture or bioadhesive material may then be used to secure a watertight closure of the conjunctival wound.

## Corneal Surgery

Scleral transplantation in corneal surgery may involve full-thickness and partial-thickness patch grafts. Full thickness scleral grafts prepared with the appropriately sized trephine may address small cornea perforations in the absence of suitable corneal tissue (Fig 6). Fine nonabsorbable sutures (9-0 or 10-0 nylon) are employed with the scleral grafts in the cornea with attention to careful coaptation of the concentric edges thereby achieving a watertight closure. The scleral inlay graft may be a temporary solution for central perforations. An optical keratoplasty may be performed later with a more favorable prognosis for a graft survival.[25] The scleral allograft may be a permanent solution for corneal perforations outside the visual axis. Partial clearing of a scleral inlay graft over time has been demonstrated in rabbits by Thomas as well as by Larsson in humans.[26,27] Maurice and Singh demonstrated with electron microscopy that progressive unraveling and replacement of scleral collagen fibers with those of recipient cornea occurs.[28] Turner et al. described a novel autologous partial thickness scleral patch graft procedure called scleral autoplasty.[29] They performed both inlay and onlay scleral autografts in eight patients with corneal perforations unresponsive to cyanoacrylate glue application.

A full thickness scleral allograft may also be used in the repair of deep or complete eye wall resections for limbal and epibulbar tumors. Shields et al. reported a successful resection of an invasive spindle cell carcinoma of the conjunctiva with a full thickness eye wall removal

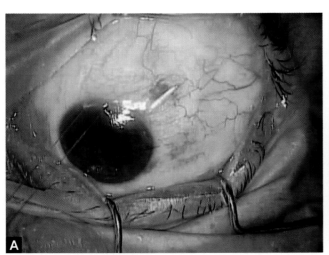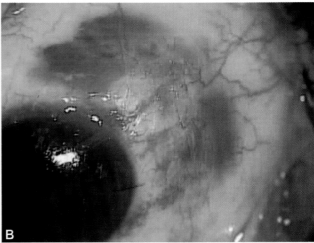

**Figs 5A and B:** Repair of exposed tube with scleral graft and tissue adhesive with conjunctivoplasty

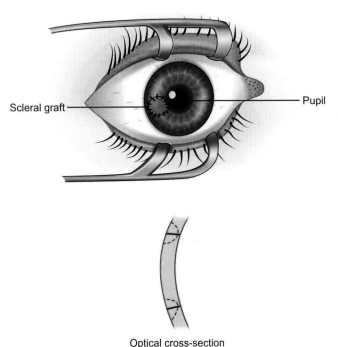

Optical cross-section

**Fig. 6:** Scleral patch graft for corneal perforation

and scleral graft replacement, which spared radiation therapy or enucleation.[30] Composite corneoscleral allografts (14+ mm) may be rarely required to address limbus to limbus infectious keratitis with perforation.[31] An onlay technique is involved over the juxtalimbal scleral bed to minimize angle closure which has been described by Cobo.[32] Shi et al. have described unique aspects of immunologic rejection in corneoscleral transplants.[33] While the visual prognosis is generally poor, Hirst has reported 14 of 23 patients with retention of the globe following heroic corneoscleral graft surgery.[31]

Lamellar scleral patch grafts may be employed in selected peripheral corneoscleral disorders, such as Mooren's ulcer and Terrien's Degeneration.[16-18,34] A long-term review of four patients with severe Terrien's degeneration over a 12–20 year period demonstrated that free hand lamellar corneal scleral grafts were successful in preventing recurrent ecstasia with irregular astigmatism. Localized thinning of the composite grafts was apparent in each patient.[18] The freehand lamellar corneoscleral graft is created using a template of the area of recipient corneoscleral thinning to customize the repair with restoration of normal globe contour and shape. The graft is secured with 9-0 or 10-0 nylon sutures and, in selected cases, with bioadhesive tissue glue.

Corneal and limbal thermal burns are now rarely seen in phacoemulsification. They result from collagen shrinkage with a gaping wound deformity. A primary wound closure with sutures will result in significant induced corneal astigmatism. A lamellar scleral allograft onlay technique may be employed to secure a watertight suture closure with less astigmatism. Alternatively, the trap door scleral autograft may be created adjacent to the limbus to effectively seal the gaping wound (Figs 7A and B).[14]

## Retinal Surgery

Retinal surgery applications of scleral transplants are similar in principle to those seen in glaucoma surgery. When silicone exoplant material is exposed due to overlying conjunctival dehiscence, an infection must be excluded or effectively treated prior to scleral patch graft application to cover the hardware.[35] A free conjunctival autograft, an adjacent conjunctival pedicle flap, or amniotic membrane tissue is required to cover the graft. Ward et al. have demonstrated the efficacy of posterior pole scleral wall support with a donor scleral band of 1 cm width in 59 eyes with degeneration myopia.[36] They achieved control of axial length over a 5-year period of observation compared to controls without surgery.

Scleral grafts have found utility in oculoplastic surgery particularly in eyelid reconstruction and prosthetic sphere coverage. Scleral allograft tissue is well-suited for tarsal replacement with eyelid reconstruction procedures. It is an effective tarsal spacer material in lid retraction surgery as well. However, due to its avascularity, it must be covered by conjunctiva or AMT on the mucosal surface to avoid scleral necrosis and sloughing. The scleral allograft may be sutured to tarsal remnants and lid retractors, respectively, with absorbable 6-0 or 7-0 vicryl. The scleral tissue effectively maintains lid shape and contour while conforming to the ocular curvature with good lid globe apposition. As mild shrinkage occurs with the scleral allograft, oversizing of the template dimensions by a factor of 3 has been recommended in thyroid disease related lid retraction by Dryden and Soll.[37] In the case of orbital sphere implant exposure and early extrusion, the homologous scleral graft is used to cover the implant prior to conjunctival repair and closure. In selected cases of enucleation, the sphere implant may be completely invested in a whole globe scleral allograft, which will also provide attachment of extraocular muscles for improved prosthetic mobility. Inkster et al. further showed that there was no need for secondary intervention

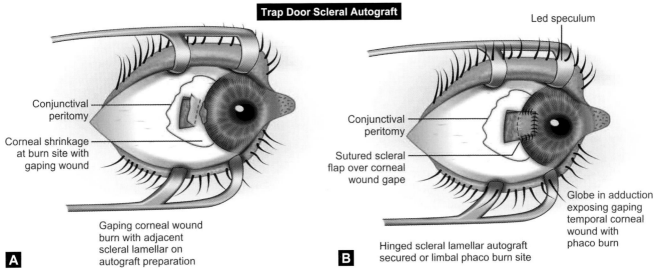

**Figs 7A and B:** Hinged scleral lamellar autograft technique for gaping limbal corneal wound following corneal burn

to address a significant conjunctival wound dehiscence rate of 33% as spontaneous closure occurred.[38]

## Dental Surgery

Sclera rarely has been used in dental surgery. When treated with glutaraldehyde, the tensile strength of the sclera is enhanced by crosslinkage. Spatzner demonstrated that freeze-dried crosslinked human sclera may successfully augment the maxillary alveolar ridge defects to facilitate prosthetic tooth fixation.[39] Effective integration of the scleral tissue has been demonstrated by Feingold in a histologic study.[40] Alternative materials have been utilized in lieu of homologous sclera in scleral transplantation procedures described above. Mehta has classified these scleral substitutes as biogenic and synthetic materials based on their origin.[41]

## ⁍ AMNIOTIC MEMBRANE

Amniotic membrane tissue (AMT) has been described as an effective material for management of partial thickness scleral defects without ectasia or staphyloma. Amniotic membrane is the innermost layer of human placenta, which consists of a basement membrane and an avascular stroma. Amniotic membrane tissue posseses anti-inflammatory and antifibrotic properties. It serves as a scaffold for rapid epithelialization following an onlay graft technique using 10-0 nylon suture fixation or bioadhesive material (Tisseel) application. A multilayered AMT graft technique has been described by Hanada, as well as Sridar with success in the management of scleral ulceration as an alternative to scleral

patch grafting.[42,43] Amniotic membrane tissue is commercially available as a cryopreserved tissue by Bio-Tissue, Inc. (Miami, Florida) and as a dehydrated tissue, AmbioDry, manufactured by Okto Ophtho (Costa Mesa, California).

## ⁍ FASCIA LATA

Fascia lata has been effectively used as a scleral substitute based on its high tensile strength. It is commercially available, preserved and sterilized by gamma sterilization (Mile High Transplantation Eye Bank). It may also be harvested from the patient's lateral thigh immediately prior to the ocular surgery. The fascia lata must be covered by conjunctival or amniotic membrane to avoid tissue necrosis. Prominent conjunctival swelling at the site of the fascia lata graft gradually resolves demonstrating good globe contour with incorporation of the graft. Torchia has reported successful use of fascial lata in the scleromalacia perforans following necrosis of prior homologous scleral graft.[44]

## ⁍ PERIOSTEUM

Periosteum has been utilized as an autologous tissue substitute for sclera. It is durable and readily becomes vascularized and incorporated as a scleral onlay graft. It must be covered by an epithelial basement membrane, such as conjunctiva, buccal mucus membrane, or amniotic membrane tissue to avoid graft necrosis. Koenig reported the use of periosteum in scleromalacia perforans and corneoscleral wound dehiscence with a 3-year follow-up.[45] After a period of local swelling and conjunctival edema, the periosteum was well incorporated with good globe contour preservation. The major drawback of the technique was the need for a general anesthetic to permit multiple site surgery. The periosteum is harvested from the anterior tibial crest.

## PERICARDIUM

Pericardium is a popular scleral substitute due to its commercial availability as a product of the proprietary tutoplast processing method.[46] It is durable and easily manipulated, however, it is thinner (0.4 mm) than scleral tissue (1.0 mm). Homologous pericardium may be used to cover drainage tube devices and exposed scleral buckles.[47] Long-term follow-up has demonstrated a significant prevalence of noninflammatory graft resorption after 7–8 months, which exposes the eye to the risk of tube erosion with endophthalmitis.[24] Bovine pericardium has also been prepared as a wrap for hydroxyapatite orbital implants. It has demonstrated a higher rate of conjunctival wound dehiscence compared to homologous sclera wraps.[48]

## DURA MATER

Dura mater has been utilized as a scleral substitute based on the durability and availability as well. It is preserved with the proprietary tutoplast process. Due to the potential for higher prion and HIV viral content in dural tissue, concerns exist as to whether complete elimination of these agents is possible.[6] Dura mater has been particularly effective as a cover for glaucoma drainage tubes.

## SPLIT THICKNESS DERMAL GRAFT

Split thickness dermal grafts have been used to cover peripheral corneal and scleral defects.[49] A powered Brown dermatome is used to create a hinged epidermal flap on the lateral aspect of the thigh of the patient. A 0.0388 mm thickness dermal graft is harvested from the dermal bed with the same dermatome. The epidermal skin layer is fenestrated and reflected over the dermal bed. It is then secured with a 4-0 chromic suture and dressed with iodoform gauze. The autologous split thickness dermal graft possesses several unique advantages. It is nonantigenic with good tensile strength. It requires no epithelial membrane coverage as a nonkeratinized epithelium is derived from dermal appendages within the graft. Significant vascularization enables its survival on avascular surfaces of the cornea and sclera. These features make the split thickness dermal grafts well-suited for large scleral defects in the presence of extensive conjunctival scarring, which prevents mobilization. Its

main disadvantage is the need for general anesthesia for multiple site surgery. Mauriello has reported success with this technique in 10 patients with corneal and scleral thinning disorders with up to 5-year follow-up.[49]

## OTHER MATERIALS

### Biologic

Other biologic substitutes for scleral transplantation include nasal septum and hard palate mucosal autografts. These materials have an epithelial surface which is well-suited for tarsal replacement in eyelid reconstruction as no conjunctival cover is required. Auricular cartilage and allograft aorta are scleral substitutes, which require conjunctival coverage. These materials are rarely used. Allograft aorta has been used in one patient with a successful repair of a scleral defect with 5-year follow-up.[50]

### Synthetic

Synthetic materials have met with variable success as scleral substitutes. Polytetrafluoroethylene (PTFE) or GoreTex has been used as a graft material in vascular surgery for 40 years. It is a porous matrix, which allows vascularization with little inflammation; however, it is poorly incorporated in tissues and requires an epithelial cover. Huang noted that PTFE covered by conjunctiva was effective in the management of necrotizing scleritis with thinning.[51] A thicker (2 mm) GoreTex graft is available for posterior eyelid reconstruction. Karesh et al. demonstrated effective application of PTFE as a spacer in the correction of lower lid retraction.[52]

Polygalactin, Dacron and Mersilene have each been formulated as a mesh suitable for a scleral substitute material.[53] Polygalactin may undergo hydrolytic degradation. It has also been used to wrap orbital implants allowing attachment of rectus muscles and vascularization. Dacron and Mersilene resist hydrolysis and have an indefinite *in vivo* presence. Dacron has been used in vascular surgery as an arterial bypass graft material, as well as suture material. Rabbit studies have suggested utility in the repair of scleral defects. Mersilene has been used as a nonabsorbable suture material, as sling materials in ptosis surgery, as a wrap for orbital implants, as well as on onlay scleral graft substitute.[54]

Resorbable matrices may have future utility in repair of scleral and corneal defects, as they may prompt surface regeneration, as well as allow engineering of replacement tissue. Recombinant collagen or a synthetic matrix would be needed to eliminate risks associated with bovine collagen currently studied.[54,55]

## CONCLUSION

Scleral transplantation has been successfully employed in multiple areas of ophthalmic surgery. It is most frequently used in support of glaucoma surgery. It remains an effective procedure in restoration of globe integrity in the presence of less frequently encountered scleral defects created by trauma and scleritis. Effective management of inflammatory or ischemic scleral melting disorders requires a thorough clinical evaluation with appropriate local and systemic medical therapy prior to and concurrent with tectonic scleral surgery. A variety of scleral substitutes have been explored with successful globe reinforcement, tube shunt coverage, as well as eyelid and socket reconstruction.

## REFERENCES

1. Foster CS, Sainzdela Maza M. The Sclera. New York: Springer–Verlay 1994. pp. 229-307.
2. Collinge J, Palmer MS, Dryden AJ. Genetic predisposition in iatrogenic Creutzfeld-Jakob disease. Lancet. 1991;337 (8755):1441-2.
3. Oh JH, Kim JC. Repair of scleromalacia using preserved scleral graft with amniotic membrane transplantation. Cornea. 2003;22(4):288-93.
4. Smith MF, Doyle JW, Tickmey JW. A comparison of glaucoma drainage implant tube coverage. J Glaucoma. 2002;11(2):143-7.
5. Brown P, Rohwer RG, Gajdusek DC. Sodium hydroxide decontamination of Creutzfeld-Jakob virus. N Engl J Med. 1984;310 (11):727.
6. Koschalzky K, Woelfel G. Inactivation of HIV-1 during preservation of dura mater tissues with sodium hydroxide, hydrogen peroxide and acetone by the Tutoplast process; 1993.
7. Lin CP, Trai MC, Wu YH, et al. Repair of a giant scleral ulcer with preserved sclera and tissue adhesive. Ophthalmic Surg Lasers. 1996;27 (12):995-9.
8. Zeppa L, Romana MR, Capasso L, et al. Sutureless human sclera donor patch graft for Ahmed glaucoma valve. Eur J Ophthalmol. 2010;20(3):546-51.
9. Johnson WA, Henderson JW, Parkhill Em, et al. Transplantation of homografts of sclera: an experimental study. Am J Ophthalmol. 1962;54:1019-30.
10. Obear MF, Winter FL. Technique of overlay scleral homograft. Arch Ophthalmol. 1964;71:837-8.
11. Blum FG, Salamoun SG. A useful surgical modification in fascia lata or scleral grafting. Arch Ophthalmol. 1963;69:287-9.
12. Sagwan VS, Jain V, Gupta P. Structural and functional outcome of scleral patch graft. Eye (Lond). 2007;21(7):930-5.
13. Rockwood EJ, Meisler DM. In: Abbott RL (Ed.). Scleritis: Surgical Intervention in Corneal and External Diseases. Orlando: Grume & Stratton; 1987. pp. 177-87.
14. Hamill MB, Krachmer J, et al. Management of scleral perforation ed. Cornea 202, volume 2. Philadelphia: Elsevier-Mosby; 2005. pp. 1863-70.
15. Esquenazi S. Autogenous lamellar scleral graft in the treatment of scleral melt after pterygium surgery. Graefes Arch Clin Exp Ophthalmol. 2007;245 (12):1869-71.
16. Stilma JS. Conjunctival excision of lamellar scleral autograft in 38 Mooren's ulcers from Sierra Leone. Br J Ophthalmol. 1983; 67(7):475-8.
17. Yang R, Guo R. The treatment of Terrien's marginal degeneration using Lamellar keratoplasty with dried corneosclera. Yan Ke Xue Bao. 2004;20 (3):140-3.
18. Pettit TH. Corneoscleral freehand Lamellar Keratoplasty in Terrien's Marginal degeneration of the cornea–long-term results. Refract Corneal Surg. 1991;7(1):28-32.
19. Rai P, Lauande-Pimentel R, Barton K. Amniotic membrane as an adjunct to donor sclera in the repair of exposed glaucoma drainage devices. Am J Ophthalmol. 2005;140 (6):1148-52.
20. Aslanides IM, Spaeth GL, Schmidt CM, et al. Autologous patch graft in tube shunt surgery. J Glaucoma. 1999;8(5):306-9.
21. Halkiadiakis I, Lim P, Moroi SE. Surgical results of bleb revision with scleral patch graft for late-onset bleb complications. Ophthalmic Surg Lasers Imaging. 2005;36 (1):14-23.
22. Nguyen QD, Foster CS. Scleral patch graft in the management of necrotizing scleritis. Int Ophthalmol Clin. 1999;39(1):109-31.
23. Au L, Wechsler D, Spencer F, et al. Outcome of bleb revision using scleral patch graft and conjunctival advancement. J Glaucoma. 2009;18(4):331-5.
24. Lama PJ, Fechtner RD. Tube erosion following insertion of a glaucoma drainage device with a pericardial patch graft. Arch Ophthalmol. 1999;117:1243-4.
25. Chaidaroon W, Sonthi W, Manassakorn A. Penetrating keratoplasty following scleral patch graft procedure. J Med Associ Thai. 2004;87 (1):53-8.
26. Thomas JWT. Transplantation of scleral tissue onto rabbits cornea. Trans Ophthalmol Soc UK. 1932;5:64-7.
27. Larsson S. Treatment of perforated corneal ulcer by autoplastic scleral transplantation. Br J Ophthalmol. 1948;32:54-7.
28. Maurice DM, Singh T. The fate of slceral grafts in the cornea. Cornea. 1996;15:204-9.
29. Turner SJ, Johnson Z, Corbett M, et al. Sclera autoplasty for the repair of corneal perforations: a case series, Br J Ophthalmol. 2010;94(5):669-70.
30. Shields JA, Eagle RC, Man BP, et al. Invasive spindle cell carcinoma of the conjunctiva managed by full thickness eye wall resection. Cornea. 2007;26 (8):1014-6.
31. Hirst LW, Lee GA. Corneoscleral transplantation for end stage corneal diseases. Br J Ophthalmol. 1998;82 (11):1276-9.
32. Cobo M, Ortiz JR, Safran SG. Sclerokeratoplasty with maintenance of the angle. Am J Ophthalmol. 1992;125:549-52.
33. Shi W, Wang T, Zhang J, et al. Clinical features of immune rejection after corneoscleral transplantation. Am J Ophthalmol. 2008;82 (11):1276-9.
34. Esquenazi S, Shihadeh WA, Abdenkadur A, et al. A new surgical technique for anterior segment ectasia: tectonic lamellar sclerokeratoplasty. Ophthalmic Surg Lasers Imaging. 2006;37(5):434-6.

35. Kittredge KL, Lonway BP. Management of the exposed scleral explant. Semin Ophthalmol. 1995;10:45-60.

36. Ward B, Tarutta EP, Mayer MJ. The efficacy and safety of posterior pole buckles in the control of progressive high myopia. Eye (Lond). 2009;23 (12):2169-74.

37. Dryden RM, Soll DB. The use of scleral transplantation in cicatricial entropian and eyelid retraction. Trans Sect Ophthalmol Am Acad Ophthalmol Otolanryngol. 1977;83 (4, pt 1):669-78.

38. Inkster CF, Ng SG, Leatherbarrow B. Primary sanked scleral patch graft in the prevention of exposure of hydroxyapatite orbital implants. Ophthalmology. 2002;109 (2):389-92.

39. Spatzner M, Deporter DA. Preprosthetic alveolar ridge correction using gluteraldehyde cross-linked lyophilized scleral allografts. Compendium. 1990;11(3):176-81.

40. Feingold JP, Chassens AL, Doyle J, et al. Preserved scleral allografts in periodontal defects in man. II. Histological evaluation. J Periodontal. 1977;48 (1):4-12.

41. Mehta JS, Franks WA. The sclera, the prion, and the Ophthalmologist. Br J Ophthalmol. 2002;86 (5):587-92.

42. Hanada VS, Jain V, Shimmuri S, et al. Multilayered amniotic membrane transplantation for severe ulceration of the cornea and sclera. Am J Ophthalmol. 2001;131 (3):324-31.

43. Sridhar MS, Bansal AK, Rao GN. Mulitlayered amniotic membrane transplantation for partial thickness scleral thinning following pterygium surgery. Eye (Lond). 2002;16:639-42.

44. Torchia RT, Dunn RE, Pease PJ. Fascia lata grafting in scleromalacia perforans. Am J Ophthalmol. 1968;66:705-9.

45. Koenig SB, Sanitato JJ, Kaufman HE. Long term follow up study of scleroplasty using autogenous periosteum. Cornea. 1990;9:139-43.

46. Schein OD. The use of processed pericardial tissue in anterior segment reconstruction. Am J Ophthalmol. 1992;113(5):533-7.

47. Weissgold DJ, Millay RH, Bochow TA. Rescue of exposed scleral buckles with cadaveric pericardial patch grafts. Ophthalmology. 2001;108:753-8.

48. Debakerr CM, Dutton JJ, Prola AD, et al. Bovine pericardium versus homologous sclera as wrapping materials for hydroxyapatite ocular implants: an animal study. Ophthalmic Plast Reconstr Surg. 1999;15:312-6.

49. Mauriello JA, Pokorny K. Use of split-thickness dermal grafts to repair corneal and scleral defects—a study of 10 patients. Br J Ophthalmol. 1993;77(6):327-31.

50. Merz EH. Scleral reinforcement with aortic tissue. Am J Ophthalmol. 1964;57:766-70.

51. Huang WJ, Hu FR, Chang SW. Clinicopathologic study of Gore-Tex patch graft in corneoscleral surgery. Cornea. 1994; 13:82-6.

52. Karesh JW, Fabrega MA, Rodriguez MM, et al. Polytetrafluoroethylene as an interpositional graft material for correction of the lower eyelid retraction. Ophthalmology. 1989; 96:419-23.

53. Tarulla EP, Andreava LD, Morkoslam GA, et al. Reinforcement of the sclera with new types of synthetic materials in progressive myopia. Vesin oftalmol. 1999;115:8-10.

54. Allon B. Closer to Nature; new biomaterials and tissue engineering in ophthalmology. Br J Ophthalmol. 1999;83:1235-40.

55. Sillinger M, Bujia J, Roller N, et al. Tissue engineering and autologous transplant formation: practical approaches with resorbable biomaterials and new culture techniques. Biomaterials. 1996;17:237-42.

# SECTION 16

# Ocular Surface Rehabilitation

## CHAPTERS

*Contd...*

# CHAPTER 71

# Corneal and Conjunctival Foreign Bodies

*Larry Ferdinand, Vanessa Ngakeng*

## ▶ BACKGROUND

Corneal and conjunctival foreign bodies are one of the most frequently encountered urgent problems that present not only to ophthalmologists but also to urgent care health professionals. There are various objects that can be embedded in the conjunctiva or cornea ranging from inorganic to organic, such as metal, glass, plastic, insect appendages, and vegetation, etc. The associated ocular discomfort and irritation experienced by the patient will naturally drive them to seek care. Therefore, it is prudent for an ophthalmologist to know how to treat these problems but also to educate fellow healthcare colleagues who usually encounter these patients first.

## ▶ CLINICAL FINDINGS AND EVALUATION

The signs and symptoms usually include complaints of foreign body sensation, tearing, epiphora, irritation, pain and redness. A comprehensive medical history along with a detailed ocular examination is required for any ocular foreign body. A good history must include the mechanism of injury, visual status before the injury, past ocular history, occupational and environmental setting at the time of injury, presence of eye protection, whether first aid or any treatment was rendered, and time of the injury. Afterwards, documentation of visual acuity is absolutely essential before any procedure is done to remove the foreign body.[1] If the patient is uncooperative with examination, topical anesthetic should help to alleviate blepharospasms and intolerable ocular pain. Also, an attentive examination of pupillary appearance and function would help to indicate if traumatic iris tear and/or angle injury is present. In some cases, gonioscopic evaluation is essential in the eye exam,

but this is usually done after the foreign body is removed. The eye and adnexa should be inspected for lacerations or debris. Segmental injection of the conjunctiva often directs the clinician to the site of injury. Conjunctival or corneal foreign bodies are best identified with a good slit lamp examination (Fig. 1). Slit-lamp examination of the conjunctiva and cornea assists to definitively locate the particulate matter and assess the degree of injury. It is important to evert the upper and lower lids, because some debris may be embedded in the tarsus, particularly if vertical track marks are observed on the cornea and

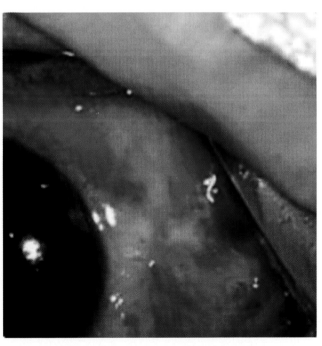

**Fig. 1:** Metallic conjunctival foreign body

highlighted with sodium fluorescein dye aided by the cobalt blue light on the slit lamp. Double eversion of the upper eyelid using a Desmarres retractor or bent paper clip to push the upper fornix can be helpful for visualization.[2] These linear abrasions are highly suggestive of a foreign body embedded in the superior palpebral conjunctiva.[1] Once the location of the foreign body is identified, the clinician should assess the depth of penetration, extension into the anterior chamber, or sclera wall and whether the foreign body is of inorganic or organic material. Sodium fluorescein used under cobalt blue helps to determine corneal epithelium disruption as well as the presence of aqueous leakage namely the 'Seidel test' at the site of injury. Finally, fundoscopic examination is necessary in all cases to look for presence or absence of intraocular foreign body, perforating, penetrating injury and contusion injury to the intraocular structures. Ultrasonography or radiography is recommended if the clinician suspects an intraocular foreign, especially if the posterior segment view is inadequate with indirect ophthalmoscopy. Once the examination is complete, the clinician should carefully document all clinical findings that include visual acuity, the degree of injury, approximation of size of abrasion, laceration and presence of anterior uveitis. Also, anterior segment photography to assist in the documentation of the conjunctival and/or corneal foreign body is recommended.

## PATHOGENESIS

Mechanical injury to the corneal epithelium creates immediate cell migration and spreading to cover the epithelial defect.[3] Stromal injury can take months to years to complete, the end results sometimes reduces corneal clarity. Excessive deposition of fibrotic repair tissue can lead to pathologies involving excessive scarring and contracture. In the cornea, fibrotic repair presents special challenges affecting both clarity and shape of the cornea.[4] Optical coherence tomography is a useful test to quantify the exact depth to cornea penetration and scarring. Foreign bodies are often birefringent and can be demonstrated on examination of tissue sections with polarized light.

Chemosis, is the translucent swelling of the conjunctiva, suggesting severe inflammation. This is usually not worrying as long as it settles.

## MANAGEMENT

Removal of any corneal or conjunctival foreign body should be done with great care and caution. However, regardless of the skill of the clinician, foreign bodies located at the level of Bowman's membrane or in the stroma will produce

scarring. Not all foreign bodies require removal. Deeply embedded nontoxic foreign bodies such as glass may best be left in the cornea, if they do not impede vision or create intolerable visual disturbance.

Firstly, irrigation should be attempted as a conservative measure to try to dislodge a superficial foreign body from the ocular surface, especially if the foreign body is located on the conjunctiva or in the fornices. Sterile irrigation solution should not be pointed directly at the foreign body but rather at a slight angle, because the pressure exerted from the irrigation stream straight onto the particle may embed it more deeply into the cornea or conjunctiva.

If irrigation is unsuccessful, instrumentation is used to dislodge the foreign body. A moistened cotton-tipped applicator may be helpful for dislodging conjunctival foreign bodies (Fig. 2), and foreign bodies found in the tear film but should not be used for corneal foreign bodies because, the cotton tip applicator may drive the particle deeper into the cornea. Before removal with any type of instrument, topical anesthetic such as proparacaine 0.5% or tetracaine 0.5% should be placed in the affected eye along with a drop of topical antibiotic. However, any treating clinician should be mindful not to dispense topical anesthetic drop to a patient for symptom relief, because these medications are toxic to the corneal epithelium if used excessively.

Corneal foreign body removal using instrumentation or needles is more precisely accomplished with biomicroscopy magnification with a slit lamp. Patient cooperation must be encouraged during the procedure because any sudden unexpected movements could worsen the injury. A wire speculum may greatly facilitate eyelid control in an anxious patient. A standard 23-gauge needle on a 5 ml syringe along

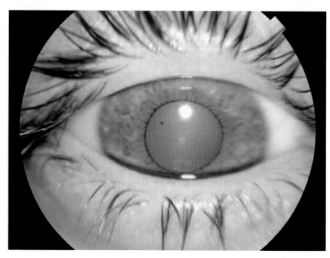

**Fig. 2:** Corneal foreign body (superior temporally)

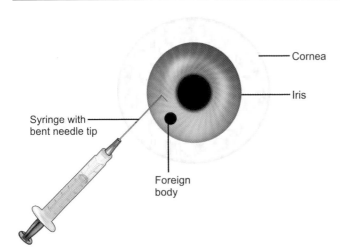

**Fig. 3:** A standard 23-gauge needle on a 5 ml syringe along with a hemostat or needle

with a hemostat or needle driver by using either one to bend 1–2 mm of the sharp tip end of the needle at a 90° angle in a fashion similar to a 'hockey stick'.[5] This makes the procedure much safer and gives the clinician better control of the device. The bent tip can now be used to flick the foreign body from the cornea (Fig. 3).

## RUST RINGS

Metal pieces represent one of the most hazardous and common foreign body materials to the eye. When an iron foreign body has been embedded in the cornea for more than a few hours an orange-brown 'rust ring' appears secondary to metal oxidation. This process stains the adjacent epithelial cells as well as Bowman's membrane. The rust may eventually diffuse into the stroma, and may continue to be a source of irritation and delay of the healing process. The rust ring can be removed using a battery powered dental burr with a sterile tip. However, care must be taken to preserve the corneal stroma. There is no need to be overly meticulous about removing all traces of rust. The remaining particles will extrude over time. If the rust ring is left intact, the stain will eventually fade, leaving a circular scar called 'Coats's ring'.[1]

Although medical therapy is a useful adjunct, a surgical approach is required for most corneal or conjunctival perforations. Depending on the size and location of the corneal perforation, treatment options include gluing, amniotic membrane transplantation, and corneal transplantation.[6]

The amniotic membrane is a biologic tissue that has been used as a graft for corneal and conjunctival reconstruction in a variety of ocular surface diseases. It is avascular and possesses antiangiogenic, antiscarring and anti-inflammatory properties. It is not a substitute but rather a substrate upon which cells can migrate and regenerate, forming new and healthy tissue.[7] Conjunctival perforations can be treated with scleral suturing or freezing with a cryoprobe.

## REMOVAL OF CORNEAL FOREIGN BODIES IN LASIK PATIENTS

Laser *in situ* keratomileusis (LASIK) is one the most common refractive surgery procedures. Porges et al. reported the outcomes of uncomplicated removal of corneal foreign bodies in patients who previously underwent LASIK surgery.[8] They reported no complications with cornea foreign body removal in 9 eyes of 8 patients. All eyes had full recovery within 24–48 hours with no subsequent decrease in visual acuity. Therefore, they concluded that corneal foreign bodies can be removed safely and effectively from corneas after LASIK and also recommended to properly instruct patients to take postoperative precautions such as using protective eyewear. However, a case report by Crowther and Ellingham documented a complication of astigmatism from corneal scar formation after corneal foreign body removal, but the removal was done by the patient's general practitioner without the aid of a slit lamp.[9]

## REMOVAL OF CORNEAL FOREIGN BODY THROUGH A LAMELLAR CORNEAL POCKET

Au et al. describes a technique for removing a small piece of glass in the posterior corneal stroma within 2 mm of the optical axis.[10] The site of entry of the foreign body was sealed and epithelialized. The patient complained of blurry vision, foreign body sensation, and decrease in vision in the affected eye. They removed the foreign body by creating lamellar corneal pocket in the operating room. The full steps of the procedure are illustrated in the article. Postoperatively, the patient achieved corrected 20/20 vision in the affected eye with no abnormality of corneal surface on topography or corneal edema and inflammation. They suggest that this is a viable technique to remove deeply embedded foreign bodies.

## TREATMENT

The goals of treatment are to remove the foreign body, relieve discomfort, avoid secondary infection, and minimize corneal scarring. Caution should be taken to avoid disruption of deeper layers of the cornea, which can lead to unnecessary scarring. Therapy following the removal of a corneal foreign body includes broad-spectrum topical antibiotics, cycloplegia with mydriatics, and the application

CHAPTER 71

of a firm pressure patch or bandage contact lens to help healing process. The Corneal Abrasion Patching Study Group evaluated the effectiveness of pressure patching in the treatment of noninfected, noncontact lens-related traumatic corneal abrasions and abrasions secondary to removal of corneal foreign bodies.[11] They found that patients with noninfected, noncontact lens-related traumatic corneal abrasions or foreign body removal-related corneal abrasions healed significantly faster and had less pain compared to patients with congruent injuries that had patching (Patching that was not pressure patching). Therefore, patients can be treated with antibiotic ointment and mydriatics alone without the need for patching.

## ⊱ FOLLOW-UP

Patients should be examined the next day to evaluate the healing of any epithelial defects on the cornea and detect any signs of infection. Foreign bodies from potentially contaminated substances such as vegetative matter deserves careful follow-up. A few hours to several days are required for complete re-epithelialization of the cornea, depending on the size of the abrasion. However, if the basement membrane has been damaged, it can take 6 weeks or more to restore firm attachments between the epithelial layer and the basement membrane.

After 24 hours, the acute symptoms should have significant resolution, but if patient continues to complain of foreign body sensation or of marked discomfort, the clinician should suspect retained foreign body particles, anterior uveitis, infection, or penetrating injury to the eye. If the corneal abrasion is resolving but still significant, patching, placing a bandage contact lens, or antibiotic ointment can be used depending on the size of defect. If anterior uveitis continues to persists, then a topical steroid regimen can be used only if the corneal epithelium has completely healed. Cycloplegic agents should be used for any symptomatic traumatic iritis.

## ⊱ COMPLICATIONS

Traumatic iritis, recurrent cornea erosion, corneal edema, corneal ulcerations, corneal stromal scarring and penetrating ocular injury are the main complications that are associated with corneal foreign bodies. Recurrent cornea erosions are rare, but can occur several months after injury. This can be usually being managed with debridement of the overlying epithelium along with placement of a bandage contact lens or patching with a regimen of hypertonic sodium chloride drops. Anterior stromal puncturing or phototherapeutic

keratectomy (PTK) can also be used to assist with the healing. Any signs of corneal ulceration warrant culture and aggressive treatment with topical fortified antibiotics. Traumatic iritis should be treated with steroids only after epithelium has completely healed along with cycloplegia with mydriatics. Finally, penetrating corneal injuries should be treated with great caution. Deep corneal foreign bodies that have penetrated into the anterior chamber or removal that may lead to perforation should be managed as an intraocular foreign body. If uncertain, ultrasonography and CT scan can help to determine if there is an intraocular foreign body present. Also, fibrin glue or cyanoacrylate can assist for small penetrations with leakage of aqueous from anterior chamber. Larger lacerations or penetrations should be evaluated and repaired in the operating room.

## ⊱ PROGNOSIS

Patients usually have full recovery after uncomplicated removal of foreign body. Visual acuity is not typically affected by noncentral cornea bodies but caution should be taken with patients with prior history of LASIK. Diagnosis, removal, treatment, and attentive follow-up produce good outcomes for foreign body injuries.

## ⊱ REFERENCES

1. Augeri PA. Corneal foreign body removal and treatment. Optom Clin. 1991;1(4):59-70.
2. Newell SW. Management of Corneal Foreign Bodies. 1985;31 (2):149-56.
3. DelMonte DW, Kim T. Anatomy and physiology of the cornea. J Cataract Refract Surg. 2011;37(3):588-98.
4. Fini ME, Stramer BM. How the cornea heals: cornea-specific repair mechanisms affecting surgical outcomes. Cornea. 2005; 24(8 Suppl):S2-S11.
5. Beyer H, Cherkas D. Corneal foreign body removal using a bent needle tip. Am J Emerg Med. 2012;30(3):489-90.
6. Jhanji V, Young AL, Mehta JS, et al. Management of Corneal Perforation. Surv Ophthalmol. 2011;56(6):522-38.
7. Gomes JA, Romano A, Santos MS, et al. Amniotic membrane use in ophthalmology. Curr Opin Ophthalmol. 2005;16(4): 233-40.
8. Porges Y, Landau D, Douieb J, et al. Removal of corneal foreign bodies following laser in situ keratomileusis. J Refract Surg. 2001;17(5):559-60.
9. Crowther KS, Ellingham RB. Complicated removal of corneal foreign bodies 18 months after laser in situ keratomeileusis. J Cataract Refract Surg. 2005;31(4):851-2.
10. Au YK, Libby C, Patel JS, et al. Removal of a Corneal Foreign Body through a Lamellar Corneal Pocket. Ophthalmic Surg Lasers. 1996;27(6):471-2.
11. Kaiser PK. A Comparison of Pressure Patching versus No Patching for Corneal Abrasions due to Trauma or Foreign Body Removal. Ophthalmology. 1995;102(12):1936-42.

# Superficial Keratectomy and Epithelial Debridement

*Julian A Procope*

## ❧ HISTORY

For greater than a century, simple debridement of loosely adherent epithelium was the treatment of choice in patients with recurrent corneal erosions.[1-5] Later, superficial keratectomy[4,6-8] developed as a more aggressive and efficacious technique, due to the inability of epithelial debridement to significantly enhance epithelial adherence, and to remove all abnormal basement membrane. Sometimes, the terms corneal epithelial debridement and superficial keratectomy may be used interchangeably. However, except for very superficial and localized corneal pathology, superficial keratectomy is generally of the two procedures, the choice in anteriorly located disease. Debridement may be most efficacious for removing a localized area of a loosely adherent sheet of epithelium in a limited number of erosion patients. This technique might only require a cotton swab or blunt instrument and is easily performed with topical anesthesia at the slit lamp. However, this procedure is limited in its efficacy due to the fact that no significant modifications are achieved at the level of Bowman's layer or deeper corneal structures to enhance epithelial adhesion. Therefore, a more aggressive approach in performing a wider superficial keratectomy, sometimes requiring the use of an operating microscope, is much more likely to be of benefit to patients with recurrent corneal erosions.

## ❧ INDICATIONS

### Anterior Dystrophies[6,9]

Primary dystrophic corneal disorders are classified into categories based on the location of the dystrophy in the cornea: anterior, stromal or posterior. Anterior basement membrane dystrophy (ABMD) is a common cause of recurrent corneal erosions.[6,9] ABMD is the most frequently encountered of the anterior dystrophies. It includes conditions such as anterior epithelial membrane dystrophy (Cogan's microcystic dystrophy, map-dot fingerprint dystrophy) (Figs 1 to 4).

### Recurrent Erosion Syndrome

Recurrent corneal erosion is a distinct clinical entity, the hallmark of which is repeated episodes of spontaneous breakdown and painful sloughing of the corneal epithelium.[2,3,7,8,10,11] The most common cause of recurrent corneal erosions is minor trauma or abrasion of the corneal epithelium that typically occurs as a result of a shallow corneal injury, such as might be produced by a fingernail.[7] Patients who have suffered spontaneous corneal erosion typically

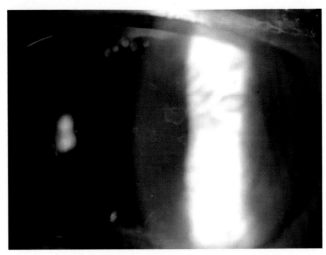

**Fig. 1:** Anterior basement membrane dystrophy
*Source:* Photo courtesy of Francis W Price

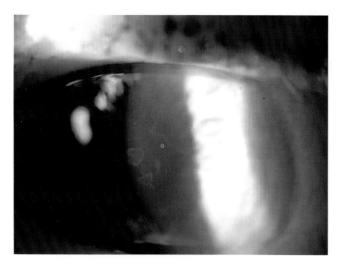

**Fig. 2:** Anterior basement membrane dystrophy
*Source*: Photo courtesy of Francis W Price

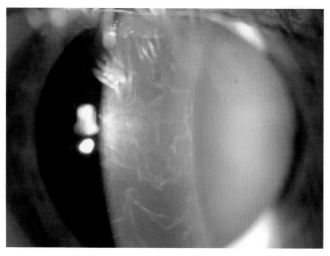

**Fig. 3:** Anterior basement membrane dystrophy
*Source*: Photo courtesy of Francis W Price

report the sudden onset of pain, foreign body sensation, epiphora and photosensitivity, most often upon opening the eye after awakening in the morning. The pathogenic mechanism is due to a disruption of the normal adhesive bonds between the corneal epithelium and the underlying stroma.[2,3,11] This abnormality may occur either as a result of abnormal epithelial basement membrane, or abnormal deposition of a normal epithelial basement membrane. Most spontaneous epithelial erosion attacks are treated quite well with either patching or the use of a bandage soft contact lens (BSCL) in concert with topical antibiotics and topical nonsteroidal anti-inflammatory drugs (NSAIDs). However, for those recalcitrant cases and for patients with recurring erosions, surgical intervention in the form of superficial

keratectomy, anterior stromal micropuncture or phototherapeutic keratectomy (PTK) is indicated. Other conditions for which superficial keratectomy has been employed include the following. In most instances, the basic surgical technique remains the same with few modifications (Figs 5 and 6).

- Band keratopathy
- Superficial pannus or scar[12]
- Salzmann's nodules (Figs 7 and 8)[13]
- Corneal dermoid
- Pterygium
- Excision of retained foreign bodies
- Harvesting of corneal tissue for microbiological or histological examination in the setting of corneal infection[14]

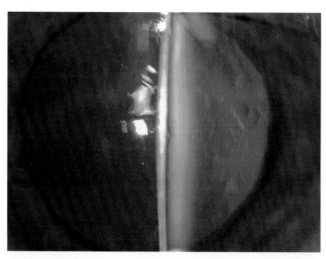

**Fig. 4:** Anterior basement membrane dystrophy in retroillumination
*Source*: Photo courtesy of Francis W Price

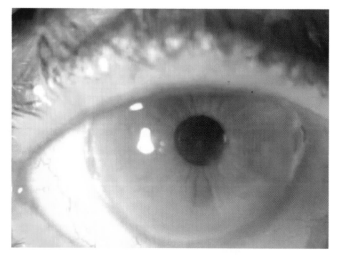

**Fig. 5:** Recurrent epithelial erosions
*Source*: Photo courtesy of Francis W Price

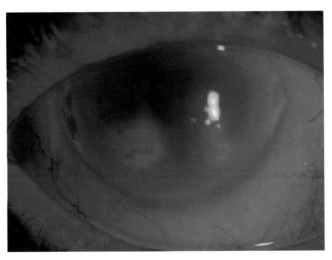

**Fig. 6:** Recurrent epithelial erosions
*Source*: Photo courtesy of Francis W Price

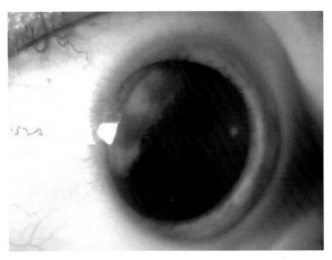

**Fig. 7:** Salzmann nodules
*Source*: Photo courtesy of Francis W Price

- Photorefractive keratectomy,[15] laser-assisted subepithelial keratectomy (LASEK) and PTK
- Prior to riboflavin-UVA collagen crosslinking.

## ⟫ TECHNIQUE

### Preoperative Procedure

Once the decision has been made to proceed with superficial keratectomy, and immediately prior to performing the procedure, the patient is brought to the slit lamp and examined with careful scrutiny of the level and nature of the corneal pathology. Depending on the preoperative diagnosis, for example whether the entity being treated is more focal in nature, such as might be seen with a trauma-induced recurrent erosion process or more diffuse in nature, as with diffuse ABMD, a decision needs to be made at this time as to performing a relatively focal or even multifocal keratectomy versus a diffuse epithelial keratectomy.

Vertical slit beam analysis to determine the depth of the pathology is similarly critical, for, if in the surgeon's judgment the pathology being addressed is more posteriorly located than that which may be effectively treated via superficial keratectomy, then consideration may need to be given to another modality such as PTK or lamellar keratoplasty.

Transillumination through the dilated pupil to determine the vertical and horizontal margins of pathology is also critical, as again the surgeon will utilize these parameters in his decision-making process as to the extent of surgery required for the pathology at hand. This is also the stage at which the surgeon must decide whether the patient, based upon the nature and the extent of pathology to be treated,

is a good candidate for operation upon at the slit lamp, or is better suited for a procedure performed supine under an operating microscope. The vast majority of patients typically encountered who require superficial keratectomy may have their pathology reliably and effectively attended to at the slit lamp.

### Instrumentation

- Topical proparacaine
- Eyelid speculum
- #57 Beaver blade
- Tooke knife (for scraping of Bowman's layer following epithelial debridement)
- Diluted (20%) alcohol
- Cellulose sponges (for brushing of Bowman's layer

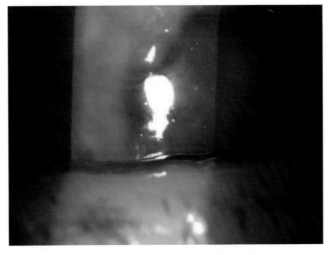

**Fig. 8:** Salzmann nodules
*Source*: Photo courtesy of Francis W Price

following epithelial debridement)
- Bandage soft contact lens
- 0.12 or Colibri forceps if dissecting a lesion off the cornea
- Diamond burr (optional) to polish Bowman's layer[16]
- Topical mitomycin-C (optional)
- Antibiotic, topical NSAID and lubricating drops with BSCL until defect re-epithelialized.

## Procedure

In the author's typical procedure for superficial keratectomy on a patient with recurrent epithelial erosions secondary to ABMD disease, povidone-iodine 5% on a cotton-tip applicator is used to sterilize the lids and lashes pre-operatively. After placing a drop of topical anesthetic in the eye, a drop of povidone-iodine 5% diluted by 50% with balanced salt solution is placed into the conjunctival fornix and allowed to sit for 60 seconds. The patient is then brought up to the slit lamp, and with the aid of a surgical assistant, a wire lid speculum is then inserted into the palpebral fissure to spread the lids apart. An 8.0 mm optical zone marker is then used to mark the corneal zone to undergo keratectomy. The planned area of treatment typically is centered around the focal point of erosive pathology. For those patients with diffuse ABMD disease in whom superficial keratectomy is being performed for the indication of decreased or fluctuating vision, the 8.0 mm optical zone marker is centered on the patient's visual axis so as to mark the central cornea as the zone for treatment. 20% ethanol on a cotton-tip applicator is then administered to the area of pathology to loosen the predetermined area of epithelium. Then, using a #57 Beaver blade without a handle keratectomy is commenced in the area of loosened

epithelium. Great caution is taken to ensure that the blade remains in cleavage plane and to avoid sharp dissection into and damage of subepithelial and Bowman's layers (Figs 9 and 10).

After lesion removal, it is paramount that the corneal bed is left as smooth as possible to facilitate epithelialization. To this end, the author will most commonly employ a blunt spatula or Tooke corneal knife to further polish Bowman's layer. Bowman's layer should not be incised but should be scraped with a blade oriented perpendicular to the surface being treated, with care being taken to avoid inducing linear defects in Bowman's layer. Alternatively, a diamond burr may be used to further polish Bowman's layer to enhance epithelial adherence. If possible, injuries to the limbal epithelium are to be avoided, as the limbal stem cells are vital for subsequent re-epithelialization.

Upon completion of the superficial keratectomy, the lid speculum is removed from the palpebral opening and the patient is allowed to recline in the exam chair. A bandage soft contact lens is placed onto the cornea and one drop each of a topical nonsteroidal anti-inflammatory agent such as nepafenac (nevanac) for pain, a topical antibiotic such as moxifloxacin (vigamox) and prednisolone acetate is then placed on to the cornea. The patient is discharged home with a pair of postmydriatic sunglasses and instructed to keep the above drops chilled at home for enhanced analgesic effect. Aggressive topical ocular lubrication with chilled artificial tears is also encouraged. The combination of topical NSAID, topical antibiotic and topical steroid is instilled four times a day, and the artificial tears at least once an hour while awake until follow-up at postoperative day three or four, at which time corneal re-epithelialization

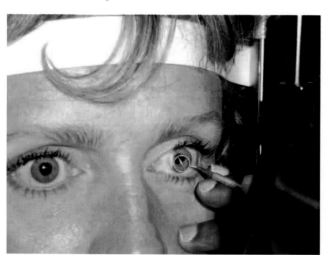

**Fig. 9:** Delineating the area for superficial keratectomy with a 5.0 mm OZ marker

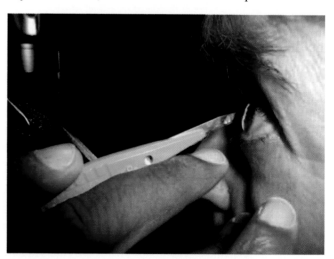

**Fig. 10:** Superficial keratectomy at the slit lamp using a #15 scalpel blade

is typically complete. Once the BSCL is removed, the patient is instructed to discontinue the topical NSAID and steroid. Topical antibiotic therapy is continued for a total of 1 week of therapy. Aggressive topical ocular lubrication is continued for several weeks postoperatively, and may sometimes be augmented with topical sodium chloride 5% ointment for additional nocturnal lubrication.

## COMPLICATIONS

Intraoperative complications in the performance of superficial keratectomy are rare. However, disruption of or creation of nicks in Bowman's layer are possible if care is not taken to maintain a perpendicular orientation and sweeping motion of the scalpel at the corneal surface.

As with any corneal procedure, there is inherent risk of corneal perforation however, because of the typically superficial nature of this keratectomy procedure, this type of complication would be extremely unlikely.

Postoperatively, the most commonly encountered complication is likely to be a slow healing persistent epithelial defect which may require prolonged BSCL wear or extended patching. Management of a persistent epithelial defect is usually centered around topical therapy to stimulate a more accelerated re-epithelialization, but may, in some cases, require the addition of oral or surgical modalities.

Postoperative topical antibiotic prophylaxis renders the development of a corneal infection in patients undergoing superficial keratectomy uncommon, and corneal scarring or development of visually significant stromal haze is unlikely. For patients who may be considered at higher risk of development of corneal haze or scarring, the use of topical mitomycin-C has found some success.[15]

## REFERENCES

1. Franke E. Uber Erkrankungen des Epithels der Hornhaut. Klin Monastsbl Augenheilkd. 1906;44:508-32.
2. Williams R, Buckley RJ. Pathogenesis and treatment of recurrent erosion. Br J Ophthalmol. 1985;69:435-7.
3. Laibson PR. Recurrent corneal erosions: diagnosis and management. In: Reinecke RD (Ed). Ophthalmology Annual. New York: Raven Press; 1989.
4. Wood TO, Griffith ME. Surgery for corneal epithelial basement membrane dystrophy. Ophthalmic Surg. 1988;19:20-4.
5. Trobe JD, Laibson PR. Dystrophic changes in the anterior cornea. Arch Ophthalmol. 1972;87:378-82.
6. Buxton JN, Fox ML. Superficial keratectomy in the treatment of epithelial basement membrane dystrophy: a preliminary report. Arch Ophthalmol. 1983;101:392-5.
7. Kenyon KR. Recurrent corneal erosion: pathogenesis and therapy. Int Ophthalmol Clin. 1979;19:169-95.
8. Galbavy EJ, Mobilia EF, Kenyon KR. Recurrent corneal erosions. Int Ophthalmol Clin. 1984;24:107-31.
9. Buxton JN, Constad WH. Superficial epithelial keratectomy in the treatment of epithelial basement membrane dystrophy. Ann Ophthalmol. 1987;19:92-6.
10. Hersh PS, Zagelbaum B, Cremers SL. Ophthalmic Surgical Procedures. Boston: Little, Brown; 1968.
11. Brown N, Bron A. Recurrent erosion of the cornea. Br J Ophthalmol. 1976;60:84-96.
12. Qian CX, Bahar I, Levinger E, et al. Combined use of superficial keratectomy and subconjunctival bevacizumab injection for corneal neovascularization. Cornea. 2008;27:1090-2.
13. Bowers PJ, Price MO, Zeldes SS, et al. Superficial keratectomy with mitomycin-C for the treatment of Salzmann's nodules, presentation at ASCRS symposium on cataract, IOL, and refractive surgery. 2002.
14. Karp Cl, Forster RK. The corneal ulcer. In: Krachmer JH, Mannis MJ, Holland EJ (Eds). Cornea. St. Louis: Mosby; 1997.
15. Khakshoor H, Zarei-Ghanavati M, Saffarian L, et al. Mechanical superficial keratectomy for corneal haze after photorefractive keratectomy with mitomycin C and extended wear contact lens. Cornea. 2011;30:117-20.
16. Forstot SL, et al. Diamond burr keratectomy for the treatment of recurrent corneal erosion syndrome. Ophthalmol Suppl: Poster. 1994.

# CHAPTER 73

# Limbal Dermoid

*Charles S Bouchard, Samir Vira*

**Keywords**: Dermoid, Choristoma, Lipodermoid, Limbal dermoid, Goldenhar syndrome, Linear sebaceous nevus syndrome

## ‣ INTRODUCTION AND OVERVIEW

Dermoids are benign, dysontogenetic, congenital tumors (choristomas) consisting of tissues not normally present in a specific location. Limbal or epibulbar dermoids generally occur in the inferotemporal limbus as well-defined, elevated masses which typically contain ectodermal tissue, such as hair follicles, sebaceous and sweat glands, with overlying squamous epithelium. These lesions are typically noted after birth but may not be diagnosed until the 2nd decade of life. Their sizes range from a few millimeters to more than 1 cm. Although more commonly unilateral, they may occur bilaterally as well. There is no gender or race predilection.

Various types of dermoids have been described.[1] Limbal dermoids tend be superficial, affecting only the anterior portion of the corneoscleral stroma, but they rarely occur only in the cornea, sparing the limbus. Occasionally, they penetrate deeply into the cornea and anterior segment. Subconjunctival lipodermoids are commonly located near the lateral limbus and the stroma and consist predominantly of adipose tissue with hair follicles and sebaceous glands which are not required findings.

## ‣ EPIDEMIOLOGY

They occur in 1–3 cases of 10,000 live births. The Armed Forces Institute of Pathology found that 7.5% of epibulbar lesions were choristomas, 52% of these epibulbar choristomas were located in the bulbar conjunctiva, 29% at the limbus, 6% on the cornea, 4% at the caruncle and 2.5% in the conjunctival fornix.[2] Another large study from the Wilmer Institute eye pathology laboratory concluded that choristomas comprise 33% of epibulbar lesions removed before the age of 16 and 2.2% of lesions in individuals 16 years or older; 19% of these choristomas were dermoids.[3]

## ‣ CLINICAL FEATURES

A dermoid usually appears as a firm, dome-shaped yellow-white limbal mass in the inferotemporal quadrant (Fig. 1). Occasionally, small cilia or hair follicles may appear from the mass. A lipid line may appear in the corneal stroma adjacent to the lesion. Small dermoids may remain asymptomatic, but larger lesions may cause ocular surface irritation, lagophthalmos, astigmatism or visual axis compromise (Fig. 2). In one case series,[4] they were shown to induce an average of 2.1 diopters of astigmatism in subjects with limbal dermoids as opposed to 1.0 diopter in those with conjunctival dermoids. Limbal dermoids more commonly occur as an isolated finding but have been associated with

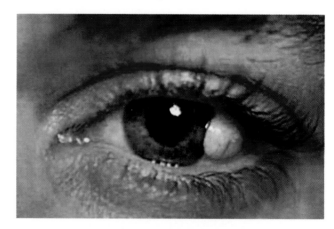

**Fig. 1:** Limbal dermoid
*Source*: Photograph courtesy of Marilyn Miller

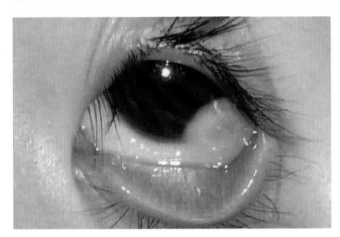

**Fig. 2:** Child with a corneal dermoid encroaching the visual axis
*Source*: Photograph courtesy of Isaac Porter

other ocular abnormalities such as eyelid and iris colobomas, and systemic abnormalities such as Goldenhar syndrome and epidermal nevus syndrome.

## Classification

Ida Mann[1] created a classification scheme for dermoids based on the depth of corneal involvement (Table 1).

### Grade I

Grade 1 is the most common form of dermoid. It is typically small, superficial and present from birth. It is usually located inferotemporally and occurs as a single lesion (Fig. 1).

### Grade II

These lesions are larger and cover a larger surface of the cornea with a variable involvement of the stroma. These dermoids generally do not involve the endothelium or Descemet's membrane.

### Grade III

The most severe and rare of the dermoids, these lesions can be extensive, often involving the entire anterior segment. Many of these patients also have microphthalmos.

## Associated Abnormalities

### Ocular

Ocular abnormalities associated with dermoids include eyelid colobomas, aniridia, aphakia, scleral and corneal staphylomas, microphthalmos and dermolipomas (more frequently seen superotemporally).[5]

### Systemic

Approximately 10% of patients with dermoid choristomas are associated with systemic abnormalities, including Goldenhar syndrome, neurofibromatosis and epidermal nevus syndrome.[3] Goldenhar syndrome is a complex presentation of the oculoauriculovertebral (OAV) spectrum. Most cases are sporadic, but familial cases with an autosomal dominant inheritance pattern have been reported. The classic triad of abnormalities includes epibulbar dermoids, preauricular appendages and pretragal fistulas. Limbal dermoids, usually Grade 1, have been noted in approximately 35% of cases and bilateral lesions occur in 25% of cases. Other ocular findings include lacrimal duct stenosis, motility disturbances including Duane syndrome, eyelid colobomas, and retinal and optic nerve abnormalities. Systemically malformations of the ear, mandible and facial muscles are noted. Ear abnormalities include microtia or anotia, deafness, and more commonly, pretragal skin tags. These skin tags have been shown to be correlated to the laterality of limbal dermoids.[4,6] Cardiac, genitourinary, neurologic and vertebral anomalies may also occur.

**73**
CHAPTER

| Table 1: Mann's classification of ocular dermoids | | | |
|---|---|---|---|
| | *Grade I* | *Grade II* | *Grade III* |
| Frequency | Most frequent | Less frequent | Rare; before the formation of the lens |
| Size | Small | Larger | Extensive |
| Location | Inferotemporal limbus | Part or entire central cornea | Entire cornea |
| Depth | Superficial | Stromal extension, not to Descemet's | Entire anterior segment |
| Associated disease | 33% associated with Goldenhar | | Microphthalmos, posterior segment disorders |

Other associated phakomatoses include neurofibromatosis and linear sebaceous nevus syndrome.[7] Linear sebaceous nevus syndrome, also known as organoid nevus syndrome, is a type of epidermal nevus syndrome characterized by a triad of midline facial skin lesions, mental retardation and seizures. Other neurologic, vascular, skeletal and ocular anomalies are common. Dermoids are the most common ocular finding in linear nevus sebaceous syndrome[8] and are often bilateral, extensive, multiple and complex.[9]

## HISTOPATHOLOGY

Histologically, dermoids are choristomas, which are congenital tumors with tissue elements not normally at the site of origin. They consist of epidermis and dermis structures, such as collagen, pilosebaceous units and nerve tissue, and are occasionally lined by keratinized squamous epithelium (Figs 3A and B). They may be classified as complex choristomas when they contain fat, lacrimal gland, cartilage, brain, or even tooth.[10,11]

## ETIOLOGY/PATHOGENESIS

Limbal dermoids result from metaplastic aberrations of the mesoblast associated with other mesodermal dysgenesis or as an isolated anomaly.[1] Another theory is a sequestration of the pluripotent cells during embryonic development of the surrounding ocular structures. The severity of the lesions may depend on the timing of the insult during gestation.

Most cases have no inheritance pattern; however, two familial forms have been reported. An isolated dermoid in an annular limbal form without any systemic findings was reported in three generations with an autosomal dominant pattern.[12] Henkind et al. first described a congenital, bilateral form with central corneal involvement in a X-linked recessive pattern of transmission.[12] The dermoids have been mapped to Xq24-qter.[13,14]

## DIFFERENTIAL DIAGNOSIS

Dermoids should always be considered in the list of diagnoses for congenital corneal opacity. Other lesions that may be confused with limbal dermoids include congenital hereditary endothelial dystrophy (CHED), congenital hereditary stromal dystrophy, Peter's anomaly, sclerocornea, congenital keloid, Salzmann's nodular degeneration, congenital glaucoma, birth trauma, corneal staphyloma, metabolic diseases (mucopolysaccharidoses, mucolipidoses), intrauterine infection with scarring and infectious or neurotrophic ulcer. Table 2 outlines the differentiating features of the more important lesions in this differential.

## MANAGEMENT

Treatment of limbal dermoids depends on size of the lesion and patient symptoms. Small, asymptomatic lesions outside the visual axis can be simply observed. Mild irritation or foreign body sensation can be treated with topical lubricants or mild steroids. Corneal dellen may occur if the lesion is raised enough and may be an indication for surgical intervention. Surgical excision is indicated for irregular astigmatism, cosmetic deformity, inadequate eyelid

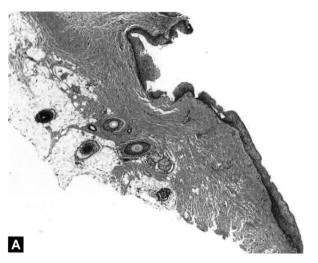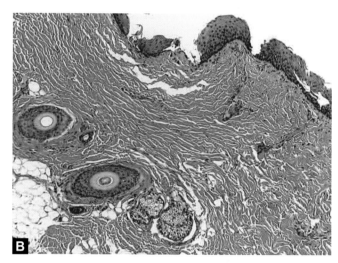

**Figs 3A and B:** (A) Histologic section of corneal dermoid demonstrating stratified squamous epithelium, underlying collagen, pilosebaceous units and adipose tissue (H&E x 40); (B) Higher magnification of the same section (H&E x 100)
*Source*: Photographs courtesy of Richard Grostern

**Table 2:** Differential diagnosis of corneal dermoid

| | Pathophysiology | Onset | Location | Description |
|---|---|---|---|---|
| Dermoid | Choristoma consisting of epithelial tissue with underlying dermal elements | Birth | Usually infer-otemporal | Unilateral, vascularized, yellow-white elevated lesion along limbus |
| Keloid | Reactive fibrous proliferation with myofibroblasts | Response to corneal injury, usually first two decades | Variable—central or peripheral | White, glistening mass of variable depth; normal anterior segment structures (lens, AC) |
| CHED | Primary dysfunction of the endothelium with abnormal Descemet's membrane secretion | CHED 1 (AD)—delayed onset within first two years of life CHED 2 (AR)—birth | Diffuse | Bilateral, diffuse corneal edema with increased thickness but normal IOP |
| Peter's anomaly | Defect in posterior stroma with absence of Descemet's membrane and endothelium | Birth | Central | Focal, central opacification ± iridocorneal adhesions with lens anomalies; often bilateral |
| Sclerocornea | Corneal stroma appears like sclera with irregular arrangement of collagen fibrils | Birth | Peripheral | Smooth, white continuation of sclera into peripheral cornea; bilateral |
| Salzmann's nodule | Thickened epithelial and scar tissue secondary to prior inflammation, contact lens trauma | Variable, not present at birth | Midperiphery | Superficial, multiple, elevated gray lesions |
| Congenital glaucoma | Immature and poorly developed trabecular meshwork | Variable, rarely present from birth | Diffuse | Bilateral, diffuse corneal edema with high IOP; Haab's striae |

closure, growth into or compromise of the visual axis and recurrence. Early intervention is indicated for management of amblyopia and to avoid dramatic growth of the tumor. Best corrected visual acuity should be determined for all patients. Evaluation with ultrasound biomicroscopy preoperatively allows for visualization of the depth of the lesion and planning for subsequent surgery (Fig. 4).[15-17]

Various surgical techniques have been described to remove dermoids and reconstruct resulting corneoscleral defects.[18-28] Superficial lesions may be removed by simple excision or keratectomies, taking care to excise the lesion flush with the corneal surface. However, this procedure may result in persistent epithelial defect, corneal vascularization, pseudopterygium, corneal scar formation and even conjunctival symblepharon formation.[18-20] For deeper dermoids, lamellar keratoplasty serves as an effective means to stabilize the surgical site with excellent visual outcomes and good cosmesis.[20-23] If the lesion does not extend to Descemet's, deep anterior lamellar keratoplasty (DALK) may be attempted in order to reduce the risk of rejection.[24] Lamellar keratoplasty does not seem to improve astigmatism.[22,23,25] Incomplete excision of the lesion

may result in recurrence. Large central lesions often require penetrating keratoplasty. More recently, amniotic membrane transplantation has been used as an adjunct after excision to

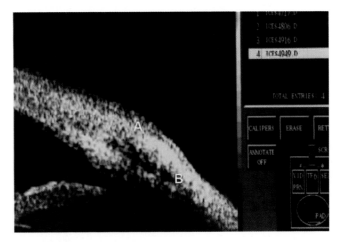

**Fig. 4:** Ultrasound biomicroscopy of limbal dermoid demonstrating high reflectivity
*Source:* Reprinted with permission from Elsevier. Grant CA, Azar D. Ultrasound biomicroscopy in the diagnosis and management of limbal dermoid. Am J Ophthalmol. 1999;128(3):365-7.

promote conjunctival and corneal re-epithelialization with reduced postoperative inflammation and scarring.[26,27] Rarely, dermoids may regress spontaneously.[29]

## ❧ REFERENCES

1. Mann I. *Developmental Abnormalities of the Eye.* 1957. pp. 357-64.
2. Ash JE. Epibulbar tumors. Am J Ophthalmol. 1950;33(8):1203-19.
3. Elsas FJ, Green WR. Epibular tumors in childhood. Am J Ophthalmol. 1975;79(5):1001-7.
4. Mansour AM, Wang F, Henkind P, et al. Ocular findings in the facioauriculovertebral sequence (Goldenhar-Gorlin syndrome). Am J Ophthalmol. 1985;100(4):555-9.
5. Mansour AM, Barber JC, Reinecke RD, et al. Ocular choristomas. Surv Ophthalmol. 1989;33(5):339-58.
6. Goldenhar M. Associations malformatives de l'oeil et de l'oreille, en particulier le syndrome dermoïde epibulbaire-appendices auriculaires-fistula auris congenita et ses relations avec la dysostose mandibulo-faciale. J Genet Hum. 1952;1:243-82.
7. Malik SR, Gupta DK. Limbal dermoid with naevus flammeus and neurofibromatosis. Eye Ear Nose Throat Mon. 1967;46(5):612-4.
8. Alfonso I, Howard C, Lopez PF, et al. Linear nevus sebaceous syndrome. A review. J Clin Neuroophthalmol. 1987;7(3):170-7.
9. Mansour AM, Barber JC, Reinecke RD, et al. Association of epibulbar choristomas with linear cutaneous nevi. Review of the literature. Ophthalmic Paediatr Genet. 1984;4(2):111-6.
10. Gorlin RJ, Cohen MM, Hennekam RCM. Syndromes of the head and neck. 4th edition. New York: Oxford University Press; 2001.
11. Spencer WH. Ophthalmic Pathology: An Atlas and Textbook. 4th edition. Philadelphia: WB Saunders; 1996.
12. Mattos J, Contreras F, O'Donnell FE. Ring dermoid syndrome. A new syndrome of autosomal dominantly inherited, bilateral, annular limbal dermoids with corneal and conjunctival extension. Arch Ophthalmol. 1980;98(6):1059-61.
13. Henkind P, Marinoff G, Manas A, et al. Bilateral corneal dermoids. Am J Ophthalmol. 1973;76(6):972-7.
14. Dar P, Javed AA, Ben-Yishay M, et al. Potential mapping of corneal dermoids to Xq24-qter. J Med Genet. 2001;38(10):719-23.
15. Lanzl IM, Augsburger JJ, Hertle RW, et al. The role of ultrasound biomicroscopy in surgical planning for limbal dermoids. Cornea. 1998;17(6):604-6.
16. Grant CA, Azar D. Ultrasound biomicroscopy in the diagnosis and management of limbal dermoid. Am J Ophthalmol. 1999;128(3):365-7.
17. Hoops JP, Ludwig K, Boergen KP, et al. Preoperative evaluation of limbal dermoids using high-resolution biomicroscopy. Graefes Arch Clin Exp Ophthalmol. 2001;239(6):459-61.
18. Panton RW, Sugar J. Excision of limbal dermoids. Ophthalmic Surg. 1991;22(2):85-9.
19. Kaufman A, Medow N, Phillips R, et al. Treatment of epibulbar limbal dermoids. J Pediatr Ophthalmol Strabismus. 1999;36(3):136-40.
20. Panda A, Ghose S, Khokhar S, et al. Surgical outcomes of epibulbar dermoids. J Peditr Ophthalmol Strabismus. 2002; 39(1):20-5.
21. Mader TH, Stulting D. Technique for the removal of limbal dermoids. Cornea. 1998;17(1):66-7.
22. Scott JA, Tan DT. Therapeutic lamellar keratoplasty for limbal dermoids. Ophthalmology. 2001;108(10):1858-67.
23. Watts P, Michaeli-Cohen A, Abdolell M, et al. Outcome of lamellar keratoplasty for limbal dermoids in children. J AAPOS. 2002;6(4):209-15.
24. Noble BA, Agrawal A, Collins C, et al. Deep anterior lamellar keratoplasty (DALK): visual outcome and complications for a heterogeneous group of corneal pathologies. Cornea. 2007;26(1):59-64.
25. Stergiopoulos P, Link B, Naumann GO, et al. Solid corneal dermoids and subconjunctival lipodermoids: impact of differentiated surgical therapy on the functional long-term outcome. Cornea. 2009;28(6):644-51.
26. Chen Z, Yan J, Yang H, et al. Amniotic membrane transplantation for conjunctival tumor. Yan Ke Xue Bao. 2003;19(3):165-7.
27. Pirouzian A, Ly H, Holz H, et al. Fibrin-glue assisted multilayered amniotic membrane transplantation in surgical management of pediatric corneal limbal dermoid: a novel approach. Graefes Arch Clin Exp Ophthalmol. 2011;249(2):261-5.
28. Choi SK, Lee D, Kim JH, et al. A novel technique: eccentric lamellar keratolimbal allografting technique using a femtosecond laser. Cornea. 2010;29(9):1062-5.
29. Roncevic MB, Doresic JP, Dorn L. Large congenital corneal dermoid with spontaneous partial regression: the first report. Cornea. 2011;30(2):219-21.

# Evaluation and Management of Eyelid and Eyelash Malposition for the Anterior Segment Surgeon

*Salman J Yousuf, Earl D Kidwell*

## ❧ INTRODUCTION

The anterior segment surgeon frequently encounters keratopathy induced by eyelid and eyelash malposition. Lubrication is often insufficient for these conditions and the underlying condition must be corrected surgically. In this chapter, we describe the classification, evaluation, and management options for ectropion, entropion, and trichiasis related keratopathy in the hands of the anterior segment surgeon.

## ❧ KERATOPATHY DUE TO EYELID MALPOSITION

### Ectropion

Ectropion is an 'outward turning'of the eyelid margin (Fig. 1). Mild cases may result in isolated eversion of the punctum. In such cases, keratopathy is mostly due to tear drainage dysfunction and to a lesser extent direct exposure. More severe cases result in complete eversion of the lid, resulting in direct corneal exposure. Ectropions are commonly classified as: involutional, paralytic, cicatricial, mechanical, or congenital.[1-6] Two types of ectropion commonly encountered by the anterior segment surgeon are involutional and paralytic lower lid ectropion. Office based corrective procedures for these two types are discussed below. These procedures are temporarily palliative and more definitive surgical procedures may be necessary. The goal of these procedures is to strengthen the lower lid tissue so that the lid margin is raised and stays apposed to the globe.

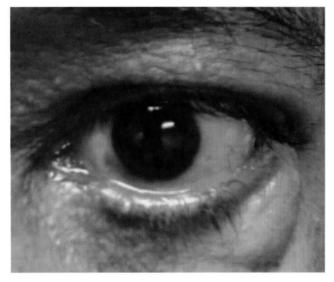

**Fig. 1:** Ectropion

A positive distraction test (eyelid margin can be pulled > 6–8 mm from the globe) and positive snapback test (eyelid margin does not return to its normal position after being pulled downward, without blinking) suggest abnormal laxity of the lid support system, consistent with an involutional etiology. For isolated medial lid eversion, cautery may be placed under the punctum in a careful manner to avoid injury to the ampulla. Alternatively, a medial spindle procedure is particularly useful in correcting isolated punctual malposition.[7] The goal of this procedure is to reposition the punctum in its natural position: aligned with the posterior eyelid margin and posteriorly angled so it is apposed to the globe. This procedure is accomplished by making a fusiform (or diamond-shaped) excision of the conjunctiva and the tarsus inferior to the punctum and placing an inverting suture. A medial spindle procedure may be performed as follows (Fig. 2):

- Administration of local anesthesia
- Identification of the lower canaliculus, so that it may be avoided during the procedure (a probe may be placed into the canaliculus as a marker)
- Fusiform (i.e. diamond-shaped) excision of conjunctiva and tarsus inferior to the punctum
- Passage of an absorbable suture through the conjunctiva, tarsus, and lower lid retractors
- Tying the knot on the conjunctiva, so that the punctum now better approximates its natural position.

In cases of more severe ectropion, both the medial and lateral eyelid becomes everted. This may be corrected with the lateral tarsal strip procedure, which corrects horizontal tarsal laxity by horizontally shortening the eyelid.[8-9] A lateral tarsal strip procedure may be performed as follows (Figs 3A to F):

- Administration of local anesthesia
- Performing a lateral canthotomy
- Incision of the inferior crus of lateral canthal tendon
- Splitting the eyelid into anterior and posterior lamellae
- Formation of the tarsal strip
- Shaving off the palpebral conjunctiva of the tarsal strip
- Excision of excess anterior lamella
- Suturing the lateral tarsal strip into the periosteum of the inner lateral orbital rim
- Closure of the lateral canthotomy wound.

Paralytic ectropion occurs in the lower lid as a result of dysfunction of the seventh cranial nerve, and forced closure of the eyelids will demonstrate weakened orbicularis muscles. When aggressive lubrication and lid taping are insufficient treatment, tarsorrhaphy or gold weight loading of the upper lid may be performed. A desirable feature of tarsorrhaphy is that it may be modified to meet the specific needs of the patient. It can be performed on the medial or lateral eyelids, or both, based on the extent of corneal exposure. It can be performed temporarily by simply placing nonabsorbable sutures through the upper and lower lid margins or by applying cyanoacrylate glue to the lateral eyelid margin. Alternatively, in patients who will not become prohibitively functionally impaired and who need a more definitive tarsorrhaphy, the marginal epithelium is removed to allow direct appositional closure of the upper and lower tarsal plates with a mattress suture. An alternative procedure for long-term correction of involutional upper lid

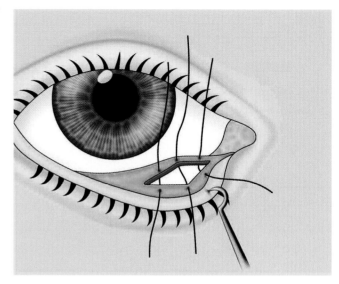

**Fig. 2:** Medial spindle procedure

ectropion involves gold weight loading.[10-12] A pocket for the weight is made by making an incision through skin and orbicularis. The gold weight is then inserted and sutured to the anterior tarsal plate.

## Entropion

Entropion is an inward turning of the eyelid margin (Fig. 4). Entropion may induce keratopathy by directly irritating the cornea or secondarily by causing tear dysfunction. Entropion are commonly classified as involutional, cicatricial, acute spastic, or congenital.[1,13-18] Acute spastic entropion is often the result of ocular irritation, inflammation, or prolonged patching; treatment of the underlying cause and aggressive lubrication are often sufficient because this condition is often transient especially when seen postoperatively. In refractory cases, botulism toxin type A may be considered.

The cicatricial type often involves the upper lid and examination of the fornix should be performed to look for symblephara, scarring and foreshortening. In contrast to involutional entropion, cicatricial entropion is not corrected by digital eyelid traction attempting to place the eyelid margin to its natural position. Treatment should include aggressive lubrication and epilation if trichiasis is present. However, definite surgical therapy should be deferred until the inciting disease process is stabilized. Trachoma remains a frequent cause of this in developing countries.

Involutional entropion is the most common type of entropion. When related to disinsertion or stretching of the lower eyelid retractors, signs include deepening of the inferior fornix, lower lid ptosis, and limited lower lid movement

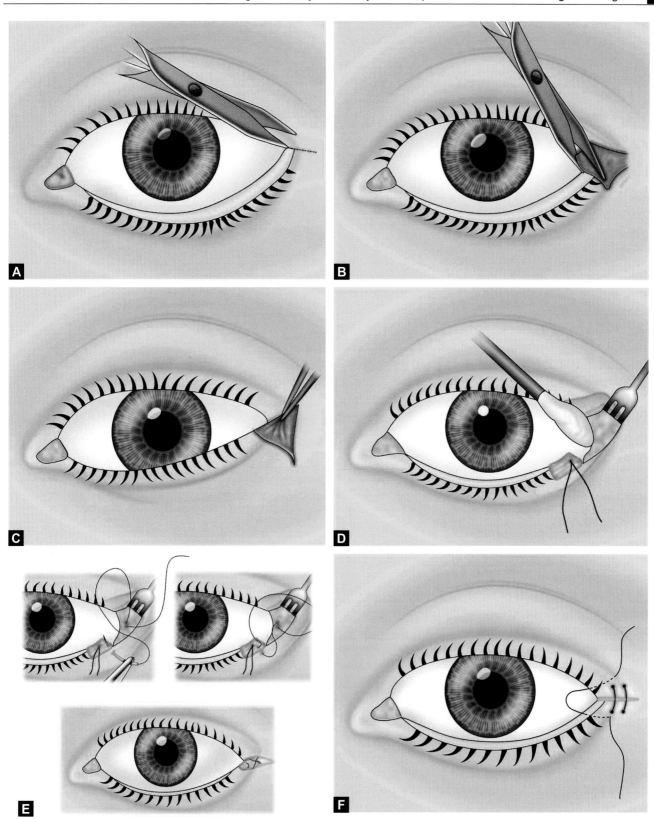

**Figs 3A to F:** Lateral tarsal strip

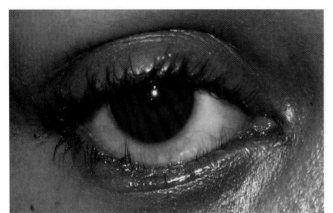

**Fig. 4:** Entropion

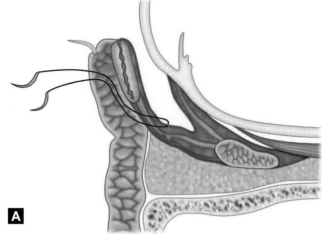

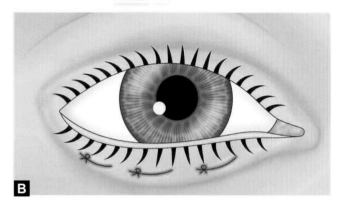

**Figs 5A and B:** Quickert suture repair

in downgaze; this may be accentuated in the postoperative setting. Other factors contributing to involutional entropion include horizontal laxity (demonstrated by poor snapback) and overriding of the pretarsal by the preseptal orbicularis muscle. Definitive treatment may require a horizontal tightening procedure (i.e. lateral tarsal strip), identification and reinsertion of lower lid retractors, or partial excision of preseptal orbicularis. However, a temporizing measure, Quickert suture repair,[15] may be tried first (Figs 5A and B):

- Administration of local anesthesia
- Everting sutures are placed horizontally along the lower eyelid by passing a suture from skin into the conjunctival fornix 2–3 mm below the lower border of the tarsal plate to include the lower retractors and then returning upward to emerge onto skin 2–3 mm below the lashes.
- Tying the suture onto skin; the tightness is titrated to desired amount of eversion.

Another suture based procedure for the management of entropion is the Weis procedure[18] (Figs 6A to D):

- Administration of local anesthesia
- A full-thickness transverse incision is made below the tarsus of the lower eyelid (approximately 4 mm below the lower eyelid margin). The length of the incision is determined by the extent of margin that is inverted.
- Retraction of the lower half of the incised eyelid. Sutures are placed only through the superior half.
- Passing double-armed nonabsorbable sutures through the anterior lamellae and tarsus, then through the lower lid retractors, and then back through the anterior lamellae. The knot is tied onto skin (with a bolster, if desired).
- Placing two additional sutures, in the same fashion
- Closing the full-thickness transverse eyelid incision

This procedure may be modified 'Reverse Weis' in the treatment of ectropion (Figs 7A and B). Weis procedures may be augmented with a lateral strep procedure if needed.

## KERATOPATHY DUE TO EYELASH MALPOSITION

Eyelash malposition may be acquired or congenital. Trichiasis, or acquired misdirection of eyelashes toward the ocular surface, results from fibrosis and cicatrization of the eyelash follicles, but the lid margin may remain in its normal position (in contrast to entropion).[19-23] A common cause of trichiasis worldwide is trachoma, and it more frequently affects the upper lid compared to other etiologies. Distichiasis, or the presence of an accessory posterior row of eyelashes, may be congenital or acquired (e.g. after eyelid trauma). If the distichiasis is asymptomatic and no keratopathy is present, the patient may be observed. If signs and symptoms are mild, lubrication may be tried. If necessary, the techniques for treatment options may be performed, as described below. Epiblepharon is

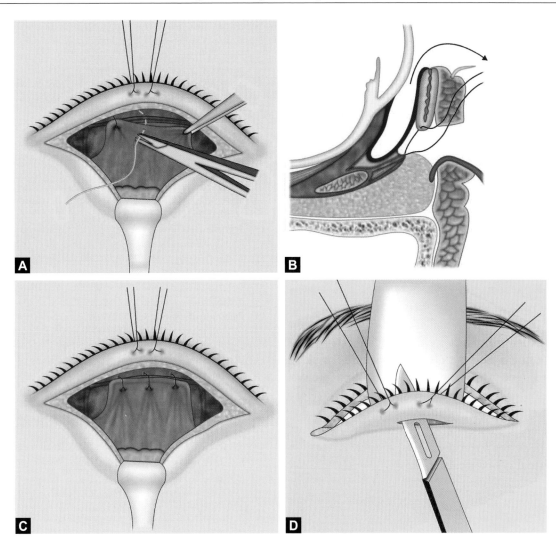

**Figs 6A to D:** Weis procedure

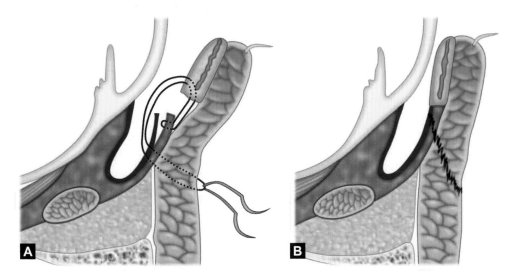

**Figs 7A and B:** Reverse Weis

another condition that involves eyelash malposition and that may be observed in the absence of keratopathy. In epiblepharon, the skin and pretarsal muscle override the lower lid margin, causing eyelash contact with the cornea, often only in downgaze. This condition is primarily seen in Asian children and often resolves spontaneously with facial development.

Epilation, or removal of eyelashes, may be performed manually with forceps if only a few cilia are misdirected. However, recurrence is the rule (typically within 2 weeks), rather than the exception. Several other, more permanent alternatives can be performed under local anesthesia. Cryotherapy (e.g. double rapid-freeze and slow thaw method) preceding mechanical epilation is effective but causes noticeable edema and erythema and possible bullae and skin depigmentation.[19] Corneal ulcer and herpes reactivation have also been reported after cryotherapy for trichiasis.[21] Radiofrequency epilation is a newer, better-tolerated alternative to epilation with standard electrolysis. Instead of using a bare needle, radiofrequency uses an insulated electrode, which is inserted 3–4 mm into the lash bulb, and a current is applied for 12 seconds to destroy the lash follicle.[24] Advantages of focal laser photocoagulation include reduced inflammation compared with cryotherapy, and it may be performed under topical anesthesia:[25]

- Administration of topical anesthesia
- Instruct patient to gaze away from laser beam
- Evert eyelid so to that eyelash root is coaxial with laser beam
- Direct laser beam to the lash base (argon blue-green laser setting: 1–2 watts of power, 50–100 µ spot size, for 0.1–0.2 seconds).

## ► REFERENCES

1. Fox SA. Ophthalmic Plastic Surgery, 3rd edition. New York: Grune and Stratton. 1963.
2. Nerad JA. Techniques in ophthalmic plastic surgery: a personal tutorial. Philadelphia: Saunders; 2009.
3. Goldberg RA, Neuhaus RW. Eyelid malpositions associated with skin and conjunctival disease. Ophthalmol Clin North Am. 1992;5:227-41.
4. Vallabhanath P, Carter SR. Ectropion and entropion. Curr Opin Ophthalmol. 2000;11:345-51.
5. Eliasoph I. Current techniques of entropion and ectropion correction. Otolaryngol Clin North Am. 2005;38:903-19.
6. Frueh BR, Schoengarth LD. Evaluation and treatment of the patient with ectropion. Ophthalmology. 1982;89(9):1049-54.
7. Nowinski TS, Anderson RL. The medial spindle procedure for involutional medial ectropion. Arch Ophthalmol. 1985;103(11):1750-3.
8. Anderson RL, Gordy DD. The tarsal strip procedure. Arch Ophthalmol. 1979;97(11):2192-6.
9. Olver JM. Surgical tips on the lateral tarsal strip. Eye (Lond). 1998;12(Pt 6):1007-12.
10. Rofagha S, Seiff SR. Long-term results for the use of gold eyelid load weights in the management of facial paralysis. Plast Reconstr Surg. 2010;125(1):142-9.
11. Townsend DJ. Eyelid reanimation for the treatment of paralytic lagophthalmos: historical perspectives and current applications of the gold weight implant. Ophthal Plast Reconstr Surg. 1992;8(3):196-201.
12. Bergeron CM, Moe KS. The evaluation and treatment of upper eyelid paralysis. Facial Plast Surg. 2008;24(2):220-30.
13. Barnes JA, Bunce C, Olver JM. Simple effective surgery for involutional entropion suitable for the general ophthalmologist. Ophthalmology. 2006;113(1):92-6.
14. Pereira MG, Rodrigues MA, Rodrigues SA. Eyelid entropion. Semin Ophthalmol. 2010;25(3):52-8.
15. Quickert MH, Rathbun E. Suture repair of entropion. Arch Ophthalmol. 1971;85(3):304-5.
16. Dresner SC, Karesh JW. Transconjunctival entropion repair. Arch Ophthalmol. 1993;111(8):1144-8.
17. Olver JM, Barnes JA. Effective small-incision surgery for involutional lower eyelid entropion. Ophthalmology. 2000;107(11):1982-8.
18. Wies FA. Spastic entropion. Trans Am Acad Ophthalmol Otolaryngol. 1955;59(4):503-6.
19. Bartley GB, Bullock JD, Olsen TG, et al. An experimental study to compare methods of eyelash ablation. Ophthalmology. 1987;94(10):1286-9.
20. Kersten RC, Kleiner FP, Kulwin DR. Tarsotomy for the treatment of cicatricial entropion with trichiasis. Arch Ophthalmol. 1992;110(5):714-7.
21. Ferreira IS, Bernardes TF, Bonfioli AA. Trichiasis. Semin Ophthalmol. 2010;25(3):66-71.
22. Choo PH. Distichiasis, trichiasis, and entropion: advances in management. Int Ophthalmol Clin. 2002;42(2):75-87.
23. Dutton JJ, Tawfik HA, DeBacker CM, et al. Direct internal eyelash bulb extirpation for trichiasis. Ophthal Plast Reconstr Surg. 2000;16(2):142-5.
24. Kezirian GM. Treatment of localized trichiasis with radiosurgery. Ophthal Plast Reconstr Surg. 1993;9(4):260-6.
25. Başar E, Ozdemir H, Ozkan S, et al. Treatment of trichiasis with argon laser. Eur J Ophthalmol. 2000;10(4):273-5.

# Pterygium Surgery

*Alfred L Anduze*

## ᴥ INTRODUCTION

A pterygium is a degenerative or proliferative fibrovascular lesion that occurs in the bulbar conjunctiva and encroaches onto the cornea. It is the result of a combination of cumulative exposure to sunlight [ultraviolet (UV)-B radiation], dehydration (in the form of altered tear film or dry eyes) and chronic inflammation. Symptoms include a gritty, foreign body sensation and mild to moderate irritation. Risk factors include geographic location in the tropics between latitude 30° north and 30° south; low-lying areas with dry-hot climates; outdoor occupations with long-term exposure to sunlight; male gender; age less than 40; photosensitizing drugs; and chemical or physical trauma.[1,2] Eyes exposed to reflective surfaces like white sandy beaches, clear waters and minimal cloud cover are more susceptible to burn than those in areas with protective cloud and tree coverage, darker volcanic sand and higher elevations.[3] On an anatomic basis, protruding eyes, those with poor quality tear film, low blink rate and red-fair pigmentation appears to be more susceptible to pterygium formation. Though abundant pigmentation was found to be protective, there is a higher prevalence in those with darker skin complexion and age more than 50 due to longer exposure times.[4] The incidence of pterygium was 11.6% in Barbados, 3.8% in rural China, and 2.8% in Australia.[5,6] Figure 1 shows a classic pterygium extending onto and into the cornea.

Visual disturbances involve anatomic obstruction with encroachment on the visual axis, induced with-the-rule astigmatism from corneal distortion and impediment of the external muscles with diplopia (Fig. 2A). A large, raised

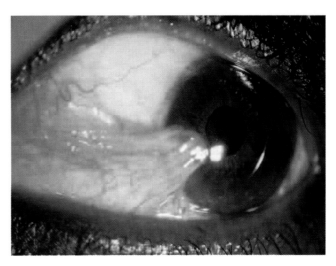

**Fig. 1:** Classic pterygium

lesion may interfere with blinking which leads to less tear film coverage, dry eyes and blurred vision.

## ᴥ PATHOGENESIS

The primary causative factor of pterygium formation is environmental. UV-B radiation and some irritants stimulate the inflammatory response in susceptible conjunctivae that leads to loss of collagenase and production of epidermal growth factors. The affected cells which change to fibroblasts through the process of epithelial mesenchymal transition (EMT), along with extracellular matrix and newly organized vascular channels, accumulate and extend onto and into the cornea. Laden with activated fibroblasts and lymphocytes, the subconjunctival tissue proceeds to damage Bowman's membrane and leads to the characteristic

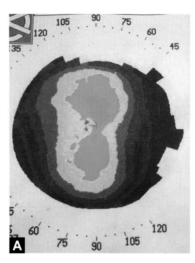
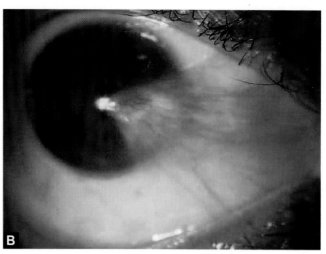

**Figs 2A and B:** (A) Induced astigmatism CT; (B) Stage V pterygium

fibrovascular lesion. Tissue factor is a transmembrane protein that interacts with coagulation factors to initiate blood coagulation. Transcription factor (TF) expression as detected by abnormal immunoreactivity in the cytoplasm of basal, suprabasal, and superficial epithelial cells may also play a role in the epithelial and fibrovascular tumor-like configuration of the pterygium. Inflammation is the key process in the proliferation of a pterygium. The presence of inflammatory cells and TF expression combine to give variations in lesion size, activity and tumor-like behavior.[7]

## PATHOLOGY

Histological examination of pterygium epithelium and subconjunctival tissue reveals basophilic degeneration with collagenization and hyalinization, or vascular proliferation with a preponderance of inflammatory cells (B- and T-lymphocytes) or a combination of the two. There is significant pleomorphism with dysplasia and hyperplasia and an increase in goblet cells in 75% of the cases. The presence

of p63-alpha-positive epithelial cell clusters suggests that pterygia develop from limbal epithelial progenitors and may be associated with preneoplastic lesions. Clinically suspicious pterygia should undergo histological examination to rule out melanoma or carcinoma.[9,10] Figure 2B shows a large active compound stage V lesion. Figure 3 shows the mixed histology of a typical pterygium. Table 1 is a classification based on clinical features.

## PREVENTION

Avoiding the peak times of sun exposure, using UV-400 sunglasses and/or a brimmed hat, umbrella, and avoidance of irritants will provide basic protection. Reduction and control of inflammation can be done with dietary measures (oral flaxseed oil) and topical applications of vasoconstrictors,

| **Table 1:** Clinical staging[8] |
| --- |
| I. Exposure conjunctivitis: Early mild congestion with increased conjunctival vessels but no formed lesion; asymptomatic |
| II. Conjunctival lesion with thickening and inflammation; symptomatic |
| III. Limbal pterygium head at or on the limbus, or just onto the cornea; mixed proliferation and/or degenerative response |
| IV. Corneal pterygium 2 mm or more into the cornea with edema, dellen or iron line; symptoms of itching, burning, irritation present |
| V. Compound pterygium with extension through Bowman's membrane into the stroma causing visual disturbances |

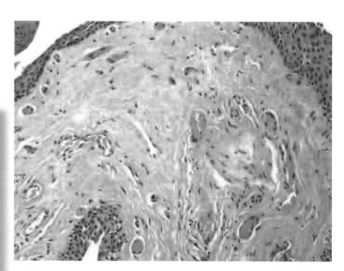

**Fig. 3:** Mixed histology with inflammatory cells and hyalinization

SECTION 16

**Table 2:** Differential diagnosis[11]

| | | | | |
|---|---|---|---|---|
| Pingueculum | Pseudopterygium | Hematoma | Phylctenule | Granuloma |
| Nodular episcleritis | Vernal keratoconjunctivitis | Limbal dermoid | Amelanotic melanoma | Squamous cell carcinoma |
| Bowen's epithelioma | Foreign body granuloma | Papilloma | Lymphoma | Conjunctival hemangioma |

decongestants, vitamin A and moderate anti-inflammatories like dexamethasone, loteprednol, cyclosporine a, and nonsteroidal anti-inflammatory agents (NSAIDs). A healthy tear film should be maintained through adequate hydration and hygienic eye care.[11-14] Table 2 is a differential diagnosis of common lesions.

## ⟩ SURGERY

Indications for surgery include cosmesis, discomfort from a large stage II, proliferative stage III, IV, and V with corneal involvement, degenerative with visual disturbances, increasing astigmatism, impending encroachment on the visual axis, and recurrences with symptomatic corneal involvement. Small asymptomatic lesions can be treated medically and/or observed. Patients with clinically significant cataract and a large corneal pterygium that may be inducing astigmatism and interfering with keratometry readings for intraocular lens calculations should have the lesion removed first, heal for a few months and then undergo cataract surgery. The calculations should be more accurate, visualization for phaco should be better and the possibility of complications from adjunctive therapy should be reduced.

Preoperative preparation in reducing inflammation is essential to achieving the best possible outcome from pterygium surgery.

Topical and local infiltration will give good anesthesia. Local stand by may also be used. The author recommends rotational conjunctival flaps for all primaries, double-headed and small recurrences; conjunctival autograft for degenerative pterygia without glaucoma and small vascular primaries; and amniotic membrane grafting for large primary lesions, degenerative, double-headed and all recurrences. All active fibrovascular primaries and recurrences should have adjunctive mitomycin C (MMC) in a single intraoperative dose. The principal objectives are the reduction of postoperative inflammation and prevention of recurrence through preoperative and intraoperative use of vasoconstrictors, less cautery, covering the sclera, sparing the muscle sheath, low dose single use MMC, and 9-0 nylon or tissue glue. Corneal healing is promoted through minimal surgical trauma to prevent dellen, reduced initial steroid use, supplemental vitamin C and zinc and tear film restoration.[15,16] Figures 4A and B show preoperative and postoperative pterygia.

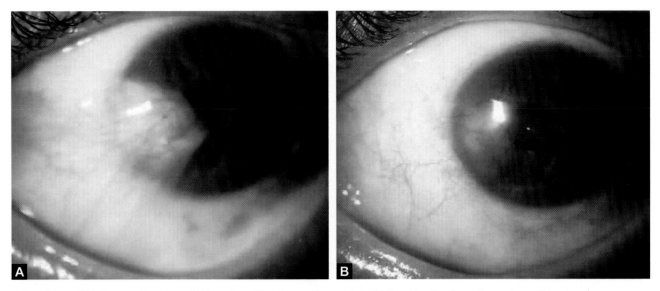

**Figs 4A and B:** Preoperative stage IV pterygium with inflammation control; (B) Good healing 3 months postoperative pterygium surgery

CHAPTER **75**

## Suggested Surgical Techniques

### Conjunctival Flaps

Conjunctival (rotational) flaps pterygium surgery can be done on six basic steps. Figure 5 is a diagramatic scheme of the conjunctival flap procedure. Figures 6A to F show the six basic steps in the conjuctival flap procedure for pterygium surgical removal. The initial incision is made with the scissors into the body of the lesion at a point 2–4 mm from the limbus. This facilitates good visibility of the head and the body. Isolate the head and allow the conjunctiva and subconjunctival tissues to retract. Use lightly applied cautery for hemostasis to avoid scleral damage. Topical phenylephrine 2.5% for vasoconstriction may also be applied. Excise the head by accessing the cleavage plane and shaving. Clean the limbus but avoid removing too much tissue as this is the nidus for re-epithelialization of the cornea and conjunctiva. Fashion the flaps by incising the conjunctiva superiorly and inferiorly in a vertical line and bring the edges together in the midline of the flaps. Suture the flaps to each other with 9-0 nylon using 3–4 short bites and 1–2 long bite traction sutures (4–6 sutures total). Nonabsorbable sutures are preferred as the inflammatory response is less than to absorbable (vicryl). The knots should be trimmed and left in the midline to give maximum comfort. The flaps should cover the sclera completely up to the limbus, orient the conjunctival blood vessels vertically away from the limbus

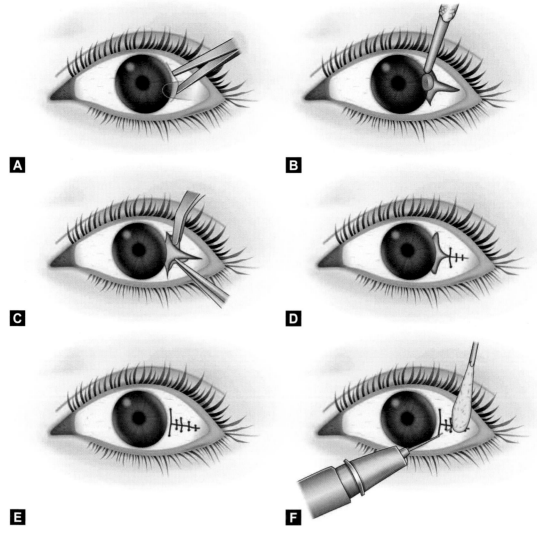

**Figs 5A to F:** Conjunctival flaps technique (six steps)*

*Source: Anduze AL. Pterygium: A Practical Guide to Management, 1st edition. New Delhi: Jaypee Brothers Medical Publishers Pvt Ltd: 2009

**16** SECTION

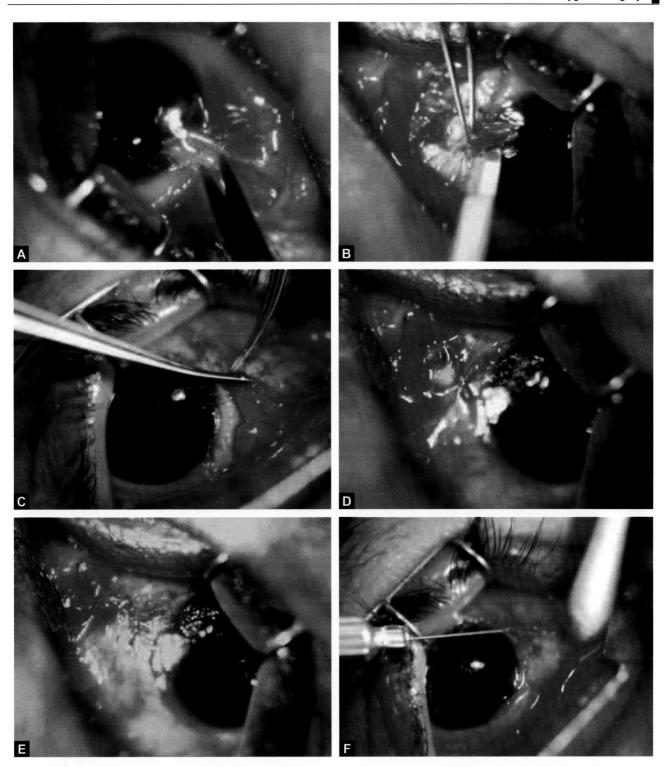

**Figs 6A to F:** Conjunctival flaps technique. (A) Initial incision; (B) Excision of head; (C) Flaps formation; (D) Initial closure; (E) Complete closure; (F) Adjunctive therapy (mitomycin C)

and act as a barrier to prevent neovascular vessels from re-entering the cornea horizontally. Use adjunctive therapy to prevent recurrence. MMC, 0.1 cc of 0.02%, is instilled under the conjunctiva and rinsed with balanced salt solution (BSS). Interval times vary from 1–5 minutes. An antibiotic ointment may be instilled for coverage and comfort. Since there is no foreign material used, steroids may be avoided for the first few days to allow adequate initial corneal re-epithelialization and faster wound healing.[16]

Conjunctival flaps technique is recommended for primary pterygium, double-headed pterygia (where there is not enough normal tissue for two free grafts), and small first time recurrences.

### Conjunctival Autograft

The initial incision is made at the distal end of the lesion, being careful not to take too much tissue. Both the head and the body are excised *en toto*. Minimal corneal dissection and lightly applied cautery is used to minimize tissue damage. Harvesting of the free graft is done in the superior quadrant and the graft slid into place to realign the limbus to its new position. The graft is fixed in place to the conjunctiva with nonabsorbable suture or to the sclera with fibrin tissue glue applied to both surfaces and positioned to cover the vacant area up to the limbus. The donor wound site is closed with nonabsorbable suture to minimize postoperative inflammation.[17] Note that vicryl is associated with prolonged inflammation during its dissolution.[18] Adjunctive therapy is then applied to the subconjunctival surface and an antibiotic-steroid combination instilled topically. Figures 7A to D show the four basic steps for conjunctival autograft or free graft which is recommended for primary pterygium and small first time recurrences.

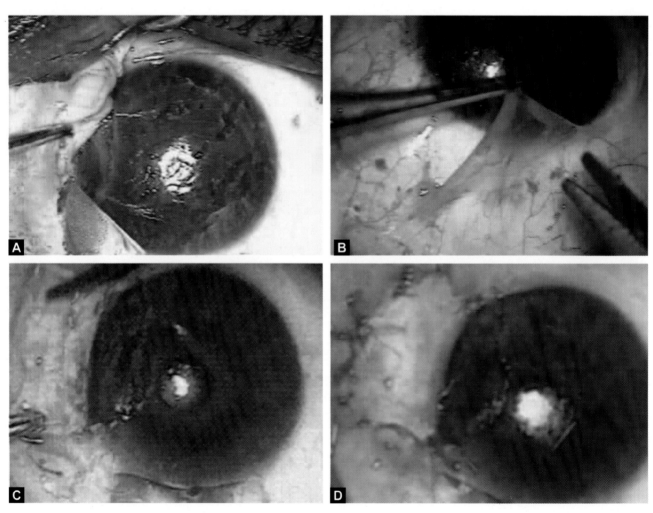

**Figs 7A to D:** Conjunctival autograft technique. (A) Lesion excision; (B) Graft harvest; (C) Graft positioning; (D) Graft fixation

## *Amniotic Membrane Graft*

The initial incision is made at the distal end and the head and body are removed together. Adequate hemostasis is desired in the area of the recipient bed in order to facilitate a smooth, even graft fixation. Some residual heme may act as additional fibrin glue. The amniotic membrane graft is positioned with basement membrane side up and fixed in place with tissue glue or nonabsorbable sutures. Re-epithelialization will occur on the surface of the graft, which acts as a basement membrane. A stable graft is essential for a successful outcome. Adjunctive therapy with MMC is applied subconjunctivally and an antibiotic-steroid combination instilled and used throughout the postoperative period. Cryopreserved human amniotic membrane tissue from donor placentas from a cornea tissue bank or freeze-dried amniotic tissue can be used. Amniotic tissue contains growth factors and anti-inflammatory proteins which promote adhesion of basal epithelial cells and suppress inflammation.[19]

Amniotic membrane grafts can be used for primary pterygium, all recurrences, double-headed pterygia and is especially indicated for large lesions with complications such as symblepharon, multiple surgeries, viral and chemical components.

To obtain the best outcome and reduce the risk of recurrence, both the conjunctival flaps and autograft should include corneolimbal stem cells in the tissue covering the sclera that is juxtaposed to the limbus;[20] minimal surgical cautery is used and adjunctive therapy with MMC, 0.05–0.1 cc of 0.02–0.04% is preferred and administered in a single subconjunctival dose. The low dosage and

avoidance of tissue damage from excessive cautery avoids many complications. Figures 8A and B show the initial placement and orientation of the amniotic graft tissue and the postoperative position and initial healing.

## Comparison of Techniques

The conjunctival flaps technique is easy to perform, has one wound site, keeps the blood supply intact and leads to faster healing. Conjunctival autograft involves two wound sites (donor and recipient) on the same eye which may lead to prolonged healing and possible scar tissue interference from the donor site for future glaucoma surgery. With the use of fibrin glue, it is less time-consuming and may provide a more comfortable postoperative experience. The amniotic tissue graft has one wound site and good healing but results are dependent on the preoperative status of the eye and size and cause of the lesion. Chemical burns and inflammatory lesions are more difficult to contain. The best technique is one with which the surgeon is most familiar and most comfortable and most appropriate for the lesion.

Conjunctival flaps without MMC have been reported to have recurrence rates of 2% and 6.9%, when compared to free graft with an average recurrence of 18.5%.[21,22]

Another comparison of the conjunctival flaps and free graft finds that both are equally safe and effective in reducing recurrence.[23] Figures 9A to C are a comparison of the three procedures relative to healing at a particular point in time.

A comparison of amniotic membrane graft, conjunctival autograft and conjunctival autograft with MMC for primary and recurrent pterygia showed them to be equally effective

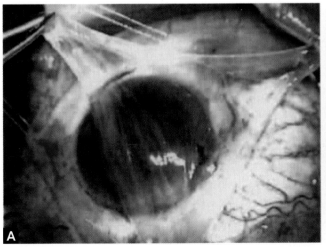
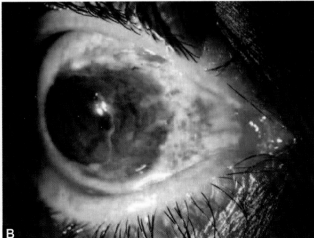

**Figs 8A and B:** Amniotic membrane grafting for a large scleral defect in pterygium surgery.
(A) Amniotic membrane graft; (B) Graft in position up to the limbus

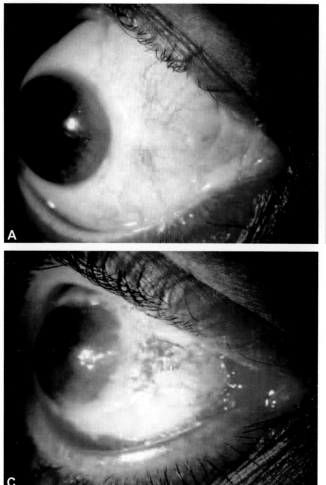

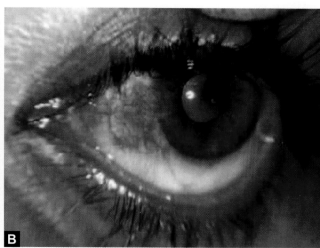

Figs 9A to C: Postoperative comparisons at 2 weeks postoperative. (A) Conjunctival flaps; (B) Conjunctival autograft; (C) Amniotic membrane graft

in preventing recurrence.[24] Amniotic membrane and conjunctival autografts give significantly better outcomes than primary closure and bare sclera techniques, with free graft and MMC having slightly better results.[25,26]

Though the functional and cosmetic results of all three are acceptable, it should be noted that since a large number of amniotic membrane grafts are done on secondary recurrences and large, high-risk primaries, there will usually be more scarring and higher risk of further recurrence.

The bare sclera technique has an unacceptably high recurrence rate of 25–50% and should not be done.[27,28] The average recurrence rate for conjunctival flaps is in the range of 2–7%. Conjunctival autografts recur at a rate of 5–25% and amniotic membrane grafts, 10–35% with adjunctive therapy. Conjunctival autografts were found to be cosmetically more pleasing than amniotic grafts.[29-31]

## ▶ COMPLICATIONS

Recurrence after pterygium surgery is due to a combination of focal intraoperative stress and persistent postoperative inflammation which results in poor wound healing and usually occurs within the first 3 postoperative months but may occur later. It may be defined as regrowth of abnormal subconjunctival fibrovascular tissue 2 mm or more onto clear cornea in the area of previous pterygium excision.[32] Risk factors for recurrence include the following: fibrovascular type, broad base and thick blunt head, continued high UV-B radiation exposure, bare sclera technique, surgical dellen, poor general health and poor wound healing, age less than 50, fair-red complexion, unusual host response, insufficient follow-up, lack of patient cooperation, and incorrect choice of surgical technique (bare sclera with MMC drops, bare sclera with irradiation, extensive tissue dissection with difficult healing).[1,33] Corneal re-epithelialization and rapid conjunctival wound healing are essential to avoid recurrence. The primary objective of the management of recurrence is the initial reduction of the inflammatory fibrovascular process through topical NSAIDs, phosphate-based steroids, cold tear film lubricants and decongestants. Promotion of corneal wound healing with optional oral supplements, adequate hydration and a bandage contact lens is helpful when indicated. An appropriate surgical approach different than the original should be planned and performed when the eye is quiet.[11]

A comparative study of recurrent pterygium surgery with limbal conjunctival autograft and conjunctival flaps with low dose MMC produced 14.6% recurrence with the former and 12.5% with the latter. Amniotic membrane grafting with MMC is most often recommended for recurrences particularly when multiple. The recurrence rate remained the same (10–12.5%) whether MMC was used or not.[34] Figures 10A and B show early and late recurrence of a pterygium.

Less ominous surgical complications include persistent hyperemia, dellen, wound dehiscence, graft slippage, granuloma, hematoma, and induced astigmatism. A persistently red, irritated eye can be treated with topical steroids and antibiotics after the cornea is sufficiently healed. Corneal dellen can be treated with a bandage contact lens until it re-epithelializes. Granuloma and hematoma can be observed or removed depending on size and symptoms. Wound dehiscence and graft slippage can be repaired or replaced as soon as detected and usually with good results.

More serious complications include scleral necrosis, graft or flap infection, symblepharon and visually significant induced astigmatism. Scleral necrosis may occur after overuse of cautery which leaves dents in the sclera. Thinning may occur after high or frequent doses of MMC or beta-irradiation, which can lead to scleral melt and necrosis. Healing usually results in irregular scarring. A patch graft is indicated if perforation is imminent. Complete covering of the sclera at the end of surgery is essential to reducing inflammation and the risk of recurrence. Poor technique, postoperative care or poor health and hygiene can lead to infection, which can potentially develop into endophthalmitis and should be treated aggressively with antibiotics. Symblepharon formation is usually associated with multiple recurrence surgery and/or excision of too much conjunctival and Tenon's tissue. Symptoms of diplopia and muscle restrictions may be present. It can be repaired with ample amniotic membrane grafting to resume the normal or near-normal anatomy. Visually significant astigmatism can be repaired with limbal relaxing incisions or excimer laser therapy after it stabilizes. Figures 11A to D show common postoperative complications of pterygium surgery. Figures 12A to C show the more serious complications of infection, scleral melt and restrictive symblepharon.

CHAPTER 75

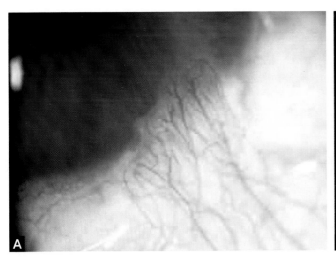 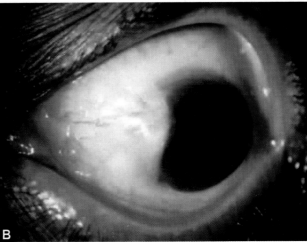

**Figs 10A and B:** Recurrence. (A) Nidus of recurrence at 5 months; (B) Established recurrence at 2 years

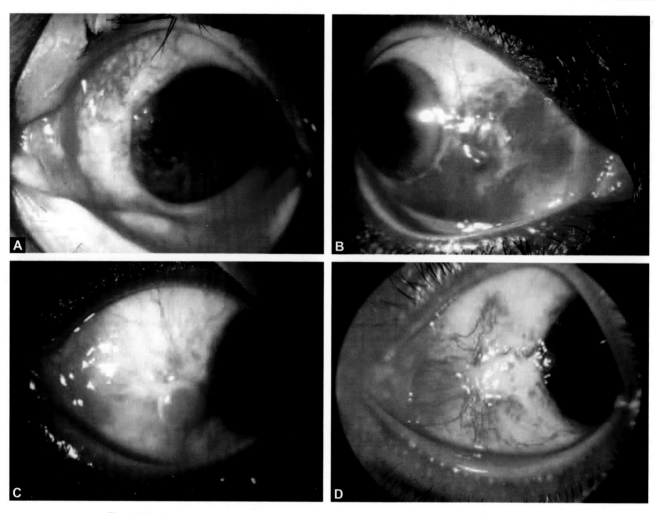

**Figs 11A to D:** Minor postoperative pterygium surgery complications. (A) Dellen; (B) Hematoma; (C) Granuloma; (D) Wound dehiscence/graft slippage

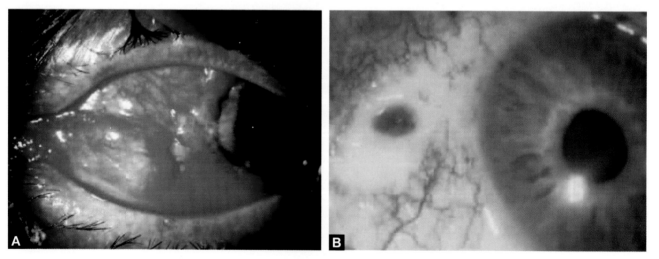

**Figs 12A and B**

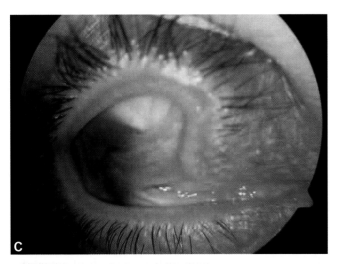

**Figs 12A to C:** Major postoperative pterygium surgery complications. (A) Acute infection; (B) Scleral melt/necrosis; (C) Symblepharon and recurrence

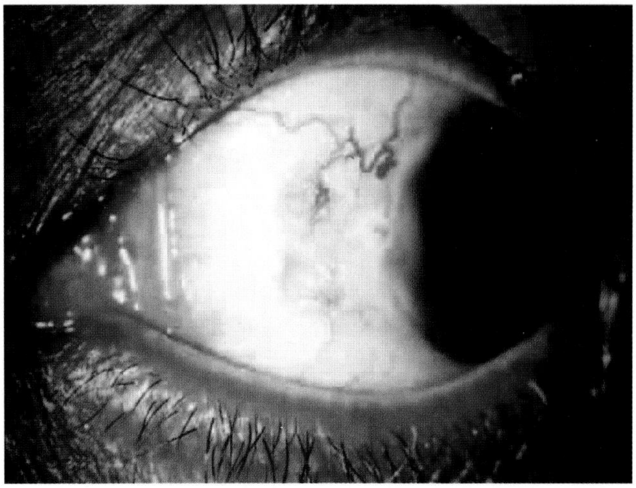

**Fig. 13:** Scleromalacia 5 years post beta-irradiation

## ADJUVANT THERAPIES

Mitomycin C is the most commonly used adjuvant therapy in pterygium surgery. It is an antimetabolite that acts by inhibiting DNA synthesis and exhibiting a modulatory effect on wound healing. It is safe and effective when used properly, i.e. not as multiple drops and not on bare sclera. In a single intraoperative low dose, placing a small amount directly to the underside of the conjunctiva prevents both corneal and conjunctival toxicity and significantly reduces the rate of recurrence. Recommended dosages are between 0.05 and 0.1 cc. of 0.02–0.04% diluted in BSS or bacteriostatic water. Long-term (10 years) evaluation for late radiomimetic effects has shown that the use of MMC is safe and effective.[35,36] A single low dose of MMC combined with free conjunctival graft, conjunctival flaps and amniotic membrane grafting for primary and recurrent pterygium, has been shown more than not to reduce the recurrence rate. Complications are dose related, occur most often with the usage of multiple drops on bare sclera, and include scleral thinning in areas of dellen formation, and reduced corneal endothelial cell counts.[40,41] These can be avoided by covering the sclera, using the proper low dosage, using minimal cautery, and rinsing the excess MMC from the tissues where it is not needed. Other complications at higher dosages (> 0.05%) include pain, prolonged discomfort and hyperemia, and tearing.[42,43]

Intraoperative 5-fluorouracil infiltration as an adjuvant treatment in pterygium surgery yielded a recurrence rate of 35% in primary and 36% in recurrent lesions. Though considered safe, the dosage and concentrations need to be adjusted.[44]

Beta-irradiation with strontium-90 delivered postoperatively with doses between 30 and 35Gy and up to five applications is effective but with variable results. Side effects include moderate conjunctivitis, local pain, visual disturbances, photophobia and epiphora.[45] Recurrence rates are comparable to surgery with MMC at between 1.7% and 12.0% for both primary and recurrent lesions, and more effective with less complications in some cases.[46,47] Late complications include scleromalacia and irregular scar tissue formation and appear to be dose-related.[48] Strontium-/yttrium-90 beta-irradiation used on primary and recurrent pterygia without prior surgery led to assize reduction in all lesions and without side effects (Fig. 13).[49]

Fibrin tissue glue or adhesive consists of two components, fibrinogen and thrombin, prepared from banked human blood. Applications to the surfaces and edges of donor and host tissues simulate the final stage of wound healing in facilitating the adherence of basement membranes and epithelial tissues through crosslinking and clot formation. It may be used either as an alternative or as a complement to sutures when securing autologous or amniotic membrane grafts to the sclera in pterygium surgery. It provides adequate adhesion of grafts to the ocular surface. Inflammation has been reported as minimal to moderate and cosmetic results are good. Though operation time, postoperative inflammation and discomfort are reported as reduced, the rate of recurrence is similar to that of using sutures.[50-53] Graft slippage from eye rubbing or poor adhesion contributes to the main complication of recurrence since it is converted to a bare sclera. The glue may cause chemical irritation in hypersensitive eyes.[54]

75
CHAPTER

Improvements in cost effectiveness, holding ability and inflammation control are needed.

Bevacizumab is an anti-angiogenic human monoclonal antibody against vascular endothelial growth factor (VEGF), which should reduce vascularity in primary pterygium and prevent neovascularization in potentially recurrent lesions. Subconjunctival injection of 0.05 ml to primary pterygia resulted in a short term decrease in irritation and vascularization, which returned to preinjection levels after several weeks.[55,56] A reduction on lesion size with a dose of 2.5 mg/0.1 ml has been reported as well tolerated but not clinically significant.[57] Multiple subconjunctival injections for advanced primary pterygium has been effective in reducing size and improving visual acuity but the clinical lesion remains.[58] After pterygium excision, a single intraoperative injection had no effect on recurrence rate or early postoperative minor complications. When administered in two doses after primary pterygium excision and a recurrence rate of 13% without other adverse effects was obtained.[59] Topical drops administered to an eye with impending recurrence produced a regression of limbal-conjunctival neovascularization in the early postoperative period.[60] Though there were no adverse effects from bevacizumab injections at low dosages, the expected dramatic improvements have not appeared.[61] Bevacizumab injections or topical eyedrops appear to be slightly but not statistically effective in reducing the risk or causing a delay in recurrence in the presence of neovascularization in the early period after pterygium excision.[62-65]

An improvement in quality of outcome over what is now available is needed in order for this adjunct to become a mainstay of treatment.

The application of adjunctive hyperbaric oxygen therapy after pterygium removal to aid in revascularization and wound healing has shown promising results. The recurrence rate is reduced, it has shown no adverse effects and can be applied after all three main surgical techniques with or without MMC. The treatment was also effective in a case of scleral necrosis. Numerous sessions (20–25) are required.[66,67]

## COMMENTS

Since great strides have been made in recent years in establishing an effective but safe dosage and application technique for MMC and beta-irradiation in the course of pterygium surgery in reducing the recurrence rate after pterygium surgery, attention has been directed toward the best cosmetic results. The cost of adjuvant therapy needs

to be reduced to make them more readily available in many countries in which pterygium is endemic.

There is still the need to address the causal factors and emphasize prevention through protection from exposure and improvement in general health and hygiene practices.

## REFERENCES

1. Luthra R, Nemesure BB, Wu SY, et al. Frequency and risk factors for pterygium in the Barbados Eye Study. Arch Ophthalmol. 2001;119:1827-32.
2. Droutsas K, Sekundo W. Epidemiology of pterygium: A review. Ophthalmologe. 2010;107:511-2, 514-6.
3. Threlfall TJ, English DR. Sun exposure an pterygium of the eye: a dose-response curve. Am J Ophthalmol. 1999;128(3):280-7.
4. Nemesure B, Wu SY, Hennis A, et al. Nine-year incidence and risk factors for pterygium in the barbados eye studies. Ophthalmology. 2008;115(12):2153-8.
5. Liang QF, Xu L, Jin XY, et al. Epidemiology of pterygium in aged rural population of Beijing, China. Chin Med J (Engl). 2010;123(13):1699-701.
6. McCarty CA, Fu CL, Taylor HR. Epidemiology of pterygium in Victoria, Australia. Br J Ophthalmol. 2000;84(3):289-92.
7. Ando R, Kase S, Ohashi T, et al. Tissue factor expression in human pterygium. Mol Vis. 2011;17:63-9.
8. Anduze AL. Pterygium staging in the Caribbean. Ann Ophthalmol. 1998;30(2):92-4.
9. Golu T, Mogoantă L, Streba CT, et al. Pterygium: histological and immunohistological aspects. Rom J Morphol Embryol. 2011;52(1):153-8.
10. Chui J, Coroneo MT, Tat LT, et al. Ophthalmic pterygium: a stem cell disorder with premalignant features. Am J Pathol. 2011;178(2):817-27.
11. Anduze AL. Prevention. Pterygium: A Practical Guide to Management. New Delhi: Jaypee Brothers Medical Publishers; 2009. pp. 38-45.
12. Pinheiro MN, dos Santos PM, dos Santos RC, et al. Oral flaxseed oil (Linum usitatissimum) in the treatment for Sjögren's syndrome patients. Arg Bras Oftalmol. 2007;70(4):649-55.
13. Villegas Becerril E, Pérula de Torres L, Bergillos Arillo M, et al. Evaluation of topical vasoconstrictors in pterygium surgery and their role in reducing intraoperative bleeding. Arch Soc Esp Oftalmol. 2011;86(2):54-7.
14. Kim EC, Choi JS, Joo CK. A comparison of vitamin a and cyclosporine a 0.05% eye drops for treatment of dry eye syndrome. Am J Ophthalmol. 2009;147(2):206-13.
15. Ringsdorf WM, Cheraskin E. Vitamin C and human wound healing. Oral Surg Oral Med Oral Pathol. 1982;53(3):231-6.
16. Anduze AL. Conjunctival flaps for pterygium surgery. Ann Ophthalmol (Skokie). 2006;38(3):219-23.
17. Kenyon KR, Wagoner MD, Hettinger ME. Conjunctival autograft transplantation of advanced and recurrent pterygium. Ophthalmology. 1985;92:1461-70.
18. Karalezli A, Kucukerdonmez C, Akova YA, et al. Fibrin glue versus sutures for conjunctival autografting in pterygium surgery: a prospective comparative study. Br J Ophthalmol. 2008;92(9):1206-10.

19. Solomon A, Pires RTF, Tseng SCG. Amniotic membrane transplantation after extensive removal of primary and recurrent pterygia. Ophthalmology. 2001;108(3):449-60.

20. Sadiq MN, Arif AS, Jaffar S, et al. Use of supero-temporal free conjunctivo-limbal autograft in the surgical management of pterygium: our technique and results. J Ayub Med Coll Abbottabad. 2009: 21(4):121-4.

21. Kaya M, Tunc M. Vertical conjunctival bridge flaps in pterygium surgery. Ophthalmic Surg Lasers Imaging. 2003;34(4):279-83.

22. Müller S, Stahn J, Schmitz K, et al. Recurrence rates after pterygium excision with sliding conjunctival flap versus conjunctival autograft. Ophthalmologe. 2007;104(6):480-3.

23. Kim M, Chung SH, Lee JH, et al. Comparison of mini-flap technique and conjunctival autograft transplantation without mitomycin C in primary and recurrent pterygium. Ophthalmologica. 2008;222(4):265-71.

24. Katircioğlu YA, Altiparmak UE, Duman S. Comparison of three methods for treatment of pterygium: amniotic membrane graft, conjunctival autograft and conjunctival autograft plus mitomycin C. Orbit. 2007;26(1):5-13.

25. Ozer A, Yildirim N, Erol N, et al. Long-term results of bare sclera, limbal-conjunctival autograft and amniotic membrane graft techniques in primary pterygium excision. Ophthalmologica. 2009;223(4):269-73.

26. Prabhasawat P, Barton K, Burkett G, et al. Comparison of conjunctival autografts, amniotic membrane grafts, and primary closure for pterygium excision. Ophthalmology. 1997;104(6):974-85.

27. Fernandes M, Sangwan VS, Bansal AK, et al. Outcome of pterygium surgery: analysis over 14 years. Eye (Lond). 2005; 19(11):1182-90.

28. Hirst LW. The treatment of pterygium. Surv Ophthalmol. 2003;48(2):145-80.

29. Memarzadeh F, Fahd AK, Shamie N, et al. Comparison of de-epithelialized amniotic membrane transplantation and conjunctival autograft after primary pterygium excision. Eye (Lond). 2008;22(1):107-12.

30. Tananuvat N, Martin T. The results of amniotic membrane transplantation for primary pterygium compared with conjunctival autograft. Cornea. 2004;23(5):458-63.

31. Küçükerdönmez C, Akova YA, Altinörs DD. Comparison of conjunctival autograft with amniotic membrane transplantation pterygium surgery: surgical and cosmetic outcome. Cornea. 2007;26(4):407-13.

32. Mutlu FM, Sobaci G, Tatar T, et al. A comparative study of recurrent pterygium surgery: limbal conjunctival autograft transplantation versus mitomycin C with conjunctival flap. Ophthalmology. 1999;106(4):817-21.

33. Ti SE, Tseng SC. Management of primary and recurrent pterygium using amniotic membrane transplantation. Curr Opin Ophthalmol. 2002;13(4):204-12.

34. Ma DH, See LC, Hwang YS, et al. Comparison of amniotic membrane graft alone or combined with intraoperative mitomycin C to prevent recurrence after excision of recurrent pterygia. Cornea. 2005;24(2):141-50.

35. Anduze AL. Pterygium surgery with mitomycin-C: ten-year results. Ophthalmic Surg Lasers. 2001;32(4):341-5.

36. Raiskup F, Solomon A, Landau D, et al. Mitomycin C for pterygium: long term evaluation. Br J Ophthalmol. 2004;88 (11):1425-8.

37. Uçakhan OO, Kanpolat A. Combined 'symmetrical conjunctival flap transposition' and intraoperative low-dose mitomycin C in the treatment of primary pterygium. Clin Experiment Ophthalmol. 2006; 34(3):219-25.

38. Segev F, Jaeger-Roshu S, Gefen-Carmi N, et al. Combined mitomycin C application and free flap conjunctival autograft in pterygium surgery. Cornea. 2003;22(7):598-603.

39. Altiparmak UE, Katircioğlu YA, Yağci R, et al. Mitomycin C and conjunctival autograft for recurrent pterygium. Int Ophthalmol. 2007;27(6):339-43.

40. Tsai YY, Lin JM, Shy JD. Acute scleral thinning after pterygium excision with intraoperative mitomycin C: a case report of scleral dellen after bare sclera technique and review of the literature. Cornea. 2002;21(2):227-9.

41. Kheirkhah A, Izadi A, Kiarudi MY, et al. Effects of mitomycin C on corneal endothelial cell counts in pterygium surgery: role of application location. Am J Ophthalmol. 2011;151 (3): 488-93.

42. Anduze AL, Burnett JM. Indications for and complications of mitomycin-C in pterygium surgery. Ophthalmic Surg Lasers. 1996;27:667-73.

43. Sharma A, Gupta A, Ram J, et al. Low dose intra-operative mitomycin C versus conjunctival autograft in primary pterygium surgery: long-term follow-up. Ophthalmic Surg Lasers. 2000;31:301-7.

44. Valezi VG, Schellini SA, Viveiros MM, et al. Safety and efficacy of intraoperative 5-fluorouracil infiltration in pterygium treatment. Arg Bras Oftalmol. 2009;72(2):169-73.

45. Isohashi F, Inoue T, Xing S, et al. Postoperative irradiation for pterygium: retrospective analysis of 1,253 patients from the Osaka University Hospital. Strahlenther Onkol. 2006;182(8):437-42.

46. Paryani SB, Scott WP, Wells JW, et al. Management of pterygium with surgery and radiation therapy. The North Florida Pterygium Study Group. Int J Radiat Oncol Biol Phys. 1994;28(1):101-3.

47. Aimsek T, Günalp I, Atila H. Comparative efficacy of beta-irradiation and mitomycin-C in primary and recurrent pterygium. Eur J Ophthalmol. 2001;11(2):126-32.

48. MacKenzie FD, Hirst LW, Kynaston B, et al. Recurrence rate and complications after beta irradiation for pterygia. Ophthalmology. 1991;98(12):1776-80.

49. Vastardis I, Pajic B, Greiner RH, et al. Prospective study of exclusive strontium-/yttrium-90 beta-irradiation of primary and recurrent pterygia with no prior surgical excision. Clinical outcome of long-term follow-up. Strahhienther Onkol. 2009; 185(12):808-14.

50. Por YM, Tan DT. Assessment of fibrin glue in pterygium surgery. Cornea. 2010;29(1):1-4.

51. Miranda-Rollón MD, Pérez-González LE, Sentieri-Omarrementería A, et al. Pterygium surgery: comparative study of conjunctival autograft with suture versus fibrin adhesive. Arch Soc Esp Oftalmol. 2009;84(4):179-84.

52. Hall RC, Logan AJ, Wells AP. Comparison of fibrin glue with sutures for pterygium excision surgery with conjunctival autografts. Clin Experiment Ophthalmol. 2009;37(6):584-9.

53. Cut and paste: a no suture, small incision approach to pterygium surgery. Koranyi G, Seregard S, Kopp ED. Br J ophthalmol. 2004;88(7):911-4.

54. Srinivasan S, Slomovic AR. Eye rubbing causing conjunctival graft dehiscence following pterygium surgery with fibrin glue. Eye (Lond). 2007;21(6):865-7.

55. Hosseini H, Nejabat M, Khalili MR. Bevacizumab (Avastin) as a potential novel adjunct in the management of pterygia. Med Hypotheses. 2007;69(4):925-7.

56. Teng CC, Patel NN, Jacobson L. Effect of subconjunctival bevacizumab on primary pterygium. Cornea. 2009;28(4):468-70.

57. Fallah Tafti MR, Khosravifard K, Mohammadpour M, et al. Efficacy of intralesional bevacizumab injection in decreasing pterygium size. Cornea. 2011;30(2):127-9.

58. Saxena S, Vishwkarma K, Khattri M, et al. Multiple subconjunctival bevacizumab for advanced primary pterygium. Ann ophthalmol (Skokie). 2010;42:28-30.

59. Razeghinejad MR, Hosseini H, Ahmadi F, et al. Preliminary results of subconjunctival bevacizumab in primary pterygium excision. Ophthalmic Res. 2010;43(3):134-8.

60. Wu PC, Kuo HK, Tai MH, et al. Topical bevacizumab eyedrops for limbal-conjunctival neovascularization in impending recurrent pterygium. Cornea. 2009;28(1):103-4.

61. Banifatemi M, Razeghinejad MR, Hosseini H, et al. Bevacizumab and ocular wound healing after primary pterygium excision. J Ocul Pharmacol Ther. 2011;27(1):17-21.

62. Leippi S, Grehn F, Geerling G. Antiangiogenic therapy for pterygium recurrence. Ophthalmologe. 2009;106(5):413-9.

63. Bahar I, Kaiserman I, McAllum P, et al. Subconjunctival bevacizumab injection for corneal neovasculrization in recurrent pterygium. Curr Eye Res. 2008;33(1):23-8.

64. Mansour AM. Treatment of inflamed pterygia or residual pterygial bed. Br J Ophthalmol. 2009;93(7):864-5.

65. Fallah MR, Khosravi K, Hashemian MN, et al. Efficacy of topical bevacizumab for inhibiting growth of impending recurrent pterygium. Curr Eye Res. 2010;35(1):17-22.

66. Assaad NN, Chong R, Tat LT, et al. Use of adjuvant hyperbaric oxygen therapy to support limbal conjunctival graft in the management of recurrent pterygium. Cornea. 2011;30(1):7-10.

67. Bayer A, Mutlu FM, Sobaci G. Hyperbaric oxygen therapy for mitomycin C-induced scleral necrosis. Ophthalmic Surg Lasers. 2002;33(1):58-61.

# CHAPTER 76

# Amniotic Membrane Transplantation

*Soosan Jacob, Amar Agarwal*

## ⦁ EMBRYOLOGY

The amniotic membrane is part of the amniotic sac inside which the human embryo develops. It is formed by the mesoderm on the outer side and the ectoderm on the inner side. The amniotic cavity appears about the 2nd week. As the blastocyst burrows into the endometrium, lacunae are formed between the inner cell mass and the cytotrophoblast which join to form the amniotic cavity. The amniotic sac continues to enlarge by cell division till about 28 weeks of gestation after which, it enlarges mainly by stretching.[1] As the amniotic cavity enlarges, the extraembryonic celom gets smaller and smaller until it is finally obliterated. At this stage, the amniotic membrane lies against the chorion to form the chorioamniotic membrane. Thus, the amniotic membrane arises from the cytotrophoblast. The amniotic sac contains the amniotic fluid which is formed from both the maternal and fetal circulation. The main function of the amniotic fluid is to form a protective cushion around the fetus as well as to regulate its body temperature.

## ⦁ ANATOMY OF THE AMNIOTIC MEMBRANE

The placenta consists of the maternal decidua and the fetal amniochorion. The amnion and the chorion are loosely fused together. The amniotic membrane has a smooth and shiny appearance and consists of a single layer of cells on a thick basement membrane. This rests on an avascular stroma that is composed of a compact layer, a fibroblastic layer and a spongy layer. It is 0.02–0.5 mm in thickness.[2] The amniotic membrane has multipotent stem cells which are of low immunogenicity.

## ⦁ PHYSIOLOGY OF AMNIOTIC MEMBRANE

The basement membrane of the amniotic membrane consists of Type I, III, IV, V and VII collagen, fibronectin and Type 1 and 5 laminin. It is thus abundant in various extracellular matrix materials.[3,4] The basement membrane side of the amniotic membrane promotes epithelial cell adhesion, migration and differentiation and prevents cellular apoptosis. It downregulates the TGF-beta system and therefore, allows normal differentiation and maintenance of cellular characteristics by corneal cells.[5]

The amniotic membrane also has anti-inflammatory and antiangiogenic properties. It expresses various growth factors and antiproteinases.[6,7] It also suppresses myofibroblast differentiation.[8,9] Because of the dual role, viz. anti-inflammatory as well as antifibrotic properties that amniotic membrane possesses, it is likely to have an antiscarring effect which can be put to good use in the cornea.

Amniotic membrane also does not have any of the HLA-A, B, C or DR antigens on their surface which is the reason they do not incite any effective immune response following amniotic membrane allograft transplantation.[10]

## ⦁ PREPARATION OF AMNIOTIC MEMBRANE

The amniotic membrane has the great advantage of being easily obtainable. When used for ophthalmological purposes, it is taken from placentas obtained via elective Cesarian section and is handled in utmost sterile conditions. The amniotic membrane is easily separated from the chorion at the level of the spongy layer of stroma by stripping off.

Once stripped it is cleaned of blood and blood clots under a laminar flow hood and is by prepared as described by Tseng et al. It is immersed in phosphate-buffered saline (PBS) containing 50 μg/ml penicillin, 50 μg/ml streptomycin, 100 μg/ml neomycin and 2.5 μg/ml amphotericin B. The membrane is then laid onto nitrocellulose filter paper with stromal side down and is cut into pieces each of which is stored in Dulbecco's modified Eagle medium and glycerol in a 1:1 ratio. The membranes are then cryopreserved till use at −80°C.[11]

The placental donor is always screened for infectious diseases such as HIV 1 and 2, HBsAg, HCV and Syphilis at the time of obtaining the placenta and then again after a window period of 3 months after cesarean section. A small section of the membrane is also sent for microbiological evaluation and culture and sensitivity for bacteria and fungi. Once all tests come negative, the membranes are released for use.

Freshly prepared amniotic membrane may also be used from the placenta obtained through elective cesarean section of serologically screened individuals. These are cleaned and prepared as described earlier and are used immediately in the patient.

## ROLE OF AMNIOTIC MEMBRANE IN OPHTHALMOLOGY

The amniotic membrane was first used by De Roth in 1940s, but it was not till 1995 that Kim and Tseng again

made its use widespread and popular.[12,13] Amniotic membrane is used for its anti-inflammatory and antiangiogenic properties as well as its ability to promote epithelial differentiation, adhesion and migration. It also has antibacterial, wound-protecting, pain-reducing and fibrosis-suppressing effects. It can be used as a graft where it fills defects and promotes epithelialization or it can be used as a patch where it is used for its anti-inflammatory and antiangiogenic properties.[14-16] It may also be used as a patch graft simultaneously according to the underlying condition being treated. The stromal side of the amniotic membrane is differentiated from the basement membrane by touching with a sponge. The stromal side is sticky whereas the basement membrane side is nonsticky.

## CORNEAL USES

### Persistent Epithelial Defect(s)

Amniotic membranes have been used in the treatment of persistent epithelial defects (PED) secondary to neurotrophic corneas, autoimmune disorders or limbal stem cell deficiency (Figs 1A and B). In these cases, amniotic membrane may act by inhibition of collagenases while at the same time providing collagen and a basement membrane for epithelial cells to grow on. The amniotic membrane also provides growth factors all of which provide a conducive atmosphere for epithelial cells to grow on.[14,17]

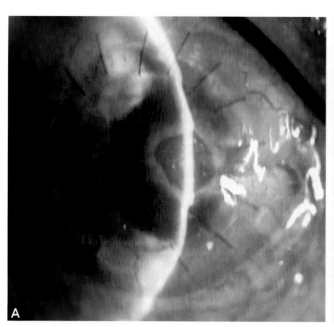 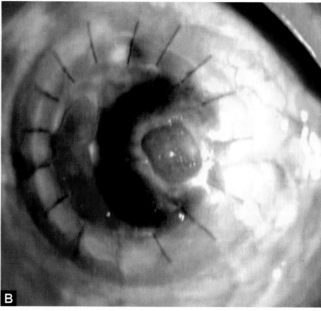

**Figs 1A and B:** Slit view and view on diffuse illumination of persistent epithelial defect in a corneal graft

## Corneal/Scleral Melts

The amniotic membrane is used as a patch graft or an inlay-onlay graft in this case. It is used to fill the defect and replace stromal matrix loss caused by the melt. This is done by using multilayered amniotic membrane. The amniotic membrane is repeatedly folded on itself using fibrin glue to stick the multiple layers to each other. Once this inlay is prepared, the base and edges of the defect are scraped and all necrotic tissue as well as loose epithelium is removed. The inlay prepared is then used to fill the defect and is stuck into place using glue as well as anchoring sutures. An amniotic membrane patch or an onlay graft is then used to cover the inlay graft in such a manner as to extend beyond the denuded epithelium. This onlay provides anti-inflammatory effects and promotes wound healing (Figs 2A to D). Confocal microscopy of the transplanted amniotic membrane filler shows its contraction, remodelling with new collagen formation and its population by corneal stroma derived cells by about 3 months implying the integration of the filler inlay graft into the corneal matrix.[18] Re-epithelialization of the amniotic membrane is essential for integration of the graft into the stroma. While in the sclera, integration into scleral

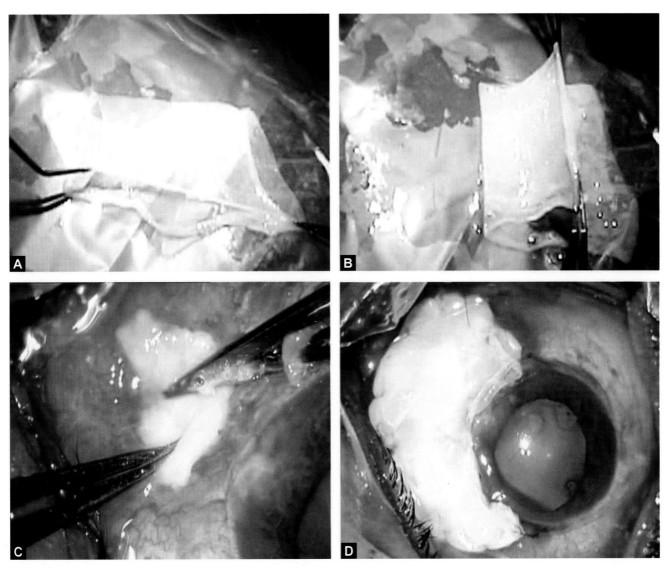

**Figs 2A to D:** (A) Amniotic membrane with fibrinogen applied on one half and thrombin on the other half. On folding together, these two constituents of fibrin glue stick layers of the folded amniotic membrane together; (B) The same is repeated again to get a four-layered amniotic membrane, all the layers being glued to each other; (C) The area of scleral melt is filled with this multilayered amniotic membrane graft cut to size and glued into place as an inlay. Any excess outside the area of melt is trimmed; (D) The entire inlay graft is covered with an onlay patch graft of amniotic membrane stroma usually halts the disease process, in the cornea, the graft persists as a scar in the stroma. Nevertheless, it still makes the cornea amenable to a future transplant in a quiet eye. Certain studies have also used this technique in very deep ulcers and Descemetoceles.[14,19]

Amniotic membrane use alone is insufficient in cases of corneal ulcer with active infection and this should be avoided. It may also not be enough by itself to provide tectonic support in cases of large areas of scleral melt with staphyloma formation or in large corneal ulcers where tissue with greater tectonic support such as a corneal or scleral tectonic graft should be used. In cases with ongoing scleral melt and necrosis, additional medical management directed at the disease pathology would also be required.

## Bullous Keratopathy

Bullous keratopathy secondary to surgery or Fuchs' dystrophy in an eye with no potential for vision can be treated with amniotic membrane grafting.[20] The amniotic membrane may be used as an isolated treatment after removing the unhealthy epithelium or in conjunction with anterior stromal puncture or phototherapeutic keratectomy. The membrane is spread out under tension and sutured under onto the cornea with the stromal side facing down. It acts as a good alternative to conjunctival hooding in these cases and also provides better cosmetic results to the patient than the conjunctival flap. It also does not decrease the chances of survival of a future keratoplasty if required unlike conjunctival flaps.

## Limbal Stem Cell Deficiency

The limbal stem cells are responsible for continuous replenishment of the corneal epithelial cells and this is proposed to occur via the X-Y-Z hypothesis of Thoft.[21]

### Partial Limbal Stem Cell Deficiency

Amniotic membrane can be used in partial limbal stem cell deficiency as an isolated treatment modality. It is spread over the corneal and conjunctival surface and anchored in place using sutures with or without fibrin glue (Fig. 3). This may be attributed to its unique property that has been identified in laboratory studies of prolonging the life span of corneal and conjunctival progenitor cells and of maintaining slow-cycling label-retaining cells.[22-24] It can thus be used to expand the surviving limbal stem cells and the transient amplifying cells (TAC) of the cornea.[25]

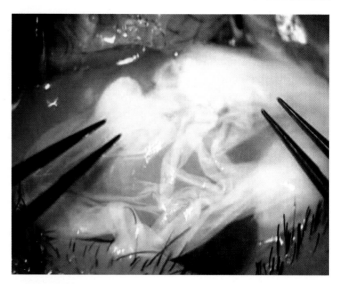

**Fig. 3:** The use of freshly prepared amniotic membrane for partial limbal stem cell deficiency

### Total Limbal Stem Cell Deficiency

In a patient with total limbal stem cell deficiency, stem cell transplantation restores the normal phenotypic corneal epithelium. It also acts as a barrier to conjunctivalization. Amniotic membrane is used in conjunction with limbal stem cell autograft (Figs 4A to F) or allograft. In all these cases, it has multiple beneficiary effects. It gives a protective cover over the transplanted stem cells and protects it from external trauma, lid movements, etc. till the stem cells have taken. Its anti-inflammatory properties as well as inhibition of angiogenesis help in suppressing graft rejection to an extent. It decreases corneal scar formation postpannus excision. It also promotes epithelial differentiation, adhesion and migration from the newly transplanted limbal stem cells.

The limbal stem cells are harvested as an autograft from the other eye of the same patient (Figs 5A and B) or are taken as an allograft. An allograft can be either a living related donor or from a cadaveric eye (Figs 6 and 7). The advantages of a cadaveric eye include the ability to transplant a much greater number of limbal stem cells which is not possible either in autograft or living related donor because of the risk of inducing iatrogenic limbal stem cell deficiency (Figs 8A and B). It is also used in those cases where the patient or the relative is not willing to be a donor. Once the host cornea is cleared of scar tissue and pannus, the limbal stem cell donor tissue is sutured onto the host limbus. The entire graft and sometimes also the entire donor cornea (depending on amount of corneal dissection) are covered with the amniotic membrane. A small central

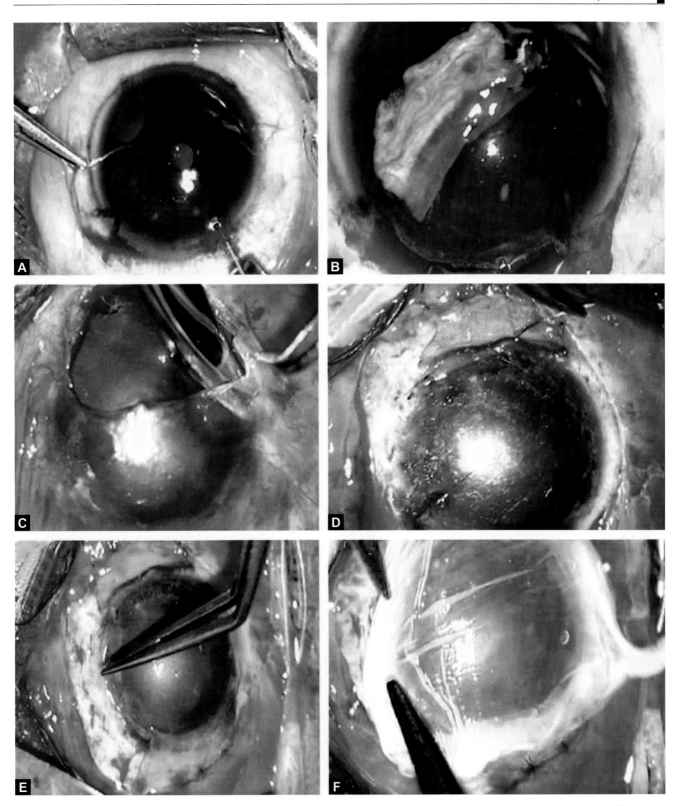

**Figs 4A to F:** (A) Conjunctival limbal autograft (CLAU) being taken from contralateral eye; (B) CLAU after harvesting. Two such grafts are harvested; (C) Unhealthy epithelium and pannus being resected off the affected eye in preparation for limbal stem cell transplantation; (D) The inferior CLAU being sutured in place; (E) The recipient eye after both grafts have been sutured in place; (F) An amniotic membrane is used to cover the entire ocular surface

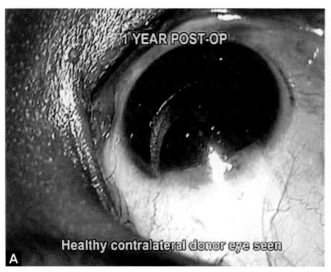
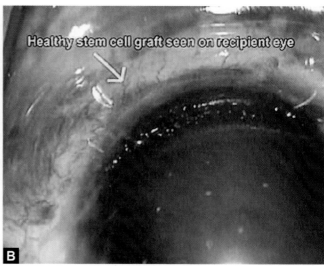

**Figs 5A and B:** Same patient as in Figure 4 at 1 year postoperative period. (A) The healthy contralateral donor eye; (B) Healthy stem cell graft in recipient eye with an improved ocular surface

hole may be cut with scissors over the pupillary area to enable the patient to see in case of one-eyed patients. The amniotic membrane because of its unique properties helps in making the perilimbal microenvironment conducive to the limbal stem cell transplantation.[26]

## CONJUNCTIVAL USES

### Pterygium Excision

Pterygia are known to be associated with a high recurrence rate and various modalities including the use of Mitomycin-C and conjunctival autografts have been reported to decrease the incidence of recurrence. Amniotic membranes have also been used in pterygium surgery, especially in surgery for large double headed pterygia and in patients with inadequate conjunctiva to perform a conjunctival autograft. Nevertheless, conjunctival autograft has been shown to have a lower incidence of postoperative inflammation and recurrence than amniotic membrane transplantation.[27,28]

The amniotic membrane graft provides anti-inflammatory effect as well as antifibrotic effect via downregulation of transforming growth factor beta and is thus of benefit in preventing recurrence (Figs 9A to D).

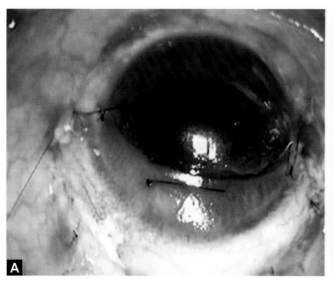
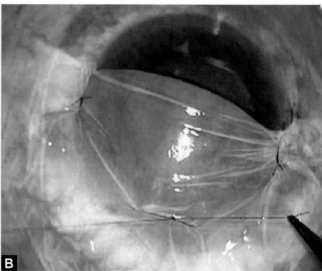

**Figs 6A and B:** (A) A cadaveric keratolimbal allograft (KLAL) performed in a patient not willing for an autograft and with no other willing donor; (B) The KLAL being covered with an amniotic membrane graft at the end of surgery. The amniotic membrane is firmly fixed at the limbus with sutures besides also being sutured at the edges

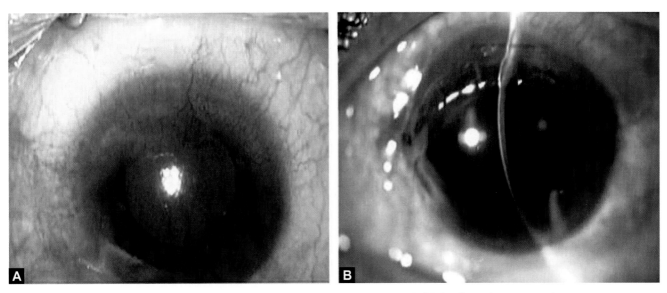

**Figs 7A and B:** (A) The preoperative appearance of the patient seen in Figure 6; (B) The 6 months postoperative appearance of the same patient. The patient is maintained on systemic and topical immunosuppressives

## Fornix Reconstruction

Many cases of symblephara, fornix foreshortening and forniceal obliteration require correction of lid deformity and reformation of fornices. Simple dissection alone even if combined with symblepharon rings may not always succeed as the raw surfaces obtained after dissection easily adhere and fuse again if allowed to be in contact with each other. Amniotic membrane may be used to cover these raw surfaces.[29,30] Once the fornix is dissected out, the affected part of the bulbar, forniceal and palpebral conjunctiva is covered with amniotic membrane which is held in place using a combination of glue and sutures. Glue alone is generally not sufficient. Fornix forming sutures are then taken where double armed sutures are passed through the fornix, through the orbital rim periosteum and tied down on the surface of the lids using bolsters (Figs 10A to C).

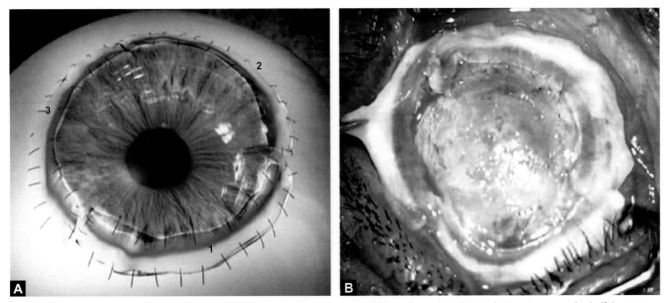

**Figs 8A and B:** (A) Illustration of a cadaveric stem cell graft which gives the ability to harvest and transplant up to one-and-a-half times more stem cells than an autograft or a living related allograft; (B) A cadaveric keratolimbal allografting being performed on a patient with severe limbal stem cell deficiency

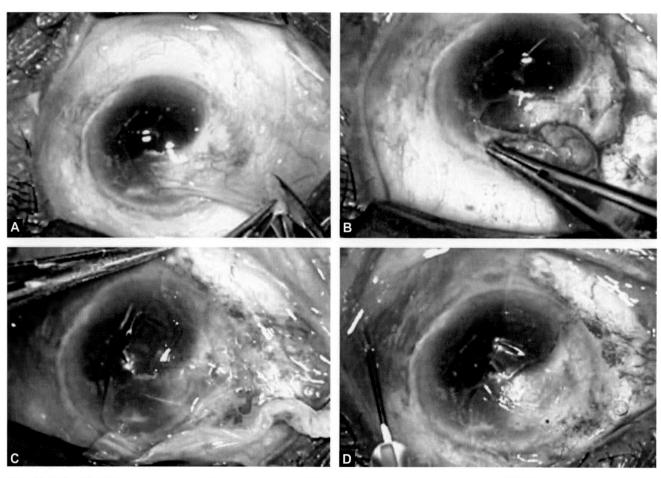

**Figs 9A to D:** (A) A large pterygium extending onto the cornea. The conjunctival component is being cut; (B) The pterygium head is being stripped off the underlying stroma; (C) An amniotic membrane graft is used to cover the conjunctival defect as well as is placed over the raw surface on the cornea; (D) The amniotic membrane is glued into place

## Surface Reconstruction

Amniotic membranes can be used for ocular surface reconstruction after removal of large lesions, such as ocular surface squamous neoplasias, large pterygia or other surgeries which result in loss of large area of the conjunctival surface with inadequate conjunctiva available for autograft (Figs 11A to C). It is also used for closing conjunctival defects in patients with pre-existing blebs or those who might require a trabeculectomy or valve surgery in the future. Placing an amniotic membrane graft in such patients leaves the superior conjunctiva untouched for possible future use.

## Acute Corneal and Conjunctival Insults

Steven Johnson syndrome (SJS), toxic epidermal necrolysis (TEN), mucous membrane pemphigoid and chemical and thermal burns can all cause extensive damage to the limbal stem cells and the conjunctiva resulting in a multitude of problems including persistent epithelial defects,

corneal ulceration, stem cell deficiency, conjunctival cicatrization, symblepharon formation, fornix foreshortening and so on (Fig. 12). In the early stages of these conditions, covering the ocular surface with an amniotic membrane graft decreases the chances of complications by means of its anti-inflammatory, antiangiogenic, antiscarring and proepithelial effects. The amniotic membrane graft also prevents symblepharon formation by acting as a physical barrier; it also likely provides a scaffold for early re-epithelialization.[31-33]

During the acute phase of SJS or TEN, amniotic membrane is used as a patch graft covering the entire ocular surface dipping into the fornix and out onto the eyelid margin. Delayed or inadequate coverage may result in substandard results. It is used in combination with intensive steroid therapy and a large diameter Kontur lens (Kontur Contact Lens Co., Richmond, CA) in order to maintain the fornices. They can also be used similarly for acute chemical and thermal burns.[34]

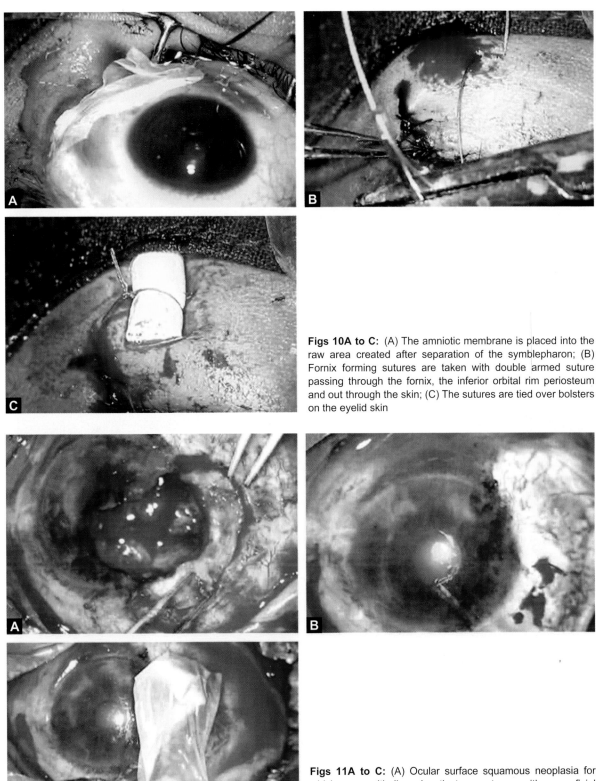

**Figs 10A to C:** (A) The amniotic membrane is placed into the raw area created after separation of the symblepharon; (B) Fornix forming sutures are taken with double armed suture passing through the fornix, the inferior orbital rim periosteum and out through the skin; (C) The sutures are tied over bolsters on the eyelid skin

**Figs 11A to C:** (A) Ocular surface squamous neoplasia for which an epithelioconjunctivotenonectomy with superficial lamellar sclerectomy is being done; (B) The eye at the end of resection of tumor; (C) The conjunctival defect as well as the de-epithelialized area of cornea being covered with an amniotic membrane graft

CHAPTER

**76**

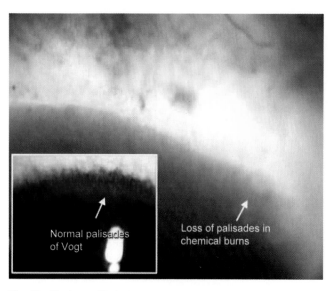

**Fig. 12:** The loss of limbal stem cells secondary to chemical burns as opposed to the normal appearances of the palisades of Vogt (inset)

## Bleb Leaks and Overfiltering Blebs

Late bleb leaks and overfiltering blebs are generally seen after application of wound-modulating agents. The conjunctiva covering the bleb is often thin and avascular. Excision of the bleb and direct resuturing, conjunctival advancement or conjunctival autografts may be used, but these depend on availability of adequate mobile conjunctiva to cover the defect without shortening the fornix. As described by Tseng et al., these blebs can be closed with amniotic membrane graft though they reported superior results with conjunctival advancement.[35] The amniotic membrane is used to cover the defect after excising the area of thin and avascular conjunctiva.

In our personal experience, we prefer performing a conjunctival advancement in conjunction with an amniotic membrane graft applied under the conjunctiva. The amniotic membrane decrease subconjunctival fibrosis and possible failure of bleb functioning (Figs 13 and 14). This is because

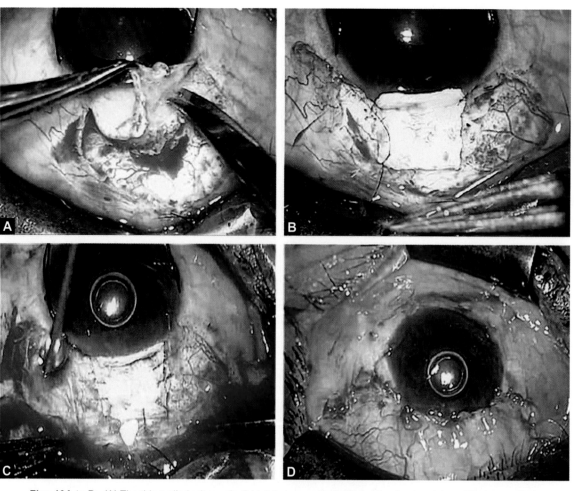

**Figs 13A to D:** (A) The thin-walled mitomycin-C bleb being excised; (B) A scleral autopatch graft being applied; (C) Amniotic membrane being applied; (D) A conjunctival advancement flap done at the end

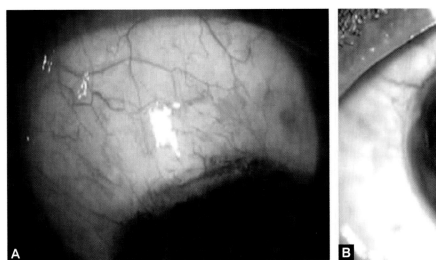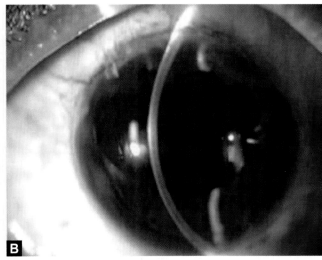

**Figs 14A and B:** (A) The same patient 6 months postoperatively after also having undergone a cataract extraction with intraocular lens implantation. The superior area of bleb is seen, the intraocular pressure remains under control; (B) Slit-lamp view of the cornea and anterior chamber

the amniotic membrane is thin and avascular similar to a bleb with antimetabolite, therefore, it is possible that there may be bleb leak and an increased risk of endophthalmitis in case of blebs reconstructed with amniotic membrane alone (as also noted by Tseng et al.).

The use of amniotic membrane under the scleral flap instead of antifibrotic agents has also been described by Fukushima et al.[36]

## TISSUE CULTURED HUMAN AMNIOTIC EPITHELIAL CELLS

Corneal collagen sheets seeded with amniotic epithelial cells obtained from human donor placentas are cultured *ex vivo* and have been used for treatment of various conditions such as persistent epithelial defects.[37] The advantage of this technique is that it is repeatable, fast, easy to perform and does not involve surgery.

## AMNIOTIC MEMBRANE SUBSTRATE FOR EX VIVO EXPANSION OF LIMBAL STEM CELLS

The amniotic membrane is nonimmunogenic and also does not contain any actively replicating cells. It also promotes epithelial adhesion and migration. Hence, it is an ideal substrate for *ex vivo* expansion of limbal stem cells obtained via a small biopsy from the patients eye.[38] Once expanded on the amniotic membrane sheet, this can be used to transfer the limbal stem cells to the patients eye. It

has the advantage of not leading to iatrogenic limbal stem cell deficiency in the donor eye as only a small biopsy is required.

## CONCLUSION

Even though various theories have been proposed regarding how amniotic membrane works in various conditions, the exact mechanism and the exact composition of this invaluable membrane is still not fully understood. It is easily obtainable, is relatively cheap and is easy to manipulate. Despite being an allograft, it has low immunogenicity and therefore, does not cause rejection.

## REFERENCES

1. Blackburn ST. Prenatal Period and Placental Physiology. Maternal, fetal and neonatal physiology: a clinical perspective, 4th edition. St Louis: Missouri, Saunders; 2007. pp. 70-120.
2. Bourne GL. The microscopic anatomy of the human amnion and chorion. Am J Obstet Gynecol. 1960;79:1070-3.
3. Fukuda K, Chikama T, Nakamura M, et al. Differential distribution of subchains of the basement membrane components type IV collagen and laminin among the amniotic membrane, cornea, and conjunctiva. Cornea. 1999;18(1):73-9.
4. Dua HS, Gomes JA, King AJ, et al. The amniotic membrane in ophthalmology. Surv Ophthalmol. 2004;49(1):51-77.
5. Boudreau N, Sympson CJ, Werb Z, et al. Suppression of ICE and apoptosis in mammary epithelial cells by extracellular matrix. Science. 1995;267:891-3.
6. Koizumi NJ, Inatomi TJ, Sotozono CJ, et al. Growth factor mRNA and protein in preserved human amniotic membrane. Curr Eye Res. 2000;20(3):173-7.

CHAPTER **76**

7. Na BK, Hwang JH, Kim JC, et al. Analysis of human amniotic membrane components as proteinase inhibitors for development of therapeutic agent of recalcitrant keratitis. Trophoblast Res. 1999;13:459-66.

8. Tseng SC, Li DQ, Ma X. Suppression of Transforming growth factor-beta isoforms, TGF-beta receptor II, and myofibroblast differentiation in cultured human corneal and limbal fibroblasts by amniotic membrane matrix. J Cell Physiol. 1999;179:325-35.

9. Lee SB, Li DQ, Tan DTH, et al. Suppression of TGF-beta signaling in both normal conjunctival fibroblasts and pterygial body fibroblasts by amniotic membrane. Curr Eye Res. 2000;20:325-34.

10. Adinolfi M, Akle CA, McColl I, et al. Expression of HLA antigens, beta 2-microglobulin and enzymes by human amniotic epithelial cells. Nature. 1982;295(5487):325-7.

11. Wang MX, Gray TG, Park WC, et al. Reduction in corneal haze and apoptosis by amniotic membrane matrix in excimer laser photoablation in rabbits. J Cataract Refract Surg. 2001;27(2):310-9.

12. de Roth A. Plastic repair of conjunctival defects with fetal membrane. Arch Ophthalmol. 1940;23:522-5.

13. Kim JC, Tseng SC. Transplantation of preserved human amniotic membrane for surface reconstruction in severely damaged rabbit corneas. Cornea. 1995;14(5):473-84.

14. Hanada K, Shimazaki J, Shimmura S, et al. Multilayered amniotic membrane transplantation for severe ulceration of the cornea and sclera. Am J Ophthalmol. 2001;131(3):324-31.

15. Colocho G, Graham WP, Greene AE, et al. Human amniotic membrane as a physiologic wound dressing. Arch Surg. 1974;109(3):370-3.

16. Talmi YP, Finkelstein Y, Zohar Y. Use of human amniotic membrane as a biologic dressing. Eur J Plast Surg. 1990;13:160-2.

17. Meller D, Tseng SC. Conjunctival epithelial cell differentiation on amniotic membrane. Invest Ophthalmol Vis Sci. 1999;40(5):878-86.

18. Nubile M, Dua HS, Lanzini M, et al. In vivo analysis of stromal integration of multilayer amniotic membrane transplantation in corneal ulcers. Am J Ophthalmol. 2011;151(5):809-22.

19. Solomon A, Meller D, Prabhasawat P, et al. Amniotic membrane grafts for nontraumatic corneal perforations, descemetoceles, and deep ulcers. Ophthalmology. 2002;109(4):694-703.

20. Pires RT, Tseng SC, Prabhasawat P, et al. Amniotic membrane transplantation for symptomatic bullous keratopathy. Arch Ophthalmol. 1999;117(10):1291-7.

21. Thoft RA, Friend J. The X, Y, Z hypothesis of corneal epithelial maintenance. Invest Ophthalmol Vis Sci. 1983;24(10):1442-3.

22. Meller D, Tseng SCG. In vitro conjunctival epithelial differentiation on preserved human amniotic membrane. Invest Ophthalmol Vis Sci. 1998;39:S428.

23. Meller D, Pires RTF, Tseng SCG. Ex vivo preservation and expansion of human limbal epithelial progenitor cells by amniotic membrane. Invest Ophthalmol Vis Sci. 1999;40:329.

24. Anderson DF, Ellies P, Pires RT, et al. Amniotic membrane tran- splantation for partial limbal stem cell deficiency. Br J Ophthalmol. 2001;85(5):567-75.

25. Tseng SCG, Prabhasawat P, Barton K, et al. Amniotic membrane transplantation with or without limbal allografts for corneal surface reconstruction in patients with limbal stem cell deficiency. Arch Ophthalmol. 1998;116(4):431-41.

26. Gomes JA, dos Santos MS, Cunha MC, et al. Amniotic membrane transplantation for partial and total limbal stem cell deficiency secondary to chemical burn. Ophthalmology. 2003;110(3):466-73.

27. Kheirkhah A, Nazari R, Nikdel M, et al. Postoperative conjunctival inflammation after pterygium surgery with amniotic membrane transplantation versus conjunctival autograft. Am J Ophthalmol. 2011;152(5):733-8.

28. Miyai T, Hara R, Nejima R, et al. Limbal allograft, amniotic membrane transplantation, and intraoperative mitomycin C for recurrent pterygium. Ophthalmology. 2005;112(7):1263-7.

29. Kheirkhah A, Blanco G, Casas V, et al. Surgical strategies for fornix reconstruction based on symblepharon severity. Am J Ophthalmol. 2008;146(2):266-75.

30. Solomon A, Espana EM, Tseng SC. Amniotic membrane transplantation for reconstruction of the conjunctival fornices. Ophthalmology. 2003;110(1):93-100.

31. Shammas MC, Lai EC, Sarkar JS, et al. Management of acute Stevens-Johnson Syndrome and Toxic Epidermal Necrolysis utilizing amniotic membrane and topical corticosteroids. Am J Ophthalmol. 2010;149(2):203-13.

32. Barabino S, Rolando M, Bentivoglio G, et al. Role of amni- otic membrane transplantation for conjunctival reconstruction in ocular-cicatricial pemphigoid. Ophthalmology. 2003;110(3):474-80.

33. John T, Foulks GN, John ME, et al. Amniotic membrane in the surgical management of acute toxic epidermal necrolysis. Ophthalmology. 2002;109(2):351-60.

34. Sridhar MS, Bansal AK, Sangwan VS, et al. Amniotic membrane transplantation in acute chemical and thermal injury. Am J Ophthalmol. 2000;130(1):134-7.

35. Budenz DL, Barton K, Tseng SC. Amniotic membrane transplantation for repair of leaking glaucoma filtering blebs. Am J Ophthalmol. 2000;130(5):580-8.

36. Fujishima H, Shimazaki J, Shinozaki N, et al. Trabeculectomy with the use of amniotic membrane for uncontrolled glaucoma. Ophthalmic Surg Lasers. 1998;29(5):428-31.

37. Parmar DN, Alizadeh H, Awwad ST, et al. Ocular surface restoration using non-surgical transplantation of tissue-cultured human amniotic epithelial cells. Am J Ophthalmol. 2006;141(2):299-307.

38. Grueterich M, Espana EM, Tseng S. Ex vivo expansion of limbal epithelial stem cells: amniotic membrane serving as a stem cell niche. Surv Ophthalmol. 2003;48(6):631-46.

SECTION 16

# Limbal Stem Cell Transplantation

*Justin D Aaker, Andrew J W Huang*

## ☞ INTRODUCTION

The ocular surface consists of the cornea, conjunctiva and a junctional zone, which is known as the limbus. This anatomical description matches the findings on a cellular level: the three epithelia that make up the ocular surface are corneal, limbal and conjunctival. Since corneal and conjunctival epithelial cells belong to two separate lineages, they have two separate sets of stem cells that make up a small fraction of the ocular surface.[1] The stem cells of corneal and conjunctival epithelia are small, quiescent and undifferentiated subpopulations of the ocular surface epithelial cells. The corneal stem cells are responsible for corneal epithelial homeostasis and wound healing, whereas the conjunctiva epithelia are renewed by conjunctival stem cells.

A healthy ocular surface is of paramount importance in the preservation of vision. Compromised tear function, conjunctival cicatrization and limbal stem cell deficiency can individually or in combination affect the overall health of the ocular surface and have an adverse effect on the level of visual acuity and the quality of vision. After diagnosing a patient with limbal stem cell deficiency, the management of the disorder must be undertaken. When medical measures fail to manage ocular surface disease, surgical intervention may be the only route to restore the ocular surface and preserve vision. Patients should be stratified based on the severity and disability of the deficiency, whether or not it is bilateral, and the need for medical or surgical therapy. Minor, unilateral deficiencies are managed in a drastically different manner than bilateral total limbal stem cell deficiency. Often, the ocular surface must be reconstructed before attention can be turned to penetrating keratoplasty for visual rehabilitation.[2-4]

## ☞ REMOVAL OF ABNORMAL TISSUE BY SUPERFICIAL KERATECTOMY

For localized and mild partial limbal stem cell deficiencies that are either unilateral or bilateral, superficial keratectomy may be employed.[5] The idea behind this treatment is that by debriding the area of cornea with abnormal conjunctival ingrowth, the normal cornea epithelium may repopulate the debrided area. This has been reported in the setting of contact lens limbal stem cell deficiency, and may be combined with amniotic membrane or other methods to aid in epithelial healing. If this method does not alleviate the condition, more aggressive methods for ocular surface reconstruction (Table 1) may need to be employed.

**Table 1:** Classification of ocular surface reconstruction

| Unilateral Damage | Bilateral Damage |
| --- | --- |
| I. Restoration of ocular surface substrate | |
| CAU | c-CAL or lr-CAL |
| AMT | AMT |
| | OMAU |
| II. Restoration of corneal stem cells | |
| CLAU | c-CLAL or lr-CLAL |
| | KLAL |
| EVELAU | EVELAU or EVELAL |

CAU: conjunctival autograft; c-CAL: cadaveric conjunctival allograft; lr-CAL: living-related conjunctival allograft; AMT: amniotic membrane transplantation; OMAU: oral mucosa autograft; CLAU: conjunctival limbal autograft; c-CLAL: cadaveric conjunctival limbal allograft; lr-CLAL: living-related conjunctival limbal allograft; KLAL: keratolimbal allograft; EVELAU: *ex vivo* expansion of limbal autograft; EVELAL: *ex-vivo* expansion of limbal allograft

## Restoration of Ocular Surface Substrate by Mucous Membrane Transplantation

### Conjunctival Transplantation

Conjunctival transplantation can be a conjunctival autograft (CAU) or a conjunctival allograft (CAL). A CAU is a patch of tissue obtained from the fellow eye or same eye (such as in pterygium surgery) that is used to replace the damaged epithelial surface in the affected eye. The idea behind this surgery is that the conjunctival epithelium would differentiate into a corneal-like epithelium, a process known as conjunctival transdifferentiation.[6-8] In general, in the absence of significant stromal inflammation, the transplanted conjunctival epithelium will spread onto the previously damaged corneal surface and redifferentiate into a cornea-like phenotype. However, some studies indicate that the resulting conjunctival epithelial cells and corneal epithelial cells do not share a similar phenotype or structure.[9-10] In fact, after conjunctival transplantation, there are reports that the epithelium has become more like conjunctival epithelium rather than corneal epithelium.[10] The main use for this procedure is pterygium with partial limbal stem cell deficiency.[11]

A living related conjunctival transplantation (lr-CAL) or a cadaveric conjunctival transplantation (c-CAL) could be used for cases of bilateral limbal deficiency associated with cicatricial conjunctival disorders such as Stevens-Johnson syndrome, mucous membrane pemphigoid (previously known as ocular cicatricial pemphigoid), or bilateral chemical injuries.[12] Rejection has been noted when there was a poor HLA match.

### Oral Mucosa Transplantation

Bilateral chronic cicatricial conjunctivitis such as Stevens-Johnson syndrome or mucous membrane pemphigoid often leads to significant conjunctival scarring and malpositioning of eyelids. Despite adequate suppression or control of inflammation during the acute phase of underlying etiology, autologous conjunctiva or limbal stem cells are usually not available for ocular surface reconstruction. Unaffected autologous mucosal membrane from oral or nasal origin contains mucin-producing goblet cells. These tissues can be considered as an alternative source for conjunctival replacement to resurface the keratinized or scarred bulbar conjunctiva or to resurface the tarsal conjunctiva for restoring the foreshortened fornix or lid malpositioning. As the procedure is an autologous graft in nature, systemic immunosuppressants are not required.

The prerequisite for the success of autologous mucosal graft is to adequately suppress the underlying ocular surface inflammation. Upon adequate control of inflammation, the dense corneal pannus or conjunctiva scars can be excised from the ocular surface with careful dissection with respect to the tissue plane. If the bulbar conjunctival appears to be wet and free of keratinization or epidermalization, it can be used to restore the tarsal conjunctiva during fornix reconstruction to minimize the need for ectopic mucosal tissue. Oral mucosal membrane can generally be obtained from the inner lip or buccal surface. Superficial oral mucosa can be ballooned up by infiltration of the tissue with saline to allow easier separation from the submucosal tissues. A thin oral mucosal layer can be dissected manually or via the assistance of a mucotome. The oral mucosa can be used as conjunctival grafts as described above.

For fornix reconstruction, the host tarsal conjunctiva is first removed up to the mucocutaneous junction and any adhesion to the globe is released by blunt dissection. The freshly harvested oral mucosa is placed on the denuded tarsal plate, fibrin tissue adhesive can be used to attach the mucosal graft to tarsus. Additional 9-0 monofilament Vicryl sutures can be used to secure the free graft borders to the deep fornix and mucocutaneous junction. A symblepharon ring or conformer is then inserted into the eye to maintain the upper and lower fornices. Postoperatively, topical corticosteroids and prophylactic antibiotic ointments are used on the ocular surface as well as the oral donor site to promote wound healing and provide better lubrication. The conformer is usually left in place for 2–3 weeks until the healing and proper adhesion of oral mucosal graft takes place.

The oral mucosa usually heals without significant inflammation and it is much thicker than typical amniotic membrane with stiffer tissue consistency. In general, oral mucosa does not readily assume the flexible conjunctival characteristics and remains more boggy and inflamed than the native conjunctiva. However, it does provide adequate lubrication for the ocular surface and proper tissue strength of the tarsal conjunctiva. In contrast to the thin amniotic membrane, oral mucosa tends to be less ideal for the replacement of bulbar conjunctiva. As oral mucosa remains vascularized and will not support corneal epithelial differentiation, the procedure is primarily indicated for mucosal replacement or fornix reconstruction. While large surface area of oral mucosa can be obtained, it may not be sufficient to cover extensive ocular surface defects. Combined use of oral mucosa and commercial amniotic membrane can be considered for advanced cicatricial conjunctivitis.

Nonetheless, neither amniotic membrane nor oral mucosa will provide limbal stem cells to maintain corneal epithelial lineage. Residual compromised ocular surface due to limbal stem cell deficiency usually needs to be further addressed as the procedure does not provide adequate source of limbal stem cells.

### Amniotic Membrane Transplantation

Amniotic membrane is the innermost layer of the placenta and consists of three layers: epithelium, basement membrane and avascular stroma. It has been demonstrated to be successful for the reconstruction of the ocular surface.[13] Amniotic membrane can be used as a bandage, as the carrier for cultivated limbal stem cells, and sometimes as primary therapy in limbal stem cell deficiency.

In patients with partial limbal deficiency with superficial corneal surface disease, amniotic membrane transplantation alone is often sufficient to restore the corneal surface by reducing inflammation or corneal vascularization and providing a substrate for the remaining stem cells to proliferate.[14] The amniotic basement membrane serves as a matrix replacement for diseased conjunctival and corneal epithelial basement membrane.[15] It may support the epithelial proliferation and facilitate the maintenance of appropriate epithelial phenotypes.[16] For complete limbal deficiency requiring allogeneic limbal transplant, adjunctive amniotic membrane transplant to replace the damaged corneal stroma may suppress perilimbal inflammation and enhance the survival of limbal allografts.[14]

Besides being used as an epithelial substrate, amniotic membrane may provide a favorable niche to expand limbal stem cells. Soluble factors derived from amniotic membrane can suppress the production of TGF-ß1, a cytokine responsible for fibroblast activation in wound healing, and may limit scar formation on the ocular surface.[17] In addition, amniotic membrane can promote the nongoblet cell differentiation of cultured rabbit conjunctival epithelial cells.[18] Other studies have suggested that removal of the amniotic epithelium to expose its basement membrane can increase connexin 43 and K3 cytokeratin expression in actively dividing limbal cells cultured on amniotic membrane.[19]

## Restoration of Corneal Stem Cells by Limbal Transplantation

Limbal transplantation procedures can be classified based on the substrate used to deliver the limbal stem cells and the source of the donor tissue. Since corneal stem cells are located at the basal limbus, they are most safely transplanted by removing the stem cells with surrounding scaffolding tissue. The scaffolding tissue may consist of conjunctiva or of the cornea with associated limbus. However, newer techniques involve using *ex vivo* cultivation and transplant of the cultivated stem cells with amniotic membrane or fibrin.[9,20-22] The stem cells can be derived from an unaffected eye of the same subject (autograft) or can be collected from another donor (allograft). Allografts can be further stratified as cadaveric tissue versus living-related tissue.[23] The success of transplantation will vary depending on the substrate and source of the transplanted cells. Newer methods of transplantation make use of fibrin glue to attach the stem cell grafts to the host.[24,25] These may improve upon the success of previous methods by increasing the yield of stem cells delivered. The essential steps in surgery regardless of the type of transplant are a 360° conjunctival peritomy, superficial keratectomy and attachment of the graft. The corneal bed may be smoothed with a diamond burr or an excimer laser to perform a phototherapeutic keratectomy.[26,27] A new technique utilizes the femtosecond laser to prepare cadaver grafts and to prepare the recipient bed.[28]

### Conjunctival Limbal Autograft

A conjunctival limbal autograft (CLAU) only works with unilateral limbal stem cell deficiencies. It requires the harvesting of healthy stem cells from a fellow unaffected eye. It uses the perilimbal conjunctiva as a carrier for the stem cells. In many cases, the 'unaffected' eye has been exposed to the inciting factor, and only has subclinical damage. This is frequently the case in asymmetric chemical burns, and patients with prior surgeries or contact lens use where this procedure would be contraindicated.[29] Theoretical risks include iatrogenic limbal stem cell deficiency in the donor eye. Animal studies have suggested that full-thickness excision of the sectorial limbus, similar to the surgery performed in a donor eye for limbal autografting, can eventually compromise corneal epithelial healing in the presence of a subsequently induced epithelial defect.[30] Even though there are no reports of serious limbal stem cell deficiency in the donor eye, this concern is one of the major limitations of this technique. Because of these potential concerns, excision of the minimal amount of tissue possible that can result in a successful graft is recommended. Traditionally, excision of less than 4 clock hours of the limbus with conjunctiva is recommended, but there are reports of using only 2 clock hours of tissue from the contralateral eye combined with amniotic membrane.[31] The donor tissue can be obtained by making a circumferential thin dissection of the conjunctiva starting 3 mm posterior to the limbus to its limbal insertion. A lamellar dissection of the limbus approximately 150 microns thick and 1 mm into the peripheral cornea is then performed to obtain the donor limbal epithelium (Fig. 1). Since the donor tissue in CLAU is autologous, there is no concern about immunological rejection of the donor tissue. Reports of success have been as high as 100% for this technique.[32]

### Cadaveric Conjunctival Limbal Allograft

When both eyes are affected with limbal stem cell deficiency, the surgeon and/or patient does not want the risk of harvesting cells from the unaffected eye, or there are no available living-related donors, a cadaveric conjunctival limbal allograft (c-CLAL) can be used. It was first described as homotransplantations of limbal stem cells by Pfister, who performed the transplantation with conjunctiva and limbus from a cadaveric corneoscleral rim in which the central donor cornea had been used for another patient.[33] When using the donor corneoscleral rim for a c-CLAL, the rim needs to be thinned, thereby yielding a thin doughnut-shaped conjunctival limbal graft and avoiding adding too much tissue thickness to the peripheral cornea of the recipient. Alternatively, lamellar dissection of the entire donor corneoscleral button using a lamellar dissecting blade or viscoelastic agents can be performed, followed by trephination of the central donor cornea to obtain a thin donor ring.

The benefits of cadaveric allografts include the potential for transplantation of 360° of limbal tissue, the lack of risk to living donors and the availability of tissue. However, significant negatives include the increased risk of allograft rejection compared to living-related donors and autografts, and the availability of viable conjunctiva. Since it is an allograft, there is increased need for potentially toxic long-term immunosuppression. Postoperatively, conjunctivolimbal injection and significant chemosis are often noted in conjunctival limbal allografts. Conjunctival vascular engorgement and hemorrhage are also observed in recipients and may represent early signs of limbal allograft rejection or reactive hyperemia from vascular anastomosis of large conjunctival vessels.[34] Conjunctival limbal allografts with proper immunosuppression may lead to a stable ocular surface and successful penetrating keratoplasty.[33]

### Living-related Conjunctival Limbal Allograft

The theoretical benefits of living-related conjunctival limbal allograft (lr-CLAL) include reduced risk of rejection compared to cadaveric transplants, and possible increased yield of viable cells and conjunctiva since the tissue is fresh. The indications for lr-CLALs are similar to those for c-CLALs or keratolimbal allografts (KLALs) when the fellow, or less involved, eye is deemed unsuitable for donating limbal stem cells. The living-related tissue has the advantage of providing better histocompatibility.

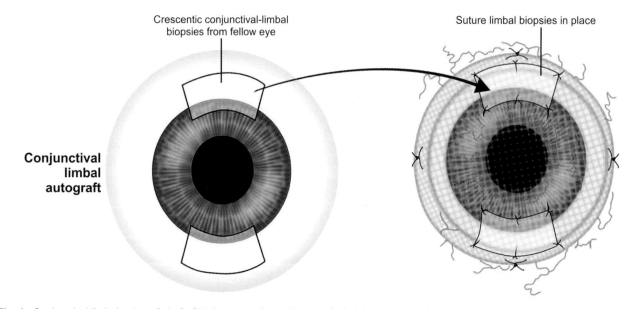

**Fig. 1:** Conjunctival limbal autograft. Left: Obtain crescentic conjunctival limbal donor tissues from the superior and inferior limbus from fellow eye. Right: After removing corneal pannus by superficial keratectomy, attach autograft tissue with fibrin glue or sutures onto the peripheral cornea with or without preplaced amniotic membrane

**SECTION 16**

In lr-CLALs, rapid transfer of freshly harvested graft from the donor to the recipient may prevent the unexpected stem cell death associated with preservation and storage of cadaveric donor tissue.[34] However, due to the risk of developing limbal deficiency in the donor eye, it has been recommended that the amount of tissue to be obtained from the living donor should be limited to 2 clock hours of limbal tissue at the superior and inferior limbus of each eye.[34] Regardless of the degree of immune histocompatibility, moderate systemic immunosuppression is still recommended to prevent limbal allograft rejection. The lr-CLAL has recently been combined with keratolimbal allograft (KLAL) as a potential method to increase the number of stem cells transplanted to the recipient.[23] This technique allows the possible benefits of HLA matching while allowing for the maximum amount of stem cells to be transferred. Theoretically, this technique should yield more successful outcomes, but as is the problem with all

of these techniques, there are inadequate numbers of subjects for randomized controlled trials.

### Keratolimbal Allograft

Because of the larger amount of corneal tissue required, only cadaveric donor tissue is suitable for KLALs. KLALs are indicated for most ocular surface disorders requiring restoration of the limbus. Several different surgical techniques for keratolimbal allotransplantation have been proposed. They include the corneoscleral ring (Fig. 2),[35] the corneoscleral crescent,[36] and homologous penetrating central limbokeratoplasty.[37,38] The use of fibrin glue to secure the transplant to the host has also been reported and may represent a less traumatic method of performing the transplant.[24,25]

Initial experience on KLALs indicated a moderate (~ 50–75%) but satisfactory success in restoring ocular surface integrity.[34,38,39] Later reviews revealed a long-term

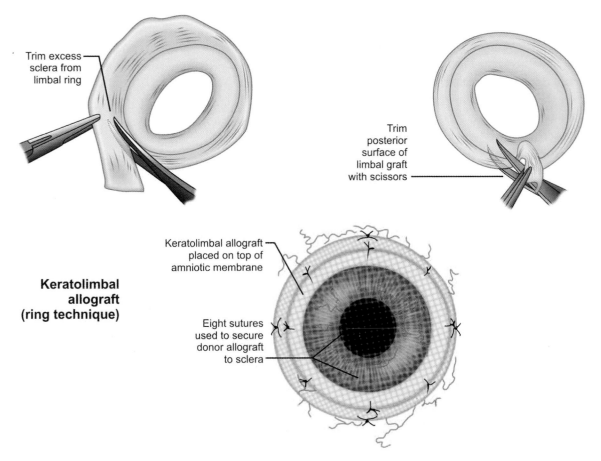

Trim excess sclera from limbal ring

Trim posterior surface of limbal graft with scissors

**Keratolimbal allograft (ring technique)**

Keratolimbal allograft placed on top of amniotic membrane

Eight sutures used to secure donor allograft to sclera

**Fig. 2:** Keratolimbal allograft. Use trephine to remove central cornea from donor corneal button and trim excess sclera from limbal ring. Trim posterior surface of limbal graft to allow better tissue approximation. Keratolimbal allograft can be placed directly on the denuded limbosclera or on top of the preplaced amniotic membrane

survival rate of less than 30% in KLALs performed for severe ocular surface disorders.[40,41] Many of the patients who received limbal allografts also required penetrating keratoplasty (PKP) for visual rehabilitation (Figs 3A and B). Patients who underwent KLAL alone seemed to fare better than those who underwent a KLAL combined with PKP. In patients who received a KLAL and PKP simultaneously, corneal graft rejection was a major complication. Within this subset of patients, rejection episodes were more frequently encountered in patients with chemical or thermal injury (69%) than in patients with inflammatory conjunctivitis such as Stevens-Johnson syndrome or mucous membrane pemphigoid (27%).[35]

Possible explanations for this observation include increased antigenic loads from the central corneal graft and peripheral keratolimbal rim. The combined procedure may have also resulted in a greater wound healing response and increased postoperative inflammation. Primary failure of the limbal stem cell transplant may lead to further conjunctivalization and vascularization of the cornea with a subsequent increase of immune sensitization and eventual rejection of the corneal graft. Consequently, some investigators have recommended PKP to be performed no earlier than 3–6 months after a KLAL.[4,36,40] The major disadvantage of a KLAL is the high risk of graft rejection. Intensive immunosuppression by systemic corticosteroids and cyclosporine has been reported to improve the survival of limbal allografts (Figs 4A and B).[42] Newer studies urged adoption of tacrolimus and mycophenolate mofetil to aid in graft survival.[25,39]

## Ex Vivo Expansion of Limbal Stem Cell (EVEL)

To generate sufficient limbal stem cells and minimize the risk of developing subsequent limbal deficiency in the donor eye, *ex vivo* expansion of the corneal epithelial stem cells by culturing limbal explants on an amniotic membrane, fibrin, or other carrier such as a hydrophilic soft contact lens has been investigated.[20,43] Only a small amount of limbal tissue (1–2 mm²) is needed from the donor eye in this technique compared to traditional conjunctival limbal auto- and allografts.[22,43] Theoretically, an eye with bilateral limbal stem cell deficiency can be treated with this method as long as one of the eyes has sufficient stem cells to be harvested for the autograft. Additionally, the risks to living-related donors may be minimized, thereby increasing availability of this source of tissue. The amount of tissue taken from the donor eye is minimized, and the potential amount of transplantable tissue is increased; this technique may decrease the risk and increase the success rate for limbal stem cell transplantation.

In the mid-1980s, corneal epithelial cell transplantation was first described.[44-46] However, cells derived from the central corneal epithelium consisted primarily of terminally differentiated cells that could not be subcultivated more than twice after senescence.[47] Transplanting cultured limbal stem cells was subsequently achieved by McCulley et al.[48,49] Following transplantation, the cultured cells formed hemidesmosomal adhesion to the underlying stroma within 24 hours.[49] Many ocular surface disorders with limbal stem cell deficiencies have been successfully managed by autologous limbal stem cells with or without amniotic membrane or additional feeder layers.[4,22,28,47,50-52]

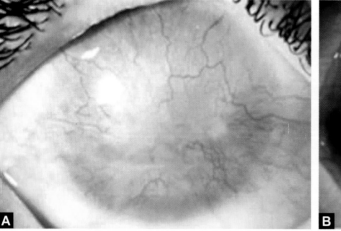 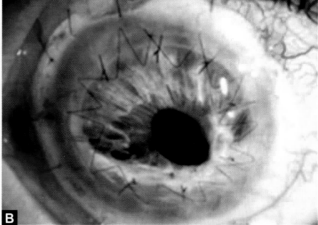

**Figs 3A and B:** Keratolimbal allograft. (A) A patient with bilateral severe chemical burns with total limbal deficiency; (B) The patient received a keratolimbal allograft followed by penetrating keratoplasty and extracapsular cataract surgery with a stable ocular surface and vision

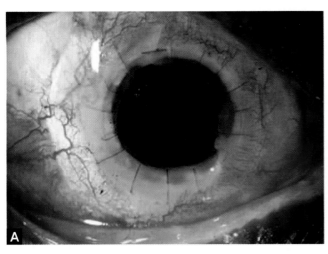 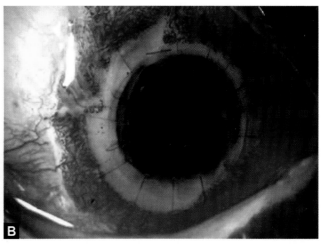

**Figs 4A and B:** Keratolimbal allograft rejection. (A) A patient received a keratolimbal allograft, followed by a penetrating keratoplasty for chemical burns; (B) Marked vascular engorgement of perilimbal vessels was noted after the patient self-discontinued the oral cyclosporine. The vascular congestion improved after systemic immunotherapy was resumed

However, variable success rates have been observed in transplanting limbal allografts cultivated on amniotic membrane.[53,54] Furthermore, the terminology of success differs between studies with success being defined by permutations of clinical, confocal microscopy, and corneal impression cytology derived definitions.[20-22] A variety of biological and immunological factors may have contributed to the variable success rates in these reported series.[53,54] One recent study reported a 68.2% success rate after only one graft, and has identified a possible marker for success; grafts with more than 3% holoclones (identified by production of p63) were more likely to survive.[22]

Despite these more recent successes, the clinical application of this technique has been significantly limited secondary to regulatory concerns. The culture technique involves placing the limbal stem cells directly on the amniotic membrane or in a suspension and then transferring the cells to amniotic membrane or other carrier medium.[21] Most of the cultures have included murine 3T3 feeder cells or have been bathed in bovine serum.[20] This has presented concerns for transfer of mouse genetic material to human cells, and risk of prion diseases in the case of bovine serum. Newer techniques that do not use 3T3 murine feeder cells and use autologous serum instead of bovine serum have been reported.[21,55] The advent of these newer techniques may speed up the way to regulatory approval and broader adoption of this technique.

The surgical method for transfer of cultured limbal stem cells is similar to any limbal stem cell transplant. A 360° conjunctival peritomy is performed followed by a superficial keratectomy. Mitomycin C may be used in the subconjunctival space to prevent the conjunctival epithelium from growing onto the cornea.[56] The cultured stem cells are sutured or glued if amniotic membrane is the substrate, or directly placed on the cornea if the substrate is fibrin.[20,21] Other aspects of improving graft survival have varied, but may include bandage contact lens, tarsorrhaphy, botulinum toxin induced ptosis, or amniotic membrane sutured over the graft. Medical management includes topical steroids and antibiotics along with systemic immunosuppression often consisting of a short course of oral prednisone in autografts; cyclosporine and sometimes cyclophosphamide are usually reserved for allografts.[20,21,43,51,56,57]

Since limbal stem cells for *ex vivo* cultivation may be harvested from autologous (EVELAU) or allogeneic (EVELAL) donor sites, this technique is applicable for nearly all types of limbal stem cell deficiency.[50,53,54] Despite the long postoperative course, *ex vivo* limbal stem cell expansion has had significant success, especially in the case of autografts, and is probably the future of limbal stem cell replacement therapy pending resolution of regulatory issues.

## OTHER SURGICAL TECHNIQUES FOR OCULAR SURFACE RECONSTRUCTION

Other techniques exist to restore vision and the ocular surface with limbal stem cell deficiency. These include placement of the keratoprosthesis and transplantation of oral mucosal grafts.

CHAPTER 77

The keratoprosthesis has been used in the case of limbal stem cell deficiency.[23,58] Complications may occur including extrusion, retroprosthetic membrane, endophthalmitis, glaucoma and additional difficulties. However, the keratoprosthesis represents a technique with quick visual rehabilitation, and may be the only option for patients that cannot tolerate systemic immunosuppression. The keratoprosthesis may also be combined with limbal stem cell transplant in order to improve sustainability.[23]

Another technique of value is oral mucosal epithelial expansion. Oral mucosal transplantation may be accomplished with *ex vivo* expansion or with placement of the graft directly onto the ocular surface as described above.[26,56,59,60] However, the expansion of oral mucosa is not readily available in the United States. Theoretical benefits include the ability to replace total bilateral stem cell deficiency with autologous mucosa without the risks of potentially toxic immunosuppression. Despite the possible benefits, corneal neovascularization frequently occurs after the procedure.[60] Furthermore, improvement in visual acuity is not particularly reliable with only 42% of patients having visual acuity improved by more than two lines at 36 months in one study.[59,60]

Both of these techniques are potential adjuncts to limbal stem cell transplantation, but both have their weaknesses. Additional work on these techniques is required before they become the *de facto* method for rehabilitation for limbal stem cell deficiency.

## ▶ MANAGEMENT OF LIMBAL STEM CELL TRANSPLANTS

Limbal stem cell transplantation is one of the later steps in a long sequence promoting visual rehabilitation. The transplanted limbal stem cells require an immunologically tolerant environment for success, but other factors that compromise the ocular surface will result in reduced survival. Therefore, modifiable conditions of the eye must be managed prior to transplant to increase the transplant's chances of success. These eyes are often associated with tear film instability due to damage of the neural reflex or lacrimal apparatus. Aqueous tear deficiency can be improved by topical lubricants or punctal occlusion. However, ocular surface inflammation should also be controlled with topical and/or oral anti-inflammatory agents, if needed. Mechanical irritations of the ocular surface from lid pathologies such as trichiasis or entropion should be properly managed to ensure the survival of newly transplanted limbal tissues.

Topical and systemic immunosuppressive agents are usually necessary for limbal allografts, regardless of the donor origin. Commonly used agents include topical and systemic corticosteroids, mycophenolate mofetil and cyclosporine or tacrolimus. The systemic cyclosporine and mycophenolate are often continued for an extended duration to prevent the rejection of limbal allografts or corneal transplants. Patients should be monitored for toxicity associated with these medications. Because of their anti-inflammatory and other supportive properties, autologous serum or plasma drops can be used to treat severe dry eye and to support the nourishment of transplanted limbal tissues.

## ▶ SUMMARY

Limbal stem cell transplantation has evolved in recent years with many iterations of the procedure. Success has improved, but lack of controlled trials and regulatory issues has led to difficulty in improving outcomes. *Ex vivo* expansion of tissue seems to provide hope for solutions less dependent on allografts and long-term immunosuppression.

## ▶ REFERENCES

1. Wei ZG, Sun TT, Lavker RM. Rabbit conjunctival and corneal epithelial cells belong to two separate lineages. Invest Ophthalmol Vis Sci. 1996;37:523-33.
2. Tseng SC. Concept and application of limbal stem cells. Eye (Lond). 1989;3:141-57.
3. Dua HS, Saini JS, Azuara-Blanco A, et al. Limbal stem cell deficiency: concept, aetiology, clinical presentation, diagnosis and management. Indian J Ophthalmol. 2000;48:83-92.
4. Basu S, Mohamed A, Chaurasia S, et al. Clinical outcomes of penetrating keratoplasty after autologous cultivated limbal epithelial transplantation for ocular surface burns. Am J Ophthalmol. 2011;152:917-24.
5. Jeng BH, Halfpenny CP, Meisler DM, et al. Management of focal limbal stem cell deficiency associated with soft contact lens wear. Cornea. 2011;30:18-23.
6. Huang AJ, Watson BD, Hernandez E, et al. Photothrombosis of corneal neovascularization by intravenous rose bengal and argon laser irradiation. Arch Ophthalmol. 1988;106:680-5.
7. Kinoshita S, Friend J, Thoft RA. Biphasic cell proliferation in transdifferentiation of conjunctival to corneal epithelium in rabbits. Invest Ophthalmol Vis Sci. 1983;24:1008-14.
8. Shapiro MS, Friend J, Thoft RA. Corneal re-epithelialization from the conjunctiva. Invest Ophthalmol Vis Sci. 1981;21:135-42.
9. Ang LP, Tanioka H, Kawasaki S, et al. Cultivated human conjunctival epithelial transplantation for total limbal stem cell deficiency. Invest Ophthalmol Vis Sci. 2010;51:758-64.
10. Tsai RJ, Sun TT, Tseng SC. Comparison of limbal and conjunctival autograft transplantation in corneal surface reconstruction in rabbits. Ophthalmology. 1990;97:446-55.

11. Kenyon KR, Wagoner MD, Hettinger ME. Conjunctival auto-graft transplantation for advanced and recurrent pterygium. Ophthalmology. 1985;92:1461-70.

12. Kwitko S, Marinho D, Barcaro S, et al. Allograft conjunctival transplantation for bilateral ocular surface disorders. Ophthalmology. 1995;102:1020-5.

13. Kim JC, Tseng SC. Transplantation of preserved human amniotic membrane for surface reconstruction in severely damaged rabbit corneas. Cornea. 1995;14:473-84.

14. Tseng SC, Prabhasawat P, Barton K, et al. Amniotic membrane transplantation with or without limbal allografts for corneal surface reconstruction in patients with limbal stem cell deficiency. Arch Ophthalmol. 1998;116:431-41.

15. Fukuda K, Chikama T, Nakamura M, et al. Differential distribution of subchains of the basement membrane components type IV collagen and laminin among the amniotic membrane, cornea, and conjunctiva. Cornea. 1999;18:73-9.

16. Grueterich M, Espana EM, Touhami A, et al. Phenotypic study of a case with successful transplantation of ex vivo expanded human limbal epithelium for unilateral total limbal stem cell deficiency. Ophthalmology. 2002;109:1547-52.

17. Tseng SC, Li DQ, Ma X. Suppression of transforming growth factor-beta isoforms, TGF-beta receptor type II, and myofibroblast differentiation in cultured human corneal and limbal fibroblasts by amniotic membrane matrix. J Cell Physiol 1999; 179:325-35.

18. Meller D, Tseng SC. Conjunctival epithelial cell differentiation on amniotic membrane. Invest Ophthalmol Vis Sci. 1999;40:878-86.

19. Grueterich M, Espana E, Tseng SC. Connexin 43 expression and proliferation of human limbal epithelium on intact and denuded amniotic membrane. Invest Ophthalmol Vis Sci. 2002;43:63-71.

20. Baylis O, Figueiredo F, Henein C, et al. 13 years of cultured limbal epithelial cell therapy: a review of the outcomes. J Cell Biochem. 2011;112:993-1002.

21. Shortt AJ, Secker GA, Rajan MS, et al. Ex vivo expansion and transplantation of limbal epithelial stem cells. Ophthalmology. 2008;115:1989-97.

22. Rama P, Matuska S, Paganoni G, et al. Limbal stem-cell therapy and long-term corneal regeneration. N Engl J Med. 2010;363:147-55.

23. Biber JM, Skeens HM, Neff KD, et al. The cincinnati procedure: technique and outcomes of combined living-related conjunctival limbal allografts and keratolimbal allografts in severe ocular surface failure. Cornea. 2011;30:765-71.

24. Sonmez B, Beden U. Fibrin glue-assisted sutureless limbal stem cell transplantation surgery for the treatment of severe ocular chemical injury. Cornea. 2011;30:296-300.

25. Nassiri N, Pandya HK, Djalilian AR. Limbal allograft transplantation using fibrin glue. Arch Ophthalmol. 2011;129: 218-22.

26. Liu J, Sheha H, Fu Y, et al. Oral mucosal graft with amniotic membrane transplantation for total limbal stem cell deficiency. Am J Ophthalmol. 2011; 152:739-47.

27. Vinciguerra P, Albe E, Rosetta P, et al. Custom phototherapeutic keratectomy and autologous fibrin-cultured limbal stem cell autografting: a combined approach. J Refract Surg. 2008;24:323-4.

28. Choi SK, Kim JH, Lee D, et al. A new surgical technique: a femtosecond laser-assisted keratolimbal allograft procedure. Cornea. 2010;29:924-9.

29. Jenkins C, Tuft S, Liu C, et al. Limbal transplantation in the management of chronic contact-lens-associated epitheliopathy. Eye (Lond). 1993;7:629-33.

30. Chen JJ, Tseng SC. Corneal epithelial wound healing in partial limbal deficiency. Invest Ophthalmol Vis Sci. 1990;31:1301-14.

31. Kheirkhah A, Raju VK, Tseng SC. Minimal conjunctival limbal autograft for total limbal stem cell deficiency. Cornea. 2008;27:730-3.

32. Miri A, Al-Deiri B, Dua HS. Long-term outcomes of autolimbal and allolimbal transplants. Ophthalmology. 2010;117:1207-13.

33. Pfister RR. Corneal stem cell disease: concepts, categorization, and treatment by auto- and homotransplantation of limbal stem cells. CLAO J. 1994;20:64-72.

34. Daya SM, Ilari FA. Living related conjunctival limbal allograft for the treatment of stem cell deficiency. Ophthalmology. 2001;108:126-33.

35. Tsubota K, Satake Y, Kaido M, et al. Treatment of severe ocular-surface disorders with corneal epithelial stem-cell transplantation. N Engl J Med. 1999;340:1697-703.

36. Croasdale CR, Schwartz GS, Malling JV, et al. Keratolimbal allograft: recommendations for tissue procurement and preparation by eye banks, and standard surgical technique. Cornea. 1999;18:52-8.

37. Sundmacher R, Reinhard T. Central corneolimbal transplantation under systemic ciclosporin A cover for severe limbal stem cell insufficiency. Graefes Arch Clin Exp Ophthalmol. 1996;234:S122-5.

38. Reinhard T, Sundmacher R, Spelsberg H, et al. Homologous penetrating central limbo-keratoplasty (HPCLK) in bilateral limbal stem cell insufficiency. Acta Ophthalmol Scand. 1999;77:663-7.

39. Liang L, Sheha H, Tseng SC. Long-term outcomes of keratolimbal allograft for total limbal stem cell deficiency using combined immunosuppressive agents and correction of ocular surface deficits. Arch Ophthalmol. 2009;127:1428-34.

40. Solomon A, Ellies P, Anderson DF, et al. Long-term outcome of keratolimbal allograft with or without penetrating keratoplasty for total limbal stem cell deficiency. Ophthalmology. 2002;109:1159-66.

41. Ilari L, Daya SM. Long-term outcomes of keratolimbal allograft for the treatment of severe ocular surface disorders. Ophthalmology. 2002;109:1278-84.

42. Tsubota K, Toda I, Saito H, et al. Reconstruction of the corneal epithelium by limbal allograft transplantation for severe ocular surface disorders. Ophthalmology. 1995;102:1486-96.

43. Colabelli Gisoldi RA, Pocobelli A, Villani CM, et al. Evaluation of molecular markers in corneal regeneration by means of autologous cultures of limbal cells and keratoplasty. Cornea. 2010;29:715-22.

CHAPTER 77

44. Friend J, Kinoshita S, Thoft RA, et al. Corneal epithelial cell cultures on stromal carriers. Invest Ophthalmol Vis Sci. 1982;23:41-9.

45. Gipson IK, Friend J, Spurr SJ. Transplant of corneal epithelium to rabbit corneal wounds in vivo. Invest Ophthalmol Vis Sci. 1985;26:425-33.

46. Geggel HS, Friend J, Thoft RA. Collagen gel for ocular surface. Invest Ophthalmol Vis Sci. 1985;26:901-5.

47. Pellegrini G, Traverso CE, Franzi AT, et al. Long-term restoration of damaged corneal surfaces with autologous cultivated corneal epithelium. Lancet. 1997;349:990-3.

48. He YG, McCulley JP. Growing human corneal epithelium on collagen shield and subsequent transfer to denuded cornea in vitro. Curr Eye Res. 1991;10:851-63.

49. He YG, Alizadeh H, Kinoshita K, et al. Experimental transplantation of cultured human limbal and amniotic epithelial cells onto the corneal surface. Cornea. 1999;18:570-9.

50. Tsai RJ, Li LM, Chen JK. Reconstruction of damaged corneas by transplantation of autologous limbal epithelial cells. N Engl J Med. 2000;343:86-93.

51. Baradaran-Rafii A, Ebrahimi M, Kanavi MR, et al. Midterm outcomes of autologous cultivated limbal stem cell transplantation with or without penetrating keratoplasty. Cornea. 2010;29:502-9.

52. Sangwan VS, Matalia HP, Vemuganti GK, et al. Clinical outcome of autologous cultivated limbal epithelium transplantation. Indian J Ophthalmol. 2006;54:29-34.

53. Shimazaki J, Aiba M, Goto E, et al. Transplantation of human limbal epithelium cultivated on amniotic membrane for the treatment of severe ocular surface disorders. Ophthalmology. 2002;109:1285-90.

54. Schwab IR, Reyes M, Isseroff RR. Successful transplantation of bioengineered tissue replacements in patients with ocular surface disease. Cornea. 2000;19:421-6.

55. Nakamura T, Inatomi T, Sotozono C, et al. Transplantation of autologous serum-derived cultivated corneal epithelial equivalents for the treatment of severe ocular surface disease. Ophthalmology. 2006;113:1765-72.

56. Shortt AJ, Secker GA, Notara MD, et al. Transplantation of ex vivo cultured limbal epithelial stem cells: a review of techniques and clinical results. Surv Ophthalmol. 2007;52:483-502.

57. Pauklin M, Steuhl KP, Meller D. Characterization of the corneal surface in limbal stem cell deficiency and after transplantation of cultivated limbal epithelium. Ophthalmology. 2009;116:1048-56.

58. Chew HF, Ayres BD, Hammersmith KM, et al. Boston keratoprosthesis outcomes and complications. Cornea. 2009;28:989-96.

59. Satake Y, Higa K, Tsubota K, et al. Long-term outcome of cultivated oral mucosal epithelial sheet transplantation in treatment of total limbal stem cell deficiency. Ophthalmology. 2011;118:1524-30.

60. Nakamura T, Takeda K, Inatomi T, et al. Long-term results of autologous cultivated oral mucosal epithelial transplantation in the scar phase of severe ocular surface disorders. Br J Ophthalmol. 2011;95:942-6.

# CHAPTER 78

# Autologous Ex Vivo Cultivated Limbal Epithelial Transplantation

*Sayan Basu, Virender S Sangwan*

## ✛ OCULAR BURNS, LIMBUS, STEM CELLS AND THERAPY

Ocular surface disease following chemical or thermal burns is a rare but severe form of corneal blindness. Initially, corneal surgeons believed that like other corneal diseases, corneal transplantation could restore corneal transparency and vision. In fact, the first successful corneal transplantation, by the Austrian surgeon Dr Eduard Zirm in 1905, was in the left eye of a farmer with bilateral chronic lime burns.[1,2] However, with experience corneal transplant surgeons realized that almost all corneal grafts performed for ocular burns failed within a year because of recurrence of epithelial defects and vascularization.[3] In the late 1970s and early 1980s Dr Richard Thoft showed in a small series of cases that autologous conjunctival transplantation as opposed to corneal transplantation was effective in stabilizing the corneal surface and moderately improving vision in eyes with ocular burns.[4] He later proposed that the limbus and not the conjunctiva was the source of corneal epithelium hinting that adult corneal epithelial stem cells could be present at that location.[5] Soon in 1986, Sun and associates actually demonstrated the presence of stem cell like cells in the basal layers of the limbus which were slow-cycling, did not express cytological markers for either the conjunctiva or the cornea and were capable of proliferation *in vitro*.[6] This discovery led to a paradigm shift in the understanding of the pathophysiology of ocular burns suggesting that limbal stem cell deficiency (LSCD) was the reason behind corneal epithelial problems in ocular burns.[7]

The obvious implication of this new knowledge was whether LSCD could be treated by performing limbal transplantation?[7] Following successful preclinical animal trials,[8] Kenyon and Tseng in 1989 provided the proof-of-principle by describing successful corneal regeneration in patients with unilateral acute and chronic chemical burns following limbal autograft transplantation.[9] This technique involved removing as much as 6 clock hours of donor limbal tissue from healthy donor eyes and transplanting it on the recipient eyes after clearing the pathological pannus covering the cornea.[9] Although this technique was extremely effective, other groups who tried to replicate the results reported rare incidents of iatrogenic LSCD in the donor eyes.[10-12] In 1997, Pellegrini and associates proposed a way around this problem by developing a technique of culturing the limbal cells *ex vivo* in a laboratory to form a transplantable sheet of epithelium from less than 1 clock hour of donor limbal tissue.[13] Following this, several large clinical trials have established the safety and efficacy of autologous *ex vivo* cultivated limbal epithelial transplantation for the treatment of unilateral LSCD.[14-17]

### Advantages of Ex Vivo Cultivated Limbal Epithelial Transplantation

Although improving the safety of limbal transplantation was probably the driving force behind its development, this technique offers several other advantages as compared to conventional limbal transplantation (Fig. 1).

*Minimal donor tissue*: Since first described in 1997, cultivated limbal transplantation has been performed in hundreds of patients with LSCD and till date there are no reports of donor site complications.[14,15] The authors specifically looked at the donor eyes in 200 cases of

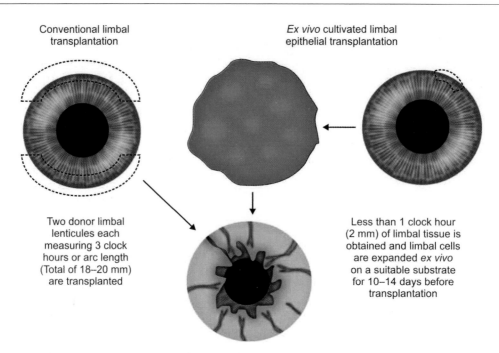

Conventional limbal
transplantation

*Ex vivo* cultivated limbal
epithelial transplantation

Two donor limbal
lenticules each
measuring 3 clock
hours or arc length
(Total of 18–20 mm)
are transplanted

Less than 1 clock hour
(2 mm) of limbal tissue is
obtained and limbal cells
are expanded *ex vivo*
on a suitable substrate
for 10–14 days before
transplantation

**Fig. 1:** This schematic diagram explains the essential difference in the technique of conventional limbal transplantation and *ex vivo* cultivated limbal epithelial transplantation. The conventional technique is called Conjunctival Limbal Autografting or CLAU when the donor tissue is obtained from the healthy fellow eye in patients with unilateral limbal stem cell deficiency (LSCD). The same technique is called Conjunctival Limbal Allografting (CLAL) or Kerato-Limbal Allografting (KLAL) when the donor tissue is obtained from living or cadaveric allogeneic donors, respectively

unilateral LSCD which underwent autologous cultivated limbal epithelial transplantation and noted that the donor-site epithelized within 2 weeks without complications.[17]

*Repeatability:* One or two repeat limbal biopsies can be safely obtained from the same donor eye if the primary procedure fails, because more than 90% of the limbus is left untouched by a single biopsy.[16,18] This is not possible in conventional limbal transplantation as the donor eye is not left with any limbal reserve.

*Early corneal epithelization:* Since a ready-made epithelial sheet is transplanted in cultivated limbal epithelial transplantation, corneal epithelization is almost immediate or is completed by the first week.[16-19] In conventional limbal transplantation, the entire cornea is epithelized only by 6 weeks.[19]

*Less surface inflammation:* Postoperative ocular surface inflammation subsides faster after cultivated limbal epithelial transplantation as compared to conventional limbal transplantation.[19]

*Less scarring:* Cultivated limbal transplantation is associated with less scarring on the recipient corneal surface and probably better visual recovery as compared to the conventional technique.[19]

*Amplification in number of transplanted stem cells:* Ex vivo cultivation results in increase in the number of limbal stem cells obtained by biopsy and this in turn can lead to better long-term survival of the graft.[14,15]

## INDICATIONS FOR AUTOLOGOUS LIMBAL TRANSPLANTATION

Any traumatic or inflammatory damage to the limbus can cause permanent functional damage to the limbal stem cells.[20,21] This leads to corneal epithelial instability, recurrent or persistent epithelial defects, invasion of the corneal surface by the surrounding opaque conjunctival tissue (conjunctivalization) and consequently severe visual loss.[21] The commonest indication of autologous limbal transplantation world over is unilateral ocular surface burns, due to chemical or thermal injury.[14,15] Earlier this procedure was performed both during the acute and chronic stages,[9] but it is presently indicated only in the chronic stage, after the ocular surface inflammation has subsided. The other rare indication is iatrogenic LSCD after multiple or extensive ocular surface surgery like excision of ocular surface squamous neoplasia (OSSN). LSCD due to Stevens Johnson syndrome (SJS), ocular cicatricial pemphigoid (OCP), severe allergic eye disease aniridia associated keratopathy have bilateral affliction and need either allogeneic limbal transplantation or keratoprosthesis surgery.[14,15] However, *ex vivo* cultivated autologous limbal epithelial transplantation can be performed in patients who have bilateral LSCD but with asymmetrical involvement having at least 1 clock hour of healthy limbus in either eye.[22]

## PREOPERATIVE CLINICAL ASSESSMENT AND COUNSELING

Selecting the proper cases is probably the most important determinant of the outcome of limbal transplantation. The first step is clinically assessing whether the affected eye has visual potential by performing simple macular function tests or electrophysiological testing. Additionally, young children developing unilateral blindness before the age of 8 years, fixing light poorly and with monocular deviation are likely to have dense amblyopia with poor visual potential. Limbal transplantation may still be performed in amblyopic eyes to provide cosmetic relief, but the poor visual prognosis must be explained to the patient or parents, as appropriate. As there is no objective way of accurately assessing ocular surface inflammation and since these eyes are heavily scarred and vascularized, some surgeons prefer to wait for 3–6 months after the acute event before performing limbal transplantation. Lid abnormalities like notches, improper closure, entropion and trichiasis also need to looked for and addressed. Eyes with severe dry eye disease, with a Schirmer's test 1 score of less than 10 mm at 5 minutes are unsuitable for this procedure and punctual occlusion may be needed prior to surgery. In summary, the ocular surface environment must be conducive for the limbal transplantation to succeed. Any cause which may inflict inflammatory damage on the grafted cells postoperatively need to be taken care of prior to planning limbal transplantation. The extent of corneal stromal scarring is also difficult to assess preoperatively and patients must be counseled that they may need additional surgery in the form of an anterior lamellar or penetrating keratoplasty (PK) for visual improvement despite a successful limbal transplantation. In the author's experience it is prudent to perform limbal and corneal transplantation as a two-stage rather than a single-stage procedure.[23]

## TECHNIQUE OF LIMBAL BIOPSY

A biopsy is taken from a healthy part of the limbus; a $2 \times 2$ mm piece of conjunctival epithelium with 1 mm into clear corneal stromal tissue at the limbus is dissected; conjunctiva is excised just behind the pigmented line (palisades of Vogt), and the limbal tissue that contained epithelial cells and a part of the corneal stroma is obtained.[24]

## TECHNIQUE OF LIMBAL CULTURE

Broadly there are two techniques of limbal cultivation, (1) The suspension culture where a cell suspension of the biopsied limbal tissue is prepared and spread over a suitable substrate; and (2) Explant culture where the limbal tissue is sectioned into smaller pieces and directly placed on the substrate without separating the epithelial cells from the stroma.[14,15] Additionally the constituents of the culture medium may or may not contain animal derived products or xenobiotic materials.[25] Xenogenic constituents of a limbal culture system can be in the form of murine feeder-cells, bovine serum, or animal derived growth factors.[25] To avoid the use of animal-derived products four groups,[26-28] including our own,[24] have independently developed completely xeno-free laboratory protocols of limbal culture.

In our technique,[24] the tissue is transported to the laboratory in human corneal epithelium (HCE) medium. HCE is composed of modified Eagle's medium/F12 medium (1:1) solution containing 10% (vol/vol) autologous serum (AS), 2mM l-glutamine, 100 U/ml penicillin, 100 µg/ml streptomycin, 2.5 µg/ml amphotericin B, 10 ng/ml human recombinant epidermal growth factor and 5 µg/ml human recombinant insulin. Under strict aseptic conditions, the donor limbal tissue is shredded into small pieces. Human amniotic membrane (hAM), prepared and preserved by our eye bank is used as a carrier. A $3 \times 4$ cm hAM sheet is de-epithelized using 0.25% recombinant trypsin and EDTA solution for 15 minutes. The shredded bits of limbal tissue are explanted over the center of de-epithelized hAM with the basement membrane side-up. A similar parallel culture is also prepared as a backup. A submerged explant culture system without a feeder-cell layer is used. We used the HCE medium to nurture the culture. The culture is incubated at 37°C with 5% $CO_2$ and 95% air. The growth is monitored daily under an inverted phase contrast microscope and the medium is changed every other day (Figs 2A to D and 3A to C). The culture is completed when a monolayer of the cells growing from the explants became confluent, typically in 10–14 days.

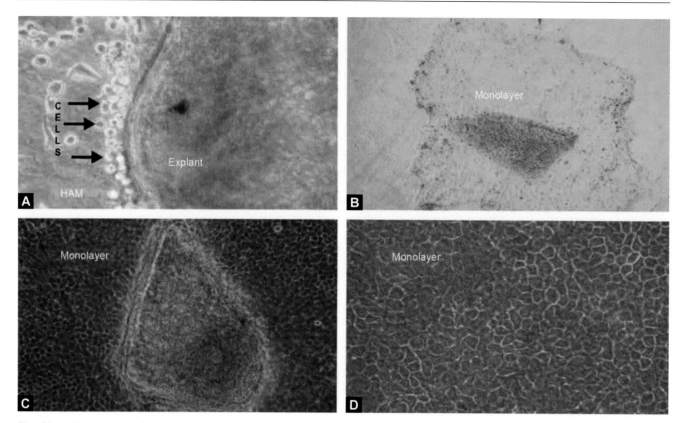

**Figs 2A to D:** Limbal cultures as seen under phase contrast microscope (Clockwise). (A) Cells proliferating from the periphery of the explant on day 2–3 (x200); (B) Monolayer of limbal cells on day 4–5 (x40); (C) Extension of monolayer through days 6–10 (x40); (D) Confluent monolayer on day 10–14 (x200); as observed under phase contrast microscope

## TECHNIQUE OF LIMBAL TRANSPLANTATION

Any symblepharon which prevented adequate separation of the lids is released to permit the insertion of a wire speculum (no additional surgery to treat the symblepharon is performed). A peritomy is performed and the corneal fibrovascular pannus is excised. If an impending or frank corneal perforation is noted at this stage a PK is performed prior to placing the limbal graft.[23] The hAM and monolayer of cultivated limbal epithelial cells is spread over the cornea, epithelial side up (See Video).[17,18] The graft is then secured to the peripheral cornea by interrupted, circumferential 10-0 nylon sutures and to the surrounding conjunctival edge by interrupted 8-0 polyglactin sutures. Alternately, using a sutureless technique, the graft is secured to underlying ocular surface with fibrin glue (TISSEEL™ Kit from Baxter AG, Austria) and the margins of the graft are tucked under the surrounding conjunctival edge. Bandage contact lenses are not applied at the end of surgery.

## POSTOPERATIVE MANAGEMENT

All patients receive 1% prednisolone acetate eyedrops eight times a day tapered to once a day in 35–42 days and 0.3% ciprofloxacin hydrochloride eyedrops four times a day for 1 week, in both the biopsied and transplanted eye. The latter are continued till the epithelial defect completely resolves. No systemic antibiotics or steroids are needed. Patients are examined on postoperative days 1, 7, 42 and at an interval of 90–180 days thereafter, as customized by the clinical appearance of the transplant. Each examination includes a complete history, visual acuity assessment with Snellen's charts, intraocular pressure measurement and detailed ocular examination with slit-lamp biomicroscopy (Figs 4A to H).

## CLINICAL OUTCOMES OF CULTIVATED LIMBAL TRANSPLANTATION

The techniques and outcomes of autologous cultivated limbal transplantation described by various groups are summarized in Table 1.[13,17,26-44] Success was defined

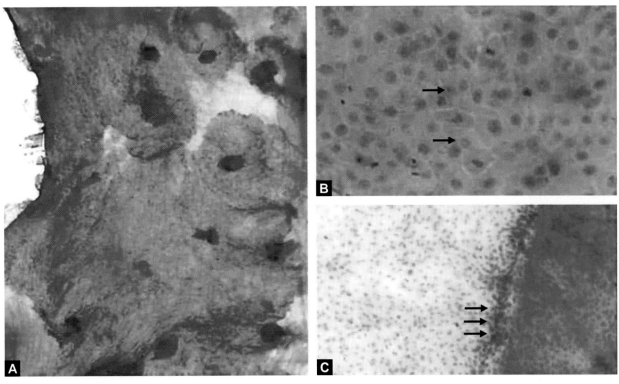

**Figs 3A to C:** (A) Whole mount preparation of the cultured limbal epithelial cells on naked eye examination revealing rings of pink darkly stained areas around the explants (arrows), (H&E); (B) Stained whole mounts as observed under microscope revealing a confluent monolayer of polygonal cells (H&E, x400); (C) which were seen originating from the edge of the explants (arrows) (H&E, x200)

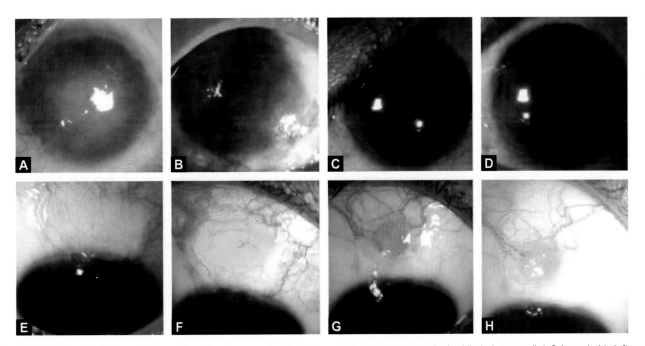

**Figs 4A to H:** Serial slit-lamp photographs of the donor and recipient eye of the same patient who had limbal stem cell deficiency in his left eye following lime burns. The top panel (A to D) shows (A) The recipient eye before surgery; (B) One month after surgery; (C) Three months and (D) 1 year after surgery. The serial images how that the clear, avascular and stable corneal epithelium is regenerated and maintained over time. The bottom panel (E to F) shows (E) The donor eye stained with sodium fluorescein at 1 day; (F) Five days; (G) Ten days and (H) Two weeks after limbal biopsy. The serial images show that by 2 weeks the limbus is completely epithelized with a resolving conjunctival epithelial defect clinically in most studies; a few studies additionally used impression cytology or symptom scoring. With our technique the hAM usually disappeared (it either disintegrates or is incorporated as a part of the corneal stroma) by 4 weeks and the recipient ocular surface stabilized by 6 weeks. The donor site completely epithelized without scarring within 2 weeks of limbal biopsy. Overall, the success rate of autologous cultivated limbal transplantation varied from 50% to 100% and a two-line improvement in visual acuity after cultivated limbal transplantation alone was seen in 22–100% cases (Table 1). More than 90% of failures occurred by the end of 1 year and more than half of these by 6 months after transplantation.[15,16]

Although on cursory review it appears that there is no clinical advantage that one culture technique holds over the other, comparing success rates among different culture techniques may be misleading as the indications for surgery, sample size and follow-up duration are variable among different studies. Shimakazi et al.[32] and Nakamura et al.[33] compared the explant and suspension culture techniques, finding no significant difference in the outcomes. It is noteworthy in this context that with similar indications for surgery, clinical criteria for success and follow-up Sangwan et al. (explant culture, 71%, 200 eyes)[17] Rama et al. (suspension culture, 68%, 107 eyes)[16] and Di Iorio et al. (suspension culture, 80%, 166 eyes)[38] reported similar and impressive success rates of cultivated limbal epithelial transplantation with mean follow-up ranging from 1.5 to almost 3 years and maximum follow-up of up to 8 years. It is noteworthy that of the various groups only Sangwan et al.[17] Kolli et al.[26] Di Girolamo et al.[27] and Zakaria et al.[28] described completely xeno-free techniques of culturing

**Table 1:** Techniques and outcomes of autologous cultivated limbal transplantation for unilateral limbal stem cell deficiency

| Author | Year | Culture Technique | Sub-strate | Culture Time | Eyes | Clinical Success (%) | 2-line visual gain (%) | Follow-up (years) Mean | Follow-up (years) Range |
|---|---|---|---|---|---|---|---|---|---|
| *Feeder-Free and Xeno-Free Cell Cultures* | | | | | | | | | |
| Sangwan et al.[17] | 2011 | Explant | hAM | 10–14 | 200 | 71 | 60.5 | 3 | 1–7.6 |
| Kolli et al.[26] | 2010 | Explant | hAM | 12–14 | 8 | 100 | 63 | 1.6 | 1–2.5 |
| Di Girolamo et al.[27] | 2009 | Explant | CL | 10 | 2 | 100 | 50 | 0.9 | 0.7–1.1 |
| *Feeder-Free but not Xeno-Free Cell Cultures* | | | | | | | | | |
| Barandan-Rafii et al.[29] | 2010 | Explant | hAM | 14 | 8 | 88 | 63 | 2.8 | 0.5–4 |
| Pauklin et al.[30] | 2010 | Explant | hAM | 14 | 30 | 77 | 73 | 2.4 | 0.8–6 |
| Shortt et al.[31] | 2008 | Suspension | hAM | 14–21 | 3 | 78 | 22 | 0.8 | 0.5–1.1 |
| Shimakazi et al.[32] | 2007 | Explant | hAM | 14.6 | 16 | 50 | 37.5 | 2.5 | 0.5–7.1 |
| Nakamura et al.[33] | 2006 | Explant | hAM | 15–16 | 2 | 100 | 67 | 1.2 | 0.5–1.6 |
| Sangwan et al.[34] | 2006 | Explant | hAM | 11–15 | 88 | 73 | 37 | 1.5 | 0.3–3.3 |
| Sangwan et al.[35] | 2003 | Explant | hAM | 10–14 | 2 | 100 | 50 | 1 | 1 |
| Grueterich et al.[36] | 2002 | Explant | hAM | 21 | 1 | 100 | 100 | 3.1 | 3.1 |
| Tsai et al.[37] | 2000 | Explant | hAM | 14–21 | 3 | 100 | 50 | 2 | 0.3–10 |
| *Neither Feeder-Free nor Xeno-Free Cell Cultures* | | | | | | | | | |
| Di Iorio et al.[38] | 2010 | Suspension | Fibrin | NA | 166 | 80 | NA | NA | NA |
| Rama et al.[16] | 2010 | Suspension | Fibrin | 14–16 | 107 | 68 | 54 | 2.9 | 1–10 |
| Gisoldi et al.[39] | 2010 | Suspension | Fibrin | 14–16 | 6 | 83 | 83 | 2 | 0.9–2.8 |
| Kawashima et al.[40] | 2007 | Explant | hAM | NA | 2 | 100 | 67 | 2.7 | 1.7–3.7 |
| Nakamura et al.[41] | 2004 | Explant | hAM | 23 | 1 | 100 | 100 | 1.6 | 1.6 |
| Rama et al.[42] | 2001 | Suspension | Fibrin | 14–16 | 18 | 74 | 33 | 1.5 | 1–2.2 |
| Schawb et al.[43] | 2000 | Suspension | hAM | 21–28 | 10 | 60 | 36 | 1.1 | 0.5–1.6 |
| Schawb et al.[44] | 1999 | Suspension | hAM | 28–35 | 17 | 76 | 16 | 0.9 | 0.2–2 |
| Pellegrini et al.[13] | 1997 | Suspension | 3T3s | 16–19 | 2 | 100 | 50 | NA | NA |

HAM: Human amniotic membrane; CL: Contact lens; NA: Data not available

limbal epithelium while others used at least one or more animal derived products for culture. None of the studies reported any donor-site complications.

Around 18–38% of all eyes treated with autologous cultivated limbal epithelial transplantation also needed a PK for visual improvement.[14,15] The authors have found that adopting a staged approach of performing limbal transplantation first, followed at least 6 weeks later by PK resulted in better clinical outcomes as compared to a single-staged approach of combined limbal transplantation and PK (Figs 5A and B).[23] Therefore, PK and limbal transplantation should not be combined unless PK is absolutely unavoidable as in the case of an impending or frank corneal perforation discovered after removal of the vascular pannus. The authors also found that a repeat limbal biopsy from the healthy eye followed by *ex vivo* cultivation and transplantation of the cultured cells on the affected eye can successfully restore the ocular surface and improve vision in at least two-thirds of cases with failure of therapy with primary autologous cultivated limbal epithelial transplantation.[18] Therefore, combining the efficacy of primary (71%) and repeat autologous cultivated limbal epithelial transplantation (67%) almost 90% of cases of unilateral LSCD can be treated successfully without any adverse impact on the healthy donor eye.[17,18]

## ▶ CONCLUSIONS

In terms of clinical efficacy there is hardly any difference between conventional and cultivated autologous limbal transplantation as treatment options for unilateral LSCD

(Table 2).[9-11,45-52] Proponents of *ex vivo* cultivation cite the safety of the donor eye as the main advantage of their technique. However, *ex vivo* cultivation requires specialized expertise and a licensed (by the Human Tissue Authority in the United Kingdom) laboratory. It can take up to 2 weeks to generate a sheet of desired dimensions, and it is expensive, costing approximately 10,300 Pounds Sterling or 12,000 Euros at current exchange rates for cultivation alone.[46] Furthermore, many groups practicing this technique continue to use xenobiotic materials for cell culture (Table 1). Not surprisingly, conventional limbal transplantations are still widely performed worldwide and cultivated limbal transplantation is restricted to few select centers around the globe.[14,15] There are, however, certain clinical scenarios where cultivated limbal epithelial transplantation can be a superior alternative to conventional limbal transplantation. For example, in patients with bilateral but asymmetrical LSCD, even 1 clock hour of healthy limbal area in either eye can be utilized to restore the ocular surface and improve vision in both eyes.[22]

The only study that compared conventional and cultivated limbal transplantation reported slower epithelization rate, prolonged ocular surface inflammation and significantly more scarring with the conventional technique.[53] However, for cultivated limbal epithelial transplantation to emerge as the more popular technique of treating unilateral LSCD the economic and logistic barriers of cell culture have to be overcome first. Moreover, the actual mechanism by which limbal transplantation works is still debated. It is unclear

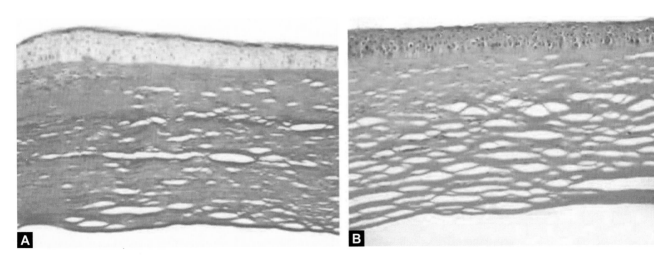

**Figs 5A and B:** (A) Periodic Acid Schiff stained and Hematoxylin and Eosin stained sections of corneal buttons obtained from eyes undergoing penetrating keratoplasty; (B) Deep anterior lamellar keratoplasty, 1 year after successful *ex vivo* cultivated limbal epithelial transplantation for unilateral limbal stem cell deficiency. The indication for keratoplasty in both cases was residual corneal stromal scarring obscuring the visual axis. Both stained sections show a multilayered corneal epithelium with absence of superficial vessels or goblet cells

**Table 2:** Clinical outcomes of conjunctival limbal autografting or conventional limbal transplantation for eyes with unilateral limbal stem cell deficiency

| Author | Year | Eyes | Clinical Success (%) | 2-line Vision gain (%) | Complications | Follow-up (months) | |
|---|---|---|---|---|---|---|---|
| | | | | | | Mean | Range |
| Miri et al.[45] | 2011 | 25 | NA | NA | Filamentary keratitis (4) | 41 | 3–127 |
| Miri et al.[46] | 2010 | 12 | 100 | 81.3 | None | 46 | 12–120 |
| Santos et al.[47] | 2005 | 10 | 80 | 61 | None | 33 | NA |
| Ozdemir et al.[48] | 2004 | 15 | 87 | 80 | None | 13.9 | 3–24 |
| Dua et al.[49] | 2000 | 6 | 100 | 83 | Filmentary keratitis (1) | 18.8 | 14–31 |
| Rao et al.[50] | 1999 | 16 | 94 | 82 | None | 19.3 | 3–45 |
| Basti et al.[10] | 1999 | 3 | 100 | 100 | LSCD in donor eye (1) | NA | 9–15 |
| Frucht-Pery et al.[51] | 1998 | 9 | 100 | 100 | None | NA | 15–60 |
| Tan et al.[11] | 1996 | 9 | 77 | 77 | LSCD in donor eye (1) | 27.1 | 2.5–46 |
| Morgan et al.[52] | 1996 | 6 | 83 | 83 | Donor site micro-perforation (1) | NA | 3–24 |
| Kenyon et al.[9] | 1989 | 26 | 77 | 65 | None | 18 | 2–45 |

NA: Data not available; LSCD: Limbal Stem Cell Deficiency.

whether this therapy replenishes the stem cell reserve[16] or revives the surviving stem cells by improving the micro-environment.[14] It is also widely accepted that the cause of failure of limbal transplantation is multi-factorial and poorly understood.[16,17] In the large clinical trials Rama et al. and Sangwan et al. investigated the cause for failure and found that eyes with more severe injuries and postoperative complications were more likely to fail.[16,17] Rama et al. also found that the proportion of holoclone forming cells (actual stem cells) in culture needed to be more than 3% of the total cell population for the transplant to have higher chances of success.[16]

In summary, the last two decades have witnessed tremendous progress in the understanding of ocular surface disease due to corneal burns and this has in turn led to therapeutic innovations, at the cutting edge of which stands *ex vivo* cultivated limbal epithelial transplantation. Stem cell based therapy for LSCD has already benefitted hundreds of patients worldwide and continuous research and medical development in this field holds promise for an even more exciting future.

## ❧ REFERENCES

1. Zirm E. Eine erfolgreiche totale Keratoplastik. Albercht von Graefes Acrh Ophthalmol. 1906;64:580-93.
2. Armitage WJ, Tullo AB, Larkin DF. The first successful full-thickness corneal transplant: a commentary on Eduard Zirm's landmark paper of 1906. Br J Ophthalmol. 2006;90(10):1222-3.
3. Brown SI, Bloomfield SE, Pearce DB. Follow-up report on transplantation of the alkali burned cornea. Am J Ophthalmol.1974;77(4):538-42.
4. Thoft RA. Conjunctival transplantation as an alternative to keratoplasty. Ophthalmology. 1979;86(6):1084-92.
5. Thoft RA, Friend J. The X, Y, Z hypothesis of corneal epithelial maintenance. Invest Ophthalmol Vis Sci. 1983;24(10):1442-3.
6. Schermer A, Galvin S, Sun TT. Differentiation-related expression of a major 64K corneal keratin in vivo and in culture suggests limbal location of corneal epithelial stem cells. J Cell Biol. 1986;103(1):49-62.
7. Cotsarelis G, Cheng SZ, Dong G, et al. Existence of slow-cycling limbal epithelial basal cells that can be preferentially stimulated to proliferate: implications on epithelial stem cells. Cell. 1989;57(2):201-9.
8. Tsai RJ, Sun TT, Tseng SC. Comparison of limbal and conjunctival autograft transplantation in corneal surface reconstruction in rabbits. Ophthalmology. 1990;97(4):446-55.
9. Kenyon KR, Tseng SC. Limbal autograft transplantation for ocular surface disorders. Ophthalmology. 1989;96(5):709-22.
10. Basti S, Mathur U. Unusual intermediate-term outcome in three cases of limbal autograft transplantation. Ophthalmology. 1999;106:958-63.
11. Tan DT, Ficker LA, Buckley RJ. Limbal transplantation. Ophthalmology. 1996;103(1):29-36.
12. Jenkins C, Tuft S, Liu C, et al. Limbal transplantation in the management of chronic contact-lens-associated epitheliopathy. Eye(Lond). 1993;7:629-33.
13. Pellegrini G, Traverso CE, Franzi AT, et al. Long-term restoration of damaged corneal surfaces with autologous cultivated corneal epithelium. Lancet. 1997;349(9057):990-3.
14. Shortt AJ, Secker GA, Notara MD, et al. Transplantation of ex vivo cultured limbal epithelial stem cells: a review of techniques and clinical results. Surv Ophthalmol. 2007;52(5):483-502.
15. Baylis O, Figueiredo F, Henein C, et al. Ahmad S.13 years of cultured limbal epithelial cell therapy: A review of the outcomes. J Cell Biochem. 2011;112(4):993-1002.

16. Rama P, Matuska S, Paganoni G, et al. Limbal stem-cell therapy and long-term corneal regeneration. N Engl J Med. 2010;363(2):147-55.

17. Sangwan VS, Basu S, Vemuganti GK, et al. Clinical outcomes of xeno-free autologous cultivated limbal epithelial transplantation: a 10-year study. Br J Ophthalmol. 2011;95(11): 1525-29.

18. Basu S, Ali MH, Sangwan VS. Clinical Outcomes of Repeat Autologous Cultivated Limbal Epithelial Transplantation for Ocular Surface Burns. Am J Ophthalmol. 2011.

19. Ang LP, Sotozono C, Koizumi N, et al. A comparison between cultivated and conventional limbal stem cell transplantation for Stevens-Johnson syndrome. Am J Ophthalmol. 2007;143 (1):178-80.

20. Tseng SC. Concept and application of limbal stem cells. Eye. 1989;3:141-57.

21. Dua HS, Saini JS, Azuara-Blanco A, et al. Limbal stem cell deficiency: concept, aetiology, clinical presentation, diagnosis and management. Indian J Ophthalmol. 2000;48(2):83-92.

22. Sangwan VS, Vemuganti GK, Iftekhar G, et al. Use of autologous cultured limbal and conjunctival epithelium in a patient with severe bilateral ocular surface disease induced by acid injury: a case report of unique application. Cornea. 2003;22(5):478-81.

23. Basu S, Mohamed A, Chaurasia S, et al. Clinical outcomes of penetrating keratoplasty after autologous cultivated limbal epithelial transplantation for ocular surface burns. Am J Ophthalmol. 2011;152(6):917-24.

24. Mariappan I, Maddileti S, Savy S, et al. In vitro culture and expansion of human limbal epithelial cells. Nat Protoc. 2010; 5 (8):1470-9.

25. Schwab IR, Johnson NT, Harkin DG. Inherent risks associated with manufacture of bioengineered ocular surface tissue. Arch Ophthalmol. 2006;124(12):1734-40.

26. Kolli S, Ahmad S, Lako M, et al. Successful clinical implementation of corneal epithelial stem cell therapy for treatment of unilateral limbal stem cell deficiency. Stem Cells. 2010;28 (3):597-610.

27. Di Girolamo N, Bosch M, Zamora K, et al. A contact lens-based technique for expansion and transplantation of autologous epithelial progenitors for ocular surface reconstruction. Transplantation. 2009;87(10):1571-8.

28. Zakaria N, Koppen C, Van Tendeloo V, et al. Standardized limbal epithelial stem cell graft generation and transplantation. Tissue Eng Part C Methods. 2010;16(5):921-7.

29. Baradaran-Rafii A, Ebrahimi M, Kanavi MR, et al. Midterm outcomes of autologous cultivated limbal stem cell transplantation with or without penetrating keratoplasty. Cornea. 2010;29:502-9.

30. Pauklin M, Fuchsluger TA, Westekemper H, et al. Midterm results of cultivated autologous and allogeneic limbal epithelial transplantation in limbal stem cell deficiency. Dev Ophthalmol. 2010;45:57-70.

31. Shortt AJ, Secker GA, Rajan MS, et al. Ex vivo expansion and transplantation of limbal epithelial stem cells. Ophthalmology. 2008;115(11):1989-97.

32. Shimazaki J, Higa K, Morito F, et al. Factors influencing outcomes in cultivated limbal epithelial transplantation for chronic cicatricial ocular surface disorders. Am J Ophthalmol. 2007;143(6):945-53.

33. Nakamura T, Inatomi T, Sotozono C, et al. Transplantation of autologous serum-derived cultivated corneal epithelial equivalents for the treatment of severe ocular surface disease. Ophthalmology. 2006;113(10):1765-72.

34. Sangwan VS, Matalia HP, Vemuganti GK, et al. Clinical outcome of autologous cultivated limbal epithelium transplantation. Indian J Ophthalmol. 2006;54(1):29-34.

35. Sangwan VS, Vemuganti GK, Singh S, et al. Successful reconstruction of damaged ocular outer surface in humans using limbal and conjunctival stem cell culture methods. Biosci Rep. 2003;23(4):169-74.

36. Grueterich M, Espana EM, Touhami A, et al. Phenotypic study of a case with successful transplantation of ex vivo expanded human limbal epithelium for unilateral total limbal stem cell deficiency. Ophthalmology. 2002;109(8):1547-52.

37. Tsai RJ, Li LM, Chen JK. Reconstruction of damaged corneas by transplantation of autologous limbal epithelial cells. N Engl J Med. 2000;343(2):86-93.

38. Di Iorio E, Ferrari S, Fasolo A, et al. Techniques for culture and assessment of limbal stem cell grafts. Ocul Surf. 2010;8(3): 146-153.

39. Colabelli Gisoldi RA, Pocobelli A, Villani CM, et al. Evaluation of molecular markers in corneal regeneration by means of autologous cultures of limbal cells and keratoplasty. Cornea. 2010;29:715-22.

40. Kawashima M, Kawakita T, Satake Y, et al. Phenotypic study after cultivated limbal epithelial transplantation for limbal stem cell deficiency. Arch Ophthalmol. 2007;125(10):1337-44.

41. Nakamura T, Inatomi T, Sotozono C, et al. Successful primary culture and autologous transplantation of corneal limbal epithelial cells from minimal biopsy for unilateral severe ocular surface disease. Acta Ophthalmol Scand. 2004;82(4):468-71.

42. Rama P, Bonini S, Lambiase A, et al. Autologous fibrin-cultured limbal stem cells permanently restore the corneal surface of patients with total limbal stem cell deficiency. Transplantation. 2001;72(9):1478-85.

43. Schwab IR. Cultured corneal epithelia for ocular surface disease. Trans Am Ophthalmol Soc. 1999;97:891-986.

44. Schwab IR, Reyes M, Isseroff RR. Successful transplantation of bioengineered tissue replacements in patients with ocular surface disease. Cornea. 2000;19(4):421-6.

45. Miri A, Said DG, Dua HS. Donor Site Complications in Autolimbal and Living-Related Allolimbal Transplantation. Ophthalmology. 2011;118(7):1265-71.

46. Miri A, Al-Deiri B, Dua HS. Long-term outcomes of autolimbal and allolimbal transplants. Ophthalmology. 2010;117(6): 1207-13.

47. Santos MS, Gomes JA, Hofling-Lima AL, et al. Survival analysis of conjunctival limbal grafts and amniotic membrane transplantation in eyes with total limbal stem cell deficiency. Am J Ophthalmol. 2005;140(2):223-30.

CHAPTER **78**

48. Ozdemir O, Tekeli O, Ornek K, et al. Limbal autograft and allograft transplantations in patients with corneal burns. Eye (Lond). 2004;18(3):241-8.

49. Dua HS, Azuara-Blanco A. Autologous limbal transplantation in patients with unilateral corneal stem cell deficiency. Br J Ophthalmol. 2000;84(3):273-8.

50. Rao SK, Rajagopal R, Sitalakshmi G, et al. Limbal allografting from related live donors for corneal surface reconstruction. Ophthalmology. 1999;106(4):822-8.

51. Frucht-Pery J, Siganos CS, Solomon A, et al. Limbal cell autograft transplantation for severe ocular surface disorders. Graefes Arch Clin Exp Ophthalmol. 1998;236(8):582-7.

52. Morgan S, Murray A. Limbal autotransplantation in the acute and chronic phases of severe chemical injuries. Eye (Lond). 1996;10(Pt 3):349-54.

53. Ang LP, Sotozono C, Koizumi N, et al. A comparison between cultivated and conventional limbal stem cell transplantation for Stevens-Johnson syndrome. Am J Ophthalmol. 2007;143:178-80.

# Modern Eye Banking: Advances and Challenges

*Jon A Konti, Prashant Garg, John J Requard, Jonathan H Lass*

## ⊁ HISTORY OF EYE BANKING

Restoring vision by replacing an opaque cornea with a clear cornea was described well over two centuries ago in France by Pellier de Quengsy in 1789.[1] Over the next century, experiments with animal corneas were performed and it was realized that homologous tissue was essential for grafts to remain clear. In 1906, Eduard Zirm performed the first successful human corneal transplant that demonstrated an improvement in the patient's vision.[1] Another half of a century would then pass after Zirm's initial work before corneal transplantation would become a routine procedure. As the procedure gained in popularity and success, it was evident that an organized system would soon be needed in order to procure, process and distribute donor corneas.[2]

In 1935, one of the most important discoveries that led to the development of eye banking was demonstrated by Filatov of Odessa, Ukraine. He demonstrated the applicability of donor tissue that was obtained postmortem.[3] The way was paved with this advance for the development of the first eye bank models in the United States. In 1944, Dr R Townley Paton founded the Eye Bank for Sight Restoration in New York with the help of his colleagues, as well as Lions Club members, and the Manhattan Eye and Ear Infirmary.[2,4] He began by obtaining eye tissue from Sing Sing Penitentiary prisoners that had just been executed, but soon realized that living persons instead could agree to give their eyes upon death to benefit the living.[4]

Earlier eye banks had been created in other countries shortly before this, but modern eye banking from Dr Paton's efforts in the 1940s helped establish the principles of eye banking as they exist today.[2] In this early period of eye banking, the entire eyeball was stored at 4–5°C in a glass bottle that contained wetted gauze, a form of so-called moist chamber storage. This allowed for only very short storage times of no more than 48 hours and mandated grafting as soon as possible after tissue became available.[2] In 1974, this practice changed with the introduction of a cold storage technique developed by McCarey and Kaufman in which the isolated cornea with scleral rim was stored in a culture medium at 4°C, suitable for transplantation up to 72 hours from death. No longer would the donor cornea after retrieval from a morgue have to be immediately transplanted as soon as possible after death or the patient have to be admitted to the hospital while awaiting the availability of a donor cornea.[2]

The American Academy of Ophthalmology and Otolaryngology realized the need to organize eye banks as their numbers increased throughout the United States. They formed an eye banking subcommittee to address issues of standardization of practice. The subcommittee's work led to the creation in 1961 of the Eye Bank Association of American (EBAA).[5] It began with only 31 members whose goal was to standardize eye banking practices. Regulation of eye banking was largely controlled by the EBAA in a self-regulated manner until 1988, when it became regulated by Health Care Financing Administration (HCFA) under the Clinical Laboratories Improvement Act (CLIA). However, 5 years later in 1993, eye banking came under the oversight of the United States Food and Drug Administration (FDA), which was consistent with the ideals of the EBAA.[5]

## ▶ GROWTH AND TRENDS IN TISSUE UTILIZATION

In the late 1960's there were 6,000 eye donations a year. By 2008 the EBAA had grown to encompass 85-member banks with 95,000 total tissue recoveries in that year alone, with approximately 52,500 distributed for keratoplasty nationally and internationally.[2,6] In 2010, the EBAA's statistical report included information for 79 United States member eye banks and reported 110,630 total tissue recoveries.[6] This was an increase of 3.1% from 107,289 in 2009, and a 13.1% increase over 2008's figures listed above. The total tissue distributed in 2010 was 92,521 (includes full-thickness and lamellar keratoplasty corneal tissue, as well as scleral and research tissue).[6] In 2010, a total of 42,642 corneas were distributed for keratoplasty including those processed for endothelial keratoplasty (EK), essentially unchanged from the 42,606 distributed in 2009.[6]

The greatest and most exciting change over the past decade has been the shift toward EK. The 2010 report indicated that 19,159 EKs were performed in 2010, which was a 5.1% increase over the 18,221 performed in 2009, and a 9.7% increase over the 17,468 EK's in 2008.[6] Only 1,429 EK's were reported nationwide in 2005.[6,7] In contrast, penetrating keratoplasties (PK's) have decreased over that same interval, from 51,500 to 32,500.[2] The 2010 EBAA statistical report indicated that 21,970 PK's were performed that year.[6] This was a 5.6% decrease from 23,269 in 2009, and a remarkable 32% decrease from 32,524 PK's reported nationally in 2008. Their report showed that the number of PK's for corneal disease in the United States has declined for the 5th straight year in a row from a high of 42,063 in 2005.[6]

The trend toward EK has also occurred internationally. The 2010 EBAA statistical report showed that 16,629 (28% of total 59,271 distributed) corneas were exported internationally that year, compared with 17,178 (29%) corneas exported in 2009, but still a significant increase over 10,835 (21%) in 2008.[6] PK's reported by nine international EBAA eye banks decreased 5% to 2,931 in 2010 compared to a 3% decrease in 2009 (to 3,088 from 3,194 in 2008).[6] EK procedures increased 38% to 1,540 in 2010. There was also a large (41%) increase in these procedures from 2008 to 2009 (from 786 to 1,112).[6]

## ▶ DONOR TISSUE SELECTION

The EBAA in the United States sets the criteria for donor selection. These criteria are in place to increase graft success rate and prevent disease transmission. The success rate is determined by healthy corneal tissue, which depends on a functional endothelium and absence of corneal pathology.

### Donor Age

The age criteria differ from one eye bank to another and from one surgeon to another and are not clearly defined by the EBAA. Besides the fact that corneal tissue from very young donors poses technical challenges during transplantation, there is no lower age limit for corneal donors.[8] Elasticity, diameter and thinness can be problems encountered when using young donor tissue.[9] Flexible corneal tissue can make suture placement difficult and the tissue may fold on itself. However, flexibility of the cornea is helpful for assuming normal curvature and for more rapid visual recovery after the surgery.[10] A small diameter cornea can make trephination difficult and it will be more prone to eccentric trephination that might lead to inclusion of sclera and possibly conjunctiva. Thin corneal tissue can make it difficult to align the donor Descemet's membrane with that of the host. It is also easy to perforate a thin donor cornea during suturing, that may lead to a wound leak and hence more chance for shallow anterior chamber and infection postoperatively.[10] Superficial sutures may cut through the tissue. However, the younger the tissue the higher the endothelial cell density (ECD) which may be of benefit for long-term graft survival.[11,12]

Corneal tissue from donors younger than 3 months is associated with a high myopic shift postoperatively because of the steepness of the cornea.[9,13] On the other hand, a study by Beltmonte and colleagues had found that corneal tissue from newborn donors led to hyperopia rather than myopia and this was due to rapid healing of the tissue which led to early loosening of the sutures.[14] Corneal tissue from newborn donors is also associated with higher risk of rejection, which is believed to be due to a higher density of endothelial cells.[14] Therefore, the use of a newborn donor cornea remains questionable due to these unpredictable refractive and immunological responses.[14]

Corneal surgeons usually accept tissue up to 75 years old.[8] However, as long as the ECD is within an acceptable limit and there are no endothelial abnormalities, theoretically there is no upper age limit. The Cornea Donor Study Group showed that the 5-year graft survival after PK at moderate risk for failure due to endothelial dysfunction was similar using corneas from donors greater than or equal to 66.0 years and donors less than 66.0 years. There was an 86%

success rate in both groups, confirming the value of the use of older donor tissue in corneal transplantation.[15] However, since endothelial cell loss was somewhat greater in the older donor age group (75% vs 69%) at 5 years,[16] the study has now been extended to 10 years to see if this difference in cell loss translates to greater graft failures in the older donors with longer follow-up.

## Infectious Diseases

As with any other organ or tissue transplantation, there is always the concern for transmission of infectious diseases. The EBAA, in conjunction with the United States FDA, has developed strict guidelines to be followed to help minimize this risk. A broad overview of the potential viruses, bacteria, fungi, *Acanthamoeba*, as well as prions that have been known to be transmitted or have theoretical implications for transmission from donor to host is discussed within this section.

Table 1 shows the United States FDA donor eligibility blood tests that are required for tissue transplantation.

### Viruses

Rabies virus has been proven to be transmitted to the host from corneal donor tissue.[17,18] Therefore, death from possible central nervous system (CNS) cause of unknown etiology is an EBAA exclusion criterion for corneal donation in order to prevent the potential for transmission of rabies.[19,20] Hepatitis B virus transmission has been reported twice following PK and in both cases the donors were indeed positive for hepatitis B surface antigen.[10] There are no documented cases of hepatitis C transmission after corneal transplantation.[10] HIV, herpes simplex virus (HSV) and cytomegalovirus (CMV) are possibly transmitted via corneal transplantation,

**Table 1:** United States FDA requires donor blood to be screened for HIV, Hepatitis B and C viruses, as well as Syphilis

Donor blood tests currently required by the United States FDA

*Human immunodeficiency virus (HIV)*:
Antibodies to HIV Type 1 and Type 2 (anti-HIV 1 and 2)
Nucleic acid test for HIV Type 1

*Hepatitis B virus*:
Hepatitis B surface antigen (HBsAg)
Antibodies to hepatitis B core antigen (anti-HBc, IgM and IgG)

*Hepatitis C virus*:
Antibodies to hepatitis C virus (anti-HCV)
Nucleic acid test for hepatitis C virus

*Treponema pallidum*:
Syphilis serology
Rapid plasma regain (RPR), FTA-ABS

but has never been proven. HIV has been transmitted by kidney transplantation, but there have been no reports of transmission via corneal transplantation.[10] However, donors with a high risk for HIV infection should be excluded as donors for corneal transplantation. If indicated, donors should be tested for HIV by enzyme-linked immunosorbent assay (ELISA) and Western blot.[19,21] Removing the epithelial layer from the donor cornea by the surgeon during transplantation has been advocated by some authors.[22] More recently, polymerase chain reaction (PCR) testing of blood of the donors for HIV has been used.[11,23]

Herpes simplex virus has only been proven to be transmitted by corneal transplantation in animals.[11] Cases of new HSV infection have been reported after corneal transplantation, but it remains unclear whether these were simply new infections as opposed to reactivation of latent viral infections within the donor corneas. PCR has also been used in more recent times to detect HSV in corneal tissue.[10] Varicella-zoster virus (HZV), on the other hand, has not been associated with transmission during corneal transplantation.[10]

Cytomegalovirus is well-known to be transmitted by major organ transplantation. CMV has been recovered from keratocytes of corneal tissue, but CMV has not been implicated in causing any clinical disease after corneal transplantation.[24]

Reye's syndrome is contraindicated by EBAA for tissue use because of suspected viral etiology.[19,20] Tissues from patients with diseases of possible viral etiology should never be used for transplantation. Examples of these diseases are subacute sclerosing panencephalitis (SSPE) and progressive multifocal leukoencephalopathy (PML).[10] Leukemia, lymphoma and Hodgkin's disease may all be caused by viruses as well. Further, the increased risks of opportunistic infections in these patients due to having inherent compromised immunity are the reasons to avoid using tissues from these patients.[11,19]

### Prions

A prion is a host-encoded protein that has been altered via an unknown mechanism. Prions are thought to be a cause for transmissible neurodegenerative disorders. These diseases remain very poorly understood. The patient usually dies within a year from CNS damage after contracting the disease. Creutzfeldt-Jacob Disease (CJD) is a well-known example of a disease caused by prions. Only one case of CJD has been proven to be transmitted by corneal transplantation.[10] Because it is difficult to screen patients for CJD, the EBAA does not accept any corneal donations from patients, who received human pituitary-derived growth hormone, which has been associated with the disease.[19,20]

### Bacteria

A positive culture from the donor rim is associated with a significantly higher incidence of infection, and according to the EBAA, corneal-scleral rim cultures can be obtained before or at the time of surgery.[10,25] Corneas from patients who died from pneumonia led to Streptococcus pneumoniae endophthalmitis in two known cases described in one study.[11] Tissue derived from donors with septicemia has led to *Pseudomonas aeruginosa* in the corneal donor tissue.[10] Sepsis in a donor should be regarded as high risk and it is better to avoid using this tissue.[20] It is important to note that the antibiotics in storage media are ineffective at 4°C and therefore the importance of warming the tissue back to room temperature prior to transplantation cannot be overemphasized.

### Fungi

Fungal infections transmitted by corneal transplantation are becoming an increasingly important issue. This is mainly because of the increased number of publications in the peer-reviewed literature on fungal infections following corneal transplantation over the last decade.[26] In reality, the rate of reported fungal infections following corneal transplantation has remained essentially stable over the past 6 years according to the EBAA.[26] In late 2010, a subcommittee was formed by the EBAA Medical Advisory Board to investigate the incidence of fungal infections following corneal transplantation. They also wanted to evaluate the need for supplementation of storage media with an antifungal agent. The subcommittee reviewed a 4-year period in which a total of 221,664 corneal transplants were performed. Over this time period, a total of 34 cases of fungal keratitis and/or endophthalmitis were reported.[26] This represents 63% of all reported infections occurring after corneal transplantation over this period of review. In 31 of the 34 reported cases, the diagnosis was based on a positive culture result from the donor and/or the recipient.[26] Candida species were the only fungi identified in either the donor or host cultures.[26] There is a perception amongst corneal surgeons that fungal infections occur more commonly after EK than after PK.[26] While the overall incidence of fungal infection transmitted by donor corneal tissue is very low, the review performed

by the subcommittee did indeed confirm this perception. They found that the number of eyes that developed fungal infection after EK (0.022%) was nearly twice that after PK (0.012%).[26] It is noteworthy to mention here that no association was found between fungal infection after EK and whether the tissue was prepared by the eye bank technician or the surgeon.[26]

Another very important finding in this large study was that approximately three-quarters of the mates of corneas that produced fungal infection in the recipient were themselves fungal culture positive, and two-thirds of these mates would themselves go on to result in fungal infection in a recipient as well. The source eye bank is therefore required to notify the surgeon who transplants the mate of a donor cornea that is known to be fungal culture positive.[27]

Several important questions were raised from this review, most importantly was whether an antifungal agent should be added to storage media. Ritterband and colleagues demonstrated that the supplementation of voriconazole (100 mg/ml) to Optisol GS reduces the rate of positive fungal rim cultures.[28] Further studies revealed, however, that voriconazole added to Optisol GS only suppressed fungal growth for 6–7 days.[26] This complicates matters because it means that the voriconazole would have to be added to the medium at the time of tissue procurement as opposed to at the time of production of the Optisol GS medium.[26] The safety of adding voriconazole to Optisol GS would need to be thoroughly evaluated as well. Ritterband and colleagues also showed Optisol GS with voriconazole (100 mg/ml) supplementation did not decrease endothelial cell viability, but they only used two pairs of corneal donor buttons, and obviously more extensive studies would have to be carried out before supplementation with an antifungal could be approved.[28]

It is also important to note that cryptococcal infection can be transmitted through corneal transplantation as well.[10,11]

### Protozoan (Acanthamoeba)

Only two cases of Acanthamoeba keratitis transmitted by corneal transplantation have been reported in the literature.[10,11]

## Noninfectious Corneal Pathology

### Neoplastic Disease

Retinoblastoma has been transmitted from the donor corneal tissue to the recipient in one known case.[10] That is the only known case reported that involved transferring a neoplastic disease through corneal transplantation.[11] Wagoner and coworkers found no evidence of transmission of neoplastic disease through corneal transplantation in their study.[29] Taking a conservative approach, the recommendation by the EBAA is to avoid use of such tissue.[19]

### Local Corneal Diseases

Local corneal diseases can theoretically be transmitted from donor to host through corneal transplantation.[10] Appropriate screening can usually identify such cases, but subtle diseases can be easily missed on routine screening. For example, early stages of keratoconus, as well as excimer laser-treated (LASIK/PRK) donor corneas may be missed.[10] Corneas with a genetic predisposition for Fuchs' endothelial corneal dystrophy may be transplanted and then later may develop changes associated with advanced Fuchs'.[11] However, these cases are likely very rare.

## ❧ TISSUE RETRIEVAL

### Pre-removal Measures

Hospitals usually refer potential donors to eye banks at the times of their death or the eye bank may be notified by an organ procurement agency since many states mandate the hospital to call only one agency to notify about a death and possible organ(s) donation.[10] The eye bank gets the consent for eye tissue removal, which is usually given by the donor, next of kin or the medical examiner.[25] When the bank receives the donor, the donor's head should be elevated to reduce factors that can affect the cornea during the postmortem period.[25] This also decreases swelling of periorbital tissues, which aids in reconstruction of the orbit by funeral home directors. The donor's eyes should be kept closed and the whole body should be cooled by refrigeration or at least ice packs should be placed on the eyes for cooling.[11]

### Donor Evaluation and Physical Inspection

The cause of death and donor's complete history, including medical and social history, should be completely reviewed before tissue retrieval.[30] Eye banks should also get autopsy information that may provide additional insight as to factors that may preclude obtaining eye tissue.[30] The eye bank technician should examine the ocular tissue with a slit lamp or penlight. They should also examine the whole body for evidence of intravenous drug abuse, tattoos, Kaposi's sarcoma, and any body piercings which can all suggest high risk for HIV, hepatitis B or C.[10]

## Blood Sample

Serology tests are performed for HIV, hepatitis and syphilis on all donors.[11] Some eye banks may require additional testing to be performed. According to a study by Challine and colleagues, cadaveric donors should not be sampled more than 12 hours after death.[31] This is because after this period the cadaveric serum will be of low quality and can yield high false-positive results.[31]

## Enucleation

The enucleation should be done by an eye bank technician or trained personnel and should be performed under aseptic conditions. Care should be given to prevent corneal endothelial damage during eye removal. Before the procedure 0.9% normal saline and antibiotic drops should be irrigated over the eye.[25] The eye is prepped in the usual fashion as for any typical eye surgery. The enucleator scrubs just as if this were any other sterile procedure. A speculum is then introduced between the lids, using caution to avoid creating a corneal abrasion. The conjunctiva around the cornea is opened at 360°. The conjunctiva and Tenon's capsule are separated from the sclera using a blunt dissection technique.[10] All the muscles are hooked and then disinserted. The optic nerve is localized and then cut.[25] Care should be taken not to perforate the sclera at any point of the procedure, as this will lead to collapse of the globe.[25] The globe is then irrigated with balanced salt solution (BSS) and antibiotics after placing it in a sterile eye jar.[25] It is important to reconstruct the donor later, which is easier to do if there is less edema in the tissue around the eye.[25] Gentle handling of the tissue during the procedure minimizes this edema and also minimizes color changes around the eye. The orbit is either filled with moist gauze or a plastic sphere.[25] This helps the funeral director to restore the normal appearance. The lids should be well-lubricated and the periorbital tissue should be cleaned.[10]

Complications can occur during the enucleation procedure, most commonly bleeding.[10] The predisposing factors to this are obesity, high blood pressure and the use of blood thinners.[10] The bleeding should be stopped by either vessel ligation or cautery, but not by pressure because this will undoubtedly force the blood into surrounding tissues and cause unwanted discoloration.[10] Another complication of enucleation is difficulty of delivering the globe out of small lid fissures such as seen in infants.[10] In these situations, vitreous can be aspirated to decrease the globe size and ease its delivery.[25] Care should be taken to avoid damaging the lids.[25]

## Donor Reconstruction

It is usually the funeral director who reconstructs the donor eye. Therefore, the person who does the enucleation should do everything possible to decrease swelling and discoloration around the eye as described above.[25]

## Corneoscleral Rim Excision

The corneoscleral rim excision is associated with risks of contamination and endothelial cell loss.[10,25] Therefore, every effort should be made to avoid these two things from occurring during the excision. This can be easily accomplished by following aseptic technique and gentle management. The excision is done either directly following the enucleation after returning to the laboratory for removal under a laminar flow hood or it is done in the field without enucleation (*in situ*).[10] When the globe has been enucleated and returned to the laboratory, povidine-iodine 5% is used for decontamination in this context.[10] The globe is immersed in it for a few minutes. The conjunctiva around the cornea is removed. Sclerotomy is performed using a blade to cut 3 mm posterior to the limbus; one or up to four incisions may be made to minimize distortion of the cornea while excising the corneoscleral rim.[10] Then, a 360° cut is performed around the globe with scissors. This excision should be done very meticulously in such a way that there is not any distortion of the cornea during the process.[11] Choroid should not be involved in the cutting. A sign that the choroid has been cut during the excision process is the occurrence of vitreous prolapse.[10] Once vitreous is noted, cutting in that area should be discontinued and then restarted in a different location.[11] The anterior chamber should be formed at all times during excision. A shallow anterior chamber will bring the iris into contact with the cornea. At the end of the excision, any tissue that is still attached to the corneoscleral rim should be removed.[10] The endothelium should be protected at all times and the rim should be placed in the storage medium after excision.[25]

*In situ* excision of the cornea is also possible.[10] Sterilization is very important here. The cornea should be evaluated carefully before removal. The conjunctiva is first removed around the eye and then the excision is performed in much the same way as described above.[10] *In situ* excision is performed, when there is a risk of bleeding after enucleation which would make donor reconstruction more difficult.[10] It is also performed in instances when the consent dictates that only the cornea can be removed.[25]

The risk of contamination with *in situ* excision is no higher and endothelial cell viability is no lower than in tissue derived from enucleated globes, provided that the excision is performed by a skilled technician and a rigorous disinfection protocol is instituted.[32,33]

## TISSUE EVALUATION

### Gross Examination

Using a penlight to provide oblique illumination, the eye should be carefully evaluated for the presence of any of the following findings: (1) Epithelial defects; (2) Trauma or foreign bodies; (3) Stromal disease/edema; (4) Presence of keratitic precipitates; (5) Corneal ectasia and (6) Status of anterior chamber (formed, shallow or presence of hyphema).[10]

### Slit-Lamp Examination

Slit-lamp biomicroscopy is performed routinely on donor corneas and can be used to obtain indirect assessments of the endothelial quality by grading the amount of stromal edema, Descemet's folds and presence of guttae.[11] The most difficult skill for technicians to acquire is the ability to adequately evaluate the endothelial layer.[10] The endothelium of whole globes or excised corneoscleral rims can be evaluated while the tissue remains in media, which is an even more difficult skill to acquire.[10]

The whole globe should be prepared in a sterile area for viewing with the slit lamp. It can be placed in a jar that can be clamped in a viewing brace attached to a slit lamp (Fig. 1). Then the anterior globe should be viewed under low magnification with a wide slit beam oriented at 45°.[10] It is easier to discern major defects using lower magnification.[11] The technician should then proceed in a systematic approach starting from the corneal epithelium and progressing back to the anterior surface of the iris, using first a broad beam, then switching to a narrower beam for each step of the examination.[10] Retroillumination should also be employed in order to detect any stromal abnormalities missed previously.[11]

### Specular Microscopy

Specular microscopy (Fig. 2) provides a more sensitive method in evaluating corneal endothelial morphology.[11] ECD alone does not always correlate with a healthy endothelium; however, a high percentage of hexagonal cells along with a lack of polymegathism have been shown

Specular microscopy can safely extend the donor age criterion by identifying older donors with normal morphological parameters. The converse is true with respect to rejecting younger donors that do not meet morphological criteria. In one series, roughly 75% of corneas from donors older than 67 years had normal endothelial cell morphology and density by specular microscopy.[11]

Specular microscopy provides the measurement of mean cell density (MCD) and mean cell area (MCA) of endothelial cells. It also provides for measurement of variations in cell size (polymegathism) expressed as coefficient of variation (standard deviation of MCD ÷ MCA) and shape (pleomorphism) expressed as percentage of hexagonal cells. These last two measurements may actually better correlate with corneal function and integrity better than MCD alone.[34] Many studies have shown that with increasing age, there is a trend toward diminished MCD, increased MCA and variations in size, as well as a decreased percentage of hexagonal cells.[34]

Modified corneal storage containers (Fig. 3) are commonly employed to examine the corneal tissue by specular microscopy. Newer designs allow the same chamber to be used for viewing and storage of the tissue, effectively decreasing the contamination risks and endothelial trauma by avoiding unnecessary manipulation of the tissue.[35] Rapid endothelial screening can be performed with high-resolution video systems without direct tissue contact.[10] It is best to perform the specular microscopy evaluation as soon as possible to avoid excessive stromal edema, which may degrade the image quality.[35] The tissue should also be at room temperature for a sufficient time for the endothelium to assume normal shape to ensure the best image quality.[35]

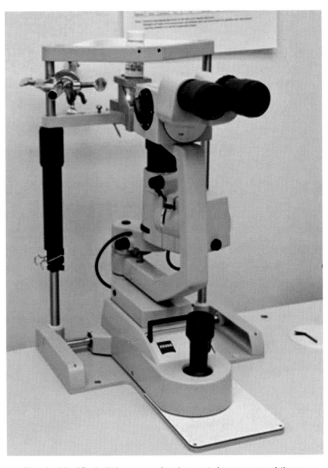

Fig. 1: Modified slit lamp used to inspect donor corneal tissue

to correlate with a healthy endothelium. These properties can only be detected by specular microscopy and when abnormal do not always show clinically significant stromal edema or guttae by slit lamp examination.

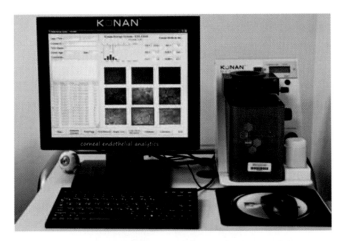

Fig. 2: Specular microscope used to analyze corneal donor endothelial morphology and density

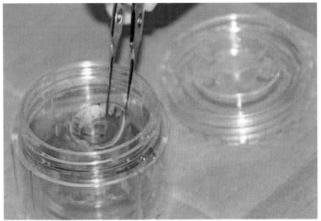

Fig. 3: Corneal storage container. Slit lamp and specular microscopy evaluation can be performed through these containers and therefore avoid unnecessary tissue manipulation

CHAPTER 79

## Histocompatibility Matching

Histocompatibility matching, ABO blood group matching, and cross-matching donors and recipients was debated for many years. The Collaborative Corneal Transplantation Studies (CCTS) addressed these questions in a multicenter study that included 419 patients that were at high risk for rejection (due to presence of vascularization or prior episode of rejection).[36] The study evaluated graft failure that occurred with donor corneas that were matched for HLA-A, HLA-B, HLA-DR, ABO blood group matching as well as donor-recipient crossmatching.[36] The study concluded that matching of the three human leukocyte antigens evaluated did not significantly reduce graft failure nor did a positive donor-recipient crossmatch substantially increase the risk of graft failure.[36] Interestingly, it showed that ABO blood group matching might be effective in reducing graft failure. Treseler et al. showed that the presence of ABO blood group antigens in the corneal epithelium may be the inciting reason for the reduction in graft failure that was seen in the CCTS patients that were ABO-matched.[36]

The issue of ABO blood group matching was revisited recently in 2009 by the Cornea Donor Study Group. They determined blood group compatibility for 1,002 donors and recipients and evaluated corneal graft survival over a 5-year period in participants of the Cornea Donor Study. The patients underwent PK for conditions that are considered low risk for rejection (Fuchs' endothelial dystrophy or pseudophakic corneal edema). The study classified episodes of graft rejection as to whether or not they were attributable to immunologic rejection.[37] Their study concluded that ABO donor-recipient incompatibility was not associated with causing graft failure of any kind, including rejection or occurrence of a rejection episode.[37] Over the 5-year follow-up period, 32 (6%) of the grafts failed in the ABO-matched group, whereas only 12 (4%) failed in the ABO-incompatible group.[37] The 5-year incidence for a definite rejection episode (regardless of whether or not graft failure ultimately occurred) was 64 (12%) for the ABO-matched group and 25 (8%) for the ABO-incompatible group.[37]

Eye banks do not offer ABO and histocompatibility matching routinely, but perhaps further research is needed to evaluate their effectiveness in high-risk circumstances.

## ▶ TISSUE PREPARATION FOR DESCEMET STRIPPING ENDOTHELIAL KERATOPLASTY

When an eye bank prepares a cornea for Descemet stripping endothelial keratoplasty (DSEK), it is called a precut cornea. The advantage to the transplanting surgeon is that there is less time spent in an operating room preparing the tissue. The surgeon also knows that prior to surgery the cornea is successfully prepared. The tissue is generally cut the day before surgery and shipped to the surgeon the same day; however, there is no defined time between tissue preparation for DSEK by the eye bank and the surgery.

To begin the process, the storage medium is aspirated with a syringe and then attached to tubing through a two-way stopcock (Fig. 4). The medium is sent through the tubing to an artificial anterior chamber until a bubble of medium is established. Once a sufficient bubble of the storage medium has built up, the cornea is mounted and centered on the artificially created anterior chamber (Fig. 5). A cup cover with attached guide ring is locked in place over the anterior chamber (Fig. 6). A screw on the base of the chamber is then wound so the cornea is held firmly in place. At this time, the cornea is placed under pressure by turning the stopcock to allow BSS to pressurize the storage medium. Pressure is

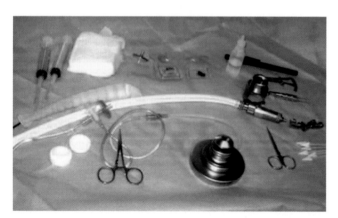

**Fig. 4:** Tray with essential instruments for performing donor corneal cutting for DSEK procedure using the Moria reusable system

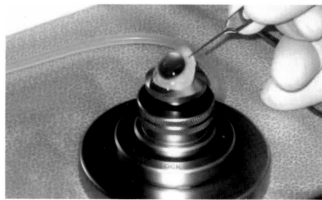

**Fig. 5:** Placing corneal donor over artificial anterior chamber using the Moria reusable cutting system

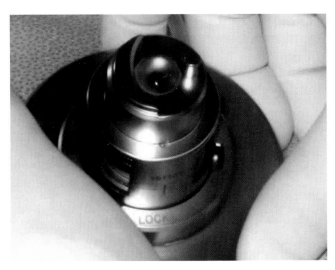

**Fig. 6:** Locking corneal donor tissue in place prior to cutting with the Moria

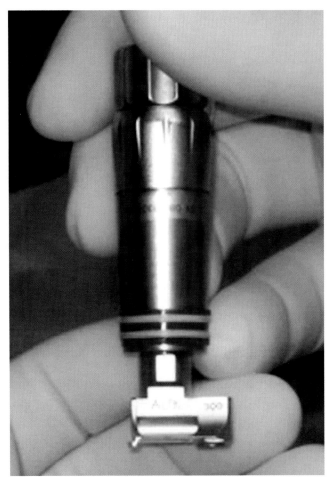

**Fig. 7:** Microkeratome blade used with the Moria reusable system. This is a 300 micrometer blade; other sizes are available depending upon pachymetry results and thinness of tissue desired for DSEK

obtained by raising the bottle of BSS to approximately 120 cm above the anterior chamber. The tubing is then clamped with a hemostat 50 cm from the entry point to the anterior chamber. There is an alternate means of pressurizing the cornea by using an air syringe. Either system is used to maintain a constant pressure on the cornea of 80–90 mm Hg.

A microkeratome attached to a unit powered by nitrogen gas is used to cut the cornea. Once the cornea has been successfully mounted and pressurized, a sonic pachymeter is used to measure the thickness of the cornea. Based on the thickness of the cornea, a microkeratome head is chosen to cut the cornea to the desired thickness (Fig. 7). A blade is placed in the head, and the head is attached to the turbine. A surgical sterile marker is used to mark the cornea. The turbine is placed in the guide track and turned on using a foot pedal. The cutting head is passed over the cornea at a constant speed for about 5–7 seconds (Fig. 8). The ultrasonic pachymeter is then used to measure the posterior bed and the anterior segment is repositioned on the cornea. The cornea is then dismounted by unscrewing the cup cover and allowing the BSS to push the cover away from the anterior chamber. Once the cover is removed it is turned upside down, and the cornea is separated from the cup cover. If an air syringe is being used, the pressure is taken off and the cornea is manually removed from the cup cover using forceps. Once the cornea is removed from the cup cover, it is placed back in the storage medium.

It should be noted that this procedure describes how a precut is done using the Moria reusable microkeratome system (Moria Inc., Doylestown, PA). There is also a disposable Horizon system that can be used (Hawken Industries, Cleveland, OH) (Fig. 9). Procedures are similar for both systems. The main difference is that the Horizon system is single use and comes sterilized, while the Moria system is reusable, but needs to be cleaned and sterilized after each use.

## ▶ STORAGE MEDIA

The EBAA estimates that 3,500–5,000 Americans wait an average of 1–2 months to undergo corneal transplantation.[34] There is a significantly longer waiting period worldwide given the greater limitation of tissue. Extensive research has been performed in order to create new storage media over the years with the goal to prolong donor storage time, while maintaining a viable endothelium. Prolonged storage times have allowed for the epic transformation of corneal transplantation into an elective procedure.[34,36]

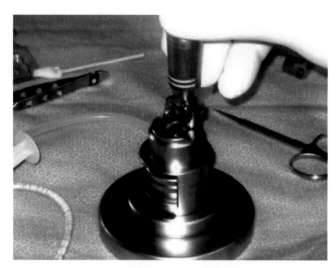

**Fig. 8:** Microkeratome blade mounted prior to making sweeping cut to remove anterior 300 micrometers of donor corneal tissue

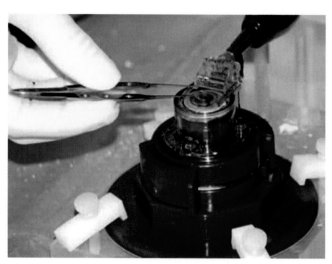

**Fig. 9:** Horizon single use disposable cutting system

Although the first successful transplant was performed by Zirm in 1906, preservation did not begin until after 1930 when Filatov of Russia first stored whole globes at 4°C for up to 56 hours.[3,10,11] Upon realizing that the corneal endothelium was the most important in maintaining a clear cornea after PK, many groups became interested in finding a technique to best preserve this critical tissue layer.[38] Among them were Eastcott, Mueller, and then ultimately Capella et al., whose group developed a cryopreservation technique of corneas excised with a rim of sclera that involved passing the tissue through a series of solutions with increasing concentrations of dimethyl sulfoxide (DMSO).[10] The tissue was then frozen under controlled conditions and had to be thawed under strict conditions. Capella's technique was used for many years in eye banks throughout the world.[10,11] (See 'Long-Term Storage' on page no. 1022 for further discussion on cryopreservation).

### Short-Term Storage

Before the advent of storage media, whole globes were simply stored in glass vials at 4°C for up to 48 hours, after which time, innate nutrients within the aqueous were depleted. This in addition to unavoidable warming during storage and/or shipping may have been important causes of primary graft failure.[35]

#### McCarey and Kaufman Medium

In 1974, McCarey and Kaufman developed the first corneal preservation medium containing tissue culture medium to maintain nutrition of the cornea.[39] This marked the modern era of corneal storage and transformed the practice of corneal transplantation surgery. It allowed for cases to be electively scheduled, rather than at the whim of the availability of tissue. They used tissue culture 199 (TC199) and also included dextran to help dehydrate the tissue, thus making transplantation easier.[39] Gentamicin was also added in high concentrations.[39] The M-K medium can preserve corneal tissue for up to 6 days, with 4 days being the recommended storage time.[39] It initially had a simple bicarbonate buffer, which was eventually replaced with the HEPES buffer. Interestingly, M-K medium was never patented and thus is available to eye banks all over the world and remains in widespread use today.[10]

### Intermediate-Term Storage

#### Chondroitin Sulfate-based Media: K-Sol, DexSol, Optisol and Optisol GS

With the development of K-Sol by Kaufman and DexSol by Lindstrom, these media marked the introduction of chondroitin sulfate into storage media.[10] Chondroitin sulfate is chemically very similar to hyaluronic acid, but it has the unique ability to prolong storage time, possibly by limiting the amount of peroxidation that can occur to cell membranes. These media were soon replaced by Optisol, which was developed in a joint effort by Lindstrom and Kaufman based on studies performed on K-Sol and DexSol.[40,41] Optisol and Optisol GS (containing streptomycin) are currently the most commonly used storage media in the United States.[10,11,34] It contains 1% dextran, as well as 2.5% chondroitin sulfate and vitamins C and B$_{12}$ (Table 2).[41]

**Table 2:** Comparison of Life4°C and Optisol GS components

*Human corneal preservation medium comparison*

| Parameter | Component | Life4°C™ | Optisol GS™ |
|---|---|---|---|
| Base medium | MEM with Earle's salts, 25 mM HEPES, 2 mM L-glutamine | X | X |
| Glycosaminoglycan | Chondroitin sulfate | X | X |
| Additional Buffering agent | Sodium bicarbonate | X | X |
| Deturgescent agent | Dextran 40 | X | X |
| Antibiotics | Gentamycin | X | X |
| | Streptomycin | X | X |
| ATP precursors | | X | X |
| Nonessential amino acids | | X | X |
| Additional cell supplements A | | X | X |
| Additional cell supplements B | Recombinant human insulin | X | None |
| | Reduced glutathione | X | None |
| | Stabilized L-glutamine | X | None |
| Additional cell nutrients | | X | None |
| Additional cell membrane stabilizers | | X | None |
| Additional cell antioxidants | | X | None |
| Trace elements (micronutrients) | | X | None |

Chondroitin sulfate containing media have a tendency to cause corneal swelling and therefore dextran was added to Optisol to counteract this tendency.[41,42] Optisol also contains precursors to ATP.[41] The antibiotic added to Optisol is gentamicin, the original antibiotic used in M-K medium.[41] Lass et al. compared Optisol to DexSol corneal storage media in 1992.[43] Although successful corneal storage had been achieved with the older chondroitin sulfate-based media such as DexSol for up to 2 weeks, issues still arose regarding corneal swelling during prolonged storage at 4°C.[10,44] Optisol was introduced as the chondroitin sulfate-based medium to better deal with this problem.[41,44] Lass et al. prospectively followed 31 pairs of donor corneas (one stored in Optisol and the other in DexSol ranging from 20 to 134 hours) that were transplanted into 62 patients.[43] All were clear at 1-year, except for one primary donor failure that occurred in the Optisol group.[43] Optisol-stored corneas were thinner during surgery than DexSol-stored corneas.[43,44] There was less lysozymal enzyme activity in the Optisol medium after tissue storage.[43] There were significantly fewer morphologic changes after 14 days in 4°C in the Optisol group; however, there were no significant differences in postoperative clinical or endothelial morphometric parameters.[43]

As mentioned previously, the current gold standard in 4°C corneal preservation media is Optisol GS (Bausch & Lomb Surgical, Inc.) (Fig. 10). This is an improved formulation of Optisol (Chiron Vision, Irvine, CA, USA), which has the addition of 200 µg/ml of streptomycin

sulfate. *Streptococcus pneumoniae* and *Propionibacterium* are known organisms to cause endophthalmitis and these bacteria are relatively resistant to gentamicin, so it was necessary to increase the antibiotic coverage in the standard Optisol formulation.[11] The addition of streptomycin to the original Optisol yielded the newer form of the medium called Optisol GS.[11]

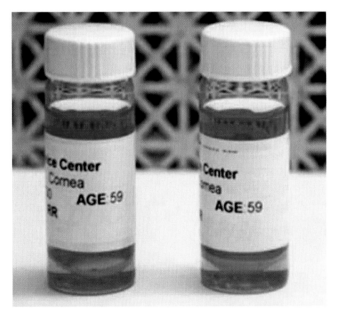

**Fig. 10:** Paired donor corneas in standard viewing chambers containing Optisol GS

Adding streptomycin to Optisol was recognized to be effective against resistant bacterial strains and was no more toxic to the endothelium than standard Optisol.[11] Tissue can be stored in Optisol GS with FDA approval for up to 14 days at 4°C.[34] The main limitation of Optisol GS is its inability to preserve corneal epithelium greater than 1 week.[34] It is important to note that 84% of the endothelium was viable even after 3 weeks of storage.[34]

A superior medium at 4°C than currently available would have to maintain cellular viability and lengthen the current storage times in order to provide for more efficient use of donor corneal tissue.[34] A new medium would also have to prevent stromal swelling at prolonged storage times in order to facilitate transplantation by the corneal surgeon.[34] The medium would also have to prevent microbiological growth.[34]

A new 4°C medium, Life4°C (Numedis, Inc.) has been FDA approved to be used for intermediate-term corneal preservation times (Fig. 11, Table 2). In an internal study, 34 paired human corneas were stored in either Life4°C or Optisol GS. The paired corneas were evaluated by specular microscopy and pachymetry both at time of arrival (2–4 days) and then again at 13–15 days postincubation.[34] The paired corneas were then placed in one of the two preservation media at 35°C for 14 additional days and then thinned down to be evaluated by specular microscopy and pachymetry again. The total incubation time for the paired corneas was 26–30 days. This extensive study demonstrated that corneas stored in Life4°C medium (in Numedis viewing chambers) were able to maintain corneal ECD statistically greater than corneas stored in commercially available Optisol GS (in Bausch & Lomb viewing chambers) at both the 14 and 28 day evaluations. Furthermore, corneas stored in Life4°C medium were able to maintain statistically greater corneal deturgescence than corneas stored in commercially available Optisol GS at both the 14 and 28 day evaluations. No statistically significant changes in endothelial cell coefficient of variation or percent hexagonality between corneas stored in Life4°C medium or Optisol GS were observed at the 14 or 28 day evaluations. All 92 paired corneas stored in both Life4°C and Optisol GS had intact corneal endothelium that could be visualized by swelling of the corneal endothelial cell borders. The ability of the corneal endothelial cells' borders to be visualized confirmed endothelial cell functionality. All 92 paired corneas stored in both Life4°C and Optisol GS had intact multilayered corneal epithelium at 28 days. All 92 paired corneas stored in both Life4°C and Optisol GS remained sterile throughout the 28-day incubation period. This extensive study with human corneas confirms that Life4°C medium (in Numedis viewing chambers) maintains corneas at 4°C substantially equivalent to corneas stored in Optisol GS (Bausch & Lomb viewing chambers). Life4°C has now been successfully introduced in the United States, where further clinical studies regarding its performance compared to Optisol GS are anticipated.

### Eusol-C

Eusol-C is manufactured by Alchimia (Abeamed, Miami, FL) as a completely synthetic medium for corneal storage at 4°C approved for storage for up to 14 days.[45] The medium contains a single antibiotic (gentamicin) at an effective dose for a higher stability of the medium. Before use, the medium can be stored at room temperature and it can withstand temperature peaks during transport.[45] It has a standard phenol red indicator which allows for a rapid visualization of variations in pH. It also features an optically clear vial bottom which allows for evaluation of the tissue with specular microscope (e.g. Konan, HAI Laboratories) without transferring it to another container.[45] Eusol-C is widely used by European eye banks and is also available in the United States.

### Long-Term Storage

#### Organ Culture

A technique called organ culture was first developed by Doughman. This technique uses organ culture media at 34°C for up to 33 days.[2,46] It provides the luxury of a greater amount of time to prove sterility and vitality of the corneal tissue prior to transplantation. This long-term storage approach also allows for the additional time that

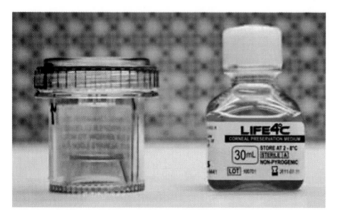

**Fig. 11:** Life4°C storage medium and Numedis viewing chamber

may be required to perform histocompatibility matching. It can facilitate the transferring of tissue between centers, including internationally.[2] Bourne et al. compared it to M-K medium and showed that postsurgical ECDs were similar between the two.[36] Stromal thickness was initially increased in the organ culture group, but this resolved and became similar to the M-K group after 3 weeks.[36] To counteract the increase in stromal thickness, Doughman later placed dextran 5% into the medium 48 hours before transplantation.[36] Organ culture, however, is logistically challenging since the medium must be changed regularly, equipment costs are high, and there is a need for well-trained technicians.[36] These disadvantages have outweighed the advantage of longer storage times and hence organ culture is seldom used in the United States. There is a modified form that is in use in the United Kingdom and in Europe.[36]

Pels and colleagues analyzed the technical and quality data for their organ culture technique that had been electronically stored since 1989 on greater than 41,000 corneas processed by the Cornea Bank Amsterdam.[47] They concluded that organ culture allows for storage of donor corneas for up to 5 weeks followed by a much shorter phase of up to a week to reverse the swelling that occurred during the initial phase of storage.[47] It is standard protocol in the regions analyzed to select corneas based on endothelial evaluation after the quarantine period, as well as perform microbiological testing of the storage solution after the quarantine period. Other technical aspects (such as endothelial cell mosaic, tissue performance and cut-off points for selection) are highly variable.[47] They emphasized that universal standards are needed to make the organ-cultured cornea a more standardized product and that this should be left up to the European Eye Bank Association (EEBA) to formulate tissue-specific regulations, training and technical guidelines.[47]

Eurosol (Bausch and Lomb Surgical, Inc.) is a serum-free organ culture medium for use at 34°C, which was developed for use in European countries. It has had limited usage.[36]

## Cryopreservation

Interests in cryopreservation of corneal tissue have recurred throughout the decades of modern eye banking. Long-term storage of corneal tissue is necessary worldwide in order to maximize use of the very limited tissue available in many countries and also to allow ample time to perform the necessary studies on the tissues prior to their transplantation. Cryopreservation is the only method of corneal preservation that can provide indefinite storage.[48] As early as the 1960s, successful corneal transplants in humans and animals had been performed using tissue that had been cryopreserved in DMSO.[48] Cryopreservation, however, causes significant endothelial cell injury, and it is a very expensive and a technically complex method of preservation. With the introduction of short-term storage at 4°C, cryopreservation failed to gain wide acceptance and its uses are frequently limited to urgent situations in which unfrozen tissue is not available.[48] Brunette and colleagues showed an increase in primary failure rate and a higher initial endothelial loss in cryopreserved corneas over a 4-year period (1986–1990) in a Montreal hospital in which they compared them to noncryopreserved controls.[49] They, therefore, concluded that cryopreserved corneas are viable, but that they should be used mainly for emergency situations in which tissue availability is an issue.[49]

Wusteman and colleagues used an interesting technique to demonstrate the importance of osmotic stresses on the corneal endothelium during cryopreservation. They devised a protocol using rabbit corneas that minimized osmotic variations on endothelial cells during cryopreservation by adding and removing the cryoprotectant, DMSO, in stages and only at room temperature, instead of adding it when the tissue was already on ice.[48] This decreased the duration of endothelial swelling during the removal phase (was not clear-cut during the addition phase), and therefore decreased the osmotic stresses on the endothelium during at least the removal stage.[48] This is in contrast to the other published methods at the time that involved adding and removing DMSO on ice, which normally reduces its tissue toxicity, but this factor is outweighed in corneal tissue by the damaging effects of osmotic stresses on the endothelium seen at removing the DMSO at colder temperatures.[48] Their method showed significant improvement in maintaining endothelial structural integrity in comparison to the prior technique, such as that popularly described by Capella. Cryopreservation, therefore, likely deserves further investigation.

## ▶ OTHER TISSUE PREPARATIONS

While a large portion of eye banking activity involves collection, evaluation, processing and supply of human corneal tissues, eye banks also collect, process and supply other tissue used in ophthalmology. Some of these tissues are human amniotic membrane, sclera and fascia lata. In this section, we will describe preparation and preservation of amniotic membrane and scleral tissues.

## Amniotic Membrane

Amniotic membrane is used extensively for various ocular surface diseases.[50] It is also used as a tissue scaffold for *in vitro* expansion of limbal stem cells.[51] Although preserved amniotic membrane tissue is available commercially, some laboratories and eye banks prepare and supply amniotic membrane tissue for human use.[52]

### Materials Required

The list of materials required for the processing and storage of amniotic membrane is given in Table 3.

### Recovery of Human Placenta

Human placenta recovered from cesarean section deliveries only is used for amniotic membrane processing. Based on the national or state requirements, the eye bank personnel must obtain a copy of the consent either from the donor or their legal heir, as well as relevant serology reports (HIV, hepatitis B and C antigen and VDRL) of the donor from the obstetrician. As soon as placenta is delivered, it is wrapped in a sterile gauzed towel and placed in a sterile plastic bag. The plastic bag containing placenta is brought to the eye bank laboratory in a thermo-flask containing ice packs.

### Processing of Amniotic Membrane from Placenta

The placenta is maintained at 4°C until processing. Two technicians need to be gowned, masked, capped and

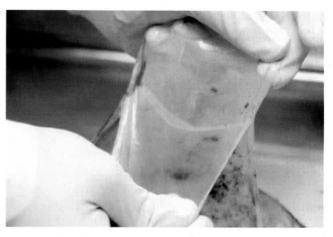

**Fig. 12:** Human placental tissue. Amnion being carefully separated from the chorion

gloved for the procedure. The placenta is transferred in a sterile stainless steel pan and washed repeatedly with antibiotic containing Ringer's lactate or normal saline until clear water is obtained. It is then transferred aseptically to another sterile pan and carried to the laminar flow hood which is precleaned and UV sterilized. After changing gloves, with the assistance of the other technician, the amniotic membrane is peeled off gently separating the amnion from the chorion (Fig. 12). The separated amniotic membrane is kept stretched during this maneuver (Fig. 13). The amnion has to be meticulously separated from the chorion without button-holing it. Once a clean transparent membrane of approximately 3" x 3" area size (7.5 x 7.5 cm) is available, the assistant attaches a precut square of nitrocellulose paper of 7 x 7 cm size on the chorion side of the membrane (Fig. 14). The amniotic membrane is then cut around the paper while rolling the edges on the other

| Table 3: Materials required for processing of amniotic membrane | |
|---|---|
| Laminar flow hood | : Biosafety class II |
| Borosil vials and caps | : 20 ml capacity |
| Nitrocellulose membrane | : 7.5 x 7.5 cm square sheets 0.45 µm pore size |
| Scissors (small, medium) | : 2 each |
| Ringer lactate solution or normal saline | : 20 liters |
| Ice packs and bin | : 1 bin, 2–3 packs |
| Large stainless steel pan | : 2 |
| −70°C deep freezer | : 1 |
| Cotton swabs | : |
| Gowns/Masks/Caps | : 3 sets |
| Towels (0.5 m²)/plastic bags | : 2 |
| Laboratory equipment, glassware, instruments | : |
| Plastic wash bottle | : 1 |

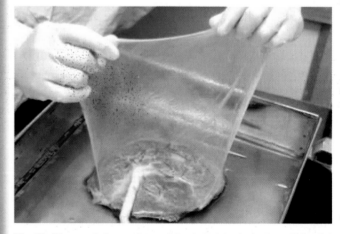

**Fig. 13:** The amniotic membrane is kept stretched prior to applying the nitrocellulose paper. Caution is taken to avoid button-holing the tissue

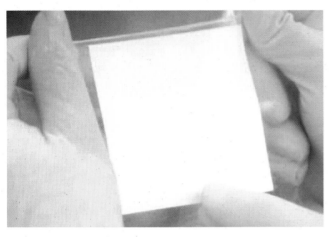

**Fig. 14:** Precut square of nitrocellulose paper being attached to chorion side of amniotic tissue

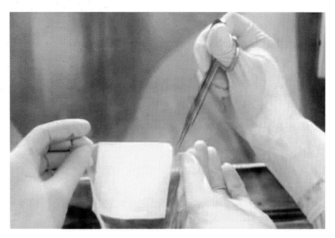

**Fig. 15:** The excess amniotic membrane is then cut from around the nitrocellulose paper

side of the paper, thereby adhering the membrane to the paper seamlessly without gaps or air bubbles (Fig. 15). The large piece of paper with amniotic membrane is then cut into smaller pieces of variable sizes and transferred into vials containing the preservation medium. Each vial is labeled appropriately and stored at −70°C in a deep freezer.

### Preservation Medium

The human amniotic membrane is preserved in a solution containing Dulbecco's Modified Eagle's Medium (DMEM), glycerol, amphotericin B, benzyl penicillin and Streptomycin. The composition of the medium is given in Table 4.

### Quality Assurance

At the end of aliquoting the medium into vials, approximately 1 ml of solution from a vial is inoculated into a tube of thioglycollate broth and then sent to microbiology laboratory for culture. At the end of the tissue preparation,

| Table 4: Composition of Dulbecco's Modified Eagle's Medium |
| --- |
| 13.4 g/L DMEM |
| 3.7 g/L sodium bicarbonate |
| 2.5 mg/L amphotericin B |
| 50 mg/L benzyl penicillin |
| 50 mg/L streptomycin |
| All dissolved in water and filtered through a 0.22 μm membrane filter and stored at 4°C |
| Equal volume of 95% glycerol |
| pH adjusted to 7.8 |

a small piece of tissue which is cut along with the nitrocellulose paper is inoculated into a tube of thioglycollate broth and sent to microbiology laboratory for culture as well. As serology report from the obstetrician should be on file for every placenta processed.

## Scleral Tissue

Pieces of preserved sclera are used for tectonic support as well as to cover glaucoma implants.[53,54]

### Processing of Sclera

Whole eyeballs are required for processing of scleral tissue. After excision of the corneal-scleral rim, the remaining posterior portion is used for processing of scleral tissue.

### Materials Required

The procedure is performed under a laminar flow hood under strict aseptic conditions. The list of materials required for processing of scleral tissue is given in Table 5.

### Preservation Medium

Scleral tissue is usually preserved in 95% ethyl alcohol.

### Processing

Initial preparation is the same as the preparation of the whole eyeball for laboratory excision of corneal-scleral rims. After excision of the corneal-scleral rim, the posterior pole is picked up with a tissue forceps and placed on sterile gauze. Remaining conjunctival tissue and any remaining ocular muscles attached at their insertion points are cut using iris forceps and scissors. All intraocular contents,

**Table 5:** Materials required for processing of scleral tissue

Laminar flow hood

Gauze pads

Scissors

Tooth forceps

Cotton tipped applicators

#10 scalpel blade

Ocular irrigation solution with gentamicin

95% ethyl alcohol

Glass vials for storage of scleral tissue

including vitreous humor, retina, choroid, and other uveal tissue are removed using a metal scoop and forceps. The inside of the posterior pole is cleaned thoroughly with cotton tipped applicators and gauze to remove all choroidal tissue and other tissue fragments. The posterior pole is placed into a specimen cup containing the sterile ocular irrigation and antibiotic solution mix such that the posterior pole is completely filled with the solution. The tissue is soaked in this solution for nearly 5 minutes, after which the solution is then drained. The posterior pole is then divided into halves, and any remaining pigments and blood vessels are removed from both surfaces of sclera by scraping with a scalpel blade such that the sclera is clean, smooth and free of any pigmentation or blood vessels. If there are any remaining pigments, it is returned into the antibiotic solution for additional soak. If the pigmentation or blood vessels cannot be removed even after the second attempt of scraping with scalpel blade, the tissue is discarded.

The scleral tissue is further divided into smaller pieces depending upon requirements and then transferred into appropriately labeled alcohol storage vials using aseptic technique. Each vial is then appropriately labeled, including the size of preserved sclera contained within them.

## ▶ INTERNATIONAL EYE BANKING

Eye banking in developed countries such as United States, Europe and Australia has achieved several notable milestones in the last 25 years. These have resulted in significant improvement in quantity and quality of corneal tissues available in these countries. Improvement in numbers of transplantable corneas is not only due to improved local eye banking procurement programs, but also to a large extent by improvements in corneal storage methods, use of specular microscopy and better networking among eye banks. The improvement in quality and standard of eye

banking has been to a large extent due to training and certification of eye bank technicians, development of procedure manuals, development and periodic revision of medical standards and accreditation of each individual eye bank.[36]

There is limited published data on the status of international eye banking. Based on the author's (Prashant Garg) knowledge of the status of eye banking in India, and his participation in regional eye banks and cornea meetings, as well as meetings of nongovernmental organizations involved in eye banking outside the United States and Europe, it appears that the status of eye banking is very different in the remaining part of the world. Nearly all countries in regions like Africa, the Middle East and Asia either do not have an established eye bank or are struggling with issues related to quantity and quality of corneal donor tissue. The current challenges for eye banking in the rest of the world are described below.

## Corneal Blindness as an Important Cause of Blindness

The World Health Organization (WHO) conducted a systematic review and analysis of all population-based surveys of blindness and low vision from 55 nations for the year 2002 and applied it to the 17 WHO epidemiological subregions.[55] As per the review, it is estimated that globally approximately 37 million people are blind and 124 million people have low vision; the prevalence of blindness is 3–4 times higher in Africa, South East Asia and the Western Pacific regions compared to the United States and Europe; and corneal scarring including that caused by trachoma is the third most important cause of blindness, accounting for 9% of total blindness. Further, there is a geographic difference in relative importance of corneal diseases as a cause of blindness.[56] Corneal diseases are more important as a cause of blindness in nations that lie within the geographic regions of Africa, the Middle East and South East Asia. These regions carry a major burden of the total blindness.[56] Further, these statistics do not reflect a much larger pool of people with unilateral disease. This is a very crucial fact in understanding challenges of eye banking in these geographical regions.

### Causes of Corneal Blindness

The epidemiology of corneal blindness is diverse and highly dependent on the ocular diseases that are endemic in each geographical area. Traditionally, important diseases responsible for corneal blindness globally include trachoma, onchocerciasis, leprosy, ophthalmia neonatorum and xerophthalmia.[57] With effective public health interventions the incidence of many of these diseases is showing a declining trend.[58,59] However, some other diseases are generating interest as causes of corneal blindness in these regions. These include corneal trauma, corneal ulceration and complications from the use of traditional eye medicines.[57]

All the above mentioned diseases result in vascularized corneal scar or adherent leukoma. Thus, it is obvious that vascularized corneal scarring is the most important cause of corneal blindness in developing countries.[60] This trend was reflected in a population-based study from India published in 2003 by Dandona et al.[61] Further, review of indications of corneal transplantation published from India, Nepal and Taiwan also suggest that corneal scarring or adherent leukoma and active microbial keratitis are the major indications for corneal transplantation in these countries.[60]

In the context of eye banking, it is important to understand the nature of corneal pathology for which transplants are performed in these geographical areas because the recipient pathology has direct bearing on the outcome of corneal transplantation surgery and thereby on demand for corneal tissue and the need for quality eye banking. The outcome data published from L V Prasad Eye Institute, a leading tertiary eye care center in India, clearly show that nearly 50% of corneal transplants fail over a 5 year period and 20% of all transplants are performed for failed grafts.[62]

## International Eye Banking Concerns

Keratoplasty is the definitive treatment for corneal blindness. Due to the high prevalence of corneal blindness coupled with overall poor outcomes, the demand for transplantable corneal tissue and efficient eye banking is very high in the geographic regions of Africa, Asia, South America as well as the Middle East. But the reality is that most of the nations in these regions either do not have any eye banking establishments or are struggling with issues related to the quality and quantity of corneal tissues. As per the data of National Program for Control of Blindness in India with a population of close to 1 billion, 46,589 donor corneas were procured in the year 2009. The requirement for donor corneas per year in India is estimated to be 200,000, i.e. nearly five times the current procurement.[63,64] This clearly shows that there is a huge gap between the supply and demand of donor corneal tissues in India and probably in other countries where corneal blindness is most prevalent. There are several causes for such a situation and these include: (1) Social: lack of

public awareness about the magnitude of corneal blindness and need for eye donation; (2) Religious: strong reservations from communities for organ donation and do not participate in eye banking; (3) Legal: lack of appropriate legislation to support eye banking in many nations; (4) Political: lack of serious efforts from governments in these regions to organize and support eye banking and (5) Organizational: most eye banks are run on charity with no defined structure or vision. The management boards of many eye banks do not have the essential understanding of the structure and function of eye banking.

The problem in these nations is not just the low number of eye banks, but the existing eye banks are also not functioning optimally. A large number of eye banks are run in one room with a refrigerator and a couple of enucleation sets; and the number of corneas collected per annum by several of these existing eye banks are in the single digits.[65]

Another important challenge in these regions is the quality of eye banking. Eye banks are manned by untrained staff. No protocols are followed for day-to-day operations. Due to lack of funds and necessary understanding, most eye banks do not have necessary infrastructure including a specular microscope and laminar flow hood. Medical standards are either not established or they are not followed strictly. In the absence of any accreditation system there is a wide variability in the quality of eye banking. Furthermore, most eye banks procure whole eyeballs and preserve them using a moist chamber method, which greatly limits the duration of its use. Most short and intermediate-term storage media are either not available or not affordable.

Due to all these factors, more than 50% of tissues collected by the eye banks in these regions are either graded as not suitable for surgical use or discarded due to exceeding the preservation time.

## Meeting the Challenges

In this background, one option for making corneas more available in these regions is supplying excess corneas from other countries, such as the United States and European nations, that have surplus tissue. But this is not a viable option to take care of corneal blindness in these regions, primarily due to the cost involved and also due to other logistics. Helping these countries to become self-sufficient by establishing self-sustaining high quality eye banks is rather a more viable option. Several organizations such as Tissue Banks International (TBI), Vision Share, Orbis International and Sightlife are working in this direction in various parts of the world.[36] Such efforts may be the catalysts to new efforts by local governments and nongovernmental organizations in bringing desired changes to eye banking in these regions.

Yet another effort in this direction can be in the formation of societies or associations of local and regional eye banks. These societies or associations can then work to provide for: (1) Cooperative efforts to enhance, regulate, and unify eye banking standards and tissue procurement guidelines; (2) Assistance in further development of current eye banks and establishment of new eye banks where they are most needed; (3) Establishment of Centers of Excellence for eye banking education and training; (4) Initiatives for tissue-sharing and (5) Promote advocacy and educational support for eye donation programs specific to regional cultures and religions.[65]

## ◆ FINANCIAL AND LEGAL CONSIDERATIONS IN EYE BANKING

### Financial

While eye banks are generally not-for-profit organizations, they must be established and operated using good business practices. This approach will ensure the best chance for program efficiency and effectiveness. There are three major avenues for eye banks to finance their operations: (1) Fundraising; (2) Charging processing fees and (3) Government healthcare system subsidization. In some cases, the first two options can operate together.

From a historical perspective, the first eye banks in the United States were funded as an adjunct of an eye hospital, or with private donations. As the eye bank movement began to grow in the 1950s in the United States, Lions Clubs provided the funding base for many eye banks. Helen Keller had challenged the Lions at their founding meeting in 1925 to become the 'Knights of the Blind' and support for eye banking and its role in sight-restoration fit very well with their mission. Many of these first 'Lions Eye Banks' were established at university ophthalmology departments since that was where corneal transplantation surgery mainly occurred during this early period. In some cases, other not-for-profit service clubs also supported eye banks, such as the American Legion and Odd Fellows. Financial support from the service clubs also set the foundation for eye banks to be not-for-profit organizations.

Eye banking was a fairly simple process then, when a donor was identified, an enucleator was contacted to go to the donor site and remove the whole donor eyes. This person was either an ophthalmology resident or funeral director.

Minimal documentation was required about the donor and there was no need for any serology testing at that time. The whole eyes were stored in a moist sterile container at about 4°C and shipped on ice. Evaluation of the donor corneas for possible therapeutic use involved gross examination of the corneas with a penlight and possibly using slit-lamp biomicroscopy. This rather simple process did not require much in terms of labor or material costs; therefore, service clubs could raise enough funds to financially support the entire service.

As eye banking technology advanced and the volume of donor corneas needed to meet patient needs increased, the cost of operating an eye bank grew as well. Full-time trained eye bank technicians had to be hired and trained to be available 24 hours, 7 days a week to recover donor eye tissue. Eye bank administrators and support staff then had to be hired to manage the technical staff and provide payroll functions. Preservation of donor corneas shifted from simple moist chamber storage to the use of tissue culture media that could preserve the donor corneas from 4 to 30 days, depending on the type of medium used.

By the mid-1970s, the funds provided by service clubs were not sufficient to support eye bank operations, so a few eye banks started charging a 'processing fee' to augment revenues and remain financially healthy. The concept of the processing fee was not to assign a cost to the donor eye tissue itself, but to help subsidize the costs related to provision of the service to provide the tissue. The processing fee concept had already been pioneered by blood banks when they started to assess a fee for the costs of recovery and processing for donated blood and blood products. The donor tissue itself thus has no intrinsic commercial value. This principle, along with eye banks being not-for-profit organizations, is important for public trust and support for altruistic donation programs in which individuals decide themselves or their families decide to donate tissues at the time of an individual's death.

In the United States, when the processing fees were first commonly used, the fee was charged to the hospital where the corneal transplant occurred. In turn, arrangements were made with insurance companies so that the hospital could include the charge on the patient's hospital bill so that the patient's medical insurance would pay for the charge. The hospital reimburses the eye bank for its invoiced fees and the insurance company pays the hospital. This approach is still used today, but most corneal transplant procedures are performed at the outpatient surgery center of a hospital or at a free-standing Ambulatory Surgery Center (ASC).

As eye banking technology became more sophisticated with the advent of specular microscopy and use of computer databases for record-keeping purposes, the costs of operating eye banks continued to increase as did the related processing fees. Processing fees became the larger source of operating funds for eye banks as opposed to money raised by service clubs. On a practical basis, the service clubs could not raise enough funds to keep up with escalating operating costs.

In the mid-1980s, with the identification of HIV, serological testing of tissue donor's serum became required, followed by testing for hepatitis B and C, and some other infectious agents in some countries. In the United States, the EBAA promulgated medical standards in the early 1980s and established an accreditation program for eye banks and certification of eye bank technicians. In 1993, the United States FDA started to regulate eye and tissue banks.[66] These federal regulations expanded at intervals that required additional staffing in order to comply with regulatory requirements. An example is that all United States eye banks are required to have in-place a quality assurance (QA) system and QA Manager to oversee the QA program.[66] These accreditation and regulatory requirements added to the overall costs of operating an eye bank.

As costs increased, by the early 1990s most eye banks had adopted processing fees as the foundation of their financial operating base. Concurrently, the donations and financial support from service clubs decreased to the point that their contribution to an eye bank's overall budget was minimal. While many American eye banks remain affiliated with Lions Clubs, the financial support from Lions generally is used for capital equipment purchases rather than for operational expenses.

Most eye banks have a Board of Directors. Some Board members will take on the responsibility of raising funds for the eye banks from corporate or private sources for capital projects such as purchasing land or a building for the eye bank, making renovations to existing eye bank laboratory space or purchasing key pieces of laboratory equipment. A new specular microscope to evaluate donor corneas for possible transplant use may cost as much as $25,000 and a microkeratome system for preparing donor corneas for EK procedures can cost as much as $50,000. Larger eye banks or eye bank networks may have full-time professional development staff to write grants to foundations for capital projects.

### Countries with National Health Systems

In those countries that have national health insurance programs, as is the case in many European countries, the financing of eye bank operations is generally tied into the national health program. Eye banks receive a set fee for providing various types of eye banking services and must operate within the financial limitations of their budgets.[67] In these situations, it is important that these eye banks have a thorough understanding of their financial operating requirements. Several developed countries continue to have a limited supply of donor eye tissue simply because they are financially limited in developing their donor programs.

### Eye Bank Funding in Developing Countries

In developing countries, when efforts are made to establish working eye banks, among the many challenges they face is not only to find funds to support start-up of the eye bank, but funding to maintain the program. This will require the eye bank organization (and its Board, if one exists) to approach all available funding sources, including general donations, international service club organizations, the national health department, and applying for grants to obtain start-up funding. An important part of these efforts is to develop an overall strategic and operational plan as to how the eye bank program will be successfully started and then maintained and grown so that it fulfills its mission. This includes how the eye bank will be funded on an ongoing basis. The organizations providing the start-up funding may not do so, if the plan does not include a well-designed and achievable strategy to have a regular revenue stream to sustain eye bank operations.

It has been common for eye banks in developed countries to provide donor eye tissue to eye banks or corneal surgeons in developing countries on a gratis basis. This practice may not be conducive to future eye bank development in the developing countries because it will promote the idea that there are no real costs involved with the establishment and operation of an eye bank. A lack of understanding of the importance of having access to start-up funding and ongoing revenues to support sustained operations can contribute to the foundation for an eye bank program not to be created in the developing nation.

Some novel approaches have been used in some developing countries to fund eye bank operations on an ongoing basis, such as having variable fees for various ophthalmic surgery procedures based on the patient's ability to pay. A wealthier patient may be charged for services at a higher rate and in return gets better accommodations for inpatient hospitalization or access to more advanced surgical equipment and procedures. The extra funds may then be used to provide care for those patients, who have very limited or no financial resources to pay for care. As a result, there may be differences in processing fees charged among patients based on their ability to pay. This approach has been used to fund donor tissue being available for patients at all levels of the socioeconomic spectrum.

### Organization of Eye Banks

The 'size' of an eye bank may be important for its ability to maintain its financial health. If an eye bank is mainly dependent on tissue processing fees to support its operations, then it must have enough demand for tissue in its service area to generate sufficient revenues in line with budgeted expenses, or be able to provide tissue to users outside their local service area to generate needed revenues.

Eye banks can be part of organ procurement organizations (OPOs) or nonocular tissue banks. This combination may reduce administrative expenses by sharing costs, but there can be a tendency for these combined organizations to put more emphasis on the organ and tissue parts of their activity since these sectors can produce much more revenue. As a result, insufficient attention may be paid to eye bank operations.

Eye banks can also financially benefit by forming networks in order to make tissue sharing more efficient and effective, as well as share costs related to common services such as accounting and human resources. These networks may also facilitate purchase of supplies or services on a group basis resulting in discounts related to large volume purchases from vendors.

### Tissue Acceptance Criteria

The tissue acceptance criteria employed by an eye bank can also have an impact on its operations. For instance, American corneal surgeons used to routinely accept donor corneas with ECDs of 2000+ cells/mm$^2$ for PK. As the supply of donor corneal tissues available for transplant has increased and improved over the years, the 'bar' at which tissues are found to be acceptable for PK has increased to 2500+ cells/mm$^2$ despite clinical evidence that has shown that initial donor ECD (or donor age) does not have a major effect on long-term graft survival. By raising the minimum acceptable limit for donor ECD or lowering the maximum acceptable donor age, corneal surgeons decrease the percentage of recovered donor tissue that is actually used for transplant, and as a result, limit the percentage of recovered tissues on which costs can be recovered. In turn, this practice can result in eye banks having to increase their processing fees in order to generate sufficient funds to

support operations. There needs to be a balance between what tissues are found to be acceptable for surgical use and the desire of the corneal surgeon to have the highest quality tissue for the benefit of his/her patients. The maintenance of this balance is especially important to eye banks that are being established in developing countries where a regular revenue stream is very important to the establishment of new eye bank programs.

### Processing Fee Variations

There are some variations in tissue processing fees based on the type of tissue and how it is prepared by the eye bank. In addition to donor corneas for transplant, sclera is also used for glaucoma valve surgery and for covering orbital implants. Donor corneas that are not suitable for PK, EK, or anterior lamellar keratoplasty (ALK) and deep anterior lamellar keratoplasty (DALK) due to scars or other defects, but are otherwise medically suitable for therapeutic use, can be preserved in anhydrous glycerin or gamma-irradiated in albumin and then used as tectonic patch grafts or for glaucoma valve surgery. The processing fees charged for scleral grafts and tectonic tissue are less than those for donor corneas used for various types of keratoplasty.

With the recent advent of EK procedures for endothelial dysfunctions, including DSEK and Descemet membrane endothelial keratoplasty (DMEK) that are prepared for the surgeon by the eye bank using a microkeratome and/or a femtosecond laser (Intralase-enabled keratoplasty, or IEK), eye banks charge an additional fee on top of the base tissue processing fee to cover the labor and material costs for these services.

### Costs of Donor Eye Tissues for Research and Teaching

Eye banks' mission also includes the provision of donor eye tissue for medical research and education. In the early years of eye banking, tissues for these purposes were provided on a no fee or gratis basis. The whole eyes or other tissues that were distributed for these purposes were generally those tissues that were not able to be used for transplant use due to poor tissue quality or medical history. However, as molecular biology research techniques advanced and improved to include genomic and proteomic research on normal physiologic versus disease pathways, access to very fresh donor eye tissue from normal donors and disease-specific donors has become extremely important. Key target eye diseases include age-related macular degeneration, diabetic retinopathy as well as glaucoma. Researchers require detailed medical and ophthalmic history on disease-specific donors for these specimens to provide maximum scientific value for genomic studies. Also, these donor eye tissues need to be recovered within 4–6 hours of cardiac death to be of maximum value.

For-profit companies developing new ophthalmic devices or surgical equipment also frequently need access to a regular supply of human donor whole eyes for research and development purposes, or for training ophthalmic surgeons to use new equipment. Ophthalmology residents also need access to fresh human donor eyes to learn and practice ophthalmic surgery procedures.

Eye banks have worked to increase the fees charged for providing research tissue since in reality, there is no difference in accrued costs when an eye bank pursues a donor specifically for research purposes as compared with transplant use. The cost of tracking down detailed medical and ophthalmic history can be costly since that process can be very labor and time intensive. To a large extent, the processing fees charged for donor corneas used for transplant have subsidized to some degree the ability of eye banks to provide donor eye tissue for research and teaching. With corneal processing fees being better defined in European nations, those eye bank programs are geared to recover mainly transplant quality tissue and put little emphasis on recovery of donor eye tissue specifically for research. Eye banks have been very challenged to have medical researchers and ophthalmic device companies understand these financial dynamics so that eye banks can be appropriately reimbursed fees that cover their costs for these services.

## Legal

An eye bank program must have a legal basis for accepting donor eye tissues from deceased persons. On a practical basis, this means that a law must exist that permits anatomical donations for the purposes of transplantation, scientific research and medical education. Eye banks do not serve exclusively as a source of tissue for transplantation; they also serve tissue needs for research and education.

Eye banks can be established in a country, state or other political entity without a law specifically authorizing an eye bank's existence, but many countries have laws and regulations that require eye and tissue banks to be registered with a government agency and comply with specific regulations related to donor screening and serological testing. For example, the United States FDA started to actively regulate eye and tissue banks in late 1993. In 2005, the FDA promulgated Good Tissue Practices (GTPs) which

defined in detail donor screening, recovery and processing requirements for human tissues intended for therapeutic use. An important note which will be referenced later is that GTPs in the United States require that a medical and social history interview be conducted with the donors' family or next of kin as a routine part of the donor screening process. These regulations are similar to Good Manufacturing Practices (GMPs) that exist for medical devices and pharmaceuticals. The European Union also has directives specifically regulating eye and tissue banking within its member states.[67]

The World Health Organization also has a forum for the development of harmonized global standards for eye and tissue banking, since eye banks are being created in a number of developing countries where they have not previously existed.[68]

The ultimate purpose of any and all regulations in regard to eye banking, based on national or local laws, is to provide recipients (patients) with donor tissues that are microbiologically safe, and physiologically and structurally functional. These laws also provide an ethical and socially-defined basis for the practice of eye and tissue banking. One of the most important aspects regarding laws relating to any type of organ or tissue donation are those related to how consent for donation is defined. This means that there must be a law(s) that authorize and define the process for the recovery of tissues and organs, including donor eye tissue, from a deceased person by an eye bank.

This process generally involves having an anatomical gift law, which defines how an individual or related party can legally make an anatomical gift at the time of a potential donor's death. The first such laws were created in the United States in 1968.[69] These laws were passed by state legislatures and are more or less uniform through an agency that works to maintain uniformity among the laws of different American states. These laws permitted an individual to execute a 'donor card' that stated that the individual wanted to donate their tissues or organs at the time of their death. The individuals' signature on the card was witnessed so that the card was considered in theory a legal document. These laws also allowed the legal next of kin (family or significant others) to donate a relative's tissues or organs at the time of death. A hierarchy was defined in the laws as to which legal next of kin had precedence to make this decision, e.g. spouse, adult children and parents. A decision by the legal next of kin was authorized in case the decedent (donor) had not made a premortem decision to donate. It is important to note here that even through the donor card was considered as a legal document, in practice, it was not used as such until many years later. This was because in practice, the donor card was not used as a legal decision to donate as intended. Respect for the wishes of the family or next of kin remained paramount concurrent with the family making all decisions about disposition of the deceased's body, i.e. type of memorial or religious service, burial versus cremation.

The decision to donate by an individual later became referred to as 'First Person Consent'. The decision to donate by the legal next of kin can be defined as 'Third Person Consent'. These definitions will be referenced later in relation to how anatomical gift laws have changed and advanced over the years.

Another approach to legalizing the donation process was to define that all citizens in a country could either opt-out as donors. The opt-out approach means that all citizens are considered as potential donors at the time of their death unless they register with the government that they do not want to be a donor. This approach requires that the government maintain a donor registry of those citizens that choose to opt-out. On a practical basis, the approach still involves the family or next of kin because the donation, if carried out, may affect funeral plans, and as stated previously, donor screening procedures require that the nearest relatives or significant others be interviewed about the medical and social history of the prospective donor.

Some countries have used an approach known as 'presumed consent' in which all citizens are considered as prospective donors so that organs or tissues can be recovered at the time of death. This practice was common in the former Soviet Union and Eastern European countries. The practice in these countries has shifted more toward those practices used in the Western European countries which involve involvement of the next of kin. In practice, tissues were recovered as part of an autopsy when performed in hospitals. The practice in these countries has shifted more toward those practices used in Western Europe which involves the next of kin as part of the donor screening process.

There was one country in which corneas could be recovered using presumed consent. The corneas were recovered from suitable donors in the hospital morgue before the body was released to the family for the funeral and burial. The families were not informed that the corneas had been removed. On one occasion, a family member noticed that the corneas had been removed and reported the practice to the news media. The news was not received well by the public and the practice was immediately suspended.

This story shows that if a presumed consent approach is going to be successfully used, the public needs to know that it is a standard practice so that there is social support for the practice. If not, the presumed consent program will end up being suspended as described above. There have been some countries with laws that have defined corneas as 'tissues', and separate from 'organ donation', so that 'informed consent' by the family or next of kin is not required. However, those presumed consent programs were never initiated. There was no public education about the law or planned practice, so that there was no social support for the donor program. We will come back to the principle of informed consent later.

Another version of presumed consent is 'legislative consent'. In the United States in 1974, the State of Maryland passed a law that allowed an eye bank to recover the corneas only from Medical Examiner's autopsies from decedents whose corneas were suitable for transplant. A Medical Examiner's Office is the same as a Coroner or District Surgeon, who performs a forensic examination of deaths for medicolegal reasons. These deaths include accidents, homicides, suicides and decedents found dead with no apparent causes. The law did not require the family or next of kin to be contacted about the recovery of the corneas so that in essence, cornea recovery for transplantation became part of the autopsy.

Similar laws for the recovery of corneas were adopted by a number of other states in the United States during the late 1970s and early 1980s. A large percentage of the American donor cornea tissue supply became available as a result of these laws during this period. Over time, the contribution these laws made to the donor corneal supply in the tissue supply waned. In 1998, the United States Federal Government passed laws that required all acute care hospitals to report each death to the regional OPO as part of a plan to increase the availability of primarily donor vascular organs such as kidneys, hearts and livers. There was a benefit to eye and tissue banks in that those decedents that were not suitable for organ donation were triaged for the eye and tissue banks that worked with the OPO in their service area and were provided access to this information. As part of the Federal law, hospitals had to work with the OPO, eye banks and tissue banks to have effective programs to provide families of identified prospective eye and tissue donors with the opportunity to donate, based on informed consent. Over the years, as these programs matured and became more effective, the percentage of donor corneas in the United States became higher from this approach, as opposed to the legislative consent/Medical Examiners approach. Also, an integral part of the donor screening process involved the medical/social history interview with the donor's family. That interview could not be performed using the legislative consent approach. In some jurisdictions that used the Medical Examiners law, if the autopsy report included a note about the corneas being recovered as part of the autopsy and without family consent, there were an increasing number of cases in which to legal next of kin complained to the authorities and news media about the practice. These public complaints resulted in the legislative consent approach falling out of favor due to lack of public support.

Most recently, in the United States, most states are adopting laws that redefine the legal status of donor cards as originally intended as a legal document. Specifically, these amendments to the anatomical gift laws state that the decision by an individual to donate tissues and organs at the time of death is an irrevocable decision.[69] What also makes this new approach to 'First Person Consent' practical is that when a citizen of a state renews their driver's license at a government office, when they state they want to be a donor, their name is entered into a 'donor registry database' that is maintained by the state. In turn, when a hospital or other agency reports a death to the regional OPO and the death report gets triaged to the eye bank, then the eye bank contacts the prospective donor's family, generally by telephone. The purpose of the call is not to obtain consent, as with a third person consent approach, but to remind the family that their relative was registered as a donor and that there is information the family needs to provide (the medical/social history interview) for the eye bank to follow through with their relative's wish to be a donor and perform the actual corneal or tissue recovery. As a result of long-term public education programs about the benefits to individuals and society of organ, eye and tissue donation, the vast majority of families support their relative's decision to be a donor and willingly provide the required medical/social history information. While this approach uses 'First Person Consent', it is also an informed consent.

A key observation at this point is that there needs to be public understanding and support for whatever type of anatomical donation laws are created and put into practice. The law, and the practice it permits, must fit with acceptable social and religious practices within a country. The movement toward harmonizing organ, eye, and tissue donation laws, as well as standards and practices on a global basis, means that the donor's family must be informed of the donation and involved in providing information about the suitability of the anatomical gifts for transplantation. Education and awareness are absolutely essential so that the practical use of the anatomical gift laws is understood and transparent to both medical professionals as well as the public.

A final note about 'brain death'—most donor vascular organs become available as a result of the donor being declared brain dead. In addition to there being neurological and physiologic criteria that must be met to declare a patient as being brain dead, this condition by necessity needs to be legally defined in any and all countries. This consideration is important for corneal or eye donation since most organ donors also qualify as eye and tissue donors.

## FUTURE THREATS IN EYE BANKING

Currently in the United States the donor tissue supply is adequate to meet domestic demand, allowing for a significant portion of the supply to be exported internationally. This is clearly not the case in other countries, as some rely largely on the United States eye banks to routinely supplement their demand for quality tissue. As discussed previously, tissue preservation methods are of utmost importance in international countries in order to have the most optimal use of their limited supplies. Landmark studies, such as the Corneal Donor Study, will also likely prove to have a major impact earlier on in international countries. This important study has demonstrated that increased donor age is not as important as once thought, and hopefully will help remove the stigma against using tissue from older donors, effectively increasing the potential donor pool.

In looking at why there are such limited supplies of donor corneal tissue internationally, one can easily find many reasons. Cultural views regarding organ/tissue donation vary greatly between nations and this may be one important factor which can greatly impact the ability to start an effective eye banking system.[70] Other factors are likely limited government support systems in place to initiate and sustain necessary institutions to effectively manage and direct organ donation awareness programs, organ and tissue harvesting, storage and distribution protocols, as well as training programs for all of these aforementioned entities. It is hoped that with the increasing success in restoring vision through more modern procedures and the ever-increasing demand for tissue, that infrastructure can be developed to allow for highly successful eye banks to be established in nations that are currently underserved.

Although United States corneal surgeons currently have some liberty in tissue selection for elective corneal transplantations, it is projected that this will not always be the case. Sheth and Van Meter presented a poster recently, wherein they retrospectively reviewed EBAA statistical reports going back to 1991, as well as United States and world population projections published by the United States government. Their observations were that tissue utilization will increase over the next 20 years faster than its rate of increase has been over the past 20 years, while the United States population rate of increase will remain essentially flat. Their data analysis concluded that the rate of tissue utilization is climbing at 35% every 5 years. The population of the United States is projected to increase by 17% over the next 5 years, which obviously would not support the increases in tissue utilization, if all other factors remain constant (consent rates, etc.). At the same time, alarming numbers of donor candidates will be unsuitable for donating corneal tissue because of an increasing number of rule-outs (due to medical/social history such as IV drug use), which have doubled over the past 5 years and accounted for about 50% of the unsuitable tissues in 2009. They concluded that we must continue to promote awareness of the importance of organ and eye donations, addressing the dismal consent rate for donation (28% in the United States in 2009), while continuing to improve preservation techniques.[70]

One example of this effort, that follows the tremendous value derived from the Cornea Donor Study findings in broadening the use of older donor tissue, is the soon to be launched National Eye Institute sponsored Cornea Preservation Time Study (CPTS). This new study will examine whether donor corneas preserved from 8 to 14 days from death-to-surgery in either Optisol GS or Life4°C have similar graft success rates and endothelial cell loss 3 years following EK surgery as compared to corneas with a death-to-surgery time of 7 days or less. If no difference is found, this will allow eye banks more time to determine tissue safety and have more donor tissue available for transplantation to meet the increasing tissue demands that Sheth and Van Meter have predicted.

## ▶ ACKNOWLEDGMENTS

This work was supported in part by NIH EY12728, EY012358, Research to Prevent Blindness, Ohio Lions Eye Research Foundation. We wish to thank Erik Hellier, CEBT, MBA for his contributions and review of this manuscript, Karen Piloto for photography and Debra Skelnik for her contributions regarding Life4°C.

## ▶ REFERENCES

1. Zirm E. Eine erfolgreiche totale keratoplastik. Graefes Arch Clin Exp Ophthalmol. 1906;64:580-93.
2. Ehlers N. Corneal banking and grafting: the background to the Danish Eye Bank System, where corneas await their patients. Acta Ophthalmol Scand. 2002;80(6):572-8.
3. Filatov VP. Transplantation of the cornea. Arch Ophthalmol. 1935;13:321-47.
4. Farge E. Eye banking: 1944 to the Present. Surv Ophthalmol. 1989;33(4):260-3.
5. Mian S, Kamyar R, Sugar A, et al. Regulation of eye banking and uses of ocular tissue for transplantation. Clin Lab Med. 2005;25(3):607-24.
6. Eye Banking Statistical Report, Washington, DC: 2010, Eye Bank Association of America.
7. Li JY, Mannis MJ. Eye banking and the changing trends in contemporary corneal surgery. Int Ophthalmol Clin. 2010;50(3):101-12.
8. Binder PS. Eye banking and corneal preservation. In: Barraquer JI (Ed). Symposium on Medical and Surgical Diseases of the Cornea—Transactions of the New Orleans Academy of Ophthalmology, St. Louis: Mosby; 1980. pp. 320-54.
9. Koenig SB, Graul E, Kaufman HE. Ocular refraction after penetrating keratoplasty with infant donor corneas. Am J Ophthalmol. 1982;94:534-9.
10. Brightbill FS. Corneal surgery: theory, technique, and tissue, 3rd edition. St. Louis: Mosby; 1999.
11. Brightbill FS. Corneal surgery: theory, technique, and tissue, 4th edition. St. Louis: Mosby; 2009.
12. Forster RK, Fine M. Relation of donor age to success in penetrating keratoplasty. Arch Ophthalmol. 1971;85(1):42-7.
13. Koenig SB. Myopic shift in refraction after penetrating keratoplasty with pediatric donor tissue. Am J Ophthalmol. 1986;101:740-1.
14. Belmonte J, Moral R, Vallcanera S, et al. Suitability of newborn donor corneal graft in penetrating keratoplasty. Arch Soc Esp Oftalmol. 2008;83(4):219-30.
15. Gal RL, Dontchev M, Beck RW, et al. The effect of donor age on corneal transplantation outcome results of the cornea donor study. Ophthalmology. 2008;115(4):620-6.
16. Lass JH, Gal RL, Dontchev M, et al. Donor age and corneal endothelial cell loss 5 years after successful corneal transplantation. Specular microscopy ancillary study results. Ophthalmology. 2008;115(4):627-32.
17. Centers for Disease Control. Human-to-human transmission of rabies by a corneal transplant—Idaho, MMWR Morb Mortal Wkly Rep. 1979;28:109-11.
18. Khalil A, Ayoub M, el-Din Abdel-Wahab KS, et al. Assessment of the infectivity of corneal buttons taken from hepatitis B surface antigen seropositive donors. Br J Ophthalmol. 1995;79:6-9.
19. Technical Manual. Washington, DC, 2010, EBAA.
20. Medical Standards, Washington, DC, 2010, Eye Bank Association of America.
21. Hassan SS, Wilhelmus KR, Dahl P, et al. Infectious disease risk factors of corneal graft donors. Arch Ophthalmol. 2008;126(2):235-9.

22. Basu PK, Ormsby HL. In vivo storage of corneal grafts. Am J Ophthalmol. 1959;47:191-5.

23. Chung CW, Rapuano CJ, Laibson PR, et al. Human immuno-deficiency virus p24 antigen testing in cornea donors. Cornea. 2001;20(3):277-80.

24. Wehrly SR, Manning FJ, Proia AD, et al. Cytomegalovirus kera-titis after penetrating keratoplasty. Cornea. 1995;14:628-33.

25. Procedures Manual/Medical Standards, Washington, DC, 2010, Eye Bank Association of America.

26. Medical Advisory Board Meeting Agenda of EBAA, Tuscon, Arizona, 6/2011. EBAA, Washington, DC.

27. Tappeiner C, Goldblum D, Zimmerli S, et al. Donor-to-host transmission of Candida glabrata to both recipients of corneal transplants from the same donor. Cornea. 2009;28:228-30.

28. Ritterband DC, Shah MK, Meskin SW, et al. Efficacy and safety of voriconazole as an additive in Optisol GS: a preservation me-dium for corneal donor tissue. Cornea. 2007;26:343-7.

29. Wagoner MD, Dohlman CH, Albert DM, et al. Corneal donor material selection. Ophthalmology. 1981;88(2):139-45.

30. Donor Evaluation Form, Washington, DC, 2010, Eye Bank Association of America.

31. Challine D, Roudot-Thoraval F, Sabatier P, et al. Serological viral testing of cadaveric cornea donors. Transplantation. 2006;82(6):788-93.

32. Garweg J, Hagenah M, Engelmann K, et al. Corneoscleral discs excised from enucleated and non-enucleated eyes are equally suitable for transplantation. Acta Ophthalmol Scand. 1997;75(5):483-6.

33. Jhanji V, Tandon R, Sharma N, et al. Whole globe enucleation versus in situ excision for donor corneal retrieval—a prospective comparative study. Cornea. 2008;27(10):1103-8.

34. US Food and Drug Administration, Center for Devices and Radiological Health (CDRH), Numedis, Inc. Life4°C, 510(k) K063304, approval letter, 12/21/2007.

35. Krachmer JH, Mannis MJ, Holland EJ, et al. Cornea. Philadelphia: Elsevier/Mosby; 2010.

36. Chu W. The past twenty-five years in eye banking. Cornea. 2000;19(5):754-65.

37. Dunn SP, Stark WJ, Stulting RD, et al. The effect of ABO blood incompatibility on corneal transplant failure in conditions with low-risk of graft rejection. Am J Ophthalmol. 2009;147(3):432-8.

38. Stocker FW. The endothelium of the cornea and its clinical implications. Trans Am Ophthalmol Soc. 1953;51:669-786.

39. McCarey BE, Kaufman HE. Improved corneal storage. Invest Ophthalmol. 1974;13:165-73.

40. Kaufman HE, Beuerman RW, Steinemann TL, et al. Optisol corneal storage medium. Arch Ophthalmol. 1991;109:864-8.

41. Lindstrom RL, Kaufman HE, Skelnik DL, et al. Optisol corneal storage medium. Am J Ophthalmol. 1992;114:345-56.

42. Halberstadt M, Bohnke M, Athmann S, et al. Cryopreservation of human donor corneas with dextran. Invest Ophthalmol Vis Sci. 2003;44(12):5110-5.

43. Lass JH, Bourne WM, Musch DC, et al. A randomized, prospective, double-masked clinical trial of Optisol vs DexSol corneal storage media. Arch Ophthalmol. 1992;110(10):1404-8.

44. Lass JH, Reinhart WJ, Skelnik DL, et al. An in vitro and clinical comparison of corneal storage with chondroitin sulfate corneal storage medium with and without dextran. Ophthalmology. 1990;97:96-103.

45. Eusol-C effectiveness as a corneal storage media. Alchimia website. http://www.alchimiasrl.com/en/alchimia-publications ?view=publication&task=show&id=33 (2011).

46. Doughman DJ, Harris JE, Schmitt MK. Penetrating keratoplasty using 37°C organ cultured cornea. Trans Sect Ophthalmol Am Acad Ophthalmol Otolaryngol. 1976;81:778-93.

47. Pels E, Rijneveld WJ. Organ culture preservation for corneal tissue. Technical and quality aspects. Dev Ophthalmol. 2009;43:31-46.

48. Wusteman MC, Boylan S, Pegg DE. Cryopreservation of rabbit corneas in dimethyl sulfoxide. Invest Ophthalmol Vis Sci. 1997;38(10):1934-43.

49. Brunette I, Le Francois M, Tremblay MC, et al. Corneal trans-plant tolerance of cryopreservation. Cornea. 2001;20(6):590-6.

50. Dua HS, Gomes JA, King AJ, et al. The amniotic membrane in ophthalmology. Surv Ophthalmol. 2004;49:51-77.

51. Higa K, Shimazaki J. Recent advances in cultivated epithelial transplantation. Cornea. 2008;27 Suppl 1:S41-7.

52. Burman S, Tejwani S, Vemuganti GK, et al. Ophthalmic appli-cations of preserved human amniotic membrane: a review of current indications. Cell Tissue Bank. 2004;5:161-75.

53. Sangwan VS, Jain V, Gupta P. Structural and functional out-come of scleral patch graft. Eye (Lond). 2007;21:930-5.

54. Halkiadakis I, Lim P, Moroi SE. Surgical results of bleb revision with scleral patch graft for late-onset bleb complications. Ophthalmic Surg Lasers Imaging. 2005;36:14-23.

55. Resnikoff S, Pascolini D, Etya'ale D, et al. Global data on visual impairment in the year 2002. Bull World Health Organ. 2004;82(11):844-51.

56. Thylefors B, Negrel AD, Pararajasegaram R, et al. Global data on blindness. Bull World Health Organ. 1995;73:115-21.

57. Whitcher JP, Srinivasan M, Upadhyay MP. Corneal blindness: a global perspective. Bull World Health Organ. 2001;79:214-21.

58. Congdon NG, Friedman DS, Lietman T. Important causes of visual impairment in the world today. JAMA. 2003;290(15): 2057-60.

59. Foster A, Resnikoff S. The impact of Vision 2020 on global blindness. Eye (Lond). 2005;19(10):1133-5. Review PubMed PMID: 16304595.

60. Garg P, Krishna PV, Stratis AK, et al. The value of corneal trans-plantation in reducing blindness. Eye (Lond). 2005;19:1106-14.

61. Dandona R, Dandona L. Corneal blindness in a southern Indian population: need for health promotion strategies. Br J Ophthalmol. 2003;87:133-41.

62. Dandona L, Naduvilath TJ, Janarthanan M, et al. Survival analysis and visual outcome in a large series of corneal transplants in India. Br J Ophthalmol. 1997;81:726-31.

63. Saini JS. Realistic targets and strategies in eye banking. Indian J Ophthalmol. 1997;45(3):141-2.

64. Rao GN. Eye banking—Are we really up to it in India? Indian J Ophthalmol. 2004;52(3):183-4.

65. Griffith FN, Valmadrid CT. International corneal supply. In: Brightbill FS (Ed). Corneal Surgery: Theory, Technique, and Tissue. St. Louis: Mosby; 1993. pp. 734-42.

66. U.S. Food and Drug Administration Eye and Tissue Banking Regulations. See www.fda.gov/BiologicsBloodVaccines/TissueTissueProducts/RegulationofTissues/ucm150485.htm

67. European Union Direcotves Regarding Eye and Tissue Banks. See website of European Eye Bank Association under 'EEBA Infopool' at www.europeaneyebanks.org

68. World Health Organization Information on Transplantation. www.who.int/transplantation/cell_tissue/en

69. Uniform Anatomical Gift Act, USA. www.nccusl.org/Act.aspx?title=Anatomical&20%Gift&20 (2006)

70. Sheth PH, Van Meter WS. Poster presentation: the cornea donor pool in 2030: where will my donor cornea come from? College of Medicine and Department of Ophthalmology, University of Kentucky. Eye Bank Association of America Annual Meeting June, 2011.

# CHAPTER 80

# Penetrating Keratoplasty: Surgical Techniques and Pre- and Postoperative Care

*John W Cowden*

## INTRODUCTION

The cornea is one of the most commonly transplanted tissues. In penetrating keratoplasty (PKP), the entire thickness of the recipient's cornea is replaced with donor cornea. In contrast, in posterior lamellar keratoplasty and endothelial keratoplasty, only the inner layers of the cornea are transplanted. Anterior lamellar keratoplasty may be superficial, mid-stromal or deep, depending on the depth of the pathology. Despite the development of these newer transplant techniques during the past decade, PKP remains the most commonly performed transplant procedure. According to statistics from the Eye Bank Association of America (EBAA), PKP accounted for 21,970 (51.5%) of the 42,642 corneal grafts performed in the United States in 2010.[1]

## INDICATIONS FOR PENETRATING KERATOPLASTY

Penetrating keratoplasty is usually required in diseases that involve both the corneal endothelium and the corneal stroma. The indications for PKP can be classified into two general categories: (1) decreased vision due to corneal opacification or corneal irregularity that is not correctable by other means, such as spectacles, contact lenses, Intacs® corneal implants, phototherapeutic keratectomy or lamellar keratoplasty and (2) any corneal condition that is likely to cause loss of the eye, if the condition is not corrected by PKP. Such conditions include impending corneal perforation or frank perforation and failed treatment of a fungal ulcer or acanthamoeba keratitis.

Clinical indications for PKP include chemical burns and other types of traumatic injury, corneal scarring or edema, Fuchs endothelial dystrophy and other corneal dystrophies, herpes simplex or herpes zoster viral keratitis, interstitial keratitis, keratoconus with deep scarring or prior hydrops, pseudophakic bullous keratopathy, re-graft, stromal dystrophies and ulcerative conditions.

The EBAA data from 2010 show that the leading indication for PKP was keratoconus, with 4,731 (21.5%) of the 21,970 PKPs in 2010 performed in patients with this disorder.[1] The second leading indication was in the EBAA category 'other causes of corneal opacification or disorder', which includes corneal scars and interstitial keratitis. This category was the indication in 4,455 PKPs (20% of all PKPs). Following the top two reasons for PKP in 2010 were repeat transplant (18% of all PKPs), postcataract surgery edema (13.9%) and corneal degenerations or dystrophies (8.5%).[1]

## DONOR TISSUE

In the United States, most donor corneas are obtained from the local eye bank and have been cleared for use according to the standards established by the EBAA.[2] Donor corneas are obtained by either enucleation or corneal excision, usually performed by an eye bank technician or trained paramedical personnel. The tissue along with the donor's medical information and blood samples are processed by the local eye bank. The corneal sclera tissue is maintained in preservation media at 4°C until the laboratory tests have been completed to verify that the tissue meets EBAA standards[2] or those of other similar organizations. Other methods may be used in other parts of the world.

The cornea is kept in a preservation solution (Optisol®, Chiron Ophthalmics, or Life4°C®, Numedis, Inc.) as a whole cornea with a 2–4 mm scleral rim (Fig. 1). The surgeon can request tissue with specific attributes that may be the best for a particular patient. For example, a patient with an alkali burn of the cornea, resulting in a highly vascularized scar with stem cell deficiency, may benefit from donor tissue that was harvested and preserved in less than 6 hours of the donor's death and has intact epithelium. Special requests for corneas for lamellar keratoplasty, such as precut tissue for an endothelial keratoplasty, can be provided by some eye banks.

The Cornea Donor Study (CDS) appears to have settled the question of whether or not donor age is a factor in graft survival.[3] The CDS data clearly show that donor age itself is not a significant factor in graft survival. Donor corneas from infants under 2 years of age, however, are often not used because of the steep curvature and pliability of the infant cornea. Human leukocyte antigen (HLA) typing for histocompatibility has not proven to be cost-effective or practical for corneal transplantation, although it may be beneficial in high-risk transplants, such as in highly vascularized corneas.[4,5]

An appropriate cornea for a PKP usually has an endothelial cell density greater than 2,000 cells per $mm^2$ and has been in storage for no longer than 1 week. However, storage of corneal tissue in preservation media may be suitable for up to 2 weeks without jeopardizing the tissue quality for

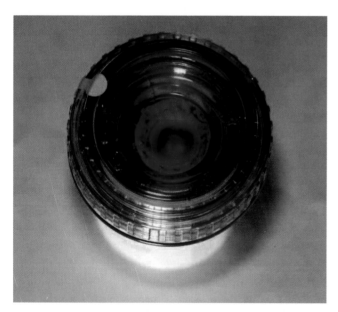

**Fig. 1:** Donor cornea in Life4°C® preservation solution

transplant.[6] In emergency circumstances, when suitable donor tissue is not immediately available, a therapeutic keratoplasty may be performed using any donor tissue, even though it may not meet the normal criteria of time or quality, provided the tissue has cleared screening tests for infectious diseases.

The process most cornea transplant surgeons use is to first schedule the PKP procedure, then notify the eye bank and request the corneal tissue for the date of the scheduled operation. At the present time, there are very few locations in the United States in which the tissue cannot be provided in a timely fashion.

When the corneal tissue is offered by the eye bank, the surgeon receives a copy of the tissue report, which documents the interval between the donor's death and corneal excision and the interval between corneal excision and processing of the tissue. The eye bank report also includes information on the endothelial cell count or density, the slit lamp appearance of the corneal tissue and pertinent history regarding the donor's age and cause of death and the results of screening tests of the tissue.

On the day of the operation, the donor tissue is delivered, in a styrofoam container filled with ice, to the transplant surgeon's office or the operating suite prior to the scheduled time of the operation. Upon receipt of the donor cornea, the styrofoam container is opened and the degree in which the ice has melted during transport is noted to make sure the tissue has been kept at the appropriate temperature. Recently introduced in the market is a freeze-sensitive indicator[6] that is affixed to the donor cornea vial and changes color if a freeze event occurred during transport. Such a device may help ensure that the donor cornea is kept at the proper temperature during transport.

The vial containing the cornea is removed from the container, and the cornea is inspected with a slit lamp or under a microscope to determine whether the information from the eye bank's slit lamp examination remains valid. The donor cornea is examined for epithelial or endothelial defects, stromal scars, the degree of arcus and the presence of folds in Descemet's membrane or the stroma. Some eye banks provide a specular microscopic photograph of the cornea that shows the endothelial cells so that the degree of polymegathism or polymorphism can be evaluated. It is not until the corneal tissue has been inspected and approved by the surgeon that the patient is transferred to the operating room.

## ▶ DISCUSSING PENETRATING KERATOPLASTY WITH THE PATIENT

After it has been determined that the patient is a candidate for a PKP, a comprehensive informed consent should be undertaken to assure that the patient knows what to expect postoperatively and can make an informed decision about whether to undergo such a procedure. The patient will want to know her/his chances of a successful outcome and how good his/her vision will be after the transplant. Too often, patients have high expectations for restoration of vision and are not made aware of the realistic potential for vision restoration after a cornea transplant. They also often do not appreciate the length of time necessary to achieve the best correction. In addition, the lifelong need for frequent examinations and medications must be emphasized to the patient. Monthly visits may be required for up to 1 year after surgery, followed by interval visits every 6–12 months for the rest of the patient's life. Patients need to understand the long-term follow-up and aftercare that are required after PKP.

Even in a procedure as relatively straightforward as PKP, the possibility exists for complications, such as hemorrhage during or after the procedure (including choroidal hemorrhage), postoperative infection, glaucoma, primary graft failure, rejection and the need for further surgery, including a repeat corneal transplant because of rejection. All of these complications need to be explained to the patient. In addition, the patient needs to be made aware of the fact that even though the transplanted cornea is clear, a high degree of astigmatism can be a significant factor and cause less than desired vision. Also it may be necessary to perform additional corneal procedures, such as an astigmatic keratomy (AK) or photorefractive keratectomy (PRK), in order to reduce the astigmatism if it cannot be corrected with glasses or contact lenses. Discussion should also include information about other forms of treatment that may provide the patient some relief from pain or may provide limited improvement in vision.

A family member should be present during the discussions in case the patient has trouble understanding what he/she has been told. The family member may be able to answer the patient's questions when the patient returns home after the visit. Although the author often sees patients for the first time in consultation for the possibility of cornea transplant or as referrals because of a need for PKP, he prefers to see patients for a second (preoperative) visit, if possible, so that both can make an informed decision together. It is helpful to provide the patient with a pamphlet and/or show a short video that describes the procedure and contains answers to many of the questions patients have about cornea transplant surgery.

The patient must also understand that a PKP type of cornea transplant requires many months of healing prior to obtaining the best possible vision. Complete recovery could take over a year before all sutures are removed and eyeglasses or contact lenses are prescribed. Patients should also understand that activities may be restricted for a significant period after the transplant. During the postoperative period, patients should not participate in contact sports or other activities that could result in direct trauma to the eye, since the cornea will always be weaker having undergone transplantation.

Discussion with the patient also should include the type of anesthesia that will be used during the operation. Anesthesia needs to be determined with input from both the patient and the anesthesiologist. If the patient is cooperative and agreeable, monitored anesthesia with a retrobulbar or peribulbar and lid block is usually done. General anesthesia is required in children, in patients with mental disabilities and in patients who are extremely apprehensive and anxious about the operation.

## ▶ THE OPERATIVE PROCEDURE

### Preparation of the Patient

Penetrating keratoplasty is usually performed as an outpatient procedure. Preparation for the procedure begins in the preoperative area with administration of antibiotic eyedrops, usually moxifloxacin (Vigamox), once every 5 minutes three times. Similarly, pilocarpine eyedrops, 2%, are administered every 5 minutes three times, if the eye is phakic or pseudophakic and if PKP is the only procedure planned. Dilating drops in the form of cyclopentolate (Cyclogel), 1%, and phenylephrine (Neo-Synephrine®), 2.5%, each administered three times, are utilized if a combined procedure is planned, such as cataract removal with intraocular lens implant or secondary posterior chamber intraocular lens implant.

The patient is taken to the operating room after slit lamp examination of the donor tissue in the preservation vial has shown that the donor cornea is acceptable for transplantation. Once the patient is positioned on the operating table in the supine position, the operating microscope is adjusted at the top of the patient's head and the retrobulbar and lid block anesthesia or general anesthesia is administered. The eyelashes are trimmed or taped out of the operative field, and the eye is prepped and draped in the usual manner for ophthalmic surgery. Intravenous cefazolin (Kefzol), 1 g, is routinely given unless the patient is allergic to penicillin, in which case vancomycin is administered.

### Donor Tissue Preparation

Approximately 1 hour before transplantation, the vial containing the donor cornea is removed from the styrofoam container and allowed to warm to room temperature. A cornea at room temperature facilitates the actions of antibiotics in the solution against bacteria that might be inadvertently attached to the corneal tissue.

Most cornea surgeons determine the proper size of the donor corneal button and the trephine diameter in the recipient by selecting a donor button size that is 0.25–0.50 mm larger than the diameter of the recipient trephine. A donor button of a larger diameter than the trephine size of the recipient's excised cornea helps provide a watertight wound closure, decrease the incidence of postoperative glaucoma in aphakic or pseudophakic eyes and provide a deeper anterior chamber. The eye, however, will be more myopic. In the case of keratoconus, however, some surgeons prefer to use the same trephine size for both the donor and the recipient corneas.

Using forceps, the donor corneal scleral tissue is carefully removed from the vial, transferred to the operating table and placed into a medicine glass or sterile specimen container along with some of the preservation media. The donor button is punched with the selected trephine after a partial-thickness trephine incision has been made in the recipient cornea, but prior to entering the anterior chamber. The donor corneal scleral tissue is placed on the concave teflon cutting block, endothelial side up, centered and punched by hand using the Castroviejo-type disposable trephine blade

with the obturator retracted (Fig. 2). A guillotine-type corneal donor punch, such as a Hessburg-Barron disposable donor trephine[7] or one of several other corneal trephine punches, may also be used (Fig. 3). The corneal button must be punched so as to be centered entirely within the limbus. To minimize astigmatism, it is important that the trephine blade be positioned to cut the cornea perpendicularly to the table. Once cut, the button is immersed with several drops of preservation media, covered and set aside until it will be sutured into the patient's eye.

Although not yet widely utilized, femtosecond laser technology is used by a few transplant surgeons to produce a variety of incision patterns that are not achievable with conventional trephines.[8,9] The femtosecond laser can be programmed to cut various incision patterns for the donor and recipient corneas, such as mushroom-shaped, top hat and zigzag patterns.

### ❧ RECIPIENT PROCEDURE

The lids are separated with a wire lid speculum, and superior and inferior rectus traction sutures are placed in phakic eyes to stabilize the globe during trephination. In pseudophakic or aphakic eyes and in infant eyes, a double Flieringa ring or the McNeill-Goldmann ring (Fig. 4) is sewn to the episclera or sclera in four to six locations in order to support the cornea. This technique is particularly important in cases of decreased scleral rigidity or in which a vitrectomy might be utilized. The diameter of the trephine to be utilized can be determined by using calipers or sizer trephine blades, in 0.25 mm increments, which were used in previous keratoplasties. In most cases, the marking or sizer trephine blade is selected to surround the central pathology adequately and to be large enough to supply adequate endothelial cells, but not extend to the limbus.

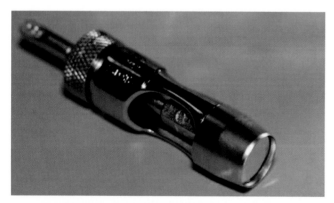

**Fig. 2:** Castroviejo corneal trephine with the obturator slightly retracted

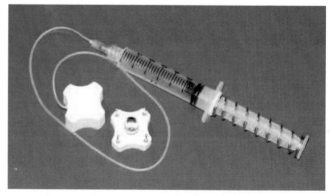

**Fig. 3:** Hessburg-Barron disposable donor corneal trephine

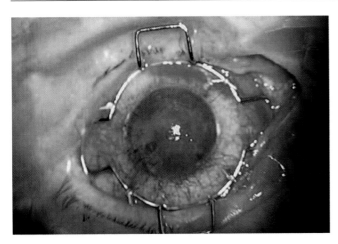

**Fig. 4:** McNeill-Goldmann ring with blepharostat is sewn to the sclera in four to six equally spaced 5-0 dacron sutures

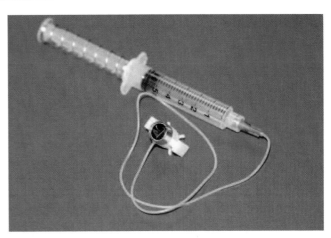

**Fig. 5:** Hessburg-Barron disposable suction recipient trephine

Trephination may be performed with the hand-held Castroviejo trephine (Fig. 2), the Hessburg-Barron disposable suction trephine (Fig. 5) or the Hanna trephine system. A partial-thickness trephination is done to approximately two thirds to three fourths of the depth of the cornea (Fig. 6). The cornea is then marked with a four- or an eight-bladed radial keratotomy marker in order to facilitate suture placement (Fig. 7). At this point, attention is directed to trephination of the donor button. Once the donor button is trephined and stored, attention is redirected to the patient's cornea. A #75 blade is used to enter the anterior chamber at the 9 o'clock position (for a right-handed surgeon) (Fig. 8). Using a sweeping motion in the previous groove, the incision is extended for about

2 o'clock hours to permit the insertion of the Katzin corneal transplant scissors. The right cutting scissors are used to complete the corneal incision inferiorly, from the 9 o'clock position and around to the 2 o'clock position (Fig. 9). The left corneal scissors are used to complete the incision superiorly. Some surgeons prefer to leave a small inner lip by tilting the scissors slightly.

Care is taken not to injure the iris or lens during entrance with the knife or while extending the incision with the scissors. A viscoelastic material may be injected into the anterior chamber to protect the iris and lens. Any necessary trimming of the recipient incision is done at this time. Once the cornea is removed, other procedures may be undertaken, such as extracapsular cataract extraction, intraocular

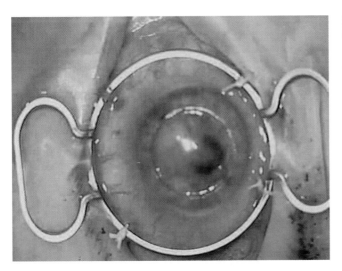

**Fig. 6:** Partial-thickness trephine incision

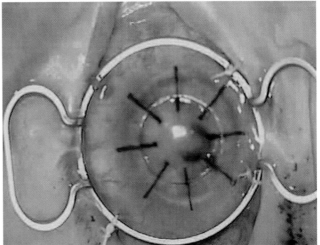

**Fig. 7:** Eight-bladed radial keratomy marker imprinted dye marks to facilitate suture placement

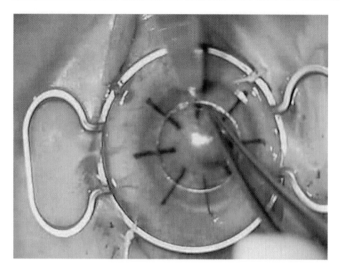

**Fig. 8:** A #75 knife blade entering the anterior chamber through the previously made partial-thickness trephine

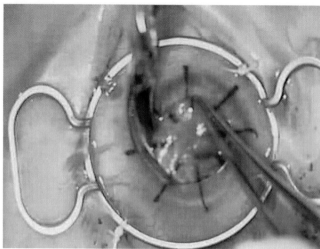

**Fig. 9:** Katzin corneal scissors cutting the recipient cornea in the groove of the partial trephine incision

lens exchange, lysis of peripheral anterior synechia and iridoplasty or iridectomy. A small amount of viscoelastic material is placed in the pupillary area, especially if an intraocular lens is in place, following which the donor cornea is brought into position using a Paton spatula.

## Suturing the Donor Cornea in Place

The Pierce Colibri forceps are used to hold the donor cornea at the 12 o'clock position. Using a forceps, the assistant stabilizes the cornea at the 6 o'clock position. The double-pronged Pollack corneal forceps can be used at 12 o'clock in lieu of an assistant holding the cornea at the 6 o'clock position. A 10-0 nylon suture on a spatula needle is placed

at the 12 o'clock position by the surgeon (Figs 10A to C). Holding the donor cornea at exactly the 6 o'clock position, the needle is passed under the forceps and through the donor and recipient corneas, utilizing the previously placed markings as a guide. The 3 and 9 o'clock sutures are placed similarly, forming in the cornea a square crease with equal sides (Fig. 11). The four interrupted cardinal sutures are placed perpendicular to the corneal surface in order to obtain a deep, 80–90% depth of the corneal thickness, with approximately a 0.75–1.0 mm bite on each side of the corneal incision. A triple throw followed by two single throws are used to tie the knot. The 6 o'clock suture is the most important for determining the degree of astigmatism and must equally bisect the cornea.

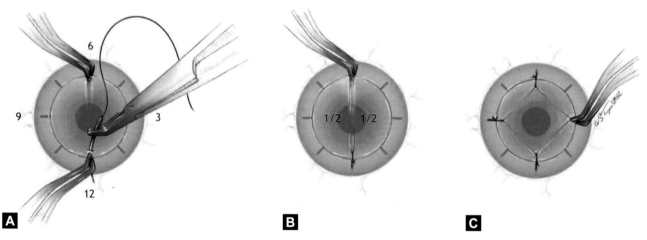

**Figs 10A to C:** Cardinal suture placement. (A) Place the needle through the donor and recipient cornea at 12 o'clock while the assistant holds the donor cornea at 6 o'clock; (B) Equally bisect the donor cornea by holding the donor cornea 180° from the first suture; (C) Complete cardinal sutures by a similar procedure at the 3 and 9 o'clock positions

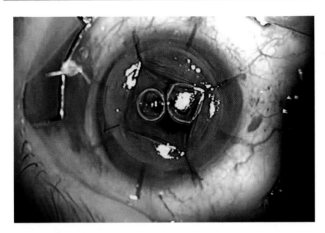

**Fig. 11:** Proper placement of the cardinal sutures, forming a square crease with equal sides

The final decision on the type of suture technique, which includes interrupted, interrupted running, double running and running techniques, is determined after the cardinal sutures are placed (Fig. 12). The suture technique utilized depends on both the surgeon's preferences and the circumstances. For infants and patients with vascularized corneas, 16 interrupted sutures are used. All knots are buried (Fig. 13). For relatively clear corneas, which are not vascularized, a single or double running suture may be appropriate, which could allow quicker visual rehabilitation. A combination of 8 or 12 interrupted sutures and a running 10-0 or 11-0 nylon suture is used by some surgeons so that astigmatism can be adjusted by early selective suture removal.

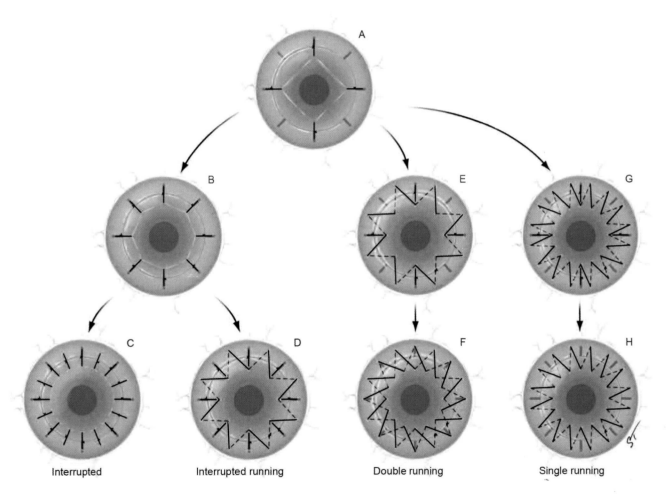

Interrupted    Interrupted running    Double running    Single running

**Fig. 12:** Suture placement techniques. (A) Cardinal sutures placed at the 3, 6, 9 and 12 o'clock markings; (B) Eight interrupted 10-0 nylon sutures; (C) Sixteen interrupted sutures with knots buried; (D) Interrupted running suture pattern with all knots buried; (E) First running 10-0 nylon suture for double running technique. Note cardinal sutures; (F) Double running, usually 11-0 nylon, for the second suture. The cardinal sutures are removed; (G) Single running 10-0 nylon suture with cardinal sutures still in place; (H) Single running 10-0 nylon sutures with cardinal sutures removed

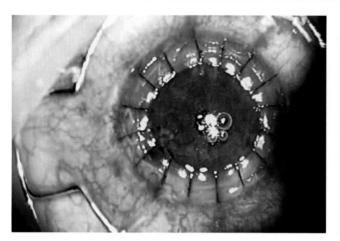

**Fig. 13:** Sixteen interrupted sutures, with all of the knots buried, in a corneal transplant patient

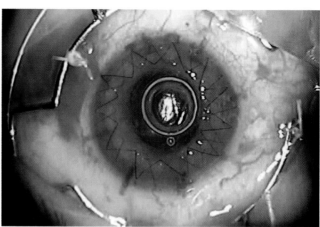

**Fig. 14:** Double running 10-0 and 11-0 nylon sutures in a cornea transplant patient

A single running nylon suture is often used in cases of keratoconus, since healing usually occurs sooner in the younger individual. A double running 10-0 and 11-0 nylon suture may be utilized in older individuals (Fig. 14), with the 11-0 sutures remaining in place indefinitely after removal of the 10-0 suture 3–6 months postoperatively, after which spectacles are prescribed. When a running suture is used, the cardinal sutures are typically removed before the running suture has been tied and adjusted. The running suture is tightened slightly, to remove any slack and to prevent any leakage of aqueous, and then tied. The knot is buried in the incision, if it was not buried when tied in the incision. Intraoperative keratoscopy is utilized to determine if significant astigmatism exists by projecting a ring of light or reflections onto the corneal surface. If any ovality of the circle is noted, the sutures are adjusted to make the circle round, tightening the area of the suture that is the longest dimension of the oval ring.

Following removal of the McNeill-Goldmann ring, an antibiotic, usually 40 mg of gentamicin or tobramycin and 80 mg of a long-acting steroid, such as methylprednisolone (Depo-Medrol), are injected below Tenon's capsule. A topical antibiotic is then applied, and the eye is patched. The patient is sent home, to be seen in the clinic the following day.

## ▶ POSTOPERATIVE CARE

On the first postoperative day, the patient's vision, with and without pinhole, is checked, along with the intraocular pressure and the corneal thickness. A slit lamp examination is performed, noting the corneal clarity, wound appearance and epithelial healing by using fluorescein dye. The wound is inspected and the Siedel test is used to rule out wound leak. The degree of cellular inflammation in the anterior chamber is noted. A thickened, hazy cornea on postoperative day 1 can be due to primary graft failure, excessive handling of the donor tissue or hypotony due to a wound leak. A crystal clear thin cornea may indicate a high intraocular pressure, in the range of 40 mm Hg. However, the pressure usually returns to normal in two or three days if the pressure elevation is secondary to the viscoelastic administered during the operation, although temporary antiglaucoma treatment should be started. A bandage soft contact lens is usually utilized to aid the re-epithelialization unless it is nearly complete. A topical fluoroquinolone and prednisolone acetate 1%, both administered four times a day, are prescribed at the first postoperative visit. To reduce the chance for graft rejection, cyclosporin A, 2%, four times daily, is given empirically for 1 year to all patients undergoing a repeat graft, in patients with highly vascularized corneas and in all young children.

The second follow-up visit occurs 1 week after the operation and then follow-up visits are scheduled monthly thereafter for at least 1 year to continue monitoring graft healing. The antibiotic drops are discontinued when complete re-epithelialization has occurred. The steroid dose is gradually tapered over 3 months, after which maintenance with fluorometholone 0.1% ophthalmic solution, once or twice daily, is continued indefinitely.

Exposed interrupted sutures should be removed or replaced, if necessary. Tight interrupted sutures may be removed at 2 or 3 months to adjust for astigmatism. However, in older individuals, the running suture may need to remain for longer than 1 year to allow for adequate healing. Too early suture removal may result in wound dehiscence that requires resuturing. Glasses or a contact lens can be prescribed after 3 months in most individuals.

## ❧ COMBINED PROCEDURES WITH PENETRATING KERATOPLASTY

### Cataract Surgery

If a visually significant cataract is present, the cataract should be removed at the time of the PKP. Cataract extraction is usually performed through an open-sky trephine incision, unless the visibility is clear enough to do a phacoemulsification procedure prior to performing PKP. The cataract is removed at the time of cornea transplant surgery for two reasons. First, the cataract will get worse following a PKP because of the steroid use and the length of time before the patient is visually rehabilitated. Second, a cataract operation following PKP will cause damage to the corneal endothelium and may incite a graft rejection or corneal decompensation. The disadvantage of a combined procedure is that the intraocular lens power is an estimation using irregular K readings from the diseased eye, K readings from the opposite eye, and/or the surgeon's experience.

### Triple Procedure: Penetrating Keratoplasty, Cataract Extraction and Intraocular Lens Implant

Penetrating keratoplasty and cataract removal with an intraocular lens implant are usually done by means of open-sky extracapsular cataract extraction because of the inability to adequately visualize the lens through an opaque cornea. After the recipient cornea is removed, any trimming of the recipient wound edge is performed and peripheral synechia are lysed. The cataract can then be removed using the extracapsular technique. A #75 blade is utilized to pierce the anterior capsule 8–10 times in a circular fashion, creating a 5–6 mm in diameter capsularhexis. Conversely, a circular capsularhexis can be performed with curved Vannas scissors. The anterior capsule is removed with forceps, and the cataractous lens is rocked back and forth to loosen the nucleus from the cortex. A lens loop and a Paton spatula or other blunt instrument are used to press on the limbus at the 6 and 12 o'clock positions, applying enough pressure to tumble the lens nucleus through the pupil, where it can be removed with the lens loop (Fig. 15). Care must be taken to avoid any pressure on the globe or lids, which would result in positive vitreous pressure.

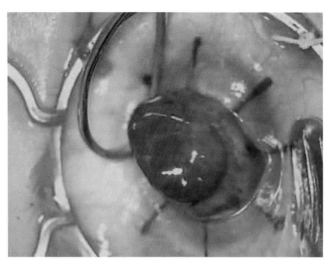
**Fig. 15:** Open-sky extracapsular cataract removal

The irrigation-aspiration handpiece of the phacoemulsification unit is used to remove the cortical remains from the equator, applying slight posterior pressure and irrigation to avoid engaging the iris or anterior capsule. It is best to use a low-aspiration suction to slowly and carefully remove the cortex from under the iris and from the lens equator in a radial fashion for 360°, watching for capsule remnants that may be caught in the opening of the irrigation-aspiration handpiece. Once all visible cortex has been removed, a viscoelastic material is placed on the posterior capsule. The intraocular lens power calculation is determined by K readings and A-scan or IOL Master® measurement in the opposite eye, reducing the power by about 2 diopters if the graft is oversized by 0.5 mm.

Using the Harms tying forceps, the intraocular lens is inserted into the capsular bag. One haptic is inserted deep below the iris into the capsular bag on one side (Fig. 16). Next, pressing down on the optic and holding it in place with the curved Harms forceps in a reversed position, the other haptic is folded centrally. While the optic is pushed posteriorly, the haptic is released under the iris and in the capsular bag. Acetylcholine chloride intraocular solution (Miochol) is instilled onto the iris surface to constrict the pupil so that the iris covers as much of the optic of the intraocular lens as possible. Viscoelastic is again placed on the surface of the intraocular lens and the donor cornea is sutured at 12, 6, 3 and 9 o'clock positions. The cardinal sutures are quickly and accurately placed, allowing the anterior chamber to be reformed with air and balanced salt solution (BSS).

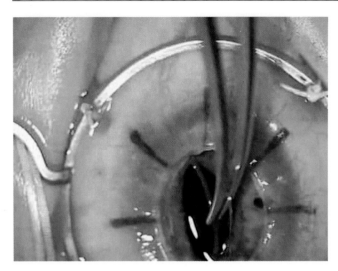

**Fig. 16:** Insertion of an intraocular lens into the capsular bag

If vitreous loss occurs during lens implantation, an open-sky vitrectomy is performed to remove the central core of vitreous, extending the vitrectomy toward the 3 and 9 o'clock positions. If the anterior capsule remains adequate for haptic support, scleral fixation is not required. However, if capsular support is inadequate, the lens haptics must be placed in the ciliary sulcus and sutured to sclera using double-armed 10-0 prolene suture on a CIF-4 needle. A limbal peritomy is made at the 3 and 9 o'clock positions, extending 2 mm posteriorly in order to cover the scleral sutures. The intraocular lens the author prefers is the CZ70BD PMMA® (manufactured by Alcon) with the eyelets on the haptic, but a 6 mm optic, three-piece acrylic lens may be used, if the surgeon prefers. If an intraocular lens with the eyelets in the haptics is used, the prolene suture is threaded through the eyelet and each needle is passed through the sclera from within the eye, 1.0–1.5 mm from the visible limbus, at the 3 or 9 o'clock positions. The sutures are then tied to each other and trimmed close to the knot. The knot is then carefully rotated into the sclera. The opposite side is done similarly. If a three-piece acrylic lens is used, a girth hitch is placed on each haptic and the prolene suture is passed and tied the same manner, except the suture ends must be trimmed flush with the knot and covered with Tenon's fascia and conjunctiva.[10]

## Uncontrolled Glaucoma

A patient with a corneal condition that requires PKP may also have uncontrolled or marginally controlled glaucoma despite receiving maximum dosages of antiglaucoma medications.

Such a patient may benefit from trabeculectomy, endolaser trabeculoplasty, transscleral cyclophotocoagulation, insertion of a valve or tube shunt. The author's preference is to perform all glaucoma procedures as a separate procedure before PKP in order to establish normal intraocular pressure. However, in rare cases, he has performed a tube shunt or a valve insertion at the time of the PKP. At the present time, he prefers the Ahmed valve because it appears to be the best way to avoid hypotony or choroid detachment following the procedure. There is, however, a higher rate of corneal decompensation with any valve or tube whether it is implanted before, during or after PKP.[11,12]

## Iris Procedures

An optical iridoplasty peripheral iridectomy or closure of an iridodialysis cleft can be done at the same time as the PKP.

## Oculoplastic Surgery

Eyelid pathology such as entropion, ectropion and exposure keratitis should be corrected before PKP. A lateral tarsorrhaphy is often necessary at the time of PKP in cases of neurotrophic keratitis. Insertion of punctal plugs or punctual cautery may also be required in patients with very dry eyes.

## Strabismus Surgery

Eye muscle surgery should be deferred until after PKP has been performed and attempts at visual correction have been made. It should not be performed immediately after suture removal. Rather, because of the possibility of wound dehiscence due to excessive pressure on the globe, eye muscle surgery should be performed prior to the final suture removal if improved corrected vision is obtained or at least 3 months after suture removal.

## INTRAOPERATIVE COMPLICATIONS

Intraoperative complications include vitreous loss, which can be due to excessive pressure on the globe or to positive vitreous pressure from fluid, including blood from a choroidal hemorrhage. If suprachoroidal hemorrhage develops, early recognition is imperative and the cornea must be immediately sutured in place with 9-0 or stronger sutures to prevent expulsion of intraocular contents. Intraoperative choroidal hemorrhage may be signaled by the onset of a progressive increase in vitreous pressure and the appearance of a black choroidal shadow. Sclerotomies to drain the suprachoroidal hemorrhage should be performed as soon as the cornea has been sewn in place. Usually, the lens is extruded and the vitreous present in the wound may be removed after the intraocular pressure is reduced by drainage of the choroidal hemorrhage.

For vitreous loss of a less serious nature, a vitrectomy can be performed to remove the vitreous in front of the iris. Removal of vitreous from the anterior chamber is aided by the injection of air if the cornea graft has been sutured in place. A dislocated intraocular lens can be replaced once an adequate vitrectomy has been performed. The intraocular lens haptics are placed in the ciliary sulcus and sewn into the sclera, as previously described for intraocular lens implant.

A wound leak after the donor cornea is sutured into place can usually be controlled by using additional interrupted sutures. On rare occasions, a leak from the suture tract occurs, which can be closed by placing a longer suture, compressing the cornea and closing the leak as the suture is tightened. The loose suture at the leak site is then removed.

## ▶ EARLY POSTOPERATIVE COMPLICATIONS

A wound leak or flat anterior chamber on postoperative day 1 requires resuturing of the graft at the leak site. This procedure can usually be accomplished in a minor surgery room without the need to take the patient to the operating suite. Another complication on the first postoperative day is an elevated intraocular pressure of 40 mm Hg or above, usually secondary to retained viscoelastic substance. However, another cause of the increased intraocular pressure can be glaucoma not controlled before the corneal transplant.

### Primary Graft Failure

Signs of primary graft failure are seen on the first postoperative day. The transplanted cornea appears thick and hazy, and its appearance fails to improve over a 2-month period despite frequent use of steroid eyedrops. If primary graft failure is diagnosed, and there is no improvement in 1–2 months, the cornea should be replaced, providing there is no contraindication for further surgery.

### Glaucoma

Significantly elevated intraocular pressure should be treated medically to lower the pressure to a normal range. Besides topical antiglaucoma drugs, acetazolamide, 500 mg twice daily, may be necessary temporarily. Steroid-induced elevated intraocular pressure can be helped by using fluorometholone in place of prednisolone acetate drops. Occasionally, transscleral cyclophotocoagulation is necessary.

Some patients who are aphakic or pseudophakic may develop high intraocular pressure postoperatively because an oversized graft was not utilized, thus compromising the anterior chamber angle.[13] This situation requires medical treatment and, occasionally, a peripheral iridectomy.

### Epithelial Defect

If a large epithelial defect is present, a bandage contact lens should be placed and frequent lubrication provided. If the epithelial defect fails to heal or improve significantly after 1 week of treatment, an additional procedure, such as lateral tarsorrhaphy, an amniotic membrane graft or ProKera ring®, may be required to stimulate healing. Other methods to promote healing include: treatment with oral doxycycline, 100 mg once daily; punctal occlusion, and dry eye therapy.

### Endophthalmitis

The presence of decreased vision, pain and increased inflammation of the eye during the early postoperative period may signify microbial endophthalmitis. If cultures taken from the cornea rim at the time of keratoplasty were positive for an organism, early treatment can be directed to that organism specifically. However, broad-spectrum antibiotic treatment of endophthalmitis, with a vitreous tap for culture at the same time, consists of intraocular vancomycin, 1.0 mg per ml, and ceftazadine, 2.0–2.25 mg per ml, with each given in the amount of 0.1 ml.

## ▶ LATE COMPLICATIONS

A corneal ulcer or suture abscess can develop at anytime during the postoperative course. After scraping and culture are obtained, and the suture at the infected site is removed, the corneal ulcer or abscess is treated with the usual antibiotic therapy.

### Corneal Graft Rejection

Although PKP is associated with an excellent long-term survival rate,[14] graft rejection may occur anytime from 1 or 2 weeks postkeratoplasty to more than 30 years following PKP.[15] The patient should be taught the symptoms of an impending graft rejection. Corneal transplant patients with symptoms of photophobia, redness and decreased vision should be evaluated as soon as possible, within 24–48 hours in order to start antirejection treatment. The diagnosis of a graft rejection is confirmed by slit lamp findings of an anterior chamber cellular reaction, an endothelial rejection line or increased corneal thickness seen by slit lamp examination, and decreased vision. The usual treatment of graft rejection consists of a sub-Tenon's injection of 80 mg of methylprednisolone, plus hourly prednisolone acetate 1% eyedrops (Pred Forte) for 12–14 days, after which the dosage is gradually reduced if a favorable response is seen. If no improvement occurs after 2 weeks of therapy, the condition is unlikely to resolve and the graft is considered rejected. In rare cases, such as a young patient with keratoconus, the corneal graft may clear over 6–12 months due to central migration of the peripheral recipient endothelium.

## Wound Dehiscence at Suture Removal

Corneal wound dehiscence at the time of suture removal may occur as a result of inadequate healing of the corneal incision. Adequate healing is seen by slit lamp examination as a fine line of scar formation in the incision 360°. Wound dehiscence requires resuturing of the corneal wound, allowing 4–6 more months of healing, with the possibility of permanent sutures.

## Astigmatism

Selective suture removal is done to reduce astigmatism as soon as 3 months postoperatively. However, removal of all sutures varies from patient to patient, depending on how much scar has formed in the wound. Scarring is age- and steroid-dependent. Older patients must heal for a year or more before all sutures can be removed safely. Once all sutures are removed, the patient may remain with high astigmatism, which may require a corneal relaxing incision or laser refractive surgery treatment for corneal astigmatism if spectacles or gas permeable contact lenses are not satisfactory.

## ▶ MAKING THE DECISION TO PERFORM REPEAT PENETRATING KERATOPLASTY

Several factors must be considered when faced with the decision of whether or not to perform a second (or a third) PKP: Does the patient still have the potential for useful vision? What was the cause of the graft failure? Was the graft failure because of an allograft rejection or was it because of corneal decompensation secondary to endothelial cell dysfunction or loss? Is there an absence of

an active disease process, such as keratouveitis, ongoing graft rejection, primary graft failure, progressive scarring from stem cell deficiency or active infection in the graft resulting in impending perforation?

If the condition has been successfully treated and stabilized to the extent that the patient's eye has a good chance for improved vision, then repeat PKP can be considered. The second operation should not be performed until the eye has remained noninflamed for at least 6 months. If the patient has excellent vision in the contralateral eye, a repeat PKP may not be indicated as a means of improving the patient's quality of life.

## ▶ ACKNOWLEDGMENTS

Preparation of this chapter was supported in part by an unrestricted departmental grant from Research to Prevent Blindness, New York, NY. Figures 10 and 12 were illustrated by Stacy Turpin, medical illustrator at the University of Missouri School of Medicine. Sharon Scott Morey assisted in the preparation of the manuscript.

## ▶ REFERENCES

1. Eye Bank Association of America, 2010. Eye Banking Statistical Report. Washington, DC: Eye Bank Association of America; 2010. pp. 5, 13.
2. Eye Bank Association of America. Medical standards. Washington, DC: Eye Bank Association of America; 2010.
3. Cornea Donor Study Investigator Group, Gal RL, Dontchev M, et al. The effect of donor age on corneal transplantation outcome: results of the Cornea Donor Study. Ophthalmology. 2008;115(4):620-6.
4. Bartels MC, Doxiadis IIN, Colen TP, et al. Long-term outcome in high-risk corneal transplantation and the influence of HLA-A and HLA-B matching. Cornea. 2003;22(6):552-6.
5. Völker-Dieben HJ, Claas FHJ, Schreuder GMT, et al. Beneficial effect of HLA-DR matching on the survival of corneal allografts. Transplantation. 2000;70:640-8.
6. Numedis, Inc., Isanti, Minn. Webpage titled Life4°C: Changing the World One Cornea at a Time. Available at: http://numedis.us/life4c_files/life4c.html. [Accessed August 15, 2010].
7. Hessberg P, Barron M. A disposable corneal trephine. Ophthalmic Surg. 1980;11:730-3.
8. Farid M, Steinert RF, Gaster RN, et al. Comparison of penetrating keratoplasty performed with femtosecond laser zig-zag incision versus conventional blade trephination. Ophthalmology. 2009; 116:1638-43.
9. Chamberlain WD, Rush SW, Mathers WD, et al. Comparison of femtosecond laser-assisted keratoplasty versus conventional penetrating keratoplasty. Ophthalmology. 2011;118:486-91.
10. Cowden JK, Hu BV. A new surgical technique for posterior chamber lens fixation during penetrating keratoplasty in the absence of capsular or zonular support. Cornea. 1988;7: 231-5.

11. McDermott ML, Swendris RP, Shin DH, et al. Corneal endothelial cell counts after Molteno implantation. Am J Ophthalmol. 1993;115:93-6.
12. Steward DH, Swendris RP, Shin DH, et al. Outcome of Molteno implantation for glaucoma associated with penetrating keratoplasty. Invest Ophthalmol Vis Sci. 1992;33(4):1273.
13. Heidemann DG, Sugar A, Meyer RF, et al. Oversized donor grafts in penetrating keratoplasty. Arch Ophthalmol. 1985;103:1807-11.
14. Thompson RW, Price MO, Bowers PJ, et al. Long-term graft survival after penetrating keratoplasty. Am J Ophthalmol. 2003;110:1396-402.
15. Cowden JW, Udell IJ. Allograft rejection reaction after 28 and 35 years (Poster). Presented at Eye Bank Association of American Scientific Sessions, 1996, and at the Second International Conference on Cornea, Eye Banking and External Disease, Prague, Czech Republic; 1996.

CHAPTER 80

# Management of Postkeratoplasty Astigmatism

*Lorenzo J Cervantes, Alex Mammen, Wan Xiao, Deepinder K Dhaliwal*

## ❧ INTRODUCTION

Astigmatism is the main refractive complication to occur following penetrating keratoplasty (PKP), and is due to a variety of different factors.[1] It is one of the major limiting parameters for visual rehabilitation of patients, even if the graft is clear, and it has been the subject of investigation and management for many years.[2-5] Average postkeratoplasty astigmatism has been reported to be between 4 and 6 diopters.[4] The amount of residual postoperative astigmatism that can be tolerated depends on the eye's visual potential, refractive status of the fellow eye, presence of binocularity, and the patient's occupation and expectations.[6]

Our paradigm for treatment of postkeratoplasty astigmatism consists of an approach that begins with preoperative planning and continues into the operating room with meticulous surgical technique. Every step of the procedure can have a lasting effect on the creation of surgically-induced astigmatism (SIA). Immediately following surgery, care to promote healing is of paramount importance. Once the epithelium has healed and the graft deturgesces, visual rehabilitation can proceed. The postkeratoplasty period can be divided into two parts regarding visual rehabilitation: before and after complete suture removal. We typically start to selectively remove sutures from postkeratoplasty eyes approximately 6 months following surgery in order to reduce keratometric and manifest astigmatism. All sutures are removed after about a year, at which time the cornea has more or less stabilized and the astigmatism can be more permanently addressed. Vision can be improved after suture removal with proper spectacle refraction or contact lens fitting. It should be noted, however, that astigmatism

can continue to evolve, especially in progressive ectatic disorders.[6] For patients who are contact lens intolerant, surgical techniques like astigmatic keratotomy or limbal relaxing incisions can be performed, as well as excimer laser treatments like laser-assisted *in situ* keratomileusis (LASIK) or photorefractive keratectomy (PRK). In severe cases of high irregular astigmatism, repeating the keratoplasty might be the only way to rehabilitate the eye.

## ❧ PREOPERATIVE FACTORS

Preoperative factors that may contribute to post-PKP astigmatism include a deep orbit, tight palpebral fissure, thin or ectatic cornea or sclera, corneal scarring, presence of an anterior chamber intraocular lens, aphakia, and high positive vitreous pressure.[7] These factors should be kept in mind both during trephination of the host cornea and suturing of the donor cornea.

## ❧ INTRAOPERATIVE FACTORS

The major intraoperative goal in decreasing post-PKP astigmatism is good wound alignment. The first step in achieving this goal is creation of the host portion of the wound. Care should be taken to avoid introducing globe distortion from eyelid, lid speculum or scleral fixation ring pressure. A fixation ring larger than the lid opening or one that is sutured too tightly, can exert pressure on the globe and induce distortion. Next, whenever possible, the graft should be centered within the host cornea. Large amounts of graft decentration, although sometimes necessary to encompass the pathology being treated, can introduce astigmatism.[8]

Trephination of the host cornea that yields a perpendicular edge minimizes astigmatism.[9] Suction trephination has a theoretical benefit of a more controlled cut with less blade tilt and therefore less astigmatism. However, the evidence to support this theory is limited to a single study showing less astigmatism (average 2.55 D) when a Krumeich-guided suction trephine was used to trephine both the donor and host corneas when compared to manual trephination of both (average 6 D) or suction trephination of just the host cornea (average 3 D).[10] Comparison of suction trephines has not shown a significant difference in refractive outcome.[11] Femtosecond laser trephination allows for customized wound creation that reduces the need for sutures and theoretically facilitates better wound alignment. However, in a 24-month-long retrospective case series of 50 eyes that underwent femtosecond laser-assisted zig-zag PKP compared to 50-age-, diagnosis-, and comorbidity-matched eyes that underwent conventional blade PKP, there was no significant difference in topographic astigmatism after the 6-month interval or best-corrected spectacle visual acuity at any time point.[12] Moreover, the current hurdles of cost and practicality with regard to the availability of lasers within or in close proximity to the operating room remain.

Significant eccentricity when punching the donor cornea can introduce astigmatism. Tissue deficiency or underride in a particular meridian will steepen it and tissue excess or override will flatten it.[13,14] Posterior punching of the donor corneal button (endothelium side up) has been shown to produce a more regular cut compared to an anterior approach with an artificial anterior chamber but no significant difference in astigmatic outcome has been shown.[15] Oversizing the corneal graft by 0.25–0.5 diopters does not affect postoperative astigmatism compared to same-sized grafts. Grafts greater than 8.75 mm, however, are associated with less astigmatism, and those less than 7.00 mm are associated with greater astigmatism. Graft sizes in between are minimally affected.[16]

Once the donor corneal button is punched, the next step is aligning the donor cornea with the host's. Prior to suturing, however, rotating the donor button until the most spherical reflex is obtained with an intraoperative keratometer may improve postoperative astigmatism.[10] When it comes to suturing, the intraoperative step that has the greatest influence on the resulting astigmatism, emphasis should be placed on epithelial alignment. Misalignment here, which usually manifests as graft-host override, can contribute to both astigmatism and problems with wound healing. The greater role that epithelial misalignment plays over endothelial misalignment is evidenced by the fact that there is no significant difference in astigmatic outcome between deep anterior lamellar and penetrating keratoplasty.[17,18] Various handheld keratometers can be used to assess intraoperative keratometry and subsequently adjust sutures following removal of the scleral fixation ring and reformation of the anterior chamber. While these keratometers are for gross inspection of astigmatism, highlighting astigmatism of about 4 diopters or greater, intraoperative suture adjustment has been shown to significantly reduce the amount postoperative astigmatism compared to postoperative adjustment.[19] However, there is no consensus on whether this difference is maintained following suture removal.[1,20]

Suturing technique can be an important intraoperative factor contributing to postoperative astigmatism. There have been a number of different suture techniques proposed, including interrupted (IR), single-running (SR), double-running (DR) and combined interrupted and running (CIR) sutures. The interrupted suture technique was thought to have the advantage of reducing astigmatism through selective removal of sutures postoperatively. In 1977, McNeill and Kaufman reported the use of double-running nylon sutures.[21] In 1982, Stainer et al. reported a greater postoperative astigmatism reduction using the combination of interrupted sutures followed by an overlay of continuous suture.[22] In 1989, McNeill and Wessels reported the use of a single continuous running suture that is adjusted in the early postoperative period accordingly, thereby helping to reduce astigmatism.[23]

Despite much literature trying to answer which technique is optimal for minimizing postoperative astigmatism, there is no clear consensus about the superiority of any one particular technique. While some studies have shown no difference between the types of suture techniques,[24-29] other studies have reported less astigmatism with single-running technique, especially prior to suture removal.[30-33] There are also studies that have reported better results with double-running[34,35] or combined techniques.[36] The picture is further clouded by the heterogeneous disease of the patient population, the number of suture bites employed, and the change in astigmatism over time before and after suture removal. The results of comparisons from existing studies are summarized in Table 1. What can be agreed upon is that symmetric placement of radial sutures with bites of equal length and tension provides the best chance of minimizing suture-induced corneal astigmatism.

**Table 1:** Suturing techniques and their effects on astigmatism

| Author | Year | Type of Study | Suture Technique | Astigmatism Postoperative (Diopters) | Astigmatism Before Suture Removal (Diopters) | Astigmatism After Suture Removal (Diopters) |
|---|---|---|---|---|---|---|
| Lin[30] | 1990 | Randomized prospective | SR (16 bites) | 6.7 ± 2.3 | 1.7 ± 0.6 | |
| | | | DR (16 + 16 bites) | 5.9 ± 2.4 (p > 0.58) | 4.8 ± 2.6 (p < 0.01) | |
| Ramirez[31] | 2001 | Retrospective | SR (24 bites) | 2.2 ± 1.9 | 3.0 ± 2.2 | |
| | | | DR (12 + 12) | 4.5 ± 2.8 (p < 0.001) | 4.2 ± 2.1 (p = 0.03) | |
| Van Meter[32] | 1991 | Retrospective | SR (20–24 bites) | 6.5 ± 4.4 | 1.5 ± 1.1 | |
| | | | CIR (12 or 16 separate + 12–16 bites) | 8.4 ± 3.8 (p = 0.18) | 3.2 ± 1.9 (p < 0.01) | |
| Filatov[33] | 1993 | Randomized prospective | SR (24 bites) | 4.6 ± 1.5 | 2.7 ± 2.2 | |
| | | | CIR (8 separate + 16 bites) | 5.3 ± 2.1 (p < 0.479) | 3.9 ± 2.5 (p < 0.02) | |
| Filatov[24] | 1996 | Randomized prospective | SR (24 bites) | | | 3.3 ± 1.3 |
| | | | CIR (8 separate + 16 bites) | | | 2.8 ± 1.5 (p < 0.46) |
| Javadi[25] | 2006 | Randomized prospective | IR (16) | 3.77 ± 1.68 | 2.69 ± 2.5 | 3.83 ± 1.65 |
| | | | SR (16–18 bites) | 5.48 ± 2.1 | 3.23 ± 1.74 | 3.37 ± 1.9 |
| | | | CIR (8 separate +16 bites) | 4.1 ± 1.79 (p = 0.015) | 3.11 ± 2.75 (p = 0.851) | 3.88 ± 2.79 (p = 0.851) |
| Acar[26] | 2011 | Retrospective (DALK) | IR (16) | 5.56 ± 1.78 | 3.82 ± 1.72 | 3.87 ± 1.38 |
| | | | SR (16 bites) | 3.79 ± 1.19 | 3.56 ± 1.52 | 3.43 ± 1.44 |
| | | | CIR (8 separate + 16 bites) | 4.21 ± 1.55 (p = 0.012) | 3.75 ± 1.56 (p = 0.846) | 3.71 ± 1.46 (p = 0.846) |
| Karabatsas[27] | 1998 | Randomized prospective | SR (24 bites) | | 7.18 ± 3.12 | 4.46 ± 3.24 |
| | | | CIR (12 separate + 24 bites) | | 6.69 ± 3.11 | 4.76 ± 2.99 (p = 0.25) |
| Spadea[28] | 2002 | Randomized prospective | SR (16 bites) | | | 2.62 ± 1.20 |
| | | | DR (8 + 8 bites) | | | 2.73 ± 1.17 (p = 0.652) |
| Solano[29] | 2003 | Retrospective | SR (24 bites) | | | 5.2 ± 3.2 |
| | | | DR (12 + 12) | | | 4.6 ± 2.7 (p = 0.72) |
| Kim[34] | 2008 | Randomized prospective | IR (16 separate) | 7.14 ± 1.60 (p = 0.006 btw IR and SR) | 6.93 ± 1.42 | 5.99 ± 1.69 (p > 0.05 btw IR and SR) |
| | | | SR (16–24 bites) | 4.92 ± 1.96 (p = 0.872 btw SR and DR) | 4.71 ± 1.21 | 5.69 ± 1.49 (p < 0.05 btw SR and DR) |
| | | | DR (12 + 12 bites) | 5.13 ± 2.08 (p = 0.006 btw DR and IR) | 4.07 ± 1.37 | 3.63 ± 1.56 (p < 0.05 btw DR and IR) |
| Assil[35] | 1992 | Retrospective | DR (12 + 12 bites) | 3.55 | 1.54 | |
| | | | CIR (12 separate + 12 bites) | 6.98 (p = 0.004) | 4.07 (p = 0.004) | |
| Musch[36] | 1989 | Randomized prospective | DR | 3.5 | 4 | |
| | | | CIR (12 separate) | 4 | 2.5 (p = 0.06) | |

CIR: combined interrupted and running; DR: double-running; IR: interrupted; SR: single-running

# ❧ POSTOPERATIVE CONSIDERATIONS

## Topographical Evaluation

From using something as simple as a washer or safety pin to reflect a placido disk off the cornea at the operating microscope or slit lamp, to topography, keratometry, photo and videokeratoscopy, and utilizing Scheimpflug imaging, corneal astigmatism can be assessed both intra- and postoperatively with a variety of different instruments, and its management can thus be planned.[37-39] The reflection of a circular ring of light off the cornea is similar to a placido disk, with an ideal shape being completely round. The circular reflection becomes an ellipse with its longer dimension perpendicular to the meridian of tight sutures or parallel to the meridian of loose sutures. Cylinder and its axis measured by refractive power maps and topography correlate well with subjective manifest cylinder and axis.[40] Differences between topographical and manifest cylinder, however, do exist. This is often the result of suture-induced irregular astigmatism, causing asymmetric keratometric powers in meridians separated by an angle other than 180°, large changes in power from the most central to peripheral areas of the graft, areas of steepening present in the graft periphery, or lenticular astigmatism.[41] This disagreement between corneal topography, keratometry and refraction can lead to confusion when planning a treatment for the offending cylinder, as well as a less than efficacious result. During selective suture removal, for example, when there is disagreement, significantly less cylinder might be corrected when compared to the amount corrected when the various methods of quantitative cylindrical measurement agree.[42]

An important concept to understand is that in a cornea naïve to relaxing incisions, central steepening corresponds to peripheral flattening in the same meridian. This can be caused by a tight suture or a series of sutures whose vector sum direction is equivalent to the meridian of interest. The tight suture pulls on the peripheral cornea, thereby steepening the central cornea, which is the area assessed by topography and keratometry. Removing the tight suture, therefore, releases tension in the peripheral cornea allowing it to steepen. This causes the central cornea in that meridian to flatten, decreasing the amount of positive cylinder. Similarly, a peripheral arcuate or tangential incision relaxes the peripheral tension, creating peripheral steepening and central corneal flattening.

## Treatment of Postpenetrating Keratoplasty Astigmatism

### Suture Tension Adjustment

The goal of suture adjustment is to reduce the amount of postoperative astigmatism while maintaining the presence of the suture to preserve the integrity of the graft-host interface as it heals. By loosening tight sutures and redistributing tension evenly across the wound, visual rehabilitation might be possible in the early postkeratoplasty period when suture removal is not advised. When performed at the slit lamp, it can save the patient the inconvenience of replacing a suture in the operating room. Any postoperative suture adjustment should utilize topical anesthetic and antibiotic drops to reduce discomfort and the risk of infection. These antibiotic drops should be continued at 3–4 times daily for 3 or 4 days afterward. Topical steroids should also be utilized at the same frequency and at least the same duration to reduce risk of graft rejection. Timing of suture adjustment is important and should occur early enough before complete wound healing. Attempting to alter suture tension after complete healing has occurred may not allow for the reduction in cylinder to be translated to the final corneal shape following suture removal. Adjustment, however, should occur late enough for the graft to deturgesce, as tension on the sutures will change as the graft thins.[43] The most effective time to adjust sutures, however, might be at the time of surgery. Serdarevic et al. suggested that intraoperative suture adjustment, as opposed to postoperative adjustment, permitted more rapid visual rehabilitation, increased safety and increased refractive stability.[19] Because of its ability to redistribute tension circumferentially around the wound, a continuous suture has certain advantages to interrupted sutures in this respect, and can lead to earlier optical stability for visual rehabilitation.[32]

### Techniques of Suture Adjustment

*Interrupted sutures:* As previously discussed, tight interrupted sutures are identified in the meridian of central steepening. After drops of topical anesthetic and antibiotic, both tips of a Jewelers forceps can be guided underneath the anterior portion of the identified suture. The tips are then lightly allowed to spread, causing the nylon suture to stretch and release tension. Care must be taken to avoid breaking the suture, which might cause wound instability and necessitate suture replacement in the early postoperative period.

*Running sutures:* Adjustment of continuous running sutures should be carefully planned and executed. Over-manipulation of the suture increases the risk of rupture and graft dehiscence, requiring immediate repair. When evaluating corneal astigmatism using topography, the flat meridian corresponds to a region of relative suture laxity, and the steep meridian corresponds to a region of relative suture tautness. Therefore, one should plan to advance the distribution of the suture from the flat meridian to the direction of the steep one. Repeating the topography during adjustment can verify the effect of the manipulations. A less accurate, but more convenient, way of assessing corneal astigmatism at the operating microscope is with a washer or round end of a safety pin held above the cornea at a plane parallel to the iris, utilizing the previously-mentioned placido disk method. The direction of suture adjustment has been described by Van Meter[44] and illustrated in Figure 1. Epithelium is broken over the area of the suture. Using forceps, the suture is carefully grasped without twisting and advanced toward the steep meridian. This is done in a stepwise fashion until the tension has been distributed effectively.

### Suture Removal

Timing of selective suture removal should allow for the graft-host interface to heal, thereby decreasing the risk of wound

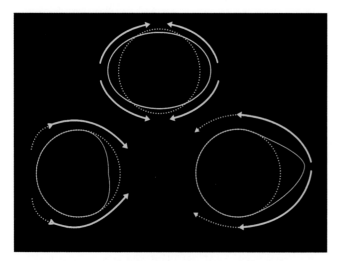

**Fig. 1:** Tension in the keratoplasty wound can be adjusted by advancing the continuous suture from the area of lower suture tension where the cornea is flat to where suture tension is higher and the cornea is steep. Thin solid lines represent astigmatic keratometer mires. Dotted lines represent spherical keratometer mires. Arrows represent direction of suture advancement.
*Source:* Reprinted from W Van Meter. The efficacy of a single continuous nylon suture for control of post keratoplasty astigmatism. Trans Am Ophthalmol Soc. 1996;94:1157-1180, courtesy of the American Ophthalmological Society

dehiscence.[45] Delaying selective suture removal until after the wound has completely healed, however, might reduce the effect of the intended astigmatic adjustment. This critical period is likely within one year following keratoplasty. Of 162 eyes that had undergone PK, there was no significant difference in astigmatic change with time when sutures were removed 1–2 years, 2–3 years, 3–4 years, and more than 4 years after surgery.[20] While many choose to leave corneal sutures in place indefinitely, spontaneous rupture of the sutures can have serious complications, including foreign body sensation, irritation, pain, suture infiltrates, corneal neovascularization, graft rejection and infection.

Single interrupted sutures should be cut as close as possible to the point where the suture turns posteriorly on the side of the graft-host interface opposite the knot. This can be done by sliding the tip of a 30-gauge needle bevel up underneath the anterior section of suture and passing it across the insertion point, meeting a slight bit of resistance as the suture breaks. This creates a long suture arm that can be easily grasped, prevents the knot from crossing the graft-host interface and inducing a wound dehiscence, and reduces the amount of potentially contaminated suture from passing through deep corneal stroma and seeding it with microorganisms. Grasping with larger caliber forceps, such as a fine tipped needle holder as opposed to fine jeweler's forceps, reduces the chance of amputating the suture arm. Provided the wound appears to be healing well, we start selective interrupted suture removal 6–9 months post keratoplasty, and continue to remove astigmatically-significant sutures every 4–6 weeks. All sutures are eventually removed after about 1 year.

Continuous running sutures can be removed in a fashion similar to that of interrupted sutures. A 30-gauge needle held bevel up can be used to fragment the running suture into multiple segments by cutting it at every other insertion site on the host side of the graft-host interface. This creates segments of the suture that can be grasped and pulled while minimizing the amount of contaminated suture pulled through the corneal stroma. Depending on the surgeon and the technique used for continuous suture placement, timing and effect of suture removal can vary. For example, using one surgeon's technique of a 10-0 nylon suture with deep bites used in conjunction with 10-0 or 11-0 suture with half-thickness bites, the deeper suture can be removed at around 6 months to reduce the amount of astigmatism. The remaining running suture has less effect on induced cylinder and serves mostly to reinforce the wound, to be removed after about a year.[46] When using double running sutures for keratoconus, removal of the first running suture can improve astigmatism or at times lead to an increase in astigmatism. Removal of the second running suture can potentially improve the situation, but this can only be performed after the wound has healed.[47]

## Corrective Wear—Spectacles/Contact Lenses

Large amounts of regular astigmatism, aniseikonia, irregular astigmatism and higher order aberrations can be challenging impediments to visual rehabilitation. In one series of patients, the optical indications for contact lens fitting after PKP included irregular astigmatism (62.9%), spherical anisometropia (57.1%), and astigmatic anisometropia (54.3%). The average time from surgery to initial contact lens fitting was 18.2 months, with spherical rigid gas-permeable lenses as the most common type of lens used. Punctal occlusion and lubrication helped to improve contact lens tolerance.[48] Based on the severity of refractive errors, spectacles and various sorts of soft, rigid gas permeable, or hybrid contact lenses may provide improved vision.[49,50]

Specially designed contact lenses may provide additional benefits to improved visual acuity. Higher order aberrations reduce visual quality and can be significant. Pantanelli et al. concluded that post-PK eyes had approximately 5.5 times more higher order aberrations, such as spherical aberration and coma, than normal eyes. Trefoil was found to be another prominent higher order aberration in eyes after PK.[51] Patients who have improved vision with rigid gas permeable lenses, but cannot tolerate them due to a compromised ocular surface, may benefit from hybrid lenses, such as SynergEyes (SynergEyes, Carlsbad, California, USA)[52,53] or a scleral contact lens such as the Boston ocular surface prosthesis (now called the PROSE lens), which does not touch the cornea and has been shown to decrease higher order aberration errors.[54]

## Incisional Techniques

*Astigmatic keratotomy and limbal relaxing incisions:* Various incisional techniques have been described and used with reasonable success for decades.[55-58] There are several incisional techniques to reduce postkeratoplasty astigmatism, which can be divided into flattening and steepening techniques. Flattening techniques include astigmatic keratotomy and limbal relaxing incisions. Steepening procedures include corneal wedge resections and compression sutures.

Results of studies examining relaxing incisions have been reviewed.[59] Wilkins et al. describe making 60° incisions of 600 μm corneal depth, leaving a 6 mm optic zone, which was able to decrease mean cylinder from $-10.99\,D \pm 4.26\,D$ to $-3.03\,D \pm 2.18\,D$, with a strong correlation between the preoperative magnitude of astigmatism and the magnitude of change in astigmatism ($R^2 = 0.76$).[60] Poole and Ficker used paired arcuate incisions of 90% corneal thickness making a 6–7 mm optical zone 0.5 mm inside the graft-host junction, and positioning them using preoperative refraction and topographic mapping and confirmed with keratoscopy. The mean cylinder was 9.13 D preoperatively and 4.85 D postoperatively, and the amount of cylinder reduction was correlated with the amount of pre-existing cylinder ($P < .001$).[61]

*Wedge resections and compression sutures:* Wedge resection can be used for higher degrees of astigmatism compared to relaxing incisions, and involves removing a wedge of tissue of approximately 90% thickness from the flat central corneal meridian of the donor cornea.[56-58] The resulting wedge defect is then sutured closed, increasing tension and peripheral corneal flattening, and inducing central corneal steepening. The resected tissue has been described to have been taken from the limbus and from the graft-host interface.[62,63] In a recent study, de la Paz et al. reported results 22 post-PK eyes with mean preoperative refractive, topographic and keratometric cylinders of 11.58 ± 3.52 D (4.5–20 D), 10.88 ± 5.03 D (2.58–21.3 D), and 11.29 ± 4.33 D (4.50–18 D), respectively, that underwent wedge resection in the host cornea. The mean postoperative refractive, topographic and keratometric cylinders at 3 years were 4.91 ± 2.48 D (0.50–10 D), 3.38 ± 2.10 D (2.05–7.1 D), and 5.31 ± 2.90 D (0.50–9 D) respectively. The percentage of correction at 3 years of follow-up was 57.5% for refractive cylinder, 68.97% for topographic cylinder and 53.01% for keratometric cylinder.[64]

Compression sutures might augment the effects of relaxing incisions. Javadi et al. made relaxing incision in the graft-host interface down to Descemet membrane on both sides of the steepest meridian, then placed interrupted 10-0 nylon compression sutures to achieve overcorrection of the astigmatism in the opposite meridian. Mean decreases in keratometric and refractive astigmatism were 5.9 D and 4.8 D respectively, using vector analysis.[65]

*Femtosecond laser incisions:* Applications for the use of femtosecond laser technology are finding a role in incisional techniques for the management of astigmatism. Some theoretical advantages are that the incisions created can be made relatively atraumatically and very accurate to a specific length and depth, thereby decreasing the chance of complications, such as microperforation, wound dehiscence, and under or overcorrection.[66] Table 2 shows a summary of studies examining these procedures. Femtosecond laser-created incisions are able to provide results similar to those

**Table 2:** *In vivo* femtosecond incisional techniques to reduce postkeratoplasty astigmatism

| Authors | Technique | Number of Eyes | Cylinder Reduction (D) |
|---|---|---|---|
| Ghanem RC, Azar DT (2006)[70] | Wedge resection: flap diameters of 6.0 mm and 7.0 mm, flap thickness of 400 µm, sutured | 1 | 14.5 |
| Bahar I, et al. (2008)[68] | Arcuate keratotomy: 60–90°, 90% depth, donor | 20 | 4.26 ± 1.72 |
| Harissi-Dagher M, Azar DT (2008)[71] | Arcuate keratotomy: donor | 2 | 4.9, 4.3 |
| Hoffart L, et al. (2009)[67] | Arcuate keratotomy: 75% depth | 10 | Refractive: 4.79 ± 2.23 Keratometric: 3.03 ± 2.42 |
| Buzzonetti L, et al. (2009)[72] | Arcuate keratotomy: 70°, 80% depth, 5.9 mm OZ, donor | 9 | Refractive: 6.00 Keratometric: 5.2 |
| Nubile M, et al. (2009)[73] | Arcuate keratotomy: 90°, 90% thickness, donor | 12 (10 PK, 2 DALK) | Refractive: 4.7 |
| Kumar NL, et al. (2010)[69] | Arcuate keratotomy: Variable length, 90% depth, donor | 37 | +7.46 ± 2.70 pre-op decreased to +4.77 ± 3.29 post-op |

D: diopters; PK: penetrating keratoplasty; DALK: deep anterior lamellar keratoplasty

of manually-created incisions. Hoffart et al. showed no significant difference in keratometric cylinder reduction when comparing laser-created astigmatic keratotomy to manual arcitome. Interestingly, in other studies, laser-created incisions appeared to be more efficacious (p = 0.011).[67] Bahar et al. found a mean cylinder reduction of 3.23 ± 4.69 D in a group who received manual AK and 4.26 ± 1.72 D in a group that had laser AK (p = 0.36).[68] In a series of 37 patients, Kumar et al. reported a decrease of mean absolute value of astigmatism from 7.46 ± 2.70 D to 4.77 ± 3.29 D over the first 3 postoperative months, with initial reduction occurring within the first 6 weeks, slight regression of the effect at 3 months, and stability between 3 and 6 months. They also report good correlation between the achieved and the intended reduction in astigmatism.[69]

### Effects on Deep Anterior Lamellar Keratoplasty

These techniques might have equal effect in eyes after deep anterior lamellar keratoplasty (DALK). In a study by Kubaloglu et al., the effect of astigmatic keratotomy was evaluated between PKP eyes and those that had undergone DALK. The surgical technique was identical in both groups in that the paired incisions were made in the steepest meridian at 90% thickness with arc lengths of 90° placed 0.5 mm inside the host cornea. The mean refractive cylinder 6 months after AK surgery decreased from 6.24 ± 0.75 D to 3.53 ± 1.62 D in the DALK group and from 6.48 ± 1.45 D to 3.31 ± 2.17 D in the PK group respectively (P < 0.001 and P = 0.001). There was no significant difference between the DALK or PK groups when comparing refractive cylinder or keratometric astigmatism after 3 or 6 months following

the procedure.[74] In a series of post-DALK eyes, Jayadi et al. sutured relaxing incisions made at the steep meridians, then selectively removed sutures to control the effect of the incisions. In these eyes, the average keratometric astigmatism was reduced by 3.8 and 5.5 D measured with subtraction and vector analysis methods respectively. Mean preoperative refractive astigmatism was 6.52 ± 1.14 D, decreasing to 3.67 ± 1.82 D postoperatively (P = 0.002).[75] Nubile et al. included two patients who had DALK in their series of 12 patients who all received femtosecond laser arcuate keratotomy for high astigmatism with promising results.[73]

### Laser Refractive Surgery

It is possible to reduce the amount of astigmatism in post-keratoplasty eyes using laser refractive surgical methods, such as LASIK and PRK, and many studies have described this (Table 3). Because of the large amounts of refractive error and irregular astigmatism present in postkeratoplasty eyes, the presurgical discussion with the patient should include realistic goals. Rather than striving for best uncorrected visual acuity, as is the case for laser vision correction in normal corneas, the goal might be to allow for visual rehabilitation and improve best corrected visual acuity.[100] Flaps created for LASIK in these eyes can be created mechanically with a microkeratome or with femtosecond laser technology. Microkeratome-created flaps can usually be made relatively safely across the graft-host interface. The scarring at the interface, however, might prevent the penetration of the femtosecond laser and risk an incomplete plane or buttonhole. Thus, the flap made in this fashion should be centered and completely contained in the graft.

**Table 3:** Reducing postkeratoplasty astigmatism with excimer laser ablation

| Author | Technique | Number of Eyes | Pre-procedure Cylinder (D) | Post-procedure Cylinder (D) |
|---|---|---|---|---|
| Amm M (1996)[76] | Excimer laser with rotating mask system to make a toric ablation | 16 PK | | 2.8 D reduction |
| Lazzaro DR (1996)[77] | PRK | 7 PK | Refractive: 5.32 Keratometry: 5.54 (1.50 to 10.00) | Refractive: 2.79 Keratometry: 4.00 (1.00 to 7.50) |
| Tuunanen TH (1997)[78] | PRK | 7 PK | Refractive: 5.98 ± 2.28 (3.50 to 11.25) | 4.28 ± 2.42 |
| Arenas E (1997)[79] | LASIK – single surgery, microkeratome | 4 PK | Refractive: 2.87 (1.00 to 5.00) | 3.50 |
| Wiesinger-Jendritza B (1998)[80] | LASIK | 23 PK | | |
| Donnenfeld ED (1999)[81] | LASIK – single surgery, microkeratome | 23 PK | Refractive: 3.64 ± 1.72 | 1.29 ± 1.04 |
| Forseto AS (1999)[82] | LASIK – single surgery, microkeratome | 22 PK | Refractive: 4.24 ± 2.28 | 1.79 ± 1.12 |
| Webber SK (1999)[83] | LASIK – single surgery, microkeratome, traditional; arcuate keratotomy for high cylinder | 18 PK | Refractive: 8.67 | 2.92 |
| Yoshida K (1999)[84] | PRK | 33 PK | | Refractive: 31.0% reduction Keratometry: 13.56% reduction |
| Bilgihan K (2000)[85] | PRK | 16 PK | Refractive: 5.62 ± 2.88 | 3.23 ± 1.70 |
| Nassaralla BR (2000)[86] | LASIK – single surgery, microkeratome | 8 PK | Refractive: 3.50 (1.50 to 5.00) | 1.25 (0.75 to 2.00) |
| Rashad KM (2000)[87] | LASIK – single surgery, microkeratome | 19 PK | Refractive: 9.21 ± 1.95 (6.50 to 14.50) | 1.09 ± 0.33 (0.50 to 1.75) |
| Koay PY (2000)[88] | LASIK – single surgery, microkeratome | 8 PK | Refractive: 6.79 (SD 3.28) | 1.93 D (SD 1.17) SIA 5.50 (SD 2.42) |
| Kwitko S (2001)[89] | LASIK – single surgery, microkeratome | 14 PK | Refractive: 5.37 ± 2.12 | 2.82 ± 2.42 |
| Lima G da S (2001)[90] | LASIK – single surgery, microkeratome | 27 PK | | |
| Hardten DR (2002)[91] | LASIK – single surgery, microkeratome | 57 PK | Refractive: 4.67 ± 2.18 | 1.94 ± 1.35 |
| Busin M (2003)[92] | LASIK – two-stage, microkeratome | 11 PK | Refractive: 6.02 ± 1.74 | After flap: 5.16 ± 1.34 After treatment: 1.77 ± 1.80 |
| Cosar CB (2006)[93] | LASIK – single surgery, microkeratome, topography guided 7.5 mm (+1.53 − 4.42 × 030°) | 1 PK | Manifest: +1.75 − 4.75 × 030° Keratometry: 44.83 × 123/39.74 × 33 | Residual: +0.25 − 0.75 × 040° |
| Mularoni A (2006)[94] | LASIK – two-stage, microkeratome, topography guided | 15 PK | Refractive: 6.68 ± 3.29 (1.0–13.0) | After flap: 6.32 ± 2.82 After treatment: 1.67 ± 1.26 (0–3.5) |
| Rajan MS (2006)[95] | LASEK – single surgery, epithelial flap, wavefront guided (maximum 7 D cylinder correction) | 15 PK | Refractive: 7.22 (2.75–13.5) | 2.72 ± 1.59 (0.5–6.5) |

*Contd...*

| Author | Technique | Number of Eyes | Pre-procedure Cylinder (D) | Post-procedure Cylinder (D) |
|---|---|---|---|---|
| Pedrotti E (2006)[96] | Transepithelial PRK, custom | 9 (6 = PK, 3 = DALK) | Range 2.00–8.00 | Range 0–2.50 |
| Kovoor TA (2009)[97] | PRK – traditional or custom | 14 PK | Refractive: 5.23 ± 2.26 | 3.21 ± 1.78 |
| | LASIK – single surgery, microkeratome or femtosecond | 9 PK | Refractive: 4.11 ± 2.38 | 2.08 ± 1.26 |
| Bahar I (2010)[98] | LASIK – femtosecond laser, astigmatic keratotomy prior to LASIK for high cylinder | 18 PK | Refractive: 3.11 ± 2.75 (2.5–6.0) | 1.3 ± 1.42 (0–3.00) |
| Dos Santos Forseto A (2010)[99] | PRK with mitomycin C, cylinder limit 6.00 D | 36 (34 = PK, 2 = DALK) | Refractive: 4.42 ± 1.69 (1.00–7.25) | 1.88 ± 1.75 (0–8.00) |

D: diopters; LASIK: laser assisted *in situ* keratomileusis; PRK: photorefractive keratectomy; PK: penetrating keratoplasty; DALK: deep anterior lamellar keratoplasty

*Laser-assisted in situ keratomileusis*: When considering LASIK, it has been observed that creating the flap alone can affect and possibly reduce astigmatism.[101-104] It has been postulated that creation of a lamellar corneal flap alone might result in circumferential release of contractile forces in the graft-host interface with a resultant change in corneal shape.[101,105] For this same reason, retraction of the flap has been reported to be a unique complication of mechanical LASIK flap creation in postkeratoplasty eyes.[106,107] This process may be responsible for changing the nature of corneal astigmatism. Lee et al. found that 60% of postkeratoplasty eyes that underwent lamellar keratotomy alone had a SIA vector of more than 1 D.[108] Pereira et al. similarly reported that SIA calculated through vector analysis was greater than 1.01 D in 52.4% of eyes that had only a flap created by mechanical microkeratome. A statistically significant correlation was found between the amount of astigmatism induced by creating the flap and the preoperative refractive astigmatism (P = 0.025).[109] Because of this effect, it has been recommended by some that postkeratoplasty LASIK be done as a two-stage procedure, with excimer laser ablation performed well after the keratometric changes of the flap creation take place.[110] Femtosecond laser-created flaps created entirely within the graft avoid the dynamic situation created by the contractile fibers of the wound. Thus, femtosecond LASIK can be performed as a single-stage procedure and with a stable refractive result.[111]

*Photorefractive keratectomy*: Photorefractive keratectomy performed in postkeratoplasty eyes circumvents the potential flap complications with LASIK. Reported problems, however, include visually significant graft haze[76,85,112,113] and graft rejection.[114] Kovoor et al. reported a retrospective study of 14 PRK and 9 LASIK procedures performed on postkeratoplasty eyes. In the PRK group, the preoperative manifest refractive cylindrical error was 5.23 ± 2.26 D, which was reduced to 3.21 ± 1.78 D (P = 0.02). In the LASIK group, the preoperative manifest refractive cylindrical error was 4.11 ± 2.38 D, which was reduced to 2.08 ± 1.26 (P = 0.03). The small size and the retrospective nature of the uncontrolled case series, however, limited the ability to detect any superiority between LASIK and PRK.[97]

## Combining Methods

The amount of astigmatism reduction with excimer laser is limited to moderate amounts and may need to be combined with other methods for greater efficacy. For patients with a large amount of postkeratoplasty astigmatism, Webber et al. combined LASIK with arcuate keratotomy.[83] For planned combined procedures, it might be reasonable to stage them to allow the individual effects to take place. Hardten et al. found that refractive cylinder for the most part stabilizes by 3 months after LASIK.[91] Bahar et al. reported performing combined astigmatic keratotomy and femtosecond LASIK as a two-stage procedure, in which the flap and the astigmatic keratotomy were performed several weeks before proceeding with the excimer laser ablation.[98]

## Repeat Keratoplasty

If the amount of astigmatism is too great to be corrected conservatively or even with nonpenetrating techniques, consideration might be given to repeat keratoplasty.[115] This option should come after a thorough discussion of the risks and benefits of performing the procedure, including the unpredictable nature of the postoperative refraction, lengthy time of visual rehabilitation, as well as the inherent risks that accompany any form of keratoplasty.

SECTION 16

## ❧ REFERENCES

1. Hoppenreijs VP, Van Rij G, Beekhuis WH, et al. Causes of high astigmatism after penetrating keratoplasty. Doc Ophthalmol. 1993;85(1):21-34.

2. Swinger CA. Postoperative astigmatism. Surv Ophthalmol. 1987;31(4):219-48.

3. Perlman EM. An analysis and interpretation of refractive errors after penetrating keratoplasty. Ophthalmology. 1981;88(1):39-45.

4. Riddle HK, Parker DA, Price FW. Management of post-keratoplasty astigmatism. Curr Opin Ophthalmol. 1998;9(4):15-28.

5. Samples JR, Binder PS. Visual acuity, refractive error, and astigmatism following corneal transplantation for pseudophakic bullous keratopathy. Ophthalmology. 1985;92(11):1554-60.

6. Langenbucher A, Naumann GO, Seitz B. Spontaneous long-term changes of corneal power and astigmatism after suture removal after penetrating keratoplasty using a regression model. Am J Ophthalmol. 2005;140(1):29-34.

7. Skeens HM. Management of postkeratoplasty astigmatism. In: Krachmer JH, Mannis MM, Holland EJ (Eds), Cornea. (3rd edition). St. Louis, MO: Mosby/Elsevier; 2011. p. 1398.

8. Van Rij G, Cornell FM, Waring GO, et al. Postoperative astigmatism after central versus eccentric penetrating keratoplasties. Am J Ophthalmol. 1985;99:317-20.

9. Verdier DD. Penetrating keratoplasty. In: Krachmer JH, Mannis MJ, Holland EJ (Eds), Cornea. (3rd edition). St. Louis, MO: Mosby/Elsevier; 2011. p. 1338.

10. Belmont SC, Zimm JL, Storch RL, et al. Astigmatism after penetrating keratoplasty using the Krumeich guided trephine system. Refract Corneal Surg. 1993;9(4):250-4.

11. Wiffen SJ, Maguire LJ, Bourne WM. Keratometric results of penetrating keratoplasty with the Hessberg-Barron and Hanna trephine systems using a double running suture technique. Cornea. 1997;16(3):306-13.

12. Chamberlain WD, Rush SW, Mathers WD, et al. Comparison of femtosecond laser-assisted keratoplasty versus conventional penetrating keratoplasty. Ophthalmology. 2011;118(3):486-91.

13. Troutman RC, Gaster RN. Effects of disparate sized graft and recipient opening. Trans New Orleans Acad Ophthalmol. 1980; 386-405.

14. Cohen KL, Tripoli NI, Pellom AC. Effect of tissue fit on corneal shape after transplantation. Invest Ophthalmol Vis Sci. 1984;25:1226-31.

15. Moshirfar M, Meyen JJ, Kang PC. A comparison of three methods of trephining donor corneal buttons: endothelial cell loss and microscopic ultrastructural evaluation. Current Eye Research. 2009;34(11):939-44.

16. Heidemann D, Sugar A, Meyer R, et al. Oversized donor grafts in penetrating keratoplasty. Arch Ophthalmol. 1985;103:1807-11.

17. Javadi MA, Feizi S, Yazdani S, et al. Deep anterior lamellar keratoplasty versus penetrating keratoplasty for keratoconus: a clinical trial. Cornea. 2010;29(4):365-71.

18. Han DC, Mehta JS, Por YM, et al. Comparison of outcomes of lamellar keratoplasty and penetrating keratoplasty in keratoconus. Am J Ophthalmol. 2009;148(5):744-51. e1. Epub 2009 July 9.

19. Serdarevic ON, Renard GJ, Pouliquen Y. Randomized clinical trial of penetrating keratoplasty. Before and after suture removal comparison of intraoperative and post-operative suture removal. Ophthalmology. 1995;102(10):1497-503.

20. Mader TH, Yuan R, Lynn MJ, et al. Changes in keratometric astigmatism after suture removal more than one year after penetrating keratoplasty. Ophthalmology. 1993;100(1):119-26.

21. McNeill JI, Kaufman HE. A double running suture technique for keratoplasty: earlier visual rehabilitation. Ophthalmic Surg. 1977;8:58-61.

22. Stainer GA, Perl T, Binder PS. Controlled reduction of post-keratoplasty astigmatism. Ophthalmology. 1982;89:668-76.

23. McNeill JI, Wessels IF. Adjustment of single continuous suture to control astigmatism after penetrating keratoplasty. Refract Corneal Surg. 1989;5:216-23.

24. Filatov V, Alexandrakis G, Talamo JH, et al. Comparison of suture-in and suture-out post-keratoplasty astigmatism with single running suture or combined running and interrupted sutures. Am J Ophthalmol. 1996;122:696-700.

25. Javadi MA, Naderi M, Zare M, et al. Comparison of the effect of three suturing techniques on post-keratoplasty astigmatism in keratoconus. Cornea. 2006;25(9):1029-33.

26. Acar BT, Vural ET, Acar S. Does the type of suturing technique used affect astigmatism after deep anterior lamellar keratoplasty in keratoconus patients? Clin Ophthalmol. 2011;5:425-8.

27. Karabatsas CH, Cook SD, Figueiredo FC, et al. Combined interrupted and continuous versus single continuous adjustable suturing in penetrating keratoplasty: a prospective, randomized study of induced astigmatism during the first postoperative year. Ophthalmology. 1998;105(11):1991-8.

28. Spadea L, Cifariello F, Bianco G, et al. Long-term results of penetrating keratoplasty using a single or double running suture technique. Graefes Arch Clin Exp Ophthalmol. 2002;240(5):415-9. Epub 2002 Apr 3.

29. Solano JM, Hodge DO, Bourne WM. Keratometric astigmatism after suture removal in penetrating keratoplasty: double running versus single running suture techniques. Cornea. 2003;22(8):716-20.

30. Lin DT, Wilson SE, Reidy JJ, et al. An adjustable single running suture technique to reduce post-keratoplasty astigmatism. A preliminary report. Ophthalmology. 1990;97(7):934-8.

31. Ramirez M, Hodge DO, Borne WM. Keratometric results during the first year after keratoplasty: adjustable single running suture technique versus double running suture technique. Ophthalmic Surg Laser. 2001;32:370-4.

32. Van Meter WS, Gussler JR, Soloman KD, et al. Post-keratoplasty astigmatism control. Single continuous suture adjustment versus selective interrupted suture removal. Ophthalmology. 1991;98:177-83.

33. Filatov V, Steinert RF, Talamo JH. Post-keratoplasty astigmatism with single running suture or interrupted sutures. Am J Ophthalmol. 1993;115:715-21.

34. Kim SJ, Wee WR, Lee JH, et al. The effect of different suturing techniques on astigmatism after penetrating keratoplasty. J Korean Med Sci. 2008;23(6):1015-9. Epub 2008 Dec 24.

35. Assil KK, Zarnegar SR, Schanzlin DJ. Visual outcome after penetrating keratoplasty with double continuous or combined interrupted and continuous suture wound closure. Am J Ophthalmol. 1992;114(1):63-71.

36. Musch DC, Meyer RF, Sugar A, et al. Corneal astigmatism after penetrating keratoplasty. The role of suture technique. Ophthalmology. 1989;96:698-703.

37. Frangieh GT, Kwitko S, McDonnell PJ. Prospective corneal topographic analysis in surgery for post-keratoplasty astigmatism. Arch Ophthalmol. 1991;109:506-10.

38. Karabatsas CH, Cook SD, Figueiredo FC. Surgical control of late post-keratoplasty astigmatism with or without the use of computerised video keratography: a prospective randomized study. Ophthalmology. 1998;105:1999-2006.

39. Solomon A, Siganos CS, Frucht-Pery J. Relaxing incision guided by videokeratography for astigmatism after keratoplasty for keratoconus. J Refract Surg. 1999;15(3):343-8.

40. Borderie VM, Touzeau O, Laroche L. Videokeratography, keratometry, and refraction after penetrating keratoplasty. J Refract Surg. 1999;15(1):32-7.

41. Maguire LJ, Bourne WM. Corneal topography of transverse keratotomies for astigmatism after penetrating keratoplasty. Am J Ophthalmol. 1989;107(4):323-30.

42. Sarhan AR, Dua HS, Beach M. Effect of disagreement between refractive, keratometric, and topographic determination of astigmatic axis on suture removal after penetrating keratoplasty. Br J Ophthalmol. 2000;84(8):837-41.

43. Van Meter W, Katz DG. Keratoplasty suturing techniques. Chapter 116. Cornea, 3rd edition. Krachmer. pp. 1355-66.

44. Van Meter W. The efficacy of a single continuous nylon suture for control of post keratoplasty astigmatism. Trans Am Ophthalmol Soc. 1996;94:1157-80.

45. Mannan R, Jhanji V, Sharma N, et al. Spontaneous wound dehiscence after early suture removal after deep anterior lamellar keratoplasty. Eye Contact Lens. 2011;37(2):109-11.

46. Musch DC, Meyer RF, Sugar A. The effect of removing running sutures on astigmatism after penetrating keratoplasty. Arch Ophthalmol. 1988;106(4):488-92.

47. Langenbucher A, Seitz B. Changes in corneal power and refraction due to sequential suture removal following nonmechanical penetrating keratoplasty in eyes with keratoconus. Am J Ophthalmol. 2006;141(2):287-93.

48. Wietharn BE, Driebe WT. Fitting contact lenses for visual rehabilitation after penetrating keratoplasty. Eye Contact Lens. 2004;30:31-3.

49. Jacobs DS. Update on scleral lenses. Curr Opin Ophthalmol. 2008;19(4):298-301.

50. Erdurmus M, Yildiz EH, Abdalla YF, et al. Contact lens related quality of life in patients with keratoconus. Eye Contact Lens. 2009;35(3):123-7.

51. Pantanelli S, MacRae S, Jeong TM, et al. Characterizing the wave aberration in eyes with keratoconus or penetrating keratoplasty using a high-dynamic range wavefront sensor. Ophthalmology. 2007;114(11):2013-21.

52. Abdalla YF, Elsahn AF, Hammersmith KM, et al. SynergEyes lenses for keratoconus. Cornea. 2010;29(1):5-8.

53. Nau AC. A comparison of synergeyes versus traditional rigid gas permeable lens designs for patients with irregular corneas. Eye Contact Lens. 2008;34(4):198-200.

54. Gumus K, Gire A, Pflugfelder SC. The impact of the Boston ocular surface prosthesis on wavefront higher-order aberrations. Am J Ophthalmol. 2011;151(4):682-90. e2. Epub 2011 Jan 26.

55. Duffey RJ, Jain VN, Tchah H. Paired arcuate keratotomy; a surgical approach to mixed and myopic astigmatism. Arch Ophthalmol. 1988;106:1130-5.

56. Lindstrom RL, Lindquist TD. Surgical correction of postoperative astigmatism. Cornea. 1988;7(2):138-48.

57. Troutman RC. Microsurgical control of corneal astigmatism in cataract and keratoplasty. Trans Am Acad Ophthalmol Otolaryngol. 1973;77(5):OP563-OP72.

58. Krachmer JH, Fenzl RE. Surgical correction of high post-keratoplasty astigmatism: relaxing incisions vs wedge resection. Arch Ophthalmol. 1980;98(8):1400-2.

59. Geggel HS. Arcuate relaxing incisions guided by corneal topography for post-keratoplasty astigmatism: vector and topographic analysis. Cornea. 2006;25(5):545-57.

60. Wilkins MR, Mehta JS, Larkin FP. Standardized arcuate keratotomy for post-keratoplasty astigmatism. J Cataract Refract Surg. 2005;31(2):297-301.

61. Poole TR, Ficker LA. Astigmatic keratotomy for post-keratoplasty astigmatism. J Cataract Refract Surg. 2006;32 (7):1175-9.

62. Frucht-Pery J. Wedge resection for post-keratoplasty astigmatism. Ophthalmic Surg. 1993;24(8):516-8.

63. Ilari L, Daya SM. Corneal wedge resection to treat progressive keratoconus in the host cornea after penetrating keratoplasty. J Cataract Refract Surg. 2003;29(2):395-401.

64. De la Paz MF, Sibila GR, Montenegro G, et al. Wedge resection for high astigmatism after penetrating keratoplasty for keratoconus: refractive and histopathologic changes. Cornea. 2010;29(6):595-600.

65. Javadi MA, Feizi S, Yazdani S, et al. Outcomes of augmented relaxing incisions for postpenetrating keratoplasty astigmatism in keratoconus. Cornea. 2009;28(3):280-4.

66. Kymionis GD, Yoo SH, Ide T, et al. Femtosecond-assisted astigmatic keratotomy for post-keratoplasty irregular astigmatism. J Cataract Refract Surg. 2009;35(1):11-3.

67. Hoffart L, Proust H, Matonti F, et al. Correction of post-keratoplasty astigmatism by femtosecond laser compared with mechanized astigmatic keratotomy. Am J Ophthalmol. 2009;147(5):779-87.

SECTION 16

68. Bahar I, Levinger E, Kaiserman I, et al. IntraLase-enabled astigmatic keratotomy for post-keratoplasty astigmatism. Am J Ophthalmol. 2008;146(6):897-904. e1. Epub 2008 Aug 30.

69. Kumar NL, Kaiserman I, Shehadeh-Mashor R, et al. IntraLase-enabled astigmatic keratotomy for post-keratoplasty astigmatism: on-axis vector analysis. Ophthalmology. 2010;117(6): 1228-35.

70. Ghanem RC, Azar DT. Femtosecond-laser arcuate wedgeshaped resection to correct high residual astigmatism after penetrating keratoplasty. J Cataract Refract Surg. 2006;32(9):1415-9.

71. Harissi-Dagher M, Azar DT. Femtosecond laser astigmatic keratotomy for post-keratoplasty astigmatism. Can J Ophthalmol. 2008;43(3):367-9.

72. Buzzonetti L, Petrocelli G, Laborante A, et al. Arcuate keratotomy for high postoperative keratoplasty astigmatism performed with the intralase femtosecond laser. J Refract Surg. 2009; 25(8):709-14.

73. Nubile M, Carpineto P, Lanzini M, et al. Femtosecond laser arcuate keratotomy for the correction of high astigmatism after keratoplasty. Ophthalmology. 2009;116(6):1083-92.

74. Kubaloglu A, Coskun E, Sari ES, et al. Comparison of astigmatic keratotomy results in deep anterior lamellar keratoplasty and penetrating keratoplasty in keratoconus. Am J Ophthalmol. 2011;151(4):637-43.

75. Javadi MA, Feizi S, Mirbabaee F, et al. Relaxing incisions combined with adjustment sutures for post-deep anterior lamellar keratoplasty astigmatism in keratoconus. Cornea. 2009;28(10):1130-4.

76. Amm M, Duncker GI, Schröder E. Excimer laser correction of high astigmatism after keratoplasty. J Cataract Refract Surg. 1996;22(3):313-7.

77. Lazzaro DR, Haight DH, Belmont SC, et al. Excimer laser keratectomy for astigmatism occurring after penetrating keratoplasty. Ophthalmology. 1996;103(3):458-64.

78. Tuunanen TH, Ruusuvaara PJ, Uusitalo RJ, et al. Photoastigmatic keratectomy for correction of astigmatism in corneal grafts. Cornea. 1997;16(1):48-53.

79. Arenas E, Maglione A. Laser in situ keratomileusis for astigmatism and myopia after penetrating keratoplasty. J Refract Surg. 1997;13(1):27-32.

80. Wiesinger-Jendritza B, Knorz MC, Hugger P, et al. Laser in situ keratomileusis assisted by corneal topography. J Cataract Refract Surg. 1998;24(2):166-74.

81. Donnenfeld ED, Kornstein HS, Amin A, et al. Laser in situ keratomileusis for correction of myopia and astigmatism after penetrating keratoplasty. Ophthalmology. 1999;106(10): 1966-75.

82. Forseto AS, Nosé RA, Francesconi CM, et al. Laser in situ keratomileusis for undercorrection after radial keratotomy. J Refract Surg. 1999;15(4):424-8.

83. Webber SK, Lawless MA, Sutton GL, et al. LASIK for post penetrating keratoplasty astigmatism and myopia. Br J Ophthalmol. 1999;83(9):1013-8.

84. Yoshida K, Tazawa Y, Demong TT. Refractive results of post penetrating keratoplasty photorefractive keratectomy. Ophthalmic Surg Lasers. 1999;30(5):354-9.

85. Bilgihan K, Ozdek SC, Akata F, et al. Photorefractive keratectomy for post-penetrating keratoplasty myopia and astigmatism. J Cataract Refract Surg. 2000;26(11):1590-5.

86. Nassaralla BR, Nassaralla JJ. Laser in situ keratomileusis after penetrating keratoplasty. J Refract Surg. 2000;16(4):431-7.

87. Rashad KM. Laser in situ keratomileusis for correction of high astigmatism after penetrating keratoplasty. J Refract Surg. 2000;16(6):701-10.

88. Koay PY, McGhee CN, Weed KH, et al. Laser in situ keratomileusis for ametropia after penetrating keratoplasty. J Refract Surg. 2000;16(2):140-7.

89. Kwitko S, Marinho DR, Rymer S, et al. Laser in situ keratomileusis after penetrating keratoplasty. J Cataract Refract Surg. 2001;27(3):374-9.

90. Lima G da S, Moreira H, Wahab SA. Laser in situ keratomileusis to correct myopia, hypermetropia and astigmatism after penetrating keratoplasty for keratoconus: a series of 27 cases. Can J Ophthalmol. 2001;36(7):391-6; discussion 396-7.

91. Hardten DR, Chittcharus A, Lindstrom RL. Long-term analysis of LASIK for the correction of refractive errors after penetrating keratoplasty. Trans Am Ophthalmol Soc. 2002;100:143-50; discussion 150-2.

92. Busin M, Zambianchi L, Garzione F, et al. Two-stage laser in situ keratomileusis to correct refractive errors after penetrating keratoplasty. J Refract Surg. 2003;19(3):301-8.

93. Cosar CB, Acar S. Topography-guided LASIK with the wavelight laser after penetrating keratoplasty. J Refract Surg. 2006;22 (7):716-9.

94. Mularoni A, Laffi GL, Bassein L, et al. Two-step LASIK with topography-guided ablation to correct astigmatism after penetrating keratoplasty. J Refract Surg. 2006;22(1):67-74.

95. Rajan MS, O'Brart DP, Patel P, et al. Topography-guided customized laser-assisted subepithelial keratectomy for the treatment of post-keratoplasty astigmatism. J Cataract Refract Surg. 2006;32(6):949-57.

96. Pedrotti E, Sbabo A, Marchini G. Customized transepithelial photorefractive keratectomy for iatrogenic ametropia after penetrating or deep lamellar keratoplasty. J Cataract Refract Surg. 2006;32(8):1288-91.

97. Kovoor TA, Mohamed E, Cavanagh HD, et al. Outcomes of LASIK and PRK in previous penetrating corneal transplant recipients. Eye Contact Lens. 2009:35(5):242-5.

98. Bahar I, Kaiserman I, Mashor RS, et al. Femtosecond LASIK combined with astigmatic keratotomy for the correction of refractive errors after penetrating keratoplasty. Ophthalmic Surg Lasers Imaging. 2010;41(2):242-9.

99. Dos Santos Forseto A, Marques JC, Nose W. Photorefractive keratectomy with mitomycin C after penetrating and lamellar keratoplasty. Cornea. 2010;29(10):1103-8.

100. Donnenfeld ED. Author's reply. Ophthalmology. 2001;107(10): 1802.

101. Dada T, Vajpayee RB, Gupta V, et al. Microkeratome-induced reduction of astigmatism after penetrating keratoplasty. Am J Ophthalmol. 2001;131(4):507-8.

102. Busin M, Arffa RC, Zambianchi L, et al. Effect of hinged lamellar keratotomy on post-keratoplasty eyes. Ophthalmology. 2001;108(10):1845-51; discussion 1851-2.

103. Vajpayee RB, Dada T. LASIK after penetrating keratoplasty. Ophthalmol. 2001;107(10):1801-2.

104. Walker NJ, Apel AJ. Effect of hinged lamellar keratotomy on post-keratoplasty astigmatism and vision. Clin Experiment Ophthalmol. 2004;32(2):147-53.

105. Kohnen T, Bühren J. Corneal first-surface aberration analysis of the biomechanical effects of astigmatic keratotomy and a microkeratome cut after penetrating keratoplasty. J Cataract Refract Surg. 2005;31(1):185-9.

106. Chan CC, Rootman DS. Corneal lamellar flap retraction after LASIK following penetrating keratoplasty. Cornea. 2004;23(6):643-6.

107. Sharma N, Sinha R, Vajpayee RB. Corneal lamellar flap retraction after LASIK following penetrating keratoplasty. Cornea. 2006;25(4):496. Comment on Cornea. 2004;23(6):643-6.

108. Lee GA, Pérez-Santonja JJ, Maloof A, et al. Effects of lamellar keratotomy on post-keratoplasty astigmatism. Br J Ophthalmol. 2003;87(4):432-5.

109. Pereira T, Forseto AS, Alberti GN, et al. Flap-induced refraction change in LASIK after penetrating keratoplasty. J Refract Surg. 2007;23(3):279-83.

110. Kollias AN, Schaumberger MM, Kreutzer TC, et al. Two-step LASIK after penetrating keratoplasty. Clin Ophthalmol. 2009;3:581-6.

111. Barequet IS, Hirsh A, Levinger S. Femtosecond thin-flap LASIK for the correction of ametropia after penetrating keratoplasty. J Refract Surg. 2010;26(3):191-6. Epub 2010 Mar 11

112. Chan WK, Hunt KE, Glasgow BJ, et al. Corneal scarring after photorefractive keratectomy in a penetrating keratoplasty. Am J Ophthalmol. 1996;121(5):570-1.

113. John ME, Martines E, Cvintal T, et al. Photorefractive keratectomy following penetrating keratoplasty. J Refract Corneal Surg. 1994;10(2 Suppl):S206-S10.

114. Hersh PS, Jordan AJ, Mayers M. Corneal graft rejection episode after excimer laser phototherapeutic keratectomy. Arch Ophthalmol. 1993;111(6):735-6.

115. Szentmáry N, Seitz B, Langenbucher A, et al. Repeat keratoplasty for correction of high or irregular post-keratoplasty astigmatism in clear corneal grafts. Am J Ophthalmol. 2005;139(5):826-30.

# CHAPTER 82

# Glaucoma Surgery in Penetrating and Nonpenetrating Keratoplasty Patients

*Oluwatosin Smith, Davinder Grover*

## ▶ INTRODUCTION

Glaucoma remains a leading cause of visual impairment after penetrating or nonpenetrating keratoplasty.[1] Much of this is due to irreversible glaucomatous optic neuropathy, but uncontrolled glaucoma is also associated with an increased risk of graft failure.[2,3] Interestingly, glaucoma is already present in approximately 15% of eyes prior to keratoplasty and another 15% of cases are diagnosed after corneal transplantation.[4] A higher incidence of elevated intraocular pressure (IOP) ranging from 29% to 80% was found after keratoplasty in patients with pre-existing glaucoma, hence these patients require an increased vigilance for postoperative IOP spikes.[5,6]

In patients post keratoplasty, elevation in IOP can be found in anywhere from 10.6% to 42.2% of cases.[6-10] Apart from preoperative glaucoma, aphakia, as well as concomitant anterior segment reconstruction and vitrectomy are risk factors for development of glaucoma postkeratoplasty.[6,7] Other risk factors include preoperative inflammatory disease and PAS.[6] An increase in glaucoma therapy was also significantly associated with pre-existing glaucoma following deep lamellar endothelial keratoplasty.[5] Given the multitude of factors leading to an increase in likelihood of IOP elevation in patients following keratoplasty with no prior history of glaucoma, all patients require vigilance for postoperative IOP spikes.

The pathophysiology of postkeratoplasty glaucoma is multifactorial and a clear understanding of the various mechanisms involved is vital when deciding on treatment options.[2] Occasionally, the primary corneal conditions can lead to an IOP elevated (inflammatory corneal diseases) and sometimes the treatment of corneal conditions can lead to elevated IOP (steroid-induced glaucoma). The causes of IOP elevation post keratoplasty vary almost as much as the glaucoma surgical procedures used to manage this condition; all of which will be addressed in the following chapter.

## ▶ PENETRATING KERATOPLASTY

Penetrating keratoplasty (PKP) is commonly complicated by glaucoma in the postoperative period. The incidence of glaucoma after PKP ranged from 9% to 31% in the early postoperative period and from 18% to 35% in the late period.[6] The average time of onset of IOP elevation was about 3 months after surgery.[9] Glaucoma or IOP elevation following a corneal transplant is a risk factor for graft rejection and must be managed aggressively in order to preserve visual function.[11] In children, pre- and/or postpenetrating keratoplasty glaucoma patients had worse 1-year graft survival rates compared to patients without pre- and/or postoperative glaucoma [32% versus 70% survival, respectively (P = 0.02)].[12] Interventions, such as using oversized graft and iris tightening procedures to reduce synechial angle closure, minimize the incidence of glaucoma and are important for long-term graft preservation.[2]

The ophthalmologist following the postoperative PKP patient must be aware of the common and less common mechanisms by which patients develop glaucoma. Eyes that undergo PKP are at risk for PAS which may lead to chronic synechial closure of the anterior chamber angle. Epithelial downgrowth is another cause of glaucoma in these patients. The epithelial tissue grows over the structures of the anterior chamber including the angle leading to elevated IOP. Rarely, implantation cysts have been noted to be a causative factor as well. Steroid-induced elevation in IOP plays a big role in postkeratoplasty glaucoma given the essential role that steroids play in the postoperative management of PKP patients.[13] Typically, steroid-induced IOP elevation occurred 3–6 months after keratoplasty in 78% of eyes,[14] although it can be observed as early as 10–14 days. The incidence of presumed steroid related IOP elevation ranges from 22% to 35%, depending on the study.[14,15]

Management of congenital corneal abnormalities is extremely challenging. For example, in conditions like aniridia and Peter's anomaly, the decision to do simultaneous or staged surgery is difficult and requires a team effort from glaucoma, corneal and pediatric anterior segment subspecialists.

## ❧ DESCEMET'S STRIPPING ENDOTHELIAL KERATOPLASTY

Descemet's stripping endothelial keratoplasty (DSEK) is becoming an increasingly popular surgical procedure for the management of endothelial disorders. From 2005 to 2008, the Eye Bank Association of America reported an increase in the number of endothelial transplants from 1,429 to 17,468. Interestingly, during the same period of time, the number of penetrating keratoplasties have decreased from 45,821 to 32,524.[16] We have already discussed the inherent surgical complications with PKPs, specifically pertaining to glaucoma. Although DSEK is less invasive and theoretically less traumatic to the eye than PKP, this procedure is still complicated by various mechanism of glaucoma. Some of these mechanisms are similar to PKP and others distinctly unique to DSEK.

Like PKP, eyes that undergo DSEK are at risk for peripheral anterior synechiae (PAS), steroid-induced glaucoma and inflammatory glaucoma. Given that the anterior segment anatomy is typically less distorted and less manipulated, the degree of postoperative PAS formation and inflammation are observed with lower frequency, when compared to PKP.[17] However, given the similar rates of rejection for DSEK when compared to PKP, the likelihood of postoperative inflammation is still a concern.[18] Despite the decreased frequency of certain complications, these mechanisms still occur and should be managed similarly to the approach described above for PKP. Rarely, epithelial downgrowth has been reported to occur after Descemet's stripping automated endothelial keratoplasty (DSAEK).[19]

Unique to DSEK is the use of an air bubble, which is injected into the anterior chamber following the surgery. The patient is placed supine and an air bubble is used to assist in graft attachment. If the air bubble is too large and occludes the entire pupillary area, pupillary block can occur. This can often times be treated medically by dilating the pupil with a long acting agent, like atropine sulfate 1% ophthalmic solution. When this does not work, a surgical intervention is often required. One can simply decrease the volume of air in the anterior chamber through manipulation at the slit lamp.[20-24] Alternatively, some authors have created an iridectomy or iridotomy preoperatively, intraoperatively or postoperatively, in an attempt to avoid pupil block. If air enters the posterior chamber intraoperatively and remains behind the iris, it can lead to an anteriorly displaced iris and PAS formation. When pupillary block glaucoma occurs, the risk of graft failure increases substantially.[21]

A specific challenge occurs when performing DSEK in a patient who has previously undergone a glaucoma filtering procedure (a trabeculectomy or glaucoma drainage implant). In these patients, the air bubble can escape through the drainage site. In these patients, one should place the air bubble and wait for the air to equilibrate between the subconjunctival space and the anterior chamber. These patients often require repeat air injections until adequate fill is obtained. Often times, these eyes have prior iridectomies, therefore one can "over" fill the eye slightly without the concern of pupillary block.[25,26]

Postoperative glaucoma management in patients having undergone DSEK is also challenging, especially in regards to measuring IOP and interpreting the pressure level. After the corneal edema has resolved postoperatively, most DSEK eyes have a central corneal thickness of around 700 micrometers.[20,27-29] Several studies have demonstrated that the thickened DSEK corneas do not artificially elevate eye pressures in the same manner that has been observed with native thick corneas. These studies also reported a good correlation between Goldmann applanation and dynamic contour tonometry and suggest that Goldmann applanation can be used to monitor IOP in glaucoma patients. Further research into this area is needed, as more and more patients with glaucoma will be undergoing DSEK and more patients having undergone DSEK may develop glaucoma.[28,29]

Several authors have reported on the management of glaucoma following DSEK. Vajaranant et al. reported on their experience with IOP management in patients having undergone DSEK with and without pre-existing glaucoma. The three groups in this study were: (1) DSEK without pre-existing glaucoma; (2) DSEK with history of glaucoma without prior glaucoma surgery and; (3) DSEK with history of glaucoma and glaucoma surgery. These authors found that the incidence of postoperative IOP elevation was 35%, 45% and 43% respectively for groups 1, 2 and 3. The elevated IOP was medically managed by initiating or increasing glaucoma medications or decreasing topical steroid use in 27%, 44% and 38% respectively in groups 1, 2 and 3. Moreover, a subsequent glaucoma procedure was required in 0.3%, 5% and 19% respectively in these groups. Vajaranant et al. also postulated that the major cause of postoperative IOP elevated was likely secondary to a steroid response and less likely attributed to scarring of the angle structures, chronic angle closure or graft rejection (which are more commonly seen in patients with PKP). As such, most of the cases of IOP elevation were able to be treated with noninvasive interventions.[28]

With regard to which glaucoma surgery should be best used to manage glaucoma in patients that have undergone DSEK, there is no general consensus. The short answer is one should perform the surgery with which they have the most experience or comfort. However, the same preoperative surgical guidelines should apply. If there is extensive conjunctival scarring, one may consider a glaucoma drainage device over a traditional trabeculectomy. There is very limited evidence on which surgery is superior in patients with DSEK. Several case reports have demonstrated safety and efficacy in both situations.[25,30-33] However, when performing a glaucoma drainage device, care should be taken to place the tube as far from the endothelium as possible. One may even consider placing the tube in the sulcus if possible. There is little data on the outcomes of newer glaucoma surgeries, such as trabectome, canaloplasty, or endocyclophotocoagulation in the setting of DSEK but given the increasing frequency of DSEK, there will surely be more studies on these newer surgical modalities.

## ❧ KERATOPROSTHESIS

Several types of keratoprosthesis (K-pro) are being utilized throughout the world to help patients with very advanced anterior segment and corneal diseases. However, regardless of the prosthesis used, glaucoma is often a concern. Based on previous studies, the prevalence of glaucoma can be as high as 76% in patients with a K-pro.[34-37] Often times, patients that have undergone a K-pro placement have had several failed corneal transplants. Therefore, these patients are at a very high risk for chronic angle closure glaucoma. In fact, one should probably assume these patients either have chronic angle closure or will develop this condition soon after the K-pro is placed.

The difficulty in managing glaucoma in the setting of a K-pro is several fold.[34-38]

- It is difficult to objectively measure the IOP.
- These patients are at high risk for glaucoma drainage device erosion.
- Topical glaucoma medications may be less effectively absorbed through the K-pro than through a normal or transplanted cornea.
- Given the small aperture of most K-pros as well as the high incidence of retroprosthetic membranes, diagnostic testing (functional and structural glaucoma evaluations) can be very challenging and may be of limited utility.

Fortunately, as long as the ophthalmologist is aware of these challenges, glaucoma can usually be successfully managed in patients with a K-pro. Studies have demonstrated that digital palpation (in a trained specialist) can be used to effectively monitor glaucoma and accurately measure IOP to within 5 mm Hg.[39-41]

Several authors have reported on the rate of glaucoma drainage device tube erosions in the setting of K-pro devices. Li et al. reported a relatively high rate of tube complications in the setting of K-pros, including tube erosion, infection and hypotony.[42] Specifically, this study found that nearly 60% of all drainage devices eroded during the follow-up period. Five of the 25 eyes with glaucoma drainage implants required device explantation. Two of the 25 eyes developed endophthalmitis. Given the higher number of complications experienced with these challenging cases, some authors have advocated for ciliary body destructive procedures like cyclophotocoagulation (CPC) or endoscopic cyclophotocoagulation (ECP).[37,43-45]

Prior to placing a K-pro in a patient, one must thoroughly evaluate the patient and assess their glaucoma status. If the patient has mild to moderate glaucoma, prior placement or concurrent placement of a glaucoma drainage implant may be beneficial. If the patient has advanced glaucomatous optic neuropathy or uncontrolled IOP, one should consider placing a nonvalved drainage implant 6–8 weeks prior to the K-pro to control the IOP prior to surgery. Alternatively, one could perform as ECP or CPC concurrently with the K-pro. There is currently no good evidence in the literature suggesting that one intervention is superior to another in this situation.

## REFRACTIVE SURGERY

Much more is understood with regard to glaucoma management and refractive surgery. Although this is beyond the scope of this chapter, one should carefully evaluate refractive surgery candidates for glaucoma. If the refractive surgeon is concerned for glaucoma, a complete glaucoma work-up is warranted including baseline IOP, gonioscopy, pachymetry, nerve fiber layer (NFL) thickness measurements, visual field testing and disk photography. Some consider the presence of glaucoma a relative contraindication for refractive surgery; however, there is no consensus in the field.[46] The patient must be followed closely postoperatively. The physician should be cognizant of the effect that refractive surgery has on central corneal thickness and should also be aware of steroid-induced glaucoma postoperatively. Additionally, they should take into account that a thinner cornea will often times underestimate the actual IOP, especially in refractive patients. Therefore, when following postrefractive surgery patients, more weight should be placed on structural and functional testing and less, per se, on the actual IOP.

## SURGICAL APPROACH

A stepwise approach to the management of the post-keratoplasty patients is required to treat the cause of IOP elevation. There are several treatment options if standard medical therapy cannot adequately control the IOP. These surgical interventions include trabeculectomy (with and without an antimetabolite), glaucoma drainage devices, or cyclodestructive procedures with Nd:YAG or diode laser.[1,2] In a comparative study, no difference was found among the three glaucoma procedures with respect to IOP control and graft failure.[47]

Laser glaucoma treatment usually has limited utility in these patients. Obviously, if pupillary block is present, a laser or surgical iridotomy with or without gonio-synechiolysis may be the procedure of choice especially following DSAEK (where one can see acute papillary block in the early postoperative period with an air bubble in the anterior chamber). Laser trabeculoplasty has been reported as a management option in the management of a subset of patients who have a normal angle anatomy with no PAS preventing the visualization of the trabecular meshwork.

In patients with elevated IOP, the use of topical glaucoma medication and antimetabolites following surgery may lead to keratopathy. These as well as uncontrolled IOP are risk factors for graft failure as well as glaucomatous optic neuropathy. It is therefore best that pre-existing glaucoma issues are addressed with the regulation of IOP prior to corneal transplantation, when possible. Some authors suggest using unpreserved glaucoma medications without proinflammatory effects following keratoplasty to minimize trauma to the graft.[4]

The clinician must always weigh the risk:benefit ratio of performing glaucoma surgery post keratoplasty as graft rejection and failure could be triggered. Glaucoma procedures are not without risk and certain sequelae of glaucoma surgery can compromise a patient's vision.[2] Among patients who develop glaucoma following keratoplasty, 19–27.3% require a glaucoma surgical intervention.[4,7,8] The most frequent glaucoma intervention is a glaucoma drainage device.[3]

## Trabeculectomy

Trabeculectomy is perhaps the most common procedure performed for chronic forms of glaucoma. It involves the creation of an opening at the limbus allowing aqueous to flow under a scleral flap into the subconjunctival space. The general features of a trabeculectomy include placement of traction suture for appropriate globe positioning, creation of a paracentesis for irrigation and reformation of the anterior chamber, conjunctival flap preparation which could be limbus or fornix based, adjuvant subconjunctival antimetabolite treatment if required, creation of scleral flap, sclerostomy formation, peripheral iridectomy, closure of scleral flap and flow titration. This surgical procedure concludes with closure of the conjunctiva in a watertight fashion. Postoperative management of trabeculectomy involves close monitoring of the healing process and suture lysis as needed to maintain aqueous outflow. Steroids are used in the postoperative period to minimize scarring (Fig. 1).

Trabeculectomy with or without an antimetabolite like mitomycin C (MMC) can be a surgical option for IOP reduction post keratoplasty. The use of antimetabolite therapy increases the success rate of trabeculectomy without severe adverse effect to the graft. One must make sure the superior conjunctiva is healthy as patients who have undergone a PKP may have extensive conjunctival scarring. Graft rejection remains a possible complication of trabeculectomy after keratoplasty, therefore, careful observation of the graft is necessary to catch early rejection. Complication of trabeculectomy as well as antimetabolite use include persistent epithelial defect, cystoid macula edema, choroidal effusions and bleb leaks.[48]

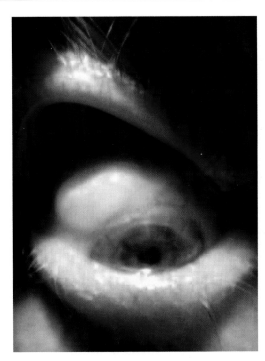

**Fig. 1:** Trabeculectomy following penetrating keratoplasty

Trabeculectomy without the use of an antimetabolite has a lower success rate compared to a trabeculectomy with MMC.[48,49] Combined trabeculectomy with MMC and keratoplasty could be considered in patients with uncontrolled glaucoma and corneal disease; however, one must be vigilant about managing postoperative inflammation as the bleb and graft could have a high risk for failure.[50,51]

Some authors have described combining a trabeculectomy with an additional glaucoma surgery. These authors argue that although a single procedure may be less stressful to the graft, there is a lower chance of long-term IOP control.[52] Cyclodialysis-augmented trabeculectomy with MMC has been described and shown to provide a safe and effective method of lowering IOP in intractable glaucoma post keratoplasty.[53]

## Glaucoma Drainage Device

A glaucoma drainage implant is often the surgery of choice when caring for patients who have undergone invasive corneal surgeries. Several studies have demonstrated the safety of glaucoma drainage devices following multiple prior eye surgeries. For example, the tube versus trabeculectomy (TVT) Study evaluated the safety and efficacy of tube-shunt surgery to trabeculectomy with MMC in eyes with previous cataract and/or unsuccessful glaucoma

surgery. The TVT Study did not demonstrate clear superiority of one glaucoma operation over the other. In fact, it demonstrated that both provided adequate IOP control and both had their unique set of complications. However, other factors must be considered when deciding which surgery is best of a specific patient. These factors include surgeon's skill and experience with both operations, the patient's willingness to undergo repeat glaucoma surgery, the health of the superior conjunctiva and the planned surgical approach should failure occur.[54]

The general surgical technique for a 350-mm² Baerveldt glaucoma implant (BGI; Abbott Laboratories Inc, Santa Ana, California, USA) has various subtle differences however, the following description is the technique preferred by the authors. A 7.0 polygalactin (Vicryl; Ethicon, Inc, Somerville, New Jersey, USA) corneal traction suture is placed in the superior temporal cornea. A 5-clock hour conjunctival peritomy is created in a fornix-based fashion. Dissection is carried out posteriorly between Tenon's space and the sclera in the superior temporal quadrant. Wet-field cautery is then applied for hemostasis. The superior and lateral rectus muscles are isolated on muscle hooks. The device is placed underneath the bellies of the superior and lateral rectus muscles in the superior temporal quadrant approximately 8 mm posterior to the limbus. The implant is then secured to the sclera using interrupted 9.0 polypropylene (Prolene Ethicon, Inc, Somerville, New Jersey, USA) sutures placed through the implant's anchoring holes with partial thickness sclera bites. The knots are then rotated into the anchoring holes. The tube is then trimmed to the appropriate length with an anteriorly-placed bevel and subsequently ligated using a 7.0 vicryl suture followed by confirmation of complete occlusion. The option of tube fenestration is patient and physician dependent. The tube is placed in the anterior chamber through a 23-guage needle tract and secured to the sclera using a 9.0 prolene suture. A partial-thickness piece of donor cornea is placed over the tube and sutured in place using interrupted 7.0 vicryl sutures. The conjunctival and tenon's tissues are reapproximated to their original position and closed in a water tight fashion using 8.0 vicryl sutures in a running, interrupted and mattress fashion (Figs 2 and 3).

## Cyclophotocoagulation

Cyclophotocoagulation or endoscopic cyclophotocoagulation are great options for lowering the IOP in complicated glaucoma cases where the risk of an incisional procedure

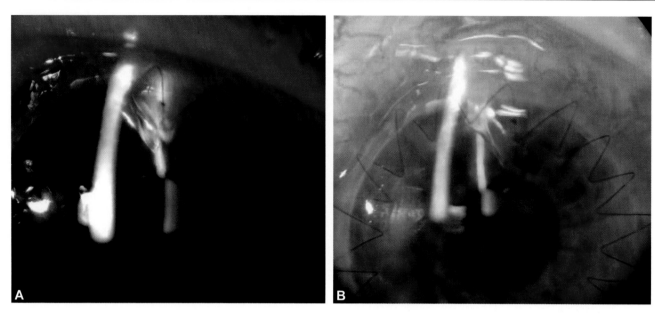

**Figs 2A and B:** Glaucoma drainage device following penetrating keratoplasty

is relatively high. Cyclophotocoagulation has long been the treatment of choice for glaucoma in cases that have not responded to other surgical interventions. The benefit of CPC is that it is minimally invasive and relatively easy to perform, even in eyes that have had several previous surgical procedures. However, because the laser is applied directly through the sclera, there is a moderate risk of collateral damage. The common side effects of CPC include hypotony, inflammation, phthisis, pain, graft failure, choroidal effusions, cataract, and macular edema. However, Rotchford et al. recently reported on the use of CPC in patients with good vision and found that 67.3% of

the studied eyes retained vision of 20/60 or better after a mean follow-up of 5.0 years. In fact, their reported visual loss is similar to that described in patient after incisional glaucoma surgeries.[55]

Endoscopic cyclophotocoagulation has also been demonstrated to be a safe and effective method for lowering IOP.[56-58] In theory, because ECP is less destructive and most effectively applies the laser energy directly to the ciliary body, there is less collateral damage to the surrounding structures.[59] Several authors report relatively good success rates (in terms of IOP control), up to 88%, in patients who have undergone ECP.[58,59] There are, as always, side effects.

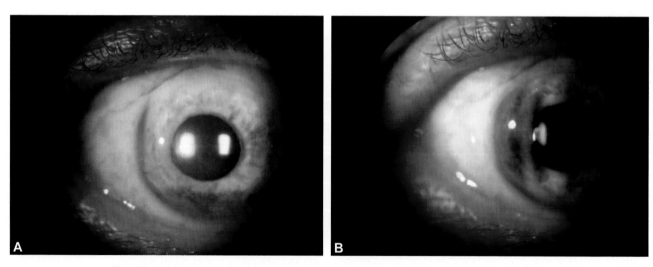

**Figs 3A and B:** Glaucoma drainage device after Descemet's stripping endothelial keratoplasty

Frances et al. found that of the five eyes with PKPs that underwent ECP, two of them had graft failure. Their study was not specifically designed to evaluate graft failure following ECP; however, this finding emphasizes the real side effect of surgical intervention in these challenging cases. To the authors' knowledge, to date, no literature has reported the safety or efficacy of ECP or CPC in the setting of DSEK.

## Laser Trabeculoplasty

Argon laser trabeculoplasty (ALT) or selective laser trabeculoplasty (SLT) can be used to treat medically uncontrolled glaucoma post keratoplasty in patients with open angles and a clear graft.[60] It has been found to reduce IOP with rare complications and stable visual function post keratoplasty. Laser trabeculoplasty is a valuable therapeutic option that limits invasive surgery for the treatment of glaucoma following PKP.[61] The major limitation of laser trabeculoplasty in patients who have previously undergone a PKP is that these eyes typically have PAS, which makes trabeculoplasty challenging and possibly contraindicated. The possibility of graft rejection could also occur following the procedure.

## Other Surgical Procedures

Newer glaucoma surgical procedures are being developed and used to manage glaucoma. Many of these newer devices and techniques are termed minimally invasive glaucoma surgery (MIGS). These include canaloplasty, Trabectome™, and the EX-press shunt™ among others. The details of these surgeries are beyond the scope of this chapter. Typically, patients who have undergone extensive corneal surgeries require more definitive and predictable glaucoma surgical interventions. The recent studies validating the efficacy of canaloplasty and trabectome suggest that these are best used in patients with healthy eyes who have mild glaucomatous changes. The EX-press shunt, a variation upon the traditional trabeculectomy is being used as an alternative to the trabeculectomy. Short-term results have demonstrated relatively good success in controlling IOP, however, long-term data in patients with extensive corneal surgery is not currently available.[62]

## ❧ SUMMARY

Glaucoma is a common complication following keratoplasty and patients should be observed closely for this possible complication. An awareness of all the potential mechanisms for IOP elevation would help aid the diagnosis and institution of appropriate treatment in this unique patient population. There are several surgical options for treatment but a stepwise approach to diagnosis and treatment is important in managing these patients. Although medical and surgical management of glaucoma may be more challenging in patients that have undergone corneal surgery, most patients do very well when managed appropriately.

## ❧ REFERENCES

1. Ayyala RS. Penetrating keratoplasty and glaucoma. Surv Ophthalmol. 2000;45(2):91-105.
2. Dada T, Aggarwal A, Minudath KB, et al. Post-penetrating keratoplasty glaucoma. Indian J Ophthalmol. 2008;56(4): 269-77.
3. Sihota R, Sharma N, Panda A, et al. Post-penetrating keratoplasty glaucoma: risk factors, management and visual outcome. Aust N Z J Ophthalmol. 1998;26(4):305-9.
4. Geerling G, Muller M, Zierhut M, et al. Glaucoma and corneal transplantation. Ophthalmologe. 2010;107(5):409-18.
5. Wandling Gr, Parikh M, Robinson C, et al. Escalation of glaucoma therapy after deep lamellar endothelial keratoplasty. Cornea. 2010;29(9):991-5.
6. Allouch C, Borderie V, Touzeau O, et al. Incidence and factors influencing glaucoma after penetrating keratoplasty. J Fr Ophtalmol. 2003;26(6):553-61.
7. Franca ET, Arcieri ES, Arcieri RS, et al. A study of glaucoma after penetrating keratoplasty. Cornea. 2002;21(3):284-8.
8. Karadag O, Kugu S, Erdogan G, et al. Incidence of and risk factors for increased intraocular pressure after penetrating keratoplasty. Cornea. 2010;29(3):278-8.
9. Prasher P, Muftuoglu O, Hsiao ML, et al. Epithelial downgrowth after descemet stripping automated endothelial keratoplasty. Cornea. 2009;28(6):708-11.
10. Rahman I, Carley F, Hillarby C, et al. Penetrating keratoplasty: indications, outcomes, and complications. Eye (Lond). 2009;23(6):1288-94.
11. Banitt M, Lee RK. Management of patients with combined glaucoma and corneal transplant surgery. Eye (Lond). 2009;23 (10):1972-9.
12. Huang C, O'Hara M, Mannis MJ. Primary pediatric keratoplasty: indications and outcomes. Cornea. 2009;28(9):1003-8.
13. Karabatsas CH, Hoh HB, Easty DL. Epithelial downgrowth following penetrating keratoplasty with a running adjustable suture. J Cataract Refract Surg. 1996;22(9):1242-4.
14. Fan JC, Chow K, Patel DV, et al. Corticosteroid-induced intraocular pressure elevation in keratoconus is common following uncomplicated penetrating keratoplasty. Eye (Lond). 2009;23(11):2056-62.
15. Erdurmus M, Cohen EJ, Yildiz EH, et al. Steroid-induced intraocular pressure elevation or glaucoma after penetrating-keratoplasty in patients with keratoconus or Fuchs dystrophy. Cornea.2009;28(7):759-64.

16. Eye Banking Statistical Report. Washington, District of Columbia, USA: Eye Bank Association of America.

17. Allan BD, Terry MA, Price FW, et al. Corneal transplant rejection rate and severity after endothelial keratoplasty. Cornea. 2007;26:1039-42.

18. Terry MA, Shamie N, Chen ES, et al. Endothelial keratoplasty: a simplified technique to minimize graft dislocation, iatrogenic graft failure, and pupillary block. Ophthalmology. 2008;115:1179-86.

19. Prasher P, Muftuoglu O, Hsiao ML, et al. Epithelial downgrowth after descemet stripping automated endothelial keratoplasty. Cornea. 2009;28(6):708-11.

20. Covert DJ, Koenig SB. New triple procedure: Descemet's stripping and automated endothelial keratoplasty combined with phacoemulsification and intraocular lens implantation. Ophthalmology. 2007;114:1272-77.

21. Lee JS, Desai NR, Schmidt GW, et al. Secondary angle closure caused by air migrating behind the pupil in Descemet stripping endothelial keratoplasty. Cornea. 2009;28:652-6.

22. Price FW, Price MO. Descemet's stripping with endothelial keratoplasty in 200 eyes: early challenges and techniques to enhance donor adherence. J Cataract Refract Surg. 2006;32: 411-8.

23. Suh LH, Yoo SH, Deobhakta A, et al. Complications of Descemet's stripping with automated endothelial keratoplasty: survey of 118 eyes at One Institute. Ophthalmology. 2008;115:1517-24.

24. Cheng YY, Hendrikse F, Pels E, et al. Preliminary results of femtosecond laser assisted Descemet stripping endothelial keratoplasty. Arch Ophthalmol. 2008;126:1351-6.

25. Ide T, Yoo SH, Leng T, et al. Subconjunctival air leakage after Descemet's stripping automated endothelial keratoplasty (DSAEK) in a post-trabeculectomy eye. Open Ophthalmol J. 2009;3:1-2.

26. Banitt MR, Chopra V. Descemet's stripping with automated endothelial keratoplasty and glaucoma. Curr Opin Ophthalmol. 2010;21(2):144-9.

27. Price MO, Price FW. Descemet's stripping with endothelial keratoplasty: comparative outcomes with microkeratome-dissected and manually dissected donor tissue. Ophthalmology. 2006;113(11):1936-42.

28. Vajaranant TS, Price MO, Price FW, et al. Intraocular pressure measurements following Descemet stripping endothelial keratoplasty. Am J Ophthalmol. 2008;145(5):780-6.

29. Bochmann F, Kaufmann C, Becht C, et al. Comparison of dynamic contour tonometry with Goldmann applanation tonometry following Descemet's stripping automated endothelial keratoplasty (DSAEK). Klin Monatsbl Augenheilkd. 2009;226(4):241-4.

30. Vajaranant TS, Price MO, Price FW, et al. Visual acuity and intraocular pressure after Descemet's stripping endothelial keratoplasty in eyes with and without preexisting glaucoma. Ophthalmology. 2009;116(9):1644-50.

31. Bahar I, Kaiserman I, Buys Y, et al. Descemet's stripping with endothelial keratoplasty in iridocorneal endothelial syndrome. Ophthal Surg Lasers Imaging. 2008;39:54-6.

32. Duarte MC, Herndon LW, Gupta PK, et al. DSEK in eyes with double glaucoma tubes. Ophthalmology. 2008;115(8):1435.

33. Esquenazi S, Rand W. Safety of DSAEK in patients with previous glaucoma filtering surgery. J Glaucoma. 2010;19(3):219-20.

34. Aldave AJ, Kamal KM, Vo RC, et al. The Boston Type I keratoprosthesis: improving outcomes and expanding indications. Ophthalmology. 2009;116(4):640-51.

35. Bradley JC, Hernandez EG, Schwab IR, et al. Boston Type I keratoprosthesis: the University of California Davis experience. Cornea. 2009;28:321-7.

36. Chew HF, Ayres BD, Hammersmith KM, et al. Boston keratoprosthesis outcomes and complications. Cornea. 2009;28(9): 989-96.

37. Rivier D, Paula JS, Kim E, et al. Glaucoma and keratoprosthesis surgery: role of adjunctive cyclophotocoagulation. J Glaucoma. 2009;18(4):321-4.

38. Banitt M. Evaluation and management of glaucoma after keratoprosthesis. Curr Opin Ophthalmol. 2011;22(2):133-6.

39. Baum J, Chaturvedi N, Netland PA, et al. Assessment of intraocular pressure by palpation. Am J Ophthalmol. 1995;119(5): 650-1.

40. Birnbach CD, Leen MM. Digital palpation of intraocular pressure. Ophthalmic Surg Lasers. 1998;29(9):754-7.

41. Rubinfeld RS, Cohen EJ, Laibson PR, et al. The accuracy of finger tension for estimating intraocular pressure after penetrating keratoplasty. Ophthalmic Surg Lasers. 1998;29(3):213-5.

42. Li JY, Greiner MA, Brandt JD, et al. Long-term complications associated with glaucoma drainage devices and Boston Keratoprosthesis. Am J Ophthalmol. 2011;152(2):209-18.

43. Kumar RS, Tan DT, Por YM, et al. Glaucoma management in patients with osteo-odonto-keratoprosthesis (OOKP): The Singapore OOKP Study. J Glaucoma. 2009;18:354-60.

44. Akpek EK, Harissi-Dagher M, Petrarca R, et al. Outcomes of Boston keratoprosthesis in aniridia: a retrospective multicenter study. Am J Ophthalmol. 2007;144:227-31.

45. Tan DT, Tay AB, Theng JT, et al. Keratoprosthesis surgery for end-stage corneal blindness in Asian eyes. Ophthalmology. 2008;115(3):503-10.

46. Shrivastava A, Madu A, Schultz J. Refractive surgery and the glaucoma patient. Curr Opin. Ophthalmol. 2011;22(4): 215-21.

47. Gilvarry AM, Kirkness CM, Steele AD, et al. The management of post-keratoplasty glaucoma by trabeculectomy. Eye (Lond). 1989;3 (Pt 6):713-8.

48. Ayyala RS, Pieroth L, Vinals AF, et al. Comparison of mitomycin C trabeculectomy, glaucoma drainage device implantation, and laser neodymium: YAG cyclophotocoagulation in the management of intractable glaucoma after penetrating keratoplasty. Ophthalmology. 1998;105(8):1550-6.

49. Figueiredo RS, Araujo SV, Cohen EJ, et al. Management of coexisting corneal disease and glaucoma by combined penetrating Keratoplasty and trabeculectomy with mitomycin-C. Opthalmic Surg. Lasers. 1996;27(11):903-9.

50. Kirkness CM, Steele AD, Ficker LA, et al. Coexistent corneal disease and glaucoma managed by either drainage surgery and subsequent keratoplasty or combined drainage surgery and penetrating keratoplasty. Br J Ophthalmol. 1992;76(3): 146-52.

51. Sihota R, Srinivassan G, Gupta V. Ab-externo cyclodialysis enhanced trabeculectomy for intractable post-penetrating keratoplasty glaucoma. Eye (Lond). 2010;24(6):976-9.

52. Nakakura S, Imamura H, NakamuraT. Selective laser trabeculoplasty for glaucoma after penetrating keratoplasty. Optom Vis Sci. 2009;86(4):404-6.

53. WuDunn D, Alfonso E, Palmberg PF. Combined penetrating keratoplasty and trabeculectomy with mitomycin C. Ophthalmology. 1999;106(2):396-400.

54. Gedde SJ, Schiffman JC, Feuer WJ, et al. Tube Versus Trabeculectomy Study Group. 'Three-year follow-up of the tube versus trabeculectomy study'. Am J Ophthalmol. 2009;148 (5):670-84.

55. Rotchford AP, Jayasawal R, Madhusudhan S, et al. Transscleral diode laser cycloablation in patients with good vision. Br J Ophthalmol. 2010;94(9):1180-3.

56. Chen J, Cohn RA, Lin SC, et al. Endoscopic photocoagulation of the ciliary body for treatment of refractory glaucomas. Am J Ophthalmol. 2010;94(9):1180-3.

57. Lima FE, Magacho L, Carvalho DM, et al. A prospective, comparative study between endoscopic cyclophotocoagulation and the Ahmed drainage implant in refractory glaucoma. J Glaucoma. 2004;13:233-7.

58. Gayton JL, VanDer Karr M, Sanders V. Combined cataract and glaucoma surgery: trabeculectomy versus endoscopic laser cycloablation. J Cataract Refract Surg. 2000;26:330-6.

59. Francis BA, Kawji, Vo NT, et al. Endoscopic cyclophotocoagulation (ECP) in the management of uncontrolled glaucoma with prior aqueous tube shunt. J Glaucoma. 2010;20(8):523-7.

60. Doyle JW, Smith MF. Glaucoma after penetrating keratoplasty. Semin Ophthalmol. 1994;9(4):254-7.

61. Van Meter WS, Allen RC, Waring GO, et al. Laser trabeculoplasty for glaucoma in aphakic and pseudophakic eyes after penetrating keratoplasty. Arch Ophthalmol. 1988;106 (2):185-8.

62. Ates H, Palamar M, Yagci A, et al. Evaluation of Ex-PRESS mini glaucoma shunt implantation in refractory postpenetrating keratoplasty glaucoma. J Glaucoma. 2010;19(18):556-60.

CHAPTER 82

# CHAPTER 83

# Pediatric Corneal Transplant Surgery

*Gerald W Zaidman*

## ⊱ INTRODUCTION

Pediatric corneal transplant surgery continues to evolve over the years. Corneal transplant surgery was first described by Eduard Zirm in 1905. For many years corneal transplant surgery in children was considered to be contraindicated because of the generally poor results. Beginning in the 1980s, however, attitudes began to change through the work of Drs George Waring, Stuart Brown[1], Doyle Stulting[2] and Peter Laibson. They began to more accurately describe and then categorize pediatric corneal diseases and assign to them the various surgical techniques that were then available. In the 1990s and 2000s the work of Drs Reza Dana,[3] Gerald Zaidman,[4] Lucy Yang[5] and David Rootman,[6] reviewed the surgical techniques used in children. Combining their original work and their reviews eventually led to increased surgical success rates and enabled corneal surgeons to reach the point at which corneal transplant surgery became a good option for children with corneal scarring or corneal disease. Therefore, what was once considered a dangerous procedure with high risks and low success rate,[7,8] has evolved so that the use of current medical and surgical techniques can provide clear corneal grafts in a majority of patients. As a result, corneal transplant surgery is now viewed as the first step in averting irreversible visual loss due to amblyopia in children with severe corneal diseases.

## ⊱ INDICATIONS

The indications for corneal transplant surgery in children can be divided into three groups—congenital etiologies, acquired nontraumatic etiologies, and trauma.[2,3,6,9-11] In North America, the congenital group is the most common. In the author's experience of nearly 300 corneal transplants in children, 65–70% were for congenital indications, acquired nontraumatic indications accounted for about 20–25% and 5–10% were due to trauma (Table 1).

There are four main causes of congenital corneal opacities (CCO) (Table 2). The most frequent cause of CCO is anterior segment dysgenesis.[12] This includes Peters' anomaly[13] Types I and II (Fig. 1), sclerocornea, corneal dermoids (Fig. 2), and congenital anterior staphyloma. This group accounts for nearly 65% of the CCO seen in North America. Congenital glaucoma (Fig. 3) is the next most common cause of CCO comprising 15% of patients. Next are the congenital corneal dystrophies such

**Table 1:** Indications for corneal transplant surgery in children

| Congenital | 65–70% |
|---|---|
| Acquired nontraumatic | 20–25% |
| Traumatic | 10% |

**Table 2:** Differential diagnosis of congenital corneal opacities

| Anterior Segment Dysgenesis (Peters' anomaly, Sclerocornea, Dermoid, Congenital Staphyloma) | 65% |
|---|---|
| CHED | 15% |
| Congenital glaucoma | 15% |
| Birth trauma, infection, metabolic | 5% |

CHED: Congenital hereditary endothelial dystrophy

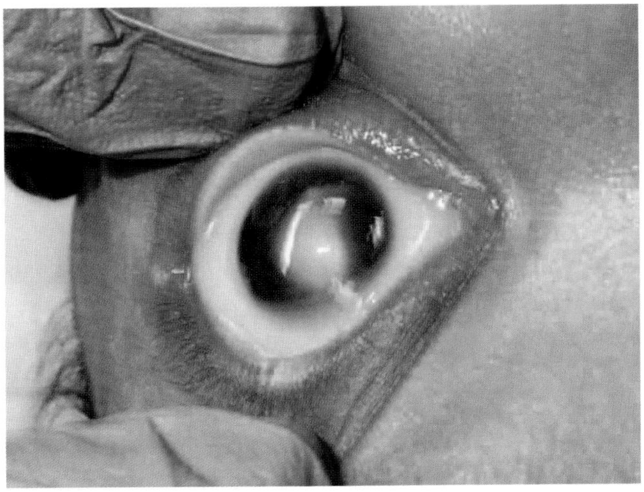

**Fig. 1:** A 3-month-old child with Peters' anomaly Type I

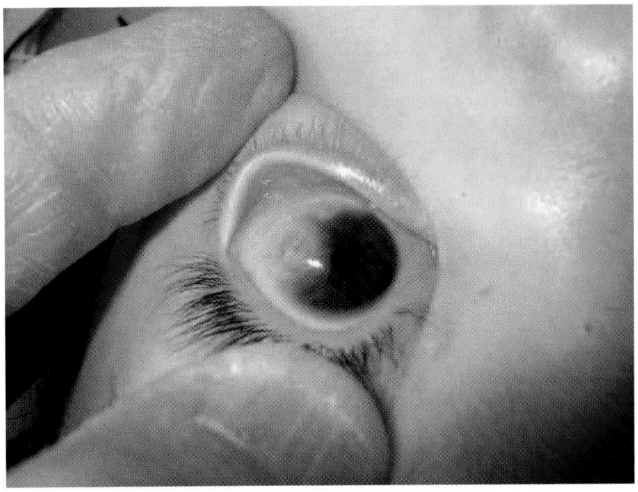

**Fig. 2:** A 7-month-old child with limbal corneal dermoid

as congenital hereditary endothelial dystrophy (CHED), (Fig. 4) congenital hereditary stromal dystrophy, and posterior polymorphous dystrophy. This group makes up approximately 15% of the patients with CCO. Finally, birth trauma, infection, and metabolic causes make up less than 5% of the patients.

In North America, acquired pediatric corneal opacities requiring corneal transplants are most frequently due to keratoconus (about 45% of the patients in this group), microbial keratitis (15%), herpes simplex keratitis (10%) and failed grafts (15%) (Table 3). Trauma (usually penetrating corneal lacerations) makes up the smallest group of children requiring corneal transplants (Fig. 5).[4,14]

## SURGERY

### Preoperative Evaluation

All children that require corneal transplants require a comprehensive preoperative evaluation. The diagnosis and treatment plan are determined after an office visit and family history, consultation with a pediatrician (to rule out systemic, genetic or metabolic disorders) and a pediatric ophthalmologist and most importantly an examination under anesthesia (EUA). This is necessary in all infants and poorly-cooperative children (generally those under 4–5 years old or those with attention deficit disorders). During the EUA, we evaluate all the parameters that can



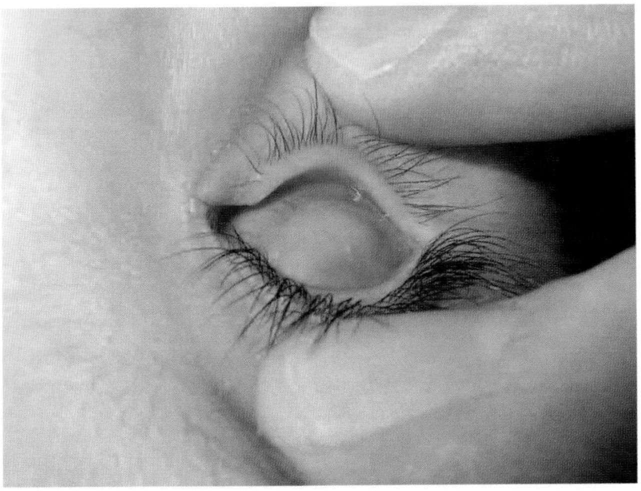

**Fig. 3:** A 10-month-old child with congenital glaucoma

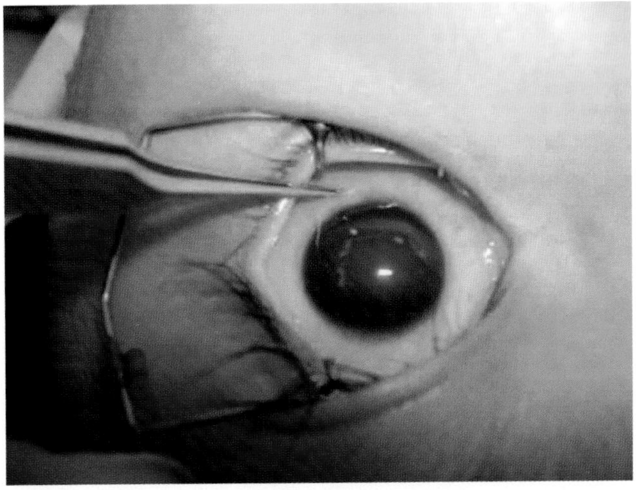

**Fig. 4:** A 6-month-old child with CHED

**Table 3:** Differential diagnosis of acquired nontraumatic corneal opacities

| | |
|---|---|
| Keratoconus | 45% |
| Microbial keratitis | 15% |
| HSV | 10% |
| Failed grafts | 15% |

HSV: Herpes simplex virus

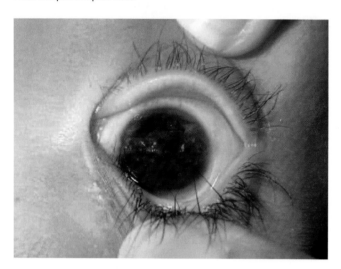

**Fig. 5:** A 3-year-old child with corneal laceration

affect the success rate of corneal transplant surgery—the severity of the corneal pathology, the intraocular pressure, and the corneal diameter. If funduscopy is not possible a B-scan sonogram is done.[15,16] Presently, ultrasound biomicroscopy (UBM) is routinely performed on all children with corneal opacities (Fig. 6).

Before surgery one other factor to be considered is the child's social situation. A stable social situation is mandatory. The child will require many years of conscientious care, therefore, supportive and motivated parents or caregivers are a necessity. In an unstable social environment, surgeries often fail and should not be undertaken.

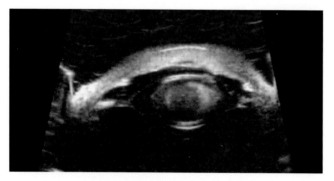

**Fig. 6:** Ultrasound biomicroscopy of an infant with Peters' anomaly and a cataract

The parents should also be counseled as to what they can reasonably expect from corneal transplant surgery in infants and children. We teach the parents about amblyopia and the necessity for comanagement with a pediatric ophthalmologist. We explain the difference between surgical success and visual development. We stress that the goal of transplant surgery is functional and ambulatory vision and not perfect vision and that many patients need spectacles or rigid gas permeable contact lenses postoperatively.

Finally, intraocular pressure control is required before corneal transplant surgery.[17,18] In the author's experience, most patients with glaucoma (except for those patients with congenital glaucoma) can usually be controlled medically (especially if the untreated intraocular pressure is less than 30 mm Hg). Patients are treated with prostaglandin inhibitors, beta-blockers, or topical or systemic carbonic anhydrase inhibitors. Brimonidine is not used because of pulmonary side effects. If medical control is unsuccessful, glaucoma surgery will be required prior to penetrating keratoplasty. In children, filtering surgery has fewer complications than tube shunts.

## Timing

Because of the small size of the neonatal eye and the high risk of intraoperative complications, a penetrating keratoplasty for a congenital corneal opacity is not done before a child is 2 months of age. In an ideal situation, the child is first seen in the office at 7–14 days of age. The EUA is scheduled for 3–6 weeks of age. In a child with a unilateral congenital opacity, the corneal transplant is then done at about 10–12 weeks of age. In a bilateral case the first transplant is done between 8 and 12 weeks of age. In a bilateral case, the more severe eye is not necessarily done first. It is often advisable to do the better eye first so that the child can begin to recover some vision. In bilateral cases, the second eye is usually done from 6 to 8 weeks after the first eye. Though this may worsen the amblyopic difference between the two eyes, this allows for several weeks of postoperative care, during which time we can remove sutures, control glaucoma, avoid infection, and validate parental compliance. For an acquired corneal opacity in a child beyond the amblyopic age, surgery can be scheduled electively, similar to an adult. In children under 8 years age, with acquired traumatic diseases, amblyopia remains a risk and surgery is performed soon after the eye has stabilized and all inflammation has resolved.

# ▸ SURGICAL TECHNIQUE

The surgery is always done under general anesthesia. The author's preference is to use donor corneal tissue between the ages of 4 and 19. Corneal donor tissue under the age of 4 is very flaccid. This makes it difficult to manipulate. A weight appropriate dose of intravenous mannitol (20%) is given before surgery commences. Children are then hyperventilated by the anesthesiologist. A pediatric speculum is inserted and a scleral support ring is sutured to the sclera. The recipient corneas are usually trephined between 5 and 7 mm and the donor cornea between 5.5 and 7.5 mm. This produces a 0.5 mm difference between the donor and recipient cornea. After trephination, the anterior chamber is entered with a Micro-Sharp #75 blade and the anterior chamber is reformed with viscoelastic. The viscoelastic or a cyclodialysis spatula is used to lyse any synechiae between the iris and the cornea. The author uses a specially designed pediatric cyclodialysis spatula (manufactured by Storz) that is smaller than the adult spatula and more easily fits into the pediatric eye. The recipient corneal button is excised with pediatric corneal transplant scissors, also designed by Storz (E3320 RL). Infants and children can develop significant amounts of positive pressure during excision of the cornea. The surgeon has to be experienced in handling this to avoid loss of the lens or vitreous loss. After the patient's cornea has been removed, (and after completion of any required anterior segment surgery) the donor graft is sutured into position with 12–16 interrupted 10-0 sutures.[19]

There are alternatives to penetrating keratoplasty. Amongst these are optical iridectomy, rotating keratoplasty, lamellar keratoplasty and Descemet's Stripping Automated Endothelial Keratoplasty (DSAEK) or keratoprosthesis.[20-24] The author's experience in rotating keratoplasties has been disappointing, resulting in large amounts of irregular astigmatism. Optical iridectomy can be performed in the rare patient with an off-centered opacity. In these cases, surgically opening the pupil may enable the child to see around the opacity. The author reported on this in the Journal of Cataract and Refractive Surgery in 1998.[21]

Lamellar keratoplasty is indicated for children with anterior stromal corneal scarring. This is typically seen in children with Herpes keratitis. The operation has a very high success rate, but it is technically demanding. Its advantages are that it avoids the problems of endothelial graft rejection, traumatic wound dehiscence and expulsive hemorrhage.[25] The last two may be especially important in active young children. However, the interface that develops between the host and donor stroma may limit best potential vision, which is problematic in children in the amblyogenic age group.

DSAEK is an operation designed for endothelial dysfunction. The indications in children would be CHED or corneal edema secondary to congenital glaucoma or a failed graft. DSAEK is a technically demanding procedure with a steep learning curve. In an infant or young child's eye, the crystalline lens is proportionally a larger structure within the eye than in an adult. Therefore, the anterior chamber will be shallower as compared to an adult which will make the operation more difficult. Additionally, children with glaucoma with tubes, shunts, or filters are problematic DSAEK cases. Visualization and stripping of Descemet's membrane is also often difficult and could require trypan blue or accessory illumination such as chandelier illumination. Perioperatively, one cannot do a slit-lamp examination on infants and young children. This makes it difficult to determine if the DSAEK disk and the air bubble are in the appropriate position. If DSAEK is going to be done on an infant or young child the surgeon should schedule an EUA under general anesthesia shortly after the DSAEK procedure. To date, the literature indicates that there have been 12 children with 19 eyes who have had DSAEK. Though, the first 2 were for corneal decompensation after cataract extraction, all of the most recent ones were for CHED. All of them were older children (with an average age of 9). The authors describe significant difficulty in stripping Descemet's membrane and a high incidence of re-bubbling in these children's eyes. Children healed with less astigmatism, but the children developed vision that was less than that of penetrating keratoplasty; only about 45% of the children saw better than 20/40.[26-29]

Keratoprosthesis (KPro) has recently been used in some children (Fig. 7). In the United States, the most commonly used keratoprosthesis is the Boston keratoprosthesis, which was approved by the FDA in 1992. The original indications for KPro were patients who were bilaterally blind (vision = 20/200 in the better eye) with a poor prognosis for successful transplant surgery if another homograft is attempted. Therefore, in children the primary indication for KPro is multiple failed corneal grafts. The postoperative management is time-consuming. The patients have to use a bandage contact lens and topical antibiotics and steroids indefinitely. Because children with a keratoprosthesis cannot have their intraocular pressure checked, many of them require a concomitant glaucoma procedure (usually a

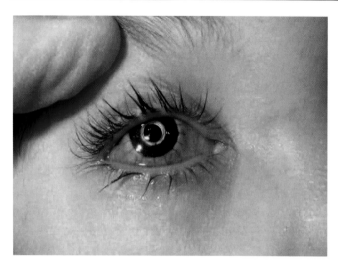

**Fig. 7:** A two and a half years old child with keratoprosthesis

tube shunt). Also there are many complications associated with keratoprosthesis including retroprosthetic membrane, severe glaucoma, infectious endophthalmitis, extrusion of the prosthesis, retinal detachment and sterile vitritis (Table 4). In comparison, children with a penetrating keratoplasty have very few of these complications, but do have significant issues with graft rejection and irregular astigmatism.

The main advantages of the keratoprosthesis are no immunologic rejection and no astigmatism. The keratoprosthesis can allow rapid visual development which can be another important advantage.

## POSTOPERATIVE MANAGEMENT

Routine postoperative care includes topical antibiotics 4 times a day, aggressive topical steroids and glaucoma therapy as needed. A topical corticosteroid (either predni-

solone acetate 1% or dorzolamide 1.5%) is used very frequently. If one is using prednisolone acetate, the drops are typically used 10 times a day for the first month, 8 times a day for the second month, 7 times a day for the next month, and then tapered by one drop per month, every month (6 times a day for 1 month, 5 times a day for 1 month, etc.). If dorzolamide is used, one can start at a lower level, usually 6 times a day for the first month and then a slow tapering regimen similar to that used by prednisolone acetate. As a result, patients are treated with topical steroids for a minimum of 10 months after surgery.

For the first month after surgery, the patient is examined 2–3 times a week; in the second month examination is done weekly (more when necessary). The frequency of the office examinations are then slowly decreased to every 6–8 weeks. Examinations under anesthesia are often performed. These are initially in the operating room and then when needed in an office setting (under chloral hydrate sedation). The first EUA is 2–3 weeks after surgery and then repeated in the operating room every few weeks until all sutures are removed. For infants, all sutures are usually removed by 5–6 weeks postoperatively (Table 5).[22] Office EUAs are done every 3–4 months using a portable slit-lamp and pneumotonometer or Tono-Pen. Finally, parents are instructed as to how to examine the grafted eye (with a light and a magnifier) to note any signs of loose sutures or graft rejection.

After all sutures are removed the patients are comanaged by a pediatric ophthalmologist who dispenses a spectacle correction and a regimen for patching the unoperated eye. Finally, the parents are warned that the graft is at risk whenever the child develops any severe febrile illness or is vaccinated. On these occasions, the corticosteroid drops are increased in frequency for a short time. For example, vaccinations are delayed until 1 year after surgery. When the child restarts vaccinations or if the child has any severe febrile illness, the corticosteroid drops are usually increased to 4 times a day for 3–5 days before and 3–5 days after the vaccination or the fever.

**Table 4:** Comparison of complication rate KPro versus penetrating keratoplasty (PKP)

| Keratoprosthesis | Keratoplasty |
|---|---|
| Retroprosthetic membrane: 30–40% | No membranes |
| Glaucoma: 20–60% (all patients get tube shunts) | Glaucoma varies |
| Infectious endophthalmitis: 9–15% | Endophthalmitis < 1% |
| Prosthesis extrusion: 0–15% | No extrusion |
| Retinal detachment: 1–10% | Retinal detachment < 2% |
| Sterile vitritis: 3–8% | Vitritis: 0% |
| No immunologic rejection | Rejection rate: 5–50% |
| No astigmatism | Irregular astigmatism frequent |

**Table 5:** Schedule of suture removal

| | |
|---|---|
| First year of life | by 5–6 weeks after surgery |
| 1–2 years olds | 2–3 months postoperatively |
| 2–3 years olds | 3–4 months postoperatively |
| 4–8 years olds | 5–6 months postoperatively |
| Children older than 8 years old require removal of all sutures by 1 year after surgery | |

# RESULTS

Older studies did not separate patients into diagnostic groups and had the tendency to combine children with a good prognosis, such as CHED or Peters' Anomaly Type I, together with children who had a poor prognosis, such as those with poorly controlled glaucoma, sclerocornea, microcornea or severely traumatized eyes. More recent studies have separated patients into diagnostic groups and have had longer follow-up. In these studies, older children usually do well. Adolescents with keratoconus have better than a 90% success rate and usually develop excellent visual results.[1,5,30] When reviewing the results in younger children, it is important to separate the children by diagnosis. Children with the milder form of Peters' anomaly, Peters' anomaly Type I and children with CHED, do best achieving success rates of 80–90%. We have reviewed our experience with Peters' anomaly Type I.[31-37] We followed our children for more than 3 years after their original transplants and noted that nearly 90% had clear grafts and that 54% of children obtained vision greater than 20/100. Similar results have been reported in a recent study from Australia and the Australian Graft Registry in which they analyzed over 700 children under the age of 20 who underwent corneal transplants between 1985 and 2009. In their study, the most common cause of corneal pathology in children under 5 years of age was Peters' anomaly and other anterior segment disorders; 56% of those children had clear grafts. Children between the age of 5 and 10 predominantly had keratoconus or corneal scarring secondary to trauma or Herpes keratitis and in those children graft clarity was present in 80% of patients. Finally, children between 13 and 19 almost exclusively had keratoconus and they had a 90% success rate of corneal transplants. The remaining children with other diagnosis (sclerocornea, Peters' anomaly Type II, severe glaucoma, or major anterior segment trauma) do less well. However, their visual potential is better with a translucent graft than if they had their original opaque or scarred cornea.

Finally, one must continuously remind the parents that visual acuity is dependent both on the status of the graft and aggressive amblyopia therapy. The child must continue to see a pediatric ophthalmologist in order to develop and maintain the best possible vision.

# CONCLUSION

Penetrating keratoplasty remains the gold standard for corneal transplantation in infants and children. In low risk eyes, very good to excellent vision can develop. With the recent development of new surgical techniques, such as DSAEK and keratoprosthesis, visual rehabilitation can be offered to additional groups of children who might have originally been poor candidates for surgery. Even with these newer techniques, however, parents must understand that corneal surgery in an infant or a child is a complex and difficult process.

To maximize the success rate, children have to be intensively managed with frequent examinations, high-dose topical steroids and aggressive control of glaucoma. Amblyopia must be comanaged with a pediatric ophthalmologist. If these conditions are met, more than 50% of the children can develop good or functional vision in their eyes.

# REFERENCES

1. Frueh BE, Brown SI. Transplantation of congenitally opaque corneas. Br J Ophthalmol. 1997;81(12):1064-9.
2. Stulting RD, Summers, KD, Cavanagh HD, et al. Penetrating keratoplasty in children. Ophthalmol. 1984;91(10):1222-30.
3. Dana MR, Moyes AL, Gomes JA, et al. The indications for and outcome in pediatric keratoplasty: a multicenter study. Ophthalmology. 1995;102(8),1129-38.
4. Zaidman G, Ramirez T, Kaufman A, et al. Successful surgical rehabilitation of children with traumatic corneal laceration and cataract. Ophthalmol. 2001;108(2):338-42.
5. Yang LLH, Lambert SR, Lynn MJ, et al. Long-term results of corneal graft survival in infants and children with Peters' anomaly. Ophthalmology. 1999;106(4):833-8.
6. Ehrlich CM, Rootman DS, Morin JD. Corneal transplantation in infants, children and young adults: experience of the Toronto Hospital for Sick Children, 1979-88. Can J Ophthalmol. 1991;26(4):206-10.
7. Castroviejo R. Selection of patients for keratoplasty. Surv Ophthalmol. 1958;3(1):1-12.
8. Leigh AG. Corneal grafting. Br J Clin Pract. 1958;12(5):329-32.
9. Michaeli A, Markovich A, Rootman DS. Corneal transplants for the treatment of congenital corneal opacities. J Pediatr Ophthalmol Strabismus. 2005;42:34-44.
10. Rezende RA, Uchoa UBC, Uchoa R, et al. Congenital corneal opacities in a cornea referral practice. Cornea. 2004;23(6):565-70.
11. Zaidman GW. Pediatric Keratoplasty Association Newsletter Vol 1, (2001). Available from www.pedkera.org/vol1.htm [Retrieved October 18, 2006].
12. Gloor P. Pediatric penetrating keratoplasty. In: Krachmer J, Mannis, M, Holland E (Eds). Cornea. Chapter 132, Elsevier, Mosby, Philadelphia, Pa, USA; 2005. pp. 1609.
13. Parmley VC, Stonecipher KG, Rowsey JJ. Peters' anomaly: a review of 26 penetrating keratoplasties in infants. Ophthalmic Surg. 1993;24(1):31-5.
14. Dana MR, Schaunberg DA, Moyes AL, et al. Outcome of penetrating keratoplasty after ocular trauma in children. Arch Ophthalmol. 1995;113(12):1503-7.

15. Bloomdahl S. Ultrasonic measurements of the eye in the newborn infant. Acta Ophthalmol (Copenh). 1979;57(6):1048-56.

16. Tucker SM, Enzenauer RW, Levin AV, et al. Corneal diameter, axial length and intraocular pressure in premature infants. Ophthalmology. 1992;99(8):1296-300.

17. Sidotti PA, Belmonte SJ, Liebmann JM, et al. Trabeculectomy with mitomycin-c in the treatment of pediatric glaucomas. Ophthalmol. 2000;107(3):422-9.

18. Feitl ME, Krupin T: Hyperosmotic agents. In: Ritch R, Shields BM, Krupin (Eds). The Glaucomas, 2nd edition. Mosby, St. Louis; 1996. pp. 1438-88.

19. Zaidman GW, Juechter K. Peter's anomaly associated with protruding corneal pseudo staphyloma. Cornea. 1998;17(2):163-8.

20. Murthey S, Bansal AK, Sridahr MS. Ipsilateral rotational autokeratoplasty: an alternative to penetrating keratoplasty in nonprogressive corneal scars. Cornea. 2001;20(5):455-7.

21. Zaidman GW, Rabinowitz Y, Forstot SL. Optical iridectomy for corneal opacities in Peters' anomaly. J Cataract Refract Surgery. 1998;24(5):719-22.

22. Zaidman GW, Brown SI. Corneal transplantation in a patient with corneal dermoid. Am J Ophthalmol. 1982;93(1):78-83.

23. Zaidman GW: Lamellar keratoplasty for anterior corneal scarring in infants and young children. In: John T (Ed): Surgical Techniques in Anterior and Posterior Lamellar Corneal Surgery, Chapter 53. Medical Publishers (P) LTD, New Delhi, India; 2006. pp. 571-8.

24. Zaidman GW. Lamellar Keratoplasty for Anterior Corneal Scarring in Infants and Young Children. In: John T (Ed). Surgical Techniques in Anterior and Posterior Lamellar Corneal Surgery. Medical Publishers (P) LTD, New Delhi, India. pp. 2005.

25. Brown SI, Salamon S. Wound healing of grafts in congenitally opaque infant corneas. Am J Ophthalmol. 1983;95(5):641-4.

26. Busin M, Beltz J, Scorcia V. Descemet-stripping automated endothelial keratoplasty for congenital hereditary endothelial dystrophy. Arch Ophthalmol. 2011;129(9):1140-6.

27. Fernandez MM, Buckley EG, Afshari NA. Descemet stripping endothelial keratoplasty in a child. J AAPOS. 2008;12(3):314-6.

28. Jeng BH, Marcotty A, Traboulsi E. Descemet stripping automated endothelial keratoplasty in a 2-year-old child. J AAPOS. 2008;12(3):317-8.

29. Pineda R, Jain V, Shome D, et al. Descemet's stripping endothelial keratoplasty: is an option for CHED. Int Ophthalmol. 2010;30(3):307-10.

30. Dana MR, Schaumberg DA, Moyes AL, et al. Corneal transplantation in children with Peters' anomaly and mesenchymal dysgenesis. Ophthalmology. 1997;104(10):1580-6.

31. Zaidman GW, Cape-Feury C, Flannagan J. Long-Term Visual Prognosis in children after corneal transplant Surgery for Peters' anomaly Type I. Am J Ophthalmology. 2007;144:104-8.

32. Comer RM, Daya, SM, O'Keefe M. Penetrating keratoplasty in infants. J AAPOS. 2001;5(5):285-90.

33. Yang LLH, Lambert SR. Peters' anomaly: a synopsis of surgical management and visual outcome. Pediatric Ophthalmology. 2001;14(3):467-77.

34. Huang C, O'Hara M, Mannia MJ. Primary pediatric keratoplasty. Cornea. 2009;28(9):1003-8.

35. Lowe MT, Keane MC, Coster DJ, et al. The outcome of corneal transplantation in infants, children and adolescents. Ophthalmology. 2011;118(3):492-7.

36. Ganekal S, Gangangouda C, Dorairaj S, et al. Early outcomes of primary pediatric keratoplasty in patients with acquired, a traumatic corneal pathology. J AAPOS. 2011;15(4):353-5.

37. Patel HY, Ormonde S, Brookes NH, et al. The indications and outcome of pediatric corneal transplantation in New Zealand: 1991-2003. Br J Ophthalmol. 2005;89(4):404-8.

**SECTION 16**

# CHAPTER
# 84

# DLEK, DSAEK, DSEK, DMEK

*Marianne O Price, Francis W Price, Arundhati Anshu*

## ⨳ INTRODUCTION

Endothelial keratoplasty (EK) is a paradigm shift in the field of corneal transplantation. Since its original description by Tillet in 1956,[1] the surgical technique has rapidly evolved, particularly in the last decade (Fig. 1). Posterior lamellar keratoplasty (later called deep lamellar endothelial keratoplasty or DLEK) as described by Melles eliminated the need for sutures to secure the graft.[2] Early results with this procedure showed promise but the technique was difficult to perform and replicate, and visual results were suboptimal.[3,4] Further pioneering work by Melles et al. led to the development of newer forms of EK techniques namely Descemet's stripping endothelial keratoplasty (DSEK)[5] and Descemet's membrane endothelial keratoplasty (DMEK).[6]

Descemet's stripping endothelial keratoplasty involves stripping of the recipient Descemet's membrane (DM) followed by transplanting a dissected posterior donor lenticule consisting of posterior stroma and DM through a small incision of usually 5 mm. Initially, donor dissection

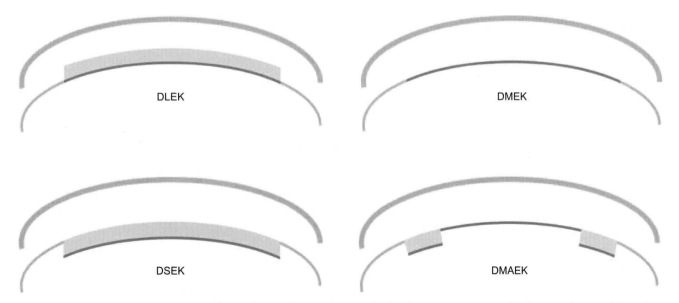

**Fig. 1:** Illustration showing how endothelial keratoplasty techniques have evolved to become more targeted in tissue replacement, from deep lamellar endothelial keratoplasty (DLEK), to Descemet's stripping endothelial keratoplasty (DSEK), to Descemet's membrane endothelial keratoplasty (DMEK), and finally the hybrid between DSEK and DMEK known as Descemet's membrane automated endothelial keratoplasty (DMAEK). For each procedure the donor tissue is represented in blue, with stromal tissue being light blue and endothelium dark blue

was manual. Later, automated, or microkeratome-assisted, donor preparation as described by Gorovoy[7] made it possible for surgeons to embrace the procedure even further. This form of automated EK technique is sometimes differentiated as Descemet's stripping automated endothelial keratoplasty or DSAEK. DSEK was quickly adopted by Price et al. in the United States, where he performed the first case of DSEK. He made modifications to the technique and played an important role in making it a popular procedure.

Descemet's membrane endothelial keratoplasty is a 'true' component lamellar surgery since it involves replacing diseased DM and endothelium with just donor DM and endothelium. Descemet's membrane automated endothelial keratoplasty or DMAEK is yet another form of EK technique described by McCauley and Price et al.[8] This is a hybrid technique that combines the donor stability and ease of insertion of DSEK along with the excellent visual results achieved with DMEK.

Descemet's stripping automated endothelial keratoplasty/ Descemet's stripping endothelial keratoplasty is the most commonly performed EK procedure today. It has gained rapid and widespread acceptance because of the advantages it offers compared to conventional full-thickness penetrating keratoplasty (PK). These advantages include reduced risk of complications like suprachoroidal hemorrhage, better structural integrity, faster and predictable visual rehabilitation, and fewer, if any, ocular surface complications (Table 1).

**Table 1:** Advantages of endothelial keratoplasty (EK) compared to penetrating keratoplasty (PK)

- Early and predictable visual rehabilitation
- Minimal refractive change
- Eyes retain more tectonic/structural integrity—greater resistance to minor trauma
- Minimal ocular surface issues—corneal innervation retained and no sutures in place to hold the graft
- Fewer activity restrictions

## ▶ INDICATIONS AND CONTRAINDICATIONS

Currently EK can be performed for any form of endothelial dysfunction (Table 2) including endothelial dystrophies like Fuchs endothelial dystrophy, iridocorneal endothelial (ICE) syndrome (Fig. 2), and pseudophakic or aphakic bullous keratopathy. With appropriate technique modifications, DSEK can also be performed in eyes with glaucoma filtration surgery, peripheral anterior synechiae (PAS) and iris abnormalities including aniridia (Fig. 3).

Also, EK can be performed in eyes with a failed PK (Figs 4 and 5) with the advantages of early visual rehabilitation, reduced follow-up visits as well as avoidance of suture-related problems. Price et al. described for the first time in 2006, the technique modifications that may help to optimize outcomes and suggested oversizing the donor graft and avoiding DM stripping unless there is DM scarring or the presence of visually significant guttae.[9] More recently,

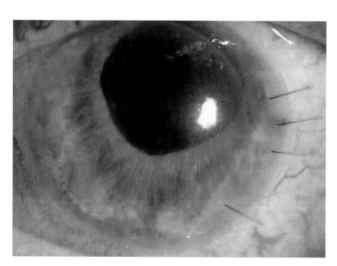

**Fig. 2:** Slit-lamp image of a Descemet's stripping endothelial keratoplasty (DSEK) graft performed to treat iridocorneal endothelial (ICE) syndrome. Peripheral anterior synechiae attached to the graft periphery between 6 and 8 clock hours

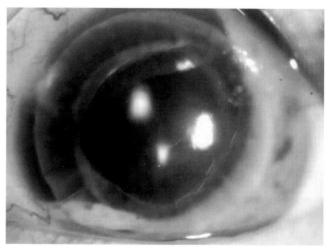

**Fig. 3:** One-week postoperative slit-lamp image of a Descemet's membrane automated endothelial keratoplasty (DMAEK) graft in an eye with iris missing between 7 and 1 o'clock following removal of an iris tumor. The central portion of the graft, consisting of just Descemet's membrane and endothelium, clears more rapidly than the peripheral stromal rim

**Table 2:** Indications and contraindications for endothelial keratoplasty

*Indications*

- All forms of endothelial dysfunction including the following:
  - Fuchs' endothelial dystrophy
  - Posterior polymorphous dystrophy
  - Congenital hereditary endothelial dystrophy
  - Pseudophakic and aphakic bullous keratopathy
  - Iridocornea endothelial (ICE) syndrome
  - Previous failed penetrating keratoplasty (PK)
  - Endothelial failure from angle closure, glaucoma drainage devices (GDD), trauma, previous surgery
- Provided there is enough room in the anterior chamber for graft insertion and placement, it can also be done in the following situations:
  - Peripheral anterior synechiae (PAS)
  - Iris abnormalities, including aniridia
  - Anterior chamber intraocular lenses (ACIOL)

*Contraindications*

- Corneal opacities or significant anterior stromal haze that would prevent achievement of good vision postoperatively
- Keratoconus and anterior stromal dystrophies
- Hypotony

Currently, it is not recommended to perform Descemet's membrane endothelial keratoplasty (DMEK) in eyes with GDD (likelihood of endothelial damage or the donor could go up the tube) or ACIOLs (high likelihood of endothelial damage) or eyes with iris abnormalities, particularly aniridia (graft could drop posteriorly into the vitreous cavity/retina)

several studies have reported good outcomes of DSEK in eyes with failed PK.[10-13] Some authors suggest oversizing the donor graft since it provides a larger endothelial cell reservoir[9,13] while others have suggested undersizing to be able to conform well to the irregular posterior profile of the PK wound.[10] Similarly, some authors suggest routine DM stripping to reduce rates of graft dislocation.[10] DM stripping needs to be carefully performed in eyes with failed PK, given the reduced tensile strength of the graft-host junction and vulnerability to wound dehiscence. Anshu et al. have reported good long-term graft survival in eyes undergoing EK under a failed PK (96% in eyes without glaucoma drainage device and 22% in eyes with a glaucoma drainage device at 4 years; p = 0.0005) with low rate of graft dislocation even without routine DM stripping.[14] Given that the reported rates of graft detachment are similar in eyes with and without DM stripping it is likely that other factors like wound leaks and hypotony may play a greater role in early graft detachment.[15]

In eyes with iris abnormalities including aniridia, DSEK can be performed as long as care is taken to prevent the donor lenticule from dropping posteriorly into the vitreous and/or retina, especially so in aphakic eyes. Some of the suggested modifications include use of a temporary fixation suture to anchor the graft,[16] or the use of suture pull through technique of donor insertion.[17] Equally important is to ensure a full air fill after donor insertion to prevent graft detachment.

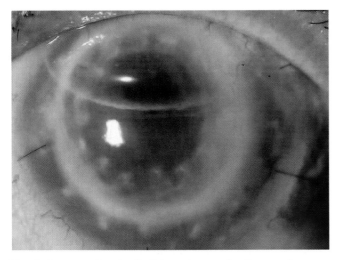

**Fig. 4:** Postoperative day-2 slit-lamp image of a Descemet's membrane endothelial keratoplasty (DMEK) graft under a failed penetrating keratoplasty. A residual air bubble from the air tamponade, used to secure the graft in place, remains in the anterior chamber and will dissipate naturally over several days

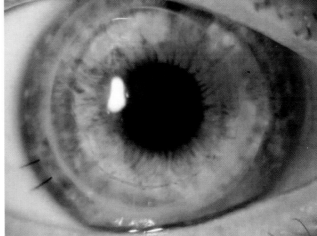

**Fig. 5:** Slit-lamp image of a Descemet's Membrane Automated Endothelial Keratoplasty (DMAEK) graft under a failed penetrating keratoplasty (PK). The DMAEK diameter is larger than that of the prior PK such that the stromal rim of the DMAEK graft straddles the prior PK incision

Donor attachment can be challenging in eyes with pre-existing glaucoma filtration surgery since the air tends to escape through the filtering bleb into the subconjunctival space. Ensuring a complete air fill is therefore critical in such eyes.

The management of eyes with anterior chamber intraocular lenses (ACIOL) is controversial. Some surgeons advocate IOL exchange with scleral or iris fixated lenses either performed concurrently with DSEK[18] or as a staged procedure. ACIOLs may be retained in the eye during DSEK as long as there is adequate space for donor insertion and manipulation.[19] However, it is important to remember that if the donor detaches in eyes with retained ACIOLs, there is a high likelihood of endothelial damage and graft failure.

In eyes with pre-existing PAS, it needs to be lysed carefully before donor insertion. If the eye has a significant amount of PAS and scarring as well as anterior chamber (AC) abnormalities where lysis or reconstruction of the AC will not result in a deep enough AC to allow graft placement without iris touch, PK might be a better alternative because it can be challenging to insert the DSEK graft in eyes with shallow AC. Tan et al. have described various measures to tackle eyes with shallow AC and high vitreous pressure; these include placement of an AC maintainer and the use of the Sheets glide or the Tan endoglide to insert the donor to maintain AC stability.[20,21]

It is important to determine the amount of lens opacity before considering EK surgery. If a patient has visually significant cataract, cataract surgery can be performed before EK, as a staged or combined procedure, or after EK surgery. Performing cataract surgery before EK provides increased space in the AC for donor insertion and manipulation and this may have bearing for surgeons during the learning curve. Combining EK and cataract surgery is a convenient option from the patient's perspective but may increase risk of endothelial damage, if the donor were to come in contact with the IOL. While not routinely done at this time, cataract surgery after EK may provide the most accurate way to calculate IOL power or treat astigmatism since several studies have shown a moderately wide range of refractive shift following EK surgery. However, cataract extraction after EK may be associated with donor graft trauma and endothelial loss.

In eyes without visually significant lens opacities, a decision on leaving the eye phakic or performing cataract extraction with EK should be made based on age of the patient, patient expectation/preference, and assessment of AC depth. Price et al. have recently demonstrated that the probability of cataract extraction was 0% and 7% at 1st and 3rd years respectively in patients 50 years and younger at the time of DSEK compared to 31% and 55% in older patients (p = 0.0005).[22] Given these findings, it would be advisable to leave the eye phakic during DSEK in patients less than 50 years of age, if no visible cataract is present. In older patients with clear lens and deep AC, an informed decision should be made based on patient's preference.

## DESCEMET'S STRIPPING AUTOMATED ENDOTHELIAL KERATOPLASTY/ DESCEMET'S STRIPPING ENDOTHELIAL KERATOPLASTY

### Surgical Technique

The surgical technique involves donor preparation, recipient preparation, donor insertion and air management. Initially the donor was hand-dissected DSEK but most surgeons prefer microkeratome dissection of the donor graft (DSAEK) since it is consistent and easy to perform, as well as provides a smoother interface with reduced risk of perforation. Precut tissue or tissue prepared by eye bank personnel is also an option for surgeons since it obviates the need to invest in costly equipment needed for automated donor preparation.

Recipient preparation involves creating a 3–5 mm scleral or corneal wound and stripping the central recipient DM under air, viscoelastic or balanced salt solution (BSS). Donor tissue is then trephined to the desired diameter (ranging from 8 mm to 9 mm) and inserted into the eye using a variety of insertion techniques that include forceps, glides (Busin glide, Sheets glide, Tan Endoglide) and inserters [e.g. cartridge inserters and closed chamber pulling injector (CCPI) system].

Using forceps, the donor is folded in a taco configuration and then inserted into the eye. Various appositional/ nonappositional forceps are available for the folding technique of donor insertion. The disadvantage of this technique is the difficulty in unfolding the donor correctly in the eye, especially for surgeons early in the learning curve of the procedure.

The glide techniques evolved to meet the challenges associated with donor unfolding with the forceps. The Busin glide enables easier donor insertion and unfolding in the eye since the donor is placed stromal side up before insertion and is already in the correct orientation. Endothelial cell loss of 25% at 6 months has been reported using Busin glide.[23]

The Sheets glide technique was developed by Mehta and Tan et al. to enable donor insertion in eyes with shallow ACs, typically seen in Asian eyes. With this technique, they reported a 1-year endothelial cell loss of 25% and significantly reduced primary graft failure (PGF) rates.[21] The Tan Endoglide incorporates the glide technique with the advantage of having a closed chamber system. This allows for greater donor control and AC stability during donor insertion. A mean endothelial cell loss of 13% and 15.6% at 6 months and 1 year respectively has been reported using the Tan Endoglide with no graft detachments or primary failure.[20]

Following donor insertion, the donor lenticule is apposed to the recipient stroma using an air bubble. Some surgeons perform an inferior peripheral iridotomy while others remove part of the air after 5–60 minutes to prevent postoperative pupil block by the air bubble.

## Visual Acuity and Refractive Outcomes

Descemet's stripping endothelial keratoplasty provides early and predictable visual rehabilitation compared to PK. The range of best-corrected visual acuity (BCVA) following DSEK averages 20/33 to 20/66 with a follow-up ranging from 3 to 30 months in several reported series (Table 3).[24-34]

A major advantage of DSEK over PK is that it causes significantly less change in the spherical equivalent or cylinder. With DSEK, most series report a mean hyperopic shift from 0.7 D to 1.5 D (Table 4).[24,25,32,35-37] This is likely related to the centrally thin and peripherally thick donor lenticule, as well as the addition of donor stroma that reduces the posterior radius of curvature and hence effective corneal power resulting in hyperopia.[38] The hyperopic shift encountered with DSEK needs to be taken into account when planning cataract surgery and IOL power calculation. Most surgeons suggest target refraction from −0.5 D to −1.5 D. This should be discussed preoperatively with the patient since the potential range of refractive shift can vary from −3.5 D to +4.0 D.[25]

Descemet's stripping endothelial keratoplasty generally causes no significant increase in astigmatism.[7,24,25,29,32,34,35,39,40] This is in sharp contrast to PK where postoperative ametropia in the form of myopia or astigmatism is common and can lead to troublesome anisometropia and suboptimal vision postoperatively as well as the need for hard contact lenses to achieve good vision.

## Endothelial Cell Density

The reported endothelial cell loss for DSEK ranges from 13% to 54% at 6 months and 15.6–61% at 1 year.[24,25] In DSEK, most of the endothelial cell loss is noted when the first postoperative measurement is taken, usually from 1 to 6 months after surgery, suggesting surgical trauma during donor preparation and/or donor insertion as the principal cause of early endothelial attrition. Subsequent cell loss occurs at a much lower rate. The median 5-year cell loss following DSEK as reported for the first time by Price et al. was 53% (range, 7.5% to 89%)[41] and this compares favorably to the 70% cell loss reported for PK in a prospective, multicenter Cornea Donor Study.[42] The DSEK 5-year cell loss study also showed that endothelial cell density was not significantly correlated with recipient gender, age or diagnosis and was weakly correlated with baseline donor endothelial cell density (p = 0.04).

## Graft Survival

The reported 1-year graft survival for DSEK ranges from 90% to 100% (Table 5)[7,14,23-25,33,35,36,41,43-45] and this is similar to that reported for PK (89% to 95%). Price et al. have reported the 5-year graft survival rate of 93% for DSEK and this is similar to PK as reported in the Cornea

**Table 3:** Visual outcomes of Descemet's stripping endothelial keratoplasty (DSEK) in reported series

| Study | Procedure | Number of Eyes | Mean Follow-up (Months) | 20/40 or Better Vision (%) |
|---|---|---|---|---|
| Price et al.,[32] 2006 | DSEK/DSAEK | 330 | 6 | 69 |
| Mearza et al.,[30] 2007 | DSEK | 11 | 12 | 65 |
| Price et al.,[26] 2008 | DSAEK | 40 | 12 | 80 |
| Basak et al.,[28] 2008 | DSEK | 75 | 3 | 83 |
| Sarnicola et al.,[33] 2008 | DSAEK | 16 | 12 | 38 |
| Kobayashi et al.,[29] 2008 | DSAEK | 14 | 6 | 100 |
| O' Brien et al.,[31] 2008 | DSAEK | 89 | Not reported | 50 |
| Bahar et al.,[27] 2009 | DSAEK | 12 | 12 | 50 |
| Terry et al.,[34] 2009 | DSAEK | 315 | 6 | 80 |

**Table 4:** Refractive outcomes of Descemet's stripping endothelial keratoplasty in reported series

| Study | Number of Eyes | Mean Spherical Equivalent Change (D) | Mean Change in Astigmatism (D) |
|---|---|---|---|
| Price and Price,[40] 2005 | 50 | Not reported | 0 |
| Price and Price,[32] 2006 | 216 | 0.7 | 0 |
| Gorovoy,[7] 2006 | 16 | | 0.6 |
| Koenig and Covert,[37] 2007 | 26 | 1.2 | 0.1 |
| Mearza et al.,[30] 2007 | 11 | | −0.4 |
| Covert and Koenig,[35] 2007 | 21 | 1.1 | 0.1 |
| Yoo et al.,[36] 2008 | 12 | 1.5 | |
| Price et al.,[26] 2008 | 40 | Not reported | 0.1 |
| Chen et al.,[39] 2008 | 100 | Not reported | 0.1 |
| Kobayashi et al.,[29] 2008 | 14 | Not reported | 0.5 |
| Terry et al.,[34] 2009 | 85 | Not reported | 0.1 |

**Table 5:** Graft survival following Descemet's stripping endothelial keratoplasty

| Study | Number of Eyes | Graft Survival (%) | | | | |
|---|---|---|---|---|---|---|
| | | 1 year | 2 years | 3 years | 4 years | 5 years |
| Anshu et al.,[14] 2011 | 60 (all DSEK under failed PK) | 98 | 90 | 81 | 74 | |
| Price et al.,[41] 2011 | 165 | 98 | 97 | 94 | 94 | 93 |
| Gorovoy,[7,46] 2011, 2006 | 51 | 94 | | | | 94 |
| Bahar et al.,[27] 2009 | 12 | 100 | 100 | | | |
| Busin et al.,[44] 2008 | 10 | 100 | | | | |
| Yoo et al.,[36] 2008 | 12 | 100 | | | | |
| Sarnicola and Toro,[33] 2008 | 16 | 100 | | | | |
| Price et al.,[45] 2008 | 263 | 100 | 99 | | | |

DSEK: Descemet's stripping endothelial keratoplasty; PK: penetrating keratoplasty

Donor Study.[41] The study also showed that 5-year graft survival was reduced significantly in eyes with pre-existing glaucoma surgery (40% vs 95% in eyes without glaucoma surgery, p = 0.0001). In a recent series of 51 eyes with DSAEK, Ratanasit and Gorovoy reported a 5-year graft survival of 94%.[46]

Letko and Price et al. have also reported on the indications for regrafting in a series of 1,050 DSEK cases.[47] The most common reason for regrafting in the 1st year was unsatisfactory vision secondary to donor folds or wrinkles, irregular donor lenticule thickness and rarely interface opacities. No DSEK eyes were regrafted because of ocular surface complications. This is in sharp contrast to PK, because ocular surface disease was found to be the most common cause of PK graft failure in the 1st year in a large series from the same center.[48]

## Complications

The commonly reported complications following DSEK include donor dislocation and PGF as shown in Table 6. Other reported complications include postkeratoplasty glaucoma, rejection, interface abnormalities and infections.

Donor dislocation results from nonadherence of the donor against the recipient stroma and remains the most commonly reported complication with rates ranging from as low as 0% to as high as 82%.[7,23-26,28,31,34,37,44,45,49] This complication is unique to EK surgery since the donor is not sutured into place; instead the donor is apposed to the recipient stroma using air tamponade. Several technique modifications have been suggested to reduce rates of graft dislocation and include good wound construction and closure massaging fluid out of the donor/host interface,[50]

**Table 6:** The various complications reported following Descemet's stripping endothelial keratoplasty in several series

| Study | Number of Eyes | Primary Graft Failure | Graft Detachment | Rejection | Glaucoma |
|---|---|---|---|---|---|
| Jordan et al.,[53-54] 2009 | 598 | | | 54 (9%) | |
| Terry et al.,[34] 2009 | 315 | 1 (0.3%) | 8 (3%) | | 1 (0.3%) |
| Bahar et al.,[23] 2009 | 63 | 1 (1.6%) | 9 (14%) | 2 (3%) | 6 (9.5%) |
| O'Brien et al.,[31] 2008 | 89 | 10 (11%) | 23 (26%) | | |
| Busin et al.,[44] 2008 | 10 | 0 | 0 | | 0 |
| Basak et al.,[28] 2008 | 75 | 1 (1%) | 6 (8%) | 1 (1%) | 2 (3%) |
| Price et al.,[26] 2008 | 40 | 0 | 4 (10%) | 2 (5%) | |
| Suh et al.,[49] 2008 | 118 | 21 (17%) | 27 (23%) | 7 (6%) | 2 (2%) |
| Allan et al.,[52] 2007 | 199 | | | 15 (7.5%) | |
| Gorovoy,[7] 2007 | 16 | 1 (6%) | 4 (25%) | 0 | |
| Koenig and Covert,[37] 2007 | 26 | 3 (11.5%) | 9 (35%) | 3 (11.5%) | 1 (4%) |

complete removal of fluid from the interface by placing mid-peripheral full-thickness venting incisions,[50] firm air fill, scraping of the peripheral recipient stromal bed[51] and advising against eye rubbing in the postoperative period.[50] Reattachment of a dislocated donor is usually achieved by reinjecting air.

Another commonly reported complication of DSEK is PGF or iatrogenic graft failure ranging from 0% to 29% in several series.[7,23-26,31,34,35,44,45,49] PGF describes a clinical situation in which the graft fails to clear as expected and usually results from suboptimal donor quality or surgically induced endothelial trauma. A high rate of PGF was reported by surgeons early in the learning curve of the procedure due to excessive donor manipulation. PGF rates are decreasing as surgeons gain more experience and the surgical technique becomes more widespread.

Allan et al. reported that EK had lower rejection rates than PK given the prolonged postoperative use of topical steroids.[52] The reported rates of allograft rejection following DSEK ranges from 0% to 45.5% with variable follow-up period.[24] In the largest reported series (598 eyes) on rejection after DSEK, the probability of a rejection episode was 7.6% at 1st year and 12% at 2nd years postoperatively.[53,54] Signs of rejection include corneal edema, keratic precipitates (Fig. 6), and an endothelial rejection line. Risk factors associated with increased risk of rejection were race and pre-existing glaucoma. A DSEK graft in the fellow eye within the prior year did not increase the risk of rejection. This is an important finding and given the rapid visual recovery, many patients prefer to have DSEK surgery in the fellow eyes a few months apart.

Postkeratoplasty glaucoma or raised intraocular pressure (IOP) following DSEK has ranged from 0% to 54%,[23-26,28,34,37,44,49] and this is similar to the range reported for PK. Some of the reported underlying mechanisms of glaucoma include steroid responsiveness, inflammation and angle closure. Studies have also shown that the presence of the donor lenticule does not alter IOP as recorded by the Goldmann applanation tonometer and since the corneal surface is not altered after DSEK, IOP can be monitored better than after PK.[55] Within the 1st year after DSEK, Vajaranant et al. reported an IOP spike in 35% of eyes without pre-existing glaucoma and in 43–45% of eyes with pre-existing glaucoma. Duration of steroid use was the only significant predictor of raised IOP.[56] More recently, Quek et al. have reported on risk factors for raised IOP and graft failure in eyes with pre-existing glaucoma.[57] They found that eyes without prior glaucoma filtration surgery and eyes

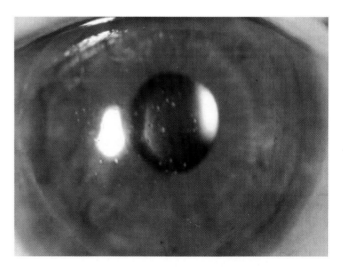

**Fig. 6:** Slit-lamp image of scattered keratic precipitates on a Descemet's stripping endothelial keratoplasty (DSEK) graft

that underwent additional intraoperative procedures during DSEK were 10 and 18 times more likely to require IOP lowering treatment after DSEK.

Another unique complication reported with lamellar corneal surgery, including EK is interface related abnormalities. In most cases, these opacities decrease over time with improvement in vision. Interface opacities that have been reported following DSEK include retained DM[49,58,59] epithelial cells[49], haem[49] and viscoelastic[60]. Retained DM with guttae, especially if in the visual axis, can result in suboptimal vision and may require regrafting.[47] Epithelial in-growth can lead to graft failure as shown in several histopathological series of graft failure.[58,59,61]

## DESCEMET'S MEMBRANE ENDOTHELIAL KERATOPLASTY

### Surgical Technique

The basic steps of DMEK surgery involve donor preparation, donor insertion and unfolding, and air management.[62-64] The SCUBA (Submerged Cornea Using Backgrounds Away) technique of donor preparation was developed by Giebel to address the handling and visualization challenges of harvesting donor DM. The details of the technique have been described in an earlier publication by Price et al.[63] In this technique, the peripheral DM is scored gently all around and then stripped away from the underlying stroma approximately half way to the center. This is followed by partial trephination of the donor cornea and separation of the centrally punched DM using nontoothed forceps. The stripped DM is then placed in tissue storage solution until the time it is transplanted into the recipient. A bimanual technique of donor harvesting has been similarly described by Kruse et al. to reduce tissue loss resulting from edge tears.[62]

Following donor preparation, the recipient DM is stripped as in DSEK and the donor is inserted into the eye using one of several injectors including a glass pipette or IOL injectors. The donor DM is then gently unfolded in the correct orientation using a combination of BSS and air. Air is then injected beneath the donor graft to enable graft attachment to the recipient stroma.

### Visual and Refractive Outcomes

Descemet's membrane endothelial keratoplasty provides excellent visual recovery and exceeds the best rates that have been reported for DSEK. More patients achieved 20/30 or better vision and this is likely due to absence of stroma in the transplanted donor tissue. As early as 1 month after surgery, patients achieved a median BCVA of 20/30 in a reported series by Price et al.[63] At one year, 97% of eyes without pre-existing ocular comorbidity saw 20/30 or better.[67] Other authors have also reported similar excellent outcomes after DMEK.[65,66]

Similar to DSEK, the refractive cylinder is unchanged after DMEK. A statistically significant hyperopic shift of 0.50 D was reported by Price et al. in DMEK single procedures.[63] Melles et al. have also reported a similar hyperopic shift following DMEK.[66]

### Endothelial Cell Loss

The reported 6 months and 1-year endothelial cell loss for DMEK was similar among the different centers reporting their results. These results mirror those of early reports of DSEK suggesting a learning curve. At 6 months, it was reported to be 32% and at 1 year it was 36%.[65-67] Melles et al. have also reported 2- and 3-year cell loss of 34% and 42% in a small cohort of patients that had complete follow-up to 2 and 3 years.[65,67-69]

### Complications

Like DSEK, graft detachment is the most commonly encountered complication following DMEK. Detachments in DMEK differ from those seen in DSEK since spontaneous reattachment as reported for DSEK does not seem to occur after DMEK. The edge of the donor has a tendency to curl inwards leading to persistent detachment as the donor edge essentially pushes away from the recipient (Fig. 7). The graft detachment rate was initially high in early DMEK series,[70,65,67] but it has dropped substantially with improved techniques.[71] Likewise, the rates of DMEK donor tissue loss and primary graft failure are dropping to levels only slightly higher than those typical of DSEK as instrumentation and methods continue to improve.[63,70,72] Importantly, the immunologic graft rejection rate has been shown to be over 10-fold lower with DMEK than it is with either DSEK or PK.[73,74]

## DESCEMET'S MEMBRANE AUTOMATED ENDOTHELIAL KERATOPLASTY

### Surgical Technique

Descemet's membrane automated endothelial keratoplasty is a hybrid technique that provides the donor stability of DSEK coupled with the visual results of DMEK. This technique entails the use of a microkeratome to perform

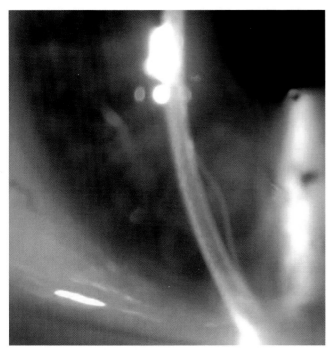

**Fig. 7:** Slit-lamp image of a Descemet's membrane endothelial keratoplasty (DMEK) graft showing a small inferior detachment

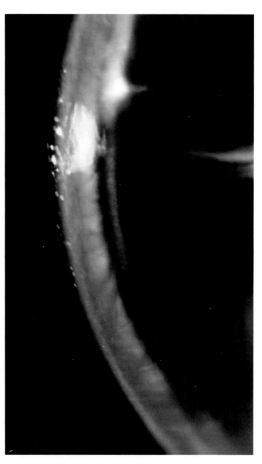

**Fig. 8:** Postoperative day-2 slit-lamp image of a Descemet's membrane automated endothelial keratoplasty (DMAEK) graft. The peripheral stromal rim is attached to the recipient cornea, but the central portion of the graft, consisting of just Descemet's membrane and endothelium, is detached

a lamellar dissection as in DSEK, big bubble formation to separate DM from stroma, excising the anterior stroma over the bubble, and trephining the donor to the desired size.[8] A microkeratome is used to perform lamellar dissection as in DSAEK and this is followed by creation of big bubble of 6–7 mm diameter to cause separation of the DM and stroma. The anterior stroma is then excised and the donor is trephined to the desired diameter in such a manner as to encompass a peripheral rim of stroma all around and bare DM in the center.

Other variations of this hybrid technique include Studeny's technique[75] called DMEK-S where the donor is dissected manually, and Busin's technique[76] that involves creating a sickle shaped area of attached stroma rather than a complete stromal ring.

Donor insertion and recipient preparation is similar to DSEK and involves creating a 3.5–5 mm corneal/scleral incision, DM stripping and donor insertion using a Busin glide as a carrier. Air is then injected to adhere the donor to the recipient cornea.

## Visual and Refractive Outcomes

Descemet's membrane automated endothelial keratoplasty also provides excellent visual recovery, like DMEK. As early as 1 month after surgery 90% of patients achieved a BCVA of 20/40 or better while at 3 and 6 months 100% achieved a BCVA of 20/40 or better with a median vision of 20/25 in a series reported by McCauley et al.[77]

## Complications and Endothelial Cell Loss

Graft detachment is one of the most common complications with DMAEK (Fig. 8), just as it is with DSEK or DMEK. Graft detachment is detected by slit lamp examination or by anterior segment optical coherence tomography (OCT) imaging and treated by reinjecting air.

McCauley et al. have reported an endothelial cell loss of 31% 6 months after DMAEK, and this is similar to that reported in initial DSEK or DMEK series from the same center.[77] Data on endothelial cell loss beyond 6 months is currently not reported but is anticipated to be similar to other EK procedures.

## CONCLUSION

Endothelial keratoplasty surgery continues to evolve both in surgical technique and instrumentation as well as in clinical outcomes. More work is needed to optimize visual outcomes and make it truly refractive neutral. Laboratory and clinical work are also needed to reduce endothelial cell loss especially so in the first 6 months. This should focus around improving donor preparation and insertion. Several inserters have been developed focusing on reducing endothelial cell loss and data from clinical studies are needed before they gain widespread acceptance. Given the scarcity of donor tissue in developing nations, focus needs to be directed towards increasing donor supply. One of the ways of achieving this goal would be the use of cultured endothelial cells. Early studies have shown some success in this area.

Long-term, prospective randomized studies are needed to evaluate the various EK techniques for endothelial cell loss and graft survival and to better compare it to conventional PK.

## REFERENCES

1. Tillett CW. Posterior lamellar keratoplasty. Am J Ophthalmol. 1956;41(3):530-3.
2. Melles GR, Eggink FA, Lander F, et al. A surgical technique for posterior lamellar keratoplasty. Cornea. 1998;17(6):618-26.
3. Terry MA, Ousley PJ. Small-incision deep lamellar endothelial keratoplasty (DLEK): six-month results in the first prospective clinical study. Cornea. 2005; 24(1):59-65.
4. Terry MA, Ousley PJ. Deep lamellar endothelial keratoplasty visual acuity, astigmatism, and endothelial survival in a large prospective series. Ophthalmology. 2005;112(9):1541-8.
5. Melles GR, Wijdh RH, Nieuwendaal CP. A technique to excise the descemet membrane from a recipient cornea (descemetorhexis). Cornea. 2004;23(3):286-8.
6. Melles GR, Lander F, Rietveld FJ. Transplantation of Descemet's membrane carrying viable endothelium through a small scleral incision. Cornea. 2002;21(4):415-8.
7. Gorovoy MS. Descemet-stripping automated endothelial keratoplasty. Cornea. 2006;25(8):886-9.
8. McCauley MB, Price FW, Price MO. Descemet membrane automated endothelial keratoplasty: hybrid technique combining DSAEK stability with DMEK visual results. J Cataract Refract Surg. 2009;35(10):1659-64.
9. Price FW, Price MO. Endothelial keratoplasty to restore clarity to a failed penetrating graft. Cornea. 2006;25(8):895-9.
10. Straiko MD, Terry MA, Shamie N. Descemet stripping automated endothelial keratoplasty under failed penetrating keratoplasty: a surgical strategy to minimize complications. Am J Ophthalmol. 2011;151(2):233-7.
11. Clements JL, Bouchard CS, Lee WB, et al. Retrospective review of graft dislocation rate associated with descemet stripping automated endothelial keratoplasty after primary failed penetrating keratoplasty. Cornea. 2011;30(4):414-8.
12. Nottage JM, Nirankari VS. Endothelial keratoplasty without Descemet's stripping in eyes with previous penetrating corneal transplants. Br J Ophthalmol. 2012;96(1):24-7.
13. Covert DJ, Koenig SB. Descemet stripping and automated endothelial keratoplasty (DSAEK) in eyes with failed penetrating keratoplasty. Cornea. 2007;26(6):692-6.
14. Anshu A, Price MO, Price FW. Descemet's stripping endothelial keratoplasty under failed penetrating keratoplasty: visual rehabilitation, complications and graft survival rate. Ophthalmology. 2011;118(11):2155-60.
15. Price FW, Price MO, Arundhati A. Descemet stripping automated endothelial keratoplasty under failed penetrating keratoplasty: how to avoid complications. Am J Ophthalmol. 2011;151(2):187-8.
16. Price MO, Price FW, Trespalacios R. Endothelial keratoplasty technique for aniridic aphakic eyes. J Cataract Refract Surg. 2007;33:376-9.
17. Macsai MS, Kara-Jose AC. Suture technique for Descemet stripping and endothelial keratoplasty. Cornea. 2007;26(9):1123-6.
18. Shah AK, Terry MA, Shamie N, et al. Complications and clinical outcomes of descemet stripping automated endothelial keratoplasty with intraocular lens exchange. Am J Ophthalmol. 2010;149(3):390-7.
19. Esquenazi S, Schechter BA, Esquenazi K. Endothelial survival after Descemet-stripping automated endothelial keratoplasty in eyes with retained anterior chamber intraocular lenses: two-year follow-up. J Cataract Refract Surg. 2011;37(4):714-9.
20. Khor WB, Mehta JS, Tan DT. Descemet stripping automated endothelial keratoplasty with a graft insertion device: surgical technique and early clinical results. Am J Ophthalmol. 2011;151(2):223-32.
21. Mehta JS, Por YM, Beuerman RW, et al. Glide insertion technique for donor cornea lenticule during Descemet's stripping automated endothelial keratoplasty. J Cataract Refract Surg. 2007;33(11):1846-50.
22. Price MO, Price DA, Fairchild KM, et al. Rate and risk factors for cataract formation and extraction after Descemet stripping endothelial keratoplasty. Br J Ophthalmol. 2010;94(11):1468-71.
23. Bahar I, Kaiserman I, Sansanayudh W, et al. Busin Guide vs Forceps for the Insertion of the Donor Lenticule in Descemet Stripping Automated Endothelial Keratoplasty. Am J Ophthalmol. 2009;147(2):220-6.
24. Lee WB, Jacobs DS, Musch DC, et al. Descemet's stripping endothelial keratoplasty: safety and outcomes: a report by the American Academy of Ophthalmology. Ophthalmology. 2009;116(9):1818-30.
25. Anshu A, Price MO, Tan DT, et al. Endothelial keratoplasty—A revolution in evolution. Survey of Ophthalmology. 2011.
26. Price MO, Baig KM, Brubaker JW, et al. Randomized, prospective comparison of precut vs surgeon-dissected grafts for descemet stripping automated endothelial keratoplasty. Am J Ophthalmol. 2008;146(1):36-41.
27. Bahar I, Sansanayudh W, Levinger E, et al. Posterior lamellar keratoplasty–comparison of deep lamellar endothelial keratoplasty and Descemet stripping automated endothelial keratoplasty in the same patients: a patient's perspective. Br J Ophthalmol. 2009;93(2):186-90.

28. Basak SK. Descemet stripping and endothelial keratoplasty in endothelial dysfunctions: three-month results in 75 eyes. Indian J Ophthalmol. 2008;56(4):291-6.

29. Kobayashi A, Yokogawa H, Sugiyama K. Descemet stripping with automated endothelial keratoplasty for bullous keratopathies secondary to argon laser iridotomy—preliminary results and usefulness of double-glide donor insertion technique. Cornea. 2008;27(Suppl 1):S62-9.

30. Mearza AA, Qureshi MA, Rostron CK. Experience and 12-month results of descemet-stripping endothelial keratoplasty (DSEK) with a small-incision technique. Cornea. 2007;26(3):279-83.

31. O'Brien PD, Lake DB, Saw VP, et al. Endothelial keratoplasty: case selection in the learning curve. Cornea. 2008;27(10):1114-8.

32. Price MO, Price FW. Descemet's stripping with endothelial keratoplasty: comparative outcomes with microkeratome-dissected and manually dissected donor tissue. Ophthalmology. 2006;113(11):1936-42.

33. Sarnicola V, Toro P. Descemet-stripping automated endothelial keratoplasty by using suture for donor insertion. Cornea. 2008;27(7):825-9.

34. Terry MA, Shamie N, Chen ES, et al. Endothelial keratoplasty for Fuchs' dystrophy with cataract: complications and clinical results with the new triple procedure. Ophthalmology. 2009;116(4):631-9.

35. Covert DJ, Koenig SB. New triple procedure: Descemet's stripping and automated endothelial keratoplasty combined with phacoemulsification and intraocular lens implantation. Ophthalmology. 2007;114(7):1272-7.

36. Yoo SH, Kymionis GD, Deobhakta AA, et al. One-year results and anterior segment optical coherence tomography findings of descemet stripping automated endothelial keratoplasty combined with phacoemulsification. Arch Ophthalmol. 2008; 126(8):1052-5.

37. Koenig SB, Covert DJ. Early results of small-incision Descemet's stripping and automated endothelial keratoplasty. Ophthalmology. 2007;114(2):221-6.

38. Dupps WJ, Qian Y, Meisler DM. Multivariate model of refractive shift in Descemet-stripping automated endothelial keratoplasty. J Cataract Refract Surg. 2008;34(4):578-84.

39. Chen ES, Terry MA, Shamie N, et al. Descemet-stripping automated endothelial keratoplasty: six-month results in a prospective study of 100 eyes. Cornea. 2008;27(5):514-20.

40. Price FW, Price MO. Descemet's stripping with endothelial keratoplasty in 50 eyes: a refractive neutral corneal transplant. J Refract Surg . 2005;21(4):339-45.

41. Price MO, Fairchild KM, Price DA, et al. Descemet's Stripping Endothelial Keratoplasty Five-Year Graft Survival and Endothelial Cell Loss. Ophthalmology. 2011;118(4):725-9.

42. Lass JH, Gal RL, Dontchev M, et al. Donor age and corneal endothelial cell loss 5 years after successful corneal transplantation. Specular microscopy ancillary study results. Ophthalmology. 2008;115(4):627-32.

43. Terry MA, Shamie N, Chen ES, et al. Precut tissue for Descemet's stripping automated endothelial keratoplasty: vision, astigmatism, and endothelial survival. Ophthalmology. 2009;116(2):248-56.

44. Busin M, Bhatt PR, Scorcia V. A modified technique for descemet membrane stripping automated endothelial keratoplasty to minimize endothelial cell loss. Arch Ophthalmol. 2008;126(8):1133-7.

45. Price MO, Price FW. Endothelial cell loss after Descemet's stripping with endothelial keratoplasty: influencing factors and 2-year trend. Ophthalmology. 2008;115(5):857-65.

46. Ratanasit A, Gorovoy MS. Long term results of Descemet's stripping automated endothelial keratoplasty. Cornea. 2011;30(12)1414-8.

47. Letko E, Price DA, Lindoso EM, et al. Secondary graft failure and repeat endothelial keratoplasty after Descemet's stripping automated endothelial keratoplasty. Ophthalmology. 2011;118(2):310-4.

48. Price MO, Thompson RW, Price FW. Risk factors for various causes of failure in initial corneal grafts. Arch Ophthalmol. 2003;121(8):1087-92.

49. Suh LH, Yoo SH, Deobhakta A, et al. Complications of Descemet's Stripping with Automated Endothelial Keratoplasty Survey of 118 Eyes at One Institute. Ophthalmology. 2008;115(9):1517-24.

50. Price FW, Price MO. Descemet's stripping with endothelial keratoplasty in 200 eyes: Early challenges and techniques to enhance donor adherence. J Cataract Refract Surg. 2006;32(3):411-8.

51. Terry MA, Hoar KL, Wall J, et al. Histology of dislocations in endothelial keratoplasty (DSEK and DLEK): a laboratory-based, surgical solution to dislocation in 100 consecutive DSEK cases. Cornea. 2006;25(8):926-32.

52. Allan BD, Terry MA, Price FW, et al. Corneal Transplant Rejection Rate and Severity After Endothelial Keratoplasty. Cornea. 2007;26(9):1039-42.

53. Jordan CS, Price MO, Trespalacios R, et al. Graft rejection episodes after Descemet stripping with endothelial keratoplasty: part one: clinical signs and symptoms. Br J Ophthalmol. 2009;93(3):387-90.

54. Price MO, Jordan CS, Moore G, et al. Graft rejection episodes after Descemet stripping with endothelial keratoplasty: part two: the statistical analysis of probability and risk factors. Br J Ophthalmol. 2009;93(3):391-5.

55. Vajaranant TS, Price MO, Price FW, et al. Intraocular pressure measurements following Descemet stripping endothelial keratoplasty. Am J Ophthalmol. 2008;145(5):780-6.

56. Vajaranant TS, Price MO, Price FW, et al. Visual acuity and intraocular pressure after Descemet's stripping endothelial keratoplasty in eyes with and without preexisting glaucoma. Ophthalmology. 2009;116(9):1644-50.

57. Quek DT, Wong T, Tan D, et al. Corneal Graft Survival and Intraocular Pressure Control after Descemet Stripping Automated Endothelial Keratoplasty in Eyes with Pre-existing Glaucoma. Am J Ophthalmol. 2011;152(1):48-54.

58. Zhang Q, Randleman JB, Stulting RD, et al. Clinicopathologic findings in failed descemet stripping automated endothelial keratoplasty. Arch Ophthalmol. 2010;128(8):973-80.

59. Shulman J, Kropinak M, Ritterband DC, et al. Failed descemet-stripping automated endothelial keratoplasty grafts: a clinicopathologic analysis. Am J Ophthalmol .2009;148(5):752-9.

CHAPTER **84**

60. Anshu A, Price MO, Price FW. A cause of reticular interface haze and its management after Descemet's stripping endothelial keratoplasty. Cornea. 2011.

61. Phillips PM, Terry MA, Kaufman SC, et al. Epithelial downgrowth after Descemet-stripping automated endothelial keratoplasty. J Cataract Refract Surg. 2009;35(1):193-6.

62. Kruse FE, Laaser K, Cursiefen C, et al. A stepwise approach to donor preparation and insertion increases safety and outcome of Descemet membrane endothelial keratoplasty. Cornea. 2011;30(5):580-7.

63. Price MO, Giebel AW, Fairchild KM, et al. Descemet's membrane endothelial keratoplasty: prospective multicenter study of visual and refractive outcomes and endothelial survival. Ophthalmology. 2009;116(12):2361-8.

64. Dapena I, Moutsouris K, Droutsas K, et al. Standardized "no-touch" technique for descemet membrane endothelial keratoplasty. Arch Ophthalmol. 2011;129(1):88-94.

65. Laaser K, Bachmann BO, Horn FK, et al. Donor Tissue Culture Conditions and Outcome after Descemet Membrane Endothelial Keratoplasty. Am J Ophthalmol. 2011;151(6):1007-18.

66. Ham L, Balachandran C, Verschoor CA, et al. Visual rehabilitation rate after isolated descemet membrane transplantation: descemet membrane endothelial keratoplasty. Arch Ophthalmol. 2009;127(3):252-5.

67. Guerra F, Anshu A, Price MO, et al. Descemet's Membrane Endothelial Kertaoplasty 1 Year Follow Up: A Prospective Multicenter Study. Ophthalmology. 2011;118(12):2368-73.

68. Ham L, van Luijk C, Dapena I, et al. Endothelial cell density after descemet membrane endothelial keratoplasty: 1- to 2-year follow-up. Am J Ophthalmol. 2009;148(4):521-7.

69. Ham L, Dapena I, Van Der Wees J, et al. Endothelial cell density after descemet membrane endothelial keratoplasty: 1- to 3-year follow-up. Am J Ophthalmol. 2010;149(6):1016-17.

70. Dapena I, Moutsouris K, Ham L, et al. Graft detachment rate. Ophthalmology. 2010;117(4):847-847.

71. Dirisamer M, Dapena I, Ham L, et al. Patterns of corneal endothelialization and corneal clearance after Descemet's membrane endothelial keratoplasty for Fuchs endothelial dystrophy. Am J Ophthalmol. 2011;152(4):543-55.

72. Kruse FE, Laaser K, Cursiefen C, et al. A stepwise approach to donor preparation and insertion increases safety and outcome of Descemet's membrane endothelial keratoplasty. Cornea. 2011;30(5):580-7.

73. Dapena I, Ham L, Netukova M. Incidence of early allograft rejection after Descemet's membrane endothelial keratoplasty. Cornea. 2011;30(12):1341-5.

74. Anshu A, Price MO, Price FW Jr. Risk of corneal transplant rejection significantly reduced with Descemet's membrane endothelial keratoplasty. Ophthalmology; 2012 (Epub ahead of print).

75. Studeny P, Farkas A, Vokrojova M, et al. Descemet's membrane endothelial keratoplasty with a stromal rim (DMEK-S). Br J Ophthalmol. 2010;94(7):909-14.

76. Busin M, Patel AK, Scorcia V, et al. Stromal support for Descemet's membrane endothelial keratoplasty. Ophthalmology. 2010;117(12):2273-7.

77. McCauley MB, Price MO, Fairchild KM, et al. Prospective study of visual outcomes and endothelial survival with Descemet membrane automated endothelial keratoplasty. Cornea. 2011;30(3):315-9.

# CHAPTER 85

# Descemet's Membrane Endothelial Keratoplasty (DMEK)

*Isabel Dapena, Vasilios S Liarakos, Martin Dirisamer, Miguel Naveiras, Ru-Yin Yeh, Ruth Quilendrino, Konstantinos Droutsas, Kyros Moutsouris, Marieke Bruinsma, Gerrit RJ Melles*

## ▶ INTRODUCTION

Nowadays, endothelial keratoplasty (EK) may have become the 'new gold standard' in the treatment of endothelial disorders in the United States. In the last decade, several EK techniques have been described for the transplantation of healthy donor corneal endothelium. Although the earliest attempts began in the 1950s,[1,2] it was not until 1998 with the introduction of 'posterior lamellar keratoplasty' (PLK),[3-5] later popularized as 'deep lamellar endothelial keratoplasty' (DLEK),[6-8] that endothelial transplantation was clinically successful. This technique later evolved into 'Descemet's stripping (automated) endothelial keratoplasty' [DS(A) EK],[9-12] procedure that became adopted by corneal surgeons all over the world. DS(A)EK was established as a safe procedure, by using a 'closed system' and by (nearly) eliminating most of the long-term complications that characterized penetrating keratoplasty (PK), like high astigmatism, suture-related complications and/or wound dehiscence.[13] Although, DS(A)EK potentially improved the clinical results of PK and DLEK, it still did not allow a complete visual rehabilitation of the eye. This was mostly due to the replacement of the diseased layers [Descemet's membrane (DM) and endothelium] by a 'thicker' posterior lamella composed of a layer of stroma, DM, and donor endothelium.[13] This 'added' layer of stroma, somehow altered the visual performance of the cornea, preventing the eye from reaching its maximal visual potential. Therefore, most DS(A)EK cases were limited to best corrected visual acuities (BCVA) of 20/40 (0.5), showing infrequently BCVA of 20/25 (0.8) or higher.[13-18]

In 2002, endothelial keratoplasty was further refined with the development of Descemet's membrane endothelial keratoplasty (DMEK),[19-21] by which the transplantation of a donor isolated DM with its endothelium devoid of stroma was accomplished. Thus, only the diseased corneal layers were substituted, providing a (nearly) normal anatomical restoration of the cornea and unprecedented visual results in the history of keratoplasty.[13,22,23]

Meanwhile, a hybrid technique between DS(A)EK and DMEK was developed. Depending on the donor being prepared manually or with the help of a microkeratome, the nomenclature used is DMEK-S (Descemet's membrane endothelial keratoplasty with a stromal rim)[24] or DMAEK (Descemet's membrane automated endothelial keratoplasty),[25,26] respectively. These techniques are based on transplanting donor tissue consisting of a peripheral rim of stroma with a central area of isolated DM and endothelium. Although results seem promising, DMEK-S/DMAEK may still face a relatively high incidence of graft detachments, often requiring a secondary air-rebubbling to achieve graft adherence.

Although DMEK was initially thought to be technically more laborious than DS(A)EK, it has dramatically increased in popularity in the last years, due to the recent developments in tissue handling, simplification of the surgical technique and low complication rates.[27-29] DMEK has now become a standardized 'no-touch' procedure,[27] designed with reproducible steps, that may be performed by the average corneal surgeon in any clinical setting and with relatively low costs. Providing the best clinical outcomes among the currently available endothelial keratoplasty techniques, DMEK may have potential to become the first treatment option for endothelial disorders.[13,28,29]

## PREOPERATIVE PREPARATION OF THE DMEK GRAFT

Several techniques have been described in order to obtain an isolated DM graft with endothelium.[20,30-35] The initially described DMEK graft harvesting technique, consisted of stripping DM from a corneoscleral rim submerged in saline.[20,30,31] This technique was proven safe and reproducible, with less than 5% of tissue loss due to inadvertent tearing, and surprisingly, no significant endothelial cell damage.[30-35] Hence, it was standardized and widely adopted by eye bank technicians and corneal surgeons.

DMEK grafts can be prepared in an eye bank or immediately before surgery itself.[34] In the authors' experience, eye bank preharvested grafts can better assure the availability of suitable DMEK-rolls for transplantation on planned surgery days. Furthermore, it may also allow a better control of donor quality, by monitoring the sterility of the transplants and the endothelial cell density after the preparation. Hence, the preparation of DMEK grafts is routinely performed in the authors' eye bank (Amnitrans Eyebank Rotterdam) 1–2 weeks prior to surgery. In short, in corneoscleral rims stored in modified minimum essential medium (CorneaMax, Eurobio, France) at 31°C within 36 hours of postmortem,[31,36] the endothelial cell morphology and viability is evaluated with an inverted light microscope (Axiovert 40, Zeiss, Göttingen, Germany) (Figs 1A to I). After provoked swelling and staining with trypan blue 0.04% (Hippocratech, The Netherlands), digital photographs are made (PixeLINK PL-A662, Zeiss, Göttingen, Germany).[19,31] Then, the corneoscleral rim is mounted endothelial side up on a custom made holder with a suction cup and the DM is loosened at the scleral spur to within the 9.0 mm central area. From the endothelial side, a superficial trephination is made to just within the posterior stroma with a 9.5-mm trephine (Ophtec, Groningen and the Netherlands). The DM is then stripped from the posterior stroma, so that a sheet of DM with its endothelial monolayer is obtained. Because of the elastic properties of the membrane, after immersion in saline a 'Descemet-roll' forms spontaneously, with the endothelium at the outer side. Immediately thereafter, the endothelial cell morphology and viability are evaluated again with inverted light microscopy and after provoked swelling and staining with trypan blue, digital photographs are made of representative areas of the endothelial cell layer.[31] Each Descemet-roll is then stored for 5–10 days in organ culture medium until the time of transplantation. Lately, this standard method for harvesting DM-grafts has been refined into a completely 'no-touch' donor preparation technique.[35]

For the preparation of donor grafts for DMEK-S/DMAEK, the technique has been modified.[24,25,37,38] DM is centrally detached by the injection of air at the donor DM-to-stromal interface and the stromal ring is then manually dissected in DMEK-S, or with the use of a microkeratome in DMAEK.[24,25,37,38]

When compared with earlier keratoplasty techniques, DMEK grafts may allow a more efficient use of the available tissue, because tissue unsuitable for PK or DS(A)EK can often be used for DMEK, and corneas with their DM stripped off are readily available for deep anterior lamellar keratoplasty procedures.[35,39,40] Moreover, as donor corneal tissue is commonly distributed as corneoscleral rims by most eye banks throughout the world, the accessibility to endothelial keratoplasty may be better with DMEK than with DS(A)EK. Even in third-world countries or in low-volume keratoplasty centers with a limited budget for equipment, DMEK may prove a feasible technique when requiring minimal financial investment.

## DESCEMET'S MEMBRANE ENDOTHELIAL KERATOPLASTY SURGICAL TECHNIQUE

In order to perform a standardized 'no-touch' DMEK procedure successfully,[27] the described steps and/or recommendations below may be followed.

### Obtaining a Soft Eye

In order to achieve a soft eye, four precautions or actions may be considered: the surgical bed should be positioned in an anti-Trendelenburg position; after retrobulbar injection (4–5 ml of ropivacain 10 mg/ml mixed with hyaluronidase 150 IE), a manual ocular massage is performed for 2–3 minutes, followed by oculopressure with a Honan's balloon for another 10–15 minutes; and during surgery, the 'tightness' of the eyelid speculum should be carefully monitored, and it may be released if the anterior chamber is shallow or if any signs of 'vitreous pressure' are observed.

### Incisions and Descemetorhexis

At the 12 o'clock surgical position, a tunnelized clear corneal incision, 3.0 mm in width, may be made with a slit-knife. Three side ports can be created at 10.30, 1.30 and 7.30 (right eye) or 4.30 o'clock (left eye) with a surgical knife.[27] Under air, the recipient's Descemet membrane is scored over 360° using a reversed Sinskey hook (Catalogue no 50.1971B, DORC International, Zuidland, The Netherlands), prior to stripping off the

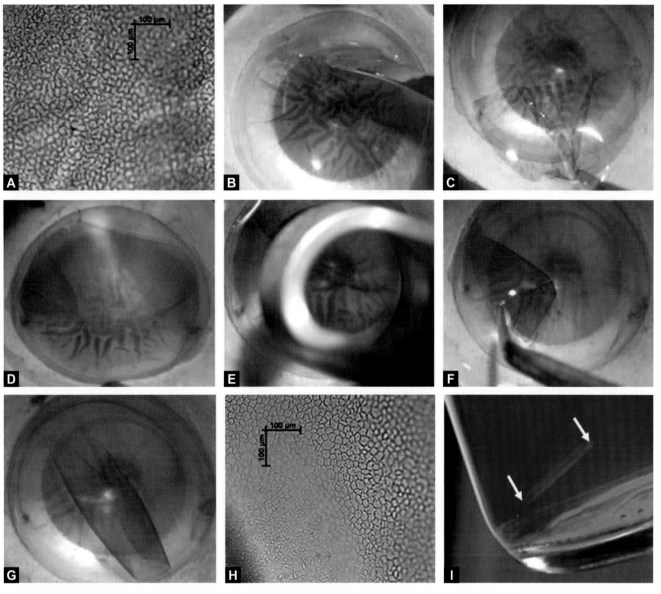

**Figs 1A to I:** (A) Light microscopy image of the endothelium just before stripping off Descemet's membrane (DM) from the posterior stroma of a donor corneoscleral rim; (B-G) Surgical view of donor tissue preparation for Descemet's membrane endothelial keratoplasty (DMEK). The donor corneoscleral rim is mounted endothelial side up onto a custom made fixation device; (B) With a hockeystick, DM is cut just anterior to the trabecular meshwork and scleral spur, and the edge of the membrane is gently pushed centrally and loosened over 180°; (C) With forceps holding its outer edge, the DM is slowly stripped off from the posterior stroma until approximately 2/3 of the stroma is denuded; (D) The entire rim is then submerged in a vial with saline to flush the DM in its original position; (E) On the fixation device, a superficial trephination is made; (F) With forceps holding its inner edge, the DM is completely stripped off from the posterior stroma; (G) After detachment, the DM rolls up spontaneously with the endothelium on the outside; (H) Light microscopy of the DMEK-roll's endothelium right after stripping off DM from the posterior stroma; (I) DMEK graft in a vial with organ culture medium. After 1–2 weeks of organ culture, during which the endothelial cell density and sterility is checked, the graft is sent off for transplantation in a DMEK procedure

membrane (descemetorhexis) with the reversed Sinskey hook or a Descemet scraper (Catalogue no 50.2118, DORC International, Zuidland, The Netherlands). During descemetorhexis, the tissue removal may be carefully monitored under air, to avoid remnant DM 'islands', that may occur in 50% of cases, since these remnants may affect the final visual acuity (VA) achieved and/or graft adherence to the posterior stroma.[41,42]

## Intraoperative Preparation of the DMEK Graft

The predissected donor DMEK graft is stored for 1 or 2 weeks in a glass vial with modified minimum essential medium (EMEM) at 31° C, until the date of transplantation (Figs 1A to I).[31] During surgery, the DMEK-roll is thoroughly rinsed (2–3 times) with balanced salt solution (BSS, Alcon Nederland BV, Gorinchem, Nederland) and stained with trypan blue 0.06% (Catalogue no VBL.10S.USA, Vision blue™; DORC International) twice for about 30 seconds, in order to ensure the visibility of the graft in the recipient anterior chamber throughout the surgery.[27] Novel surgeons starting out with DMEK may want to apply a direct flow on top of the tissue with BSS, to 'open up' the roll and to create a 'double-roll', like the plastic tubes of an electrical chord, to further facilitate unfolding of the tissue after implantation in the recipient anterior chamber. If the blue staining of the membrane fades away during the surgery, the graft can be re-stained by a few drops of trypan blue 0.06% injected in the anterior chamber, followed by rinsing out the excess dye.

## Implantation of the DMEK Graft

After staining, the DMEK-roll is sucked into a custommade glass injector (DMEK inserter; DORC International) and under the surgical microscope, the injector is turned so that the 'double-roll' is 'facing-upwards', i.e. with the hinge down.[27] Note that on the DMEK-roll, endothelial cells are located on the outer surface. For that reason, it may be advocated to avoid the use of plastic intraocular lens inserting devices, and to preferably use validated glass injectors, since glass surfaces are much smoother than those of plastic and glass injectors can be manufactured without sharp molding edges.[28,43]

Using the glass injector, the DMEK-roll is then inserted into the anterior chamber through the main incision at 12 o'clock.

## Orientating the DMEK Graft

Once implanted, the graft can be easily manipulated by gentle strokes or 'tapping' of a cannula over the outer corneal surface or the sclera overlying the iris root, rotating and/or slightly opening the roll in order to facilitate the maneuver to check the orientation of the graft in the anterior chamber (Figs 2A to I). The orientation of the graft can then be checked by positioning the tip of a 30G cannula on top of the membrane and underneath one of the peripheral curls: if the graft is correctly oriented (endothelium facing toward the iris), the tip of the cannula should be 'embraced' by one

of the rolls, becoming slightly blue as the curl overlays the cannula (Moutsouris sign) (Figs 3A and B). If the graft is oriented 'upside-down' (endothelium facing the cornea), the tip of the cannula will not turn blue, since it can not 'find' an upward curl, as the graft will be curling toward the iris, i.e. away from the cannula. If oriented upside-down, the graft may be 'rolled over' by gently flushing it within the anterior chamber.[27,44] If the graft is turned over, its orientation may be confirmed using the Moutsouris sign.

## Unfolding the DMEK Graft

Once the DMEK graft is oriented correctly with the edges facing upward, a small air-bubble is injected in between the double-roll(s), or on top of the membrane inside a curl (Figs 2A to I). If the graft is orientated upward, the air-bubble will be 'caught' in between the rolls, and it may be manipulated to further unfold the graft by 'rolling' the air on top of the membrane, using a cannula on the outer corneal surface (Dapena technique). When further unfolded, the air-bubble is enlarged until the central part of the DMEK graft is flattened over the iris.

Obtaining a correctly oriented 'double Descemet-roll' in the recipient anterior chamber may therefore be the most essential step in facilitating further unfolding of a Descemet-graft, because it allows to continue in a standardized fashion, i.e. to complete the surgery as a 'no-touch DMEK' procedure. However in a few cases, a 'double Descemet-roll' may not be obtained,[44] most often because the Descemet-graft might be either 'too loose' or 'too tight'. If 'too loose', the donor Descemet appears to lack sufficient elasticity to maintain a configuration as a 'double-roll'. Inside the recipient anterior chamber, the donor tissue shows a tendency to unfold by itself, which can be facilitated by gently moving a cannula over the outer surface of the recipient cornea that may finally unfold the graft, a maneuver named 'single sliding cannula technique'.[44] A Descemet-roll that is 'too tight', i.e. tissue with too much elasticity to maintain a 'double-roll', may be more challenging. These cases can virtually always be managed by applying gentle taps onto the recipient outer corneal surface (Droutsas taps), through which the Descemet-roll is loosened until an outer curl 'falls back' onto the iris. Once obtained, the outer curl can be fixated in position by applying downward pressure on the corneal surface with a cannula, 'sandwiching' the membrane between the stroma and the iris, and further unfolded by sliding a second cannula on the corneal surface to unroll the graft, mimicking the unrolling of a carpet (Dirisamer technique).[44] The maneuver of the second cannula can also

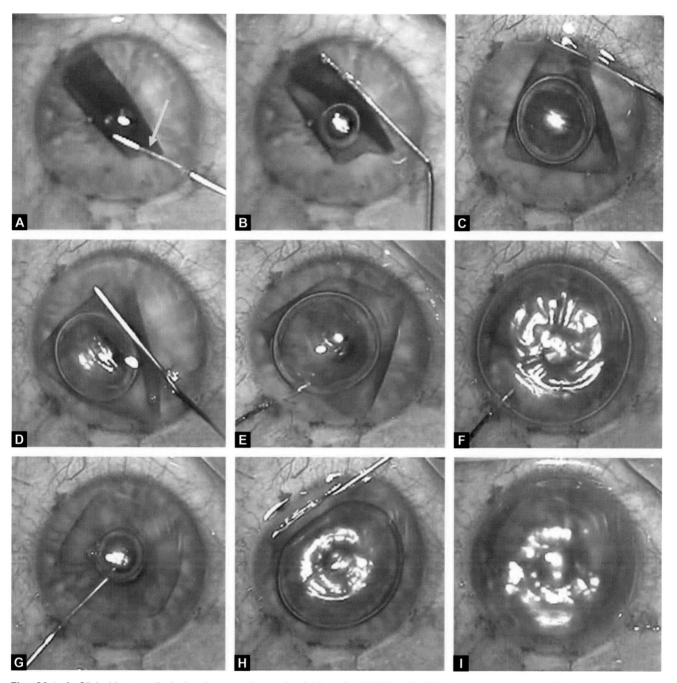

**Figs 2A to I:** Clinical images displaying the centration and unfolding of a DMEK graft within the anterior chamber. (A) A small air-bubble is positioned in between the 'double-rolls' of the DMEK graft. Note the blue coloration halfway the cannula, indicating that the cannula is in part positioned 'inside' one of the rolls (Moutsouris sign, arrow); (B and C) By applying gently strokes with the cannula onto the outer corneal surface, the DMEK graft is rotated. To unroll the DMEK-roll, light taps onto the corneal surface (Droutsas taps), as well as manipulations with the small air-bubble are used (Dapena maneuver); (D) Using the cannula at the outer corneal surface, the graft is centered; (E and F) The air-bubble is enlarged to completely unfold the DMEK graft, and to position it onto the iris (air-bubble in between graft and cornea). After approximately 10 seconds, the air-bubble is aspirated; (G) The cannula is positioned underneath the graft to inject air at the pupillary margin (air in between iris and graft); (H) An 'inward fold' of the DMEK graft is visible at the 4 o'clock surgical position, that is repositioned, i.e. unfolded, using a 'Bubble-bumping maneuver': pushing the air-bubble away from the fold induces an aqueous flow that unfolds the graft's peripheral edge; (I) Once completely unfolded, the anterior chamber is filled with air for approximately 45–60 minutes. Please note that all rotating, centering, unfolding, appositioning and fixating maneuvers may be performed with a standard 30G cannula that is bent in such a way that the distal end of the cannula measures approximately 8 mm in length

CHAPTER 85

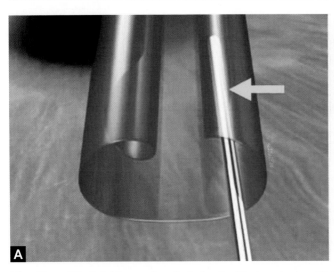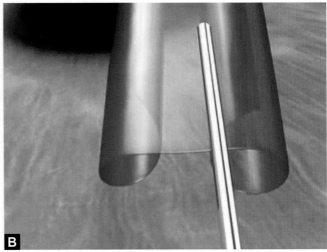

**Figs 3A and B:** Artist impression displaying the Moutsouris sign. (A) When the DMEK graft is oriented correctly within the anterior chamber (edges facing upward), the tip of the cannula can be positioned 'inside' a peripheral curl, so that the tip appears blue (arrow) because of the overlying blue colored donor tissue (Moutsouris sign positive); (B) When the graft is positioned 'upside-down' (edges facing downward), the tip of the cannula does not 'find' the curls, so the tip will not change in color (Moutsouris sign negative)

be facilitated by positioning a small air-bubble inside the curl that can be 'rolled' to flatten the graft over the iris (Dapena technique). With experience, all of these techniques can readily be used in any combination considered most suitable for the actual surgical situation, without affecting the final clinical outcome.[44]

## Centering the DMEK Graft

After unfolding, the graft can then be centered inside the anterior chamber by gentle strokes with the cannula over the outer corneal surface (Figs 2A to I). Alternatively, manual centration with an air-cannula at the very edge may be required sometimes. Slightly decentered grafts that cover the central cornea may be accepted, as clinical observation shows that a gap between the recipient Descemet's membrane peripheral rim and the decentered DMEK graft is commonly repopulated by migrating donor and/or recipient endothelial cells,[45,46] and decentration does not seem to relate to final visual outcome. If so, excessive manipulation to center the graft may be avoided to minimize donor endothelial cell damage.

## Appositioning the DMEK Graft

After centration, the air-bubble on top of the DMEK graft may be enlarged to fully flatten the transplant over the iris. After approximately 10 seconds, the air is aspirated from the anterior chamber, the cannula can then be slowly positioned

at the pupillary area underneath the transplant and a small air-bubble may be injected underneath the DMEK graft, to lift the transplant upward toward the recipient cornea. Then the air-bubble may be slowly enlarged, while carefully observing the edges of the transplant. Not infrequently, peripheral 'inward folds' may be present, i.e. an inward curl with the endothelium facing the recipient stroma. These folds should be flattened out because they tend to 'spring away' from the host cornea after surgery, causing a partial graft detachment. With a 'bubble-bumping maneuver', i.e. gentle 'Droutsas taps' with the cannula on the outer corneal surface overlying the fold,[27,44] a flow of aqueous will be created forcing the remnant folds to disappear.[27] Once the DMEK graft is completely unfolded, the anterior chamber may be completely filled with air, to position the transplant onto the recipient posterior stroma.

## Fixating the DMEK Graft

To avoid postoperative graft detachment, it is advocated to have the anterior chamber completely filled with air for at least 45–60 minutes, at approximately 20 mm Hg. A partial air-BSS exchange may be performed thereafter, to leave the eye pressurized with a 30–50% air-fill in the anterior chamber. After surgery, the patient should be instructed to maintain a supine position for 24 hours, to further secure the position of the DMEK graft against the recipient posterior stroma.

## ▶ VISUAL REHABILITATION RATE AND REFRACTIVE OUTCOME

### Visual Acuity

With 'no-touch' DMEK, about 80% of cases reach a best corrected visual acuity (BCVA) of greater than or equal to 20/25 ( $\geq$ 0.8) at 6 months postoperatively, with about 50% reaching greater than or equal to 20/20 ( $\geq$ 1.0).[28,29,47-49] Furthermore, it is not infrequent to achieve a VA of 20/20 (1.0) already at 1 week after surgery, suggesting that DMEK could provide 'instant visual recovery', approaching the results of phacoemulsification.[13]

To the best of the authors' knowledge, no other surgical technique for corneal transplantation described in literature, may compete with the visual outcomes after DMEK. After PK, only 40–50% of cases may reach a BCVA greater than or equal to 20/40 ( $\geq$ 0.5) at 1 year after surgery.[50] After [DS(A)EK], that may be the most widely performed endothelial keratoplasty technique today, the BCVA may be on average 20/40 (0.5) at 6 months postoperatively, with only few cases reaching 20/25 (0.8) or better.[13-18] Moreover, DMEK may provide a near-perfect restoration of the corneal anatomy and a better quality of the cornea than earlier endothelial keratoplasty techniques.[19,20] Thus, the visual outcome in DMEK may not be reduced by graft thickness, smoothness of the donor lenticule surface, and/or presence of a stromal interface between the posterior recipient cornea and the graft as in DS(A)EK or DLEK,[13,51,52] but mainly by the quality of the anterior portion of the receiving cornea prior to surgery. Furthermore, the rate of visual rehabilitation may also be faster after DMEK, with most patients reaching their maximal visual potential in 1–3 months,[53,54] compared to 6–12 months following DS(A)EK and PK.[12-18,50,55,56]

### Refractive Change and Stability

After DMEK, both the spheric equivalent (SE) and the cylindrical error may be within 1.0 D from the preoperative refractive error. Pachymetric and refractive data suggest that the transplanted cornea stabilizes approximately 3 months after DMEK, so that new glasses can commonly be prescribed at this time point, until which most patients are able to continue wearing their 'own' glasses.[29]

### Hyperopic Shift in DMEK and Lens Power Calculation for Cataract Surgery

A hyperopic shift of about +0.24 to +0.4 D has been observed after DMEK.[29,49] In contrast, a +1.5 D shift has been documented after DS(A)EK,[57-64] probably resulting from the 'negative lenticle' effect of the stroma carried by the endothelial transplant (being thinner centrally than at its peripheral flange). Since only an isolated donor DM is transplanted in DMEK, the hyperopic shift cannot be explained by the same mechanism. Hence, the authors suggested that the refractive shift in DMEK may result from the pre to postoperative difference in recipient corneal hydration and the associated posterior corneal curvature change.[29,65] Because the change in anterior corneal power after DMEK is only about −0.3 D, falling within the margin of intra- ocular lens power calculation, established nomograms may be used to calculate the intraocular lens power for cataract surgery at any time prior to DMEK.[65]

## ▶ ENDOTHELIAL CELL DENSITY AND GRAFT SURVIVAL

As with other endothelial keratoplasty techniques, DMEK may be associated with a drop in donor endothelial cell density (ECD) in the early postoperative phase. If performed as a 'no-touch' technique, endothelial cell damage to the isolated DMEK graft may be minimized, so that an endothelial cell density of about 1800 cells/mm² at 6 months after DMEK may be obtained. Hence, about a 30% decrease relative to the preoperative endothelial cell density; followed by a slower decrease of approximately 10% per year over 4 years may be observed after DMEK.[13,30,66,67] These findings agree with an approximate 30% decrease in ECD within 6 months after DLEK and DS(A)EK, followed by an 8% decrease between 6 and 24 months after surgery.[13,17,68-71] After PK, a cell loss up to 40–55% has been described at 1 year after surgery, with a higher than the physiological decrease in ECD continuing up to 20 years.[72-74] Hence, the biphasic decrease in ECD after DMEK may not exceed that after other types of keratoplasty.

Furthermore, in DMEK the graft diameter can be of 9.0 up to 11.0 mm, resulting in the transplantation of a far greater endothelial cell surface compared to PK/DLEK/DS(A)EK (7.0–9.0 mm). Although the correlation between the diameter of the graft and its survival has not been demonstrated, it could be expected that a larger graft in DMEK, i.e. the transplantation of more endothelial cells, would benefit the long-term survival of the transplant.

## ▶ COMPLICATIONS

The standardization of DMEK surgery into a 'no-touch' procedure after the learning curve, allowed for the transplantation of DMEK grafts in a controlled and reproducible

CHAPTER 85

fashion, decreasing the number of complications and allowing the comprehension of its preferred management. The main complications encountered after DMEK, are given below.

## Graft Detachment

### Graft Detachment Rate

Graft detachment may be the most frequently observed complication after endothelial keratoplasty. After DS(A)EK, graft detachments may occur in up to 0–82% of cases,[12,16,56,75-79] and have been associated with lower endothelial cell densities. Similarly, an initial graft detachment rate up to 20–60% has been reported after DMEK.[26-29,49,80,81] However, it may be important to better define a 'graft detachment', because especially in DMEK, small and temporary detachments of a peripheral flange, with little clinical significance, are frequently seen. If 'graft detachment' is defined as a lack of adherence of the donor DM to the recipient posterior stroma, reducing visual outcome and/or necessitating secondary intervention, the detachment rate in the authors' series was 12%. When clinically insignificant detachments were also included, the overall detachment rate was 24%. Furthermore, with clinical experience the number of clinically significant detachments decreased from 20% (when evaluating the first 75 cases operated on) to 4% (in the next 75 patients that underwent DMEK surgery).[28,80,81]

### Graft Detachment Diagnosis

In the presence of diffuse corneal edema, it might be difficult to discern between a DMEK graft detachment and delayed corneal clearance. As a result, it may be challenging to decide whether a secondary intervention is required or contraindicated, since the graft may become functional at a later time.

Optical coherence tomography has proven to be the most effective noncontact imaging tool to determine the position of the Descemet graft in the presence of corneal edema (Figs 4A to E),[82] being especially useful in cases with a flat detachment, that is, a positioning of the Descemet graft just posterior to the corneal stroma. However, in eyes with a completely detached Descemet graft, i.e. a Descemet-roll formed in the anterior chamber, slit-lamp biomicroscopy and Scheimpflug imaging may be sufficient to visualize the detachment, even though the cornea may be very edematous.[82]

## Graft Detachment Management

Given the observation that rebubbling may be less effective than expected and that several eyes cleared 'spontaneously' despite the presence of a (nearly) complete graft detachment with visual rehabilitation up to 20/20 (1.0) (Figs 4A to E),[46] the authors changed their decision-tree for management of detachments after DMEK (Fig. 5). Hence, depending on (1) the extent of the detachment and (2) interference with VA, they adopted the following intervention guidelines:[81]

*Peripheral graft detachments less than or equal to one-third not affecting the visual acuity*: These detachments have the tendency to recover by themselves at 3–6 months postoperatively, generally due to spontaneous reattachment of the graft and/or endothelialization of the recipient posterior stroma. Hence, it may be advocated to await 'spontaneous clearing', rather than performing a secondary intervention.

For these relatively benign, peripheral detachments, two main causes have been identified:

1. 'Inward folds' of the edge of the Descemet graft, left *in situ* at termination of the surgery, that may be associated with peripheral detachments because the tissue tends to 'spring away' from the stroma within the first postoperative week. Once recognized, this complication can easily be avoided by so-called 'bubble-bumping' during surgery or performing 'Droutsas-taps'.[27]
2. 'Graft-to-iris adhesions' between the outer flange of the Descemet graft and the recipient peripheral iris, which may result in a progressive detachment due to contraction of the Descemet graft after surgery that tends to 'stretch' the detachment. To avoid such a situation, it may be advocated to completely fill the recipient anterior chamber with air after graft positioning, and to check if the chamber angle is open over 360°.

*Graft detachments greater than one-third affecting the visual acuity*: In this case, decision making may be more complex, depending on the type of detachment and may be managed on a more individual basis. According to the patient's preferences, either a reoperation or awaiting spontaneous clearance may be offered as valid treatments. In case of persistent corneal edema over the detachment, a secondary DS(A)EK[28,29,83] or re-DMEK can be performed in the midterm follow-up with good results.

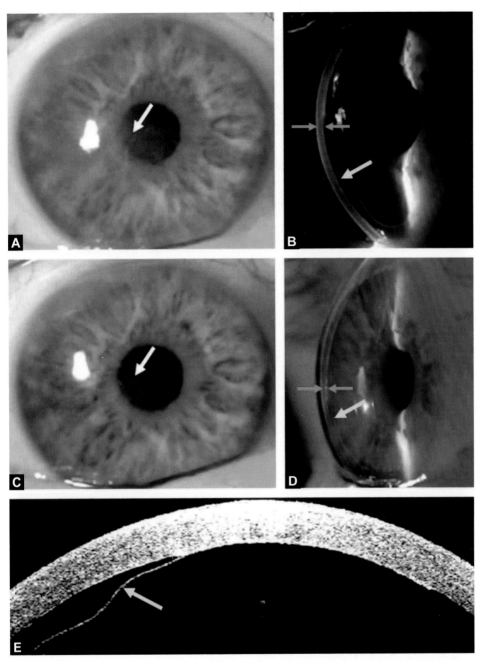

**Figs 4A to E:** Slit-lamp pictures. (A and B) 1 month; (C and D) Six months after DMEK, respectively; (E) Optical coherence tomography (OCT) at 6 months postoperatively. Note that even though the inferior half of the graft was detached (B, D and E; yellow arrows), the cornea still cleared. Observe the progressive thinning of the cornea (B and D; green arrows) and the spontaneous improvement in corneal transparency (A and C; white arrows) between 1 and 6 months, in the detached area also

In the authors' series, the large or complete detachments appeared to be associated with the presence of 'vitreous pressure' during surgery and/or improper judgment of graft orientation.[27-29] It may therefore be advocated to obtain a soft eye before commencing surgery, to minimize the risk of posterior pressure. The orientation of the graft can be determined by the 'Moutsouris-sign' and/or marking the graft.[27,84]

We previously described that the use of any plastic and/or viscoelastic materials may be avoided in DMEK surgery, to minimize the risk of graft detachment.[13,28,43] Performing the descemetorhexis under air may have the advantages that remnant host Descemet fragments are more easily identified, and that the negative imbibition pressure facilitating graft adherence is better preserved (by avoiding

**Step-ladder approach in the management of Descemet graft detachments**

Check during surgery:
- Descemetorhexis 'under air'—avoid stromal overhydration
- Avoid use of viscoelastic and plastic materials contacting graft
- Upward orientation Descemet graft (Moutsouris sign/ tissue marking)
- Proper centration Descemet graft—avoid PAS
- Complete unfolding Descemet graft—avoid 'inward folds'
- 50% air-fill in AC in pseudophakic eyes, 25% air-fill in phakic eyes

↓

After surgery: Keep supine position for 24 hours

↓

1st day postoperative: If incomplete attachment, continue supine position for 1-2 days

↓

1st week postoperative: if incomplete attachment

No interference with BCVA    Interference with BCVA

Partial detachment    Free Descemet-roll in AC

Explain options to patient:
- Await spontaneous clearance
- Re-operation

Wait for 3 months

Persistent corneal edema over detachment

Re-operation:
- Re-bubble quick or not at all
- DSEK/DSAEK
- Re-DMEK

Spontaneous clearance
Spontaneous re-attachment

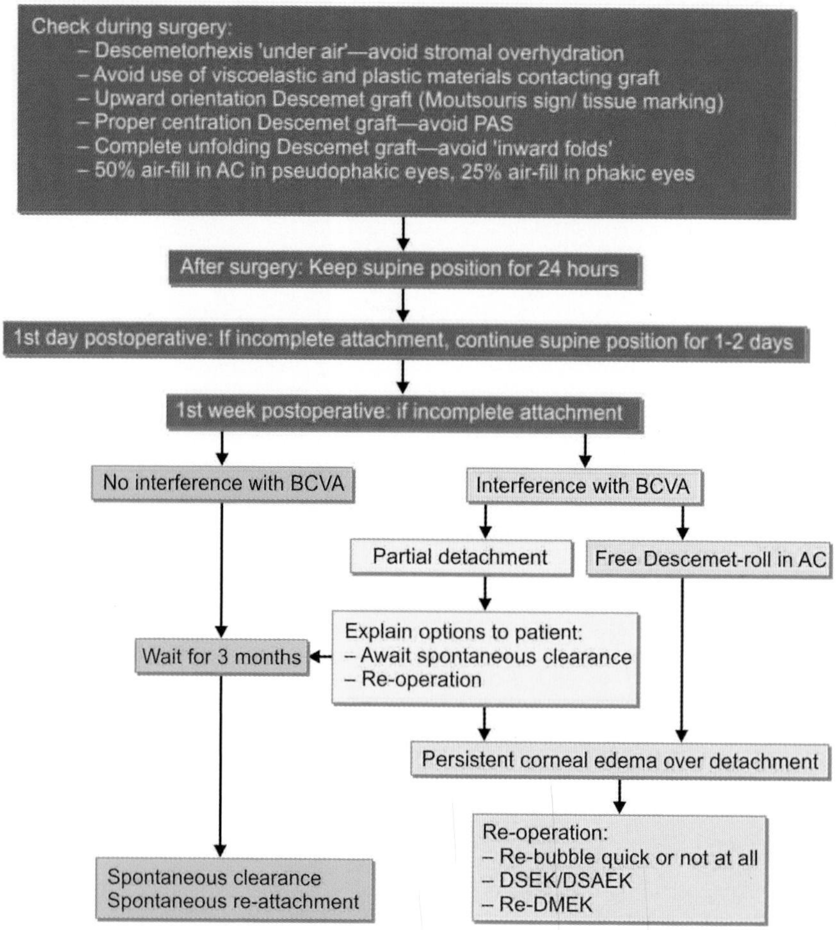

**Fig. 5:** Diagram displaying recommendations to prevent detachments in DMEK, and a decision tree in the event of a Descemet graft detachment

stromal overhydration with the use of balanced salt solution in combination with an anterior chamber maintainer). Furthermore, sufficient air-bubble support for 45–60 minutes at termination of the surgery may be a prerequisite for proper Descemet graft adhesion.[13,28,43]

Thus, graft detachment may be further reduced to less than or equal to 4%, by minor surgical adjustments and/ or additional maneuvers.[13,27,80] Furthermore, proper patient selection may be important: aphakic or postvitrectomy eyes, or eyes with a large sector iridectomy, glaucoma tube, extensive corneal decompensation, or tendency to postoperative ocular hypotonia, may be prone to Descemet graft detachment due to a lack of air-bubble support, and may be managed with a modified surgical technique.[85]

## Secondary Glaucoma

Glaucoma may be one of the most serious but least tangible complications after keratoplasty, potentially affecting long-term graft survival as well as the overall condition of the eye. Published literature reports have described an incidence of glaucoma ranging from 15–35% or even higher, after PK or earlier types of endothelial keratoplasty, i.e. DLEK and DS(A)EK.[86-91] Although the authors expected a higher incidence of glaucoma, given the literature and because of the prolonged air-bubble time in DMEK, only 6.5% of patients presented an episode of glaucoma in their series.[86] This relatively low percentage could primarily be explained by the authors' topical steroid regime (Table 1), as well as the predominantly Caucasian population. Because the incidence of steroid-induced glaucoma may be as high as 60% after PK,[89] and 35% after DS(A)EK,[86,88] their routine medication schedule includes topical 0.1% dexamethasone for just the first postoperative month, and switching to fluorometholone thereafter (Table 1), because the risk of allograft rejection in DMEK may be relatively low.[92] Furthermore,

| Table 1: Topical steroid regime after DMEK | |
|---|---|
| **Steroid regime after DMEK** | |
| *Postoperative Time Interval* | *Steroid Prescribed* |
| 1st month | Dexamethasone 0.1%, 4 times daily |
| 2nd–3rd month | Fluorometholone 0.1%, 4 times daily |
| 4th–6th month | Fluorometholone 0.1%, 3 times daily |
| 7th–9th month | Fluorometholone 0.1%, 2 times daily |
| 10th–12th month | Fluorometholone 0.1%, 1 time daily |
| >12 months | Fluorometholone 0.1%, every other day |

the authors routinely perform a prophylactic Yttrium Aluminium Garnet (YAG) laser iridotomy at 12 o'clock prior to surgery, that theoretically avoids the appearance of immediate postoperative pupillary block.

Overall, the postkeratoplasty IOP elevations after DMEK could be categorized in two groups for its etiology:[86]

### Exacerbation of pre-existing glaucoma (2.5%)

This group of eyes may be recognized before surgery to be 'at risk', as one-fourth of eyes with history of glaucoma may show an exacerbation up to 40 mm Hg, within the first 3 months after DMEK.[86] The IOP may initially be normalized after switching from dexamethasone to fluorometholone and/or adjusting (additional) topical medication.

### De novo glaucoma or surgically-induced ocular hypertension (4%)

This group may unexpectedly present with glaucoma, due to different mechanisms.[93,94]

*Mechanical angle closure glaucoma less than 24 hours after surgery (2%)*: In the authors' series, this complication occurred only in phakic eyes (in 11% of the phakic cases). The 50% air-bubble left in the recipient anterior chamber after surgery, apparently may cause a 'backward' tilt of the crystalline lens, displacing the inferior part of the iris diaphragm forward, resulting in a mechanical closure of the angle (Fig. 6). With pupillary dilation, topical 1% apraclonidine and 250 mg acetazolamide orally, and by laying the patient down in a supine position for 1–2 hours, the glaucomatous crisis may be reversed.

This relatively high incidence of glaucoma in phakic eyes (Figs 7A and B) induced a change in our surgical protocol; by which the air-fill at termination of surgery was reduced to only a 20–30% (instead of 50%) in eyes conserving their own crystalline lens.

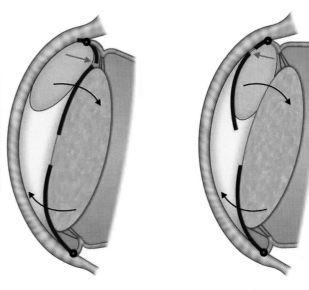

**Fig. 6:** Schematic diagram illustrating the hypothesized mechanism of air-bubble induced angle closure glaucoma due to a tilt of the crystalline lens, either by (left) an air-bubble in front of, or (right) behind the iris. Since the mechanism is different from a pupillary block glaucoma (i.e. not induced by aqueous, but air), note that the peripheral iridotomy (red arrow) is not effective in closure of the chamber angle due to the crystalline lens tilt

*Delayed postoperative ocular hypertension (2%)*: In our series, these cases occurred because of response to topical steroids, peripheral anterior synechiae form- ation or to unknown cause. The IOP was managed by steroids tapering and/or prescribing additional anti-glaucoma medication. In only one case, filtering surgery with a Baerveldt tube was needed in order to control the IOP.

### Allograft Rejection

The allograft rejection rate is less than or equal to 1% in an average postoperative follow-up of 2 years after DMEK. Hence, the incidence of allograft rejection after DMEK, would seem considerably lower than those reported after PK when similar postoperative time intervals are considered. In low-risk PK, allograft rejection has been observed in up to 5–15% of cases.[50,95-98] In DS(A)EK, it could be argued that the afferent pathway is less effective in the presence of an endothelial graft (because there is no exposure of the posterior donor tissue to the anterior antigen presenting cells. However, rejection episodes have been described after DS(A)EK in about 10% of cases.[56,87,99] Thus, although the risk of allograft rejection may be similar or somewhat lower in DS(A)EK than PK, the authors' series showed a far lower incidence of rejection after DMEK.

CHAPTER 85

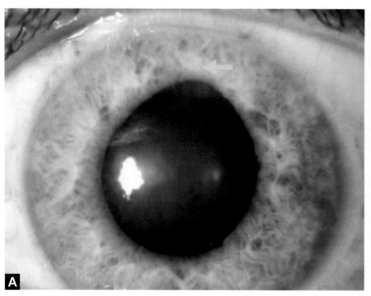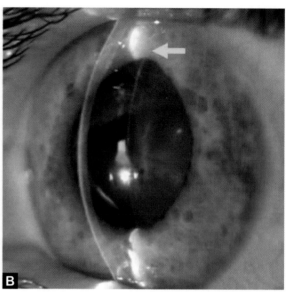

**Figs 7A and B:** Slit-lamp images of an eye 1 week after DMEK, displaying the typical appearance of the iris-diaphragm after air-bubble capture behind the iris at the first postoperative day. Note the irregular, dystonic shape of the iris at 12 o'clock (arrow)

## ❧ DESCEMET MEMBRANE ENDOTHELIAL KERATOPLASTY AND CATARACT

If both cataract extraction and DMEK surgery are required, it may be advocated to first perform phacoemulsification and DMEK as a secondary operation for two reasons. First, the use of a viscoelastic may be avoided in an endothelial keratoplasty procedure, since it may relate to a higher risk of postoperative graft detachment.[13,27,43] Second, after cataract extraction, 10–30% of patients may be satisfied with the visual improvement achieved, so that DMEK can be postponed. If the crystalline lens is clear, the pupil may be constricted with pilocarpine 2% prior to commencing DMEK, to avoid iatrogenic cataract formation due to air or surgical trauma.[27,28] Consequently, about one fourth of the phakic eyes may present mild anterior subcapsular lens opacities or a Vossius ring (iris pigment imprint onto the outer lens capsule), possibly due to mechanical air-bubble trauma induced by the complete air-fill of the anterior chamber during the surgery. These opacities or pigment deposits usually disappear with time and may not affect the final VA (Figs 8A to F). However, in one case with an air-bubble capture behind the iris, a more pronounced anterior lens opacification developed, eventually requiring phacoemulsification but resulting in optimal clinical outcomes.[100] Hence, the advantage of preserving accommodation in relatively young patients may outweigh the risk of inadvertent (iatrogenic) cataract development, because phacoemulsification after DMEK seems a viable treatment option in such cases.

## ❧ FUTURE PERSPECTIVES

Recently, the authors reported on several DMEK eyes that showed corneal clearance with visual recovery improving up to 20/20, despite subtotal graft detachment.[46,101] A similar observation after DSAEK has been reported by other authors.[102] Since specular and confocal microscopy showed repopulation of the recipient posterior stroma with endothelial cells, it may be speculated that massive endothelial migration occurs, by donor or host cells, or both.[103-105] If so, a simplified surgical technique, tentatively named 'Free-DMEK' or 'Descemet membrane endothelial transfer' (DMET),[85] in which donor tissue is merely injected into the recipient anterior chamber after descemetorhexis, could be effective in the management of corneal endothelial disease.[106] DMET could be associated with major advantages over any type of keratoplasty procedure. Obviously, perfect anatomical restoration, potentially complete visual recovery, and elimination of virtually all intra and postoperative complications associated with keratoplasty, while requiring limited surgical skills, would greatly facilitate corneal endothelial replacement. If the rate of corneal clearance could be further improved with

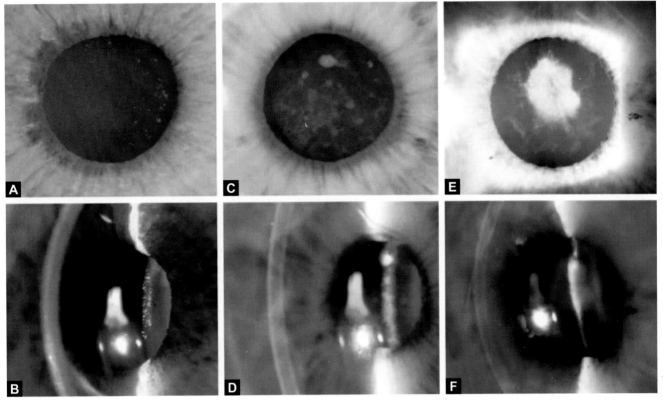

**Figs 8A to F:** Slit-lamp photographs displaying crystalline lens-related changes associated with DMEK. Probably due to mechanical pressure exerted by the air-fill of the anterior chamber during surgery, an 'imprint' of iris pigment (partial Vossius' ring) (A and B) or subtle subcapsular opacities (C and D) may be observed in the early postoperative phase after DMEK. Both these changes tend to largely resolve over a period of months. In the authors' series, only one eye developed a clinically significant subcapsular cataract (E and F) following secondary angle closure glaucoma due to entrapment of air behind iris on the first postoperative day. After phacosurgery, the BCVA improved from 20/40 (0.5) to 20/20 (1.0)[100]

*in vitro* graft modifications (Melles, unpublished observations 2010), and 'graft survival' or long-term efficacy of DMET would approach that of endothelial keratoplasty, DMET could become an alternative, 'no-keratoplasty' treatment for corneal endothelial disorders.

## ▶ REFERENCES

1. Tillett CW. Posterior lamellar keratoplasty. Am J Ophthalmol. 1956;41(3):530-3.
2. Barraquer JI. Lamellar keratoplasty (Special techniques). Ann Ophthalmol. 1972;4(6):437-69.
3. Melles GRJ, Eggink FA, Lander F, et al. A surgical technique for posterior lamellar keratoplasty. Cornea. 1998;17(6):618-26.
4. Melles GR, Lander F, Beekhuis WH, et al. Posterior lamellar keratoplasty for a case of pseudophakic bullous keratopathy. Am J Ophthalmol. 1999;127(3):340-1.
5. Melles GR, Lander F, Nieuwendaal C. Sutureless, posterior lamellar keratoplasty: a case report of a modified technique. Cornea. 2002;21(3):325-7.
6. Terry MA, Ousley PJ. Deep lamellar endothelial keratoplasty in the first United States patients: early clinical results. Cornea. 2001;20(3):239-43.
7. Terry MA, Ousley PJ. Deep lamellar endothelial keratoplasty visual acuity, astigmatism, and endothelial survival in a large prospective series. Ophthalmology. 2005;112(9):1541-8.
8. Ousley PJ, Terry MA. Stability of vision, topography, and endothelial cell density from 1 year to 2 years after deep lamellar endothelial keratoplasty surgery. Ophthalmology. 2005;112(1):50-7.
9. Melles GR, Wijdh RH, Nieuwendaal CP. A technique to excise the descemet membrane from a recipient cornea (descemetorhexis). Cornea. 2004;23(3):286-8.
10. Price FW, Price MO. Descemet's stripping with endothelial keratoplasty in 50 eyes: a refractive neutral corneal transplant. J Refract Surg. 2005;21(4):339-45.
11. Azar DT, Jain S, Sambursky R, et al. Microkeratome-assisted posterior keratoplasty. J Cataract Refract Surg. 2001;27(3):353-6.
12. Gorovoy MS. Descemet-stripping automated endothelial keratoplasty. Cornea. 2006;25(8):886-9.
13. Dapena I, Ham L, Melles GR. Endothelial keratoplasty: DSEK/DSAEK or DMEK-the thinner the better? Curr Opin Ophthalmol. 2009;20(4):299-307.
14. Bahar I, Kaiserman I, McAllum P, et al. Comparison of posterior lamellar keratoplasty techniques to penetrating keratoplasty. Ophthalmology. 2008;115(9):1525-33.

CHAPTER **85**

15. Chen ES, Terry MA, Shamie N, et al. Descemet-stripping automated endothelial keratoplasty: six month results in a prospective study of 100 eyes. Cornea. 2008;27(5):514-20.

16. Mearza AA, Qureshi MA, Rostron CK. Experience and 12-month results of Descemet-stripping endothelial keratoplasty (DSEK) with a small-incision technique. Cornea. 2007; 26(3):279-83.

17. Terry MA, Shamie N, Chen ES, et al. Precut tissue for Descemet's stripping automated endothelial keratoplasty: vision, astigmatism, and endothelial survival. Ophthalmology. 2009;116(2):248-56.

18. Wylegala E, Tarnawska D. Management of pseudophakic bullous keratopathy by combined Descemet-stripping endothelial keratoplasty and intraocular lens exchange. J Cataract Refract Surg. 2008;34(10):1708-14.

19. Melles GR, Lander F, Rietveld FJ. Transplantation of Descemet's membrane carrying viable endothelium through a small scleral incision. Cornea. 2002;21(4):415-8.

20. Melles GR, Ong TS, Ververs B, et al. Descemet membrane endothelial keratoplasty (DMEK). Cornea. 2006;25(8):987-90.

21. Melles GR, Ong TS, Ververs B, et al. Preliminary clinical results of Descemet membrane endothelial keratoplasty. Am J Ophthalmol. 2008;145(2):222-7.

22. Melles GR. Posterior lamellar keratoplasty: DLEK to DSEK to DMEK. Cornea. 2006;25(8):879-81.

23. Fernandez MM, Afshari NA. Endothelial Keratoplasty: from DLEK to DMEK. Middle East Afr J Ophthalmol. 2010;17(1): 5-8.

24. Studeny P, Farkas A, Vokrojova M, et al. Descemet membrane endothelial keratoplasty with a stromal rim (DMEK-S). Br J Ophthalmol. 2010;94(7):909-14.

25. McCauley MB, Price FW, Price MO. Descemet membrane automated endothelial keratoplasty: hybrid technique combining DSAEK stability with DMEK visual results. J Cataract Refract Surg. 2009;35(10):1659-64.

26. McCauley MB, Price MO, Fairchild KM, et al. Prospective study of visual outcomes and endothelial survival with Descemet membrane automated endothelial keratoplasty. Cornea. 2011; 30(3):315-9.

27. Dapena I, Moutsouris K, Droutsas K, et al. Standardized 'no touch' technique for Descemet membrane endothelial keratoplasty (DMEK). Arch Ophthalmol. 2011;129(1):88-94.

28. Dapena I, Ham L, Droutsas K, et al. Learning curve in Descemet's membrane endothelial keratoplasty: first series of 135 consecutive cases. Ophthalmology. 2011;118(11):2147-54.

29. Dirisamer M, Ham L, Dapena I, et al. Efficacy of Descemet membrane endothelial keratoplasty (DMEK): clinical outcome of 200 consecutive cases after a 'learning curve' of 25 cases. Arch Ophthalmol. 2011;129(11):1435-43.

30. Price MO, Giebel AW, Fairchild KM, et al. Descemet's membrane endothelial keratoplasty: prospective multicenter study of visual and refractive outcomes and endothelial survival. Ophthalmology. 2009;116(12):2361-8.

31. Lie JT, Birbal R, Ham L, et al. Donor tissue preparation for Descemet membrane endothelial keratoplasty. J Cataract Refract Surg. 2008;34(9):1578-83.

32. Zhu Z, Rife L, Yiu S, et al. Technique for preparation of the corneal endothelium: Descemet membrane complex for transplantation. Cornea. 2006;25(6):705-8.

33. Ignacio TS, Nguyen TT, Sarayba MA, et al. A technique to harvest Descemet's membrane with viable endothelial cells for selective transplantation. Am J Ophthalmol. 2005;139(2):325-30.

34. Kruse FE, Laaser K, Cursiefen C, et al. A stepwise approach to donor preparation and insertion increases safety and outcome of Descemet membrane endothelial keratoplasty. Cornea. 2011; 30(5):580-7.

35. Groeneveld-van Beek E, Lie J, van der Wees J, et al. Standardized 'no-touch' donor tissue preparation for DALK and DMEK: harvesting undamaged anterior and posterior transplants from the same donor cornea. Acta Ophthalmol; 2012 June 6 (Epub ahead of print).

36. Nieuwendaal CP, Lapid-Gortzak R, van der Meulen IJ, et al. Posterior lamellar keratoplasty using descemetorhexis and organ cultured donor corneal tissue (Melles technique). Cornea. 2006;25(8):933-36.

37. Kymionis GD, Yoo SH, Diakonis VF, et al. Automated donor tissue preparation for Descemet membrane automated endothelial keratoplasty (DMAEK): an experimental study. Ophthalmic Surg Lasers Imaging. 2011;42(2):158-61.

38. Venzano D, Pagani P, Randazzo N, et al. Descemet membrane air-bubble separation in donor corneas. J Cataract Refract Surg. 2010;36(12):2022-27.

39. Heindl LM, Riss S, Laaser K, et al. Split cornea transplantation for 2 recipients-review of the first 100 consecutive patients. Am J Ophthalmol. 2011;152(4):523-32.

40. Lie JT, Groeneveld-van Beek EA, Ham L, et al. More efficient use of donor corneal tissue with Descemet membrane endothelial keratoplasty (DMEK): two lamellar keratoplasty procedures with one donor cornea. Br J Ophthalmol. 2010;94(9):1265-6.

41. Kymionis GD, Suh LH, Dubovy SR, et al. Diagnosis of residual Descemet's membrane after Descemet's stripping endothelial keratoplasty with anterior segment optical coherence tomography. J Cataract Refract Surg. 2007;33(7):1322-4.

42. Dapena I, Ham L, Moutsouris K, et al. Incidence of recipient Descemet membrane remnants at the donor-to-stromal interface after descemetorhexis in endothelial keratoplasty. Br J Ophthalmol. 2010;94(12):1689-90.

43. Ham L, van der Wees J, Melles GR. Causes of primary donor failure in descemet membrane endothelial keratoplasty. Am J Ophthalmol. 2008;145(4):639-44.

44. Liarakos V, Dapena I, Ham L, et al. Intraocular graft unfolding techniques in Descemet membrane endothelial keratoplasty (DMEK). Arch Ophthalmol. (In press).

45. Dirisamer M, Dapena I, Ham L, et al. Patterns of corneal endothelialization and corneal clearance after Descemet membrane endothelial keratoplasty for Fuchs endothelial dystrophy. Am J Ophthalmol. 2011;152(4):543-55.

46. Balachandran C, Ham L, Verschoor CA, et al. Spontaneous corneal clearance despite graft detachment in Descemet membrane endothelial keratoplasty. Am J Ophthalmol. 2009; 148(2):227-34.

47. Droutsas K, Ham L, Dapena I, et al. Visual acuity following Descemet-membrane endothelial keratoplasty (DMEK): first 100 cases operated on for Fuchs endothelial dystrophy. Klin Monbl Augenheilkd. 2010;227(6):467-77.

48. Ham L, Dapena I, van Luijk, et al. Descemet membrane endothelial keratoplasty (DMEK) for Fuchs endothelial dystrophy. Review of the first 50 consecutive cases. Eye. 2009; 23(10):1990-8.

49. Guerra FP, Anshu A, Price MO, et al. Descemet's membrane endothelial keratoplasty prospective study of 1-Year visual outcomes, graft survival, and endothelial cell loss. Ophthalmology. 2011;118(12):2368-73.

50. Williams KA, Muehlberg SM, Lewis RF, et al. How successful is corneal transplantation? A report from the Australian Corneal Graft Register. Eye. 1995;9(Pt 2):219-27.

51. Moutsouris K, Ham L, Dapena I, et al. Radial graft contraction may relate to subnormal visual acuity in Descemet stripping (automated) endothelial keratoplasty. Br J Ophthalmol. 2010; 94(7):951-3.

52. Ham L, Dapena I, van der Wees J, et al. Secondary DMEK for poor visual outcome after DSEK: donor posterior stroma may limit visual acuity in endothelial keratoplasty. Cornea. 2010;29(11):1278-83.

53. Ham L, Balachandran C, Verschoor CA, et al. Visual rehabilitation rate after isolated descemet membrane transplantation: descemet membrane endothelial keratoplasty. Arch Ophthalmol. 2009;127(3):252-5.

54. Dapena I, Dapena L, Dirisamer M, et al. Visual acuity and endothelial cell density following Descemet membrane endothelial keratoplasty (DMEK). Arch Soc Esp Oftalmol. 2011;86(12): 395-401.

55. Price MO, Price FW. Descemet's stripping endothelial keratoplasty. Curr Opin Ophthalmol. 2007;18(4):290-4.

56. Koenig SB, Covert DJ, Dupps WJ, et al. Visual acuity, refractive error, and endothelial cell density six months after Descemet stripping and automated endothelial keratoplasty (DSAEK). Cornea. 2007;26(6):670-4.

57. Dupps WJ, Qian Y, Meisler DM. Multivariate model of refractive shift in Descemet stripping automated endothelial keratoplasty. J Cataract Refract Surg. 2008;34(4):578-84.

58. Rao SK, Leung CK, Cheung CY, et al. Descemet stripping endothelial keratoplasty: effect of the surgical procedure on corneal optics. Am J Ophthalmol. 2008;145(6):991-6.

59. Yoo SH, Kymionis GD, Deobhakta AA, et al. One-year results and anterior segment optical coherence tomography findings of descemet stripping automated endothelial keratoplasty combined with phacoemulsification. Arch Ophthalmol. 2008; 126(8):1052-5.

60. Esquenazi S, Rand W. Effect of the shape of the endothelial graft on the refractive results after Descemet's stripping with automated endothelial keratoplasty. Can J Ophthalmol. 2009;44(5):557-61.

61. Scorcia V, Matteoni S, Scorcia GB, et al. Pentacam assessment of posterior lamellar grafts to explain hyperopization after Descemet's stripping automated endothelial keratoplasty. Ophthalmology. 2009;116(9):1651-5.

62. Holz HA, Meyer JJ, Espandar L, et al. Corneal profile analysis after Descemet stripping endothelial keratoplasty and its relationship to postoperative hyperopic shift. J Cataract Refract Surg. 2008;34(2):211-4.

63. Jun B, Kuo AN, Afshari NA, et al. Refractive change after Descemet stripping automated endothelial keratoplasty surgery and its correlation with graft thickness and diameter. Cornea. 2009;28(1):19-23.

64. Lombardo M, Terry MA, Lombardo G, et al. Analysis of posterior donor corneal parameters 1 year after Descemet stripping automated endothelial keratoplasty (DSAEK) triple procedure. Graefes Arch Clin Exp Ophthalmol. 2010;248(3):421-7.

65. Ham L, Dapena I, Moutsouris K, et al. Refractive change and stability after Descemet membrane endothelial keratoplasty (DMEK). J Cataract Refract Surg. 2011;37(8):1455-64.

66. Ham L, Dapena I, Van Der Wees J, et al. Endothelial cell density after Descemet membrane endothelial keratoplasty: 1- to 3-year follow-up. Am J Ophthalmol. 2010;149(6):1016-7.

67. Parker J, Dirisamer M, Naveiras M, et al. Endothelial cell density after Descemet membrane endothelial keratoplasty: 4-year follow-up. Am J Ophthalmol. 2011;151(6):1107.

68. Price FW, Price MO. Does endothelial cell survival differ between DSEK and standard PK? Ophthalmology. 2009;116(3): 367-8.

69. Terry MA, Wall JM, Hoar KL, et al. A prospective study of endothelial cell loss during the 2 years after deep lamellar endothelial keratoplasty. Ophthalmology. 2007;114(4):631-9.

70. Price MO, Price FW. Endothelial cell loss after Descemet stripping with endothelial keratoplasty influencing factors and 2-year trend. Ophthalmology. 2008;115(5):857-65.

71. Van Dooren BTH, Mulder P, Nieuwendaal CP, et al. Endothelial cell density after posterior lamellar keratoplasty (Melles technique); 3 years follow-up. Am J Ophthalmol. 2004;138(2):211-7.

72. Borderie VM, Boelle PY, Touzeau O, et al. Predicted long-term outcome of corneal transplantation. Ophthalmology. 2009;116 (12):2354-60.

73. Patel SV, David O, Hodge MS, et al. Corneal endothelium and postoperative outcomes 15 years after penetrating keratoplasty. Am J Ophthalmol. 2005;139(2):311-9.

74. Ing JJ, Ing HH, Nelson LR, et al. Ten-year postoperative results of penetrating keratoplasty. Ophthalmology. 1998;105(10):1855-65.

75. Basak SK. Descemet stripping automated endothelial keratoplasty in endothelial dysfunctions: three-month results in 75 eyes. Indian J Ophthalmol. 2008;56(4):291-6.

76. Busin M, Bhatt PR, Scorcia V. A modified technique for Descemet membrane stripping automated endothelial keratoplasty to minimize endothelial cell loss. Arch Ophthalmol. 2008;126(8):1133-37.

77. Koenig SB, Covert DJ. Early results of small-incision Descemet stripping and automated endothelial keratoplasty. Ophthalmology. 2007;114(2):221-6.

78. Mehta JS, Por YM, Poh R, et al. Comparison of donor insertion techniques for Descemet stripping automated endothelial keratoplasty. Arch Ophthalmol. 2008;126(10):1383-8.

79. Terry MA, Shamie N, Chen ES, et al. Endothelial keratoplasty: a simplified technique to minimize graft dislocation, iatrogenic graft failure, and pupillary block. Ophthalmology. 2008;115(7):1179-86.

80. Dapena I, Moutsouris K, Ham L, et al. Graft detachment rate. Ophthalmology. 2010;117(4):847.

81. Dirisamer M, van Dijk K, Dapena I, et al. Prevention and management of graft detachment in Descemet membrane endothelial keratoplasty (DMEK). Arch Ophthalmol. 2012;130 (3):280-91.

82. Moutsouris K, Dapena I, Ham L, et al. Optical coherence tomography, Scheimpflug imaging, and slit-lamp biomicroscopy in the early detection of graft detachment after Descemet membrane endothelial keratoplasty. Cornea. 2011;30(12):1369-75.

83. Dapena I, Ham L, van Luijk C, et al. Back-up procedure for graft failure in Descemet membrane endothelial keratoplasty (DMEK). Br J Ophthalmol. 2010;94(2):241-4.

84. Bachmann BO, Laaser K, Cursiefen C, et al. A method to confirm correct orientation of Descemet membrane during Descemet membrane endothelial keratoplasty. Am J Ophthalmol. 2010;149(6):922-5.

85. Dirisamer M, Ham L, Dapena I, et al. Descemet membrane endothelial transfer (DMET): 'Free floating' donor Descemet implantation as a potential alternative to keratoplasty'. Cornea. 2012;31(2):194-7.

86. Naveiras M, Dirisamer, Parker J, et al. Causes of glaucoma after Descemet membrane endothelial keratoplasty (DMEK). Am J Ophthalmol. 2012;153(3):958-66.

87. Lee WB, Jacobs DS, Musch DC, et al. Descemet's stripping endothelial keratoplasty: safety and outcomes: a report by the American Academy of Ophthalmology. Ophthalmology. 2009; 116(9):1818-30.

88. Vajaranant TS, Price MO, Price FW. Visual acuity and intraocular pressure after Descemet's stripping endothelial keratoplasty in eyes with and without preexisting glaucoma. Ophthalmology. 2009;116(9):1644-50.

89. Erdurmus M, Cohen EJ, Yildiz EH, et al. Steroid-induced intraocular pressure elevation or glaucoma after penetrating keratoplasty in patients with keratoconus or Fuchs dystrophy. Cornea. 2009;28(7):759-64.

90. Frost NA, Wu J, Lai TF, et al. A review of randomized controlled trials of penetrating keratoplasty techniques. Ophthalmology. 2006;113(6):942-9.

91. Wandling GR, Parikh M, Robinson C, et al. Escalation of glaucoma therapy after deep lamellar endothelial keratoplasty. Cornea. 2010;29(9):991-5.

92. Dapena I, Ham L, Netukova M, et al. Incidence of early allograft rejection following Descemet membrane endothelial keratoplasty (DMEK). Cornea. 2011;30(12):1341-5.

93. Greenlee EC, Kwon YH. Graft failure: III. Glaucoma escalation after penetrating keratoplasty. Int Ophthalmol. 2008;28(3): 191-207.

94. Allen MB, Lieu P, Mootha VV, et al. Risk factors for intraocular pressure elevation after Descemet stripping automated endothelial keratoplasty. Eye Contact Lens. 2010;36(4):223-7.

95. Thompson RW, Price MO, Bowers PJ, et al. Long-term graft survival after penetrating keratoplasty. Ophthalmology. 2003; 110(7):1396-1402.

96. Maguire MG, Stark WJ, Gottsch JD, et al. Risk factors for corneal graft failure and rejection in the Collaborative Corneal Transplantation Studies. Ophthalmology. 1994;101(9):1536-47.

97. Coster DJ, Williams KA. The impact of corneal allograft rejection on the long-term outcome of corneal transplantation. Am J Ophthalmol. 2005;140(6):1112-22.

98. Küchle M, Cursiefen C, Nguyen NX, et al. Risk factors for corneal allograft rejection: intermediate results of a prospective normal-risk keratoplasty study. Graefes Arch Clin Exp Ophthalmol. 2002;240(7):580-4.

99. Allan BDS, Terry MA, Price FW, et al. Corneal transplant rejection rate and severity after endothelial keratoplasty. Cornea. 2007;26(9):1039-42.

100. Dapena I, Ham L, Tabak S, et al. Phacoemulsification after Descemet membrane endothelial keratoplasty. J Cataract Refract Surg. 2009;35(7):1314-5.

101. Price FW, Price MO. Comment on 'Spontaneous corneal clearance despite graft detachment after descemet membrane endothelial keratoplasty'. Am J Ophthalmol. 2010;149(1):173-4.

102. Zafirakis P, Kymionis GD, Grentzelos MA, et al. Corneal graft detachment without corneal edema after Descemet stripping automated endothelial keratoplasty. Cornea. 2010;29(4): 456-8.

103. Jacobi C, Zhivov A, Korbmacher J, et al. Evidence of endothelial cell migration after Descemet membrane endothelial keratoplasty. Am J Ophthalmol. 2011;152(4):537-42.

104. Lagali N, Stenevi U, Claesson, M, et al. Donor and recipient endothelial cell population of the transplanted human cornea: a two-dimensional imaging study. Invest Ophthalmol Vis Sci. 2010;51(4):1898-904.

105. Stewart RM, Hiscott PS, Kaye SB. Endothelial migration and new Descemet membrane after endothelial keratoplasty. Am J Ophthalmol. 2010;149(4):683.

106. Dirisamer M, Yeh RY, Van Dijk K, et al. Recipient endothelium may relate to corneal clearance in Descemet membrane endothelial transfer. Am J Ophthalmol; 2012;154(2):290-6.

# CHAPTER 86

# Deep Anterior Lamellar Keratoplasty

*David D Verdier*

## ᐅ INTRODUCTION

Deep Anterior Lamellar Keratoplasty (DALK) is a partial thickness corneal transplant procedure in which the patient's central corneal epithelium and stroma is replaced with donor epithelium and stroma, retaining host Descemet's membrane and endothelium. Optimal vision and interface clarity are achieved with complete removal of host central stroma and baring of Descemet's membrane. Descemetic DALK (dDALK) and maximum depth DALK (MD-DALK) are terms used to describe this preferred result. Predescemetic DALK (pre-dDALK) denotes a procedure that achieves deep but not full-depth stromal removal. This differentiation is important, as dDALK eyes achieve similar visual results to penetrating keratoplasty (PK) eyes, with quicker return of vision and often one or two line better visual acuity, compared to pre-dDALK.[1-5]

## ᐅ HISTORY

The first successful human corneal transplant with retained transparency of the graft was a lamellar procedure performed by Von Hippel in 1886, in which a full-thickness rabbit cornea was placed into a human recipient corneal lamellar bed.[6] In 1905, Zirm performed the first successful PK, but was never able to reproduce his initial result.[7] For the first half of the 20th century, lamellar keratoplasty (by this time utilizing human tissue) was the more successful and preferred corneal transplant procedure. During the second half of the 20th century, PK eclipsed lamellar keratoplasty due to better visual quality from lack of interface issues, along with increasing success from better understanding of endothelial function and rejection, availability of steroids, and surgical developments including improved suture materials, the operating microscope and viscoelastics.

The 21st century has been accompanied by a resurgence in lamellar keratoplasty. With improving surgical techniques, visual results following lamellar surgery are similar or superior to full thickness keratoplasty while allowing preservation of nondiseased corneal layers. Penetrating keratoplasty is no longer the gold standard for corneal transplantation. DALK affords visual results similar to PK for patients with intact Descemet's membrane and viable endothelium, while avoiding the problems of endothelial rejection and highly accelerated rate of endothelial cell loss.[2,8] And endothelial keratoplasty has overtaken PK for endothelial replacement, with better visual results and quicker rehabilitation.[9-11]

## ᐅ PATIENT AND PROCEDURE SELECTION

Deep Anterior Lamellar Keratoplasty is the preferred corneal transplant procedure for patients with compromised corneal stroma, intact Descemet's membrane and healthy endothelium. Indications include keratoconus, post-refractive surgery ectasia, corneal stromal dystrophies and corneal stromal scarring.[5,12-15] If Descemet's membrane is compromised by past hydrops, perforation or other forms of scarring, deep dissection techniques such as the big-bubble technique of Anwar are likely to result in Descemet's rupture and conversion to PK; these patients may benefit from a pre-dDalk procedure with manual dissection.[16]

Advantages of DALK over PK include absence of endothelial rejection, improved endothelial cell survival (Fig. 1)[17] and (Fig. 2)[8] reduced risk of choroidal hemorrhage and endophthalmitis, and decreased steroid load with

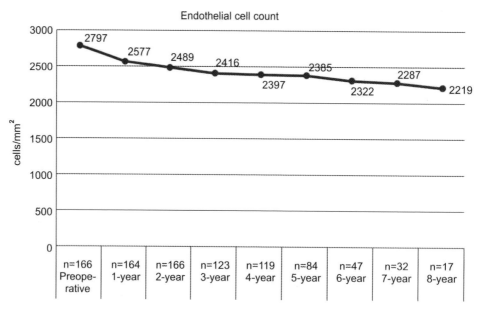

**Fig. 1:** Endothelial cell loss following DALK[17]

less steroid-associated glaucoma, cataract and infection. The incidence and severity of ruptured globe is likely reduced.[18,19]

## ▶ ESTABLISH REALISTIC EXPECTATIONS

In DALK patients, as with PK, vision is limited by unpredictable refractive error including irregular astigmatism.

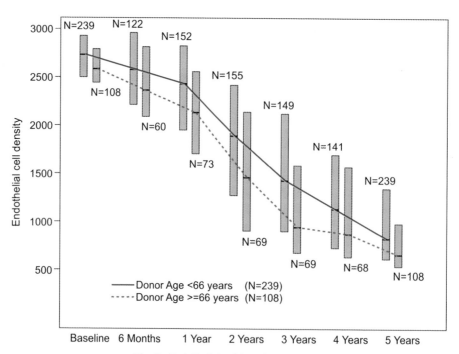

**Fig. 2:** Endothelial cell loss following PK[8]

Irregular astigmatism often improves once all sutures are out, but this may take up to 1 year or longer. Duration of visual rehabilitation and quality of vision issues should be discussed with the patient and family members before surgery.

## ▶ DONOR TISSUE SELECTION

Deep Anterior Lamellar Keratoplasty donor tissue can be lamellar grade, without demand on the eye bank for healthy endothelium. However, PK quality tissue should be readily available due to potential need to convert to PK should significant Descemet's membrane rupture occur. One donor graft can potentially be split for separate Descemet's membrane endothelial keratoplasty (DMEK) and DALK procedures.[20]

## ▶ SURGICAL VENUE AND ANESTHESIA

Deep Anterior Lamellar Keratoplasty can be safely performed in an outpatient surgical suite. Retrobulbar or peribulbar anesthesia and a lid block are routinely employed, using a relatively long-acting drug such as bupivicaine or a combination of bupivicaine and mepivacaine or lidocaine. Given the fragility of Descemet's membrane, surgeon anxiety and procedure success improve with patient comfort and akinesis. General anesthesia may be beneficial for circumstances such as youth, deafness, aphasia, language barriers, or mental impairment.

## ▶ SURGICAL STEPS IN DALK: BIG-BUBBLE TECHNIQUE

Surgical principles for achieving optimal visual results for anterior lamellar keratoplasty were well described 40 years ago by Jose Barraquer[21] and include the following: obtain clean and smooth surfaces for the graft-host interface; leave a posterior layer of uniform thickness; and achieve the deepest possible interface. The big-bubble technique described by Anwar and Teichmann[22] most easily and safely accomplishes these objectives. The big-bubble technique takes advantage of injected air seeking the path of least resistance through the less densely packed posterior stroma, to form a cleavage plane and air bubble between posterior stroma and Descemet's membrane.

### Determination of Size and Centration of Lamellar Bed and Graft

Lamellar bed diameter is typically 8.0–8.25 mm, ranging from less than or equal to 7.75 mm if host corneal

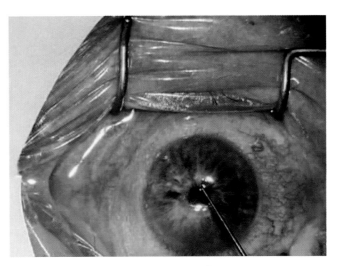

**Fig. 3:** Marking center of cornea

horizontal white-to-white measurement is 11.5 mm or less, to greater than or equal to 8.50 mm if white-to-white is 12.5 mm or more. Large or decentered grafts may be required to encompass the area of pathology. For patients with keratoconus or high axial myopia, donor and lamellar bed diameters are matched; for other patients, donor diameter is 0.25 mm larger. The donor graft is usually centered on the host cornea, or over the pupil axis which is often displaced slightly nasal. If there is much disparity between these positions, a compromise position may be chosen. In keratoconus care must be taken to encompass the entire extent of the cone, which is often inferiorly displaced and may require a larger and/or inferiorly decentered graft. The center of the recipient lamellar bed is marked with gentian violet on a Sinskey hook to guide trephine placement (Fig. 3).

### Trephination

The recipient cornea is trephined 60–80% stromal depth (Fig. 4). A Hessburg-Barron vacuum trephine (Barron Precision Instruments) with eight quarter turns achieves a depth of approximately 400 µ (Fig. 4). If the trephination groove is shallow, it can be cautiously manually deepened with a 15° blade or 2.3 mm curved crescent blade (Alcon) in the area of anticipated needle placement.

### Big-Bubble Formation (Figs 5A to D)

A 27-guage 5/8-inch needle is prepared by making a 60° bend 5 mm from the tip, bevel down, and attaching it to a 5 cc syringe with air. The needle is placed bevel down at the level of deepest dissection in the trephine groove

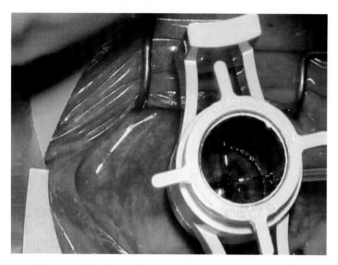

**Fig. 4:** Trephination with Hessburg-Barron vacuum trephine

and directed parallel to the corneal plane, 3–4 mm into the stroma, to a paracentral location. Extreme care must be observed to avoid tilting the needle posteriorly; a direct view away from the microscope can sometimes give a better perspective of needle plane orientation prior to insertion. Approximately 0.5 cc of air is injected to form a silver white sheen in a central disk pattern until it extends to near the trephine edge. A sudden easing of resistance may occur as the bubble forms. A feathery ring may outline the bubble, and the central cornea may dome slightly anterior. An unsuccessful big-bubble air injection can create focal dense stromal whitening without a sharp circular outline and with irregular fibrillary extensions. Air in the anterior chamber can occur with perforation of Descemet's membrane, but can also result from peripheral dissection of air through the trabecular meshwork. If the initial air

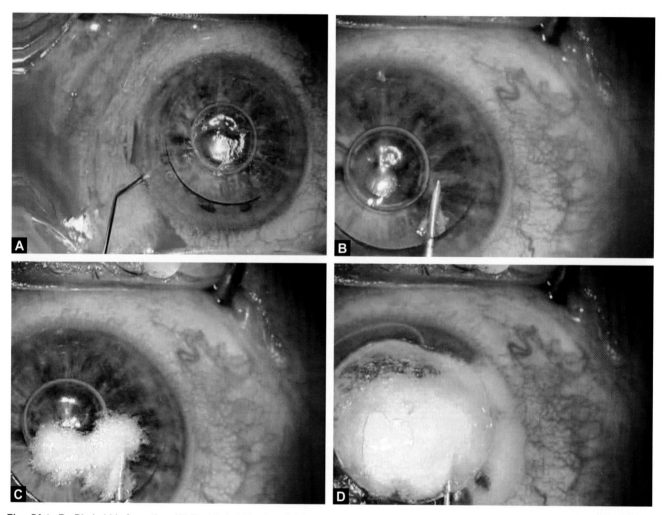

**Figs 5A to D:** Big-bubble formation. (A) Double-bubble placed in anterior chamber prior to big-bubble formation; (B) 27-guage needle placed in cornea stroma prior to big-bubble air injection. Note central location of double-bubble; (C) Big-bubble air injection in progress; (D) Completion of air injection with successful formation of big-bubble. Note peripheral displacement of double-bubble

16
SECTION

injection fails to form a big-bubble, air can be injected again from another spot, as long as there remains an area of relatively clear paracentral cornea to allow sufficient visualization of needle placement and bubble formation. After two failed attempts, risks of big-bubble failure and perforation increase such that conversion to manual dissection should be considered. Should the big-bubble fail, excellent results can still be obtained with manual dissection DALK or with conversion to PK. Even in the hands of accomplished corneal surgeons, unsuccessful big-bubble formation occurs in 7–43% of cases, Descemet's membrane perforation in 4–32% of cases, and conversion to PK in 2–18% of cases.[3,14,23]

Some surgeons have replaced needle entry with a specialized spatula (Sarnicola DALK Spatula, ASICO AE-2900) to first create a stromal tunnel, followed by injection of air through a companion cannula (Sarnicola DALK 27G Cannula, ASICO AE-7821) to form the big-bubble.[24]

### (Optional) Double-Bubble Technique to Confirm Presence of the Big-Bubble (Figs 5A to D)

A small approximately 0.1 cc air bubble is injected with a 27-guage needle into the anterior chamber directly through the limbus, or via cannula through a small limbal self-sealing paracentesis. If the big-bubble is present, it will occupy much of the central anterior chamber space, confining the small air bubble to the peripheral anterior chamber; in the absence of a big-bubble, the small bubble will center.[25,26] The paracentesis and air injection should be made sufficiently peripheral and directed more perpendicular than horizontal to the cornea to minimize risk of perforating the big-bubble. Many surgeons prefer to make the paracentesis after the big-bubble is formed, due to concern that air might extend the break in Descemet's membrane at the paracentesis site or leak into the anterior chamber and prevent the big-bubble from forming. Alternatively, the small air bubble can be placed prior to big-bubble formation, and has been advocated by Shimazaki[27] as a way to facilitate needle placement depth for the big bubble.

### Debulking/Lamellar Dissection of Recipient Anterior Stroma (Figs 6A to C)

A 2.3 mm angled crescent blade (Alcon) is placed deep in the trephine groove and maintaining a lamellar plane approximately 2/3–3/4 stromal depth, the anterior stroma

circumscribed by the trephine groove is removed. If the trephine groove is shallow, it can be cautiously focally deepened with a 15° or crescent blade prior to lamellar dissection. A lamellar plane can be maintained with a gentle sideways sweeping motion of the crescent blade parallel to the corneal plane. Avoid posterior direction, especially when approaching areas of corneal thinning.

### Fluid Release from Anterior Chamber to Lower Intraocular Pressure

In preparation for entering the big-bubble, intraocular pressure is lowered by a small release of aqueous through a self-sealing limbal paracentesis site. Be careful to direct instruments entering the paracentesis site posterior rather than central to avoid perforation of the big bubble. A softer eye allows slower and more controlled collapse of the big-bubble, with less chance of perforating Descemet's membrane as it moves anterior.

### Brave Slash

A 15° blade (Alcon) is used to make a nick incision through the central corneal stromal surface which is the roof of the big bubble, extending just deep enough to enter the big bubble. Entry should be confident and the blade withdrawn quickly [Dr Donald Tan aptly describes this as a 'brave slash' (Fig. 7)] to avoid the rapidly anteriorly displaced Descemet's membrane. Placing a glob of viscoelastic on the anticipated entry site may slow down the big bubble collapse and reduce the risk of inadvertent Descemet's perforation. Marking the blade with gentian violet improves subsequent visualization of the entry site. A successful big-bubble entry is signaled by air escape, corneal flattening and an intact well-formed anterior chamber. If air bubbles were present in the anterior chamber, they will move from a peripheral to central location as the bubble collapses.

### Baring of Descemet's Membrane/Posterior Stromal Dissection (Figs 8A to D)

A blunt-tip cyclodialysis spatula enters the nick incision site and is gently guided between remaining stroma and Descemet's membrane to form a groove from the central cornea to the 6 o'clock trephine edge. The cyclodialysis spatula is withdrawn and redirected to extend the groove from central to the 3 o'clock trephine edge, then to the 12 and 9 o'clock edges, to divide the stroma into four quadrants. Viscoelastic can be injected with a blunt-tip cannula to help dissect the space between Descemet's membrane and

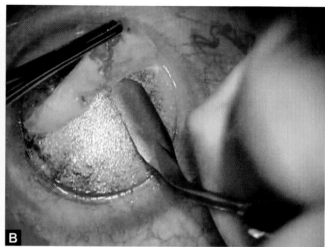

**Figs 6A to C:** Debulking/lamellar dissection of anterior stroma

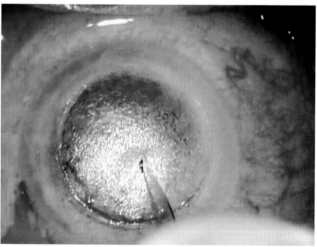

**Fig. 7:** 'Brave slash' nick incision

stroma. A gentle sideways wiggling motion of the cyclo-dialysis spatula along the corneal plane may facilitate the gentle, never forceful forward movements. The roof of the grooves are severed with blunt-tip curved Vannas scissors (Duckworth and Kent, 1-111B) from center to trephine edge to expose underlying bare Descemet's membrane. Each of the four quadrants of remaining stroma is dissected from Descemet's membrane with a cyclodialysis spatula or other blunt-tip dissecting instrument (I prefer the Tan Marginal Dissector, ASICO AE-2549), using a nonforceful gentle sideways sweeping motion with great care not to perforate Descemet's membrane. Blunt-tip corneal DALK scissors [Folga scissors right, (Storz E-3217R) or Folga scissors left (Storz E3217L)] are placed at the interface and oriented perpendicular to the corneal plane along the trephine edge to remove the stromal wedges. Avoid

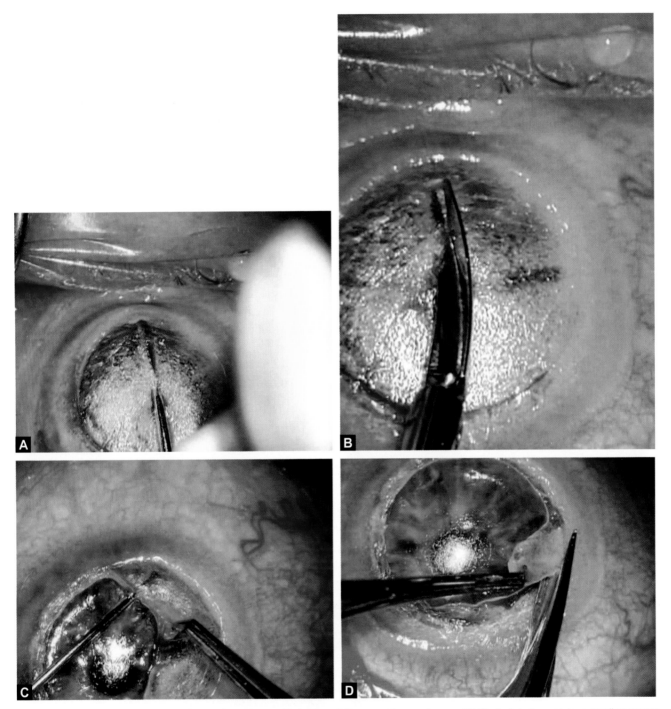

**Figs 8A to D:** Lamellar dissection of posterior stroma with baring of Descemet's membrane. (A) Cyclodialysis spatula extending groove between stroma and Descemet's membrane; (B) Unroofing groove to expose Descemet's membrane; (C) Quadrant dissection separating stroma from Descemet's membrane using Tan Marginal Dissector; (D) Final quadrant removal

downward pressure or touching Descemet's membrane with anything sharp such as toothed forceps. If there appears to be thin or multiple layers of remaining stroma rather than bare Descemet's membrane, with discretion the Tan Marginal Dissector can be used to enter and dissect the deepest interface. Be mindful that a small amount of remaining stroma is acceptable, Descemet's membrane is fragile, and the enemy of good is perfect.

If perforation of Descemet's membrane occurs, two options exist: (1) If the perforation is too large to maintain anterior chamber depth or allow for adequate removal of stromal tissue, the case is converted to PK; (2) Most cases involving perforation can be salvaged by continuing lamellar dissection away from the area of perforation and leaving the area surrounding the perforation slightly thicker. Air can be injected into the anterior chamber to tamponade a small defect but can risk extending the defect, especially if overinflation occurs prior to securing the donor graft. Perforation increases the risk of postoperative double anterior chamber and is associated with increased endothelial cell loss.[28]

### Donor Tissue Preparation

Donor tissue is placed on the trephine punch block epithelial side down and the endothelium is covered with trypan blue for 1 minute. After removing trypan blue, the tissue is submerged in balanced salt solution. Peripheral Descemet's membrane is scored 360° with a blunt-tip Sinskey hook. Descemet's membrane is removed by grasping a peripheral edge and extending central, regrasping at multiple sites should peripheral tears occur (Fig. 9). Alternatively, a dry Wexcell sponge can be used to establish an edge and dissect Descemet's membrane with a gentle pushing motion. Avoid engaging stroma. The donor tissue is trephined to the desired diameter (same diameter as recipient bed for keratoconus or high axial myopia, 0.25 mm larger for other pathology).

### Placement of Donor Tissue in Recipient Lamellar Bed

Recipient and donor surfaces are closely inspected and any debris removed with irrigation. The donor tissue is placed in the lamellar bed epithelial side up and secured with 16 interrupted 10-0 nylon sutures. (My preference. No studies to date have shown any convincing superiority of running, interrupted, combination running/interrupted, or adjustable suture techniques). To mitigate the tendency for graft-host junction override, sutures can be passed slightly more anterior through the graft tissue than host tissue, with care to avoid going too deep and perforating Descemet's membrane. Meticulous suture placement can help reduce astigmatism. The second suture location has the greatest effect on tissue alignment, and should be replaced should donor tissue not appear to be equally distributed after it is tied (Fig. 10). Suture knots are buried, facilitated by a quick flicking motion and a tightly formed anterior chamber (Fig. 11).

Antibiotic and corticosteroid drops of choice are placed, followed by lid speculum removal and application of pressure patch and shield.

### ► ALTERNATIVE TECHNIQUE TO BIG-BUBBLE DALK: MANUAL DISSECTION

If a big-bubble dissection cannot be accomplished due to multiple failed air injection attempts, or is precluded by inadequate visualization or previous Descemet's

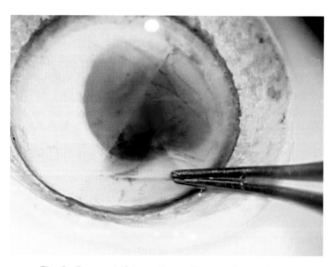

**Fig. 9:** Removal of donor tissue Descemet's membrane

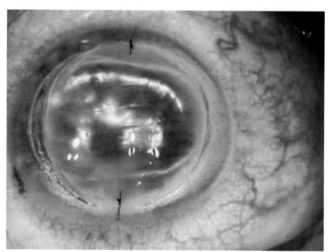

**Fig. 10:** Proper alignment of second suture is critical to insure even tissue distribution

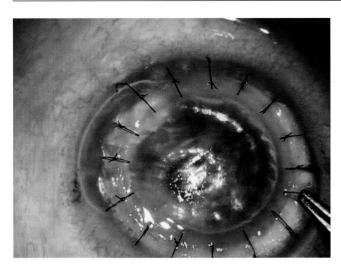

**Fig. 11:** Burying suture knots

membrane scarring or disruption, deep anterior stromal dissection can be accomplished by freehand layer-by-layer manual dissection. A crescent blade can be used to achieve increasingly deep levels of dissection, with the Tan Marginal Dissector or blunt-tip cyclodialysis spatula assisting dissection at each lamellar plane. Air, saline solution, or viscoelastic can be injected into the stroma to thicken and delaminate stroma.[22,29-31] As Descemet's membrane is approached the remaining tissue becomes less resistant to dissection and increasingly transparent and fragile. The goal in manual dissection is to obtain a smooth and intact deep lamellar surface. Attempts to achieve bare Descemet's membrane exposure will likely result in perforation.

## ▸ POSTOPERATIVE CARE

### Medications

There is no consensus for post-DALK antibiotic or anti-inflammatory regimens. Most clinicians employ both topical antibiotics and corticosteroids. Steroid regimens are usually less intense than used for PK patients, due to the absence of endothelial rejection. My protocol includes the use of a broad-spectrum antibiotic such as polymyxin B/trimethoprim or current generation fluoroquinolone, four times per day for 1 week. Prednisolone acetate 1% is given four times per day for the 1st month, three times a day for the 2nd month, two times a day for the 3rd month, then once a day for the remainder of the first 6–12 months.

Loteprednol etabonate 0.2% or fluorometholone 0.1% is substituted for glaucoma or steroid responders. Intraocular pressure should be checked at every postoperative visit! Patients with herpes simplex ophthalmicus are maintained on acyclovir 400 mg twice a day to reduce recurrence.[32,33]

### Follow-up Visits

Patients are routinely seen at 1 day postoperative, 5–7 days postoperative, 1 month postoperative, 3 months postoperative, 6 months postoperative, 1 year postoperative, then every 1–2 years.

### Anticipate Corneal Surface Problems

As with PK, the DALK corneal surface is stressed by hypesthesia (the nerves have been severed 360°), irregular tissue alignment with compromised tear coverage, and medicamentosa. Keratoconus patients are especially prone to filamentary keratitis and punctate keratitis.[34,35] A non-preserved lubricating gel or ointment is used four times per day for at least the 1st month, and often for the 1st year. If a graft epithelial defect persists or does not heal within a matter of days, treatment should quickly escalate to options including pressure patching or bandage soft contact lens trial, punctal occlusion and tarsorrhaphy. Patients with severe keratitis sicca or neurotrophic keratitis, including herpetic eyes, may benefit from surgery done during a more humid time of year.

### Suture Removal

Broken or eroding sutures should be removed. Most functional sutures should be left in place for 6–12 months. 270° wound dehiscence has been reported in a patient with all sutures out at 5 months.[36]

### Rejection

Endothelial rejection is avoided in DALK. Stromal, subepithelial and epithelial rejection can occur in DALK grafts and are usually readily reversed with increased topical corticosteroid treatment.[37,38] Stromal rejection occurs in up to 10% of cases, with most series reporting resolution without vision loss.[34,39] Stromal rejection can occasionally result in graft neovascularization, scarring and failure.[38] Subepithelial rejection has been reported in 24% of cases in one series with all cases fully resolving with topical corticosteroid treatment.[40]

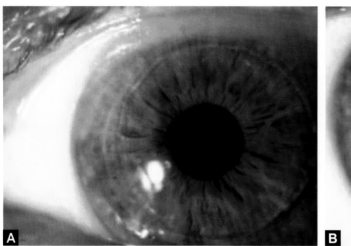
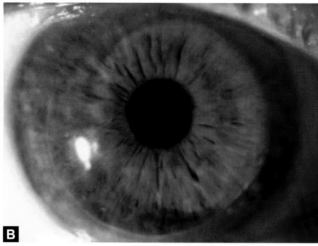

**Figs 12A and B:** Patient 's eyes appear almost identical. (A) Eye on left is 7 years postoperative PK; (B) eye on right is 18 months postoperative DALK

## Refractive Error

Refractive outcome is unpredictable following DALK, with results similar to PK. With sutures out, mean keratometric astigmatism ranges from 2.9 to 4.3 diopters, and mean spherical equivalent from −1.63 to −5.5 diopters.[1,5,39-41] Irregular astigmatism and quality of vision may improve following final suture removal. High corneal astigmatism can be effectively treated with relaxing incisions, with or without compression sutures.[42] Preliminary data suggests photorefractive keratectomy combined with Mitomycin C may offer relatively safe and effective treatment for post-DALK astigmatism and myopic error.[43]

## ❧ LONG-TERM PROGNOSIS

Regardless of surgeon compensation and time, the final reward for a DALK procedure is a patient with visual results comparable to PK but a graft that is far more likely to last a lifetime. The patient in Figures 12 A and B has equally good vision in each eye, and even to a corneal specialist the eyes appear almost identical. But his DALK eye on the right has a better long-term prognosis than his PK eye on the left (Figs 12A and B).

## ❧ REFERENCES

1. Ardjomand N, Hau S, McAlister JC, et al. Quality of vision and graft thickness in deep anterior lamellar and penetrating corneal allografts. Am J Opthalmol. 2007;143:228-35.
2. Han DCY, Mehta JS, Por YM, et al. Comparison of outcomes of lamellar keratoplasty and penetrating keratoplasty in keratoconus. Am J Ophthalmol. 2009;148:744-51.
3. Reinhart WJ, Musch DC, Jacobs DS, et al. Deep anterior lamellar keratoplasty as an alternative to penetrating keratoplasty. Ophthalmology. 2011;118:209-18.
4. Fontana L, Parente G, Sincich A, et al. Influence of graft-host interface on the quality of vision after deep anterior lamellar keratoplasty in patients with keratoconus. Cornea. 2011;30(5): 497-502.
5. Fontana L, Parente G, Tassinari G. Clinical outcomes after deep anterior lamellar keratoplasty using the big-bubble technique in patients with keratoconus. Am J Ophthalmol. 2007;143: 117-24.
6. Von Hippel A. Eine neue methode der hornhauttransplantation. Archiv Ophthalmol. 1888;34:I.
7. Zirm E. Eine erfolgreiche totale Keratoplastik. Graefes Arch Ophthalmol. 1906;64:580-93.
8. Cornea Donor Study Investigator Group. Donor age and corneal endothelial cell loss 5 years after successful corneal transplantation. Ophthalmology. 2008;115:627-32.
9. Bahar I, Kaiserman I, McAllum P, et al. Comparison of posterior lamellar keratoplasty techniques to penetrating keratoplasty. Ophthalmology. 2008;115:1525-33.
10. Price MO, Fairchild KM, Price DA, et al. Descemet's stripping endothelial keratoplasty: Five-year graft survival and endothelial cell loss. Ophthalmology. 2011;118:725-9.
11. Chen ES, Terry MA, Shamie N, et al. Descemet-stripping automated endothelial keratoplasty: Six-month results in a prospective study of 100 eyes. Cornea. 2008;27(5):514-20.
12. Javadi MA, Feizi S. Deep anterior lamellar keratoplasty using the big-bubble technique for keratectasia after laser in situ keratomileusis. J Cataract Refract Surg. 2010;36:1156-60.
13. Vajpayee RB, Tyagi J, Sharma N, et al. Deep anterior lamellar keratoplasty by big-bubble technique for treatment corneal stromal opacities. Am J Ophthalmol. 2007;143:954-7.
14. Sarnicola V, Toro P, Gentile D, et al. Descemetic DALK and predescemetic DALK: outcomes in 236 cases of keratoconus. Cornea. 2010;29:53-9.

15. Anshu A, Parthasarathy A, Mehta JS, et al. Outcomes of therapeutic deep lamellar keratoplasty and penetrating keratoplasty for advanced infectious keratitis: A comparative study. Ophthalmology. 2009;116:615-23.

16. Chew ACY, Mehta JS, Tan DTH. Deep lamellar keratoplasty after resolution of hydrops in keratoconus. Cornea. 2011;30(4):454-9.

17. Kubaloglu A, Sari ES, Unal M, et al. Long-term results of deep anterior lamellar keratoplasty for the treatment of keratoconus. Am J Ophthalmol. 2011;151:760-7.

18. Lee WB, Mathys KC. Traumatic wound dehiscence after deep anterior lamellar keratoplasty. J Cataract Refract Surg. 2009;35:1129-31.

19. Kawashima M, Kawakita T, Shimmura S, et al. Characteristics of traumatic globe rupture after keratoplasty. Ophthalmology. 2009;116:2072-6.

20. Heindl LM, Riss S, Bachmann BO, et al. Split cornea transplantation for 2 recipients: A new strategy to reduce corneal tissue cost and shortage. Ophthalmology. 2011;118:294-301.

21. Barraquer J. Lamellar keratoplasty (special techniques). Ann Ophthalmol. 1972;4:437-69.

22. Anwar M, Teichmann KD. Deep lamellar keratoplasty: Surgical techniques for anterior lamellar keratoplasty with and without baring of Descemet's membrane. Cornea. 2002;21(4):374-83.

23. Tan DTH, Mehta JS. Future directions in lamellar corneal transplantation. Cornea. 2007;26:S21-8.

24. Sarnicola V, Toro P. Blunt cannula for descemetic deep anterior lamellar keratoplasty. Cornea. 2011;30(8):895-8.

25. Fontana L, Parente G, Tassinari G. Simple test to confirm cleavage with air between Descemet's membrane and stroma during big-bubble deep anterior lamellar keratoplasty. J Cataract Refract Surg. 2007;33:570-2.

26. Parthasarathy A, Por YM, Tan DTH. Use of a "small bubble technique" to increase the success of Anwar's "big-bubble technique" for deep lamellar keratoplasty with complete baring of Descemet's membrane. Br J Ophthalmol. 2007;91:1369-73.

27. Shimazaki J. Double-bubble technique to facilitate Descemet membrane exposure in deep anterior lamellar keratoplasty. J Cataract Refract Surg. 2010;36:193-6.

28. Leccisotti A. Descemet's membrane perforation during deep anterior lamellar keratoplasty: prognosis. J Cataract Refract Surg. 2007;33:825-9.

29. Archila EA. Surgical Techniques: Deep lamellar keratoplasty dissection of host tissue with intrastromal air injection. Cornea. 1984-1985;3:217-8.

30. Sugita J, Kondo J. Deep lamellar keratoplasty with complete removal of pathological stroma for vision improvement. Br J Ophthalmol. 1997;81:184-8.

31. Manche EE, Holland GN, Maloney RK. Deep lamellar keratoplasty using viscoelastic dissection. Arch Ophthalmol. 1999;117:1561-5.

32. Uchoa UBC, Rezende RA, Carrasco MA, et al. Long-term acyclovir use to prevent recurrent ocular herpes simplex virus infection. Arch Ophthalmol. 2003;121:1702-4.

33. Ghosh S, Jhanji V, Lamoureux E, et al. Acyclovir therapy in prevention of recurrent herpetic keratitis following penetrating keratoplasty. Am J Ophthalmol. 2008;145:198-202.

34. Feizi S, Javadi MA, Jamali H, et al. Deep anterior lamellar keratoplasty in patients with keratoconus: Big-bubble technique. Cornea. 2010;29:177-82.

35. Rotkis WM, Chandler JW, Forstot SL. Filamentary keratitis following penetrating keratoplasty. Ophthalmology. 1982;89 (8):946-9.

36. Mannan R, Vishal J, Namrata S, et al. Spontaneous Wound Dehiscence After Early Suture Removal After Deep Anterior Lamellar Keratoplasty. Eye and Contact Lens: Science and Clinical Practice. 2011;37(2):109-11.

37. Alldredge OC, Krachmer JH. Clinical types of corneal transplant rejection: Their manifestations, frequency, preoperative correlates, and treatment. Arch Ophthalmol. 1981;99:599-604.

38. Watson SL, Tuft SJ, Dart JKG. Patterns of rejection after deep lamellar keratoplasty. Ophthalmology. 2006;113:556-60.

39. Noble BA, Agrawal A, Collins C, et al. Deep anterior lamellar keratoplasty (DALK): Visual outcome and complications for a heterogeneous group of corneal pathologies. Cornea. 2007;26:59-64.

40. Javadi MA, Feizi S, Yazdani S, et al. Deep anterior lamellar keratoplasty versus penetrating keratoplasty for keratoconus: A clinical trial. Cornea. 2010;29:365-71.

41. Watson SL, Ramsay A, Dart JKG, et al. Comparison of deep lamellar keratoplasty and penetrating keratoplasty in patients with keratoconus. Ophthalmology. 2004;111:1676-82.

42. Javadi MA, Feizi S, Mirbabaee F, et al. Relaxing incisions combined with adjustment sutures for post-deep anterior lamellar keratoplasty astigmatism in keratoconus. Cornea. 2009;28:1130-4.

43. Leccisotti A. Photorefractive keratectomy with Mitomycin C after deep anterior lamellar keratoplasty for keratoconus. Cornea. 2008;27:417-20.

CHAPTER 86

# Intacs Intracorneal Ring Segments and Keratoconus

*Adel Barbara, Lamis Abdel Aziz, Ramez Barbara*

## ❧ INTRODUCTION

There are four kinds of intracorneal ring segments (ICRS) available and various reports in the ophthalmic literature describe their effectiveness in treating keratoconus. The four types of ICRS are: (1) Intacs (Addition Technology Inc); (2) Intacs SK (Addition Technology Inc); (3) Ferrara Rings (Ferrara Ophthalmics) and (4) Kerarings (Mediphacos). The latter two have the same design and diameters, but are produced by different companies. In general, the ICRS differ in design, diameter, optical zone and length of arc, thus inducing different effects: the smaller the optical zone, the greater the effectiveness and the greater the ring segment diameter, the stronger is the effect obtained, and vice versa.

In this chapter, the author shall discuss the use of Intacs ICRS for treating keratoconus.

The author believes that a surgeon should master all of the surgical techniques of ICRS implantation and be aware of the various kinds of rings, because each ring has its specific characteristics and we should adopt specific rings for each patient rather than match the patient to the ring. The author personally performs implants using the four kinds of ICRS, selecting for each patient the rings which are most likely to provide the best improvement of visual acuity (VA).

A 35-year-old male with keratoconus seeks your services as a cornea specialist. The patient's vision in his only left eye is unsatisfactory with glasses, and he has already tried the whole range of contact lenses, but can no longer tolerate any of them. His cornea is clear, his average K reading is 49 diopters (D), and the central

corneal thickness is 470 microns. He lost all vision in his right keratoconic eye, due to complications following penetrating keratoplasty (PKP). What do you do?

The author hopes to convince you, the reader, to try ICRS before suggesting another corneal surgery.

The author has been using ICRS for a period of 9 years, with very satisfactory results, sparing many keratoconus patients the need for PKP and dramatically changing their quality of life for the better. The rate of complications decreased with time.

The concept of inserting polymethyl methacrylate (PMMA) segments as corneal inserts was first introduced by Fleming in 1987.[1,2] The aim at that time was myopia correction. The design of the rings developed, from a single 360° ring to two semicircular 150n° rings of hexagonal shape, with an inner diameter of 6.7 mm, an external diameter of 8.1 mm, and variable thicknesses, ranging from 0.25 mm to 0.45 mm with 0.05 mm (50 microns) increments. In the United States, 0.25 mm, 0.275 mm, 0.30 mm, 0.325 mm and 0.35 mm segments are available for use; outside of the United States, 0.40 mm and 0.45 mm-sized segments are also available[3] (Fig. 1).

Intrastromal corneal ring segments Intacs were initially designed to correct low degree myopia, by flattening the central corneal curvature.[4] Using the ICRS as a spacer between the corneal lamellae produces a shortening of the central arc length proportional to the ring thickness;[5] the peripheral portion of the anterior corneal surface is flattened and the peripheral area adjacent to ring insertion is displaced forward.[2,6] The Intacs were approved by the FDA for the correction of low myopia, between 1 and 3 D in 1996.[7]

Intacs are used to correct myopia of up to 4.5 D with no more than 1 D of astigmatism, according to the company nomograms. However, their use for the correction of myopia proved very limited, while vision correction by excimer laser, either by photorefractive keratectomy (PRK) or by laser-assisted keratomilieusis (LASIK), gained wide acceptance and popularity, by ophthalmologists and the myopic community alike, due to its safety, predictability and efficacy. Intacs produce comparable results for the correction of myopia,[8] and their clinical safety and efficacy have been shown to be comparable to those of other refractive procedures such as PRK and LASIK.[9]

The mechanism of myopia correction by Intacs is very logical and thus appealing. The cornea can be flattened without removing tissue from its center (as in myopia correction by excimer laser), tissue is added to the cornea, the center of the cornea remains untouched, the surgery is reversible, the cornea regains its former preoperative shape after the removal of Intacs, with refraction and visual acuity essentially returning to preoperative levels within 1–7 weeks.[10] Asbell et al. reported on the easy and safe removal of Intacs, whereby eyes returned to preoperative refractive status within 3 months.[11]

The position of the Intacs in the cornea is adjustable, and the rings can be replaced by thinner or thicker rings as needed. Increasing the rings' thickness increases the flattening effect on the cornea and vice versa. Exchange procedures, in which ring segments are exchanged for larger or smaller sizes, were successful in improving uncorrected visual acuity (UCVA).[10]

Intacs were used for the correction of myopia after LASIK and PRK with satisfactory, safe, stable and predictable results, like in 'virgin' myopic eyes.[12]

So why is laser surgery preferred over Intacs as the gold standard for myopia lower than 4.5 D?

Intacs do not correct the astigmatism which accompanies myopia, whereas the laser procedure does. Furthermore, manual Intacs implantation (the original method of implantation) is more demanding as there is a learning curve, meaning that it is not as easy for the surgeon to perform as is the laser technique. The introduction of femtosecond laser-assisted Intacs implantation technique became available many years after Intacs entered the market, and the femtosecond laser's high cost limits its availability. Another limiting factor is the high cost of the Intacs; a pair of Intacs costs the surgeon almost the same as the cost of laser surgery to the patient.

All the upper-mentioned reasons made the use of Intacs for low myopia unpopular among refractive surgeons.

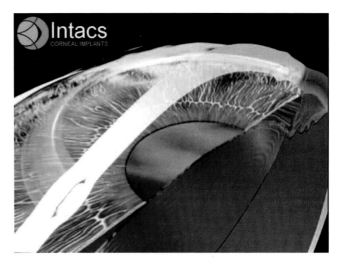

**Fig. 1:** Cross-section view of cornea showing the hexagonal shape of the ring segment

The other kind of intrastromal corneal rings is the Ferrara Ring, which was developed at a period parallel to the introduction of Intacs. Ferrara Rings have a pyramid shape, 160° length and a 5 mm optical zone, whereas Intacs have a 7 mm optical zone. The Kerarings, which are similar to the Ferrara Rings, come in arc lengths of 90, 120, 160 and 210 degrees. Both the Kerarings and the Ferrara Rings have thicknesses of 0.15–0.35 mm, with 0.05 mm increments. Recently, Ferrara et al. published positive clinical outcomes regarding the use of a new arc length of 210° in keratoconus patients.[13]

The first generation of Bisantis intrastromal segmented perioptic implants were sold by Optikon 2000 SpA and Soleko SpA (Rome, Italy). The differentiating element of this model was the number of implants. The first phase tested implantation of either three or four segments, both having 60° with a circular shape. All rings had a thickness of 150 μm and were placed in a 3.5 mm optical zone diameter. At present, four segments of 80°, each with an oval cross section, a vertical diameter of 250 μm and a horizontal diameter of 200 μm are inserted. The only variable parameter is the curvature of the inserts in order to obtain optical zone parameters of 3.5, 4.0 and 4.5 mm.[14]

The author has not seen any published papers on the clinical results of procedures using these rings nor have they been presented at the international congresses which he has attended.

An additional ICRS is the myoring which is a round ICRS inserted in a corneal pocket created by a special automated microkeratome.

## INTACS IN CORNEAS WITH SUSPECTED KERATOCONUS

In many cases when we encounter suspected keratoconus in corneas with low myopia, we hesitate to perform laser surgery. The implantation of Intacs in these low myopic eyes may be a safe and predictable procedure. Intacs were used as an alternative to laser surgery in patients with forme fruste keratoconus or with extremely thin corneas whose refractive error was less than 3.00 D.[17] Satisfactory results were reported on Intacs for the correction of myopia of less than 4.5 D in 39 eyes of 21 patients, in patients excluded from laser surgery because of abnormal topography and forme fruste keratoconus. In one patient, the Intacs were removed because of unsatisfactory results; in 7 eyes, the rings were exchanged for thicker ones because of undercorrection.[18]

The author has implanted Intacs in myopic patients with thin, steep and asymmetric corneas, and the results have been comparable to normal myopic eyes (unpublished data). A most recent case concerns a 23-year-old male with a stable refraction of −1.75 in both eyes, normal corneal reflex and central corneal thickness (CCT) of 437 microns in the right eye and 435 microns in the left eye. The author implanted 300 microns Intacs in the patient's right eye, and 3 months postoperatively, UCVA is 20/25. The patient is satisfied with the outcome and planning for the same surgery in his left eye (Figs 2A and B).

## INTACS AND KERATOCONUS

In 2004, Intacs received FDA approval under the Humanitarian Device Exemption (HDE) process for the treatment of myopia and astigmatism in patients with keratoconus, when specific criteria are met. The HDE process, which is available for devices treating conditions that affect less than 4,000 Americans per year, does not require the manufacturer to provide data confirming the efficacy of the device, but rather data supporting its 'probable' benefit.

The first Intacs implantation for improving VA in a keratoconic patient was performed by Joseph Colin in 1997.[19] Intacs were inserted in a contact lens intolerant patient with unsatisfactory visual acuity. As a result of the Intacs implantation, the astigmatism and the corneal steepening were reduced. This patient completed a 10-year follow-up with stable results. Since then, many studies have been published in the literature confirming the positive results of Intacs implantation in keratoconic eyes.

## Indications for Corneal Rings in Keratoconus

Indications for treating keratoconus by corneal ring insertion include:

- Unsatisfactory VA with glasses
- Contact lenses intolerance
- Mild to moderate keratoconus
- K reading less than 58 D
- Clear cornea and optical zone with no corneal scarring
- Patients who desire modest improvements in their visual acuity
- Corneal thickness greater than 450 μm in the area of the proposed tunnels, where Intacs are expected to be implanted, as marked by the marker and measured by pachymetry.[20,21]

Expectations should be discussed thoroughly with the patient. Many keratoconic patients come to refractive surgery centers hoping to find a total remedy for their condition, and upon hearing of the ICRS procedure, they expect results similar to those experienced by patients who underwent laser surgery. Therefore, the author discusses with them their situation: if they are contact lens intolerant with unsatisfactory VA with glasses and have a clear cornea, he offers them the Intacs option and explains that they will continue to use glasses, contact lenses, probably soft keratoconus lenses after the procedure. However, they may expect improvement of UCVA and best spectacles corrected visual acuity (BSCVA). Most importantly, by opting for this procedure, they may delay or even avoid the need for PKP.

In one particularly memorable case, the author was treating a young lady who had a very low UCVA and BSCVA, and she tolerated well the rigid gas permeable contact lenses that he had fitted for her. However, she complained that when her baby woke up at night asking for the bottle, she was unable to function because of her low vision, and she had no time to put on her contact lenses. The author was just beginning to use Intacs and he was reluctant to perform the surgery, yet he could not very well listen to her complaints without offering her a solution. Finally, he decided to agree to implant Intacs in her cornea in one eye, and later, once she was happy with the results of her first eye, into her other eye. Since then, he agrees to implant ICRS even in contact lens tolerant patients who in their daily functioning need some independence from their lenses, at least in one eye.

The mechanism of the Intacs' effect is well-reported by Kaiserman et al. They describe optical coherence tomography of a keratoconic cornea in which asymmetric Intacs

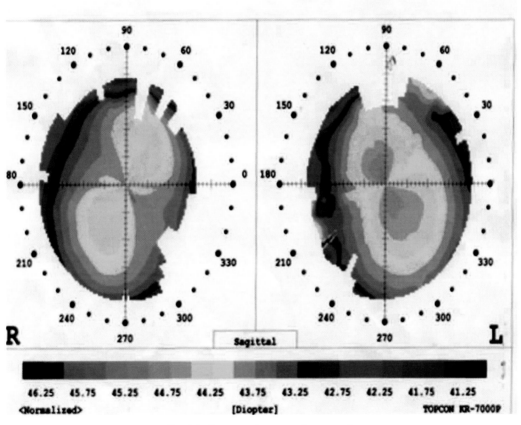

Serial No.:0072   PD:65.0   VD:12.00

[OD(Right) Data]
<Ref Data>
S:- 1.75   C:- 0.50   A:145

<Kerato Data>
```
           D      MM    A
H  : 43.75   7.71   141
V  : 44.50   7.59    51
Ave: 44.12   7.65
         CYL: - 0.75   141
```

<Peripheral Data>

N.A.

[OS(Left) Data]
<Ref Data>
S:- 1.75   C:- 0.50   A:  7

<Kerato Data>
```
           D      MM    A
H  : 44.12   7.65    22
V  : 44.75   7.54   112
Ave: 44.37   7.60
         CYL: - 0.62    22
```

<Peripheral Data>

N.A.

Sagittal

```
46.25  45.75  45.25  44.75  44.25  43.75  43.25  42.75  42.25  41.75  41.25
```
<Normalized>                    [Diopter]                    TOPCON KR-7000P

**Fig. 2A:** Preoperative corneal topography

CHAPTER
87

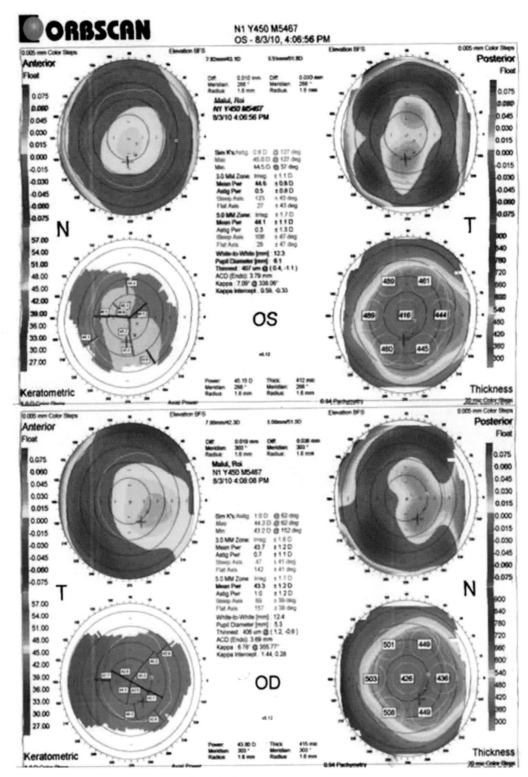

**Fig. 2B:** Preoperative Orbscan II

were implanted and conclude that the main effect of the Intacs seems to be an elevation of the corneal stroma above the inferior segment, creating a flattening of the corneal surface in that area, with no change in the apical thickness of the cone but a change in the cone's apex position.[22]

## Poor Candidates for Intacs

Poor candidates for Intacs are individuals with central or paracentral scarring, although satisfactory results were reported in eyes with central scars.[23] Nevertheless, we avoid implanting rings in scarred corneas, i.e. patients whose corneas are thinner than 450 μm at the site of placement of the Intacs and patients who expect excellent uncorrected acuity after surgery.

Alio et al. demonstrated that corneas with average K readings of less than 55 D have better results after Intacs implantation than do corneas steeper than 55 D.[24] Intacs provided better results in terms of visual acuity improvement and the regularization of corneal topography and significantly reduced the spherical equivalent in keratoconic eyes with relatively low mean K values ($\leq$ 53 D) and a relatively low spherical equivalent. In advanced keratoconus (mean K reading $\geq$ 55 D), poor results can be anticipated.[25] This was confirmed by the work of Kannelopollous, who illustrates the potential for a high rate of complication in patients with advanced disease.[26]

In contrast, Rohit Shetty et al. reported on Intacs implanted in 14 eyes with advanced keratoconus. Results after follow-up of 1 year were mean K greater than 53 D with 100% safety, and fewer complications than previously reported with Intacs for advanced keratoconus. Younger age, male sex, and minimum central pachymetry of more than 400 mm seemed to be associated with better outcomes, including improvement in K readings, astigmatism and manifest refraction spherical equivalent (MRSE) as well as improvement in UCVA and BCVA. The MRSE was reduced from −9.13 D ± 5.62 to −4.93 D ± 3.19 (P = 0.01), and the average keratometry decreased from 53.01 D ± 3.70 to 49.42 D ± 3.79 (P < 0.05). The results remained stable between 6 months to 1 year of follow-up. The procedure showed 100% safety, and more than 60% of the patients tolerated contact lenses.[27]

## ▶ OPERATION TECHNIQUES

Intacs are implanted in a circumferential corneal channel created in the corneal stroma. A small incision is created at 70% of the corneal thickness, as measured by ultrasound pachymetry, as an entry point through which the stromal rings are inserted into the channel. The incision and the tunnels are created either mechanically by surgical dissection or with the use of femtosecond laser.

## The Mechanical Technique

The center of the cornea is located for use as a reference point. A special marker is then used to mark the sites of the Intacs tunnels and the incision points. The incision site is set on the steep axis of the cornea.

Ultrasound pachymetry is performed to measure the corneal thickness at the incision site and the marked Intacs tunnels position. The calibrated diamond knife is set to a depth between 70% (recommended by the producer of Intacs) and 80%.

A 1.2–1.8 mm radial incision is created in the marked position. Pocketing hooks create corneal pockets on each side at the bottom of the incision, then a special glide is inserted on both sides in order to check the pocket depth.

A semiautomated suction ring is placed around the limbus and the vacuum system is started. The vacuum system has two grades of suction: the low suction (400–500 mbar) and high (600–667) is applied first, and once contraction of the suction ring is ascertained, the higher level of suction can be applied (Over the last 4 years, the author has been using only the low suction). Attention should be taken not to exceed 3 minutes of suction, as mentioned by Rabinowitz, in order not to compromise the blood supply to the posterior pole of the eye. The author tries not to exceed 1 minute of suction.

Two semicircular dissectors are placed (one clockwise and the other counterclockwise) into the pocket after inserting the special glide. The dissectors, which should pass under the glide, in order to ascertain the proper depth, are advanced by rotational movement, creating two semicircular tunnels with specific diameters, which are ready to accept the ring segments, one in each tunnel.

Now the Intacs are inserted and placed at least 1 mm away from the incision. In the past, one had to be inserted clockwise and the other counterclockwise, because there was only one hole in each segment and the hole had to be close to the wound for facilitating the manipulation or its explantation of the ring segment, if needed. Recently however Intacs have two holes, so that each can be inserted either clockwise or counterclockwise into the tunnels (See Surgical Technique—Figures 3A to I).

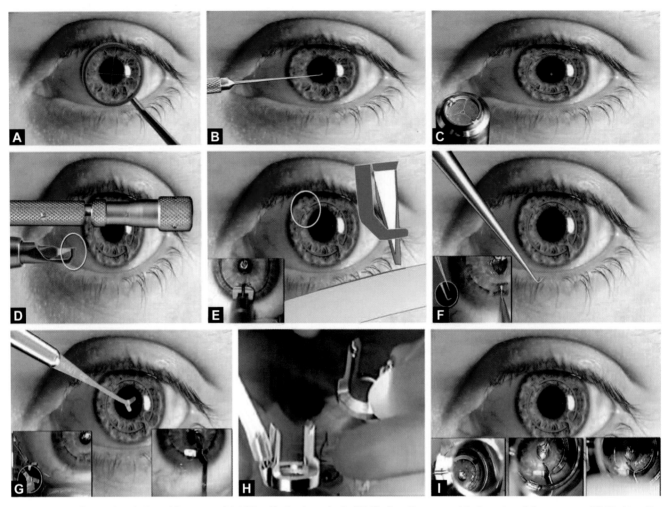

**Figs 3A to I:** Surgical technique (Courtesy of Addition Technology, Inc). (A) Finding the geometrical center of the cornea; (B) Marking the geometrical center of the cornea; (C) Marking the incision site and tunnels' position; (D) Setting the knife for the appropriate incision depth after pachymetry; (E) The incision; (F) Pocketing; (G) Glide insertion; (H) Suction ring is centered on the cornea and suction is applied; (I) Clockwise tunnelling after suction; the dissector should be inserted under the glide to ensure appropriate depth of tunnel

The incision is closed by one 10-0 nylon suture. Note that if after surgery completion the edges of the incision have closed, a suture may be unnecessary. The author finds that in his experience, this is normally the case, and he no longer sutures the wound.

## The Femtosecond Laser Technique

The femtosecond laser is an infrared laser, which works with a wavelength of 1052 nm. It sends ultrashort laser pulses of 0.001 mm diameter. A femtosecond is equivalent to a trillion seconds (10–15 sec). Focused at the required corneal depth, the femtosecond laser induces an optical breakdown in the corneal tissues without thermal or shockwave damage to surrounding tissues.[16] A microbubble consisting of carbon dihydrate and water (diameter 5–12 micrometers) is created; as it expands, it separates

the corneal tissue that surrounds it. Thousands of these photodisruptive laser pulses separate the corneal tissue during the preparation of the intrastromal ring tunnels used for insertion of Intacs and other kinds of ICRS.[28]

Here are the steps for performing the procedure:[16]

- A reference point on the center of the cornea is marked, and the corneal thickness is measured by pachymetry at the area of the ring insertion.
- The suction ring is centered, and the eye is fixated by applanation of a disposable glass lens to the cornea. This maintains a precise distance between the laser head and the focal point.
- The entry point is created, and the corneal tunnel is created at 70–80% of the corneal thickness, and then the ring segments are inserted in the tunnel.

The following settings are recommended by Rabinovitz:[3]

## For Intacs

- Incision site temporal
- Depth: 400 μm
- Incision length: 1 mm
- Incision width: 1 mm.

Channel size should be 6.6 × 7.4 mm, which gives you a 0.4-mm channel that is 0.05 mm larger than the Intacs. The outer diameter of the channel can be reduced to increase the effect, if necessary.

Here the author has to comment on the issue of 'channel size': it is assumed that Intacs topographically flatten and center the keratoconic cone, as they flatten and stretch the corneal apex. Thus, inserting the Intacs segments into smaller and tighter corneal channels should enhance their effect.[22] Ertan et al. retrospectively compared the outcomes of two channel sizes for Intacs implantation, using an Intralase femtosecond laser in 159 eyes with keratoconus and found similar refractive results in two groups of patients with different channel dissection sizes (wide: 6.7 mm × 8.2 mm; and narrow: 6.6 mm × 7.6 mm). At 6-month follow-up, the UCVA and BCVA had significantly improved in 63.9% and 70.1% of eyes, respectively, in the wide-channel group (97 eyes of 65 patients), and 72.5% and 75.8% of eyes, respectively, in the narrow-channel group (62 eyes of 38 patients). The changes in mean BCVA and in mean UCVA in both groups were statistically significant. There was no difference between the two groups in terms of the improvement in manifest spherical refraction, cylindrical refraction, manifest refractive spherical equivalent, or mean K readings.[29] However, the rate of complications was higher among the small size channel group. Epithelial plug, yellow-white deposits, tunnel haze around segments and upward movement of the inferior segment without extrusion were observed more frequently in the narrow-channel group than in the wide-channel group. The authors concluded that the VA results were similar, but the complications were higher in the narrow channel group.

Tunnel dissection by femtosecond laser results in precise tunnel and keratotomy depth, width, and location, as well as in a uniform 360° channel; haze, edema and surgical complications are minimized.

Some technical difficulty may be encountered when implanting Intacs in channels created by femtosecond laser; as the entry cut is vertical, it can be a bit tricky to advance the Intacs through the channel. To facilitate this, it is important to hydrate the cornea, identify the lip of the circular incision with a sinskey hook, and then while exerting upward pressure on the sinskey hook to keep the lip open, place the Intac and advance it under the sinskey hook, all that while keeping the lip elevated; this will prevent the Intacs from being hung on the lip of the incision.[3]

Sometimes, advancing the Intacs can be difficult due to uncut stromal fibers in the channels. To overcome this problem, the blades of the mechanical spreader can be used to open up the tunnels.[3]

## Incision, Ring Position and Nomograms

Many combinations of Intacs can be implanted:
- Two symmetrical segments
- Two asymmetrical segments
- One segment.

The location of the incision determines the placement of the Intacs, which subsequently affects the corneal shape. These decisions are made according to the surgeon's evaluation. The following factors should be considered: the grade of keratoconus, the type of the conus, and the degree of myopia and astigmatism, i.e. the spherical equivalent (SE).

In the following paragraphs, we review several approaches as reported by outstanding experts.

Colin et al. placed incisions temporally.[19,21] They implanted symmetrical Intacs of 0.4 mm or 0.45 mm according to the spherical equivalent. In 2006, Colin[30] used a nomogram that was based on the SE, location of the cone, and asymmetric astigmatism induced by keratoconus. The treatment nomograms described in Table 1 were used to determine the appropriate inserts' placement.[15]

Rabinowitz recommends making the incision on the steepest keratometric meridian, so that the Intacs will bisect the thinnest part of the cornea, which will make the cornea physiologically normal by thickening the thin area. In almost all of the cases of oval and central cones, this placement turns out to entail a temporal incision.[3]

| Table 1: Thickness nomograms as recommended by Colin[15] | | |
|---|---|---|
| **Recommended thickness (mm)** | | |
| *Type of cone* | Preop: SE < −3.00 D | Preop: SE > −3.00 D |
| Asymmetrical | 0.25 / 0.30 | 0.25 / 0.35 |
| Moderately asymmetric | 0.35 / 0.40 | 0.40 / 0.45 |
| Highly asymmetric | 0.25 / 0.40 | 0.25 / 0.45 |
| Global | 0.40 / 0.40 | 0.45 / 0.45 |
| Central | 0.40 / 0.40 | 0.45 / 0.45 |

SE: Spherical equivalent

The asymmetry of the Intacs is probably more significant than the location of the entry incision. In centrally located cones in which a maximum flattening effect is wanted, it is best to use symmetrical Intacs, if the patient is not severely myopic; smaller size symmetrical Intacs could be used so as not to overcorrect and induce hyperopia. In typical oval type cones, most surgeons follow Colin's original concept of putting in asymmetric Intacs 0.25 mm above and 0.45 mm below outside of the United States and 0.25 mm above and 0.35 mm below, in the United States. In very mild cones that do not cross the horizontal meridian, a single Intac often suffices.[3]

Alio et al. reported on unsatisfactory visual results when thicker Intacs were implanted superiorly and the thinner inferiorly, and improvement of vision when the Intacs position was exchanged.[31] A similar result was reported by Chan et al. in a case of a 33-year-old woman with keratoconus and contact lens intolerance who underwent Intacs surgery in the left eye (not at the authors' institution).[32] Two segments were used: a thinner one (0.25 mm) below the cone and a thicker one (0.35 mm) above the cone. Two months postoperatively, the patient presented to the authors with BSCVA reduced from 20/20 to 20/30. The superior Intacs segment was explanted, the inferior segment was exchanged for a thicker one (0.35 mm), and collagen cross-linking (CXL) with riboflavin treatment was performed. This resulted in visual, topographic, and refractive improvement with BSCVA returning to 20/20. They analyzed the possible reasons for the initial unsuccessful results:

- Shifting the cone centrally will shift an irregular part of the cornea into the visual axis. If the cone was a symmetrical sphere, this would have the effect of inducing myopia, but as it is an irregular shape, it will likely worsen the distortions
- The topography of a cone has two areas, a steep area below and a flat area above. Placing a segment in the upper half will further flatten an already flat area. Placing the thicker segment will flatten it further still and heighten the asymmetry.

The implantation of a thicker Intacs superiorly was based on the assumption that stretching the cone can also be performed from above.[22]

Ertan et al. report on two cases of vertical Intacs implantation for temporal cones: in two patients, a 0.45 mm segment and a 0.25 mm segment were inserted in the temporal segment and nasal segment, respectively. The incision was put at 12 o'clock, a position chosen for easy manipulation when inserting the Intacs segment vertically. The incision site was not determined according to the axis of the astigmatism. One year postoperatively, UCVA improved by 2.0 and 2.5 Snellen lines in case 1 and case 2, respectively; BCVA improved 1 and 4 Snellen lines, respectively.[33]

The ideal position for the corneal incision is on the steepest corneal meridian, to reduce the corneal power at the steepest meridian. As reported in the review of Pinero et al. and Rabinowitz, this type of incision minimizes the corneal and manifest astigmatism.[3,16] However, different surgeons use different reference points. In 2006, Kanellopoulos et al. reported making the incision temporal and at the 1 o'clock position, superior to the horizontal middle meridian of the cornea.[26] The corresponding center of the rings was also positioned to adjust to the center of the cone; therefore, the center of the virtual circle created by the two rings was positioned inferotemporally by 0.5–1.5 mm towards the center of the cone and not the geometric center of the cornea.

Guel et al. reported on the use of different modalities of Intacs implantation in 46 eyes: two symmetric segments were implanted in 19 eyes (41.3% eyes), two segments of different thickness in 23 eyes (50% eyes), and one inferiorly implanted segment in 2 eyes (4.34%).[4,34] In the eyes with an inferior or central cone, the incision was made at a 90° angle, the segments were placed nasally and temporally and then pushed until the inferior extremes were touching, as if embracing the cone, in an attempt to push the cone up, similar to the reported by Rabinowitz.[3] With this approach, the two segments act as if they are a whole inferior segment of 280°. In the eyes with oblique corneal astigmatism, two inserts of different thickness were implanted through an incision placed at the flattest meridian. The thickest segment was placed inferiorly, in the steepest axis. In cases with a SE less than –0.5 D, a single inferior segment was implanted.[34]

Wachler et al. used a combination of a 0.25 mm segment superiorly and 0.30 mm segment inferiorly for SE less than –3 D, and a combination of a 0.25 mm segment superiorly and 0.35 mm segment inferiorly for a SE greater than –3.00 D. In this study, which did not exclude patients with central scarring, the results demonstrated improvement in UCVA and BCVA, and the reduction of irregular astigmatism.[23]

A positive correlation was found between ring thickness and the change in K values; that is, the thicker the ring, the greater the flattening effect on the cornea.[35]

In summary, although the author tried to show you the different approaches reported, the findings of the prospective, comparative and randomized studies indicate a lack of scientific clarity regarding the position of the incision, and the combination of Intacs.

The question of implantation of a single versus two segments merits further probing and discussion. While most studies inserted double segment corneal rings, a few studies inserted single segment rings and compared that with double segment insertion: the latter reported no statistically significant differences between the two groups in terms of visual outcome.[3]

Rabinowitz et al. analyzed patients who had a single Intacs inserted and a group that had two Intacs inserted and reported no statistically significant differences between the two groups under any outcome measure.[19] In an unpublished series he reported on (approximately) 50 eyes treated by his team, which found a 60% success rate in improving both the UCVA and BCVA using a single inferior Intac.

Sharma et al. compared the effect of implanting a single inferior segment to the implantation of two segments in peripheral cones in 37 eyes of patients with keratoconus and post-LASIK ectasia, which were classified into two groups: a single-segment group (17 eyes, 11 patients) and a double-segment group (20 eyes, 17 patients).[36] They reported obtaining better visual and keratometric results when a single inferior segment was inserted. According to their study, single segments induced localized flattening inferiorly and steepening in the upper cornea, which leads to a greater decrease in I-S ratio. The improvement in UCVA was greater (nine lines) in the single segment group than in the double segment group (2.5 lines, $P < .01$). Best spectacles corrected visual acuity in the single segment group improved by 2.5 lines compared to $< 1$ line in the double-segment group ($P < .01$). Steep K values in the single segment group diminished by 2.76 D $\pm$ 2.68 compared to 0.93 D $\pm$ 2.01 in the double segment group ($P = .02$); I-S ratio in the single-segment group decreased by 9.51 $\pm$ 7.49 compared to 4.22 $\pm$ 4.82 in the double-segment group ($P = .01$); and there was greater cylinder decrease after Holladay vector analysis in the single segment group (5.69 D $\pm$ 3.10) than in the double segment group (1.58 D $\pm$ 3.09, $P < .01$).

Alio et al. retrospectively studied and evaluated eyes with keratoconus that had single or double Intacs implantation.[24] The patients were divided into two groups according to the results of the preoperative corneal topography: Group I included 11 eyes of 8 patients in whom the preoperative corneal topographic findings revealed steepening not involving the 180° meridian of the cornea (inferior cone).

In these eyes, only 1 segment of 0.45 mm thickness was implanted inferiorly to flatten the inferior cone. Group II included 15 eyes of 11 patients, in whom preoperative corneal topography revealed steepening extending at least 1 mm above and beyond the 180° meridian of the cornea (central cone). In this group, two segments were implanted: 0.45 mm segment inferiorly to lift the inferior cone and produce maximum flattening and 0.25 mm segment superiorly. In both groups, there was an improvement in UCVA and BCVA, reduction of astigmatism and corneal steepening, with no significant differences between the groups.

Recently, there has been a trend towards implanting only a single Intac inferiorly in the oval cones, because it is felt that this is the best way to maximize reduction of the astigmatic effect.[3] Unsatisfactory visual results were obtained in cases in which two Intac segments were implanted: these patients often saw better and were happier once the superior Intac was removed.[3]

Joaquim Murta reported better results in terms of myopia and astigmatism reduction in inferior cones implanted with one ring than with two asymmetric rings[37].

## Results and Long-Term Follow-Up

We evaluate the results of Intacs implantation in terms of the following categories:

- Uncorrected visual acuity improvement
- Best spectacles corrected visual acuity improvement
- Astigmatism reduction
- Myopia reduction
- Lowering of keratometry readings
- Increased tolerance of contact lens
- Reduction of the high order aberrations (HOA).

The results depend on the degree of the keratoconus: the more moderate the conus the less satisfactory are the results.

Table 2 summarizes the results from the literature review presented by Ertan and Colin and by Pinero et al.[15,16] Changes (mean) were achieved in spherical equivalent, sphere, cylinder and keratometry are shown. In addition, the percentage of eyes that gained lines of BSCVA is also reported. Caution must be taken when comparing these outcomes, because different samples of keratoconus eyes were evaluated and additionally different nomograms were used for ICRS implantation.

Rabinovitz in his review on Intacs for treating keratoconus states, "Most studies to date show an average of 2 to 3 D of flattening accompanied by 2 to 3 lines of gain

**Table 2:** Outcomes of ICSR treatment for keratoconus

| Study | Eyes | Yr | F/U | Surgical Procedure | Incision Site | Technique/ Implantation Criteria | Visual Acuity Change | Mean Refractive Change |
|---|---|---|---|---|---|---|---|---|
| *Intacs Rings* | | | | | | | | |
| Colin | 10 | 2000 | 6 M | Mechanical | Temporal | 0.35/0.45 | | Mean change in SE 2.12 D, mean change in sph 1.75 D, mean change in cyl 1.5 D, mean change in ker 4.85 D |
| Colin | 10 | 2001 | 1 Y | Mechanical | Temporal | Asym (0.25-0.45 mm) | BCVA improved 2 lines | Cylinder decreased from –4.00 D to –1.30 D |
| Siganos | 33 | 2002 | 11.3 M | Mechanical | @ ax 90 | Sym (0.45 mm) | 6% and 12% eyes lost lines of UCVA and BCVA; 25 of 33 (75.75%) gained 1 to 6 lines of BCVA | Change in K-values: 1.94 ± 3.51 D; mean MRSE reduction: 1.82 ± 3.03 D |
| Boxer-Wachler | 74 | 2003 | 9 M | Mechanical | @ ax 90 (manifest refraction) | Asym (0.25/0.35 mm) SE < –3.00 D: 0.25/0.30 SE > –3.00 D: 0.25/0.35 | UCVA improved 4 lines, 45% gained lines of BCVA | MRSE decreased from –3.89 D to –1.46 D |
| Alio | 26 | 2005 | 12 M | Mechanical | Temporal | Inferior corneal steepening not involving the 180° meridian: 1 inferior segment 0.45 | 81.81% of 1-segment group gained lines of BCVA, 86.67% of 2-segment group gained lines of BCVA | Mean change in SE 3.27 D in 1-segment group and 1.92 D in 2-segment group, mean change in cyl 2.47 D in 1-segment group and 2.39 D in 2-segment group, mean change in ker 4.69 D in 1-segment group and 5.27 in 2-segment group |
| Hellstedt | 50 | 2005 | 6.3 M | Mechanical | Temporal | Asym (0.25/0.45 mm) | BCVA improved from 20/78 to 20/43, 76.7% gained lines of BCVA | Keratometric astigmatic change of 2.90 D, mean change in SE 2.67 D, mean change in ker 4.20 D |
| Ibrahim | 186 | 2006 | 5 Y | | Steep meridian | Sym or asym (0.25-0.45 mm) | 85.23% and 87.9% gained lines of UCVA and BCVA | K-values improved from 52.53 D to 48.05 D |
| Colin | 57 | 2006 | 6 M | Mechanical | Temporal | Sym or asym (0.25-0.45 mm) | 78% gained lines of UCVA; 62% gained 2 to 8 lines of BCVA | MRSE 3.1 ± 2.5 D and K-values 4.3 ± 2.8 D improved, mean change in SE 1.53 D, mean change in cyl 2.88 D, mean change in ker 3.70 D |

*Contd...*

| Study | Eyes | Yr | F/U | Surgical Procedure | Incision Site | Technique/ Implantation Criteria | Visual Acuity Change | Mean Refractive Change |
|-------|------|-----|------|--------------------|---------------|-----------------------------------|----------------------|------------------------|
| Alio | 13 | 2006 | 48 M | Mechanical | Temporal | Asym (0.25/0.45 mm) Corneal steepening extending at least 1 m above and beyond 180° meridian | BCVA increased from 20/50 to 20/30, despite fluctuation in K-values, refraction and BCVA remained constant at 36 and 48 months | MRSE improved from–5.40 D to –3.95 D;Mean change in SE 1.45 D, mean change in sph 0.43 D, mean change in cyl 2.07 D, mean change in ker 2.56 D |
| Alio | 25 | 2006 | 6 M | Mechanical | @ ax 90 | Single/double (0.25/0.45 mm) Inferior corneal steepening not involving the 180° meridian: 1 inferior segment 0.45 | 80% gained 3 lines BCVA, when steep K<55, BCVA +3 lines; when steep K>55, BCVA -1 line; in 3 of the 5 eyes that worsened, only 1 segment was used | In eyes gaining BCVA: mean change in SE 2.81 D, mean change in sph 2.11 D, mean change in cyl 1.50 D, mean change in ker 2.14 D.In eyes losing BCVA: mean change in SE 2.25 D, mean change in sph 1.40 D, mean change in cyl 1.71 D, mean change in ker 4.23 D |
| Ertan | 118 | 2006 | 1 Y | Femtosecond | Temporal | Asym (0.25/0.45 mm) | 81.3% and 73.7% gained lines of UCVA and BCVA, respectively | MRSE improved by > 2.00 D in 70.3% of eyes, mean change in SE 3.85 D, mean change in sph 2.97 D, mean change in cyl 1.7 D, mean change in ker 2.95 D |
| Kanellopoulos | 20 | 2006 | 12 M | Mechanical | Temporal and superior to the horizontal meridian | Asym (0.25/0.45 mm) | UCVA improved from 20/154 to 20/28 BCVA improved from 20/37 to 29/22 | Spheric refraction decreased from –3.38 D to –1.15 D, mean change in SE 3.46 D, mean change in sph 1.92 D, mean change in cyl 2.50 D, mean change in ker 2.95 D |
| Colin | 100 | 2007 | 2 Y | | Temporal | Sym (0.45/0.40 mm) | 80.5% and 68.3% gained lines of UCVA and BCVA, respectively | Mean MRSE improved from –6.93 D to –4.01 D |
| Zare | 30 | 2007 | 6 M | Mechanical | Temporal | SE 0-2 D 0.25/0.35; SE 2-3 D: 0.25/0.40; SE 3-5 D 0.25/0.45; SE 5-8 D: 0.35/0.45; SE > 8 D: 0.40/0.45 | 73.3% gained lines of BCVA | Mean change in SE 3.64±3.16 D, mean change in sph 3.02 D, mean change in cyl 0.75 D, mean change in ker 2.13±2.35 D |

CHAPTER 87

*Contd...*

| Study | Eyes | Yr | F/U | Surgical Procedure | Incision Site | Technique/ Implantation Criteria | Visual Acuity Change | Mean Refractive Change |
|---|---|---|---|---|---|---|---|---|
| Kymionis | 36 | 2007 | 60 M | Mechanical | | Central ectasia: 0.45 temporal/ 0.45 nasal | 59% gained lines of BCVA | Mean change in SE 2.52 D, mean change in ker 1.57±2.18 D |
| Shetty | 14 | 2008 | 12 M | Mechanical | Steep topographic meridian | | 69.23% gained lines of BCVA | Mean change in SE 5.00 D, mean change in sph 4.06 D, mean change in cyl 1.87 D, mean change in ker 3.98 D |
| Ertan | 306 | 2008 | 4 M | Femto-second | Temporal | | | Mean change in SE 3.09 D, mean change in sph 2.95 D, mean change in cyl 0.29 D, mean change in ker 2.79 D |

Asym: Asymmetrical; ax: Axis; BCVA: Best corrected visual acuity; cyl: Cylinder; FU: Follow-up; MRSE: Mean refractive spherical equivalent; SE: Spherical equivalent; Sph: Sphere; Sym: Symmetrical; UCVA: Uncorrected visual acuity
*This table summarizes the results reported in refs 15 and 16

in best-corrected vision. However, the range is large and variable ranging from 2 lines of loss of BCVA to a gain in 8 BCVA. ... 70% to 80% of the patients treated in all the studies noted an improvement in the best-corrected and uncorrected vision."[3]

Decrease in higher order aberrations has been shown by Rabinowitz and by other groups.[3]

Alio et al. compared the results of 13 eyes at 6, 12, 24 and 36 months follow-up (6 eyes with a 48 month follow-up) after Intacs implantation to evaluate stability of the outcomes and report refractive stability without a significant difference.[38] Mean BSCVA increased from 20/50 preoperatively to 20/30 postoperatively. Mean decrease of inferior–superior (I-S) asymmetry was 2.81 D. Mean difference between 6 and 36 months (stability) showed no significant difference regarding BSCVA and I-S asymmetry, despite the significant decrease in the average K values at 6 months. The decrease was not stable: when the results at 6 months were compared to the 36 month results, a significant average increase of 1.67 D was noticed at 36 months in the keratometry, but without reaching the initial preoperative value.[38] This is the only study that showed a decrease in the K reading values over an extended period of time. In contrast, Colin presented data on 35 Intacs implanted patients with a 5-year follow-up and reported refractive stability and no long-term complications.[15]

Ibrahim et al. reported on a study of 186 eyes with a 5-year follow-up after Intacs implantation, in which 63.5% of eyes were bilaterally implanted and 36.5% (68 eyes)

received unilateral Intacs implantation.[39] Preoperative mean keratometric reading was 52.53 D (range, 47.00–55.60 D), 15.6% of patients gained more than three lines and 69.7% gained one to three lines, meaning a total of 85.3% of patients gained lines compared with their preoperative UCVA. At the 5 year postoperative evaluation, the findings were 11.9%, 73.3% and 85.2%, respectively (P < .01). In terms of BCVA, 19.7% of patients gained more than three lines and 68.2% of patients gained one to three lines. A total of 87.9% of patients gained lines compared with their preoperative BCVA. Results at 5 years postoperative were 13.2%, 72.9% and 86.1%, respectively (P < .01). Corneal topographic surface quality indices suggested that surface regularity improved, and surface asymmetry was reduced. The postoperative minimum simulated keratometric readings were approximately 4.00 D less than the baseline. High order aberration showed a decrease in both lower and higher order aberrations.

Another study reported 9 years of postoperative stability in a bilateral keratoconic patient.[40] Nine years postoperatively, spherical equivalent refraction changed from preoperative −0.75 and −2.25 to +0.75 and −1.25 for the right and the left eyes, respectively. Uncorrected visual acuity improved from 20/50 to 20/25 in the right and from 20/200 to 20/32 in the left eye. Best spectacles corrected visual acuity of 20/20 in the right eye remained stable in comparison with the pre-Intacs BSCVA, while BSCVA improved from 20/25 to 20/20 in the fellow eye. No early or late complications were observed.

Guel et al. presented results of a 4-year follow-up: the keratoconus was of Grade II of Krumeich's classification, mean spherical equivalent (SE) and mean keratometry decreased by 2 D.[34] Uncorrected visual acuity improved in 43 eyes (93.4%), and BSCVA remained stable or improved in 38 eyes (82.6%). Eight eyes (17.4%) lost one line of BSCVA. Both BSCVA and SE refraction improved progressively during the first 6 months, and remained stable over the 4-year follow-up period. The authors reported that cylinder results were unpredictable. No intraoperative complications occurred.

Colin and Mallet reported on 100 eyes after 2 years of follow-up: the UCVA and BCVA improved in 80.5% and 68.3% of eyes, respectively (P < .001). The proportion of eyes with a BCVA greater than or equal to 20/40 increased from 22.0% at baseline to 51.2% and 53.7% at 1 year and 2 years, respectively (P < .001). The manifest refraction spherical equivalent improved from a mean of −6.93 D +/− 3.91 (SD) preoperatively to −4.01 +/− 3.16 D at 1 year and −3.80 +/− 2.73 D at 2 years (P < .001). The mean keratometry readings decreased from 50.1 +/− 5.6 D preoperatively to 46.4 +/− 5.3 D at 1 year and 46.8 +/− 4.9 D at 2 years (P < .001). Contact lens tolerance was restored in over 80% of cases. Postoperative slit lamp observations revealed no clinically significant issues.[41]

Colin reported on 8 years follow-up results in 65 eyes. According to his report, the results demonstrated that Intacs segments are a safe and efficacious option for the treatment of patients with moderate to severe keratoconus who are contact lens intolerant. The improved functional vision associated with this treatment modality can defer or potentially eliminate the need for corneal transplantation. He also noted that penetrating keratoplasty could be carried out if necessary, as was the case for five patients in his study.[42]

Kymionis et al. reported on 17 eyes of 15 keratoconic patients who had completed 5 years of follow-up (mean follow-up ± SD, 67.2 ± 7.5 months; range, 58–78 months). Two Intacs segments of 0.45 mm thickness were inserted in the cornea of each eye, so as to embrace the keratoconus area to try to achieve maximal flattening. No late postoperative complications occurred in this series of patients. At 5 years, the SE error reduction was statistically significantly, from pre-Intacs mean ± SD −5.54 ± 5.02 D (range: −12.50 to 3.63 D) to −3.02 ± 2.65 D (range: −8.25 to 1.88 D; P = .01). Pre-Intacs UCVA was 20/50 or worse in all eyes (range: from counting fingers to 20/50), whereas, at the last follow-up examination, 10 (59%) of 17 eyes had UCVA of 20/50 or better (range: from counting fingers to 20/32).

Six eyes (35%) maintained the pre-Intacs best BSCVA and one eye lost three lines of BSCVA, whereas the rest of the 10 eyes (59%) experienced a gain of one up to eight lines. There was no evidence of progressive sight-threatening complications.[43]

## Mechanical versus Intralase

Similar postoperative outcomes are reported in both approaches, as we may see from the literature review.

In a retrospective noncomparative case series,[44] Ertan et al. studied 118 eyes of 69 patients with keratoconus who had Intacs segments implanted with the femtosecond laser. Intacs were successfully implanted in all eyes. At the end of the first postoperative year, 81.3% of the eyes had improved UCVA and 73.7% had improved BCVA. The mean keratometry decreased from 51.56 D to 47.66 D, and the mean SE decreased from −7.57 D to −3.72 D.

Carrasquillo et al. evaluated the efficacy of ICRS implanted using either mechanical dissection (17 eyes) or a femtosecond laser (16 eyes) for treating keratoconus and post-LASIK keratectasia in 29 patients (total of 33 eyes). Mean follow-up was 10.3 months. Mean UCVA improved from 20/200 to 20/80; BSCVA improved from 20/40 to 20/30; MRSE decreased from −9D ± 4 to −7D ± 4; refractive cylinder (RC) decreased by 0.5 D or more in 62% of eyes; best contact lens corrected visual acuity (BCLVA) improved from 20/30 to 20/25 and contact lens tolerance improved in 81% of eyes. These researchers concluded that there was no statistically significant difference in outcomes between mechanical dissection and femtosecond laser-assisted techniques.[45]

However, another study reported statistically significant differences in visual or refractive results between femtosecond laser and mechanical tunnel creation.[20] Intacs were implanted in 10 eyes using the mechanical spreader to create the channels and subsequently in another 20 eyes using the femtosecond laser. Both groups showed significant reduction in the average of the following parameters: keratometry (K), SE, BSCVA, UCVA, surface regularity index (SRI), and surface asymmetry index (SAI). The laser group performed better in all parameters except change in SRI. Statistical analysis, however, did not reveal any statistically significant differences between the two groups for any single parameter studied. The biggest improvement in the laser group versus the mechanical group was BSCVA (P = .09). Overall success, defined as contact lens or spectacles tolerance, was 85% in the laser group and 70% in the mechanical group.

CHAPTER 87

The laser-assisted procedure is easier for the surgeon, more patient-friendly, and ensures accurate depth of placement of the Intacs, which cannot be guaranteed using the mechanical spreader.[20] Many corneal surgeons, who had abandoned the surgical technique with the mechanical spreader due to technical difficulties experienced with the device supplied by the manufacturer, have now once again started carrying out this procedure using the Intralase to create the channels in which the Intacs are inserted, due to the high degree of certainty of the depth of placement of the Intacs.[3]

The results of a comparative retrospective two-center outpatient study comprising 205 consecutive keratoconic eyes of 150 patients were recently reported.[15] Patients were classified into two groups according to channel dissection method: mechanical (Group 1: 100 consecutive keratoconic eyes of 82 patients) or femtosecond laser (Group 2: 105 eyes of 68 patients). Improvement in UCVA (Snellen lines) in Group 1 and Group 2 was, respectively, 1.29 G 1.78 and 1.91 G 1.93. Improvement in the BCVA (Snellen lines) in Group 1 and Group 2 was, respectively, 1.20 G 1.77 and 1.83 G 2.11. Improvement in the mean BCVA and improvement in the mean UCVA were significantly better in Group 2. The major limitation of the study was the use of a sample from two separate centers, due to the use of different devices and nomograms in each. This led to a large number of patients.[15] The author claims that femtosecond laser channel creation provides precise tunnel and keratotomy depth, width, and location (rarely requiring suture placement); minimal channel haze or edema; a uniform 360° channel; minimum risk for epithelial defect and stromal edema; low risk for infectious keratitis due to the absence of a foreign element placed in the cornea; advantages in deep eyes; and completion within seconds without manipulation of the cornea.[15]

## Reposition and Reimplantation of Intacs

In some cases, when the visual results obtained are unsatisfactory, the Intacs position should be adjusted to improve the visual outcomes. Pokroy and Levinger noted that they were able to improve the results in 8 of 58 patients who initially had a poor result.[46] After the initial Intacs surgery, six of these eyes had UCVA 20/100 and one had UCVA of 20/50. After the final Intacs adjustment, three eyes achieved UCVA 20/40, five achieved UCVA 20/70, and two remained less than 20/200. The indications for Intacs adjustments were increased astigmatism in

four eyes, induced hyperopia (overcorrection) in three, and undercorrection in one. One eye had both surgically-induced astigmatism and hyperopia. Induced astigmatism and hyperopia were most often managed by removing the superior segment. The undercorrected eye, having initially received a single inferior segment, was treated by implanting a superior segment. These authors concluded that approximately 10% of keratoconic eyes managed with Intacs may require Intacs adjustment surgery, which often has a good outcome. Guel et al. reported on two eyes (4.3%) that required repositioning of a segment that had been implanted too deeply in the corneal stroma. One month after surgery, the Intacs inserts were exchanged for thicker segments in one (2.1%) eye due to unexpected undercorrection. Exchange surgery was uneventful.[34]

Alio et al.[47] reported on significant visual and refractive improvements achieved by implanting a new ICRS combination after previous unsuccessful ICRS, which were explanted due to either poor visual results or extrusion. Twenty-one eyes were followed for 6 months postoperatively. All eyes were examined prior to and 1 month after initial ICRS implantation, before ICRS explantation, and 1 month and 6 months after implantation of the new ICRS.

They found a significant improvement in uncorrected distance visual acuity and thus a significant improvement in manifest refraction 1 month after implantation of the new ICRS. There was a statistically significant difference in keratometry readings and a significant improvement in corneal aberrometry between preoperatively and 6 months after the second surgery. There was no statistically significant difference in any parameter (visual, refractive, keratometric or aberrometric) between eyes that had ICRS explantation for segment extrusion and eyes that had explantation for poor visual outcomes.[47]

## ‣ COMPLICATIONS

Although ICSR surgery has so far shown positive results, complications can occur, both intraoperatively and postoperatively.

### Intraoperative Complications

Intraoperative complications during ICRS implantation are rare, as the study by Ibrahim et al., which reported zero intraoperative complications in 186 eyes, demonstrates.[39] Nevertheless, the following intraoperative adverse events have been described in relation to the mechanical procedure for corneal channelization, but always as isolated and rare events: segment decentration, asymmetry of the implants, inadequate depth of channel, and superficial channel dissection with anterior Bowman's layer perforation. Other complications include mechanical epithelial defects at the keratotomy site, extension of the incision towards the central visual axis or towards the limbus, shallow placement and/or uneven placement of the Intacs segments, and posterior corneal perforation during channel creation.[15,16]

Preoperative sphere and cylinder proved to be statistically significant parameters associated with intraoperative decentration, which can occur also with femtosecond assisted channel dissection in Intacs implantation.[48] The mechanism of the decentration, as reported by Ertan et al., is that during applanation for Intacs correction by a femtosecond laser, the cornea and pupil are not in their natural position, which leads to decentration and misalignment of the segments.[49]

## Postoperative Complications

Kanellopoulos et al. report a 35% postoperative complication rate in 20 eyes operated. This is the highest postoperative complication rate reported. It included segment movement and exposure as well as corneal melting. There was one case of anterior chamber perforation; six eyes had ring exposure secondary to corneal thinning over the implants at 3 and 6 months follow-up, and a dense corneal infiltrate developed in one patient at 7 months postoperatively.[26]

Other postoperative complications reported include segment extrusion, corneal neovascularization, infectious keratitis, mild channel deposits around Intacs ring segment, segment migration, epithelial plug at the incision site, corneal haze around segments or at the incision site, corneal melting, night halos, chronic pain (only one case described, additional details follow) and (only one case of) focal edema around segments.[16]

In the report by Ferrer et al. on explantation of ICRS, there were more complications numerically in the Intacs group in those cases in which the channels were created by femtosecond than mechanically.[50] This fact contradicts—at least in terms of postoperative complications—the claim that femtosecond assisted Intacs implantation is safer than the mechanical Intacs implantation procedure. Complaints of halo and glare that occur more frequently at night are not uncommon, because the procedure is frequently performed in younger patients with pupils of 7 mm (larger than the inner diameter of Intacs, which is 6.7 mm). Alphagan drops may be tried in these cases.

Unexplained loss of BSCVA 1 year after Intacs implantation necessitated PKP in a case reported by Guel et al.[34]

Pannus may compromise the results of PKP by increasing the chance of rejection. Personally, the author has seen a few cases of superficial or deep pannus, especially in the incision area after Intacs implantation. Regression of deep pannus was reported by Cosar et al.[51] They reported on a case of late deep corneal vascularization noted 3 years after intrastromal corneal ring segments (Intacs) implantation for the treatment of keratoconus, which necessitated the removal of the rings. The pannus subsided 10 days after rings' removal and topical treatment with corticosteroids. Ibrahim et al. report on one case of corneal vascularization (0.53%), which appeared 18 months post-Intacs implantation in a patient who used soft contact lenses.[39] Lovisolo et al. reported on Intacs removal due to neovascularization around the edge of one Intac and extrusion 1 year postoperatively.[52] Topography-guided PRK followed by CXL was performed 6 months after the removal of Intacs. Six months after the novel PRK and CXL, the patient's UCVA was 20/25 and BCVA 20/20 and the blood vessels disappeared.

### Extrusion

The most frequent postoperative complication is extrusion, which leads to explantation (removal of the segment implants). Explantation may be performed if the patient is dissatisfied with the visual postoperative outcomes.

Explantation rate varies significantly among studies, ranging from 0.98% to 30%.[15] Colin reported explantation in 12% of eyes implanted with Intacs, due to dissatisfaction with visual symptoms.[30] ICRS can be safely and easily explanted, with visual, refractive and topographic features returning to near the preimplantation levels.[53] Ibrahim et al. reported on two explanted rings (1.07%), one due to direct ocular trauma 6 weeks post surgery and the other due to continued progression of the cone 1 year post surgery. Both Intacs were easily removed under topical anesthesia through the original incision. Both patients underwent a successful deep anterior lamellar keratoplasty 4 weeks post-Intacs removal. No eyes lost any lines compared to their preoperative UCVA and BCVA.[39]

Ferrer et al. reported on the main reasons for explantation of ICRS (which included Intacs and Ferrara Rings) over a period of 9 years (between 2000 and 2008) and the relationship with microscopic findings on the ICRS surface.[50] Intrastromal corneal ring segments were explanted from 58 eyes (47 patients) of 250 implanted ICRS, a rate of

CHAPTER **87**

22.8%. The main cause was extrusion (48.2% of explanted segments); consequently, 10% of the ICRS implanted were removed due to extrusion, followed by unsatisfying refractive outcome (37.9%), keratitis (6.8%; 3.7% culture positive), and corneal melting and perforation (6.8%). The mean interval in all cases was 7.65 months (range 0.1–82.0 months). Thirty-seven of the 58 eyes had Intacs: 18 Intacs were removed because of extrusion, 12 because of refractive failure. All cases of corneal melting were in eyes with Intacs (two had tunnel creation by femtosecond laser and one by mechanical dissection) and in all cases, the clinician observed melting before extrusion occurred and extracted the ICRS to prevent further melting. In four cases (three of them Intacs), ICRS were removed because of suspected infection, in two cases (3.4%) the cultures were positive (*Staphylococcus aureus* and *Streptococcus mitis*) and in two cases negative. It is likely that the longer implantation-to-explantation time (years) was caused by stromal thinning over time and that the shorter time was due to incorrect positioning. Kugler et al. reported in an observational retrospective case series on four cases of corneal melting after insertion of ICRS for the treatment of ectasia. Each of the four cases of corneal melt occurred in an eye with a corneal incision overlying the ICRS, three of them in eyes after radial keratotomy (RK).[54]

The rate of ICRS explantation and its correlation to the surgical technique, type of segment, and year of implantation will be the focus of an upcoming study by the same authors.[55] Colin reported on explanation of the ICRS from four (4%) eyes without complications or sequela.[41]

In the author's experience, most cases of extrusion occur usually at the edge of the Intac on the incision side. He explants the Intac, cuts it and reinserts it. In the majority of these cases, patients whom he has followed for several years had no extrusion recurrence and the visual results were not compromised.

Shallow implantation is one of the causes of extrusion. It has been associated with ring superficialization, stromal thinning and epithelial breakdown.[56-59] Lai et al. performed optical coherence tomography (OCT) to examine the depth of Intacs implanted in the corneal stroma. OCT performed between 7 days and 43 days after implantation demonstrated that the position of the distal portions of the ring segments was shallower than that of the portion closer to the insertion site ($P = .003$). They reported that segments placed in the inferior cornea ($P = .008$) experienced more distal shallowing. Shallower depth was associated with greater fractional anterior stromal compression ($P = .04$).

The authors claimed that greater tensile strain on the anterior stroma could lead to gradual stromal breakdown in a process similar to keratoconus disease progression. In addition, these regions may experience more forward bowing of the anterior corneal surface over the implant. The greater anterior surface curvature may explain the epithelial breakdown. Superficially placed segments also may compromise diffusion of nutrients to the epithelium.[60]

Kamburgolu et al. used Pentacam to assess the depth of Intacs implanted by femtosecond laser and reported decreased depth of Intacs at the end of the first postoperative year in all measured points, and the change was statistically significant at the superior, inferior and temporal sides of the Intacs. The degree of change was not correlated with size of the Intacs, preoperative central corneal thickness or mean keratometric values.[61]

A Visante OCT scan showed Intacs partially bulging into the anterior chamber and partially compressing the stroma above them, in a case with two Intacs segments: one implanted 0.25 mm superiorly and 0.45 inferiorly in a keratoconic eye. The thicker Intacs segment appeared to compress the overlying stroma.[22] Toroquetti and Ferrara, in a letter of comment on the article of Ferrer on causes of ICRS explantation, wrote that there are two major causes of ICRS extrusion: superficial implantation of a segment and the placing of a segment too close to the incision. They claimed that as a general rule, the thickness of the implanted ICRS should not be more than 50% of the corneal thickness in the ring track. Moreover, the incision depth should preferentially be set at 80% of the corneal thickness. Deeply located ICRS produce better results and also leave a greater amount of corneal stroma between the ICRS and the corneal epithelium, which could theoretically protect from extrusion related to progressive stromal thinning. Only rarely does an extrusion begin in the middle of the segment or far from the incision. An ICRS that is placed close to the incision, especially if implanted superficially, is predisposed to adjacent corneal thinning and melting and subsequent extrusion.[62]

### Keratitis Post Intacs

According to the literature, the incidence of infectious keratitis after Intacs implantation for the treatment of myopia is low, ranging from 0.2% (48) to 0.63%.[56]

Keratitis was reported after Intacs inserted with either implantation technique. Proper management of this condition requires ICRS explantation and intensive topical antibiotics. Keratitis was reported in two of 134 eyes implanted with Intacs for treating keratoconus, one case of Intacs implanted mechanically and one femtosecond laser-assisted implantation.[63] Levy et al. reported on keratitis in a case which developed weeks after femtosecond laser-assisted implantation of Intacs, and they state that it was reported at least in one other case.[64] However, based on the literature review, the number of cases is greater than two.[50]

Chaudhry et al. reported on a 20-year-old woman who developed bilateral severe infectious keratitis 11 days after uncomplicated implantation of ICRSs for keratoconus. Cultures obtained at the time of initial presentation yielded *Streptococcus viridans*. The patient responded well to the treatment and was left with stromal scars in both corneas. The authors concluded that early recognition of infection, aggressive treatment with antibiotics and, in some cases, removal of ICRSs may be necessary to prevent serious sight-threatening complications following this refractive procedure.[65] Infection most commonly occurs as a result of a loose stitch or as a result of wound gape from migration of the Intacs to the site of the wound.[3] Culturing the Intacs might be helpful in isolating the organism.[3] Anthony et al. reported on a case of traumatic shattering of intrastromal segments due to blunt trauma, with successful removal of the fragments.[66] The authors reported that the eye was white, the cornea clear, three fractures lines were visible in the upper Intac and two in the lower one. They hypothesized that the shattered segments had sharp edges and there was a concern of anterior or posterior erosion of the fragments through the cornea, yet they report that they removed the segments also at the patient's insistence.

Removing the segments due to the patient's insistence is beyond discussion, whereas the possible removal of the ring segments because of an unverified hypothesis that keeping the segments might cause anterior or posterior erosion merits a comment. Given that there has been no report in the literature concerning this type of case, and furthermore, the 10% incidence of extrusion that has been reported was not associated with damaged edges of the segments.[50]

The author has been implanting Intacs for more than 9 years and Ferrara rings for more than 8 years, and there were cases of extrusion, especially in the first few years. If the extrusion occurs at the end of the segment and the rest of it is deep in the cornea, he removes the segment, puts it in sterile polydine 4%, washes it with saline, cuts it with precision scissors and reinserts it in the channel. He follows up on most of these cases for years; the positive refractive results are usually maintained. The ends where the segments are cut are uneven; nonetheless, they do not erode either anteriorly or posteriorly if they are deep in the cornea.

In cases of extrusion, part of the segment may still do the job sufficiently, especially in the case of the inferior one. Thus, if the end of an inferior segment extrudes, cutting it or inserting a smaller segment (if available) should be considered, rather than totally removing the segments.

## Pain after Intacs

Randleman reported chronic pain after Intacs implantation and persistent discomfort caused by direct contact between the segment and corneal nerve, which did not improve with topical medication or a bandage contact lens. After removal of the segments, the pain resolved. Confocal microscopy demonstrated a corneal nerve in direct contact with the inferior Intacs segment. One day after the removal, the patient reported complete resolution of pain, and she remained pain free.[67]

## Infiltrates

Rau et al. reported a 13.3% prevalence of corneal infiltrates.[68] Ruckhofer et al. reported the frequency of intrastromal deposits after Intacs implantation in myopic eyes at 24 months: 213 (74%) of 359 myopic eyes had deposits and the incidence of deposits increased with ring thickness and duration.[69] However, these deposits do not appear to affect the performance of the segment rings or the progression of keratoconus.

Reporting on the results of Intacs implantation using two different channel sizes created by femtosecond laser, Ertan et al. found yellow-white deposits in 10 eyes (10.30%) of the large channel group and in 29 eyes (46.77%) of the narrow channel group.[29]

Guel reported on a case of sterile infiltration along one segment that required the extraction of one of the inserts. This infiltration was probably related to underlying rosacea that was diagnosed postoperatively.[34]

Ertan et al.[29] observed an epithelial plug at the incision site in 15.2% of eyes. This may have been the result of trauma during Intacs placement and a temporary gap at the unsutured incision site. Over 6 postoperative months, a few granulomatous particles around the Intacs segment were observed in 8.5% of the 118 eyes.[29]

Other rare complications include persistent inflammation, persistent fluctuation of vision, intraocular inflammation, photophobia, loss of uncorrected and best-corrected visual acuity and vascularization of the wound.[3]

CHAPTER **87**

Park et al. describe a case of a 53-year-old woman with keratoconus who presented with a dislocated Intacs in the anterior chamber 3 weeks after surgery. The Intacs were removed.[70]

In a unique report of corneal Intacs migration following implantation using the Femtosecond laser, Feldman et al. described a case where postoperatively, both rings migrated inferiorly and overlapped each other in a double-stacked formation. This migration led to a dramatic improvement in VA. Thicker segments may provide enhanced anatomic and visual effects in some keratoectatic patients.[71]

Despite the reported complications, Intacs implantation in keratoconic eyes remains a safe, adjustable and reversible procedure.

## ▶ HISTOLOGY AND DEPOSITS

### Anterior Channel Fibrosis and Increased Scattering

Microdeposits and abnormal lamellar structure adjacent to Intacs were seen using confocal microscopy.[40] Deposits on or adjacent (both inward and outward) to the segments are most probably related to intracellular lipids accumulation or morphologically abnormal cellular structures.[4,72] The incidence of intrastromal deposits (intracellular lipids) in the corneal tunnel can be as high as 60% (Figs 4A and B).[69] A case report by Twa et al. studied morphological characteristics of lamellar channel deposits in the human eye next to an Intac implant. Extracellular matrix (ECM) components typically associated with fibrosis were observed. The keratoconus cases displayed typical Bowman layer breaks and subepithelial fibrosis with deposition of various ECM components. In all cases, some keratocytes around Intacs were positive for specific proteinases associated with stromal remodelling.[73]

Another study showed that ring segments induced keratocyte apoptosis, but these changes are reversible after implant removal.[69]

Samimi et al. reported on the histopathological findings of keratoconus buttons at the time of keratoplasty following Intacs implantation.[74] This retrospective study involved eight patients who had PKP after removal of Intacs inserts, because of a poor refractive outcome or insert extrusion. Conventional histology showed hypoplasia of the epithelium immediately surrounding the channel. There was no evidence of an inflammatory response or foreign-body granuloma. Keratocyte density was decreased above and below the tunnel. All samples stained negatively with a smooth muscle actin, indicating that myofibroblasts were not present. These changes were no longer visible after PKP was performed, more than 6 months after Intacs explantation. The authors concluded that histological changes seemed to be entirely reversible after implant removal.[74]

Ly et al. assessed the structure and location of intrastromal lipid deposits after implantation of Intacs, using *in vivo* confocal microscopy in seven eyes of six patients, examined 5 years (n = 6) or 2 months (n = 1) after uncomplicated implantation of Intacs for the correction of mild myopia.[75] In the peripheral cornea of eyes examined 5 years after surgery, epithelial and endothelial cell layers appeared normal. Stromal haze was seen surrounding the

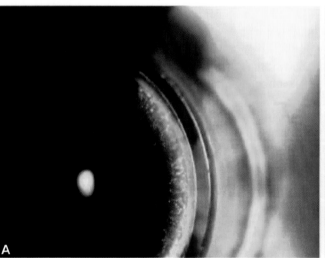
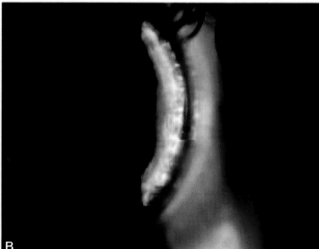

**Figs 4A and B:** (A) Deposits; (B) Crystal-like deposits

implants in all eyes examined, but no keratocyte activation was noted. Reflective amorphous or crystalline structures consistent with lipid deposition were detected in all eyes with long-term implantation of Intacs. Deposits were localized to the inner and outer edges of Intacs segments and to the region anterior to the implant. Confocal microscopy did not show any deposits in the eye examined 2 months after surgery, although the region anterior to the implant appeared hazy and edematous. Areas central to the implant appeared normal in all eyes.

Ruckhofer et al. performed confocal real-time microscopy on a total of 21 eyes from 11 patients.[76] Seventeen eyes from 10 patients who underwent uncomplicated ICRS surgery to correct myopia and were examined after surgery (average 8.6 months; range 2–15 months). Three patients had the ICRS implanted into only one eye, and those eyes were compared with the untreated fellow eyes. One eye of another patient was examined 1 and 6 months after ICRS removal. In the central cornea, the researchers found normal morphologic features at all layers. In peripheral sections, epithelial cells with highly reflective nuclei in the basal cell layer were observed in 6 of 17 eyes (35%) implanted with ICRS. They found an intact corneal nerve plexus and undisturbed corneal endothelium immediately underneath the ICRS. Around the ICRS, moderate fibrosis was seen. In one eye, linear structures in bamboo-like orientation were detected after ICRS removal in the last keratocyte layer underneath the collapsed tunnel. Concluding that the central corneal zone appeared unchanged, the corneal stroma adjacent to the ICRS was observed, which displayed a slight but distinct activation of wound healing. Epithelial cells with highly reflective nuclei in this region may be an indicator of increased biologic stress caused by the device.[76]

Ferrer et al. found no inflammatory material on the surface of any ICRS explanted for refractive failure (poor refractive outcome), showing the biocompatibility of PMMA in the area of ICRS implantation. They found macrophages and deposits only in cases of extrusion, but not in cases of ICRS removal due to refractive failure. The deposits, unlike in other reports, were in the inner curvature, along the ICRS, or near the extruded end; in addition, the deposits appeared more diffuse. In most cases (68.8%) of extruded segments, they observed inflammatory infiltrate that was larger near the wound, although deposits were seen at the segment edge. This indicates that epithelial breakdown and close contact between the corneal stroma and the tear film play a role in triggering this reaction.[50]

Migration of macrophages to the wound site, localized edema, and activation of keratocytes to fibroblast and myofibroblast phenotypes would be consistent with normal tissue response to surgical trauma. The lipid drops that were found on the surface of extruded ICRS were reported to be a consequence of trauma that occurred during implantation surgery or corneal suturing.[50]

The process of lipid accumulation might have been the result of host rejection, or it might have occurred because the superficial part of the stroma thinned over time causing the extrusion. Although the second option seems more plausible, additional studies are required to substantiate this claim.[50] The authors concluded that lack of inflammatory reaction in cases of ICRS explanted for refractive failure confirms the biocompatibility of PMMA segments in the corneal stroma.[50] Accumulation of foamy histiocytes along the lamellar channels was reported.[77]

Torquetti and Ferrara[62] believe that the inflammatory cells and cell debris found in cases of extrusion are the consequence—rather than the cause—of the extrusion. The progressive epithelial and stromal thinning can lead to segment exposure, which in turn can lead to a local inflammatory reaction, triggering corneal melting around the segment, with subsequent extrusion.

## Corneal Biomechanics and Intacs

Once the segments are inserted, the curvature is decreased centrally, including the region of the cone. As curvature is decreased in this region, the stress is redistributed, and the decompensatory biomechanical cycle of keratoconus is broken.[78] Attempts are made to measure *in vivo* the biomechanical characteristics of the cornea.

Corneal hysteresis (CH) and corneal resistance factor (CRF) are new terms which are supposed to report on the corneal biomechanics. These terms are part of the measurements made by the ocular response analyzer (ORA, Reichert). Dauwe et al. reported on the biomechanical and morphological corneal response to placement of intrastromal corneal ring segments for keratoconus treatment. They state that although ICRS significantly decreased corneal curvature, with preoperative values predicting magnitude of change, it did not alter the viscoelastic biomechanical parameters of CH and CRF.[79]

In the author's practice he has not seen any significant change in CH or CRF after Intacs implantation (unpublished data). Not only the data remain unchanged but also the graph pattern remains constant, reflecting the changes typical in keratoconus cases (see chapter on ORA and keratoconus).

## ADDITIONAL PROCEDURES TO ENHANCE INTACS' EFFECTS

### Intacs Combined with Intraocular Lenses

In some cases, although Intacs reduce astigmatism and myopia and improve corneal irregularity, high ametropia—uncorrectable by glasses—remains. In cases of high ametropia, in patients unable to tolerate or unwilling to wear contact lenses, phakic intracorneal rings can be considered to improve uncorrected refractive error or pseudophakic intraocular lenses (IOL) in patients with cataract.

The corneal rings are usually inserted 3 months before the intraocular lens insertion.[3] Good outcomes have been reported when used in combination with both the Visian ICL and the Verisyse Phakic IOL.[20,80-83] This is a reversible procedure that is less invasive than penetrating keratoplasty. Kamburoglu et al. reported on Artisan toric phakic IOL implantation after Intacs, to correct residual myopic and astigmatic refractive errors. Five months postoperatively, the UCVA was 0.6 and the BCVA was 0.7.[82]

Budo et al. implanted Artisan toric phakic intraocular lenses (pIOLs) in both eyes of three patients with keratoconus. Postoperatively, four of the six eyes were within 1.00 D of emmetropia.[84]

Colin and Velou implanted an anterior chamber pIOL after Intacs implantation in a patient with keratoconus. The refractive results were satisfactory; there was minimal residual myopia.[85]

Toric pIOLs may be preferred in eyes with high astigmatic refractive errors. Controlled randomized studies with longer follow-up are needed to decide which type of lens to use and to evaluate safety, predictability and stability.[15]

El-Raggal et al. conducted a 24-month follow-up of six patients (eight keratoconic eyes) who had maximum k values of 60 D and underwent sequential Intacs and a Verisyse pIOL implantation for refractive improvement.[80] All eyes achieved UCVA of 20/40 or better. The final spherical error ranged from −1.75 D to 1.00 D and the cylindrical error ranged from 1.25 to 2.50 D. No eye lost lines of preoperative BCVA. These results were relatively stable throughout the follow-up period. The authors concluded that the procedure was safe, stable and effective in selected cases of keratoconus.

Guell implanted in two eyes of the same patient toric phakic iris-claw Artisan (Ophtec BV Groningen, The Netherlands) IOL to correct the remaining refractive error in keratoconic patients who had Intacs implantation.[34] Moshirfar et al. reported on simultaneous and sequential implantation of Intacs and Verisyse phakic intraocular lens for refractive improvement in keratectasia.[86] They collected data from 19 eyes of 12 patients (5 eyes, postlaser in situ keratomileusis ectasia and 14 eyes, keratoconus). Intacs segments were implanted followed by the insertion of a phakic Verisyse lens at the same session (12 eyes) in the 'simultaneous group', or several months later (7 eyes) in the 'sequential group'.

No intraoperative or postoperative complications were observed. At the last follow-up (19 ± 6 months), in the simultaneous group, mean spherical error was −0.79 ± 1.0 D (range, −2.0 to +1.50 D) and cylindrical error +2.06 ± 1.21 D (range, +0.5 to +3.75 D). In the sequential group, at the last follow-up, at 36 ± 21 months, the mean spherical error was −1.64 ± 1.31 D (range, −3.25 to +1.0 D) and cylindrical error +2.07 ± 1.03 D (range, +0.75 to +3.25 D). There was no significant difference in mean uncorrected visual acuity or BSCVA between the two groups preoperatively or postoperatively. No eye lost lines of preoperative BSCVA.

### Photorefractive Keratectomy Following Intacs

Photorefractive keratectomy was reported as successful for the correction of residual refractive error with Intacs intrastromal corneal ring segments in place.[87] Hirsh et al. performed LASEK (laser-assisted epithelial keratomileusis) on four patients with stable keratoconus 6 months after Intacs implantation, to correct residual myopia and astigmatism.[88] The mean refraction prior to LASEK was myopia of −0.2D and astigmatism of −2.71 D. The mean follow-up period after LASEK was 8 months. Prior to both surgeries, the mean UCVA was 6/240 (range, count fingers to 6/60) and at the final postoperative visit 6/12 (range 6/10–6/18). The preoperative mean BSVCA was 6/15 (range 6/10–6/24) and at the final postoperative follow-up visit 6/9 (range 6/8.5–6/12). They concluded that wavefront-guided LASEK for correction of residual myopia and astigmatism in keratoconus patients after Intacs insertion and stable refraction provided excellent visual outcome, with no loss of visual acuity and no complications.

Guell reported on one eye that underwent PRK after Intacs implantation.[34] Intracorneal ring segments implantation followed by same-day photorefractive keratectomy and corneal collagen cross-linking in keratoconus in five eyes of four patients was reported by Iovieno A et al., all patients first underwent femtosecond laser-enabled placement of ICRS. Six months after Intacs plus PRK/CXL, significant improvements were noted for UCVA, BCVA, spherical equivalent refraction, keratometry and total aberrations. No patient lost lines of CDVA or developed haze.[89]

## Intacs and Collagen Corneal Crosslinking

Corneal collagen crosslinking is a relatively new therapy using ultraviolet A (UVA) with a photosensitizer riboflavin to increase corneal stiffness. It has been shown that CXL is effective in arresting the progression of keratoconus. Intacs are an effective tool for improvement of VA in keratoconic patients.

Most of the patients suffering from keratoconus are confused and ask us for advice, whether to do only CXL or only intrastromal corneal ring segment implantation (ICRS) to combine both. The author hopes that this section will shed some light on this issue.

Chan et al.[90] observed that CXL without Intacs placement induced flattening largely over the cone itself[91] and they assumed that Intacs and CXL may have an additive effect.[90] In their retrospective nonrandomized comparative case series of 25 eyes, one group was treated with a single inferior Intacs (12 eyes of 9 patients), and the other group (13 eyes of 12 patients) with a single inferior Intacs combined with CXL. The two groups were matched preoperatively. The incision was done in the steep axis of manifest refraction. Corneal collagen crosslinking with riboflavin was performed after the Intacs segments were inserted. The authors demonstrated that the combination of CXL with Intacs led to better results than Intacs insertion alone, as they obtained greater reductions in manifest cylinder, K steep, and K average, and there was a greater than twofold reduction in steep and average keratometric values. Their explanation for this increased effect was that a biomechanical coupling occurs due to local collagen changes around the Intacs segment. They observed that the riboflavin solution pooled in the contiguous area above the superior edge of the Intacs segment and also appeared to penetrate the channel of the Intacs, and assumed that this may produce increased riboflavin concentration in that area and as a consequence the crosslinking in that area may increase. The biomechanical changes induced by the Intacs insertion may facilitate the changes caused by CXL.

All of the long-term studies on Intacs show stability of the results. Only one work, that of Alio, which demonstrated a mean increase of 1.67 in mean K readings between 6 and 36 months of follow-up suggests that the improvement obtained after Intacs implantation decreased over time.[38] Although Intacs produce a certain biomechanical effect, they do not treat the cause of the disease, which is the weakness of the collagen fibers. This 'job' is done by CXL. Therefore, the combination of the two treatments is logical.

As shown in this chapter, Intacs are occasionally explanted. The combined procedure may give us some confidence that even if the Intacs are removed due to possible complications, the cornea will be stronger and more stable because of the CXL. This is important in patients who have a progressing keratoconus. The young modulus increased 4.5 folds after CXL.[92] The possibility of a more than a simple additive effect was supported by a study (by L Cadarso et al. reported in 14) in porcine eyes. In the study, three pigs had one eye randomized to crosslinking with Intacs and 1 eye treated with only CXL. The Intacs were removed 3 weeks postoperatively. The eyes that had both treatments continued to show additional flattening compared with eyes in the crosslinking group, even after the Intacs segments were removed. Thus, crosslinking can be used in conjunction with Intacs insertion to attain stability if further progression occurs after Intacs insertion or to achieve further flattening.[15]

Kamburoglu and Ertan demonstrated the additive effect of CXL after Intacs SK in a case of post-LASIK ectasia.[93] They implanted Intacs SK in both eyes of a patient suffering from bilateral post-LASIK ectasia; in the left eye, transepithelial CXL was performed. At one day post operation, Intacs SK inserts were placed horizontally in the right eye, using a superior ring of 400 μm, and an inferior one of 450 μm. Three days after Intacs SK implantation, UCVA improved to 20/60 and BSCVA improved to 20/25, with a manifest refraction of −2.50 −2.50 × 170 in the right eye. Keratometric readings were 43.60/51.10 D (mean: 47.10 D). At 1 month follow-up, UCVA decreased to 20/100 and BSCVA to 20/40, with a manifest refraction of −5.00 −3.00 × 170, and keratometric values of 46.80/51.70 D (mean: 49.20 D). At 8 months post CXL, UCVA was 20/30 and BSCVA was 20/25 with a cylinder refraction of −1.50 × 170. Keratometry was 45.00/49.50 D (mean: 47.20 D).

Ertan et al. reported on 25 eyes of 17 patients with bilateral keratoconus who underwent Intacs implantation with subsequent CXL. The results in Intacs only group were compared with those obtained after Intacs combined with CXL. Patients' mean age was 25.14 ± 7.11 (range 16–39) years. Mean time between implantation of Intacs and CXL was 3.98 months. Collagen crosslinking after

Intacs resulted in an additional improvement in UCVA, BCVA, sphere, cylinder and keratometry. Intacs alone resulted in an improvement of 1.9 Snellen lines (P < 0.05) of UCVA and 1.7 Snellen lines (P < 0.05) of BCVA. Collagen crosslinking performed after Intacs treatment yielded an additional 1.2 Snellen lines (P < 0.05) of UCVA and 0.36 Snellen lines (P < 0.05) of BCVA. After Intacs treatment, the decrease in spherical, cylindrical, mean K, and steepest K values was 2.08 D (P < 0.05), 0.47 D (P > 0.05), 2.22 D (P < 0.05), and 1.27 D (P < 0.05), respectively. An additional 0.5 D (P < 0.05), 0.15 D (P > 0.05), 0.35 D (P > 0.05), and 0.76 D (P < 0.05) of improvement was gained after CXL in each respective parameter. These results led to the conclusion that collagen crosslinking had an additive effect on Intacs implantation in these eyes and may be considered as an enhancement and stabilizing procedure.[94]

Coskunseven et al. performed Intacs implantation and collagen corneal crosslinking combined, but in a different sequence, in two groups of patients, and the two groups were followed for 13 months ± 1.[95] In Group 1, CXL was performed and then followed by Intacs implantation, while in Group 2, the rings were implanted and then CXL was performed. The interval between the treatments was 7 months ± 2, in both groups. The mean UCVA and BCVA improved in both groups; the mean SE, cylinder, and mean K values decreased in both groups. Overall, there was more improvement in BCVA, SE and mean K in Group 2 than in Group 1. Overall, there was more improvement in CDVA, SE, and mean K in Group 2 than in Group 1. These results confirm what we already know from our experience. Corneal rings have a greater effect on a keratoconic cornea than on a normal cornea and the cornea without crosslinking is weaker than one with crosslinking; therefore, the effect of the rings should be stronger prior to crosslinking. The author personally performs ring implantation and then CXL when he performs both treatments. Since 2006, he implants the rings first, and only then removes the epithelium and does the CXL.

Guell et al. state that CXL performed after Intacs implantation in keratoconic eyes has provided better results and has a more logical rationale than Intacs insertion alone, as evidenced by greater reductions in manifest cylinder and keratometry readings.[18]

Vincente et al. contradicted the conclusion of Alio et al. regarding the unsatisfactory results of Intacs implantation in advanced keratoconus, as they showed that worse preoperative vision (BCVA and spherical equivalent) and K-average values resulted in greater improvement in BCVA. They performed the combined Intacs and CXL procedure and explained that the augmented improvement in the more severe cases of keratoconus was due to the effect of transepithelial crosslinking. It might also have been that worse cases have greater improvement from baseline compared with patients with milder keratoconus. The findings suggested that patients with more advanced keratoconus still benefited from the combined approach, as they obtained greater improvement in visual parameters compared to the milder cases, even though their final BCVA was not as good as for milder cases.[96]

These are the 3-year results reported by the above-mentioned group: mean preoperative BCVA was 0.24, and spherical equivalent of −2.95 ± 3.29 (range −12.50 to +2.12). These were found to be correlated with the amount of improvement in BCVA after combined Intacs and crosslinking, using simple regression analysis. In addition, the UCVA, spherical value and K-average were also found to have direct correlation with postoperative BCVA. The mean BCVA after 3 years improved to 0.16; all keratometry values improved significantly. K-steep improved from 48.37 ± 2.94 preoperatively to 45.86 ± 4.06 postoperatively; K-flat improved from 43.29 ± 3.13 preoperatively to 42.21 ± 3.31 postoperatively; K-average improved from 45.83 ± 2.45 (range 39.85–50.76) to 44.03 ± 3.58 (range 34.85–50.47) postoperatively, (p = 0.0023); and K-power improved from 47.33 ± 2.81 (range 44.57–55.18) preoperatively to 45.04 ± 3.32 (range 39.50–54.43) postoperatively.[96]

Lovisolo et al. implanted Intacs in 12 eyes immediately before CXL. No specific complication was seen in any of the patients. Their experience of CXL application after Intacs surgery confirms the conclusion that cross-linking with riboflavin augments the positive effects of Intacs surgery.[97]

Over the last 4 years, the author has performed CXL following Intacs implantation in a few cases that suffered a regression. The cornea was stabilized by this added procedure (unpublished data). He also performed Intacs implantation with CXL immediately following the implantation. He removes the epithelium and starts the procedure of CXL.

Barbara R et al. published a case report on CXL after post-PRK ectasia followed by the implantation of one Intac with improvement of UCVA, BSCVA and reduction of astigmatism.[98]

## Contact Lenses after Intacs

Intacs implantation improves contact lens tolerance in patients with keratoconus.[3]

A study of 12 contact lens intolerant keratoconic eyes that underwent Intacs implantation with no intra- or postoperative complications found improved measures in UCVA, BCVA and K readings. Eight eyes were then able to wear contact lenses.[99] A different study, which followed 14 patients (24 keratoconic eyes) for a period of 1 year after Intacs implantation, found that 60% of the patients tolerated contact lenses.[27]

Guel et al. reported on one patient who was successfully fitted with a soft contact lens after Intacs implantation for treatment of keratoconus.[34]

Most of the studies mentioned in this chapter report better tolerance of contact lenses after Intacs, because the cornea is flattened and more regular after the procedure. The author has fitted patients following Intacs implantation with soft contact lenses, keratoconus soft contact lenses, and gas permeable contact lenses, with no special requirements from the manufacturers of the lenses. Some patients who had been intolerant of RGP contact lenses became tolerant to normal soft or keratoconus soft contact lenses, while others were able to tolerate again RGP contact lenses.

Smith et al. reported on a case of a keratoconic patient with Intacs fitted with a high-Dk piggyback contact lens system. The patient was able to wear the piggyback contact lenses comfortably 12–18 hours per day and was corrected to 20/25 (OD), 20/30 (OS) and 20/20 (OU)).[100]

Patients were fitted with a soft contact lens for visual rehabilitation 5 months after Intacs placement.[101] Nepmuceneo reported on fitting contact lenses after Intacs implantation in three eyes: two were fitted with larger than usual lens designs made of rigid gas-permeable material, and one eye was fitted with a toric soft lens. Fitting contact lenses for keratoconus patients who have Intacs inserts is feasible and has a role in augmenting their vision.[102]

Lovisolo et al. reported on several patients who had been "absolutely contact lens intolerant" and subsequently were comfortable wearing RGP contacts on a daily basis some months after Intacs implantation followed by CXL. They claimed that the regularization of the anterior corneal surface, which follows this combined treatment, might explain the positive shift.[52] The same authors also reported that overnight corneal molding by RGP contact lens lasted longer in these patients than in 'vergine keratoconic eyes'. The surface reshaping in virgin keratoconic eyes does not last longer than 2–3 hours after contact lens wear is suspended, due to unexplained biomechanical changes in the cornea after Intacs implantation.[52]

Mini scleral rigid lens design was used successfully in a case of advanced keratoconus after implantation of Intacs.[103]

Kymionis G et al. reported on severe central corneal neovascularization after prolonged use of RGP contact lens in an eye treated with Intacs implantation that recessed 1 month after discontinuing contact lens use. In the fellow eye of the same patient in which no Intacs were implanted, only mild peripheral neovascularization was observed.[104]

## Kerarings Post Intacs

Coskunseven reported on three eyes (two keratoconic patients) with previous Intacs implantation that underwent adjuvant single Keraring (Mediphacos) intrastromal corneal ring segment implantation.[105] Uncorrected visual acuity, BCVA improved significantly, and K readings were reduced.

The author implanted Ferrara rings in a similar case. After initial satisfactory results following Intacs implantation, the patient regressed in terms of UCVA and MRSE. The author implanted a pair of Ferrara rings, but a few months later the patient developed severe keratitis, and the superior Intac and the superior Ferrara segment were explanted. The patient remained with two inferior segments: one Intac and one Ferrara segment, with satisfactory UCVA and BSCVA. A few years later he regressed, and the author performed CXL, and stability was achieved.

Lovisolo et al. described an anecdotal case in which a 'LASIK-on keratoconus' eye received four ring segments: a pair of 450 μm Intacs 2 years after excimer surgery, and a pair of 250 μm Ferrara Rings, 3 years postoperatively.[52] Eight years after the original surgery, the same eye was treated with CXL. Two years after cross linking and 10 years after the original surgery, the eye showed topographic and refractive stability; the patient complied well with a 20/90 uncorrected visual acuity, and a 20/30 spectacle corrected acuity was obtained with glasses. Only for night driving did the patient require a custom-made rigid gas permeable (RGP) contact lens, which restored 20/20 vision.

## ▶ INTACS COMPARED WITH OTHER SURGICAL PROCEDURES

### Intacs versus Kerarings

Pinero et al. reported on two groups of keratoconic patients treated using either Intacs (Group A) or Kerarings

(Group B).[106] The corneal tunnels were created mechanically or with a femtosecond laser. Group A comprised 100 eyes and Group B 68 eyes. The postoperative increase in UCVA and BCVA was statistically significant in both groups (P < 0.05). Group A had greater improvement in BCVA than Group B at 6 months and at 1 year (both P < 0.001). At 1 year, the mean maximal decrease in K power was statistically significant in Group A: from 51.27 D (4.46 SD) to 47.87D (3.39 SD) and in Group B, from 51.12D (4.54 SD) to 47.58D (3.66 SD; P < .05). The mean reduction in maximum K reached greater statistical significance in Group A than in B, at 6 months and 1 year.

The authors concluded that both ICRS models were effective and safe in managing keratoconus; the Keraring ICRS led to more improvement in BCVA and UCVA and a greater reduction in the maximum K value.[106]

In a retrospective study, 16 eyes that had been implanted with Intacs ICRS and 17 eyes implanted with Ferrara ICRS were evaluated. Pre- and postoperative examinations were performed 1 year postoperatively. The study reported a significant decrease noted in spherical equivalent refractive error of 3.76 ± 0.39 D and 3.42 ± 0.88 D and keratometry of 3.43 ± 0.24 D and 3.28 ± 0.78 D in the Intacs and Ferrara groups, respectively; and increase in mean in UCVA and BCVA of 0.18 ± 0.04 and 0.21 ± 0.05, respectively, in the Intacs group and 0.21 ± 0.09 and 0.26 ± 0.08, respectively, in the Ferrara group (P < .01 for all). The postoperative increase in UCVA and BCVA and decrease in keratometry readings were not significantly different between groups (P > .05 for all). Mean higher order aberrations decreased in the Intacs group and increased in the Ferrara group (P > .05 for both). Postoperatively, a significant decrease was noted in scotopic contrast sensitivity when glare was introduced in the Ferrara group, which was positively correlated with pupil diameter.[107]

## Intacs versus Penetrating Keratoplasty

In 2005, Yahalom et al. evaluated the major indications in 1681 PKP cases over the previous 40 years in Israel; keratoconus was the leading indication in 24.1% of cases.[108] A study conducted in Venezuela, which assessed 511 PKP cases between 1996 and 2002, found keratoconus to be the leading indication in 41.80% cases (unpublished data cited by Rodriguez).[109]

Rodriguez et al. performed a nonrandomized comparative study and analysis of retrospective data of 17 patients who had PKP in one eye and Intacs implantation in the other eye.[109] Patients were classified into two groups:

asymmetric (different grade of keratoconus in each eye; eight patients) and symmetric (same grade of keratoconus in both eyes; nine patients). The follow-up was 24 months for the PKP and more than 10 months for Intacs. The results indicated more rapid recovery in the Intacs group, and no intra- or postoperative complications were noted in the eyes with Intacs. Complications in eyes with PKP included cataract, graft rejection and elevated intraocular pressure. The main difference between the procedures was that it took less time for Intacs eyes to achieve their potential visual acuity.

In the same reported study, three of the eyes with PKP had adverse reactions, including graft rejection, vascularization, a significant decrease in endothelial cell count, and a need for long-term steroid therapy. One patient had an elevation in intraocular pressure in the PKP eye and required glaucoma treatment. Two PKP patients required cataract surgery. No eye with Intacs required PKP or explantation of the segments. The authors compared the outcomes of the two techniques in an adolescent (14-year-old) patient. The PKP eye had two episodes of graft rejection, due to the patient's age-related highly sensitive immune system. These rejections were successfully controlled with steroid treatment. The keratoconus eye with Intacs in this patient had no complications over a 10-month follow-up.[109]

Despite the convincing long-term survival rates, endothelial failure, immunologic graft rejection, and ocular surface disease are persistent risks that can appear any time after surgery. Therefore, there is a need for follow-up throughout the patient's life.[110] In a longitudinal review of 3992 eyes that had PKP at a large tertiary care center, Thompson et al. found an 82% 10-year survival rate of first-time grafts.[110]

The incidence of high astigmatism after keratoplasty varies from 10% to 20%.[111,112] One way of managing high astigmatism is by fitting contact lenses; however, they can compromise corneal transplant survival if vascularization of the graft occurs. Other surgical options for managing post-PKP astigmatism include astigmatic keratotomy, compression sutures, wedge excision, and LASIK.[113]

## Sample Case Report 1

The author includes this case as a typical example of the implantation of Intacs for treating keratoconus. Moreover, this was his first case using this treatment, and one in which long-term follow-up was possible. The patient, a 54-year-old woman, was operated in her right eye to treat keratoconus. Preoperative data were as follows: UCVA

2 meter finger count; BSCVA 20/60+pin hole 20/50; refraction −6.5 ≈ −7, cylinder 33°; K 53.0 D – 60.37 D, K average 56.5 D; central corneal thickness (CCT) 409 microns.

The surgery was performed on October 2, 2001. A pair of symmetric Intacs of 0.45 mm thickness were implanted through a temporal incision at 70% of corneal thickness, as measured by pachymetry.

Data obtained at the most recent follow-up examination, on January 14, 2010, i.e. more than 8 years after the procedure were as follows: UCVA 20/200; BSCVA 20/33 partial; refraction −4.5 ≈ −3.5, cylinder × 30°; K 50.25 D −58.0 D, K average 53.87 D. These data, which as mentioned are not atypical, confirm the long-term benefits of this procedure (Figs 5A and B).

## NEW DESIGN OF INTACS: INTACS SK

Intacs SK (SK means severe keratoconus) are a new design of ICRS developed by Addition Technology Inc. They are indicated for the treatment of moderate to severe keratoconus (SK) with steep keratometric values greater than 55.00 D. These are oval-shaped rings with a diameter of 6 mm and a thickness of 0.40 and 0.45 mm. Two nomograms are used to determine the thickness of the intracorneal ring segment that is needed, one is keratometry based and the other is cylindrical based (Fig. 6).

Intacs SK corneal rings seem to offer a compromise between the traditional Intacs with the 7 mm diameter and the Ferrara rings which are 5 mm in diameter, since the diameter is inversely proportional to effectivity (Table 3).

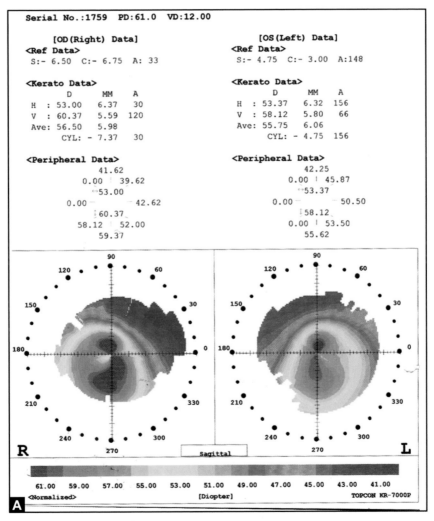

Fig. 5A

CHAPTER 87

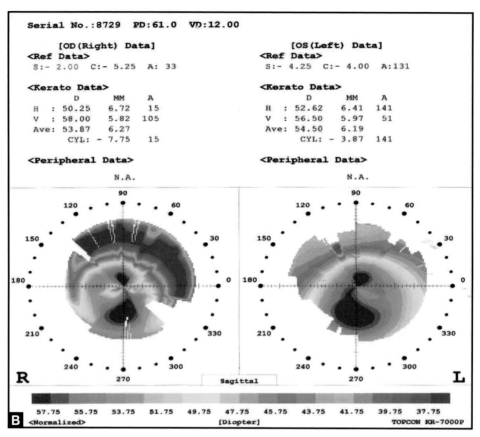

**Figs 5A and B:** Case report 1-pre- (A) and postoperative (B) corneal topography

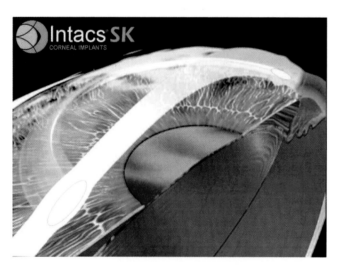

**Fig. 6:** Cross-section view of cornea with Intacs SK implant

**Table 3:** Nomogram for ICRS Intacs SK based on keratometry and cylinder

| Cylinder | Mean keratometry | Segment thickness |
|----------|------------------|-------------------|
| < 5D | 55–62 | 400 μ |
| > 5D | > 62 | 450 μ |

Like Intacs, they can be implanted mechanically with a slight difference in the marker, which marks 6 mm tunnels, and in the dissectors, which are designed like the Intacs dissectors but differ in the diameter. The rest of the procedure is exactly like that used in Intacs implantation.

Channel diameters for the channel dissection by the femtosecond laser, as recommended by Rabinowitz for Intacs SK, are 6.0 × 6.8 mm, whereas the other laser parameters are the same as with regular Intacs.[3]

There are few reports in the literature regarding the use of Intacs SK for keratoconus treatment. Sansanayudh et al. reported on Intacs SK in 10 eyes with a minimum follow-up of 6 months. There was improvement in UCVA and BCVA. There was better contact lens tolerance postoperatively. The median age was 28 years. The mean UCVA was significantly better 6 months postoperatively than preoperatively (0.66 logMAR ± 0.21 [SD] versus 1.19 ± 0.57 logMAR) ($P = 0.004$), as was the mean BCVA (0.25 ± 0.15 logMAR versus 0.51 ± 0.20 logMAR) ($P = 0.018$). The mean spherical equivalent refractive error was −8.08 D preoperatively and −5.03 D at 6 months ($P = 0.65$); the mean refractive astigmatism was −5.05 D and −3.90 D,respectively (P = 0.22); and the mean simulated keratometry value was 57.94 D and 50.07 D, respectively (P = .15). The mean total aberration improved significantly, from 13.48 ± 4.64 mum preoperatively to 9.42 ± 1.80 mum postoperatively (P =0.007). There were no complications.[114] A retrospective study reported on two groups of patients suffering from keratoconus, Group 1 included 16 eyes of 16 patients who underwent 150° single-segment Intacs SK implantation, and Group 2 included 16 eyes of 12 patients who underwent asymmetric shorter arc length 90°/120° Intacs SK implantation. Patients younger than 35 years were crosslinked. Both groups demonstrated significant improvement in UCVA, BCVA, SE and manifest cylinder after the surgery. Comparison of change (post-pre) in UCVA, BCVA and SE at the 1- and 9-month postoperative visits demonstrated significant improvement without statistically significant difference between the two groups. However, change in manifest cylinder at 1 month was statistically significantly higher in Group 2 (4.65 ± 2.21 D) versus Group 1 (2.29 ± 1.57 D) (P = 0.001). At the 9-month visit, change in manifest cylinder continued to be higher at 3.43 ± 1.79 D in Group 2 versus 2.58 ± 1.29 D in Group 1; however, this difference was not statistically significant (P = 0.17). Implantation of asymmetric shorter arc length 90°/120° Intacs SK segments achieved 33% higher correction of astigmatism compared with 150° single-segment Intacs SK implantation. Improvement in UDVA, CDVA and SE was comparable.[115]

Intacs SK were used in post-LASIK ectasia with and without CXL with favorable results.[116,117]

## Sample Case Report 2

This example of using Intacs SK for treating keratoconus concerns a 23-year-old female, who was operated in her left eye on June 26, 2008, to treat keratoconus. Preoperative data were as follows: UCVA 20/200; BSCVA 20/60p; refraction +2.00 ≈ −8.00 cylinder 140°; K readings as recorded by Orbscan II were 44.1 D to −55.3D, K average 49.7; CCT 412 microns; topography was not recordable.

Intacs SK of 0.4 mm were implanted through an incision placed along the steepest axis.

Postoperative UCVA at 9 months was − 20/25; partial correction by glasses did not improve her VA. K readings were 42.75 D to −49.12 D, K average was 45.75.

A few months after the implantation as a result of trauma to the eye, the wound was opened and pannus developed in the wound area. The patient, however, did not come for a check up immediately after the trauma (Figs 7A to C).

## Sample Case Report 3

This is a case of a 26-year-old female patient who was operated in her left eye, in order to treat keratoconus. Preoperative data were as follows: UCVA 1 meter finger count; BSCVA 20/50 partial; refraction −6.00 ≈ −10.0, cylinder 90°; K −61.12 D to −64.00 D, K average 62.62 D; CCT 420 microns.

On February 2, 2010, the patient underwent surgery. A pair of 0.45 mm Intacs SK was implanted through an incision created along the steepest axis. Immediately after surgery, the epithelium was removed from the central 8 mm of the cornea and CXL was performed.

The patient's most recent follow-up visit was conducted almost 1 year postoperatively, when the following data were obtained: UCVA 20/200; BSCVA 20/33; refraction plano ≈ −4 cylinder 130°. Haze was pronounced around the tunnels and the wound area in this case, probably due to the pooling of the riboflavin in the tunnels and the wound area, suggesting a synergistic effect of Intacs and CXL (Figs 8A to D).

## ✷ INTACS AND OTHER ECTATIC DISEASES OF THE CORNEA

### Intacs and Pellucid Marginal Corneal Degeneration

Pellucid marginal degeneration (PMD) is a progressive, noninflammatory, peripheral corneal ectatic disorder characterized by a band of thinning ranging from 1.0 – 2.0 mm in width. The area of thinning is typically found in the inferior cornea, extending from the 4 to the 8 o'clock positions.[118] For the differential diagnosis of keratoconus and PMD, see the chapter on *Diagnosis* in this textbook. Patients usually present in their fourth to fifth decades of life with reduced visual acuity and against-the-rule astigmatism.[119] VA cannot be improved by glasses to a satisfactory level, and RGP contact lenses are rarely tolerated in advanced cases, due to inferior decentration of the contact lens caused by the 'beer belly' shape of the cornea (Fig. 9).

A number of surgical procedures have been suggested to improve VA in PMD, including thermokeratoplasty, epikeratophakia, total lamellar keratoplasty, crescentic lamellar or full thickness resection, large eccentric penetrating keratoplasty, central penetrating keratoplasty, crescentic lamellar keratoplasty and a combination of the last two procedures.[120-125] All of these procedures require extensive surgery with unpredictable visual results.

CHAPTER 87

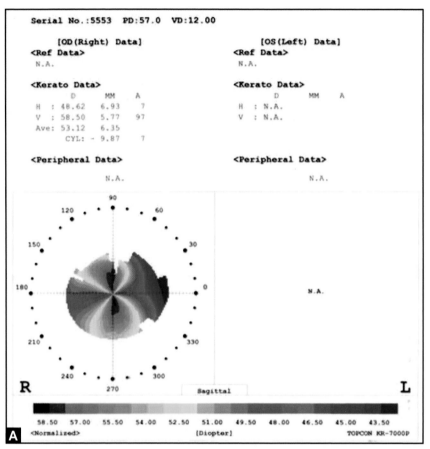

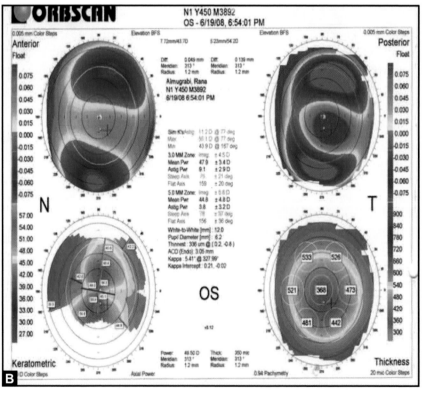

**Figs 7A and B**

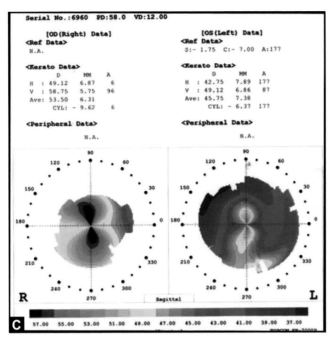

**Figs 7A to C:** Case report 2: (A) Preoperative corneal topography could not be recorded for patient's left eye; (B) Preoperative Orbscan II topography of left eye; (C) Postoperative topography

Decentered grafts have been tried in an attempt to remove as much of the affected lower cornea as possible; however, the proximity of the graft to the limbus and its blood vessels increases the rejection rate, and the inferior decentration of the graft causes a large degree of astigmatism.[126]

These procedures are not as efficient as PKP or DLK are for the treatment of keratoconus, which are considered the gold standard surgical treatments for keratoconus. Due to the complexity and unsatisfactory results with the available treatments for PMD, the ICRS have a great value in treating this progressive frustrating disease. As expected, Intacs improve UCVA and BCVA in patients suffering from PMD.[127,128] Occasionally, implanting one Intacs segment can be sufficient, as in the author's published case report,[128] in which he implanted only one segment in the upper part. He chose this alternative because (after marking and pachymetry) the inferior segment was supposed to pass in a very thin area of the cornea. As reported, good results were obtained in terms of UCVA and BCVA.

Mularoni et al. reported 1-year data of eight eyes with PMD that were treated with asymmetrical Intacs insertion, using the mechanical method.[129] Six eyes (75%) had BCVA of 20/25; the mean postoperative SE was −1.52 D (3.01 SD).

Ertan and Bahadir treated nine eyes with PMD with Intacs that were implanted using the femtosecond laser. Uncorrected visual acuity improved in all eyes; the BCVA improved in eight eyes, and remained unchanged in one eye.[130]

In a retrospective, consecutive case series, Pinero et al. reported on refractive and corneal aberrometric changes after intracorneal ring implantation in corneas with pellucid marginal degeneration. This study included 21 eyes of 15 patients with a diagnosis of PMD, whose ages ranged from 21 to 73 years and who were treated in four ophthalmologic centers. Intacs were implanted in only 3 eyes, whereas Kerarings in 18 eyes. Postoperative visits were scheduled for the first postoperative day and for months 1, 3, and 6 postoperatively. Incision was located on the steepest meridian of the anterior corneal surface in all patients. A tunnel created by femtosecond laser, with inner and outer diameters of 6.6 and 7.8 mm, respectively, was consistently planned for the Intacs implantation.[131]

No complications occurred intraoperatively. Segment ring explantation was performed in a total of four eyes (19.0%), due to significant visual deterioration during the follow-up; all of the explanted ring segments were Kerarings. A statistically significant reduction was found in sphere and cylinder after ICRS implantation. On average,

CHAPTER 87

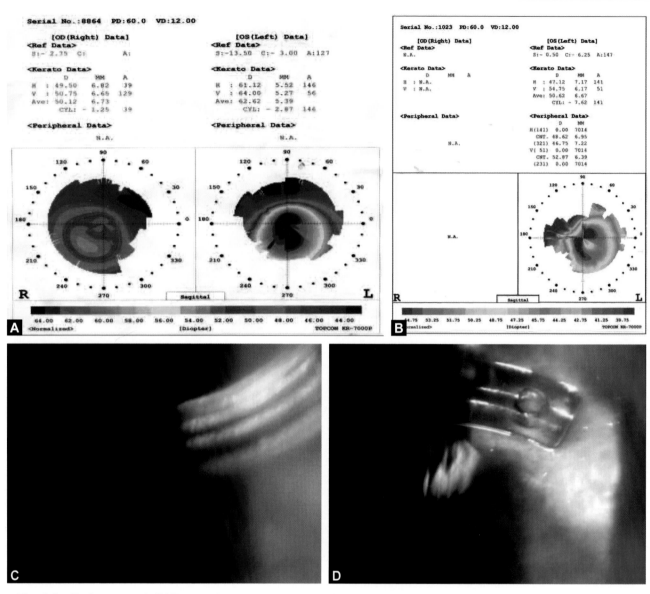

**Figs 8 Ato D:** Case report 3: (A) Preoperative corneal topography; (B) Postoperative corneal topography; (C) Haze around the tunnels; (D) Haze in the wound area and around the tunnels

manifest astigmatism was reduced with the implants by 50%. Also, mean corneal curvature was significantly reduced with the ICRS. The authors assume that the flattening effect was due to the significant reduction of curvature that occurred in the steepest meridian. This could be explained by the combination of two flattening factors, the insertion of the midperipheral implants, and the weakening effect induced by the corneal incision. Significant reduction was observed in the sphere and in the inferosuperior symmetry, along with relative centration of the peripheral corneal protrusion.

A significant change was also found in corneal asphericity, with a trend towards oblateness. The study reported anterior corneal aberrometric outcomes after ICRS implantation: astigmatism, higher order residual, and coma-like aberrations were significantly reduced with surgery. All of these changes in corneal aberrations were consistent with the improvement in BSCVA (55.55% of eyes gained lines of BSCVA). The authors used asymmetric Intacs and implanted the thick one inferiorly and the thinner one superiorly. No extrusion occurred in the Intacs group. The study does not deal with Intacs and Kerarings

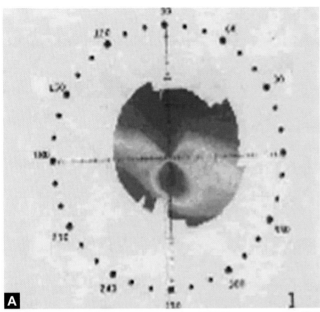

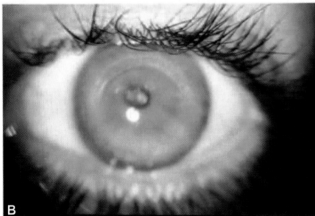

**Figs 9A and B:** (A)Topography of PMD; (B) Colored photograph of the cornea showing the Intac in the upper half of the cornea

separately, but rather provided global results; nevertheless, it confirms the beneficial effect of Intacs and Kerarings in treating PMD.

Intacs have an important role in treating PMD and may be used as an alternative to the other available previously-mentioned surgical options.

## Intacs and Post-LASIK Ectasia

Post-LASIK ectasia is equivalent to iatrogenic keratoconus with all of the visual disturbances of keratoconus. It was first reported in 1998.[132] It consists of a progressive corneal steepening, usually inferiorly, with an increase in myopia and astigmatism, loss of UCVA and BSCVA, and a significant increase in corneal aberrations. The causes of post-LASIK ectasia are beyond the scope of this chapter.

Keratoconus and post-LASIK ectasia share the same treatment options, except that the typical post-LASIK ectasia patient opts for the treatment, comes with high expectations and is consequently extremely disappointed from the treatment outcome. Such patients typically undergo laser refractive surgery to improve their UCVA and get rid of their glasses, and instead they find themselves with low UCVA and reduced BSCVA. These were patients who prior to the procedure had enjoyed excellent VA with glasses and most of them had excellent UCVA after LASIK.

Ectasia does not occur only after LASIK; few cases of ectasia were reported after PRK.[133-136] One case was reported by the author's group as mentioned before.

Improvement in visual acuity and reduction in sphero-cylindrical error and keratometry have been reported after ICRS implantation in post-LASIK ectasia[36,137-141] even in severe cases[137] with long-term favorable results and refractive stability even after 5 years.[142]

Several studies have shown the beneficial effect on UCVA and BCVA of implanting a single inferior Intac in patients with post-LASIK ectasia.[143,144] Favorable results were obtained by implanting Intacs SK.[145]

A 60% success rate in improving both UCVA and BCVA by implanting a single inferior Intac was reported on 50 post-LASIK ectasia patients.[3] It reduces the anisometropia between the two eyes and also improves contact lens tolerance in these patients.

Rabinowitz[3] states that carrying out Intacs implantation in such patients can be tricky and should only be carried out by experienced surgeons, as it is very easy to create your channel in the plane of the LASIK flap, thereby dislocating the flap and getting minimal effect. The key is to go deep and make sure your Intacs are inserted well below the plane of the flap.

Personally, the author has not faced intraoperative complications implanting Intacs in post-LASIK patients[12] or in cases of post-LASIK ectasia.

The postoperative complications are the same as in keratoconus patients. Further complications were reported by Abad et al. on two cases of flap slippage months after Intacs implantation, because of post-LASIK ectasia.[146] The cases were managed by suturing the flap 300° except the hinge, with (1 case) or without (1 case) removing one of the segments. Visual rehabilitation and refractive stability were achieved. Based on the experience in Case 1, the slippage of the flap was thought to be due to the inability of the poorly healed flap edge to withstand the remodelling effect of the segments. Since Intacs act by pushing the corneal tissue at the body of the segment inward, and the healing process is weakest at the edge of the flap, the flap could easily slip over the stromal bed where the body of the segment is located.

Like in keratoconus, the Intacs can be used in combination with intraocular lenses and CXL.

Except for the previously-mentioned postoperative flap slippage and the possible intraoperative difficulties, there is no significant difference in Intacs implantation outcomes between post-LASIK ectasia and keratoconus; in both, Intacs improved UCVA and BCVA, and reduced astigmatism and MRSE.

## ▶ CONCLUSION

Intacs are an effective way for treating keratoconus; the surgery is safe and has an adequate biocompatibility. The procedure is adjustable and reversible and, most importantly, effective in improving UCVA, BCVA. It reduces the MRSE and keratometry readings, improves contact lens tolerance, and reduces the anisometropia between the two eyes. Intacs have a positive impact on the quality of life in keratoconic patients.[35]

The nomograms need to be evaluated in prospective studies; a computer model taking into account refraction, keratometry, corneal thickness and biomechanical data needs to be developed in order to customize Intacs implantation, so as to further improve the results. The femtosecond laser facilitates the implantation, but renders results comparable to those attained using the mechanical technique. Although this procedure is highly dependent on the surgeon's manual dexterity and experience, recent studies report a low incidence of complications. If Intacs implantation fails because of extrusion or unsatisfactory visual acuity results, and the patient elects to undergo a corneal transplant, the Intacs can safely be removed at the time of the corneal transplant, without affecting the ultimate outcome of the transplant.[3] Big bubble-assisted DALK procedure was performed at the time of Intacs removal in two eyes with unsatisfactory visual outcome; no intra- or postoperative complications occurred.[147]

Intacs constitute an alternative to penetrating keratoplasty in many patients, and they should be offered to keratoconic patients with unsatisfactory UCVA and BCVA who are contact lens intolerant.

## ▶ REFERENCES

1. Fleming RL, Schanzlin DJ. The intrastromal corneal ring: two cases in rabbits. J Refract Sug. 1987;3:227-32.
2. Fleming JF, Lee Wan W, Schanzlin DJ. The theory of corneal curvature change with the intrastromal corneal ring. CLAO J. 1989;15:146-50.
3. Rabinowitz YS. Intacs for Keratoconus. Int Ophthalmol Clin. 2010;50(3):63-76.
4. Schanzlin DJ, Asbell PA, Burris TE, et al. The intrastromal corneal ring segments: Phase II results for the correction of myopia. Ophthalmology. 1997;104:1067-78.
5. Silvestrini T, Mathis M, Loomas B, et al. A geometric model to predict the change in corneal curvature from the intrastromal corneal ring (ICR). Invest Ophthalmol Vis Sci. 1994;35:2023.
6. Patel S, Marshall J, Fitzke FW. Model for deriving the optical performance of the myopic eye corrected with an intracorneal ring. J Refract Surg. 1995;11:248-52.
7. Schanzlin DJ. Studies of intrastromal corneal ring segments for the correction of low to moderate myopic refractive errors. Trans Am Ophthalmol Soc. 1999;97:815-90.
8. Schanzlin DJ, Abbott RL, Asbell PA, et al. Two-year outcomes of intrastromal corneal ring segments for the correction of myopia. Ophthamology. 2001;108:1688-94.
9. Suiter BG, Twa MD, Ruckhofer J, et al. A comparison of visual acuity, predictability, and visual function outcomes after intracorneal ring segments and laser in situ keratomileusis. Trans Am Ophthalmol Soc. 2000;98:51-5.
10. Chan SM, Khan HN. Reversibility and exchangeability of intrastromal corneal ring segments. J Cataract Refract Surg. 2002;28:676-81.
11. Asbell PA, Uçakhan ÖÖ, Abbott RL, et al. Intrastromal corneal ring segments: reversibility of refractive effect. J Refract Surg. 2001;17:25.
12. Barbara A, Shehadeh-Masha'our R, Garzozi HJ. Intacs after laser in situ keratomileusis and photorefractive keratectomy. J Cataract Refract Surg. 2004;30(9):1892-5.
13. Ferrara P, Torquetti L. Clinical outcomes after implantation of a new intrastromal corneal ring with a 210 degrees arc length J Cataract Refract Surg. 2009;35(9):1604-8.
14. Lovisolo CF, Fleming JF, Pesando PM. Nomograms for intrastromal inserts. In: Lovisolo CF, Fleming JF, Pesando PM (Eds). Intrastromal Corneal Ring Segments. Canelli, Italy: Fabiano Editore; 2002.pp.31-4.
15. Ertan A, Colin J. Intracorneal rings for keratoconus and keratectasia. J Cataract Refract Surg. 2007;33:1303-14.
16. Piñero DP, Alio JL. Intracorneal ring segments in ectatic corneal disease. Clin Exp Ophthalmol. 2010;38:154-67.
17. Rabinowitz YS. Intacs for keratoconus. Int Ophthalmol Clin. 2006;46(3):91-103.
18. Güell JL, Morral M, Salinas C, et al. Intrastromal corneal ring segments to correct low myopia in eyes with irregular or abnormal topography including forme fruste keratoconus: 4-year follow-up. J Cataract Refract Surg. 2010;36(7):1149-55.

19. Colin J, Cochener B, Savary G, et al. Correcting keratoconus with intracorneal rings. J Cataract Refract Surg. 2000;26: 1117-22.

20. Rabinowitz YS, Li X, Ignacio TS, et al. INTACS inserts using the femtosecond laser compared to the mechanical spreader in the treatment of keratoconus. J Refract Surg. 2006;22:764-71.

21. Colin J, Cochener B, Savary G, et al. Intacs inserts for treating keratoconus: one-year results. Ophthalmology. 2001;108: 1409-14.

22. Kaiserman I, Bahar I, Rootman DS. Optical coherence tomography provides insight into the effect of Intacs in keratoconus. Arch Ophthalmol. 2008;126(4):571-2.

23. Boxer Wachler BS, Chandra NS, Chou B, et al. Intacs for keratoconus. Ophthalmology. 2003;110:1031-40; errata, 1475.

24. Alio JL, Artola A, Hassanein A, et al. One or two Intacs segments for the correction of keratoconus. J Cataract Refract Surg. 2005;31:943-53.

25. Alio JL, Shabayek MH, Belda JI, et al. Analysis of results related to good and bad outcomes of Intacs implantation for keratoconus correction. J Cataract Refract Surg. 2006;32:756-61.

26. Kanellopoulos AJ, Pe LH, Perry HD, et al. Modified intracorneal ring segment implantations (INTACS) for the management of moderate to advanced keratoconus: efficacy and complications. Cornea. 2006;25:29-33.

27. Shetty R, Kurian M, Anand D, et al. Intacs in advanced keratoconus. Cornea. 2008;27:1022-9.

28. The FEMTO LASIK Professionals site (in German), www. femto-lasik-pro.com. [Accessed February 2011].

29. Ertan A, Kamburoglu G, Akgün U. Comparison of outcomes of 2 channel sizes for intrastromal ring segment implantation with a femtosecond laser in eyes with keratoconus. J Cataract Refract Surg. 2007;33:648-53.

30. Colin J. European clinical evaluation: use of Intacs prescription inserts for the treatment of keratoconus. J Cataract Refract Surg. 2006;32:747-55.

31. Alio JL, Shabayek MH. Intracorneal asymmetrical rings for keratoconus: where should the thicker segment be implanted? J Refract Surg. 2006;22:307-9.

32. Chan CC, Wachler BS. Reduced best spectacle-corrected visual acuity from inserting a thicker Intacs above and thinner Intacs below in keratoconus. J Refract Surg. 2007;23:93-5.

33. Ertan A, Bahadır M. Topography-guided vertical implantation of Intacs using femtosecond laser for the treatment of keratoconus. J Cataract Refract Surg. 2007;33:148-51.

34. Güell JL, Morral M, Salinas C, et al. Four-year follow-up of intrastromal corneal ring segments in patients with keratoconus. J Emmetropia. 2010;1:9-15.

35. de Freitas SPJ, Avila MP, Paranhos A, et al. Evaluation of the impact of intracorneal ring segments implantation on the quality of life of patients with keratoconus using the NEI-RQL (National Eye Institute Refractive Error Quality of life) instrument. Br J Ophthalmol. 2010;94(1):101-5.

36. Sharma M, Boxer Wachler BS. Comparison of single-segment and double-segment Intacs for keratoconus and post-LASIK ectasia. Am J Ophthalmol. 2006;141:891-5.

37. Murta JN. Ocular Surgery News Europe/Asia-Pacific Edition. 2007.

38. Alio JL, Shabayek MH, Artola A. Intracorneal ring segments for keratoconus correction: long-term follow-up. J Cataract Refract Surg. 2006;32:978-85.

39. Ibrahim TA. After 5 years follow-up: do Intacs help in keratoconus? Cataract Refract Surg. 2006;1:45-8.

40. Kymionis GD, Grentzelos MA, Diakonis VF, et al. Nine-year follow-up of Intacs implantation for keratoconus. Open Ophthalmol J. 2009;8(3):77-81.

41. Colin J, Malet FJ. Intacs for the correction of keratoconus: two-year follow-up. J Cataract Refract Surg. 2007;33:69-7.

42. Colin at the XXVI Congress of the European Society for Cataract and Refractive Surgery (ESCRS 2007) during a special clinical research symposium on keratoconus. http://myeurotimes. blogspot.com/2008_09_01_archive.html. [Accessed Feb 2011].

43. Kymionis GD, Siganos CS, Tsiklis NS, et al. Long-term follow-up of Intacs in keratoconus. Am J Ophthalmol. 2007;143: 236-44.

44. Ertan A, Kamburoğlu G, Bahadir M. Intacs insertion with the femtosecond laser for the management of keratoconus: one-year results. J Cataract Refract Surg. 2006;32(12):2039-42.

45. Carrasquillo KG, Rand J, Talamo JH. Intacs for keratoconus and post-LASIK ectasia: mechanical versus femtosecond laser-assisted channel creation. Cornea. 2007;26(8):956-62.

46. Pokroy R, Levinger S. Intacs adjustment surgery for keratoconus. J Cataract Refract Surg. 2006;32:986-92.

47. Alió JL, Piñero DP, Söğütlü E, et al. Implantation of new intracorneal ring segments after segment explantation for unsuccessful outcomes in eyes with keratoconus. J Cataract Refract Surg. 2010;36:1303-10.

48. Ertan A, Karacal H. Factors influencing flap and INTACS decentration after femtosecond laser application in normal and keratoconic eyes. J Refract Surg. 2008;24(8):797-801.

49. Ertan A, Kamburoğlu G. Analysis of centration of Intacs segments implanted with a femtosecond laser. J Cataract Refract Surg. 2007;33(3):484-7.

50. Ferrer C, Alió JL, Montañés AU, et al. Causes of intrastromal corneal ring segment explantation: clinicopathologic correlation analysis. J Cataract Refract Surg. 2010;36(6):970-7.

51. Cosar CB, Sridhar MS, Sener B. Late onset of deep corneal vascularization: a rare complication of intrastromal corneal ring segments for keratoconus. Eur J Ophthalmol. 2009;19(2): 298-300.

52. Lovisolo CF, Mularoni A, Mazzolani F. Combining Intacs implantation with other refractive and non-refractive procedures. J Emmetropia. 2010;1(3) Update/Review.

53. Alió JL, Artola A, Ruiz-Moreno JM et al. Changes in keratoconic corneas after intracorneal ring segment explantation and reimplantation. Ophthalmology. 2004;111:747-51.

54. Kugler LJ, Hill S, Sztipanovits D, et al. Corneal melt of incisions overlying corneal ring segments: case series and literature review. Cornea. 2011;30(9):968-71.

55. Ferrer C, Alió JL. Reasons for intrastromal corneal ring segment explantation. J Cataract Refract Surg. 2010;36(11):2014-5.

56. Apuano CJ, Sugar A, Koch DD, et al. Intrastromal corneal ring segments for low myopia: a report by the American Academy of Ophthalmology. (Ophthalmic Technology Assessment) Ophthalmology. 2001;108:1922-8.

CHAPTER 87

57. Ruckhofer J, Stoiber J, Alzner E, et al. One year results of European multicenter study of intrastromal corneal ring segments. Part 2: complications, visual symptoms, and patient satisfaction; the Multicenter European Corneal Correction Assessment Study Group. J Cataract Refract Surg. 2001;27:287-96.

58. McDonald JE, Deitz DJ. Removal of Intacs with a fractured positioning hole. J Refract Surg. 2004;20:182-3.

59. Hofling-Lima AL, Branco BC, Romano AC, et al. Corneal infections after implantation of intracorneal ring segments. Cornea. 2004;23:547-9.

60. Lai MM, Tang M, Andrade EM, et al. Optical coherence tomography to assess intrastromal corneal ring segment depth in keratoconic eyes. J Cataract Refract Surg. 2006;32(11):1860-5.

61. Kamburoglu G, Ertan A, Saraçbasi O. Measurement of depth of Intacs implanted via femtosecond laser using Pentacam. J Refract Surg. 2009;25(4):377-82.

62. Torquetti L, Ferrara P. Reasons for intrastromal corneal ring segment explantation. J Cataract Refract Surg. 2010;36(11):2014.

63. Mulet ME, Pérez-Santonja JJ, Ferrer C, et al. Microbial keratitis after intrastromal corneal ring segment implantation. J Refract Surg. 2010;26(5):364-9.

64. Levy J, Lifshit T. Keratitis after implantation of intrastromal corneal ring segments (Intacs) aided by femtosecond laser for keratoconus correction: case report and description of the literature. Eur J Ophthalmol. 2010;20(4):780-4.

65. Chaudhry IA, Al-Ghamdi AA, Kirat O, et al. Bilateral infectious keratitis after implantation of intrastromal corneal ring segments. Cornea. 2010;29(3):339-41.

66. Liu A, Manche EE. Traumatic shattering of intrastromal corneal ring segments. J Cataract Refract Surg. 2010;36(6):1042-4.

67. Randleman JB, Dawson DG, Larson PM, et al. Chronic pain after Intacs implantation. J Cataract Refract Surg. J Cataract Refract Surg. 2006;32(5):875-8.

68. Rau M, Dausch D. Intrastromal corneal ring implantation for the correction of myopia: 12-month follow-up. J Cataract Refract Surg. 2003;29:322-8.

69. Ruckhofer J, Twa MD, Schanzlin DJ. Clinical characteristics of lamellar channel deposits after implantation of Intacs. J Cataract Refract Surg. 2000;26:1473-9.

70. Park S, Ramamurthi S, Ramaesh K. Late dislocation of intrastromal corneal ring segment into the anterior chamber. J Cataract Refract Surg. 2010;10:2003-5.

71. Feldman BH, Kim T. Enhanced effect of double-stacked intrastromal corneal ring segments in keratoconus. J Cataract Refract Surg. 2010;36(2):332-5.

72. Twa MD, Ruckhofer J, Kash RL, et al. Histological evaluation of corneal stroma in rabbits after intrastromal corneal ring implantation. Cornea. 2003;22:146-52.

73. Twa MD, Kash RL, Costello M, et al. Morphological characteristics of lamellar channel deposits in the human eye: a case report. Cornea. 2004;23:412-20.

74. Samimi S, Leger F, Touboul D, et al. Histopathological findings after intracorneal ring segment implantation in keratoconic human corneas. J Cataract Refract Surg. 2007;33:247-53.

75. Ly LT, McCulley JP, Verity SM, et al. Evaluation of intrastromal lipid deposits after Intacs implantation using in vivo confocal microscopy. Eye Contact Lens. 2006;32(4):211-5.

76. Ruckhofer J, Böhnke M, Alzner E, et al. Confocal microscopy after implantation of intrastromal corneal ring segments. Ophthalmology. 2000;107:2144-51.

77. Mohammad Al-Amry, Hind M Alkatan. Histopathologic findings in two cases with history of intrastromal corneal ring segments insertion. Middle East Afr J Ophthalmol. 2011;18 (4):317-9.

78. Colin J, Ertan A. Intracorneal ring segments and alternative treatments for corneal ectatic diseases. Ankara: Kudret Eye Hospital 2007:164.

79. Dauwe C, Touboul D, Roberts CJ, et al. Biomechanical and morphological corneal response to placement of intrastromal corneal ring segments for keratoconus. J Cataract Refract Surg. 2009;35(10):1761-7.

80. El-Raggal TM, Abdel Fattah AA. Sequential Intacs and Verisyse phakic intraocular lens for refractive improvement in keratoconic eyes. J Cataract Refract Surg. 2007;33:966-70.

81. Piñero DP, Alió JL, El Kady B, et al. Corneal aberrometric and refractive performance of 2 intrastromal corneal ring segment models in early and moderate ectatic disease. J Cataract Refract Surg. 2010;36:102-9.

82. Kamburoglu G, Ertan A, Bahadir M. Implantation of Artisan toric phakic intraocular lens following Intacs in a patient with keratoconus. J Cataract Refract Surg. 2007;33:528-30.

83. Ertan A, Karacal H, Kamburoglu G. Combined Intacs and posterior chamber toric implantable Collamer lens implantation for keratoconic patients with extreme myopia. Am J Ophthalmol. 2007;144:387-9.

84. Budo C, Bartels MC, van Rij G. Implantation of Artisan toric phakic intraocular lenses for the correction of astigmatism and spherical errors in patients with keratoconus. J Refract Surg. 2005;21:218-22.

85. Colin J, Velou S. Implantation of Intacs and a refractive intraocular lens to correct keratoconus. J Cataract Refract Surg. 2003;29:832-4.

86. Moshirfar MF, Carlton R, Meyer JJ, et al. Simultaneous and sequential implantation of Intacs and Verisyse phakic intraocular lens for refractive improvement in keratectasia. Cornea. 2011;30(2):158-63.

87. Tan BU, Purcell TL, Nalgirkar A, et al. Photorefractive keratectomy for the correction of residual refractive error with Intacs intrastromal corneal ring segments in place. J Cataract Refract Surg. 2008;34:909-15.

88. Hirsh A, Barequet IS, Levinger S. Wavefront-guided LASEK after Intacs in eyes with stable keratoconus. Harefuah. 2006;145: 181-2 (In Hebrew).

89. Iovieno A , Legare ME , Rootman DB, et al. Intracorneal ring segments implantation followed by same-day photorefractive keratectomy and corneal collagen cross-linking in keratoconus. Refract Surg. 2011;27(12):915-8.

90. Chan CC, Sharma M, Wachler BS. Effect of inferior-segment Intacs with and without C3-R on keratoconus. J Cataract Refract Surg. 2007;33(1):75-80.

91. Wollensak G, Spoerl E, Seiler T. Riboflavin/ultraviolet-A-induced collagen crosslinking for the treatment of keratoconus. Am J Ophthalmol. 2003;135:620-7.

92. Wollensak G, Spoerl E, Seiler T. Stress-strain measurements of human and porcine corneas after riboflavin-ultraviolet-A-induced cross-linking. J Cataract Refract Surg. 2003;29:1780-5.

93. Kamburoglu G, Ertan A. Intacs implantation with sequential collagen cross-linking treatment in postoperative LASIK Ectasia. J Refract Surg. 2008;24:S726-9.

94. Ertan A, Karacal H, Kamburoğlu G. Refractive and topographic results of transepithelial cross-linking treatment in eyes with Intacs. Cornea. 2009;28(7):719-23.

95. Coskunseven E, Jankov MR, Hafezi F, et al. Effect of treatment sequence in combined intrastromal corneal rings and corneal collagen crosslinking for keratoconus. J Cataract Refract Surg. 2009;35(12):2084-91.

96. Vicente LL, Boxer Wachler BS. Factors that correlate with improvement in vision after combined Intacs and trans-epithelial corneal crosslinking. Br J Ophthalmol. 2010;94(12):1597-601.

97. Lovisolo CF, Calossi A. C3-R combined with intrastromal ring segments and RGP contact lens molding in progressive corneal ectatic disorders. In: Garg A, Pinelli R, O'Brart D, Kanellopoulos AJ, Lovisolo CF (Eds). Mastering corneal collagen cross linking techniques. New Delhi, India: Jaypee Brothers Publishers; 2009.

98. Barbara R, Zadok D, Pikkel J et al. Collagen corneal cross-linking followed by Intac implantation in a Case of post-PRK ectasia. The International Journal of Keratoconus and Ectatic Corneal Diseases. 2012;1;68-72.

99. Shetty R, Narayana KM, Mathew K, et al. Safety and efficacy of Intacs in Indian eyes with keratoconus: an initial report. Indian J Ophthalmol. 2009;57(2):115-9.

100. Smith KA, Carrell JD. High-Dk piggyback contact lenses over Intacs for keratoconus: a case report. Eye Contact Lens. 2008;34(4):238-41.

101. Ucakhan OO, Kanpolat A, Ozdemir O. Contact lens fitting for keratoconus after Intacs placement. Eye Contact Lens. 2006;32:75-7.

102. Nepomuceno RL, Boxer Wachler BS, Weissman BA. Feasibility of contact lens fitting on keratoconus patients with Intacs inserts. Cont Lens Anterior Eye. 2003;26:175-80.

103. Dalton K, Sorbara L. Fitting an MSD (mini scleral design) rigid contact lens in advanced keratoconus with INTACS. Cont Lens Anterior Eye. 2011;34(6):274-81.

104. Kymionis GD, Kontadakis GA. Severe corneal vascularization after Intacs implantation and rigid contact lens use for the treatment of keratoconus. Semin Ophthalmol. 2012;27(1-2):19-21.

105. Coskunseven E, Kymionis GD, Grentzelos MA, et al. Intacs followed by KeraRing intrastromal corneal ring segment implantation for keratoconus. J Refract Surg. 2010;26(5):371-4.

106. Piñero DP, Alió JL, El Kady B, Pascual I. Corneal aberrometric and refractive performance of 2 intrastromal corneal ring segment models in early and moderate ectatic disease. J Cataract Refract Surg. 2010;36(1):102-9.

107. Kaya V, Utine CA, Karakus SH, Kavadarli I, Yilmaz OF. Refractive and visual outcomes after Intacs vs Ferrara intrastromal corneal ring segment implantation for keratoconus: a comparative study. J Refract Surg. 2011;27(12):907-12.

108. Yahalom C, Mechoulam H, Solomon A, et al. Forty years of changing indications in penetrating keratoplasty in Israel. Cornea. 2005;24:256-8.

109. Rodrıguez LA, Guillen PB, Benavides MA, Garcia L, Porras D, Daqui-Garay RM. Penetrating keratoplasty versus intrastromal corneal ring segments to correct bilateral corneal ectasia: preliminary study. J Cataract Refract Surg. 2007;33:488-96A.

110. Thompson RW, Price MO, Bowers PJ, et al. Long-term graft survival after penetrating keratoplasty. Ophthalmology. 2003; 110:1396-402.

111. Troutman RC. Microsurgical control of corneal astigmatism in cataract and keratoplasty. Trans Am Acad Ophthalmol Otolaryngol. 1973;77:563-72.

112. Troutman RC, Swinger C. Relaxing incision for control of postoperative astigmatism following keratoplasty. Ophthalmic Surg. 1980;11:117-20.

113. Hardten DR, Chittcharus A, Lindstrom RL. Long term analysis of LASIK for the correction of refractive errors after penetrating keratoplasty. Cornea. 2004;23:479-89.

114. Sansanayudh W, Bahar I, Kumar NL, et al. Intrastromal corneal ring segment SK implantation for moderate to severe keratoconus. J Cataract Refract Surg. 2010;36(1):110-3.

115. Abad JC, Arango J, Tobon C. Comparison of astigmatism correction using shorter arc length 90°/120° asymmetric Intacs severe keratoconus versus 150° single-segment Intacs severe keratoconus in asymmetric keratoconus. Cornea. 2011; 30(11):1201-6.

116. Kamburoglu G, Ertan A. Intacs implantation with sequential collagen cross-linking treatment in postoperative LASIK ectasia. J Refract Surg. 2008;24(7):S726-9.

117. Kymionis GD, Bouzoukis DI, Portaliou DM, et al. New Intacs SK implantation in patients with post-laser in situ keratomileusis corneal ectasia. Cornea. 2010;29(2):214-6.

118. Krachmer JH, Feder RS, Belin MW. Keratoconus and related noninflammatory corneal thinning disorders. Surv Ophthalmol. 1984;28:315-22.

119. Karabatsas CH, Cook SD. Topographic analysis in pellucid marginal corneal degeneration and keratoglobus. Eye. 1996;10: 451-5.

120. Fronterre A, Portesani GP. Epikeratoplasty for pellucid marginal corneal degeneration. Cornea. 1991;10:450-3.

121. Kremer I, Sperber LT, Laibson PR. Pellucid marginal degeneration treated by lamellar and penetrating keratoplasty. Arch Ophthalmol. 1993;111:169-70.

122. Duran JA, Rodriguez-Ares MT, Torres D. Crescentic resection for treatment of pellucid corneal marginal degeneration. Ophthalmic Surg. 1991;22:153-6.

123. Dubroff S. Pellucid marginal corneal degeneration: report on corrective surgery. J Cataract Refract Surg. 1989;15:89-93.

124. Speaker MG, Arentsen JJ, Laibson PR. Long-term survival of large diameter penetrating keratoplasties for keratoconus and pellucid marginal degeneration. Acta Ophthalmol Suppl. 1989;192:17-9.

125. Schanzlin DJ, Sarno EM, Robin JB. Crescentic lamellar keratoplasty for pellucid marginal degeneration. Am J Ophthalmol. 1983;96(2):253-4.

126. Varley GA, Macsai MS, Krachmer JH. The results of penetrating keratoplasty for pellucid marginal corneal degeneration. Am J Ophthalmol. 1990;110:149-52.

CHAPTER 87

127. Rodriguez-Prats J, Galal A, Garcia-Lledo M, et al. Intracorneal rings for correction of pellucid marginal degeneration. J Cataract Refract Surg. 2003;29:1421-4.

128. Barbara A, Shehadeh-Masha'our R, Zvi F, et al. Management of pellucid marginal degeneration with intracorneal ring segments. J Refract Surg. 2005;21:296-8.

129. Mularoni A, Torreggiani A, di Biase A, et al. Conservative treatment of early and moderate pellucid marginal degeneration: a new refractive approach with intracorneal rings. Ophthalmology. 2005;112:660-6.

130. Ertan A, Bahadir M. Intrastromal ring segment insertion using a femtosecond laser to correct pellucid marginal corneal degeneration. J Cataract Refract Surg. 2006;32:1710-6.

131. Piñero DP, Alio JL, Morbelli H, et al. Refractive and corneal aberrometric changes after intracorneal ring implantation in corneas with pellucid marginal degeneration. Ophthalmology. 2009;116(9):656-64.

132. Seiler T, Koufala K, Richter G. Iatrogenic keratectasia after laser in situ keratomileusis. J Refract Surg. 1998;14(3):312-7.

133. Navas A, Ariza E, Haber A, et al. Bilateral keratectasia after photorefractive keratectomy. J Refract Surg. 2007;23(9):941-3.

134. Reznik J, Salz JJ, Klimava A. Development of unilateral corneal ectasia after PRK with ipsilateral preoperative forme fruste keratoconus. J Refract Surg. 2008;24(8):843-7.

135. Malecaze F, Coullet J, Calvas P, et al. Corneal ectasia after photorefractive keratectomy for low myopia. Ophthalmology. 2006;113(5):742-6.

136. Leccisotti A. Corneal ectasia after photorefractive keratectomy. Graefes Arch Clin Exp Ophthalmol. 2007;245(6):869-75. Epub 2006 Dec 20.

137. Uceda-Montanes A, Tomás JD, Alió JL. Correction of severe ectasia after LASIK with intracorneal ring segments. J Refract Surg. 2008;24:408-13.

138. Güell JL, Velasco F, Sánchez SI, et al. Intracorneal ring segments after laser in situ keratomileusis. J Refract Surg. 2004;20:349-55.

139. Kymionis GD, Siganos CS, Kounis G, Astyrakakis N, Kalyvianaki MI, Pallikaris IG. Management of post-LASIK corneal ectasia with Intacs inserts. One-year results. Arch Ophthalmol. 2003;121:322-6.

140. Siganos CS, Kymionis GD, Astyrakakis N, Pallikaris IG. Management of corneal ectasia after laser in situ keratomileusis with INTACS. J Refract Surg. 2002;18:43-6.

141. Alió JL, Salem TF, Artola A, Osman A. Intracorneal rings to correct corneal ectasia after laser in situ keratomileusis. J Cataract Refract Surg. 2002;28:1568-74.

142. Kymionis GD, Tsiklis NS, Pallikaris AI, Kounis G, Diakonis VF, Astyrakakis N, et al. Long-term follow-up of Intacs for post-LASIK corneal ectasia. Ophthalmology. 2006;113:1909-17.

143. Piñero DP, Alio JL, Uceda-Montanes A, El Kady B, Pascual I. Intracorneal ring segment implantation in corneas with post-laser in situ keratomileusis keratectasia. Ophthalmology. 2009;116:1665-74.

144. Pokroy R, Levinger S, Hirsh A. Single Intacs segment for post-laser in situ keratomileusis keratectasia. J Cataract Refract Surg. 2004;30:1685-95.

145. Rodriguez LA, Villegas AE, Porras D, et al. Treatment of six cases of advanced ectasia after LASIK with 6-mm Intacs SK. J Refract Surg. 2009;25:1116-9.

146. Abad JC. Management of slipped laser in situ keratomileusis flap following intrastromal corneal ring implantation in post-LASIK ectasia. J Cataract Refract Surg. 2008;34:2177-81.

147. Titiyal JS, Chawla B, Sharma N. Deep anterior lamellar keratoplasty with Intacs explantation in keratoconus. Eur J Ophthalmol. 2010;20(5):874-8.

# CHAPTER 88

# UVA-light and Riboflavin Mediated Corneal Collagen Crosslinking

*Erik Letko, William B Trattler, Roy S Rubinfeld*

## ▶ BACKGROUND

Keratoconus and other corneal conditions associated with progressive stromal thinning and ectasia including post-LASIK keratectasia and pellucid marginal degeneration represent therapeutic challenges. Until recently, available therapies including contact lenses, epikeratoplasty, intrastromal corneal ring segments (Intacs) and corneal transplantation targeted, in principle, the abnormal shape of the cornea by mechanical means. The underlying molecular pathogenic mechanisms of corneal ectasia were not addressed with any of these therapies until the introduction of corneal collagen crosslinking (CXL) to clinical practice in 1999.[1] This breakthrough clinical application was the result of multiple laboratory observations and discoveries made over preceding decades.

Early experiments of Cannon and Foster[2] showed that degraded normal collagen or synthesis of abnormal collagen might play a role in the pathogenesis of keratoconus. This concept was later confirmed by subsequent clinical and experimental studies. Keratoconus was characterized by progressive stromal thinning and ectasia[3] as a result of increased expression of lysosomal and proteolytic enzymes[4-7] and decreased concentration of protease inhibitors,[5,8] which result in corneal thinning and altered configuration of corneal collagen lamellae.[9,10] Due to the young age of onset, typically in the second decade of life, and progressive nature, keratoconus has a negative impact on quality of life.[11] The Collaborative Longitudinal Evaluation of Keratoconus Study[12,13] found a significant decline in visual acuity within 8 years, an increase in astigmatism, subepithelial scarring, and corneal thinning in untreated keratoconus. In fact, keratoconus was the most common indication for corneal transplant in the past decades.[14]

The idea of therapeutically targeting the underlying pathogenic mechanisms of keratoconus was explored in the 1990s by Khadem et al. who pursued the identification of biologic glues that could be activated by heat or light to increase the resistance of stromal collagen.[15] It was discovered that the gluing effect was mediated by oxidative mechanisms associated with hydroxyl radical release. A similar mechanism related to active glycosylation of age dependent tropocollagen was shown in aging corneas.[16] The phenomenon of collagen crosslinking after UVA-light exposure was reported by Kligman and Gebre[17] in 1991 when the authors observed biochemical changes in the skin of hairless mice after chronic exposure to UVA radiation. Their experiments rendered collagen highly resistant to pepsin digestion indicating increased collagen crosslinking induced by UVA.

Subsequent studies using corneal tissue showed a similar effect on corneal collagen after exposure to riboflavin and UVA-light.[18] In experimental studies using rabbit and porcine eyes an increase in corneal rigidity by approximately 70% in untreated versus treated corneas[19] after collagen crosslinking by combined riboflavin/UVA treatment was shown. After developing collagen crosslinking using the photosensitizer riboflavin and UVA similar to photopolymerization in polymers,[20] Wollensak et al. was the first to clinically induce UVA-light and riboflavin mediated CXL initially in a patient with non-seeing eyes in 1998 and later in a series of patients with keratoconus.[1]

## ➤ UVA-LIGHT AND RIBOFLAVIN

The solar spectrum represents a band of radiation including UVC (220–290 nm), UVB (290–320 nm) and UVA (320–340 nm), infrared radiation and visible light. UVC is blocked by the ozone layer in the stratosphere of the earth. UVA and UVB penetrate to the surface of the earth and are known, in some circumstances, to cause damage to ribonucleic acids. Ultraviolet-A radiation alone can induce corneal endothelial cell damage after a relatively high surface dose of 42.5 J/cm$^2$.[21,22] The typical UVA surface dose clinically used for CXL is only 5.4 J/cm$^2$, which, based on one study,[23] would be an estimated dose received by the cornea in 15–20 minutes of sun exposure during a summer day.

Animal studies showed that the threshold endothelial cytotoxic dose is 0.65 J/cm$^2$.[24] The currently used treatment parameters are set so that the anterior 250–350 microns of corneal stroma are treated[25] thus preventing damage to corneal endothelium. With current treatment parameters, the endothelial cytotoxic dose could only be delivered in human corneas thinner than 400 microns.[24] For patients with corneas thinner than 400 microns, a hypo-osmolar riboflavin solution has traditionally been used to increase the corneal thickness.[26] The conventional hypo-osmolar 0.1% riboflavin solution is prepared by diluting vitamin B$_2$-riboflavin-5-phosphate 0.5% with physiological salt solution (sodium chloride 0.9% solution) to achieve osmolarity of 310 mOsmol/L.[26] In the conventional iso-osmolar solution vitamin B$_2$-riboflavin-5-phosphate 0.5% is diluted in Dextran T500 20% to achieve osmolality of 402.7 mOsmol/L.

Riboflavin plays a critical role during exposure of the cornea to UVA. Riboflavin saturated cornea increases UVA absorption in the cornea to 95%[19] compared to 32% without riboflavin,[27] therefore enhancing the collagen crosslinking effect in the corneal stroma on one hand and reducing the exposure of the endothelium and intraocular tissues to UVA on the other (Fig. 1). The CXL results in an increase in biomechanical rigidity (stiffening) of human corneas. It has been postulated in the literature that this could possibly be caused by an increase in the collagen fiber diameter due to intrafibrillar[28,29] and interfibrillar crosslinks.[29] Surprisingly, interlamellar cohesive force does not increase after CXL.[29] The crosslinking effect is strongest in the anterior 300 microns of the corneal stroma,[30] which has been previously found to play a significant role in maintaining the corneal curvature.[31] Consequently, collagen crosslinking

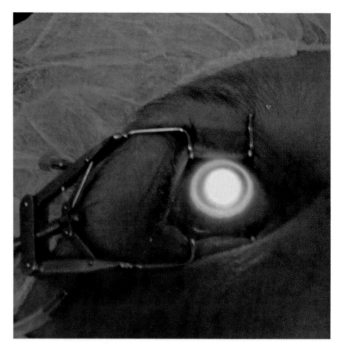

**Fig. 1:** Epithelial-on crosslinking showing the cornea saturated with riboflavin during UV-light treatment

has been seen to cause corneal flattening and reduction of spherical error.

The mechanism of CXL is not completely understood. Riboflavin is known to generate active oxygen species (singlet oxygen ($^1O_2$) and superoxide anion radicals ($O_2^-$), which have been shown to contribute to enzyme inactivation.[32,33] However, Kato et al.[34] showed that the active oxygen species do not seem to contribute to collagen crosslinking. Instead, riboflavin-sensitized photodynamic modification of collagen is responsible for collagen aggregation, which is accompanied by the loss of tyrosine and the formation of dityrosine.[34] Another study suggested that photo-oxidized histidine and lysine might contribute to collagen crosslinking as well.[35] Much speculation exists regarding these mechanisms and controversy and lacunae in understanding the science in this area remain. Further experiments are needed to better understand the mechanism of CXL.

### Clinical Application of Corneal Collagen Crosslinking

#### Keratoconus

In 2003, Wollensak et al. reported on the first series of patients with progressive keratoconus treated with CXL and showed that the procedure was not only able to halt progression in all eyes, but regression was noted in 70%

of the eyes.[1] Their results showed the mean decrease in maximum K was 2.01 D and the mean decrease in refractive error was 1.14 D over a mean follow-up period of 23 months. These clinical observations were later confirmed by multiple other reports.[36-54] Figure 2 shows an improvement of keratometry readings after CXL in a patient with keratoconus.

Caporossi et al.[39] showed mean K reduction of 2.1 D in the central 3.0 mm, which was associated with increase of uncorrected visual acuity (UCVA) by 3.6 lines, sphere spectacle corrected visual acuity (SSCVA) by 1.85 lines, and best spectacle corrected visual acuity (BSCVA) by 1.66 lines at 6 months after the treatment and a reduction of 2.5 D in the mean spherical equivalent.

Raiskup-Wolf et al.[38] reported on a large cohort of 480 eyes of 272 keratoconus patients treated with CXL and followed for up to 6 years (mean 26.7 months). Their results showed a mean decrease in maximum K by 2.68 D in the 1st year, 2.21 D in the 2nd year and 4.84 D in the 3rd year suggesting that there is a trend towards continued improvement for at least 3 years after the treatment. One or more lines of improvement in BSCVA were noted in 53%, 57% and 58% during the first, second and third postoperative year, respectively. The authors also reported on two of their patients whose keratoconus progressed despite crosslinking and who required a repeated application of UVA/riboflavin.

Wittig-Silva et al.[37] conducted a randomized controlled trial of collagen crosslinking in progressive keratoconus. Their preliminary results showed a decrease in maximum K by an average 0.74 D at 3 months, 0.92 D at 6 months and 1.45 D at 12 months in treated eyes. In contrast, the control eyes showed gradual increase in maximum K by 1.28 D at 12 months.

Grewal et al.[36] reported on 1 year follow-up data on 102 patients with progressive keratoconus. None of the patients showed progression after crosslinking. Their results revealed a mean reduction of 1.43 D in spherical equivalent, reduction in keratometry readings and improvement in BCVA. However, none of the parameters followed showed a statistical significance compared to preoperative data. The authors also examined central corneal thickness, corneal volume, lens density, foveal thickness and retinal nerve fiber layer, none of which showed statistically significant difference during the follow-up for up to 1 year after surgery. The authors pointed to a tendency towards decrease in foveal thickness and cautioned that this observation should be studied further.

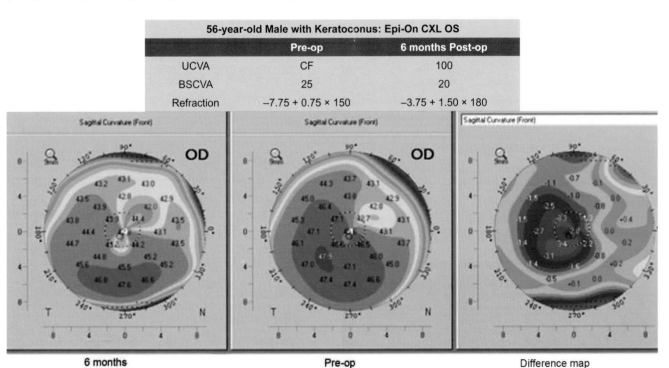

| 56-year-old Male with Keratoconus: Epi-On CXL OS | | |
|---|---|---|
| | Pre-op | 6 months Post-op |
| UCVA | CF | 100 |
| BSCVA | 25 | 20 |
| Refraction | −7.75 + 0.75 × 150 | −3.75 + 1.50 × 180 |

**Fig. 2:** A 56-year-old male with mild keratoconus underwent epithelial-on crosslinking. The patient experienced improvement in both uncorrected and best spectacle-corrected vision, as well as a significant reduction in refractive error. The pentacam difference map shows significant central flattening

CHAPTER 88

Another study by Hersh et al.[53] examined 1-year results after CXL for keratoconus or post-LASIK ectasia and showed improvement in UDVA, CDVA, the maximum and average K values. The authors also noted that both CDVA and the maximum K value worsened between baseline and 1 month after the procedure, which was followed by improvement between 1, 3 and 6 months and stabilization thereafter.

Coskunseven et al.[41] compared the results of CXL in patients with keratoconus to their fellow untreated eyes and found a significant improvement in UCVA and BSCVA, and significant decrease in spherical equivalent and astigmatism in treated eyes during a mean follow-up period of 9 months. Similar results were reported by Vinciguera et al.[42,43] and Agrawal.[44] More convincing than Grewal et al. data, these studies showed a statistically significant improvement in UCVA, BSCVA, and keratometry readings. Corneal wavefront measurements in some studies did not appear to change significantly within the first 6–9 months after the procedure,[44,45] but a significant change was noted at 12 months.[43] On the other hand, a significant reduction in coma can be seen earlier, at 6 months after crosslinking according to one report.[44]

Combining CXL with other surgical procedures to correct corneal ectasia has been explored in several clinical studies. Chan et al. compared clinical outcomes of 13 eyes with keratoconus treated with Intacs combined with transepithelial CXL to 12 eyes treated with Intacs without CXL.[46] They found that the patients treated with Intacs and CXL had a significantly greater reduction in cylinder than the Intacs-only group. Another study made similar observations.[47] Coscunseven et al. compared two groups of patients with reversed sequence of Intacs implantation and CXL with the mean interval between the two treatments of 7 months.[48] Their results showed a greater improvement in corrected distance visual acuity (CDVA), spherical error (SE), and mean K in the group treated with Intacs implantation first and with subsequent CXL later. Combining intrastromal ring implantation with CXL may offer an advantage of saturating the corneal stroma by riboflavin via the stromal pocket, hence avoiding the epitheliopathy typically seen first days after CXL.[54] Photorefractive keratectomy (PRK) is another surgical procedure that has been combined with CXL to treat keratoconus. Kanellopoulos compared a group of 127 eyes treated with topography guided PRK followed by CXL 6 months later in a group of 198 eyes treated with both procedures on the same-day and found that the same-day

group had statistically significantly better improvement in vision and K readings.[49] Kymionis et al. also showed some benefit of combining PRK and CXL in a smaller cohort of patients who received both procedures on the same-day.[50] An improvement in vision was reported in one eye with keratoconus treated with CXL and followed by topography guided PRK 12 months later.[51] Unlike the combination of PRK or Intacs implantation with CXL, the effect of same-day conductive keratoplasty combined with CXL according to one study resulted in regression 3 months after the procedures.[52]

## Post-LASIK Ectasia

Halting the progression of keratectasia in a patient after LASIK using CXL was initially reported by Kohlhaas et al.[55] Hafezi et al. reported later on a case series of 10 patients with post-LASIK ectasia treated with crosslinking.[56] The authors observed that progression of keratectasia was arrested in 5 patients and in the remaining 5 patients keratectasia regressed during the postoperative follow-up of up to 25 months. Similar results were reported by Saldago et al.[57] According to one case report, the initial improvement in SE and K values in a patient with post-LASIK keratectasia treated with Intacs, was followed by regression, which was subsequently successfully reversed using CXL (Fig. 3).[58]

## Other Indications for Corneal Collagen Crosslinking

Several authors examined the effect of UVA-light and riboflavin application in patients with infectious keratitis and found that the progression of ulcers was stopped and corneal re-epithelialization and resolution of the infectious process was observed.[59-61] Persistent corneal edema is another previously studied indication for CXL.[62-66] Improvement in pain, corneal transparency, and a decrease in central corneal thickness were typically seen initially, but return to preoperative levels within months suggested that the procedure might not have a long lasting effect in patients with corneal edema. Despite this limitation, it might be a suitable alternative for patients with pain symptoms and poor visual prognosis.[67] Kymionis et al. treated two patients with pellucid marginal degeneration with simultaneous PRK and collagen crosslinking. The authors noted in both patients a remarkable improvement of visual acuity along with significant reduction of keratometry readings.[68,69] A summary of the reported indications for CXL is in Table 1.

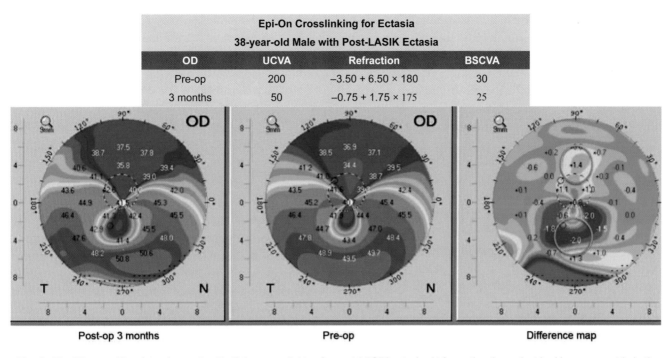

| Epi-On Crosslinking for Ectasia | | | |
|---|---|---|---|
| 38-year-old Male with Post-LASIK Ectasia | | | |
| OD | UCVA | Refraction | BSCVA |
| Pre-op | 200 | −3.50 + 6.50 × 180 | 30 |
| 3 months | 50 | −0.75 + 1.75 × 175 | 25 |

Post-op 3 months     Pre-op     Difference map

**Fig. 3:** The 38-year-old male underwent epithelial-on crosslinking for post-LASIK ectasia. At 3 months, the patient had improvement in both uncorrected vision and best-corrected vision. The difference map shows flattening inferiorly and steepening superiorly

## Complications

Although riboflavin and UVA application is considered to be a safe and well-tolerated procedure, complications can occur (Table 2). Endothelial cytotoxicity is always a concern with any corneal surgery. Animal studies showed when a cornea less than 400 microns thick is irradiated with a standard dose of 5.4 J/cm² (3 mW/cm²), the endothelial dose can reach cytotoxic levels (≥ 0.65 J/cm² = 0.36 mW/cm²) and cause significant necrosis and apoptosis of endothelial cells within 24 hours of application.[24] Therefore, caution must be exercised in patients with central corneal thickness of less than 400 microns. In these patients, application of hypotonic riboflavin to cause corneal swelling to levels above 400 microns or reduction

of UVA dose have been used. One animal study showed that 2 mW/cm² was the lowest dose that produced a significant mechanical stiffening effect[70] and an increase in resistance to enzymatic digestion.[18] With this low irradiance level the endothelial UVA dose is only 0.54 J/cm² (0.3 mW/cm²), well below the threshold of the endothelial cytotoxic dose.

According to a large study involving 117 eyes of 99 patients, the complication rate defined as loss of 2 or more Snellen lines was 2.9% and the failure rate defined as continued progression of keratectasia was 7.6%.[40] A

**Table 1:** Reported indications for UVA and riboflavin mediated corneal collagen crosslinking

| Diagnosis | References |
|---|---|
| Keratoconus | 36–54 |
| Post-LASIK ectasia | 55–58 |
| Infectious keratitis | 59–61 |
| Corneal edema | 62–67 |
| Pellucid marginal degeneration | 68,69 |

LASIK: Laser-assisted *in situ* keratomileusis

**Table 2:** Reported complications of UVA and riboflavin mediated corneal collagen crosslinking

| Complication | References |
|---|---|
| Stromal haze | 72–74 |
| Infection | |
|   Bacterial keratitis | 79–82 |
|   Acanthamoeba keratitis | 83 |
|   HSV keratitis and uveitis | 84 |
| Sterile inflammation | |
|   Keratitis and corneal scarring | 75 |
|   Stromal infiltrates and melt | 76,77 |
|   Diffuse lamellar keratitis | 78 |

HSV: Herpes simplex virus

CHAPTER 88

preoperative maximum keratometry reading of 58.0 D or more was a significant risk factor for failure. Interestingly, the authors also found that the procedure was more likely to fail in females when compared to their male counterparts. This study used the traditional protocol in which epithelial removal was performed. Sterile infiltrates were seen in 7.6% eyes and central stromal scarring was noted in 2.8% eyes. The authors found that a preoperative maximum K reading of less than 58.0 D may reduce the rate of failure to less than 3% and restricting patient age to younger than 35 years may reduce the complication rate to 1%. During UVA/riboflavin application approximately 7% of the UVA passes the cornea.[1] In the eye, UVA is absorbed primarily by the crystalline lens, which also contains riboflavin and hence, although very unlikely, lenticular crosslinking can potentially occur. To date, no case of CXL induced cataract formation has been reported in the literature over more than a decade since the first use of CXL. Systemic conditions such as pregnancy[71] and neurodermatitis[38] have been proposed to be risk factors for progression of keratectasia despite the application of CXL.

Postoperative corneal haze that does not limit vision can be seen after UVA/riboflavin crosslinking.[72] However, visually significant corneal haze, with or without stromal infiltration, has been also reported. According to one study in a series of 163 eyes, clinically significant stromal haze persisting for 1 year after crosslinking developed in 8.6% of eyes (n=14) of 13 patients.[73] The authors proposed that, based on their data, preoperative increased K value at corneal apex and decreased corneal thickness may possibly represent risk factors for persistent clinically significant stromal haze. Hersh et al.[74] examined the natural history of CXL associated corneal haze using Scheimpflug densitometry and slit-lamp biomicroscopy. The authors found that the corneal haze was greatest at 1 month, plateaued at 3 months, and decreased significantly between 3 and 12 months after CXL. They also noted that the corneal haze did not correlate with clinical outcome. Koppen et al. reported on 4 patients who developed multiple white stromal infiltrates and ciliary injection following crosslinking, which responded to topical and subconjunctival steroids. The infiltrates resolved with stromal scars and in some patients caused reduction of the visual acuity.[75] Sterile infiltrates that resulted in stromal melt were observed after CXL by some authors.[76,77] Additionally, in one patient with post-LASIK keratectasia a diffuse lamellar keratitis developed after CXL.[78]

Infectious keratitis is a known complication associated with epithelial corneal defects and/or bandage contact lens wear, both of which are present after the traditional CXL with epithelial debridement is typically performed in order to facilitate penetration of the riboflavin into the corneal stroma. A spectrum of microorganisms causing infectious keratitis after CXL including bacteria.[79-82] Acanthamoeba[83] and Herpes simplex virus[84] have been reported.

## SUMMARY

Despite the lack of large multicenter prospective randomized trials, CXL has gradually become a first line treatment for keratoconus and related corneal conditions. Although available data suggest that CXL administered with the currently widely adopted treatment parameters is safe, effective and well tolerated, further improvements are likely to come in the future. One of the improvements is development of protocols that do not require epithelial removal, which will likely lead to reduction of risk for infectious keratitis, stromal scarring and haze, and increase in patient comfort. Delivery of riboflavin into the cornea through intact epithelium[46,47,85] or through a femtosecond laser created pocket[86] could become an alternative to currently widely accepted administration of riboflavin that requires removal of the corneal epithelium (Fig. 4).

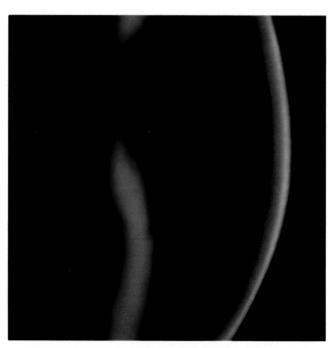

**Fig. 4:** The cornea saturated with riboflavin without epithelial removal

Reduction of procedure time will further enhance the patient comfort. A method named 'flash-linking' was recently studied in porcine eyes as an alternative to traditional administration of CXL.[87] Flash-linking used a customized photoactive crosslinking agent and only 30 seconds of UVA-light exposure time, at the same power and wavelength as currently accepted treatment parameters. Flash-linking showed a corneal stiffening effect comparable to traditional crosslinking in porcine eyes. Another improvement might come from changing the riboflavin solution. Recent experiments by McCall et al. suggested that if riboflavin is dissolved in deuterium oxide the concentration of riboflavin could be decreased or the effect could be significantly enhanced, since deuterium oxide is known to increase the half-life of singlet oxygen species.[88]

Ultimately, development of topical medications capable of inducing CXL that could be self-administered would further revolutionize treatment of keratoconus and related conditions. Several drugs including genipin,[89] glutaraldehyde[90], glyceraldehydes[91] and aliphatic beta-nitro alcohols[92] were identified, but further investigations are needed before any of these compounds could be introduced to clinical practice.

In refractive surgery, which is considered elective and required to have the highest standards for safety, a complication is defined as a loss in CDVA of 2 or more Snellen lines[93] within 6–12 months postoperatively. A refractive surgical procedure is deemed to be safe if a complication rate is lower than 5%.[94] Although the exact rate of complications after CXL has not been established in larger multicenter clinical trials, the reported success rates suggest that the procedure should invariably be considered at the very least for patients with progressive keratectasia elective, since presently it is the only treatment shown to have the ability of halting or reversing the natural course of this condition.[40] A good argument could also be made that, considering the risk of no treatment and subsequent progression of keratoconus, CXL should be considered in any patient diagnosed with forme fruste or clinically significant keratoconus or similar corneal ectatic condition.

## ❧ REFERENCES

1. Wollensak G, Spoerl E, Seiler T. Riboflavin/Ultraviolet-A-induced collagen crosslinking for the treatment of keratoconus. Am J Ophthalmol. 2003;135(5):620-7.
2. Cannon DJ, Foster CS. Collagen crosslinking in keratoconus. Invest Ophthalmol Vis Sci. 1978;17(1):63-5.
3. Krachmer JH, Feder RS, Belin MW. Keratoconus and related noninflammatory corneal thinning disorders. Surv Ophthalmol. 1984;28(4):293-322.
4. Rehany U, Lahav M, Shosan S. Collagenolytic activity in keratoconus. Ann Ophthalmol. 1982;14(8):751-4.
5. Kao WW, Vergnes JP, Ebert J, et al. Increased collagenase and gelatinase activities in keratoconus. Biochem Biophys Res Commun. 1982;107(3):929-36.
6. Sawaguchi S, Yue BY, Sugar J, et al. Lysosomal enzyme abnormalities in keratoconus. Arch Ophtahlmol. 1989;107 (10):1507-10.
7. Zhou L, Sawaguchi S, Twining SS, et al. Expression of degradative enzymes and protease inhibitors in corneas with keratoconus. Invest Ophthalmol Vis Sci. 1989;39(7):1117-24.
8. Kenney MC, Nesburn AB, Burgeson RE, et al. Abnormalities of the extracellular matrix in keratoconus corneas. Cornea. 1997;16(3):345-51.
9. Daxer A, Fratzl P. Collagen fibril orientation in the human corneal stroma and its implication in keratoconus. Invest Ophtahlmol Vis Sci. 1997;38(1):121-9.
10. Meek KM, Tuft SJ, Huang Y, et al. Changes in collagen orientation and distribution in keratoconus corneas. Invest Ophthalmol Vis Sci. 2005;46(6):1948-56.
11. Kymes SM, Walline JJ, Zadnik K, et al. Quality of life in keratoconus: the Collaborative Longitudinal Evaluation of Keratoconus (CLEK) Study Group. Am J Ophthalmol. 2004; 138(4):527-35.
12. Barr JT, Wilson BS, Gordon MO, et al. Estimation of the incidence and factors predictive of corneal scarring in the Collaborative Longitudinal Evaluation of Keratoconus (CLEK) Study; the CLEK Study Group. Cornea. 2005;25(1):16-25.
13. Davis LJ, Schechtman KB, Wilson BS, et al. Longitudinal changes in visual acuity in keratoconus; the Collaborative Longitudinal Evaluation of Keratoconus (CLEK) Study; the CLEK Study Group. Invest Ophtahlmol Vis Sci. 2006;47(2): 489-500.
14. Maeno A, Naor J, Lee HM, et al. Three decades of corneal transplantation: indications and patient characteristics. Cornea. 2000;19(1):7-11.
15. Khadem J, Truong T, Ernest JT. Photodynamic biologic tissue glue. Cornea. 1994;13(5):406-10.
16. Daxer A, Misof K, Grabner B, et al. Collagen fibrils in the human corneal stroma: structure and aging. Invest Ophthalmol Vis Sci. 1998;39(3):644-8.
17. Klingman LH, Gebre M. Biochemical changes in hairless mouse skin collagen after chronic exposure to ultraviolet-A radiation. Photochem Photobiol. 1991;54(2):233-7.
18. Spoerl E, Wollensak G, Seiler T. Increased resistance of riboflavin/UVA-treated cornea against enzymatic digestion. Curr Eye Res. 2004;29(1):35-40.
19. Spoerl E, Schreiber J, Hellmund K, et al. Untersuchungen zur Verfestigung der Hornhaut am Kaninchen. Ophthalmologe. 2000;97(3):203-6.
20. Hettlich HJ, Lucke K, Kreiner CF. Light induced endocapsular polymerization of injectable lens refilling materials. Ger J Ophthalmol. 1992;1(5):346-9.

21. Pitts DG, Gullen AP, Hacker PD. Ocular effects of ultraviolet radiation from 295 to 365 nm. Invest Ophthalmol Vis Sci. 1977; 16(10):932-9.

22. Ringvold A, Davanger M, Olsen EG. Changes of the cornea endothelium after ultraviolet radiation. Acta Ophthalmol. 1982;60(1):41-53.

23. Kimlin MG, Prisi AV, Downs NJ. Human UVA Exposures Estimated from Ambient UVA Measurements. Photochem Photobiol Sci. 2003;2(4):365-9.

24. Wollensak G, Spoerl E, Wilsch M, et al. Endothelial cell damage after riboflavin-ultraviolet-A treatment in the rabbit. J Cataract Refract Surg. 2003;29(9):1786-90.

25. Spoerl E, Mrochen M, Sliney D, et al. Safety of UVA-riboflavin cross-linking of the cornea. Cornea. 2007;26(4):385-9.

26. Hafezi F, Mrochen M, Iseli HP, et al. Collagen crosslinking with ultraviolet-A and hypo-osmolar riboflavin solution in thin corneas. J Cataract Refract Surg. 2009;35:621-4.

27. Michael R. Development and repair of cataract induced by ultraviolet radiation. Ophthalmic Res. 2000;32(suppl 1).

28. Wollensak G, Wilsch M, Spoerl E, et al. Collagen fiber-diameter after riboflavin/UVA induced collagen crosslinking in the rabbit cornea. Cornea. 2004;23(5):503-7.

29. Wollensak G, Sporl E, Mazzotta C, et al. Interlamellar cohesion after corneal crosslinking using riboflavin and ultraviolet light. Br J Ophthalmol. 2011;95(6):876-80.

30. Wollensak G, Spoerl E, Seiler T. Stress-strain measurements of human and porcine corneas after riboflavin-ultraviolet-A-induced cross-linking. J Cataract Refract Surg. 2003;29(9): 1780-5.

31. Muller LJ, Pels E, Vrensen GF. The specific architecture of the anterior stroma accounts for maintenance of corneal curvature. Br J Ophthalmol. 2001;85(4):437-43.

32. Krass W, Schiebel G, Eberl D, et al. Blue light induced reversible inactivation of the tonoplast-type $H^+$-ATPase from corn coleoptiles in the presence of flavins. Photochem Photobiol. 1987;45:837-44.

33. Gotor C, Marquez AJ, Vega JM. Studies on in vitro $O_2$-dependent inactivation of NADH-glutamate synthetase from Chlamydomonas reinhardii stimulated by flavins. Photochem Photobiol. 1987;45:353-8.

34. Kato Y, Uchida K, Kawakishi S. Aggregation of collagen exposed to UVA in the presence of riboflavin: A plausible role of tyrosine modification. Photochem Photobiol. 1994;59(3):343-9.

35. Dilon J, Chiesa R, Wang RH, et al. Molecular changes during the photooxidation of α-crystallin in the presence of uroporphyrin. Photochem Photobiol. 1993;57(3):526-30.

36. Grewal DS, Brar GS, Jain R, et al. Corneal collagen crosslinking using riboflavin ad ultraviolet-A light for keratoconus. One-year analysis using Scheimpflug imaging. J Cataract Refract Surg. 2009;35(3):425-32.

37. Wittig-Silva C, Whiting M, Lamoureux E, et al. A randomized controlled trial of corneal collagen cross-linking in progressive keratoconus: preliminary results. J Refract Surg. 2008;24: S720-5.

38. Raiskup-Wolf F, Hoyer A, Spoerl E, et al. Collagen crosslinking with riboflavin and ultraviolet-A light in keratoconus: Long-term results. J Cataract Refract Surg. 2008;34(5):796-801.

39. Caporosi A, Baiocchi S, Mazzotta C, et al. Parasurgical therapy for keratoconus by riboflavin-ultraviolet type. A rays induced cross-linking of corneal collagen. Preliminary refractive results in an Italian study. J Cataract Refract Surg. 2006;32(5):837-45.

40. Koller T, Mrochen M, Seiler T. Complication and failure rates after corneal crosslinking. J Cataract Refract Surg. 2009; 35(8):1358-62.

41. Coskunseven E, Jankov MR, Hafezi F. Contralateral eye study of corneal collagen crosslinking with riboflavin and UVA irradiation in patients with keratoconus. J Refract Surg. 2009;25(4):371-6.

42. Vinciguerra P, Albe E, Trazza S, et al. Intraoperative and postoperative effects of corneal collagen cross-linking on progressive keratoconus. Arch ophthalmol. 2009;127(10): 1258-65.

43. Vinciguerra P, Albe E, Trazza S. Refractive, topographic, tomographic, and aberrometric analysis of keratoconic eyes undergoing corneal cross-linking. Ophthalmology. 2009;116 (3):369-78.

44. Agrawal VB. Corneal collagen cross-linking with riboflavin and ultraviolet-a light for keratoconus in Indian eyes. Indian J Ophthalmol. 2009;57(2):111-4.

45. Baumeister M, Klaproth OK, Gehmlich J, et al. Changes in corneal first-surface wavefront aberration after corneal collagen cross-linking in keratoconus. Klin Monbl Augenheilkd. 2009; 226(9):752-6.

46. Chan CC, Sharma M, Wachler BS. Effect of inferior-segment Intacs with and without C3-R on keratoconus. J Cataract Refract Surg. 2007;33(1):75-80.

47. Ertan A, Karacal H, Kamburoglu G. Refractive and topographic results of transepithelial cross-linking treatment in eyes with intacs. Cornea. 2009;28(7):719-23.

48. Coskunseven E, Jankov MR, Hafezi F, et al. Effect of treatment sequence in combined intrastromal corneal rings and corneal collagen crosslinking for keratoconus. J Cataract Refract Surg. 2009;35(12):2084-91.

49. Kanellopoulos AJ. Comparison of sequential vs same-day simultaneous collagen cross-linking and topography-guided PRK for treatment of keratoconus. J Refract Surg. 2009;25(9):S812-8.

50. Kymionis GD, Kontadakis GA, Kounis GA, et al. Simultaneous topography-guided PRK followed by corneal collagen cross-linking for keratoconus. J Refract Surg. 2009;25(9):S807-11.

51. Kanellopoulos AJ, Binder PS. Collagen cross-linking (CCL/CXL) with sequential topography-guided PRK: a temporizing alternative for keratoconus to penetrating keratoplasty. Cornea. 2007;26(7):891-5.

52. Kymionis GD, Kontadakis GA, Naoumidi TL, et al. Conductive keratoplasty followed by collagen cross-linking with riboflavin-UV-A in patients with keratoconus. Cornea. 2010;29(2): 39-43.

53. Hersh PS, Greenstein SA, Fry KL. Corneal collagen crosslinking for keratoconus and corneal ectasia: One-year results. J Cataract Refract Surg. 2011;37(1):149-60.

54. Daxer A, Mahmoud HA, Venkateswaran RS. Corneal cross-linking and visual rehabilitation in keratoconus in one session without epithelial debridement: new technique. Cornea. 2010; 29(10):1176-9.

55. Kohlhaas M, Spoerl E, Speck A, et al. A new treatment of keratectasia after LASIK by using collagen with riboflavin/UVA light cross-linking. Klin Monbl Augenheilkd. 2005;222(5):430-6.

56. Hafezi F, Kanellopoulos J, Wiltfang R, et al. Corneal collagen crosslinking with riboflavin and ultraviolet A to treat induced keratectasia after laser in situ keratomileusis. J Cataract Refract Surg. 2007;33(12):2035-40.

57. Salgado JP, Khoramnia R, Lohman CP, et al. Corneal collagen crosslinking in post-LASIK keratectasia. Br J Ophthalmol. 2011;95(4):493-7.

58. Kamburoglu G, Ertan A. Intacs implantation with sequential collagen cross-linking treatment in postoperative LASIK ectasia. J Refract Surg. 2008;24:S726-9.

59. Iseli HP, Thiel MA, Hafezi F, et al. Ultraviolet A/riboflavin corneal cross-linking for infectious keratitis associated with corneal melts. Cornea. 2008;27(5):590-4.

60. Moren H, Malmsjo M, Mortensen J, et al. Riboflavin and ultraviolet a crosslinking of the cornea for the treatment of keratitis. Cornea. 2010;29(1):102-4.

61. Micelli Ferrari T, Leozappa M, Lorusso M, et al. Escherichia coli keratitis treated with ultraviolet A/riboflavin corneal cross-linking: a case report. Eur J Ophthalmol. 2009;19(2):295-7.

62. Krueger RR, Ramos-Esteban JC, Kanellopoulos AJ. Staged intrastromal delivery of riboflavin with UVA-cross-linking in advanced bullous keratopathy: laboratory investigation and first clinical case. J Refract Surg. 2008;24(7):S730-6.

63. Ghanem RC, Santhiago MR, Berti TB, et al. Collagen crosslinking with riboflavin and ultraviolet-A in eyes with pseudophakic bullous keratopathy. J Cataract Refract Surg. 2010;36(2):273-6.

64. Bottos KM, Hofling-Lima AL, Barbosa MC, et al. Effect of collagen cross-linking in stromal fibril organization in edematous human corneas. Cornea. 2010;29(7):789-93.

65. Cordeiro Barbosa MM, Barbosa JB, Hirai FE, et al. Effect of cross-linking on corneal thickness in patients with corneal edema. Cornea. 2010;29(6):613-7.

66. Ehlers N, Hjortdal J. Riboflavin-ultraviolet light induced cross-linking in endothelial decompensation. Acta Ophthalmol. 2008;86(5):549-51.

67. Wollensak G, Aurich H, Wirbelauer C, et al. Potential use of riboflavin/UVA cross-linking in bullous keratopathy. Ophthalmic Res. 2009;41(2):114-7.

68. Kymionis GD, Karavitaki AE, Kounis GA, et al. Management of pellucid marginal corneal degeneration with simultaneous customized photorefractive keratectomy and collagen cros-llinking. J Cataract Refract Surg. 2009;35(7):1298-301.

69. Kymionis GD, Grentzelos MA, Portaliou DM, et al. Photorefractive keratectomy followed by same-day corneal collagen crosslinking after intrastromal corneal ring segment implantation for pellucid marginal degeneration. J Cataract Refract Surg. 2010;36(10):1783-5.

70. Spoerl E, Huhle M, Seiler T. Induction of cross-links in corneal tissue. Exp Eye Res. 1998;66(1):97-103.

71. Hafezi F, Iseli HP. Pregnancy-related exacerbation of iatrogenic keratectasia despite corneal collagen crosslinking. J Cataract Refract Surg. 2008;34(7):1219-21.

72. Mazzotta C, Balestrazzi A, Baiocchi S, et al. Stromal haze after combined riboflavin-UVA corneal collagen cross-linking in keratoconus: in vivo confocal microscopic evaluation. Clin Exp Ophthalmol. 2007;35(6):580-2.

73. Raiskup F, Hoyer A, Spoerl E. Permanent corneal haze after riboflavin-UVA-induced cross-linking in keratoconus. J Refract Surg. 2009;25(9):S824-8.

74. Greenstein SA, Fry KL, Bhatt J, et al. Natural history of corneal haze after collagen crosslinking for keratoconus and corneal ectasia: Scheimpflug and biomicroscopic analysis. J Cataract Refract Surg. 2010;36(12):2105-14.

75. Koppen C, Vryghem JC, Gobin L, et al. Keratitis and corneal scarring after UVA/riboflavin cross-linking for keratoconus. J Refract Surg. 2009;25(9):S819-23.

76. Angunawela RI, Arnalich-Montiel F, Allan BDS. Peripheral sterile corneal infiltrates and melting after collagen crosslinking for keratoconus. J Cataract Refract Surg. 2009;35(3):606-7.

77. Eberwein P, Auw-Hadrich C, Birnbaum F, et al. Corneal melting after cross-linking and deep lamellar keratoplasty in a keratoconus patient. Klin Monatsbl Augenheilkd. 2008;225(1):96-8.

78. Kymionis GD, Bouzoukis DI, Diakonis VF, et al. Diffuse lamellar keratitis after corneal collagen crosslinking in a patient with post-laser in situ keratomileusis corneal ectasia. J Cataract Refract Surg. 2007;33(12):2135-7.

79. Pollhammer M, Cursiefen C. Bacterial keratitis early after corneal crosslinking with riboflavin and ultraviolet-A. J Cataract Refract Surg. 2009;35(3):588-9.

80. Sharma N, Maharana P, Singh G, et al. Pseudomonas kertitis after collagen crosslinking for keratoconus: case report and review of literature. J Cataract Refract Surg. 2010;36(3):517-20.

81. Perez-Santonja JJ, Artola A, Javaloy J, et al. Microbial keratitis after corneal collagen crosslinking. J Cataract Refract Surg. 2009;35(6):1138-40.

82. Zamora KV, Males JJ. Polymicrobial keratitis after a collagen crosslinking procedure with postoperative use of a contact lens: a case report. Cornea. 2009;28(4):474-6.

83. Rama P, Di Matteo F, Matuska S, et al. Acanthamoeba keratitis with perforation after corneal collagen crosslinking and bandage contact lens. J Cataract Refract Surg. 2009;35(4):788-91.

84. Kymionis GD, Portaliou DM, Bouzoukis DI, et al. Herpetic keratitis with iritis after corneal crosslinking with riboflavin and ultraviolet A for keratoconus. J Cataract Refract Surg. 2007;33(11):1982-4.

85. Kissner A, Spoerl E, Jung R, et al. Pharmacological modification of the epithelial permeability by benzalkonium chloride in UVA/Riboflavin corneal collagen crosslinking. Curr Eye Res. 2010;35(8):715-21.

86. Kanellopoulos AJ. Collagen cross-linking in early keratoconus with riboflavin in a femtosecond laser-created pocket: initial clinical results. J Refract Surg. 2009;25(11):1034-7.

87. Rocha KM, Ramos-Esteban JC, Qian Y, et al. Comparative study of riboflavin-UVA crosslinking and "flash-linking" using surface wave elastometry. J Refract Surg. 2008;24(7):S748-51.

88. McCall AS, Kraft S, Edelhauser HF, et al. Mechanisms of corneal tissue cross-linking in response to treatment with topical riboflavin and long-wavelength ultraviolet radiation (UVA). Invest Ophthalmol Vis Sci. 2010;51(1):129-38.

89. Avila MY, Navia JL. Effect of genipin collagen crosslinking on porcine corneas. J Cataract Refract Surg. 2010;36(4):659-64.

90. Doillon CJ, Watsky MA, Hakim M, et al. A collagen-based scaffold for a tissue engineered human cornea: physical and physiological properties. Int J Artif Organs. 2003;26(8):764-73.

91. Wollensak G, Iomdina E. Crosslinking of scleral collagen in the rabbit using glyceraldehyde. J Cataract Refract Surg. 2008;34(4):651-6.

92. Paik DC, Wen Q, Braunstein RE, et al. Initial studies using aliphatic beta-nitro alcohols for therapeutic corneal cross-linking. Invest Ophthalmol Vis Sci. 2009;50(3):1098-105.

93. Stulting RD, Carr JD, Thompson KP, et al. Complications of laser in situ keratomileusis for the correction of myopia. Ophthalmology. 1999;106(1):13-20.

94. United States Food and Drug Administration. Center for Devices and Radiological Health. Checklist of information usually submitted in an investigational device exemptions (IDE) application for refractive surgery. Available from www.fda.gov/cdrh/ode/2093.html.

# 89

# Phototherapeutic Keratectomy

*John W Josephson, Jay M Lustbader*

## ⯈ INTRODUCTION

Excimer laser phototherapeutic keratectomy (PTK) is a viable alternative to standard keratectomy and keratoplasty techniques for the treatment of a variety of diseases of the anterior cornea. Phototherapeutic keratectomy uses the energy generated by the excimer laser to disrupt molecular bonds in corneal tissue, in a process known as ablation, to help treat corneal pathology. This technique allows for precise cuts at the desired depths for many anterior corneal diseases.

Since the initial Food and Drug Administration (FDA) approval for PTK in the United States in 1995, there has been no published data on trends in the use of PTK versus standard therapies. Anecdotally, doctors believe that the use has been stable over many years.

The US FDA approved PTK in 1995 for patients with the conditions noted in Table 1. The device is indicated for patients with decreased best corrected visual acuity

(BSCVA) and/or with disabling pain that are the result of superficial corneal epithelial irregularities or stromal scars in the anterior one-third of the cornea. The patients must have failed with alternative treatment options. For safety, the residual corneal thickness should not be less than 400 microns after the PTK. Many surgeons use PTK for other conditions as well, particularly recurrent corneal erosions.[1-4] Despite its widespread use, no controlled clinical study has directly compared PTK with standard keratectomy techniques.

## ⯈ CANDIDACY

The US FDA guidelines state that the condition treated must be of the anterior one-third of cornea, and the remaining stromal bed should remain greater than approximately 400 microns. The best candidates are eyes with elevated or anterior stromal opacities (i.e. Salzmann's nodules, keratoconus nodules, Reis Bucklers, etc.). Patients with deep opacities or corneal thinning would be poor candidates for this procedure.

## ⯈ CLINICAL USES

Ayres and Rapuano reviewed 1,006 patients who underwent PTK and separated patients into four broad categories.[5] These categories are anterior corneal scars, dystrophies of epithelium and Bowman's membrane, anterior corneal stromal dystrophies, and elevated corneal lesions.

Anterior corneal scars (Figs 1A and B) related to trauma, or in postsurgical eyes, can be successfully treated with PTK if the anterior 10–20% of the cornea is mainly involved. *Herpes simplex virus* (HSV) and other forms of infectious

| Table 1: FDA-approved indications for PTK |
|---|
| • Corneal scars and opacity (from trauma and inactive infections) |
| • Dystrophies (Reis-Buckler's, granular, and lattice) |
| • Thygeson's superficial keratitis |
| • Irregular corneal surfaces associated with filamentary keratitis and Salzmann's nodular degeneration |
| • Residual band keratopathy after unsuccessful EDTA treatment |
| • Scars subsequent to previous (not concurrent) pterygium excision |

*Note*: Indications for PTK as outlined by FDA guidelines in 1995

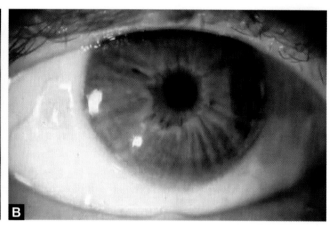

**Figs 1A and B:** (A) Patient presented with irregular anterior corneal scar; (B) Patient was treated with PTK with near resolution of scar

keratitis have also been treated successfully with PTK if anterior, though many of these lesions also involve deeper areas of the cornea. In addition, use of the excimer laser in patients with a history of HSV infection is controversial due to the risk of reactivation of herpes infection from the ultraviolet exposure. Recently, many case reports have also been published using PTK for early stages of *Acanthamoeba* keratitis. These reports show good resolution as long as infection was limited to anterior one-third of cornea.[6,7]

Dystrophies of the epithelium and Bowman's membrane have been successfully treated with many modalities including topical drops, epithelial debridement and anterior stromal puncture. In recalcitrant recurrent erosions, PTK has been found to be a useful alternative. In many studies comparing these different modalities, no statistically significant differences were found between the techniques.[2,4,8]

However, in a recent review by Das and Seitz, PTK was found to be most effective in overall treatment particularly in post-traumatic recurrent erosions.[9] Some authors recommend that though recurrent erosions may only be in a localized area, it is imperative that one treats the entire visual axis.[2] Phototherapeutic keratectomy has also been studied in small case reports following laser-assisted *in situ* keratomileusis (LASIK) to manage flap striae and other flap complications.[4,10] These studies are not comparative but show improvement in symptoms and moderate shift in refraction in both directions of hyperopia and myopia in an unpredictable fashion.

Anterior corneal stromal dystrophies including granular, lattice, and Schnyder's dystrophy (Figs 2A and B) and dystrophies of Bowman's layer (i.e. Reis-Bucklers) are particularly challenging diseases and in many instances

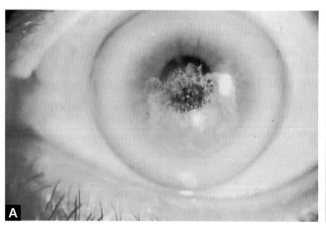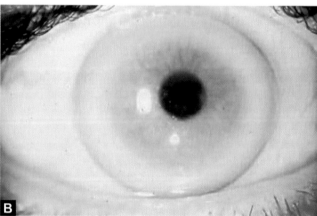

**Figs 2A and B:** (A) Patient with long standing Schnyder's crystalline dystrophy;
(B) Treated with successful PTK. Please note the residual deeper lesions postoperatively not treated

require lamellar or penetrating keratoplasty. Phototherapeutic keratectomy has been successful in treating these dystrophies, if involving the anterior 10–20% of the cornea. If deeper lesions exist, only the anterior portion is treated, leaving residual changes in the deeper stroma. Macular corneal dystrophy may also be treated, if there is significant anterior involvement.[11]

Elevated corneal lesions such as Salzmann's nodular degeneration and keratoconus nodules removed by PTK allow for a smooth surface after removal. These nodules can be removed manually but if Bowman's layer or anterior stroma is involved, a scar or irregular surface may be left. Elahn et al. discussed fifteen eyes with keratoconus and contact lens intolerance that underwent PTK to remove keratoconus nodules.[12] There were no recurrences of nodule formation in most patients, and patients had improved contact lens tolerance. Therefore, patients were able to delay or avoid more invasive surgery, such as penetrating keratoplasty.

## RESULTS

Phototherapeutic keratectomy allows corneas with opacities or scars to potentially obtain a smooth clear surface. In general, most anterior pathology as discussed above may be treated successfully with PTK. An article from a large center in India reported on 203 consecutive eyes of 191 patients who underwent PTK. They reported the data for all the indications for PTK and subcategorized for bullous keratopathy alone (53% of patients). They reported a statistically significant improvement in visual acuity in a majority of patients (79% of patients). In the bullous keratopathy patients, there was improvement in 73% of patients, but the gain was less dramatic than other corneal pathology.[13] In most studies, however, there is a mild to severe hyperopic shift depending on the degree of treatment. The hyperopic shift may be as high as four diopters.[1,14] In a study by Cavanaugh et al. a statistically significant correlation between the number of pulses applied and the degree of induced hyperopia was found.[15] This is due to flattening of the cornea that occurs as the pathology is being ablated. In some reports on treatment of recurrent erosion syndrome no refractive change was found.[4] The degree of improvement in vision or pain is mainly based on the pre-existing pathology, including its size and depth. Most reports show an improvement in symptoms of anterior corneal pathology with minimal short-term discomfort with PTK, rather than other more invasive techniques particularly when the pathology is focal and anterior.[2,3]

## CONTRAINDICATIONS AND COMPLICATIONS

Phototherapeutic keratectomy should not be used in treating deep corneal pathology (lesions in the posterior two-thirds of the cornea). In the literature, it is recommended that PTK may be beneficial in deeper corneal pathology if an anterior component is also present.[1,16] The surgeon would still treat only the anterior portion. Active inflammation or infection is also a contraindication to PTK surgery. Case reports have challenged this notion by treating early active acanthamoeba keratitis with PTK with impressive results and resolution of this debilitating infection.[6,7]

Hyperopic shift and unpredictable irregular astigmatism are the main complications seen after PTK.[1,3] Scarring or corneal haze may also be seen. However, the widespread use of mitomycin C with PTK ablation has significantly reduced its incidence.[17] Postoperative discomfort is common in the immediate few days after the surgery. This can be treated with a bandage contact lens, topical nonsteroidal drops and oral analgesics.

## SURGICAL TECHNIQUE

Once patients have given informed consent and realistic goals have been established the procedure can be performed. Although each surgeon will have individualized surgical techniques, the following is a standard approach to the procedure. After proper anesthesia is obtained through the application of topical drops, a lid speculum is inserted. Mechanical debridement of epithelium is performed. In the treatment of recurrent corneal erosion, the epithelium over the involved area can usually be removed with a surgical sponge. In other types of corneal pathology, a surgical blade or brush is needed for debridement. Debridement is performed only over the area of pathology being treated. After the epithelium is removed, the ablation is performed based on the goal of treatment. Generally, for recurrent erosion syndrome, less ablation is required (approximately 20–30 laser pulses) while a dense corneal scar would often require over 100 pulses. After the desired ablation, the patient is brought to the slit lamp and examined. It is not uncommon to have a patient returned to the laser for more treatment after this examination, if a large amount of corneal disease still remains. After the procedure a bandage contact lens is placed and antibiotic, steroid, and nonsteroidal drops are started. The goal of the surgery is to remove as little tissue as possible, while still reducing the scar or irregularity to improve vision and reduce pain. The epithelium will usually heal in 3–4 days, at which time the bandage contact lens is removed. The antibiotic and nonsteroidal drops are usually used for 1 week, while the steroid drops can be used for up to 1 month postoperatively.

One of the newer strategies in PTK is the use of masking agents. The goal is to reduce the irregular astigmatism which is one of the major obstacles in performing this procedure, by providing a smooth surface for the laser ablation. In an ablation of an irregular corneal surface, the agent will mask the deeper tissue while exposing protruding abnormalities. Some important considerations for the type of masking agent are the absorbance at 193 nm and the viscosity. In a study of masking fluids in an animal model, a solution of moderate viscosity and high absorbance at 193 nm appears to facilitate the PTK treatment.[18] Currently, many surgeons are using saline or viscous artificial tears with limited success though many new agents are being studied.[1,19] Many articles have disputed the notion that the use of a masking agent may be the source for the hyperopic shift seen in many ablations.[20-23] There are many promising technologies attempting to design an agent that can better mold the shape of the treated cornea to decrease the incidence of irregular astigmatism.[1,24]

## FUTURE TRENDS

Excimer laser PTK is a well-established and effective technique for the treatment of anterior corneal pathology. In the international literature there has been much recent focus on combining PTK with other established modalities.

Alessio et al. studied eyes that underwent PRK with resultant irregular astigmatism due to decentration of the ablation zone.[25] These eyes were treated with topography-driven PTK. Thirty-two eyes were included in the study and results were very promising, with 87.5% within one diopter of desired refraction. Postoperative topography showed well-centered treatments. As more of these studies are performed PTK may become an important modality in improving irregular astigmatism.

Another example is the work of Alio et al. who attempted to use superficial lamellar corneal excision with femtosecond laser followed by PTK and a masking substance to treat corneal leukomas.[26] Twelve patients with corneal haze or scarring underwent confocal microscopy then femtosecond laser to create a flap. Phototherapeutic keratectomy with a masking agent (0.25% sodium hyaluronate) was then performed and patients were followed up to 12 months. Eighty-three percent of eyes gained 3 or more lines in BSCVA and the remaining eyes gained 1 line of BSCVA. The authors concluded that lamellar excision with a femtosecond laser followed by masked PTK is a viable alternative to penetrating keratoplasty (PKP) and deep anterior lamellar keratoplasty (DALK) for these conditions.

An additional area of research in the international literature involves combining collagen crosslinking prior to the use of the excimer laser for PTK. Currently, the literature consists of case reports and anecdotal data.[21,22] Further studies will help delineate the role of corneal stabilization with collagen crosslinking prior to PTK.

## CONCLUSION

Phototherapeutic keratectomy with the excimer laser is a valuable treatment modality in selected patients with anterior corneal pathology. Further innovations will continue to expand its usefulness in the future.

## REFERENCES

1. Rapuano CJ. Excimer laser phototherapeutic keratectomy. Curr Opin Ophthalmol. 2001;12(4):288-93.
2. Rapuano CJ. Phototherapeutic keratectomy: who are the best candidates and how do you treat them? Curr Opin Ophthalmol. 2010;21(4):280-2.
3. Stasi K, Chuck RS. Update on phototherapeutic keratectomy. Curr Opin Ophthalmol. 2009;20(4):272-5.
4. Garcia-Gonzalez M, Teus MA. Early phototherapeutic keratectomy for basement membrane dystrophy after laser in situ keratomileusis. J Cataract Refract Surg. 2009;35(2):389-92.
5. Ayres BD, Rapuano CJ. Excimer laser phototherapeutic keratectomy. Ocul Surf. 2006;4(4):196-206.
6. Kandori M, Inoue T, Shimabukuro M, et al. Four cases of Acanthamoeba keratitis treated with phototherapeutic keratectomy. Cornea. 2010;29(10):1199-202.
7. Taenaka N, Fukuda M, Hibino T, et al. Surgical therapies for Acanthamoeba keratitis by phototherapeutic keratectomy and deep lamellar keratoplasty. Cornea. 2007;26(7):876-9.
8. Kampik D, Neumaier K, Mutsch A, et al. Intraepithelial phototherapeutic keratectomy and alcohol delamination for recurrent corneal erosions—two minimally invasive surgical alternatives. Klin Monbl Augenheilkd. 2008;225(4):276-80.
9. Das S, Seitz B. Recurrent corneal erosion syndrome. Surv Ophthalmol. 2008;53(1):3-15.
10. Steinert RF, Ashrafzadeh A, Hersh PS. Results of phototherapeutic keratectomy in the management of flap striae after LASIK. Ophthalmology. 2004;111(4):740-6.
11. Hafner A, Langenbucher A, Seitz B. Long-term results of phototherapeutic keratectomy with 193-nm excimer laser for macular corneal dystrophy. Am J Ophthalmol. 2005;140(3):392-6.
12. Elsahn AF, Rapuano CJ, Antunes VA, et al. Excimer laser phototherapeutic keratectomy for keratoconus nodules. Cornea. 2009;28(2):144-7.
13. Sharma N, Prakash G, Sinha R, et al. Indications and outcomes of phototherapeutic keratectomy in the developing world. Cornea. 2008;27(1):44-9.

14. Rao SK, Fogla R, Seethalakshmi G, et al. Excimer laser photo-therapeutic keratectomy: indications, results and its role in the Indian scenario. Indian J Ophthalmol. 1999;47(3):167-72.

15. Cavanaugh TB, Lind DM, Cutarelli PE, et al. Phototherapeutic keratectomy for recurrent erosion syndrome in anterior basement membrane dystrophy. Ophthalmology. 1999;106(5): 971-6.

16. Paparo LG, Rapuano CJ, Raber IM, et al. Phototherapeutic keratectomy for Schnyder's crystalline corneal dystrophy. Cornea. 2000;19(3):343-7.

17. Ayres BD, Hammersmith KM, Laibson PR, et al. Phototherapeutic keratectomy with intraoperative mitomycin C to prevent recurrent anterior corneal pathology. Am J Ophthalmol. 2006;142(3):490-2.

18. Kornmehl EW, Steinert RF, Puliafito CA. A comparative study of masking fluids for excimer laser phototherapeutic keratectomy. Arch Ophthalmol. 1991;109(6):860-3.

19. Fasano AP, Moreira H, McDonnell PJ, et al. Excimer laser smoothing of a reproducible model of anterior corneal surface irregularity. Ophthalmology. 1991;98(12):1782-5.

20. Dogru M, Katakami C, Yamanaka A. Refractive changes after excimer laser phototherapeutic keratectomy. J Cataract Refract Surg. 2001;27(5):686-92.

21. Liu C. Hyperopic shift and the use of masking agents in excimer laser superficial keratectomy. Br J Ophthalmol. 1992;76(1): 62-3.

22. Amm M, Duncker GI. Refractive changes after phototherapeutic keratectomy. J Cataract Refract Surg. 1997;23(6):839-44.

23. Fantes FE, Hanna KD, Waring GO, et al. Wound healing after excimer laser keratomileusis (photorefractive keratectomy) in monkeys. Arch Ophthalmol. 1990;108(5):665-75.

24. Stevens SX, Bowyer BL, Sanchez-Thorin JC, et al. The BioMask for treatment of corneal surface irregularities with excimer laser phototherapeutic keratectomy. Cornea. 1999;18(2):155-63.

25. Alessio G, Boscia F, La Tegola MG, et al. Topography-driven excimer laser for the retreatment of decentralized myopic photorefractive keratectomy. Ophthalmology. 2001;108(9): 1695-703.

26. Alio JL, Agdeppa MC, Uceda-Montanes A. Femtosecond laser-assisted superficial lamellar keratectomy for the treatment of superficial corneal leukomas. Cornea. 2011;30(3):301-7.

# CHAPTER 90

# Keratoprosthesis Surgery

*Gina M Rogers, Kenneth M Goins*

## ❧ INTRODUCTION

Corneal blindness is the fourth leading cause of blindness globally after cataract, glaucoma and age-related macular degeneration with estimates of 8 million blind from corneal disease worldwide.[1] The etiologies of corneal blindness vary across regions of the world, with trachoma being the leading cause of corneal blindness worldwide. In the United States, an array of etiologies lead to corneal blindness including chemical injury and trauma, infection/ulceration, which are commonly attributable to contact lens wear, herpes simplex virus, dystrophies, autoimmune diseases and graft failure. Regardless of the etiology, corneal scarring that leads to visual impairment is often addressed with keratoplasty.

The outcome of penetrating keratoplasty depends on the underlying disorder and availability of good donor tissue. In many patients, a full-thickness corneal graft provides good visual recovery and longevity. In other cases, such as cicatrizing diseases or repeat graft failure, a penetrating keratoplasty has a poorer outcome. A keratoprosthesis is an artificial cornea and can be considered as an alternative for transplantation in cases where conventional penetrating keratoplasty has failed or has a very low probability of success.

Many credit that the idea of an artificial cornea was first proposed in 1789 by French ophthalmologist Guillaume Pellier de Quengsy.[2,3] He suggested implantation of a glass lens held within a silver ring into the opaque cornea to restore vision. Over the years, many attempts of different materials, designs and insertion techniques but many of these experiments were fraught with high rates of complication. After the first successful human-to-human corneal transplantation was performed in 1906 by Zirm,

attention shifted to improving these outcomes and away from keratoprosthesis development. Research into development of the keratoprosthesis was renewed after World War II. After the war, the interest of many ophthalmologists was piqued when it was noted that pilots who sustained ocular injuries where polymethyl methacrylate (PMMA) was retained, tolerated this material well. This realization led to the development of PMMA intraocular lenses. Other applications of this material were studied, particularly by Cardona,[4,5] who attempted to use this inert plastic for keratoprosthesis designs. His keratoprosthesis procedure was laden with complications and did not gain widespread support.

In recent years, there have been great advances in the success of keratoprosthesis surgery and is still a very evolving procedure. There are many devices available worldwide, but this chapter will focus on the keratoprostheses most commonly utilized: the Boston keratoprosthesis (Massachusetts Eye & Ear Infirmary, Boston, MA), the AlphaCor™ (Addition Technology Inc., Des Plaines, IL) and the osteo-odonto-keratoprosthesis also known as the 'OOKP' (originally described by Strampelli, modified by Falcinelli).

## ❧ PREOPERATIVE EVALUATION

Preoperative selection is very important as studies suggest that the success of any keratoprosthesis is more often related to the underlying preoperative pathology. Examination should start with the external adnexa. Ability to blink fully and adequate lid closure, as well as adequate tear production are important considerations. Lid disease should be addressed. Assessment of the fornices is important, as postoperatively some devices need to be protected with a soft contact lens. Estimates of visual acuity and visual potential should be assessed. No light perception vision (NLP) is usually a contraindication to keratoprosthesis surgery and an indication of irreversible visual loss. Macular function can be assessed by examining preoperative visual acuity, determining if the patient can maintain central fixation to a moving muscle light, assessing color vision or even visual evoked potential. Given the severity of corneal disease and opacification, examination of intraocular structures may be limited. Complete examination of all visible intraocular structures should be performed to the best of ability. Ultrasound biomicroscopy (UBM), if available can be used as an adjunct in assessing anterior segment anatomy (Figs 1A to C). The keratoprostheses that will be discussed are designed for aphakia or pseudophakia, so, determination of the lens status is important in terms of ordering the proper device and in the surgical plan. Preoperative A-scan is necessary as axial eye length is needed for ordering the appropriate Boston KPro. Preoperative B-scan ultrasonography is also very useful in assessing the poorly

visible posterior pole. B-scan ultrasonography can aid in determining, if there is presence of any posterior segment pathology, such as retinal or choroidal detachments, posterior staphyloma or other retinal pathology. B-scan ultrasonography is also particularly useful in examining the optic nerve for excavation, which would suggest advanced optic neuropathy and possibility of a poorer visual outcome (Fig. 2). Assessment of glaucomatous optic neuropathy can be very difficult to determine in the preoperative setting because the view of the optic nerve be compromised, and intraocular pressure determination by applanation tonometry of diseased corneas is notoriously unreliable. The Diaton™ tonometer, which assesses intraocular pressure by taking measurements through the eyelids, may be of some utility (Figs 3A and B). In addition to examination for optic nerve excavation with B-scan ultrasonography, the visual field should be determined to the best of the examiners capability, even if only verifying the patient can identify projection of lighting to a given quadrant.

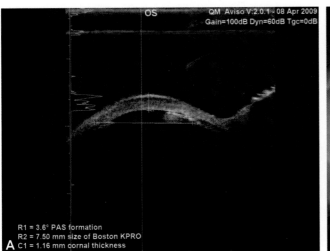

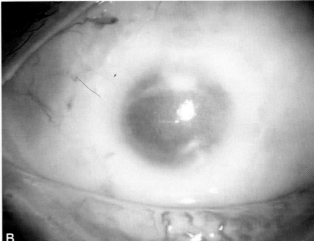

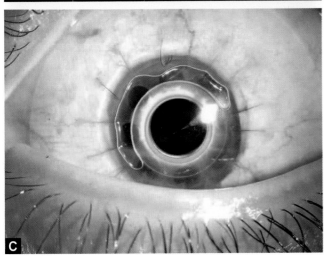

**Figs 1A to C:** Preoperative assessment of anterior segment anatomy with ultrasound biomicroscopy. Angle-to-angle measurements were approximately 7.5 mm. This monocular patient had a complex history including sclerocornea, congenital cataracts, and a small eye in which placement of a Type I Boston keratoprosthesis (7.0 mm back plate) improved vision from hand motions to 20/200

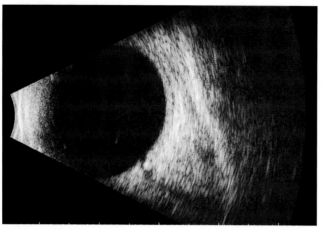

**Fig. 2:** B-Scan ultrasonography demonstrating excavation of the optic nerve head secondary to advanced glaucomatous optic neuropathy

## ⮞ TYPES OF KERATOPROSTHESIS

### Boston Keratoprosthesis

The Boston keratoprosthesis (Massachusetts Eye & Ear Infirmary, Boston, MA) was developed under the leadership of Claes Dohlman and was approved by the United States Food and Drug Administration (FDA) for marketing in 1992 (Figs 4A and B).[6,7] This procedure has gained acceptance in recent years; in 1995, only 15 procedures were performed in contrast to 2009 where 1,161 procedures were performed. To date, more than 4,500 procedures have been performed worldwide.[8]

There are two types of the device, Type I and Type II, where the Type II is utilized through the lid (Figs 5 and 6). Each type requires mounting the complex onto a donor

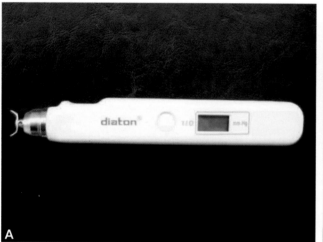
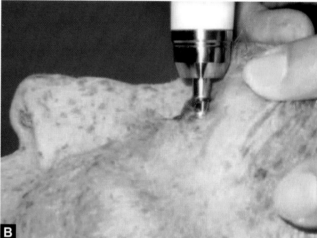

**Figs 3A and B:** Diaton tonometry. The apparatus obtains an intraocular pressure measurement through the eyelids

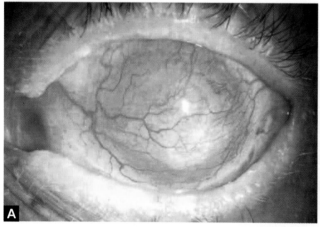
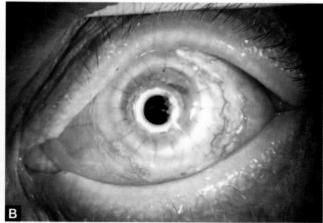

**Figs 4A and B:** Pre- and postoperative photographs, vision was restored from hand-motions to 20/20 after successful surgical intervention with the Type I Boston keratoprosthesis

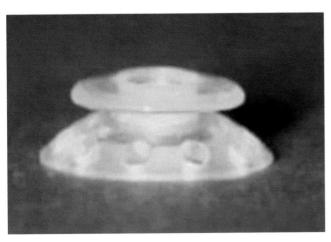

**Fig. 5:** Type I Boston keratoprosthesis (note this is the device without donor cornea)

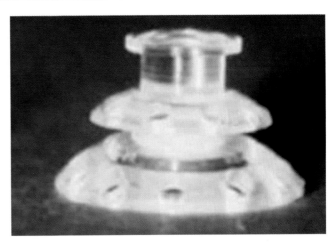

**Fig. 6:** Type II Boston keratoprosthesis (without the donor cornea)

corneal button. The Type I Boston keratoprosthesis has the shape of a collar button, with a front-plate diameter of 5.0 mm, a stem diameter of 3.4 mm and a back-plate diameter of 7.0 or 8.5 mm. The back plate now has a standard 16 holes, each 1.5 mm in diameter, to facilitate nutrition and hydration of the endothelium. The back plate is available in either clear plastic or titanium.[9] A titanium locking ring is affixed to the back plate to prevent the device from disassembly. The Type II Boston keratoprosthesis, which is implanted through the closed eyelid in eyes with severe ocular surface disease, is similar in shape, but has an additional 2.0 mm anterior nub for through-the-eyelid implantation (Figs 7A and B).[10] Researchers in Boston are working on improving the design of the Type II KPro and at the time of this writing, the new Type II prototype was not available. Both types of Boston keratoprostheses are intended for use in aphakic and

pseudophakic eyes. The remainder of the discussion will focus on the Type I.

The assembly of the Type I Boston keratoprosthesis involves preparing donor corneal tissue and assembling the device. The donor cornea is trephined using an 8.5 or 9 mm trephine to ensure that the donor corneal button is larger than the recipient corneal rim and posterior plate. Typically, a 3.0 mm dermatology skin punch is used to remove the central 3.0 mm of cornea from the donor button. It is important to make this punch centrally into the donor tissue, as the device will be centered within this opening. After the donor tissue is prepared satisfactorily, the tissue is ready to be affixed to the device. The prosthetic stem of the keratoprosthesis is placed with the anterior surface down on the adhesive mount that comes with the device. Care should be taken that the device is secure at this time so that it is stable for

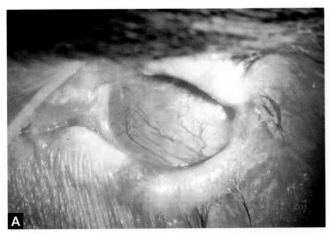

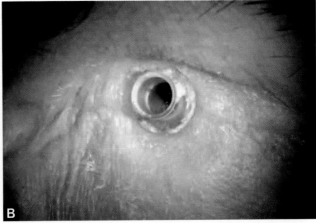

**Figs 7A and B:** Preoperative photograph of a patient with severe corneal and conjunctival scarring secondary to ocular cicatricial pemphigoid. He underwent implantation of the Type II Boston keratoprosthesis and regained visual acuity of 20/50

the remainder of the assembly. The donor button is placed over the stem, followed by the back plate of the device. The back plate is then advanced onto the posterior portion of the donor tissue, sandwiching the donor cornea in between the anterior portion of the stem and the back plate. A titanium locking ring is lastly used to secure the posterior plate onto the central cylinder by snapping the ring into place with the plunger that comes with the keratoprosthesis.

Once the device is assembled, the Type I Boston KPro has the advantage in that insertion is similar to penetrating keratoplasty (Figs 8 to 10). The donor cornea for this type of procedure may be tectonic-quality tissue, since healthy corneal endothelium is not needed for clear vision. In countries where the availability or cost of a well-tested corneal tissue is not accessible, the patient's own excised corneal tissue can serve as a carrier for the Boston KPro. The recipient cornea is then trephined using an 8.0–8.5 mm trephine. If the eye is phakic, a lens extraction is required. If the posterior capsule is intact, it is generally left in place. Vitrectomy may be performed at the time of surgery or as needed. There is no consensus as to superiority of a unicameral versus two-chamber eye in the success of the Boston keratoprosthesis. The donor button/keratoprosthesis complex is sutured into place using either 9-0 or 10-0 nylon sutures, typically between 16–24 sutures, in an interrupted fashion. Suture-induced astigmatism is not an issue, as the rigid PMMA cylinder is not deformed by suture tension.

## AlphaCor™

The AlphaCor™ keratoprosthesis is a 7 mm diameter, one-piece, nonrigid synthetic cornea. The AlphaCor™ (Addition Technology Inc., Des Plaines, IL) gained FDA approval for implantation in 2002. This device was previously called the Chirila KPro.[11] The one-piece convex keratoprosthesis is composed of central transparent optic and an opaque outer skirt that is entirely manufactured from poly 2-hydroxyethyl methacrylate (PHEMA). The outer skirt is a high water content, PHEMA sponge. The porosity of the sponge was designed to promote biointegration with host tissue. The central optic core is a transparent PHEMA gel and provides a refractive power similar to that of the human cornea. There are two types of devices available: one for phakic or pseudophakic patient and a second type for aphakic patients.

The surgical technique for implantation is a two-stage procedure and can be a bit challenging. In Stage 1, an intrastromal trephine is used to remove the central posterior corneal lamellae for insertion of the device. A corneal incision is made and dissection instruments are used to continue the corneal dissection throughout the circumference of the corneal graft, thereby creating an intralamellar pocket. An AlphaCor™ sizer, used to test the size and centration, is inserted into the intralamellar pocket followed by removal of the posterior disk via a 3.5 mm intrastromal trephine. The device is then inserted into the pocket. The device can be protected by the creation of a conjunctival flap or covered with amniotic membrane (Fig. 11). Stage 2 is usually performed 3 months later and involves trephination and removal of the central 3 mm diameter disk of anterior corneal tissue covering the device (Fig. 12). The removal of the tissue exposes the optic portion of the device, while the peripheral skirt remains integrated into the corneal lamellae (Fig. 13). Postoperative refractive correction with high oxygen permeability contact lenses, that also provide surface protection, can be used.

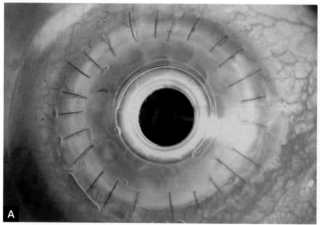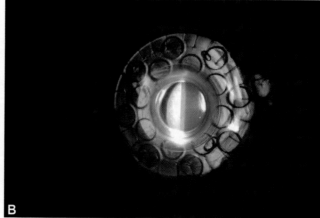

**Figs 8A and B:** Implanted Type I Boston keratoprosthesis with plastic back plate

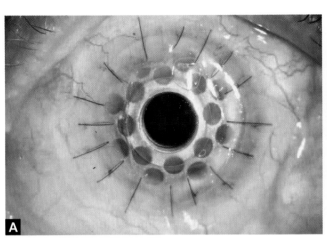
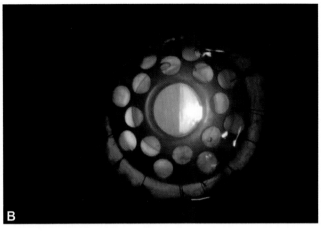

**Figs 9A and B:** Implanted Type I Boston keratoprosthesis with titanium back plate

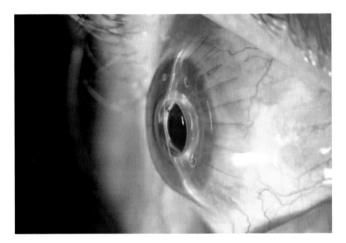

**Fig. 10:** Side profile of Type 1 Boston keratoprosthesis

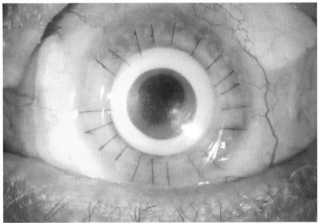

**Fig. 11:** Implanted AlphaCor™ Stage 1 (note this patient is wearing a bandage contact lens)

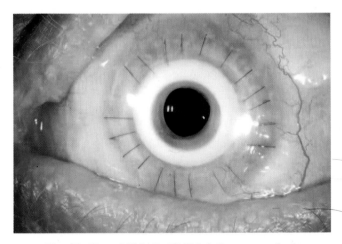

**Fig. 12:** Stage 2 AlphaCor™. This is the same patient, photographed 3 months later

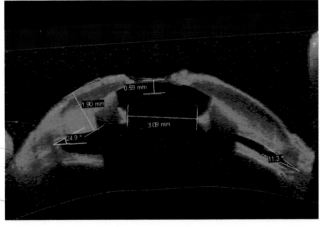

**Fig. 13:** Anterior segment OCT imaging of implanted AlphaCor™

## Osteo-Odonto-Keratoprosthesis

Osteo-odonto-keratoprosthesis is an integrated keratoprosthesis where a central optical cylinder made of PMMA is fashioned into a matrix derived from the patient's own tooth and surrounding alveolar bone. The device is then covered by buccal mucosa, allowing this prosthesis to withstand a severely damaged, dry or keratinized surface with lower rates of extrusion compared to keratoprostheses supported by nonbiological materials (Fig. 14).

The oseto-odonto-keratoprosthesis was developed in Italy by Strampelli in the 1960s[12] and modified by the works of Falcinelli.[13] This procedure is gaining acceptance as the procedure of choice for patients with severe, bilateral disease and damaged ocular surface compromised by inflammatory disease and not appropriate candidates for the less invasive Type I Boston keratoprosthesis or AlphaCor™.

Osteo-odonto-keratoprosthesis surgery is also a two-stage procedure. The first stage has two portions: preparing the ocular surface and preparing the full-thickness buccal mucous membrane graft, which houses the PMMA optic and suturing this to place onto the recipient eye. The second stage involves removing the osteodental-acrylic (ODA) complex from its subcutaneous pocket and affixing it to the ocular surface.

The first stage includes the preparation of: (1) the bulbar anterior surface and (2) the ODA complex. Surface preparation of the anterior bulbar surface differs depending upon the conjunctival status: normal versus severe damaged or scarred. In cases with normal conjunctiva, a 360° limbal peritomy is performed and the conjunctiva is detached from the sclera by removing, if necessary, any scar tissue up to the insertion of the extraocular rectus muscles.

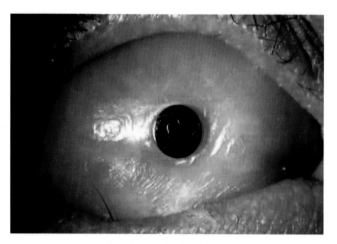

**Fig. 14:** Implanted OOKP
*Source*: Photo courtesy of Jodhbir S Mehta

Recti can be isolated with 5-0 silk threads to rotate the eyeball when needed. Next, a lamellar keratectomy is performed starting from the limbus and involving Bowman's membrane, removing any overlying scar tissue. In cases with conjunctival damage, more extensive dissection is necessary. If no surgery for symblepharon had been performed prior, then the tarsal surface is detached from the cornea at the border between the two eyelids. Tissue separation is continued up to the insertion of the recti, followed by the lamellar keratectomy. Anterior bulbar surface preparation is then continued by covering the cornea and sclera, up to the muscle insertions, by a flap of oral mucosa harvested from the cheek. The mucosal flap should be large enough to cover the surface without significant traction and is usually about 2 mm thick. It is sutured to the sclera with 6-0 polyglactin sutures. The edges of the detached conjunctiva are sutured to the periphery of the mucosal flap.[14,15]

The preparation of the device, or ODA complex, requires the assistance of an oral maxillofacial surgeon. A single-root tooth is chosen on the basis of preliminary clinical and radiological evaluation. Typically, the most suitable tooth for the preparation of the osteodental lamina is the superior canine because it had the longest and largest root with the greatest quantity of alveolar bone. The selected tooth, surrounding bone and soft tissue are extracted with a surgical saw. The osteodental lamina is then shaped to an approximately rectangular lamina of 9–10 mm (width) by 14.5–16 mm (length) with a thickness of 2.5–3.25 mm. The center is trephined to make an opening approximately 3.7 mm in diameter. A PMMA optical cylinder (Schalcon, Rome, Italy) is inserted into the opening and glued to the osteodental lamina by a biocompatible acrylic resin. The complex is inserted under the skin in a 'subcutaneous pouch' below the inferior orbital rim for approximately 3 months.[13,14]

The second stage of the procedure involves removal of the ODA complex. After 3 months' time the tissue is vascularized and secure but is verified at the time of removal. The cheek mucosal graft covering the cornea is partially detached, leaving its attachment below the limbus in place. A Flieringa is secured to the globe, followed by full-thickness trephination of the cornea corresponding to the diameter of the PMMA optic. Next, the iris and lens are removed followed by open-sky anterior vitrectomy. The posterior part of the PMMA optical cylinder is inserted and the ODA complex secured over the cornea and sutured to the sclera with at least 12, 6-0 or 7-0 polyglactin sutures. Air is injected with a 30-gauge needle to restore physiological intraocular pressure. The mucosal flap is repositioned over the complex and a hole trephined in the area of the optic. The mucosa is secured with sutures. The patient remains supine for 5–6 days after the procedure until the air is resorbed. These patients require 1–2 yearly CT scans to assess dentine resorption.[14,16]

## OUTCOMES OF KERATOPROSTHESES

Data is evolving and varies widely between the underlying pathology and type of keratoprosthesis used. In recent years, improvements in the design of the Boston Type I KPro has showed promise in restoration of visual acuity in a variety of pathologies, but long-term viability and results are in process. The AlphaCor™ has been fraught with high rates of extrusion and melt. Although the OOKP surgery is extensive and very invasive, it has a reputation for long-term stability and low rates of infection.[17] The Boston Type I keratoprosthesis study group[18] compared Kaplan-Meier survival curves for the different keratoprostheses. It reports 5-year survival of corneal allograft after one failed graft to be approximately 28% and almost none surviving after 60 months in cases of allograft after multiple failed grafts.[19] Two-year survival data for the AlphaCor™ is estimated to be approximately 50% without use of medroxyprogesterone and just over 60% with the use of medroxyprogesterone.[11] At the time of the keratoprosthesis study group's publication in 2006, 3-year survival outcome of the Type I Boston keratoprosthesis was 85%.[18]

## COMPLICATIONS AND CONSIDERATIONS

Of course, the best management of a complication is not to have one in the first place, however, complications are common in the setting of keratoprosthesis surgery and the surgeon must be aware of potential complications and how to manage these once they occur. In recent years, there has been a paradigm shift in the management of the keratoprosthesis in the postoperative period. Most keratoprosthesis surgeons agree that these measures have added greatly to the success of these procedures and include: long-term antibiotic coverage, intra and postoperative use of corticosteroids, maintenance of a bandage contact lens indefinitely and aggressive glaucoma management. Keratoprosthesis patients require close, life-long follow-up. Typically, patients are evaluated on the first postoperative day, at 1 week, at 1 month, and then monthly for the first few months before extending to follow-up to every few months indefinitely.

Long-term antibiotic coverage represents a shift in conventional thinking that the chronic use of antibiotics will lead to antibiotic resistance. Prior to the routine use of prophylactic antibiotics, it was common that intraocular gram-positive infections would occur. Current recommendations include a fourth-generation fluoroquinolone plus/minus topical vancomycin.[20]

There is no role for a contact lens in the OOKP, however, it is used in some cases of the AlphaCor™, and is highly recommended with the Boston KPro (Fig. 15). Maintenance of a bandage contact lens indefinitely, whenever possible in the Boston Type I keratoprosthesis, creates a layer of protection against the eyelids against the keratoprosthesis, provides a moist environment and diffuses evaporation. It is felt that the maintenance of the contact lens leads to less extrusion and melt and provides improved viability of remaining corneal tissue or carrier donor tissue.[21] Commonly, the Kontur contact lens (Kontur Kontact Lens, Co. Inc., Hercules, CA) is favored (available in 16 mm diameter/9.8 mm base curve and the larger and tighter 18 mm diameter/8.3 base curve), but other soft contact lenses can be used. These lenses are prone to developing protein build-up and should be removed and cleaned on a regular basis and replaced as needed. The author's typical regimen includes either replacing the contact lens or cleaning the lens monthly with MiraFlow Extra Strength Daily Cleaner (Ciba Vision) or CVS Brand Extra Strength Daily Cleaner for soft contact lenses. If the contact lens cannot be maintained, consideration of placement of lateral or even nasal tarsorrhaphies should be made.

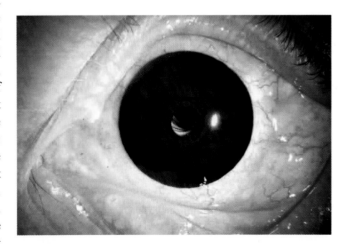

**Fig. 15:** Many keratoprosthesis patients experience bothersome glare symptoms. This is an example of an occlusive contact lens that is being worn over the Type 1 Boston keratoprosthesis

In addition to cleaning or replacement of the contact lens, the fornices of the Boston Type I keratoprosthesis patient are rinsed with dilute betadine every 3 months. Five percent betadine is mixed with an equal amount of sterile saline and withdrawn into a 3 ml syringe. After topical anesthetic is placed on the eye and any contact lenses removed, both the upper and lower fornices are irrigated with the solution. This is believed to decrease the pathogenic colonization of the fornices. The patients should be instructed that the eye might be sore or irritated for a few days after this procedure.

## Tissue Necrosis, Melt, and Extrusion

Persistent corneal defects may be the first sign of keratolysis. This patient needs to be monitored closely and managed with aggressive lubrication, maintenance of a bandage contact lens, and placed on oral doxycycline. Tarsorrhaphy may be necessary to protect the keratoprosthesis. Any sign of cornea melt or extrusion of the implant necessitates return to the operating room for reconstruction or replacement of the prosthesis (Fig. 16). Melt and extrusion are more common with the AlphaCor™ than the Boston KPro.

The rate of melt with the AlphaCor™ is quite high and studies estimate incidence of 30–60%.[11,22] The use of medroxyprogesterone was found to be beneficial in increasing the time to developing a corneal melt.[22] The multicenter Boston Type I keratoprosthesis study group found that the retention rate was 90% overall and 95% amongst nonautoimmune, nonchemical burn patients.[18]

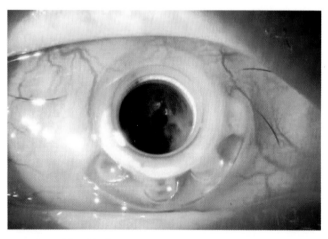

**Fig. 16:** Type I Boston keratoprosthesis with melt/extrusion of the device

## Inflammation

Postoperative inflammation may be related to the preoperative inflammatory status, and chronic postoperative inflammation is frequently encountered in the setting of autoimmune disease, such as ocular cicatricial pemphigoid, Stevens Johnson syndrome, graft versus host disease, etc. Chronic inflammation in the setting of autoimmune disease is a major factor for poorer outcomes in these patients. Inflammation can lead to a variety of vision-threatening complications, such as retroprosthetic membranes, epiretinal membranes, vitreous opacities, angle closure glaucoma and retinal detachment. Corticosteroids are the mainstay of treatment, typically topically, at times periocular, and less commonly systemic. Inflammation should be managed as best as possible.

## Glaucoma

Escalation of glaucoma in any keratoplasty is well-known to occur. In keratoprosthesis surgery, glaucoma can be a major vision-threatening comorbidity to the underlying pathology that necessitates keratoprosthesis surgery for visual rehabilitation or postoperative complication. Particularly vulnerable are severe chemical burn patients and patients with autoimmune disease. Those with pre-existing glaucoma are also at increased risk. The pathogenesis of glaucoma is probably multifactorial, but gradual closure of the anterior chamber angle is the most likely cause. Intraocular pressure monitoring is challenging in the keratoprosthesis patient and often only estimates of intraocular pressure by digital palpation of the globe can be exercised. The Diaton™ tonometer, which measures intraocular pressure through the eyelid, may be of some utility, but conventional applanation tonometry is useless. Clinical monitoring of the optic nerve head, optical coherence tomography of the retinal nerve fiber layer and visual field testing should be used in monitoring the progression of glaucomatous optic neuropathy.[23,24] Concomitant monitoring with a glaucoma specialist is advised. Many surgeons are implanting Ahmed valves at the time of Boston keratoprosthesis surgery. Glaucoma medications do penetrate into the eye and are effective. If medical therapy is inadequate in controlling progression, placement of an Ahmed valve shunt or cyclophotocoagulation may be indicated.[25]

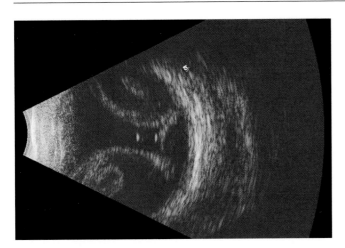

**Fig. 17:** Choroidal detachments that developed early in the postoperative period secondarily to an overfiltering glaucoma shunt. The tube of the glaucoma shunt needed to be tied off

## Posterior Segment Complications

Posterior segment abnormalities in association with a keratoprosthesis may be present prior to placement (as a consequence of injury, previous ocular disease, or complication of prior surgical intervention), may develop intraoperatively during placement of the KPro or may occur postoperatively (Fig. 17). Management of these complications may be difficult and vitreoretinal surgery challenging. The anterior segment anatomy is frequently foreshortened and with fibrosis and contracture in the area of the iris root and ciliary body. Incisions for pars plana vitrectomy are often placed as anteriorly as possible. A publication from Massachusetts Eye & Ear experience of posterior segment complications reports of 110 cases of Boston Type I and II KPro surgery yielded 22 cases in 18 patients with posterior segment complications, with retinal detachment being the most common complication requiring surgery (13 cases).[26]

## Retroprosthetic Membranes

Estimates suggest approximately 30% of eyes will eventually develop retroprosthetic membranes. Histopathologic evaluation revealed that these membranes are comprised of dense, relatively avascular fibrous tissue with numerous fibroblasts surrounded by collagen. This is most likely thought to represent corneal stromal downgrowth around the stem of the KPro.[26,27] Inflammation and vitreous hemorrhage can be inciting factors for the development of these membranes. Some authors suggest steroid injections (peribulbar triamcinolone 20–40 mg) at the first sign of membrane formation. Once formed, most of the membranes are amendable to Nd: YAG laser treatment (Figs 18A to C).[28] Laser pulses with energy above 2.0–3.0 mJ are inadvisable because it could crack or damage the prosthesis.[29] In some cases, the retroprosthetic membrane will become very thick and surgical interventional is the preferred management. These membranes can be extensive and span over vast portions of the posterior segment (Figs 19A and B).

## Retinal Detachment

Retinal detachments can develop in isolation or in conjunction with other retinal pathology, such as cyclitic membranes, epiretinal membranes, proliferative vitreoretinopathy, subretinal fibrosis, inflammation or infection. The vitreoretinal surgeon can successfully perform surgery with some potential modifications of technique given the situation.[26] Visual recovery will depend upon the extent and concurrent pathology and of course with any surgical intervention, there is the potential of complication.

## Vitreous Hemorrhage

Vitreous hemorrhage can occur at any point in the postoperative period. The severity can range from mild to very dense. Mild vitreous hemorrhages are often encountered in the immediate postoperative period as a result of surgical manipulation of tissues during the placement of the keratoprosthesis, placement of the tube shunt or more extensive surgical procedures. These will often resolve spontaneously. Dense vitreous hemorrhages may need to be surgically cleared with a vitrectomy. Development of a vitreous hemorrhage later in the postoperative course necessitates careful examination as to determine the etiology of hemorrhage.

## Vitreous Inflammation/Sterile Uveitis-Vitritis

A sudden massive vitritis reducing vision to hand motions visual acuity has been reported to occur.[30] This mimics infectious endophthalmitis but there is typically no associated pain, tenderness or redness. Given the severity of infectious endophthalmitis, a tap and inject of antibiotics is often performed. Close clinical follow up is maintained and when pathogens are not isolated, topical and peribulbar steroids are initiated. The inflammation typically resolves within a few weeks, but may take months. Vision often returns to baseline. The etiology is speculated to be a sterile autoimmune reaction.

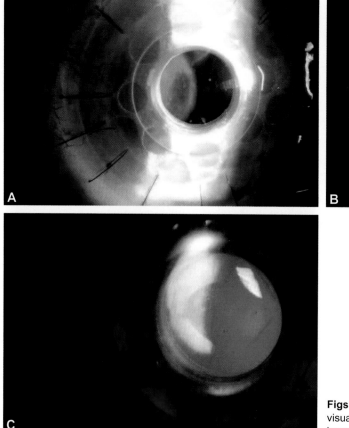

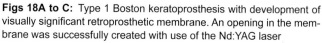

**Figs 18A to C:** Type 1 Boston keratoprosthesis with development of visually significant retroprosthetic membrane. An opening in the membrane was successfully created with use of the Nd:YAG laser

## Epiretinal Membrane and Cystoid Macular Edema

Epiretinal membrane and cystoids macular edema can develop and limit visual potential (Fig. 20). It is difficult to discern if the keratoprosthesis surgery itself, chronic inflammation or development of cystoid macular edema leads to the formation of the epiretinal membrane. Mild epiretinal membranes that do not cause distortion or traction on the macula can be monitored; more severe epiretinal membranes may need to be addressed with removal by a vitreoretinal surgeon. If an underlying cause of cystoid macular edema can be identified, it should be addressed. Treatment with corticosteroids, anti-inflammatories, and other modalities may need to be employed.

## Infectious Endophthalmitis

Development of infectious endophthalmitis often leads to devastating visual loss (Fig. 21). Depending on the infectious agent, spread can occur rapidly with permanent loss of vision within 24 hours.[31] Most commonly the infectious agent is bacterial but fungal or atypical bacterial etiologies

should be considered (Fig. 22). Should infectious endophthalmitis occur, aggressive management with a multispecialty approach should occur.[20] Urgent tap and injection should be performed. Typically an aqueous sample can be obtained by passing a 27-gauge needle through the limbus. Additional sample can be obtained by aspirating vitreous fluid, followed by injection of vancomycin, amikacin, and dexamethasone.[31] Other regimens include ceftazadime or gentamycin, depending on the culture results.

## ▶ CONCLUSION

Keratoprosthesis surgery is an evolving procedure that in recent decades has demonstrated improving outcomes as a result of improved design and postoperative management. It is a valid alternative to restore vision in eyes with the most severe corneal disease not amendable or with high risk of failure with traditional penetrating keratoplasty (Table 1). Continued research and experience with these devices and new emerging designs show promise for visual rehabilitation in these cases.

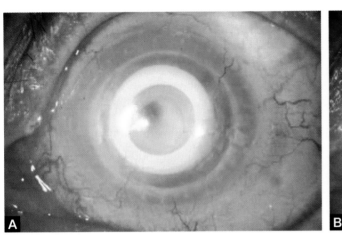
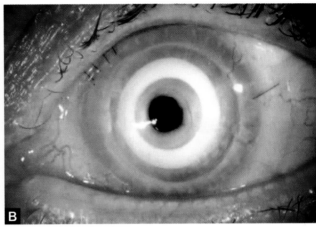

**Figs 19A and B:** AlphaCor™ with visually significant retroprosthetic membrane that had to be removed surgically

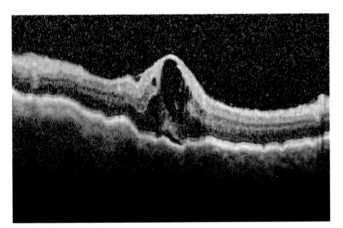

**Fig. 20:** Massive cystoid macular edema (CME) as evidenced on Heidelberg OCT

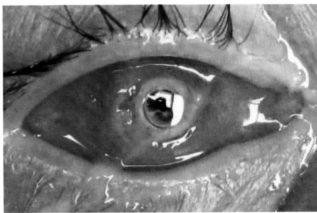

**Fig. 21:** Infectious endophthalmitis that developed in a patient that was noncompliant with recommended medications, contact lens use, or follow-up

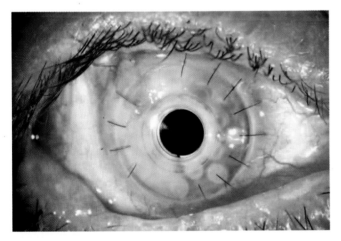

**Fig. 22:** This patient developed yeast keratitis around the stem. Any infiltrate in a keratoprosthesis must be treated immediately and closely monitored. This patient was treated emergently and the infection cleared without sequelae

| Table 1: Prognosis for successful keratoprosthesis |
| --- |
| *Maintenance*: Best to Worst |
| Noninflammatory conditions |
| Infectious |
| Chemical injuries |
| Autoimmune disease |

## ▶ REFERENCES

1. The World Health Organization. International Classification of Disease (ICD). Available at http://www.who.int/classifications/icd/en/. Chapter VII. Diseases of the eye and adnexa (H00:H59). Visual disturbances and blindness (H53-H54). [Accessed April 2011].

2. Pellier de Quengsy G. Précis au cours d'operations sur la chirurgie des yeux. Paris: Didot; 1789.

3. Chirila TV, Hicks CR. The origins of the artificial cornea: Pellier de Quengsy and his contribution to the modern concept of keratoprosthesis. Gesnerus. 1999;56(1-2):96-106.

4. Cardona H. Keratoprosthesis: acrylic optical cylinder with supporting intralamellar plate. Am J Ophthalmology. 1962;54:284-94.

5. Cardona H, DeVoe AG. Prosthokeratoplasty. Trans Acad Ophthalmol Otolaryngol. 1977;83:271-80.

6. Dohlman CH, Harissi-Dagher M, Khan BF, et al. Introduction to the use of the Boston keratoprosthesis. Expert Rev Ophthalmol. 2006;1(1):41-8.

7. Dohlman CH, Dudenhoefer E, Khan BF, et al. Protection of the ocular surface after keratoprosthesis surgery: the role of soft contact lenses. CLAO J. 2002;28(2):72-4.

8. Klufas MA, KA Colby. The Boston keratoprosthesis. Int Ophthalmol Clin. 2010;50(3):161-75.

9. Todani A, Ciolino JB, Ament JD, et al. Titanium back plate for a PMMA keratoprosthesis: clinical outcomes. Graefes Arch Clin Exp Ophthalmol. 2001 (electronic version).

10. Dohlman JG, Foster CS, Dohlman CH. Boston keratoprosthesis in Stevens-Johnson syndrome: a case of using infliximab to prevent tissue necrosis. Digital Jo Ophthalmol. 2009;15(1).

11. Hicks CR, Crawford GJ, Dart JKG, et al. Alphacor clinical outcomes. Cornea. 2006;25(9):1034-42.

12. Strampelli B. Osteo-odontokeratoprosthesis. Ann Ottalmol Clin Ocul. 1963;89:1039-44.

13. Hille K, Grabner G, Liu C, et al. Standards for modified osteodontokeratoprosthesis (OOKP) surgery according to Strampelli and Falcinielli: the Rome-Vienna Protocol. Cornea. 2005;24(8):895-908.

14. Falcinelli G, Falsini B, Taloni M, et al. Modified osteo-odontokeratoprosthesis for treatment of corneal blindness: long-term anatomical and functional outcomes in 181 cases. Arch Ophthalmol. 2005;123:1319-29.

15. Liu C, Herold J, Sciscio A, et al. Osteo-odonto-keratoprosthesis surgery. Br J Ophthalmol. 1999;83:127.

16. Falcinelli G, Barogi G, Taloni M. Osteoodontokeratoprosthesis: present experience and future prospects. Refract Corneal Surg. 1993;9:193-4.

17. Marchi V, Ricci R, Pecorella I, et al. Osteo-odontokeratoprosthesis: description of surgical technique with results in 85 patients. Cornea. 1994;13:125-30.

18. Zerbe LB, Belin MW, Joseph B, et al. Boston Type 1 Keratoprosthesis Study. Ophthalmology. 2006;113(10):1779-84.

19. Bersudsky V, Blum-Hareuveni T, Rehany U, et al. The profile of repeated corneal transplantation. Ophthalmology. 2001;108:461-9.

20. Fintelmann RE, Maguire JI, Ho AC, et al. Characteristics of endophthalmitis in patients with the Boston keratoprosthesis. Cornea. 2009;28:877-8.

21. Harissi-Daguer M, Beyer J, Dohlman CH. The role of soft contact lenses as an adjunct to the Boston keratoprosthesis. Int Ophthalmol Clin. 2008;48:43-51.

22. Hicks CR, Crawford GJ. Melting after keratoprosthesis implantation: the effects of medroxyprogesterone. Cornea. 2003;22(6):497-500.

23. Banitt M. Evaluation and management of glaucoma after keratoprosthesis. Curr Opin Ophthalmol. 2011;22:133-6.

24. Falcinelli GC, Falsini B, Taloni M, et al. Detection of glaucomatous damage in patients with osteo-odonto-keratoprosthesis. Br J Ophthalmol. 1995;79:129-34.

25. Rivier D, Paula JS, Kim E, et al. Glaucoma and keratoprosthesis surgery: role of adjunctive cyclophotocoagulation. J Glaucoma. 2009;18:321-4.

26. Ray S, Khan BF, Dohlman CH, et al. Management of vitreoretinal complications in eyes with permanent keratoprosthesis. Archives of Ophthalmol. 2002;120(5):559-66.

27. Stacy RC, Jakobiec FA, Michaud NA, et al. Characterization of retrokeratoprosthetic membranes in the Boston type 1 keratoprosthesis. Arch Ophthalmol. 2011;129(3):310-6.

28. Chak G, Aquavella JV. A Safe Nd: YAG Retroprosthetic membrane removal technique for keratoprosthesis. Cornea. 2010;29:1169-72.

29. Bath PE, Fridge DL, Robinson K, et al. Photometric evaluation of YAG-induced polymethylmethacrylate damage in a keratoprosthesis. J Am Intraocul Implant Soc. 1985;11(3): 253-6.

30. Nouri M, Durand ML, Dohlman CH. Sudden reversible vitritis after keratoprosthesis: an immune phenomenon? Cornea. 2005;24(8):915-9.

31. Nouri M, Terada H, Alfonso EC, et al. Endophthalmitis after keratoprosthesis: incidence, bacterial causes, and risk factors. Arch Ophthalmol. 2001;119:484-9.

SECTION 16

# Infant Keratoprosthesis

*James V Aquavella, Garrick Chak*

## ❧ INTRODUCTION

Neonatal corneal opacity may be congenital and the result of Peters' anomaly,[1,2] nonspecific dysgenesis, sclerocornea, Congenital hereditary endothelial dystrophy (CHED), and glaucoma.[3] The noncongenital forms are associated with birth canal injury, infection, forceps delivery or other forms of trauma.

While CHED and glaucoma are well established and readily verified diagnostic entities, the differentiation between those conditions associated with dysgenesis may be more tenuous. Thus, a clinical differentiation between Peters' anomaly (Fig. 1), sclerocornea, and nondescript dysgenesis is often unclear.[4,5]

Regardless of the specific pathology, it is essential that diagnostic evaluation and therapeutic steps be initiated quickly in order to prevent amblyopia. While it is generally accepted that therapy should be initiated within the first few months of life, the level of visual deprivation is variable from case to case,[6] different degrees of inherent brain plasticity are present and therapeutic uncertainties all combine to make it difficult to set an age limit beyond which therapy will not be fruitful. Timely visual restoration is imperative. In many instances of severe pathology intervention may be warranted despite dismal prognosis. Even small amounts of visual perception can be extremely beneficial to development.

The condition may be unilateral or bilateral (Fig. 2). Most agree that the potential for development of irreversible amblyopia is greater in unilateral cases. In some cultures, there is a reluctance to treat unilateral blindness, whether it be due to simple congenital cataract or more complex

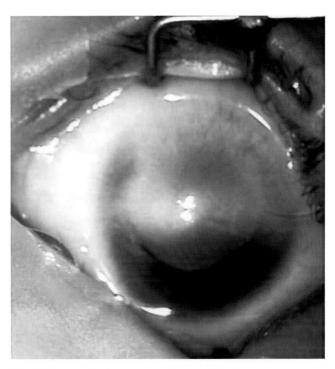

**Fig. 1:** Preoperative Peters' anomaly: note scleral-cornea appearance

dysgenesis, given the anticipated poor prognosis. Some feel that the expenditure of significant fiscal resources is not warranted in view of the fact that a reasonably normal life can be achieved with only one eye. One problem with this philosophy is that it is difficult to predict normality in newborns. Astigmatism, high refractive error, glaucoma and macular disease are difficult to diagnose in this age group and the potential for the future development of disease in an eye which has been considered 'normal' is

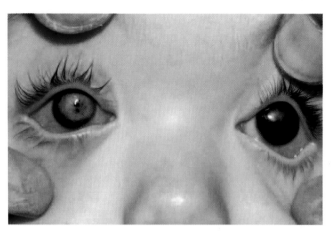

**Fig. 2:** Bilateral involvement with dense right cornea opacity

even more difficult to predict. In some the full expression of the disease, is progressive over the first several months of life. Thus, particularly in cases of dysgenesis vitreoretinal pathology and glaucoma may develop overtime, in one or both eyes. Limited amounts of vision in the weaker eye may become significant should the 'normal' eye become diseased or injured.

At the Flaum Eye Institute, we make every effort to preserve and restore vision in both monocular and binocular disease.

Traditional therapy involves patching or other forms of visual deprivation in the stronger eye. In cases in which the visual axis is obscured, not only by the corneal opacity, but by pupillary displacement, an optical iridectomy may be considered. When these methods are not indicated or have not been productive, penetrating keratoplasty has been the only remaining therapeutic approach. Penetrating keratoplasty in infants continues to be a very controversial subject. Infant cornea transplants are associated with a high incidence of allograft rejection, graft opacification, reoperation and other complications.[3,7-13] Most recently, Mannis and colleagues reported a 67% graft survival at 1 year for pediatric penetrating keratoplasty in patients with Peters' anomaly.[12] However, a clear graft per se may not be sufficient to avoid amblyopia in the infant since penetrating keratoplasty results in regular and irregular astigmatism which may still require patching and contact lens wear for management of amblyopia. When grafts fail, repeat grafting has been found to carry a dismal prognosis. In one study, all repeat grafts failed within 5 years.[14-16] Severe cases may be judged inoperable for penetrating keratoplasty thus influencing the success rate in a particular series. The literature on penetrating keratoplasty in infants

has not been compelling. A 2008 series of 40 procedures in 32 patients showed a 22% graft survival at 2 years. Another series of 144 penetrating keratoplasty procedures in 72 eyes in 47 patients a year later, showed only 29% had 20/400 visual acuity or better at a minimum 3 years follow-up. One of the problems with objective analysis of the value of corneal transplants is the fact that differing metrics are used in the published reports: graft clarity, graft rejection and visual performance are cited interchangeably. The diagnosis of a clear graft in an infant is subjective given the fact that comprehensive slit-lamp examination cannot be performed. Apparently clear grafts may be thick and mild anterior chamber inflammation and the presence of synechiae which indicate future decompensation may be missed.

Other difficulties in comparison exist, thus there is a general feeling that smaller eyes with reduced axial length are less amenable to graft survival. The age at which corneal transplantation is initiated can also be a significant variable factor. One confounding fact is that while some surgeons feel Peters' anomaly carries a relatively 'good' prognosis for penetrating keratoplasty, others feel it is dismal. Peters' anomaly in some can be associated with minimal amounts of dysgenesis producing an occasional narrow based anterior synechiae, while in others there is significant compromise of anterior chamber details, iris abnormalities, vitreous and pupillary membranes, persistent hyperplastic primary vitreous, and colobomas of the retina, etc. Many surgeons will not attempt to place a penetrating keratoplasty in such severe cases; reserving attempts at corneal transplantation to those less severe cases which they feel have a better chance of success. In the final analysis, variations in age, comorbidity, disease severity, eyeball size, patient selection and surgeon biases, all combine to create difficulties in interpretation of the existing literature.

In our series of over 75 infant eyes, 60% of the pathology has been ascribed to Peters' anomaly. Sclerocornea, glaucoma, dermoid cyst and other forms of dysgenesis have contributed to the remaining 40%. We have encountered only one case of CHED. Peters' anomaly is a rare form of anterior segment dysgenesis characterized by central or paracentral corneal opacity. Cataract, corneal lenticular adhesion, iris synechiae, pupillary and angle malformations, and pupillary irregularities are often present. The condition is named after Alfred Peters and is often described as presenting with a nonvascularized corneal opacity. In severe cases, however, the level of pannus and associated conjunctival overgrowth with vascularization render this distinction dubious. Peters' anomaly involves the *PAX 6* gene with manifestations occurring in weeks 10–16 of the first trimester which is when anterior segment formation and cleavage of the anterior chamber occur embryologically.[17] Peters' anomaly may be associated with other abnormalities, including myopia, aniridia, iris coloboma, choroidal edema, persistent hyperplastic primary vitreous, optic disk hypoplasia, as well as systemic abnormalities (including trisomy 13–15, partial deletion of chromosome 11Q, and Norrie Disease)[2,18] Peters' Plus syndrome is characterized by having additional organ involvement, such as cardiac abnormalities, genitourinary malformations, neural abnormalities, growth delays, or head and neck malformation in association with severe ocular malformations (thinning of the posterior cornea, iridocorneal adhesions). The diagnosis of Peters' Plus is often based on molecular genetic testing of the BGALTL gene.[19-22]

While there may be numerous facets to the visual deprivation, the traditional therapy has been patching, optical iridectomy, or penetrating keratoplasty. Our group at Flaum considers the poor prognosis associated with infant keratoplasty to contraindicate the procedure. We recognize the literature has not been compelling and a significant degree of controversy continues to exist.

In our series, 30% of the eyes present with existent vitreoretinal pathology or develop vitreoretinal problems over the 1st year or more of life. Glaucoma is associated with 15% of our cases. The underlying degree of dysgenesis and microphthalmia vary from case to case.

## HISTORICAL PERSPECTIVE

While keratoprosthesis has been utilized in adults since the mid-20th century,[23-27] the indications were mostly limited to otherwise inoperable adult cases and long-term visual results were poor. The situation changed significantly with the introduction of the Boston 1 device in the 21st century. Following our favorable experiences with this new device in adults, coupled with our unfavorable results with infant keratoplasty, we performed the first infant keratoprosthesis procedure in 2003. The device has been widely described[28,29] and involves the use of a ring of donor cornea tissue mounted between an optical front plate and a fenestrated back plate.[30,31] A titanium locking ring secures the device which then may be implanted in the recipient bed in standard corneal transplant fashion (Fig. 3).

Since the success of the procedure does not depend on clarity of the donor stromal material, some surgeons feel that endothelial viability should not be a matter of concern in selection of the tissue to be utilized. Indeed, recent advances in sterilized corneal tissue supplied by Tissue Banks International are used in a significant number of our keratoprosthesis cases. This tissue is sterilized and shipped at room temperature with a viability expiration date of 12–24 months. The tissue is acellular and may be ordered in specific diameters or prepunched with the central 3 mm opening. Special forms of the tissue are available for use in secondary surgical procedures or repairs.

There are a number of inherent considerations which must be understood prior to undertaking the use of keratoprosthesis in congenital corneal opacity. These are not just small eyes in newborn infants. The active infant immune system is a constant source of potential inflammatory response. The degree of dysgenesis with concurrent ocular pathology can be formidable[21] and ultimately the ever present prospect of amblyopia creates pressure for both the parents and the surgeons. While timing is imperative, there are a number of steps which must be taken to determine the extent of the disease and the potential for obtaining useful visual acuity following a keratoprosthesis procedure.

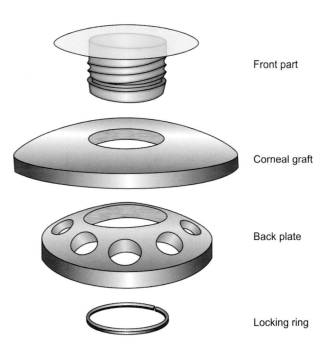

**Fig. 3:** Schematic of device (current design of the back plate includes 2 rows of fenestrations)

Front part

Corneal graft

Back plate

Locking ring

Obtaining the history is not a simple process. Often, several consultants have been involved (neonatologists, ophthalmologists, pediatric ophthalmologists and corneal surgeon) and examination under anesthesia performed. In some instances, early glaucoma procedures and even penetrating keratoplasty have been performed. While we invariably perform our own studies, the process of receiving records from multiple physicians and institutions is time consuming. Intraocular pressure, A and B-scans, as well as any objective evaluations are helpful, but not definitive. Irregular corneas with thickening or edema do not yield accurate intraocular pressure readings. Varying degrees of corneal opacity and conjunctival overgrowth render the estimation of corneal diameter difficult. On more than one occasion, a total retinal detachment was discovered during the course of surgery, having been missed by the original consultant, as well as by our own vitreoretinal team.

We insist that arrangements be in place for appropriate follow-up prior to accepting the case. Our team must be available for both preliminary evaluation, as well as the surgical procedure, and travel plans must be in place. Thus, scheduling can be complex. Insurance and financial planning must be consistent with institutional policy with prior authorization often required even in those cases where the third party carriers have a policy in place enabling reimbursement. Visual-evoked responses, brain scan, ordering of the appropriate powered device, eye bank tissue and consultation with a neonatal anesthesiologist are all part of the logistical complexities. Thus, while we prefer to operate at 6 weeks of age in eyes which have not undergone prior therapy, delays are not infrequent. Some cornea surgeons prefer to perform a single cornea transplant and recommend the use of keratoprosthesis only after failure of an initial keratoplasty.

## OUR TEAM

Cornea, vitreoretinal surgeon, pediatric ophthalmologist and glaucoma specialists are in place to review the documentation. We feel strongly that this team approach is mandatory for both initial evaluations, as well as for the subsequent surgical procedure, and the long-term follow-up. Clinical coordinators, ophthalmic technicians and surgical schedulers are important members of our team as well. Often follow-up data must be collected by the clinical coordinator and derived from a variety of practitioners, as well as from the family members. Compliance with postoperative recommendations must be assessed and documented.

## SURGICAL PROCEDURE

After general anesthesia has been obtained, we institute the prepping and draping procedures advocated by the Vitreoretinal Service. Thus, additional re-prepping or draping is not required after the first stage of surgery is completed and the vitreoretinal team proceeds. Sufficient exposure must be obtained so that a variety of different size pediatric speculums should be available. Photography, bilateral examination under anesthesia may be in order if routine examination under anesthesia has not been performed within a reasonable period of time. In microphthalmic eyes, a lateral canthotomy may be helpful. Depending on the degree of dysgenesis and existent pannus, a total peritomy can help determine limbal features. Often there is significant pannus which must be dissected carefully. If sufficient anterior segment details are still obscure, the use of a light pipe may assist in determination of the central corneal area to be trephined. We utilize a Flieringa ring in all cases, not only to provide stability to the anterior segment, but also to assist in alignment and exposure during the suturing process (Fig. 4). Where possible, a trephine (Fig. 5) is centered over the area of pathology and a nonpenetrating outline is performed, followed by cauterization of the vessels with a needle cautery to achieve hemostasis (Fig. 6). This step is extremely important in that bleeding into the anterior chamber with subsequent clot formation can impede the process of visual restoration. Guarded entry into the anterior chamber is performed (Fig. 7), followed by careful dissection with the aid of a cyclodialysis spatula and fine corneal scissors, to avoid damage to the underlying

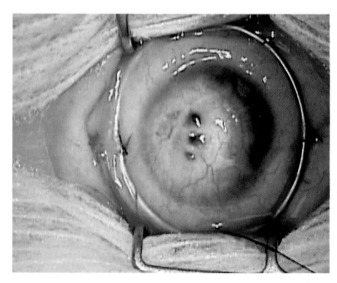

**Fig. 4:** Flieringa ring in place: Note wide exposure

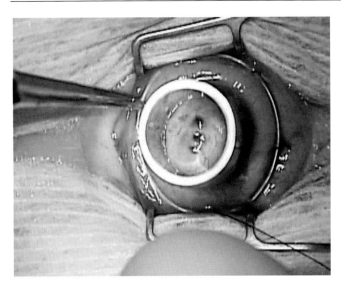

**Fig. 5:** Nonpenetrating trephination

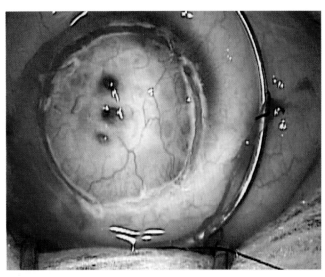

**Fig. 6:** Following cauterization of vessels to achieve homeostasis

iris (Fig. 8). Attention must be paid to existent anterior and posterior synechiae, so that they may be lysed with sharp dissection during the removal of the pathological cornea (Fig. 9). The pathological cornea is not removed until the device has been completely assembled. We do this in order to minimize the open sky time. Anesthesiologists are alerted to the necessity for paralyzing of the patient to avoid elevated pressure during the open sky interval.

## ▶ DEVICE ASSEMBLY

While the front plate and optical cylinder diameters are fixed the device has been ordered in powers commensurate with the estimation of preoperative axial length, the back

plates are available in two diameters: 7.0 and 8.5 mm. It is wise to have both size back plates available. The surgeon must also select the outer diameter of the donor tissue to be utilized. A diameter of less than 7 mm will be difficult to suture due to the limitation of space afforded by the anterior flange of the optical cylinder. Even in microphthalmic eyes with a short axial length and restricted corneal diameter, trephination of 6.5 mm can be accomplished. These smaller eyes can be expected to be associated with maximal dysgenesis and a corresponding more dismal prognosis. The degree of dysgenesis and dissociation of anterior and even posterior segment features can be often detected on preliminary B-scan and if deemed to be significant,

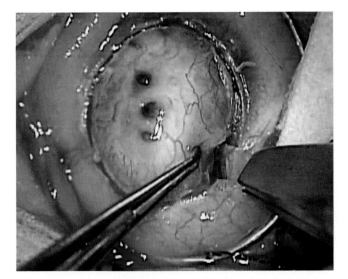

**Fig. 7:** Deepening of trephine incision and guarded entry into anterior chamber

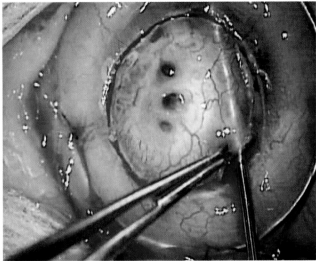

**Fig. 8:** Cyclodialysis spatula utilized to sweep angle avoiding iris damage

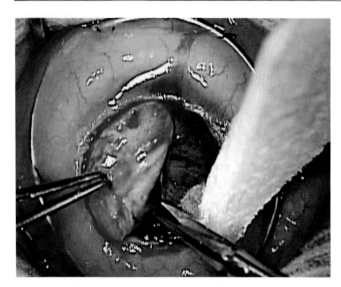

**Fig. 9:** Sharp dissection of anterior synechia adherent to endothelium

these infants are not candidates for the procedure. When possible, we prefer to select an 8.5 mm or 8.75 mm donor tissue diameter when assembling a device with a backplate of 8.5 mm. The larger backplate may impede the growth of tissue at the wound margin which can contribute to the formation of retroprosthetic membranes. The composition of the backplate has been polymethylmethacrylate, but a recent modification utilizes backplates composed of titanium which may be more inert and better tolerated. One of the significant advances of the current model of the Boston Type I KPro has been the addition of 2 rows of fenestrations in the posterior plate to enable the passage of nutrients into the stroma. (Figs 10A and B)

We thus recommend complete assembly of the device and placement in sterile saline prior to excision of the pathological cornea, reducing the potential for intraoperative complication. Lensectomy must be accomplished in all cases and the keratoprosthesis has been ordered with an appropriate aphakic power. The lensectomy may be intracapsular or extracapsular. (Fig. 11) Pupillary membranes and vascularized, anterior vitreous membranes can be excised at this time as well. Iridotomies, iris plasty and identification and formation of an adequate anterior chamber angle for 360° with viscoelastic substance using a cyclodialysis spatula is usually accomplished at this point. (Fig. 12) We feel strongly that the creation of a single chamber eye is imperative in these infants and consequently the next stage of the procedure is accomplished with the recognition that a pars plana vitrectomy will be performed subsequently. Following lensectomy and the completion of any anterior segment repair or preparation two options are available. The assembled keratoprosthesis device can be placed and sutured into final position or if the vitreoretinal team is uncomfortable working through the 3.2 mm optic, a temporary prosthesis can be placed with temporary sutures (Fig. 13). In either event, pars plana vitrectomy 360° retinal inspection with repair or endolaser coagulation may be performed as indicated. If retina repair is necessary the placement of oil in the posterior chamber is not contraindicated. If a temporary prosthesis has been utilized, the corneal surgeon must return to the operating suite to remove the initial prosthesis and insert the permanent assembled device for completion of the procedure. We feel this intervention by a vitreoretinal surgeon is important to

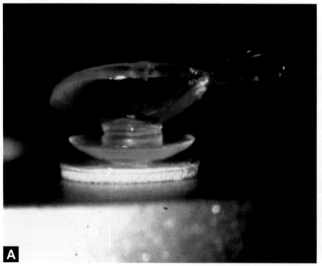

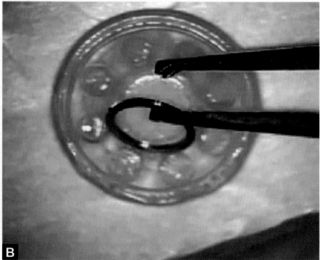

**Figs 10A and B:** (A) Placement of donor tissue on front plate; (B) Securing titanium locking ring

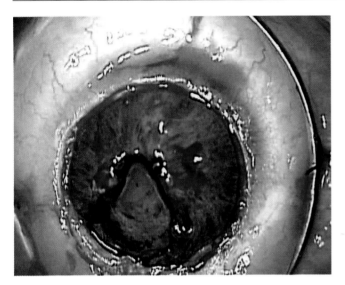

**Fig. 11:** Iridectomy to assist subsequent lensectomy

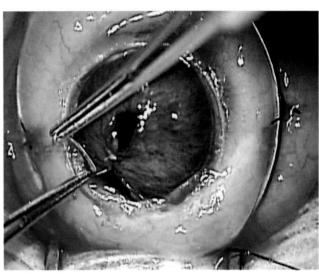

**Fig. 12:** Repair of iridectomy

ensure the long-term visual prognosis. Even in the absence of frank vitreoretinal disease, such as hemorrhage or retinal detachment, areas of peripheral thinning, inflammation and adhesions are not infrequently encountered and repaired by our retinal team, avoiding future complication. Also, the process of secondary placement and ultimate functional survival of an aqueous shunt is facilitated by the pars plana vitrectomy procedure.

The decision to implant a shunt often can be made on the basis of the findings at surgery combined with the history of previous findings and treatment. Assessment of the intraocular pressure in a newborn infant is not simple. With the further complication of corneal thinning, edema,

or anterior segment irregularity, the process becomes more challenging. With cloudy corneas, there is no opportunity to assess the optic nerve. At surgery, however, scleral depression can often confirm significant elevations or reductions of intraocular pressure and thus in cases of well-identified glaucoma often with previous surgical intervention, the decision can be made to implant a shunt concurrent with the keratoprosthesis procedure.

Once the KPro has been implanted and vitrectomy performed, there is an excellent view of the optic nerve. Our preference, in the absence of severe optic nerve cupping is, to have a pediatric glaucoma specialist involved in the future decision-making process. A secondary shunt procedure, once keratoprosthesis and vitrectomy has been performed, is relatively simple. Other confounding factors can be the presence of buphthalmos, often, but not always, an indication of uncontrolled intraocular pressure. In instances of dysgenesis, scleral rigidity can be compromised resulting in an enlarged globe despite relatively normal intraocular pressure. (Fig. 14)

At the close of the procedure, removal of the Flieringa ring and repair of conjunctival incisions precede placement of the hydrophilic bandage lens. A 9.6 mm curvature, 16 mm diameter Kontur bandage lens is supplied with the keratoprosthesis device and will fit most infant eyes.[16,31,32] If no other parameters are available in the operating room, a standard cosmetic disposable lens can be used as long as it is stable over the ocular surface. If Sub-Tenon's injections are to be employed, it is very important to place the bandage lens first, prior to swelling of the conjunctiva secondary to the injections.

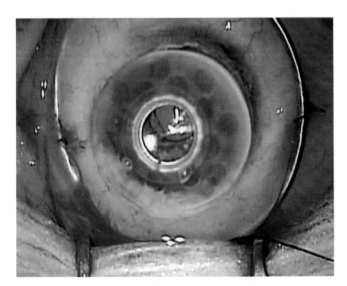

**Fig. 13:** Placement of assembled keratoprosthesis

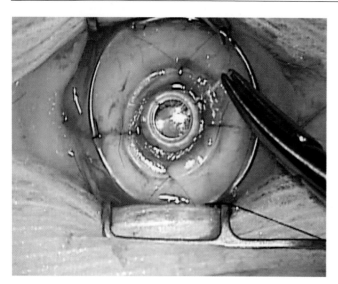

**Fig. 14:** 10-0 nylon suturing of donor rim

While bandage lenses are advocated following all keratoprosthesis procedures, the fitting and maintenance of the lens is particularly important in infants (Fig. 15). If the lens is expulsed for any reason, it must be refitted and reinserted. This process of refitting or reinsertion may not be too difficult in very young infants despite the small lid aperture, but depending on a variety of factors, anesthesia may be necessary. We find a cellulose sponge to be invaluable to contact lens insertion (Weck cell). If there is difficulty in maintaining the lens, a partial lateral tarsorrhaphy may be necessary. The development of surface irregularities and thinning are associated with inappropriate or inadequate lens wear. A simple eyepad and shield can be applied with one strip of tape before the infant is extubated. In cases of significant inflammation, a peribulbar injection of steroid may be indicated. Some

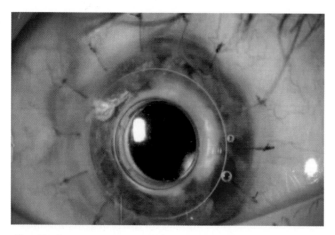

**Fig. 15:** One-year postoperative appearance: Contact lens in place

surgeons routinely instill 400 mcg of dexamethasone in the anterior chamber at the close of the procedure. Others will instill a prophylactic intraocular antibiotic and still others prefer to use peribulbar injection of prophylactic antibiotics. Our anesthesiologists recommend placement of a Tylenol suppository at the close of the case with no further pain medication being given. These babies are comfortable the next morning and usually do not require any additional systemic medication.

## POSTOPERATIVE CARE

The morning following surgery the patch and shield are removed and not replaced. The lids may be cleansed with sterile saline. Most infants will begin to open the eyes spontaneously if not on the first morning, within the first day or two. We caution the parents to take care with drop instillation and only move one lid just enough to apply the drop. Forceful opening of one or especially both lids simultaneously may result in expulsion of the bandage lens if the infant attempts to squeeze the lids closed. For all infants, we prescribe 14 mg/ml vancomycin to be instilled twice daily along with a fluoroquinolone drop. For the first 2 weeks, this antibiotic prophylaxis can be maintained, following which we routinely reduce the instillation to one drop of each medication daily. Anti-inflammatory therapy consisting of 1% methylprednisolone is also instilled three to four times daily. Examination under anesthesia should be planned for 1 month and, thereafter, at 3 month intervals for the 1st year. The vancomycin and fluoroquinolone should be maintained for the 1st year. Prophylactic antibiotic therapy may be modified thereafter if the ocular surface is normal, but must be instilled daily for the indefinite future. If there is evidence of haze or retroprosthetic membrane formation, steroids can be increased, and after the 1st year may be slowly tapered. During examinations under anesthesia, the bandage lens is removed, cleansed and disinfected prior to reinsertion. Betadine solution should be flushed over the ocular surface, examination conducted with the microscope, direct and indirect ophthalmoscopy, intraocular pressure determination with a blunt muscle hook, and A-scan and B-scans as necessary. Tonometer readings are obtained, although we recognize that they may not be accurate. The power of the contact lens may be adjusted according to a formula based on changes in axial length. Examination under anesthesia should be performed by both anterior and posterior segment specialists. Amblyopia therapy should be in place and conducted as indicated by the pediatric ophthalmologist. After the 1st year, examinations under anesthesia are usually advocated at 6 month intervals until the child is able to be examined comfortably in an office setting. Surprisingly, sutures do not need to be removed at any given time. Most likely because of the bandage lens, the sutures do not become loose until many months following the surgical procedure. When a loose suture is apparent, it can be removed. Should medications be indicated for control of intraocular pressure, any standard medication can be used in conjunction with the bandage lens and the prosthesis. In cases where it becomes difficult to maintain the hydrophilic bandage lens, antievaporative measures may be important, such as frequent instillation of lubricating drops, or the use of tight-fitting moist chamber type goggles and as mentioned earlier, lid sutures (Fig. 16).

## ❖ COMPLICATIONS

Despite our initial team approach, the multifaceted pathology demands intense and dedicated follow-up to avoid complications and to deal with any difficulties that arise. Elevation of intraocular pressure may be difficult to diagnose due to the presence of the rigid prosthesis. Scleral depression with a muscle hook combined with repeated axial length measurements and observation of the optic nerve are the best methods to diagnose glaucoma. We favor the implantation of an Ahmed aqueous shunt in cases where a single drop of topical antihypertensive medication does not result in stabilization of optic nerve changes. If pars plana vitrectomy has not been performed with the original KPro surgery, then it should be incorporated into any subsequent shunt procedure. Retention of the bandage contact lens may be adversely affected by the shunt requiring refitting of the lens.

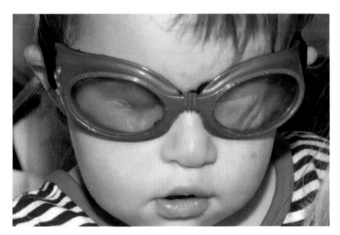

**Fig. 16:** Moist chamber goggles in place

The most dreaded complication is endophthalmitis.[33] In our experience, this is associated with noncompliance with the established prophylactic antibiotic regimen. The importance of compliance must be stressed at every available opportunity. One factor may be the difficulty in obtaining the specially prepared 14 mg/cc topical vancomycin. Arrangements with the appropriate compounding pharmacy should be in place to enable mailing of the supplies directly to the parents on a periodic basis. Consideration may be given to replacement of the vancomycin with Polytrim after the 1st year with the absence of ocular surface disease, however my recommendation is that vancomycin and quinolone be used for the first few years of life in all cases. When the ocular surface is compromised the vancomycin should be maintained. For parents who reside outside of the United States, chloramphenicol is an excellent long-term prophylactic antibiotic. Flushing of the eye with 5% Betadine solution during the course of each examination under anesthesia is a procedure which can reduce the development of fungal surface disease. Office or EUA examinations should include Betadine after the removal of the bandage contact lens (BCL), with disinfection of the BCL prior to reinsertion. Similar to the adult situation, a differential diagnosis of sterile vitreitis must be made. The absence of swelling or redness of the lids and conjunctiva, and associated pain and edema can be a major factor in this diagnosis, while the presence of these symptoms are more commonly associated with frank endophthalmitis.

Difficulty in maintaining the bandage contact lens is a not infrequent occurrence. The contact lens is critical to the prevention of ocular surface melting. Refitting with larger diameter lenses or placement of a lateral tarsorrhaphy may be necessary. Soft-skirt lenses with a rigid optic may also be considered. If the ocular surface becomes dry, the soft lens parameters will become altered. Frequent instillation of artificial tear substitutes or the use of a close-fitting goggle may be helpful in such circumstances. Maintaining the contact lens is the most important prophylactic measure that can be taken to avoid erosion or melting of the surface tissues surrounding the optic. If erosion or melting persists, a repair must be initiated.[32] The use of amniotic membrane and/or mobilization of the conjunctiva may be effective. In more extensive cases, we utilize a sterile prefabricated cornea tissue supplied by Tissue Bank International. This is a 200 micron thick 8.5 mm diameter corneal donor button with a central 3 mm trephination. By placing a radial slit, a 'horse collar' of tissue is formed. This may then be fitted and placed around the optical cylinder and tucked under the flange. The plate of tissue then is sutured closed and onto the ocular surface where it may subsequently be covered with amniotic membrane and/or conjunctiva. If this is not feasible, the entire prosthesis can be trephined and replaced.

Retroprosthetic membranes are noted to occur in about 30% of the infants (Fig. 17). Prophylactic measures include maintaining the instillation of 1% prednisolone acetate instilled three or four times daily for at least a year following the surgical procedure. YAG laser capsulotomy performed under anesthesia is the preferred treatment (Fig. 18). Focal bursts of energy around the optic in a can-opener fashion with powers not exceeding 1–1.5 millijoules are recommended.[34] Usually, one treatment is sufficient. The recurrence rate following the first treatment is approximately 15%. We have never had to utilize more than two treatments in order to permanently resolve the situation. The intraocular surgical approach is also available, but is associated with a greater level of invasiveness and potential complications, and should be used only in cases where YAG laser treatment has failed or the membrane is vascularized.

Vitreoretinal complications include inflammation, hemorrhage, retinal tears and detachments. With a planned initial pars plana vitrectomy, the incidence of these complications has lessened. But a complete fundus examination, including B-scan, should be performed at every examination under anesthesia. We must recognize that the full expression of dysgenesis related vitreoretinal occurrences has not always been completed in the first few weeks of life, but may increase in intensity and precipitate complications over the first several postoperative months.

## ▶ RESULTS

Our first infant keratoprosthesis was performed in 2003. We now have a total of 75 eyes in 60 babies, 50% of which are female and 50% males. The overall results are directly related to the severity of the disease process. We have two cases of endophthalmitis in the infant population, both of which are related to inadequate antibiotic prophylaxis. One case of bilateral phthisis involved an infant born with bilateral corneal perforations forwarded to us following two failed attempts at surgical repair. The level of dysgenesis was associated with the severe recurrent vitreoretinal pathology requiring multiple posterior segment interventions. Retinal detachments repairs, endolaser photocoagulation, and ultimately bilateral funnel detachments and phthisis were the final result. We have repaired the surface as a result of thinning and erosion six times including one case of Stevens-Johnson disease, bilaterally. The ultimate visual acuity in population of children over 4 years has varied from hand motions to 20/30.

## ▶ CONCLUSION

Neonatal corneal opacity is most frequently associated with dysgenesis of variable intensity and expression relating to a widely different prognosis for surgical correction. While some may feel that in less severe cases a single attempt at penetrating keratoplasty is warranted, we feel strongly that deployment of a multispecialty team and the placement of initial keratoprosthesis associated with a lensectomy and pars plana vitrectomy is the procedure of choice and has the best chance of providing useful vision in these desperate

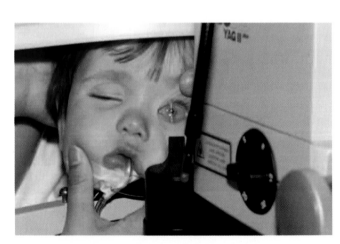

**Fig. 17:** Incipient right retroprosthetic membrane after one year      **Fig. 18:** Operating room–YAG laser procedure

cases. Long-term follow-up is mandatory. Perhaps the most important long-term benefit of this work has been recognition that these cases do not merely involve small eyes with cloudy corneas, but demand a comprehensive ongoing ocular multispecialty approach if useful vision is to be maintained.

## ❧ REFERENCES

1. Stone DL, Kenyon KR, Green WR, et al. Congenital central corneal leukoma (Peters' anomaly). Am J Ophthalmol. 1976; 81:173-93.

2. Traboulsi EI, Maumenee IH. Peters' anomaly and associated congenital malformations. Arch Ophthalmol. 1992;110: 1739-42.

3. Dana MR, Moyes AL, Gomes JA, et al. The indications for and outcome in pediatric keratoplasty. A multicenter study. Ophthalmology. 1995;102:1129-38.

4. Peters A. Ueber angeborene Defektbildung der Descemetschen Membran. Klin Mbl Augenheilk. 1906;44:27-40.

5. Senthikumar M, Darlong V, Punj J, et al. Peters' Anomaly–Anesthetic Management. In J Anesthesia. 2009;53(4):501-3.

6. Gollamudi SR, Traboulsi EI, Chamon W, et al. Visual outcome after surgery for Peters' anomaly. Ophthalmic Genet. 1994;15: 31-5.

7. Cowden JW. Penetrating keratoplasty in infants and children. Ophthalmology. 1990;97:324-8.

8. Stulting RD, Sumers KD, Cavanagh HD, et al. Penetrating keratoplasty in children. Ophthalmology. 1984;91:1222-30.

9. Schanzlin DJ, Goldberg DB, Brown SI. Transplantation of congenitally opaque corneas. Ophthalmology. 1980;87: 1253-64.

10. Hicks CR, Fitton JH, Chirila TV, et al. Keratoprosthesis: advancing toward a true artificial cornea. Surv Ophthalmol. 1997;42:175-89.

11. Yang LL, Lambert SR, Drews-Botsch C, et al. Long-term visual outcome of penetrating keratoplasty in infants and children with Peters anomaly. J AAPOS. 2009;13(2):175-80.

12. Huang C, O'Hara M, Mannis MJ. Primary pediatric keratoplasty: indications and outcomes. Cornea. 2009;28:1003-8.

13. Brown SI, Salamon SM. Wound healing of grafts in congenitally opaque infant corneas. Am J Ophthalmol. 1983;95:641-4.

14. Ma JJ, Graney JM, Dohlman CH. Repeat penetrating keratoplasty versus the Boston keratoprosthesis in graft failure. Int Ophthalmol Clin. 2005;45:49-59.

15. Yaghouti F, Nouri M, Abad JC, et al. Keratoprosthesis: preoperative prognostic categories. Cornea. 2001;20:19-23.

16. Berudsky V, Blum-Hareuveni T, Rehany U, et al. The profile of repeat corneal transplantation. Ophthalmology. 2001;108: 461-9.

17. Hanson IM, Fletcher JM, Jordan T, et al. Mutations at the PAX6 locus are found in heterogeneous anterior segment malformations including Peters' anomaly. Nat Genet. 1994;6: 168-73.

18. Beauchamp GR. Anterior segment dysgenesis keratolenticular adhesion and aniridia. J Pediatr Ophthalmol Strabismus. 1980; 17:55-8.

19. Baltimore MD. (2003). Online Mendelian Inheritance in Man, OMIM(TM). Johns Hopkins University. Available from www.ncbi.nlm.nih.gov/omim.

20. Heon E, Barsoum-Homsy M, Cevrette L, et al. Peters' anomaly. The spectrum of associated ocular and systemic malformations. Ophthalmic Paediatr Genet. 1992;13(2):137-43.

21. Ozeki H, Shirai S, Nozaki M, et al. Ocular and systemic features of Peters' anomaly. Graefes Arch Clin Exp Ophthalmol. 2000; 238(10):833-9.

22. Aubertin G, Kriek M, Lesnik Oberstein SAJ. Peters plus syndrome. In: Pagon RA, Bird TD, Dolan CR, Stephens K (Eds). Gene Reviews. Seattle (WA): University of Washington, Seattle; 1993.

23. Cardona H. Keratoprosthesis; acrylic optical cylinder with supporting intralamellar plate. Am J Ophthalmol. 1962;54:284-94.

24. Choyce DP. Results of keratoprosthesis in Britian. Ophthalmic Surg. 1973;4:23-32.

25. Rao GN, Blatt HL, Aquavella JV. Results of keratoprosthesis. Am J Ophthalmol. 1979;88:190-6.

26. Aquavella JV, Qian Y, McCormick GJ, et al. Keratoprosthesis: current techniques. Cornea. 2006;25(6):656-62.

27. Stone W, Yasuda H, Refojo MF. A 15-year study of the plastic artificial cornea basic principles. In: King JH, McTigue JW (Eds). The Corena World Congress. Washington (DC): Butterworths; 1965. pp. 654-71.

28. Aquavella JV, Qian Y, McCormick GJ, et al. Keratoprosthesis: the Dohlman-Doane device. Am J Ophthalmol. 2005;140(6): 1032-38.

29. Khan BF, Harissi-Dagher M, Khan DM, et al. Advances in Boston keratoprosthesis: enhancing retention and prevention of infection and inflammation. Int Ophthalmol Clin. 2007;47: 61-71.

30. Yaghouti F, Dohlman CH. Innovations in keratoprosthesis: proved and unproved. Int Ophthalmol Clin. 1999;39:27-36.

31. Aquavella JV, Shaw EL. Hydrophilic bandages in penetrating keratoplasty. Ann Ophthalmol. 1976;8:1207-19.

32. Saini JS, Rao GN, Aquavella JV. Post-keratoplasty corneal ulcers and banadage lenses. Acta Ophthalmol (Copenh). 1988; 66(1):99-103.

33. Ramchandran RS, Diloreto DA, Chung MM, et al. Infectious Endophthalmitis in Adult Eyes Receiving Boston Type I Keratoprosthesis. Ophthalmology. 2012.

34. Chak G, Aquavella JV. A safe Nd: YAG retroprosthetic membrane removal technique for keratoprosthesis. Cornea. 2010;29(10):1169-72.

CHAPTER 91

# Boston Keratoprosthesis in the Management of Limbal Stem Cell Failure

*Christina R Prescott, James Chodosh*

## ‣ BACKGROUND

The idea of a 'keratoprosthesis' or synthetic, or partly synthetic cornea was first proposed by Pellier de Quengsy in 1789.[1] The Boston keratoprosthesis was developed by Dr Claes Dohlman over the last 5 decades,[2] and since approval for marketing by the US Food and Drug Administration in 1992, over 6,000 Boston keratoprostheses have been implanted (Claes H Dohlman, personal communication). The basic design is comprised of four parts, including a single front plate and stem containing the optic, a corneal graft (allo- or auto-), which carries the device and allows suturing to the eye as with a routine corneal transplant, a polymethyl methacrylate (PMMA) backplate, and a titanium locking ring.[3,4] The Boston keratoprosthesis has been continuously improved upon since inception. Important changes since 1992 include the transition from a threaded backplate to a snap-in design, the addition of holes to the backplate, and most recently, the change from a PMMA to a titanium backplate.[5] Other advances include the use of prophylactic topical vancomycin[6] and long-term soft contact lenses.[7,8] Based on these advances and the improved outcomes they have brought about, the Boston keratoprosthesis is now the most commonly used artificial cornea in the western world.

The most commonly used model of the Boston keratoprosthesis is the Boston keratoprosthesis Type I, which is implanted in patients with intact eyelids, blink and tear film. In contrast, the Boston keratoprosthesis type II is designed with an anterior extension that protrudes through the eyelids; the lids are closed surgically at the time of implantation.[9] The Type II device is utilized in situations where the ocular surface and adnexa are so damaged that a Type I device is unlikely to be successful.[10] Candidate patients typically have ocular surface keratinization, severe aqueous tear deficiency, symblepharon and foreshortening of the conjunctival fornices.[11]

## ‣ LIMBAL STEM CELL FAILURE AND OCULAR SURFACE DISEASE

The corneal limbus serves multiple functions, acting as a barrier between corneal and conjunctival epithelium, and containing stem cells that are the source of corneal epithelial cells.[12,13] Limbal stem cell failure can be defined scientifically and clinically.[14] Scientifically, limbal stem cell failure is characterized by the intrusion of conjunctival goblet cells onto the cornea, and identified by periodic acid Schiff (PAS) staining of goblet cells or K13 cytokeratin expression of epithelium upon impression cytology or biopsy. K13 is a marker for conjunctival differentiation and has recently been shown to be an indicator of ocular surface disease severity.[15] The presence of goblet cells and conjunctival epithelial markers signifies replacement of the corneal epithelial phenotype by a conjunctival epithelial phenotype. Clinically, limbal stem cell deficiency can be visualized at the slit lamp as coarse, regional or diffuse, and sometimes delayed fluorescein staining of the corneal epithelium, often 'streaming' in from the limbus, corneal neovascularization, corneal scarring, conjunctivalization of the cornea and poor corneal epithelialization with persistent or recurrent epithelial defects.[12]

Patients with limbal stem cell deficiency can present with a wide spectrum of symptoms ranging from mild irritation associated with modest blurring of vision to severe pain and near total loss of vision.[16] There are many causes of limbal stem cell failure, including but not limited to aniridia; neurotrophic keratopathy; chronic corneal inflammation; chemical, thermal or radiation burns; ocular surgery; contact lens overuse; drug-induced keratopathy (medicamentosa); Stevens Johnson syndrome/toxic epidermal necrolysis (SJS/TEN) and mucus membrane pemphigoid (MMP).[17,18] Some ocular surface disease and associated limbal stem cell failure is idiopathic. In this chapter, we will focus on aniridia, chemical burns, MMP and SJS/TEN as distinct paradigms for limbal stem cell deficiency in which Boston keratoprosthesis implantation may be indicated.

Aniridia is the most common congenital cause of limbal stem cell deficiency, with an incidence of between 1:64,000 and 1:96,000.[19] It has been linked to multiple mutations in the paired box gene 6 (*PAX6*) and can be inherited in either an autosomal dominant (2/3) or sporadic fashion (1/3).[20] The defining feature of aniridia is hypoplasia of the iris, which can vary from subtle changes to near total absence. Corneal findings occur in approximately 20% of patients and are related to alterations in cell adhesion, and glycoconjugate and corneal cytokine expression due to limbal stem cell deficiency.[21] Clinical findings include vascular pannus with underlying stromal scarring, persistent epithelial defects and Salzmann's nodular degeneration. In addition to the anterior segment findings, both optic nerve and foveal hypoplasia are associated with aniridia and limit patients' visual potential.[22]

Because of a limited capacity to generate a corneal epithelium, patients with aniridia have a high failure rate with traditional penetrating keratoplasty.[23] Because of the bilateral nature of the illness, such patients are not usually candidates for contralateral limbal autografts. Therefore, treatment options are limited. One option for aniridics is keratolimbal allograft, which uses cadaveric tissue or tissue from a living related donor, and requires systemic immunosuppression.[24] One widely used immunosuppression regime combines oral mycophenolate mofetil, tacrolimus and prednisone.[24] Keratolimbal allograft followed by penetrating keratoplasty led to an average visual improvement from 20/1000 to 20/165 in one published case series.[24] An emerging option for patients with aniridia is the Boston keratoprosthesis, with relatively good visual outcomes[21,25] and which does not require systemic immunosuppression.

Chemical, thermal or electrical burns can all lead to severe ocular injury. Of all chemical injuries, alkali burns generally cause the most devastating injuries.[26] Sequential sectoral epitheliectomy may be an option for partial limbal stem cell deficiency after chemical injury.[27] This is performed by removing abnormal epithelium to enable unaffected limbus to repopulate the area with healthy epithelium. It can be combined with amniotic membrane transplantation to help promote healing.[28] If the injury is predominantly confined to one eye, the patient may be a candidate for contralateral conjunctival limbal autograft, followed if necessary by traditional penetrating keratoplasty.[29] However, many chemical injuries are bilateral, though

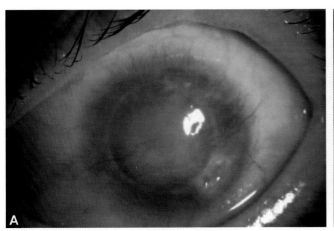 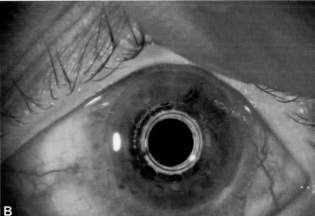

**Figs 1A and B:** (A) Anterior segment photograph of the left eye of a 37-year-old male following a severe alkali burn to both eyes, and a failed corneal transplant to the left eye. The visual acuity in the left eye was hand motion and the visual acuity in the right eye was no light perception; (B) The left eye of the same patient 6 months after implantation of a Boston keratoprosthesis type I. More than 5 years from surgery, the uncorrected visual acuity remained 20/25

CHAPTER 92

often asymmetric, and such patients would require an allograft, necessitating systemic immunosuppression.[30] Progress has been made on the cultivation of corneal limbal stem cells for use in transplantation, and it is possible that use of cultivated limbal cells will play a larger role in the future.[14] For patients who are not candidates for stem cell transplantation, an alternative treatment may be oral mucosal graft in conjunction with amniotic membrane reconstruction; however, this technique can be associated with vision limiting corneal neovascularization.[31] Patients with limbal stem cell failure after chemical injury may be candidates for the Boston keratoprosthesis (Figs 1A and B).

Mucous membrane pemphigoid (MMP) is a severe autoimmune cicatricial disease, which characteristically causes end stage dry eye, symblepharon, keratinization of the ocular surface, corneal scarring and vascularization, and sometimes ulceration and perforation.[32] MMP is typically a bilateral disease. The severity and bilaterality allow limited potential treatment options for patients with MMP. Traditional penetrating keratoplasty has a poor success rate in MMP.[33] Implantation of a Boston keratoprosthesis type I can restore vision, but one can expect to encounter significant difficulties and potential complications, principally due to MMP-associated symblepharon and severe tear deficiency. For example, bandage contact lenses are important following Boston keratoprosthesis type I implantation to keep the cornea around the keratoprosthesis well hydrated, but soft contact lenses are difficult to retain in the setting of symblepharon and forniceal foreshortening. Staged surgery, consisting

of limbal stem cell transplantation followed by a Boston keratoprosthesis type I has been attempted[34], but patients with MMP are typically elderly and may not tolerate multi-agent immune suppression. Alternatively, these patients maybe candidates for the Boston keratoprosthesis type II (Figs 2A and B), which is implanted through the closed eyelid and therefore does not require contact lens wear.[11]

Stevens-Johnson syndrome/toxic epidermal necrolysis (SJS/TEN) is a spectrum of severe, immune mediated, mucocutaneous epithelial drug reactions, characterized by vesicular eruptive lesions of skin and mucosal surfaces.[35] The distinction between SJS and TEN is primarily based on the extent of total body surface area affected (less than 10% in SJS, greater than 30% in TEN, and 10–30% in SJS/TEN "overlap").[36,37] The pathogenesis of SJS/TEN is not well understood, but the disorder may represent an innate immune response to reactive metabolites of a systemic medication.[38] The annual incidence of SJS/TEN is between 0.6 and 10 cases per million persons per year. Between 43% and 81% of patients have acute (within the first 2 weeks) ocular involvement.[39] These patients typically require care in an intensive care/burn unit and the mortality rate is significant.[37,40-44]

Patients with SJS/TEN typically suffer from acute ulceration of the eyelid margin, tarsal and bulbar conjunctiva, and corneal epithelium, which can lead to significant, long-term, cicatricial changes.[45] Even after the acute phase of the illness has past, chronic inflammation of the conjunctiva and eyelid margin may lead to limbal stem cell deficiency and chronic ocular surface disease.

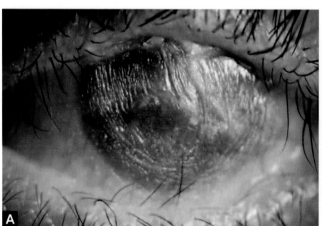 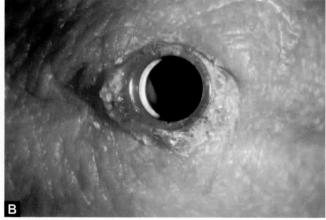

**Figs 2A and B:** (A) Anterior segment photograph of the left eye of a patient with a history of MMP and a dry keratinized ocular surface. Visual acuity was light perception; (B) The left eye of the same patient 2 years after implantation of the Boston type II keratoprosthesis. Visual acuity was 20/60 with correction

Long-term ocular complications, including cicatricial scarring and corneal blindness, occur in approximately 35% of patients.[37] In addition to chronic conjunctivitis, eyelid margin abnormalities, including loss of meibomian glands, abnormal lid margin contour and entropion with trichiasis or frank distichiasis are a major cause of long-term ocular morbidity, including corneal epithelial breakdown, ulceration, scarring and sometimes, perforation.[39]

Traditionally, ophthalmic interventions during the acute stage of SJS/TEN were limited to aggressive lubrication, prophylactic topical antibiotics, lysis of conjunctival membranes and topical corticosteroids. Recent use of cryopreserved amniotic membrane in the acute phase of SJS/TEN is very promising[39,46] and will hopefully improve the long-term visual prognosis of these patients. Briefly, a graft of amniotic membrane, the innermost layer of the placenta, and composed of a thick basement membrane and an avascular stroma, is applied to the entire ocular surface, including the lid margins, and left in place until the membrane dissolves. In the chronic phase, those patients with severe eyelid margin and corneal involvement may be managed with mucus membrane grafts[47] and/or sclera contact lenses.[48] However, patients in the late stages with severe, chronic, cicatricial corneal blindness from SJS/TEN have limited treatment options, and may be candidates for the Boston keratoprosthesis Type II. It is important to note that of all disease groups, SJS/TEN patients have the worst long-term prognosis with respect to retention of a Boston keratoprosthesis.[3,49]

## ▶ KERATOPROSTHESIS IMPLANTATION FOR SEVERE LIMBAL STEM CELL DEFICIENCY

The Boston keratoprosthesis is one of many keratoprosthesis designs.[50] For example, in patients with the most severe ocular surface diseases, the modified osteo-odonto keratoprosthesis (MOOKP), developed by Strampelli and modified by Falcinelli, represents an effective means of visual restoration.[51] However, for all patients needing a keratoprosthesis, the Boston keratoprosthesis is the most widely used of the many keratoprosthesis designs. The most common indication for keratoprosthesis surgery in general is failed corneal transplant,[52,53] but keratoprosthesis implantation may be indicated as initial surgery for patients with limbal stem cell deficiency, particularly in aniridia or in those with MMP or SJS/TEN, in whom corneal allograft surgery is expected to fail. Patients requiring keratoprosthesis surgery, and with mild to moderate tear dysfunction are candidates for Type I keratoprosthesis implantation, but patients with absent tear function, ocular surface keratinization or significant cicatricial conjunctival disease can be considered for a Boston Type II keratoprosthesis, which in such cases may have a better outcome[3] or a MOOKP. Patients with limbal stem cell deficiency, especially those with aniridia or prior chemical injuries, often present with glaucoma, which can be difficult both to control and to evaluate. Corneal opacification makes it difficult to accurately assess the appearance of the optic disk and to perform visual field tests. In a case series of SJS/TEN patients who underwent Boston keratoprosthesis surgery, 75% of eyes had pre-existing glaucoma.[3] Because patients with aniridia have an increased incidence of glaucoma,[19] concurrent implantation of a glaucoma drainage device is usually recommended. Glaucoma surgery should also be considered in patients requiring keratoprosthesis after chemical injury (especially alkali), MMP and SJS/TEN. A glaucoma drainage valve can be implanted prior to, in conjunction with, or subsequent to the keratoprosthesis.[54]

Some patients benefit from having other additional surgeries performed in conjunction with implantation of the keratoprosthesis, including pars plana vitrectomy, pupilloplasty and/or intraocular lens (IOL) removal. In patients who are phakic, lens removal is necessary at the time of keratoprosthesis surgery. Placement of an IOL is optional, but may be beneficial in maintaining a two-chambered eye in anticipation of possible future glaucoma drainage device implantation. Since the refractive power needed in the keratoprosthesis must be determined prior to surgery, in phakic patients undergoing keratoprosthesis and lens extraction for whom an IOL is desired, a plano IOL is recommended because it allows the surgeon to defer IOL placement if there is insufficient capsular support. If the patient is pseudophakic, the IOL must be carefully evaluated for stability. If the lens is unstable, it should be removed. Sometimes stability of an existing IOL cannot be determined prior to surgery which makes choosing the desired keratoprosthesis power challenging. However, any residual refractive error is easily corrected by a powered contact lens. In a comparative case series of patients with posterior chamber IOLs who underwent Boston type I keratoprosthesis surgery, including mostly patients without significant limbal stem cell deficiency, removal of the posterior chamber IOL with placement of an aphakic Boston keratoprosthesis type I resulted in significantly less postoperative refractive error, though best corrected visual acuity was similar in the two groups.[55]

Additional perioperative choices must be considered in Boston keratoprosthesis Type II implantation, including preoperative and postoperative immune suppression, for example mycophenolate at low doses. Lensectomy, iridectomy, pars plana vitrectomy and Ahmed valve implantation are generally recommended in conjunction with Boston keratoprosthesis type II implantation in all SJS/TEN patients, modified based on prior surgeries.[11]

## ▸ POSTOPERATIVE CARE FOLLOWING BOSTON KERATOPROSTHESIS IN LIMBAL STEM CELL DEFICIENCY

The duration and frequency of postoperative corticosteroids in patients undergoing Boston keratoprosthesis implantation for severe limbal stem cell deficiency is not very different from that in patients receiving a Boston keratoprosthesis for other indications. Because of local complications of topical corticosteroids, patients with severe alkali burns and SJS/TEN may be better served by low dose, single agent and systemic immune modulation. Many patients who need a keratoprosthesis have a compromised ocular surface, and persistent epithelial defects are common.[52] In this setting, excessive use of topical corticosteroids can also be harmful. Contact lens retention can be especially challenging in patients with conjunctival scarring and symblepharon, such as in MMP and SJS/TEN. Patients who have difficulty with lens retention may benefit from lateral tarsorrhaphy. For patients that can retain a lens, those with aqueous tear deficiency may develop excessive protein deposition on their soft contact lenses. In these cases, use of a hybrid contact lens can eliminate protein deposition in the central portion of the lens and leave the visual axis undisturbed.[56]

## ▸ COMPLICATIONS

The most common postoperative complication following keratoprosthesis implantation is formation of a retro-prosthetic membrane (RPM), with an incidence rate of 35–44%, and an average time of onset of 4 months postoperative.[52,53] RPM is even more common in patients with autoimmune causes such as MMP and SJS/TEN, as well as in chemical burn patients.[5] The risk of RPM formation increases with combined intraocular procedures, and appears most closely associated with postoperative inflammation. In a small series of cases, the replacement of the PMMA backplate with one made of medical grade titanium reduced RPM formation from

31.2% to 13.0%.[5] For those that develop RPM, yttrium-aluminum-garnet (YAG) membranotomy or capsulotomy may be indicated, and can be performed even through a type II keratoprosthesis.

Following severe chemical injury, damage to the cornea is usually the most obvious manifestation, but other coexisting ocular pathology may be even more important, particularly glaucoma. Patients with chemical injuries, especially alkali burns, are at high risk of glaucomatous visual loss after keratoprosthesis,[57] and may have an increased risk of retinal detachment. These patients must be followed closely with serial digital palpation, visual fields and optic nerve photos.[58] Ideally, patients should be co-managed with a glaucoma specialist.

Endophthalmitis is thankfully an uncommon late complication after Boston keratoprosthesis implantation. In a retrospective study performed at the Mass Eye and Ear Infirmary, the rate of bacterial endophthalmitis dropped from 4.13% per patient-year to 0.35% in patients using topical daily vancomycin drops.[6] In patients with severe ocular surface disease, normal antimicrobial barriers may be reduced or nonexistent. In addition, topical corticosteroids and/or systemic immunosuppressive agents may further predispose to infection. In these patients, chronic antibiotic prophylaxis, reduction to the lowest possible dose and frequency of topical corticosteroids, and intermittent topical antifungal prophylaxis should be strongly considered.

Intraocular infection must be distinguished from sterile postoperative vitritis, an idiopathic condition associated with keratoprosthesis implantation. Sterile vitritis occurred in 7–10% of patients in several published series[49,52,53] and presents with decreased vision and vitreous cells, with no other evidence for infection. If left untreated, chronic vitritis can contribute to both retroprosthetic and epiretinal membranes, and theoretically to tractional retinal detachments, and angle closure glaucoma. Sterile vitritis is treated with corticosteroids (topical and/or retrotenons) and followed closely.[59] If there is any concern for infectious endophthalmitis, the patient should be evaluated by a vitreoretinal surgeon and a vitreous tap should be performed with concomitant antibiotic (and possibly antifungal) injections.

Retinal detachment rates range from 3.5% to 12%.[53,60] Because the Boston keratoprosthesis limits visualization of the most peripheral retina, some retinal pathology may go undetected until retinal detachment ensues. It remains to be determined whether pars plana vitrectomy at the time of keratoprosthesis surgery will reduce retinal detachment rates, but theoretically, reduction of vitreous traction by subtotal vitrectomy would be expected to reduce the risk of detachment later.

## VISUAL OUTCOMES AFTER BOSTON KERATOPROSTHESIS IN LIMBAL STEM CELL DEFICIENCY

Recovery and retention of vision in patients with limbal stem cell deficiency patients receiving a Boston keratoprosthesis varies by indication for surgery. For example, in one study of 15 patients with aniridia and a mean follow-up of 17 months, the average change in visual acuity was an improvement from count fingers to 20/200.[25] In a series of 15 patients with SJS/TEN who underwent Boston keratoprosthesis implantation, of those who achieved greater than equal to 20/200 vision, one half maintained it for at least 5 years (mixture of 6 type I and 10 type II keratoprosthesis cases).[3] In another series of 11 patients with SJS/TEN treated with the Boston keratoprosthesis type II, again half of those who recovered greater than equal to 20/200 vision after surgery maintained it for at least 5 years.[11] Eyes that failed to improve to 20/200 or lost vision during follow-up had end stage glaucoma, previous occult or new retinal detachment or age related macular degeneration.

## Retention of the Boston Keratoprosthesis

The retention rate in the Multicenter Boston Type I Keratoprosthesis Study with an average 8.5 months of follow-up (2006) was 95%. Corneal stromal necrosis was a principal indication for replacement, and occurred in 16% of patients in one large series.[52] Corneal necrosis occurs more commonly in patients with underlying autoimmune pathology, including SJS/TEN and MMP.[10] In a series of patients with SJS/TEN receiving a Boston keratoprosthesis type I or II, 25% developed aqueous leakage at some time after implantation, leading to removal or replacement of the device.[3] In 6 patients with SJS/TEN treated with the Boston keratoprosthesis type I, retention rate for first keratoprosthesis was dramatically lower (0 at 5 years postoperatively) than in patients with other causes of limbal stem cell failure.[49] In 11 patients with SJS/TEN treated with the Boston keratoprosthesis type II, half the patients had retained their first device at 5 years postoperatively.[11]

## CONCLUSION

Limbal stem cell failure encompasses a wide spectrum of diseases, with varying severity but sometimes limited treatment options. Patients with severe unilateral disease may do well with a limbal autograft, sometimes in combination with a traditional corneal transplant. For patients with bilateral disease, limbal allograft is an option, but typically requires three drug systemic immunosuppression. The Boston keratoprosthesis represents an alternative treatment option for patients with severe limbal stem cell failure, does not require systemic immunosuppression in most patients, and can be managed with low dose single agents in others. The prognosis for successful long-term implantation of the Boston keratoprosthesis in severe limbal stem cell failure depends on the etiology. Patients with aniridia do comparatively well with Boston keratoprosthesis implantation. Patients with severe chemical injuries, particularly due to alkali agents, are at increased risk of glaucoma and retinal detachment after a Boston keratoprosthesis. Those with MMP are thought to have a guarded prognosis with implantation of a Boston keratoprosthesis, but of all the patient populations discussed above, those with SJS/TEN have the worst prognosis with keratoprosthesis implantation.[33,61]

Visual potential in some forms of limbal stem cell failure may be limited by posterior segment pathology, most notably glaucoma. Associated posterior segment pathology can also be difficult to detect before surgery because of corneal opacification. Due to a relatively high rate of glaucoma in most patient populations with limbal stem cell failure, simultaneous glaucoma drainage implantation should be considered at the time of keratoprosthesis surgery. Co-management with a glaucoma specialist is an important aspect of postoperative care in many of these patients. It is difficult to accurately measure intraocular pressure following keratoprosthesis implantation, so visualization and documentation of the optic nerve and regular visual fields are especially important.

MMP and SJS/TEN, along with severe alkali injuries are those least likely to retain their first device, and most likely to suffer permanently blinding complications of keratoprosthesis surgery. Single agent immunosuppressive therapy, if combined with careful antimicrobial prophylaxis, can potentially modify and delay adverse outcomes in such patients. The Boston keratoprosthesis type II is a viable option for corneal blindness from severe cicatricial ocular surface disease, but like the MOOKP, should be reserved

16 SECTION

for patients with no other options and a strong desire to regain their vision. Informed consent should include the possible need to replace the device at some time after surgery, especially in patients with MMP and SJS/TEN.

# ☞ REFERENCES

1. G.PDQ. Accurate during operations on eye surgery. Paris: Didot. 1789.
2. Dohlman CH, Mannis MJ. Corneal transplantation: a history in profiles. In: Mannis AA, Mannis MJ. Belgium: JP Wayenborough. 1999; volume 6.
3. Sayegh RR, Ang LP, Foster CS, et al. The Boston keratoprosthesis in Stevens-Johnson syndrome. Am J Ophthalmol. 2008;145(3): 438-44.
4. Khan BF, Harissi-Dagher M, Khan DM, et al. Advances in Boston keratoprosthesis: enhancing retention and prevention of infection and inflammation. Int Ophthalmol Clin. 2007;47 (2):61-71.
5. Todani A, Ciolino JB, Ament JD, et al. Titanium backplate for a PMMA keratoprosthesis: clinical outcomes. Graefes Arch Clin Exp Ophthalmol. 2011;249(10):1515-8.
6. Durand ML, Dohlman CH. Successful prevention of bacterial endophthalmitis in eyes with the Boston keratoprosthesis. Cornea. 2009;28(8):896-901.
7. Klufas MA, Colby KA. The Boston keratoprosthesis. Int Ophthalmol Clin. 2010;50(3):161-75.
8. Dohlman CH, Dudenhoefer EJ, Khan BF, et al. Protection of the ocular surface after keratoprosthesis surgery: the role of soft contact lenses. CLAO J. 2002;28(2):72-4.
9. Barnes SD, Dohlman CH, Durand ML. Fungal colonization and infection in Boston keratoprosthesis. Cornea. 2007;26(1):9-15.
10. Ciralsky J, Papaliodis GN, Foster CS, et al. Keratoprosthesis in autoimmune disease. Ocul Immunol Inflamm. 2010;18(4): 275-80.
11. Pujari S, Siddique SS, Dohlman CH, et al. The Boston keratoprosthesis type II: The Massachusetts Eye and Ear Infirmary experience. Cornea. 2011;30(12):1298-303.
12. Cauchi PA, Ang GS, Azuara-Blanco A, et al. A systematic literature review of surgical interventions for limbal stem cell deficiency in humans. Am J Ophthalmol. 2008;146(2):251-9.
13. Schermer A, Galvin S, Sun TT. Differentiation-related expression of a major 64K corneal keratin in vivo and in culture suggests limbal location of corneal epithelial stem cells. J Cell Biol. 1986;103(1):49-62.
14. Nakamura T, Sotozono C, Bentley AJ, et al. Long-term phenotypic study after allogeneic cultivated corneal limbal epithelial transplantation for severe ocular surface diseases. Ophthalmology. 2010;117(12):2247-54.
15. Poli M, Janin H, Justin V, et al. Keratin 13 immunostaining in corneal impression cytology for the diagnosis of limbal stem cell deficiency. Invest Ophthalmol Vis Sci. 2011;52(13):9411-5.
16. Kruse FE, Cursiefen C. Surgery of the cornea: corneal, limbal stem cell and amniotic membrane transplantation. Dev Ophthalmol. 2008;41:159-70.
17. Liu J, Sheha H, Fu Y, et al. Oral mucosal graft with amniotic membrane transplantation for total limbal stem cell deficiency. Am J Ophthalmol. 2011;152(5):739-47.
18. Echevarria TJ, Di Girolamo N. Tissue-regenerating, vision-restoring corneal epithelial stem cells. Stem Cell Rev. 2011;7(2): 256-68.
19. Brauner SC, Walton DS, Chen TC. Aniridia. Int Ophthalmol Clin. 2008;48(2):79-85.
20. Kokotas H, Petersen MB. Clinical and molecular aspects of aniridia. Clin Genet. 2010;77(5):409-20.
21. Lee H, Khan R, O'Keefe M. Aniridia: current pathology and management. Acta Ophthalmol. 2008;86(7):708-15.
22. Lee H, Meyers K, Lanigan B, et al. Complications and visual prognosis in children with aniridia. J Pediatr Ophthalmol Strabismus. 2010;47(4):205-10.
23. Kremer I, Rajpal RK, Rapuano CJ, et al. Results of penetrating keratoplasty in aniridia. Am J Ophthalmol. 1993;115(3): 317-20.
24. Holland EJ, Djalilian AR, Schwartz GS. Management of aniridic keratopathy with keratolimbal allograft: a limbal stem cell transplantation technique. Ophthalmology. 2003;110(1): 125-30.
25. Akpek EK, Harissi-Dagher M, Petrarca R, et al. Outcomes of Boston keratoprosthesis in aniridia: a retrospective multicenter study. Am J Ophthalmol. 2007;144(2):227-31.
26. Rozenbaum D, Baruchin AM, Dafna Z. Chemical burns of the eye with special reference to alkali burns. Burns. 1991;17(2): 136-40.
27. Dua HS. The conjunctiva in corneal epithelial wound healing. Br J Ophthalmol. 1998;82(12):1407-11.
28. Tseng SC, Prabhasawat P, Barton K, et al. Amniotic membrane transplantation with or without limbal allografts for corneal surface reconstruction in patients with limbal stem cell deficiency. Arch Ophthalmol. 1998;116(4):431-41.
29. Pires RT, Chokshi A, Tseng SC. Amniotic membrane transplantation or conjunctival limbal autograft for limbal stem cell deficiency induced by 5-fluorouracil in glaucoma surgeries. Cornea. 2000;19(3):284-7.
30. Liang L, Sheha H, Tseng SC. Long-term outcomes of keratolimbal allograft for total limbal stem cell deficiency using combined immunosuppressive agents and correction of ocular surface deficits. Arch Ophthalmol. 2009;127(11):1428-34.
31. Liu J, Hosam Sheha, Yao Fu, et al. Update on amniotic membrane transplantation. Expert Rev Ophthalmol. 2010;5(5):645-61.
32. Kirzhner M, Jakobiec FA. Ocular cicatricial pemphigoid: a review of clinical features, immunopathology, differential diagnosis, and current management. Semin Ophthalmol. 2011; 26(4-5):270-7.
33. Tugal-Tutkun I, Akova YA, Foster CS. Penetrating keratoplasty in cicatrizing conjunctival diseases. Ophthalmology. 1995;102 (4):576-85.
34. Biber JM, Skeens HM, Neff KD, et al. The cincinnati procedure: technique and outcomes of combined living-related conjunctival limbal allografts and keratolimbal allografts in severe ocular surface failure. Cornea. 2011;30(7):765-71.
35. Wetter DA, MJ Camilleri. Clinical, etiologic, and histopathologic features of Stevens-Johnson syndrome during an 8-year period at Mayo Clinic. Mayo Clin Proc. 2010;85(2):131-8.
36. Del Pozzo-Magana, Lazo-Langner A, Carleton B, et al. A systematic review of treatment of drug-induced Stevens-Johnson syndrome and toxic epidermal necrolysis in children. J Popul Ther Clin Pharmacol. 2011;18:121-33.

37. Shay E, Kheirkhah A, Liang L, et al. Amniotic membrane transplantation as a new therapy for the acute ocular manifestations of Stevens-Johnson syndrome and toxic epidermal necrolysis. Surv Ophthalmol. 2009;54(6):686-96.

38. Bellon T, Blanca M. The innate immune system in delayed cutaneous allergic reactions to medications. Curr Opin Allergy Clin Immunol. 2011;11(4):292-8.

39. Shammas MC, Lai EC, Sarkar JS, et al. Management of acute Stevens-Johnson syndrome and toxic epidermal necrolysis utilizing amniotic membrane and topical corticosteroids. Am J Ophthalmol. 2010;149(2):203-13.

40. Valeyrie-Allanore L, Bastuji-Garin S, Guégan S, et al. Prognostic value of histologic features of toxic epidermal necrolysis. J Am Acad Dermatol. 2011.

41. Finkelstein Y, Soon GS, Acuna P, et al. Recurrence and outcomes of Stevens-Johnson syndrome and toxic epidermal necrolysis in children. Pediatrics. 2011;128(4):723-8.

42. Zajicek R, Pintar D, Broz L, et al. Toxic epidermal necrolysis and Stevens-Johnson syndrome at the Prague Burn Centre 1998-2008. J Eur Acad Dermatol Venereol. 2011.

43. Barvaliya M, Sanmukhani J, Patel T, et al. Drug-induced Stevens-Johnson syndrome (SJS), toxic epidermal necrolysis (TEN), and SJS-TEN overlap: a multicentric retrospective study. J Postgrad Med. 2011;57(2):115-9.

44. Yamane Y, M Aihara, Z Ikezawa. Analysis of Stevens-Johnson syndrome and toxic epidermal necrolysis in Japan from 2000 to 2006. Allergol Int. 2007.56(4):419-25.

45. Fu Y, Gregory DG, Sippel KC, et al. The ophthalmologist's role in the management of acute Stevens-Johnson syndrome and toxic epidermal necrolysis. Ocul Surf. 2010;8(4):193-203.

46. Gregory DG. Treatment of acute Stevens-Johnson syndrome and toxic epidermal necrolysis using amniotic membrane: a review of 10 consecutive cases. Ophthalmology. 2011;118(5):908-14.

47. Fu Y, Liu J, Tseng SC. Oral mucosal graft to correct lid margin pathologic features in cicatricial ocular surface diseases. Am J Ophthalmol. 2011;152(4):600-8.

48. Rosenthal P, Cotter J. The Boston Scleral Lens in the management of severe ocular surface disease. Ophthalmol Clin North Am. 2003;16(1):89-93.

49. Sejpal K, Yu F, Aldave AJ. The Boston keratoprosthesis in the management of corneal limbal stem cell deficiency. Cornea. 2011;30(11):1187-94.

50. Gomaa A, Comyn O, Liu C. Keratoprostheses in clinical practice-a review. Clin Experiment Ophthalmol. 2010;38(2):211-24.

51. Falcinelli G, Falsini B, Taloni M, et al. Modified osteo-odonto-keratoprosthesis for treatment of corneal blindness: long-term anatomical and functional outcomes in 181 cases. Arch Ophthalmol. 2005;123(10):1319-29.

52. Aldave AJ, Kamal KM, Vo RC, et al. The Boston type I keratoprosthesis: improving outcomes and expanding indications. Ophthalmology. 2009;116(4):640-51.

53. Zerbe BL, Belin MW, Ciolino JB, et al. Results from the multicenter Boston Type 1 Keratoprosthesis Study. Ophthalmology. 2006;113(10):1779.

54. Dohlman CH, Grosskreutz CL, Chen TC, et al. Shunts to divert aqueous humor to distant epithelialized cavities after keratoprosthesis surgery. J Glaucoma. 2010;19(2):111-5.

55. Utine CA, Tzu J, Dunlap K, et al. Visual and clinical outcomes of explantation versus preservation of the intraocular lens during keratoprosthesis implantation. J Cataract Refract Surg. 2011;37(9):1615-22.

56. Beyer J, Todani A, Dohlman C. Prevention of visually debilitating deposits on soft contact lenses in keratoprosthesis patients. Cornea. 2011;30(12):1419-22.

57. Cade F, Grosskreutz CL, Tauber A, et al. Glaucoma in eyes with severe chemical burn, before and after keratoprosthesis. Cornea. 2011;30(12):1322-7.

58. Rivier D, Paula JS, Kim E, et al. Glaucoma and keratoprosthesis surgery: role of adjunctive cyclophotocoagulation. J Glaucoma. 2009;18(4):321-4.

59. Nouri M, Durand ML, Dohlman CH. Sudden reversible vitritis after keratoprosthesis: an immune phenomenon? Cornea. 2005;24(8):915-9.

60. Ray S, Khan BF, Dohlman CH, et al. Management of vitreoretinal complications in eyes with permanent keratoprosthesis. Arch Ophthalmol. 2002;120(5):559-66.

61. Yaghouti F, Nouri M, Abad JC, et al. Keratoprosthesis: preoperative prognostic categories. Cornea. 2001;20(1):19-23.

CHAPTER **92**

# Preoperative Considerations: Patient Selection and Evaluation

*Naazli M Shaikh, Stephen C Kaufman, Jamal M Mohsin*

**Keywords:** Keratorefractive surgery, Contraindications, Food and Drug Administration (FDA), Systemic disease and Keratorefractive surgery, Diabetes mellitus, Hormonal fluctuations, Immunosuppression, HIV, Autoimmune disease, Atopy, Keloid, Psoriasis, Ocular conditions and Keratorefractive surgery, Refractive stability, Large pupils, Phorias/ Tropias, Blepharitis, Dry eyes, Corneal dystrophy, Corneal ectasia, Corneal warpage, Retinal holes, Glaucoma, Cataract, Refractive intraocular lenses, Monofocal/Multifocal, Toric

*The modern refractive patient has numerous options for keratorefractive and refractive lens surgery. Systemic disease and ophthalmic conditions can affect the final outcome of keratorefractive surgery and must be considered in the preoperative evaluation. The FDA and the Academy of Ophthalmology provide guidance on the absolute and relative contraindications of keratorefractive surgery. When controlled, however, patients with most types of systemic and ocular conditions may still be considered for keratorefractive surgery. Those patients who are not candidates for or beyond the limits of keratorefractive surgery may pursue refractive lens surgery instead or in combination with the former.*

*This chapter describes the limitations and contraindications of various types of keratorefractive and refractive lens surgeries, providing insight into appropriate selection of patients based on their expectations and medical conditions, while matching them to the most suitable refractive surgery options.*

## ❧ INTRODUCTION

Keratorefractive surgery modifies the contour of the cornea using blade, corneal implants, or laser ablation, with the intent of changing the refractive error of the eye. Several keratorefractive surgical and laser procedures exist for the correction of myopia, hyperopia and astigmatism.

The United States Food and Drug Administration (FDA) established a list of absolute and relative contraindications for refractive surgery (Table 1), specifically for photorefractive keratectomy (PRK), which included ocular and systemic diseases. Among the systemic diseases are autoimmune and connective-tissue disorders such as rheumatoid arthritis (RA), systemic lupus erythematosus (SLE), ankylosing spondylitis, psoriatic arthritis, Sjögren's syndrome and other systemic vasculitides. Diabetes mellitus, antecedent keloid formation, immunosuppression and treatment with some drugs are relative contraindications. Recently atopy and allergic conjunctivitis were also included as relative contraindications. It was thought that these conditions could induce a postoperative inflammatory response, leading to corneal melting or scarring, especially in PRK in which the

corneal stroma is exposed for an extended period of time until reepithelialized.

Laser *in situ* keratomileusis (LASIK), despite less inflammation and quicker healing, carries the same FDA guidelines. The American Academy of Ophthalmology (AAO), however, categorized most of the aforementioned systemic conditions as relative contraindications, if well controlled and only uncontrolled conditions as absolute systemic contraindications. Moreover, systemic disease as a contraindication for refractive surgery has been supported only by reports of isolated cases, small series and animal studies, each with differing conclusions. Little literature can be found on contraindications or complications with newer procedures like LASEK. Most physicians, nevertheless, err on the side of caution and continue to exclude patients with these systemic diseases even if well controlled. Positive outcomes in keratorefractive surgery require careful examination and preparation on the part of the surgeon and a comprehensive understanding of several mitigating ocular and systemic disease factors. Although many conditions may be relative or absolute contraindications for keratorefractive surgery, most procedures can still be performed effectively and safely in selected patients.[1] Those patients not qualifying for keratorefractive surgery may be candidates for other refractive procedures such as specialty intraocular lenses (IOLs).

Today's refractive surgeon must have an understanding of the different refractive procedures and their risks and benefits as part of a more comprehensive approach to the surgical correction of refractive errors. This includes proficiency in both keratorefractive and intraocular lens implant surgery. Preoperative considerations for refractive surgery are predicated upon physical findings in the preoperative examination and patient's expectations.

## ▶ SELECTING THE RIGHT KERATOREFRACTIVE PROCEDURE

Radial keratectomy (RK) has been a surgical procedure that corrects myopia by making radial incisions in the peripheral cornea. Another surgical procedure that corrects myopia is intrastromal rings or INTACS, which are placed in the stromal layer of the midperipheral cornea to flatten the central cornea. Both surgical procedures have limitations in the amount of myopia that can be corrected and long-term stability. Other technology for correction of myopia uses the excimer laser to ablate the central cornea leading to flattening of the corneal curvature. Laser *in situ* keratomileusis (LASIK) surgery, creates a flap of epithelium and anterior stroma prior to laser ablation. In laser-assisted surface epithelial keratectomy (LASEK), an epithelium-only flap is created before ablation is performed and replaced afterwards to decrease pain and improve healing. In PRK, the epithelium is debrided completely and the surface reepithelializes on its own after laser surgery. Because healing in PRK, and to a lesser degree LASEK, is generally delayed, postoperative discomfort may be significant and visual recovery may be delayed. Because theoretically a 250 micron residual stromal bed must remain after the procedure, for safety and reduced risk of ectasia, PRK and LASEK are generally reserved for patients who do not have enough corneal tissue for the creation of a flap or those with irregular or loose surface epithelium who are at risk of epithelial slides, flap irregularity or high-risk of flap dislocation associated with LASIK. Moreover, PRK may prove beneficial to those who cannot tolerate elevated intraocular pressures induced during LASIK, i.e. those at risk of retinal detachments or advanced glaucoma (Table 2).

Alternatively, correction of hyperopia requires steepening of the cornea with surgery or laser. When the cornea is steepened, the eye becomes less hyperopic. Conductive keratoplasty uses radiotherapy to temporarily shrink the peripheral stromal collagen at several evenly spaced radial spots in the mid peripheral cornea, causing a flattening of peripheral and steepening of central cornea to induce myopia. No tissue is removed in conductive keratoplasty. LASIK corrects hyperopia by ablating the peripheral cornea into a ring pattern causing a relative steepening of central cornea.

## ▶ SYSTEMIC CONSIDERATIONS

### Diabetes Mellitus

Patient with diabetes mellitus are at increased risk for complications after keratorefractive surgery including glaucoma, impaired corneal healing, iris neovascularization, cataracts and neuropathies.[2,3] In patients with elevated HbA1c levels, precautions should be taken before surgery in order to minimize systemic morbidity such as cerebrovascular or cardiac events. Tear film break-up time testing and Schirmer's test values have been shown to be significantly lower in diabetic patients as compared to controls.[4] In addition to poor tear film, the most significant consideration in diabetic patients is a greater risk of poor wound healing due to increased corneal epithelial fragility and decreased epithelial function.[5] Studies have suggested that matrix metalloproteinases in diabetic patients are overactive and may be responsible for the poor corneal wound healing.[6] Corneal sensitivity is also greatly impaired in diabetics due to the neuropathic effects of the disease, which can result in neurotrophic keratitis with corneal ulceration.[7]

### Hormonal Fluctuations

The cornea is sensitive to hormonal changes, in particular estrogen. The corneal thickness can vary during the menstrual cycle. The central corneal thickness is found to be the most susceptible, changing significantly throughout different stages of the menstrual cycle. Estrogen receptors found on human corneas can cause corneal thickness variations that may result in incorrect ablation calculations and keratectasia, a serious potential complication of refractive surgery.[8] In pregnancy, estrogen is upregulated by a factor of 20 but the change is counteracted by the upregulation of progesterone. This phenomenon is important in differentiating the risk which may present for pregnant women as opposed to the risk experienced by women on hormone replacement therapy. The corneal instability occurring as a result of unopposed estrogen is much greater than increased estrogen accompanied by increased progesterone.

**Table 1:** FDA contraindications and precautions for keratorefractive surgery

*Absolute Contraindications (Not recommended to have surgery)*

- Pregnant or nursing
- Diseases that affect the body from healing collagen vascular disease (e.g. rheumatoid arthritis), autoimmune diseases (e.g. lupus), immunodeficiency diseases (e.g. AIDS)
- Corneal ectasia/degeneration (i.e. keratoconus or any other condition that causes a thinning of cornea)
- Medications with ocular side effects, e.g. Isotretinoin (Accutane®[1][1]), Amiodarone hydrochloride (Cordarone®[2][2])

*Relative Contraindications (Can have keratorefractive surgery if condition is treated and stabilized)*

- Diabetes
- Herpes simplex or herpes zoster ocular infection that has affected your eyes
- Dry eye syndrome
- Severe allergies
- Blepharitis

*Uncertain Contraindications (Precaution should be taken due to uncertain outcomes with these conditions)*

- Large pupils
- Corneal disease or abnormality
    - Corneal dystrophy
    - H/O corneal scar from infection or inflammatory condition
- History of uveitis/iritis of the eye
- Corneas are too thin
- History of glaucoma or have had IOP greater than 23 mm Hg
- Taking medicines that may affect wound healing
- Younger than 18 years of age or over 65 years of age, because it is unknown whether LASIK is safe and effective for this age group
- Unstable eyes that have changed in their visual acuity more than 0.5 diopters in nearsightedness or astigmatism in the last 12 months
- Nearsightedness worse than XX Diopters (depending on FDA approved device) or astigmatism worse than XX Diopters (depending on FDA approved device)
- History of injury or surgery to the center of the cornea (e.g. previous RK, PRK, LASIK or other surgery on the eye)

Proinflammatory cytokines and matrix metalloproteinases may play a role in estrogen-induced corneal instability after corneal refractive surgery, and therefore precautions should be taken when dealing with patients with high levels of unopposed estrogen.[9] Furthermore, changes in retinal thickness may be present during pregnancy and during breastfeeding, which can alter the effective axial length of the eye and affect the refractive state of the eye. Pregnant women are advised to wait 6 months after delivering their baby and 3 months after nursing before considering keratorefractive surgery.

## HIV/Immunocompromised Patients

Immunocompromised patients are at a higher risk of developing postoperative infections and thus immunocompromised status is a relative contraindication for refractive surgery. HIV and immunosuppressed patients are not excluded from receiving elective surgery, like cataract surgery, when their white blood cell count or CD4 levels are sufficient. Therefore, with sufficient cell counts, such patients can also selectively receive refractive surgery. Regardless, infection can still occur and patients must be followed closely.[10]

## Autoimmune Conditions

Autoimmune conditions, such as rheumatoid arthritis, Sjögren's disease, Lupus, Behcet's disease, Reiter's disease, ankylosing spondylitis and inflammatory bowel diseases, are responsible for a spectrum of inflammatory responses in the eye from dry eye syndrome to keratitis and uveitis.[11,12] Neutrophils and CD4+ T helper (Th1) cells are upregulated in the eye after keratorefractive surgery and can cause inflammation and impaired healing. Patients with autoimmune diseases undergoing LASIK may be at risk for an exaggerated postoperative inflammatory response. This may present as interface haze and inflammation after LASIK, called diffuse lamellar keratitis (DLK), or in the form of corneal melts and stromal scarring after PRK. Patients with severe atopy are also at risk of developing DLK and should be treated systemically prior to keratorefractive surgery.[13,14]

## Keloid Formation

Individuals who are prone to keloid formation and hypertrophic scars are classified by the Food and Drug Administration as contraindicated to have excimer PRK surgery due to the potential risk for corneal scarring.[15] In keloids, excessive amounts of collagen deposit in tissues undergoing postsurgical or traumatic repair. Despite this risk, several studies have proven keratorefractive surgery, namely PRK, LASIK, and EpiLASEK, to be safe and effective in dermatologic keloid patients.[16,17,18]

## Psoriasis

Psoriasis is a cutaneous autoimmune condition with recurrent flare-ups of inflammatory plaques on the skin, mediated by a T-cell response. Psoriasis can manifest in the eye as punctate keratitis, episcleritis, nonspecific conjunctivitis or uveitis. Despite the few case reports on onset of psoriatic epithelial keratitis after LASIK, it seems to be a relatively safe condition to receive refractive surgery.[19] However one must not treat with excimer during an active episode, or "flare-up," of psoriasis.

## ▶ OCULAR CONSIDERATIONS

## Refractive Stability

It is recommended that patients should be at least of 18 years age. Refraction should be stable (equal or less than .50 diopters) over a period of one year. Patients wearing soft or rigid contact lenses should discontinue their lenses for 3 weeks prior to refractive surgery evaluation for accurate refraction and surgical planning.[20] If these criteria are not met, it is advised for the patient to be rechecked at a later date until stability is achieved.

## Refractive Error and Corneal Curvature Limitations

Depending upon the manufacturer of the ophthalmic excimer laser, myopia and hyperopia and astigmatism can be corrected up to a certain degree, corneal thickness permitting. Patients with particularly high refractive errors may not be candidates for laser-based keratorefractive

surgery due to an insufficient amount of corneal tissue. Also PRK, or LASIK and its variants should not be done if the resulting postoperative cornea would end up flatter than 36 diopters or steeper than 50 diopters (Fig. 1). These extremes create optical aberrations that most people cannot tolerate. Therefore, the preoperative K's and the planned treatment can be used to estimate the postoperative K's. These patients may be more suited to receiving refractive IOLs or toric IOLs alone or in combination with LASIK or PRK for residual refractive errors.

## Orbital Anatomy

Anatomic variations, like deep-set eyes, small palpebral fissures or tight eyelids, can create significant resistance and the inability to fit a microkeratome ring or femtosecond laser vacuum ring on the surface of the eye. This can cause inadequate vacuum suction of the keratome ring and can lead to an incomplete or irregular flap. A lateral canthotomy can be performed in the case of tight palpebral fissures to allow the microkeratome to fit for LASIK. These patients may benefit from PRK or LASEK instead. Prominent forehead and brows can be compensated for by tipping the forehead back and chin up while having the patient fixate on the target, changing the plane of the prominent brow.

## Phorias/Tropias

Mild phorias and tropias should not pose a risk to final outcome in keratorefractive surgery. With older excimer lasers, a patient's inability to fixate with a non-dominant or amblyopic eye often lead to decentered ablations and visual compromise. Current technology with pupil tracking software uses corneal vertex and center of pupil targets to help control ablation in an eye that loses fixation. Tracker systems do, however, depend on stability of the pupil during treatment and may lose tracking in eyes with varying pupil size. Additionally, it may be wise to perform a contact lens trial to make certain that the patient can tolerate the correction on the corneal plane without diplopia. Regardless, some surgeons regard any strabismus or phoria as a contraindication to laser-based refractive surgery.

## Large Pupils

Patients with large pupils are at risk of postoperative night time visual disturbances like glare, haloes and blurry vision. Although pupil size is linearly correlated with age,

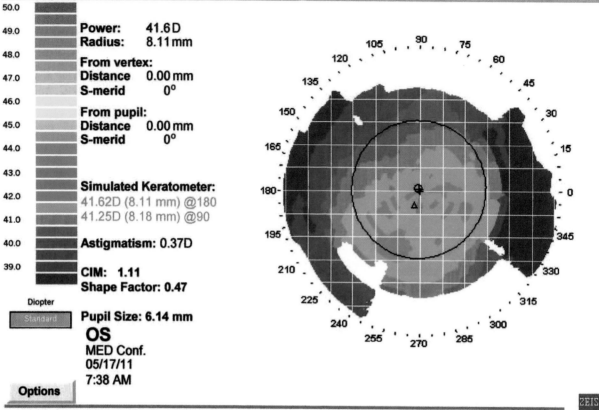

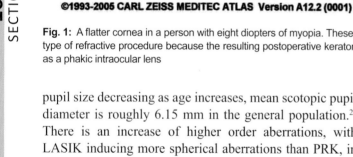

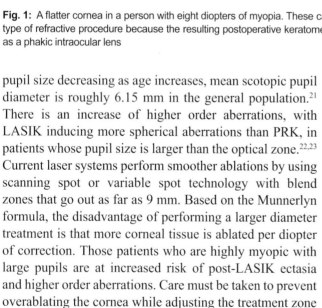

**Patient:**

# Axial Map

| Diopter | |
|---|---|
| 50.0 | |
| 49.0 | **Power:** 41.6 D |
| | **Radius:** 8.11 mm |
| 48.0 | |
| 47.0 | **From vertex:** |
| | **Distance** 0.00 mm |
| 46.0 | **S-merid** 0° |
| 45.0 | **From pupil:** |
| | **Distance** 0.00 mm |
| 44.0 | **S-merid** 0° |
| 43.0 | |
| 42.0 | **Simulated Keratometer:** |
| | 41.62D (8.11 mm) @180 |
| 41.0 | 41.25D (8.18 mm) @90 |
| 40.0 | **Astigmatism: 0.37D** |
| 39.0 | **CIM: 1.11** |
| | **Shape Factor: 0.47** |

Standard

**Pupil Size: 6.14 mm**

# OS
MED Conf.
05/17/11
7:38 AM

Options

ZEISS

©1993-2005 CARL ZEISS MEDITEC ATLAS  Version A12.2 (0001)          **Extrapolated 1 mm**

**Fig. 1:**  A flatter cornea in a person with eight diopters of myopia. These cases are rare but do occur. This person should not have a cornea flattening type of refractive procedure because the resulting postoperative keratometry will be too flat. Appropriate refractive surgery may include options such as a phakic intraocular lens

pupil size decreasing as age increases, mean scotopic pupil diameter is roughly 6.15 mm in the general population.[21] There is an increase of higher order aberrations, with LASIK inducing more spherical aberrations than PRK, in patients whose pupil size is larger than the optical zone.[22,23] Current laser systems perform smoother ablations by using scanning spot or variable spot technology with blend zones that go out as far as 9 mm. Based on the Munnerlyn formula, the disadvantage of performing a larger diameter treatment is that more corneal tissue is ablated per diopter of correction. Those patients who are highly myopic with large pupils are at increased risk of post-LASIK ectasia and higher order aberrations. Care must be taken to prevent overablating the cornea while adjusting the treatment zone in accordance to pupil diameter.

## Herpes Simplex Virus/Corneal Scars

Patients with known history of herpes simplex virus (HSV) keratitis or corneal scars of uncertain etiology can be at risk of reactivation of HSV with excimer laser or any ocular surgery. In case reports, LASIK has proven to be safe patients with a history of ocular herpes; without recurrences during the follow-up period. However, candidates should be selected with caution and surgery performed only in eyes in which the herpes has been inactive for one year before surgery, without stromal disease, and with regular topography and pachymetry maps and normal corneal sensitivity. Patients must be treated prophylactically with antiviral medications prior to and after ocular surgery, and particularly prior to keratorefractive surgery.[24]

## Blepharitis and Rosacea

Patients with evidence of blepharitis are at a higher risk of infectious and inflammatory keratitis after LASIK and PRK. Chronic blepharitis and meibomian gland dysfunction may trigger inflammation resulting in sporadic cases of catarrhal infiltrates after LASIK and diffuse lamellar keratitis.[25] Sterile peripheral infiltrates have been described under the LASIK flap, similar to marginal keratitis.

Rosacea is a skin condition, characterized by telangiectasia and course skin. Rosacea patients also suffer from blepharitis, itchy eyelids and dry eyes, and are not optimal patients for refractive surgery; although with local treatment may pursue surgery. Treatment for postoperative infection may involve lifting the flap, culturing, the use of topical steroids and/or antibiotics (refer chapter 97 LASIK complication: Etiology, Prevention and Management). To date, the most common isolated organisms from infectious keratitis after LASIK are *Staphylococcus* species and *Mycobacterium* species. Many times sources cannot be identified. Patients with significant blepharitis, nonetheless, should be instructed on lid hygiene and prophylactic use of antibiotic drops and topical steroid treatment days prior to the procedure to reduce bacterial load and toxin related inflammation.

## Dry Eyes

All candidates for refractive surgery should be screened for preexisting dry eyes. Dry eye is the most common complaint after keratorefractive surgery. It is associated with irritation, photophobia, burning, and blurred vision.[26] Women tend to be affected more than men because of hormonal changes that accompany pregnancy, menstruation and menopause, and lead to decreased tear production. Dry eye is also prevalent in men, and increases with age, hypertension, BPH and antidepressant use.[27]

The tearing reflex pathway can be disrupted in both PRK and LASIK. In LASIK, when a corneal hinged flap is cut or when corneal tissue is ablated, superficial corneal nerve damage occurs that leads to a decreased afferent signal from the cornea and decreased efferent signaling sent towards tear producing glands in the eyes.[28] Corneal sensation often returns to near normal function regardless of the method of keratorefractive surgery, many times much earlier than the actual regeneration of nerve fibers.[29,30] Dry eyes and decreased corneal sensation can remain a long-term complication after keratorefractive surgery.

## Corneal Dystrophies

Corneal dystrophies can present before or after refractive surgery and may be a major obstacle to proper healing and clarity of the cornea. Corneal dystrophy involvement spans from the anterior basement membrane to the endothelium. In anterior basement membrane dystrophy, the main pathological feature of the disease is the basement membrane which becomes thick and irregular. Slit lamp exam will reveal an irregular pattern of cysts, ridges, and whirls within this layer. These patients are at risk of developing an epithelial slide, an irregular flap cut, or irregular astigmatism during flap creation with an automated keratome in LASIK surgery.[31] Such patients should be considered as candidates for femtosecond excimer flap creation or PRK which doesn't require the automated microkeratome. In fact, PRK ablation through basement membrane may help to decrease recurrent erosion occurrence by stimulating the formation of new basement membrane which may have better adhesion to epithelial cells.

Stromal dystrophies like Avellino or granular dystrophy can often recur or worsen with corneal surgery. Case reports have shown a recurrence or increase of deposits under the LASIK flap up to months after keratorefractive surgery causing worsening of glare symptoms.[32,33,34,35] For this reason, LASIK surgery is not recommended on patients with such dystrophies.

In patients with Fuchs endothelial corneal dystrophy, extracellular deposits in the corneal endothelium, called guttatae, and endothelial cell loss give rise to symptoms of glare and blurred vision. These patients should receive particular attention because any type of refractive surgery can accelerate endothelial loss resulting in an increase in corneal edema and worsening of symptoms.[36,37] Moreover, preoperative fluctuations in corneal thickness due to swelling in the stroma can lead to inaccurate target calculations and imprecise outcomes with excimer laser.

## Corneal Ectasia

Keratoconus causes progressive corneal ectasia with instability of refraction and visual acuity. Keratoconus generally presents after puberty and progresses over many years before finally stabilizing. Figure 2 demonstrates a corneal topographic map of a patient with keratoconus. It can lead to symptoms of ghosting, distortions and glare. It is a major contraindication to keratorefractive surgery which can further the progression of this disease and worsen

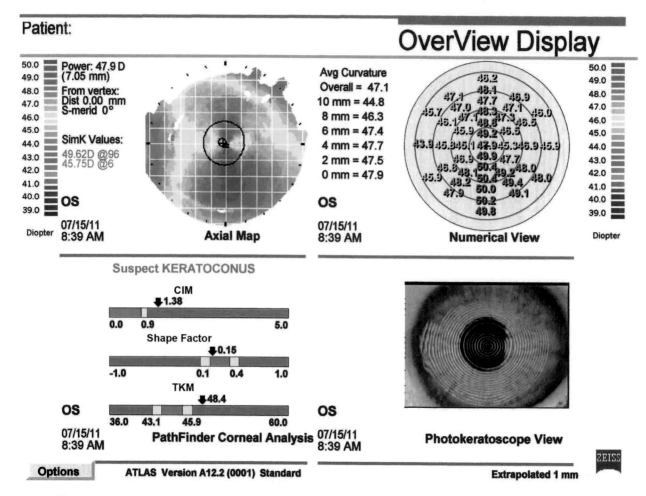

**Fig. 2:** An example of the corneal topographic map of a cornea with keratoconus. Notice that the software says 'suspect' but there is no doubt that this is keratoconus. Do not exclusively rely upon the software for a diagnosis or analysis

symptoms.[38] Forme fruste keratoconus is a very mild form of keratoconus that can present at any time throughout life. This form of keratoconus may often go undetected due to the absence of clinical symptoms. On topographical study, diagnostic signs, such as asymmetrical inferior corneal steepening and/or asymmetrical bowtie topographic patterns with skewed steep radial axes above and below the horizontal meridian, are highly indicative of increased risk for progression to keratoconus and ectasia post-LASIK. Patients that exhibit these signs preoperatively should avoid keratorefractive surgery.

Corneal pellucid marginal degeneration is also a major contributor to high astigmatism and irregular astigmatism. This condition occurs when the lower cornea becomes thinner and the optic surface of the cornea becomes irregular. Patients with inferior crab claw pattern on topography accompanied by central flattening are at risk

for the development of pellucid marginal degeneration. Corneal ectasia can be avoided by properly screening for conditions such as these preoperatively. Other factors which may result in corneal ectasia are high myopia, low residual stromal bed thickness from excessive ablation or thick flap creation and collagen disorders.

## Corneal Warpage

Corneal warpage may be induced by long-term use of contact lenses. Changes associated with contact lens wear include corneal curvature and thickness alterations. Although corneal warpage may occur in a significant amount of patients who wear contact lenses, it is important to note that most of the warpage is temporary. The time required for the cornea to stabilize varies for each patient. Warpage may also mimic keratoconus on topographic and pachymetric study.[39] Extra precautions should be taken in contact lens users during preoperative examination of the cornea due to transient changes in corneal topography induced by the contact lens. Prior to refractive surgery, patients should discontinue contact lens wear and corneal topography should be examined regularly until corneal warpage has resolved.

## Retinal Holes or Myopic Degeneration

Degenerative myopia is characterized by marked fundus changes, generalized scleral thinning, an abnormal vitreo-retinal border interface, and decreased ocular rigidity creating a posterior staphyloma. The increased axial length induced and posterior vitreous separation induced by surgery can adversely affect an already thinned and atrophic retina. In one study, axial length increased after application of the suction ring, whereas anterior chamber depth showed no significant difference, suggesting the anterior movement of the vitreous base may be causing traction of the anterior retina.[40] This type of anterior displacement may predispose already susceptible eyes to possible anterior retinal tears after LASIK.[41] Candidates with any preexisting retinal pathology, including the retinal changes associated with myopic degeneration, should be evaluated by a retinal surgeon. These patients may benefit from prophylactic laser or other appropriate retinal therapy. Myopes with retinal findings who choose to undergo keratorefractive surgery, may benefit from the use of modalities, such as PRK or LASEK, that do not increase pressure on the eye leading to pathological vitreous disinsertion.

## Glaucoma

Corneal ablation of approximately 90 microns reduces Goldmann applanation tonometry readings by 3.0 mm Hg after LASIK surgery.[42,43] Several published reports have confirmed that postoperative intraocular pressure (IOP) readings after corneal refractive surgery for myopia as well as hyperopia are reduced with Goldman applanation tomnometry[43-45] This may be due to the fact that Goldmann applanation tonometry overestimates IOP in patients with thicker corneas and underestimates it in those with thinner corneas. The reduced IOP after excimer laser refractive surgery is considered to be a false low reading by Goldmann applanation tonometry due to a thinner post operative cornea rather than a real decrease in IOP. In contrast to Goldmann applanation tonometry, contact pneumotonometry measures the IOP more reliably after laser *in situ* keratomileusis.[45]

Patients who are glaucoma suspects must have a complete baseline examination performed before LASIK. Postoperatively pachymetry must be performed by ultrasound and the nomogram adjusted for IOP measurement.[46] Failure to detect appropriate IOP in the postoperative period can lead to severe vision loss. IOP rise in the postoperative period may lead to interface fluid accumulation which also can falsely underestimate IOP measurement and miss or misdiagnose acute steroid response glaucomatous changes.[47] It must also be remembered that the microkeratome and femtosecond vacuum rings increase the intraocular pressure. Patients with fragile optic nerves or more advanced glaucoma may be better served by PRK, which does not increased IOP.

## Cataracts

Patients with cataracts were traditionally advised against keratorefractive surgery due to the difficulty in accurately calculating IOL power once the corneal contour had been altered. With time, better mathematical formulas have been developed to achieve more precise calculations for the selection of lens implants after keratorefractive surgery. Because of this, early nuclear sclerotic cataracts are no longer a contraindication for keratorefractive surgery. Patients with more advanced cataracts that are visually significant should be considered for presbyopic, accommodating, or toric IOLs depending on their refractive errors and personal preference. Usually these patients will be middle or upper age, presbyopic and may have a significant amount of lenticular and corneal astigmatism.

| Table 2: Preoperative factors favoring PRK or LASEK over LASIK |
|---|
| • Narrow palpebral fissures |
| • Deep set eyes/high brow |
| • Irregular conjunctival surface or pinguecula |
| • Corneal vascularization or pterygium |
| • Anterior basement membrane corneal dystrophy or history of recurrent erosions |
| • Thin corneas or high refractive error |
| • Certain cases of extreme irregular topography |
| • Excessively steep or flat corneas |
| • Large pupils |
| • H/O retinal holes or tears |
| • Certain cases of advanced glaucoma |

CHAPTER 93

# ❧ REFRACTIVE INTRAOCULAR LENSES

For nonconventional keratorefractive surgery patients or those who are limited by anatomical considerations, refractive IOLs may be an option (Table 3). The advantage of refractive IOLs over keratorefractive surgery is the ability to improve near vision in addition to distance vision, and the ability to correct large refractive errors and high astigmatism. This procedure can then be combined with corneal procedures like limbal relaxing incisions and or PRK/LASIK surgery for residual astigmatism or refractive errors.

For early cataract patients, monofocal lens implants provide permanent improvement in distance visual acuity by correcting hyperopia and myopia. Presbyopia was often corrected with the monovision method, which places one lens for distance correction in the dominant eye, and one lens for near correction in the nondominant eye. Although the monofocal system provides patients with some independence from glasses, most patients lose depth of perception and still require glasses for distance and near for more demanding tasks like driving or reading small print.

Multifocal IOLs can correct myopia or hyperopia for distance vision and provide several diopters of accommodation for intermediate and near vision by allowing light to meet at multiple focal points favorable to near vision, either by diffraction, refraction or anterior movement of lens. Patients, however, should be carefully selected to receive these lenses. Those with macular disease or glaucoma should be excluded. Those with high expectations, or who are happy with reading glasses, would not be good candidates for these lenses. Also, any tear in capsulorhexis or the use of sulcus fixation of lens during surgery would exclude these patients from receiving this lens due to the risk of decentration and monocular diplopia and ghosting/glare. Several specialty IOL designs exist, each with their limitations and each requiring careful patient selection and education. Pupil size can affect vision with diffractive type IOLs. Myopes may not benefit from multifocal lenses as much as hyperopes in that they may lose some accommodative capacity after receiving the lens. Regardless of proper centration of the lens, most patients will experience glare or haloes at night, and this may be particularly difficult for patients sensitive to

these symptoms or who depend on night driving for their livelihood. Although there is a longer adaption period compared to monofocal lenses, patients experiencing ghosting and haloes usually do neuroadapt over time.

Uncorrected astigmatism with multifocal lens surgery can lead to distance blur and glare/ghosting postoperatively and failure to perceive an improvement in uncorrected vision from the multifocal lens implant. Residual astigmatism can be corrected by limbal relaxing incisions at the time of cataract surgery for up to 2 diopters of astigmatism. However, limbal relaxing incisions carry the risk of a neurotrophic cornea and associated dry eye and epithelial problems. The estimated correction is not exact and many times loses its effect over time. Toric lens calculations however are very accurate, stable and predictable and can treat larger amounts of diopters of astigmatism. Greater than 0.75 diopters of astigmatism seen preoperatively should be considered for receiving a toric IOL. Future specialty lenses will likely include the combination multifocal toric lens.

With a spectrum of keratorefractive and refractive procedures, it is important for today's refractive surgeon to do a careful preoperative assessment of the patient's ocular and systemic health and their expectations, in order to provide the most appropriate treatment regimen for each individual. For patients who do not qualify for keratorefractive surgery, other options can be considered, such as the specialty IOL. Doing so would provide each patient a truly custom surgical experience, with maximized safety and superior outcome.

---

**Table 3:** Preoperative factors favoring refractive IOLs

- Patient's desire to correct presbyopia
  (multifocal or accomodating presbyopic IOLs)
- High astigmatism beyond excimer limits (Toric IOL)
- High myopia or high hyperopia beyond excimer limits
- Relatively thin corneas
- Irregular corneal surface, history of corneal scar or infection, in some cases, may be better with an IO
- When corneal surgery is contraindicated (i.e. keratoconus, corneal dystrophy, corneal degeneration, large pupils, systemic disease, etc.)
- When the resulting cornea after keratorefractive surgery would be flatter than 36 diopters or steeper than 50 diopters

# ❧ REFERENCES

1. Cobo-Soriano R, Beltrán J, Baviera J. LASIK outcomes in patients with underlying systemic contraindications: a preliminary study. Ophthalmology. 2006;113(7):1118.e1-8.

2. Ghanbari H, Ahmadieh H. Aggravation of proliferative diabetic retinopathy after laser *in situ* keratomileusis. J Cataract Refract Surg. 2003;29(11):2232-3.

3. Fraunfelder FW, Rich LF. Laser-assisted *in situ* keratomileusis complications in diabetes mellitus. Cornea. 2002;21(3):246-8.

4. Dogru M, Katakami C, Inoue M. Tear function and ocular surface changes in noninsulin-dependent diabetes mellitus. Ophthalmology. 2001;108(3):586-92.

5. Ozdemir M, Buyukbese MA, Cetinkaya A, et al. Risk factors for ocular surface disorders in patients with diabetes mellitus. Diabetes Res Clin Pract. 2003;59(3):195-9.

6. Takahashi H, Akiba K, Noguchi T, et al. Matrix metalloproteinase activity is enhanced during corneal wound repair in high glucose condition. Curr Eye Res. 2000;21(2):608-15.

7. Midena E, Brugin E, Ghirlando A, et al. Corneal diabetic neuropathy: a confocal microscopy study. J Refract Surg. 2006;22(9 Suppl):S1047-52.

8. Spoerl E, Zubaty V, Raiskup-Wolf F, et al. Oestrogen-induced changes in biomechanics in the cornea as a possible reason for keratectasia. Br J Ophthalmol. 2007;91(11):1547-50.

9. Suzuki T, Sullivan DA. Estrogen stimulation of proinflammatory cytokine and matrix metalloproteinase gene expression in human corneal epithelial cells. Cornea. 2005;24:1004-9.

10. Hovanesian JA, Faktorovich EG, Hoffbauer JD, et al. Bilateral bacterial keratitis after laser *in situ* keratomileusis in a patient with human immunodeficiency virus infection. Arch Ophthalmol. 1999;117(7):968-70.

11. Cua IY, Pepose JS. Late corneal scarring after photorefractive keratectomy concurrent with development of systemic lupus erythematosus. J Refract Surg. 2002;18(6):750-2.

12. Díaz-Valle D, Arriola-Villalobos P, Sánchez JM, et al. Late-onset severe diffuse lamellar keratitis associated with uveitis after LASIK in a patient with ankylosing spondylitis. J Refract Surg. 2009;25(7):623-5.

13. Boorstein SM, Henk HJ, Elner VM. Atopy: a patient-specific risk factor for diffuse lamellar keratitis. Ophthalmology. 2003;110(1):131-7.

14. Myrowitz EH. Laser-assisted intrastromal keratomileusis in a patient with systemic mastocytosis. Optometry. 2008;79(2):95-7.

15. Girgis R, Morris DS, Kotagiri A, Ramaesh K. Bilateral corneal scarring after LASIK and PRK in a patient with propensity to keloid scar. Eye (Lond). 2007;21(1):96-7.

16. Tanzer DJ, Isfahani A, Schallhorn SC, et al. Photorefractive keratectomy in African Americans including those with known dermatologic keloid formation. Am J Ophthalmol. 1998;126(5):625-9.

17. Artola A, Gala A, Belda JI, et al. LASIK in myopic patients with dermatological keloids. J Refract Surg. 2006;22(5):505-8.

18. Lee JY, Youm DJ, Choi CY. Conventional Epi-LASIK and lamellar epithelial debridement in myopic patients with dermatologic keloids. Korean J Ophthalmol. 2011;25(3):206-9.

19. Rodriguez-Prats JL, Morbelli H, Rodriguez-Chan JM, et al. Psoriatic intraepithelial keratitis after laser *in situ* keratomileusis treatment. J Cataract Refract Surg. 2011;37(1):194-7.

20. Tsai PS, Dowidar A, Naseri A, et al. Predicting time to refractive stability after discontinuation of rigid contact lens wear before refractive surgery. J Cataract Refract Surg. 2004;30(11):2290-4.

21. Oshika T, Klyce SD, Applegate RA, et al. Comparison of corneal wavefront aberrations after photorefractive keratectomy and laser *in situ* keratomileusis. Am J Ophthalmol. 1999;127(1):1-7.

22. Bühren J, Kühne C, Kohnen T. Influence of pupil and optical zone diameter on higher-order aberrations after wavefront-guided myopic LASIK. J Cataract Refract Surg. 2005;31(12):2272-80.

23. De Rojas Silva V, Rodríguez-Conde R, Cobo-Soriano R, et al. Laser *in situ* keratomileusis in patients with a history of ocular herpes. J Cataract Refract Surg. 2007;33(11):1855-9.

24. Ambrósio R, Periman LM, Netto MV, et al. Bilateral marginal sterile infiltrates and diffuse lamellar keratitis after laser *in situ* keratomileusis. J Refract Surg. 2003;19(2):154-8.

25. De Paiva CS, Chen Z, Koch DD, et al. The incidence and risk factors for developing dry eye after myopic LASIK. Am J Ophthalmol. 2006;141(3):438-45.

26. Schaumberg DA, Dana R, Buring JE, et al. Prevalence of dry eye disease among US men: Estimates from the Physicians' Health Studies. Arch Ophthalmol. 2009;127(6):763-8.

27. Donnenfeld ED, Solomon K, Perry HD, et al. The effect of hinge position on corneal sensation and dry eye after LASIK. Ophthalmology. 2003;110(5):1023-9; discussion 1029-30.

28. Patel SV, McLaren JW, Kittleson KM, et al. Subbasal nerve density and corneal sensitivity after laser *in situ* keratomileusis: femtosecond laser vs mechanical microkeratome. Arch Ophthalmol. 2010;128(11):1413-9.

29. Stachs O, Zhivov A, Kraak R, et al. Structural-functional correlations of corneal innervation after LASIK and penetrating keratoplasty. J Refract Surg. 2010;26(3):159-67.

30. Pérez-Santonja JJ, Galal A, et al. Severe corneal epithelial sloughing during laser *in situ* keratomileusis as a presenting sign for silent epithelial basement membrane dystrophy. J Cataract Refract Surg. 2005;31(10):1932-7.

31. Awwad ST, Di Pascuale MA, Hogan RN, et al. Avellino corneal dystrophy worsening after laser *in situ* keratomileusis: further clinicopathologic observations and proposed pathogenesis. Am J Ophthalmol. 2008;145(4):656-61. Epub 2008 Feb 19.

32. Lee WB, Himmel KS, Hamilton SM, et al. Excimer laser exacerbation of Avellino corneal dystrophy. J Cataract Refract Surg. 2007;33(1):133-8.

33. Banning CS, Kim WC, Randleman JB, et al. Exacerbation of Avellino corneal dystrophy after LASIK in North America. Cornea. 2006;25(4):482-4.

34. Kim TI, Kim T, Kim SW, et al. Comparison of corneal deposits after LASIK and PRK in eyes with granular corneal dystrophy type II. J Refract Surg. 2008;24(4):392-5.

35. Vroman DT, Solomon KD, Holzer MP, et al. Endothelial decompensation after laser in situ keratomileusis. J Cataract Refract Surg. 2002;28(11):2045-9.

36. Dastjerdi MH, Sugar A. Corneal decompensation after laser *in situ* keratomileusis in Fuchs' endothelial dystrophy. Cornea. 2003;22(4):379-81.

CHAPTER **93**

37. Binder PS, Lindstrom RL, Stulting RD, et al. Keratoconus and corneal ectasia after LASIK. J Cataract Refract Surg. 2005;31:2035-8.

38. Tseng SS-Y, Hsiao JC-J, Chang DC-K. Mistaken diagnosis of keratoconus because of corneal warpage induced by hydrogel lens wear. Cornea. 2007;26:1153-5.

39. Flaxel CJ, Choi YH, Sheety M, et al. Proposed mechanism for retinal tears after LASIK: An experimental model. Ophthalmology. 2004;111(1):24-7.

40. Arevalo JF. Posterior segment complications after laser-assisted *in situ* keratomileusis. Curr Opin Ophthalmology. 2008;19(3):177-84. 43.

41. Agudelo LM, Molina CA, Alvarez DL. Changes in intraocular pressure after laser *in situ* keratomileusis for myopia, hyperopia, and astigmatism. J Refract Surg. 2002;18(4):472-4.

42. Kaufmann C, Bachmann LM, Thiel MA. Intraocular pressure measurements using dynamic contour tonometry after laser in situ keratomileusis. Invest Ophthalmol Vis Sci. 2003;44(9):3790-4.

43. Vakili R, Choudhri SA, Tauber S, et al. Effect of mild to moderate myopic correction by laser-assisted *in situ* keratomileusis on intraocular pressure measurements with goldmann applanation tonometer, tono-pen, and pneumatonometer. J Glaucoma. 2002;11(6):493-6.

44. Duch S, Serra A, Castanera J, et al. Tonometry after laser *in situ* keratomileusis treatment. J Glaucoma. 2001;10(4):261-5.

45. Suzuki S, Oshika T, Oki K, et al. Corneal thickness measurements: scanning-slit corneal topography and noncontact specular microscopy versus ultrasonic pachymetry. J Cataract Refract Surg. 2003;29(7):1313-8.

46. Shaikh NM, Shaikh S, Singh K, et al. Progression to end-stage glaucoma after laser *in situ* keratomileusis. J Cataract Refract Surg. 2002;28(2):356-9.

47. Schnitzler EM, Baumeister M, Kohnen T. Scotopic measurement of normal pupils: Colvard versus Video Vision Analyzer infrared pupillometer. J Cataract Refract Surg. 2000;26(6):859-66.

16 SECTION

# Preoperative Considerations:
# Corneal Topography

*Stephen D Klyce, Edgar M Espana, George O Waring IV*

## ‣ INTRODUCTION

Corneal topography plays a critical role in the evaluation and management of corneal disease and the detection of corneal ectasia. Mastering of corneal topography is indispensable for the practice of refractive surgery where particular attention is given to the early detection of risk factors for development of ectatic corneal disorders and to the corneal changes induced by contact lens wear. Information obtained from corneal topographers not only provides diagnostic information, but also can be linked to the excimer laser for topography-guided ablations.

## ‣ DEVELOPMENT OF THE CORNEAL
## TOPOGRAPHER

Corneal topography is based on the computerized analysis of corneal images obtained using a Placido's disk. The Placido's disk concept has been adapted and is now the most widely used technology in modern corneal topographers. This instrument, originally introduced by Antonio Placido, consists of a circular target of alternating concentric light and dark mires, with a central aperture through which a virtual image reflected from the tear film surface can be obtained for further analysis. Steep surfaces minify the image while flat surfaces magnify it. However, unlike keratometers that assume a spherocylindrical corneal shape and take measurements from only four positions on the anterior corneal surface, approximately 3 or 4 mm apart, topography mires can be projected over a broad area of the cornea, allowing corneal curvature assessment at different positions on large corneal area.

Modern corneal topographers have excellent accuracy and reproducibility in anterior corneal curvature measurement. Corneal topography is the gold standard device to map the corneal surface and curvature. However, limitations of the device include the following: the quality of tear film is critical since the images are reflected from the tear film and in very steep areas of the corneal surface mires can merge and not be tracked leaving blank or interpolated segments. Caveat: it is useful to have a routine benchmark with which to occasionally test a corneal topographer to ensure calibration is being maintained. Optimally, this would involve the measurement of a test surface, particularly if screening reveals an unusual incidence of a particular pattern or artifact.

When corneal transplantation became a more refined surgical procedure, surgeons became aware that astigmatism was the main limitation for visual rehabilitation. Experienced corneal surgeons developed surgical keratoscopes based on the Placido's disk principle that were mounted directly on the operating microscope and were helpful for suture placement and tension adjustment during surgery.[1] Rowsey et al. were pioneers in the development of the photokeratoscope that photographed Placido's disk images projected onto the corneal surface and were captured with an instant film camera.[2] Using this technique, cornea surgeons were able to analyze 70–95% of the total corneal surface including paracentral and peripheral areas. In 1981, Doss et al.[3] scanned corneascope photographs to calculate corneal powers from mire size and the shape of the projected rings. In 1984, Klyce demonstrated a method for reconstructing corneal shape and power by digitizing mires from Nidek photokeratoscope photographs.[4] In this work, graphical plots using three-dimensional wire mesh models were used to depict corneal topography, as condensing the thousands of data points collected from the photokeratoscope photographs was necessary to permit clinical utility. The final graphical presentation form of these data, which has become the international standard, was the color-coded contour map of corneal powers introduced by Maguire et al.[5]

Placido-based anterior corneal topography analysis is the standard of care for preoperative patient screening before keratorefractive surgery. Its importance was underscored by the association of keratoconus and the development of ectasia after laser-assisted *in situ* keratomileusis (LASIK)[6] and photorefractive keratectomy (PRK).[7] Methods to detect moderate keratoconus have been available for sometime and obvious changes in corneal shape and thickness can be detected with corneal topography and pachymetry. However, the subtle corneal anterior surface curvature changes that can accompany keratoconus suspect can escape notice without careful evaluation. It is the purpose of this chapter to assist the clinician in recognizing the earliest signs of keratoconus and the associated stromal degenerative condition—pellucid marginal degeneration (PMD). Both conditions involve stromal thinning and it is the specific pattern of thinning that differentiates the two, but in the 'suspect' earliest phase of both conditions, abnormal thickness changes may not be evident even with the sophisticated multiple slit imaging or Scheimpflug based devices available.

### Myth: Photorefractive Keratectomy is Safe and Effective in Corneas with Abnormal Topography

Before turning to methods to improve recognition of the keratoconus suspect, it is important to dispel the myth that it is safe and effective to manage refractive error of the keratoconus suspect cornea with laser surface ablation as suggested in numerous articles.[8] A review of the literature through 2008 reveals 13 articles in the peer reviewed literature reporting 32 eyes that developed ectasia after laser surface ablation procedures (Fig. 1). With ongoing active research to explore the biomechanics of the cornea, it is clear that corneas that have the keratoconus or PMD defect, have a weakened stromal structure that allows the lamellae to separate and move away from one another in a radial motion (known as lamellar creep) to produce a warping distortion that leads to steepening in one part of the cornea and flattening in another. Smolek et al.[9] contend that the surface area of the cornea in progressive keratoconus remains relatively constant so that the steepening is the

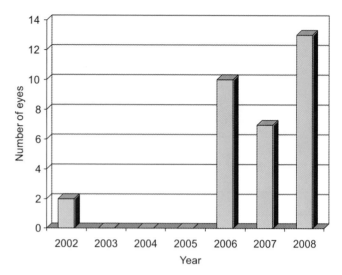

**Fig. 1:** Eyes that developed ectasia after laser surface ablation procedures—literature reports 2002–2008

result of surface warping rather than stretching, at least in the early phases of the disease. Abnormal topography is the primary risk factor for the development of ectasia after laser refractive surgery[10] and this risk remains even for surface ablation procedures. Future advances in biomechanical analytics and diagnostics will enhance the clinician's ability to differentiate corneas at risk for the development of ectasia.

### CORNEAL TOPOGRAPHY DISPLAYS AND SCALES

As corneal topography and tomography devices evolve, most have developed complex displays with large amounts of data, making a practical and clinically relevant analysis tedious. While an expert might understand how to use and analyze all this information easily, much of it is time consuming and irrelevant for routine clinical care. Because each manufacturer justifies the need for the varied representation of the corneal surface offered by his instrument, choosing the best default display is often difficult.

In clinical practice, a display of corneal topography that includes an axial power color-coded contour map alongside familiar measures such as pupil diameter and simulated keratometry should be sufficient (Fig. 2). The color-coded contour map is widely accepted now and is very helpful to conceptualize the corneal contour and shape. The palette of colors uses green for normal corneal curvature, low dioptric corneal curvature are shown in blue and high corneal curvatures are represented in red color. This color-coded contour map display is also helpful for evaluation of the

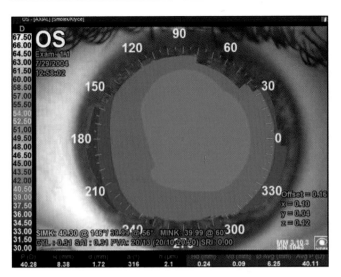

**Fig. 2:** Standard axial map presentation for routine clinical evaluation. K readings, Potential visual acuity (PVA), pupil size and position and average power within the pupil (Avg P) for intraocular lens calculations are given. Eye image underlying the color-coded contour map is essential for orientation

effects of laser ablation on the corneal shape, optical zone size, the centration of the laser ablation and for the recognition of characteristic patterns. For example, corneal cylinder displays as a 'bow tie' pattern, keratoconus as a local area of steepening and PMD with its characteristics of a claw or 'C'-shaped pattern of steepening and 'negative' bow tie (discussed below).

In 1999, the American National Standards Institute (ANSI) released a report dictating the standards in corneal topography development, research and practice.[11] The report, 'Corneal Topography Systems-Standard Terminology, Requirements', defined terminology and requirements for measurement and display of corneal topography and tests for accuracy and precision of corneal topographers. Generally, a 'standard' should define specifics of a measurement. For corneal topography, a single color palette with specific fixed intervals should be defined to facilitate the accurate comparison of data obtained with corneal topographers from different manufacturers. Unfortunately, the early ANSI standard failed to define a single specific scale for curvature maps and instead suggested the use of three different corneal diopter intervals: 0.5 D, 1.0 D or 1.5 D and color palettes with continuously varying hues. It failed to provide a default palette and scale that would be useful in clinical practice. For example, Wilson et al.[12] found an axial map scale with 1.5 D intervals to be adequate to recognize abnormal corneal topography. Maps using dioptric intervals of less than 1 D showed irrelevant details that made it difficult to interpret in the diagnosis of visually significant topographic anomalies.

However, after Smolek et al.[13] proposed a universal standard corneal topography scale, this was adopted in the next revision of the ANSI standard.[14] This scale (used in Figure 2 and in most illustrations in this chapter) combines an axial power map with a color palette of contrasting colors with a 1.5 D interval; this scale can be found on a number of corneal topographers and is suggested to be used as the default scale for routine clinical use. That is not to say that higher resolution scales and alternate methods for displaying corneal curvature should not be used in certain circumstances. For example, using a 0.5 D scale with a tangential (also called 'instantaneous') curvature display is helpful to delineate the optical zone in a keratorefractive surgical procedure.

## CORNEAL TOPOGRAPHER DISPLAYS

### Photokeratoscope View

This view displays the image of the Placido's rings projected on the cornea. It provides important information when assessing the quality of the tear film, image focus, freedom from blink or motion artifact and the accuracy with which the mires are analyzed (Fig. 3). It is good practice to have a quick look at this when taking the examination.

### Axial Map

Also known as the sagittal map, the axial map displays corneal power calculated in the manner used in keratometry, a radius of curvature approach (Fig. 4A). Importantly, corneal topographers are set to report total corneal power using the keratometric index (usually 1.3375). To obtain the corneal anterior surface radius of curvature, $R_C$, from axial power, $P_A$, the relationship $R_C = 1.3375/P_A$ can be used. Hence, the axial radius of curvature for any point on the corneal surface is defined by the radius of a sphere fit to that point and centered on the instrument axis. This is the original and most commonly used map, and has the advantage of presenting a color map of the cornea that shows the periphery of the cornea as being flatter (longer radius of curvature) than the central region.

### Refractive Power Map

While the axial power transition from center to periphery is consistent with shape data, a better estimate of the true surface power variation can be presented with the refractive power map (Fig. 4B). The refractive power map is used in conjunction with a whole eye refraction map produced

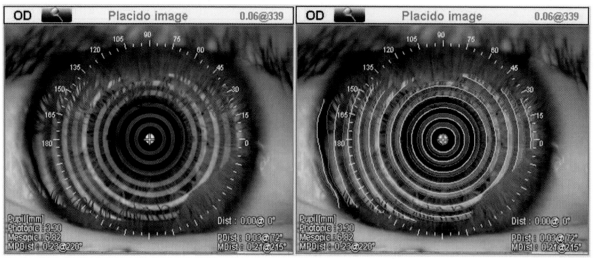

**Fig. 3:** Placido image of the eye (left panel). The margin of each mire is determined by image analysis. Especially on irregular corneas, it is prudent to look for poor tracking which will present as artifact in the color-coded map

by aberrometry to determine separately the corneal surface aberrations as well as the internal aberrations of the eye (Fig. 5). A disadvantage of the refractive power map, when used for screening, is that it can obscure subtle inferior steepening that can accompany keratoconus in its mildest presentation (Figs 6A and B).

## Tangential Power Map

Also known as the instantaneous radius of curvature (IROC) map, the tangential power display shows local changes of curvature (Fig. 4C); tangential maps do not force the center of curvature of the best fitting sphere to align to the instrument axis as does the axial map. This map is very useful in detecting local irregularities, corneal ectatic diseases, or surgically induced changes including boundaries of previous ablation treatments (optical zones).

## Elevation Map

An average cornea may have as much as 250 μm of sagittal depth from the corneal apex to the periphery; as such a direct display of corneal elevation will mask the subtle variations in elevation that produce significant changes in corneal power. Hence, the elevation map displays corneal height or elevation relative to a reference surface, often a best fit sphere or ellipsoid depending on the topographer (Fig. 4D). It is important to note that the elevation display depends on reference surface size, shape, alignment and fitting zone, and also that its colors do not represent curvature in elevation maps, but rather the distance between the

corneal surface and the reference shape. This allows amplification of the surface distortion to be visualized. The elevation data underlying this map contains the surface coordinates of the three-dimensional shape of the cornea and is used to determine the amount of tissue that must be removed by a procedure to achieve a prescribed refractive power change.

## Difference Map

The difference map is used to show changes or differences in time between two topographic maps. For example, subtraction of preoperative and postoperative axial maps are used to show surgically induced changes (Figs 7A to C), while a similar approach can be used to demonstrate stability of a postoperative result such as obtained with corneal crosslinking or the amount of progression of ectasia with keratoconus. Additionally, difference maps are useful to show the course of recovery from contact lens-induced warpage.

## ❯ QUANTITATIVE DESCRIPTORS OF CORNEAL TOPOGRAPHY

Corneal topographers are equipped with algorithms that are designed to analyze corneal topography data and to display specific clinically relevant indices that can be used to assess and to track certain quantitative aspects of corneal topography. The color coded maps are based upon quantitative measurements of the corneal surface curvature, but with these alone, it is nearly impossible to

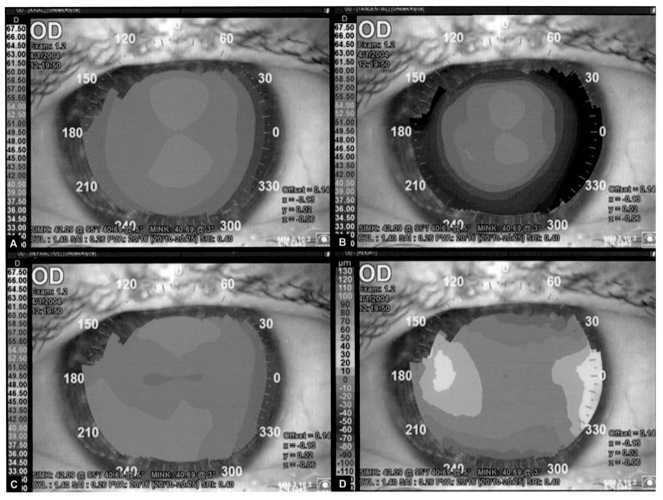

**Figs 4A to D:** Standard corneal topographer color-coded maps all produced from the same single examination. (A) The axial power map is most useful for routine clinical examination; (B) The tangential or instantaneous power map is useful to examine the transition zone after refractive surgery; (C) The refractive power map is used to difference the whole eye refraction map for internal aberrations; (D) Elevation map provides height data to drive laser ablations

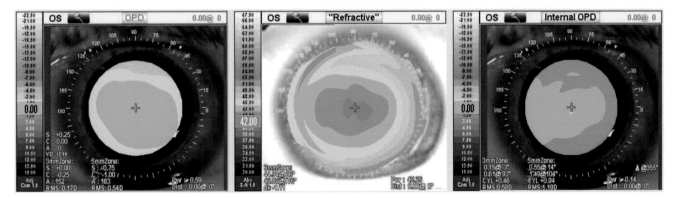

**Fig. 5:** Corneal topography and aberrometry together yield internal aberrations. The NIDEK OPD-Scan III displays the whole eye refraction map (left panel), the refractive power map (center panel), and the difference map (right panel), which shows a radially uniform prolate configuration

CHAPTER **94**

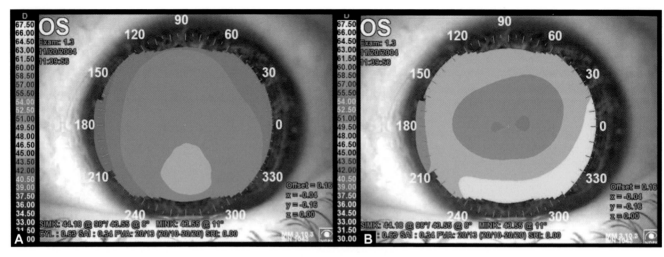

**Figs 6A and B:** Cornea with mild inferior steepening is relatively obscured when using a refractive power map. (A) Axial map; (B) Refractive power map

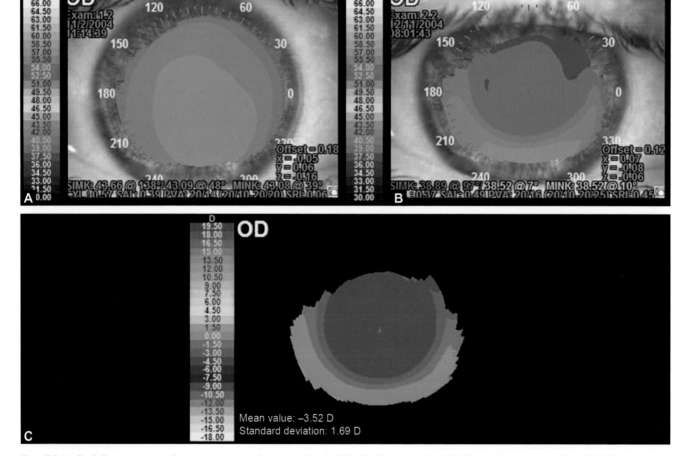

**Figs 7A to C:** Difference map of normal cornea before and after LASIK. (A) Preoperative; (B) Six weeks postoperative; (C) Difference map showing large uniform, well-centered ablation. Mean value is the average change within the pupil. Note topography indices are color-coded here. Green for within normal limits, yellow 2–3 standard deviations from the normal average and red for outliers beyond 3 standard deviations from the normal

assess the potential visual acuity of a given cornea. The most commonly used quantitative descriptor is Simulated keratometry (SimK). The SimK values simulate a traditional keratometer measurement, i.e. the K values of the steepest and flattest meridian along diameters of 3–4 mm. It is known that SimK and clinical keratometry correlate well.[15] Cylinder and spherical equivalent can be calculated using SimK indices.

Another useful quantitative descriptor is the Surface Regularity Index (SRI) that measures central corneal regularity and is useful to correlate the impact of corneal irregularities on vision.[15] The SRI correlates well with best corrected visual acuity in normal eyes and those with irregular corneal surfaces if other eye structures are intact. This correlation is used to estimate the Potential Visual Acuity (PVA) Index in Snellen chart format. The Corneal Ecentricity Index (CEI) was developed to illustrate eccentricity in the cornea.[16] Use of this index is helpful when fitting contact lenses and differentiating between normal prolate corneas and oblate corneas flattened by myopic refractive surgery. The CEI indicates how the curvature changes from the center to the periphery of the cornea. A normal cornea is prolate (i.e. becomes flatter toward the periphery) has an asphericity (Q value) of –0.26. A prolate surface has negative Q values while an oblate surface has a positive value by convention. Myopic laser vision corrections can change the anterior corneal surface from prolate to oblate, but evidence has shown that maintaining a prolate profile within the treatment zone is beneficial to maintain compensation for spherical aberration.[17]

## CORNEAL TOPOGRAPHY AND TEAR FILM

The initial and most important refractive element in the eye is the tear film which smoothly coats the anterior surface of the cornea. The front surface of the cornea and the tear film provide two-thirds of the refractive power of the eye. Placido topographers require an intact epithelial surface and tear film. Without tears, severe optical degradation of images would result, and the Placido mires would become distorted and not able to be tracked. In reality, corneal topographers actually measure the shape of the tear film. Disruptions in the tear film or the smoothness of the underlying epithelium may induce irregularities in corneal shape that degrade the optical quality of the cornea, and reduce visual acuity. If a patient has dry eyes or has been given medicated drops before the examination, irregularities in topography will be recorded that are temporary artifacts

and do not represent the true shape or optics of the cornea. To avoid this, it is important that the operator brings the patient to the corneal topography device first. Asking patients to blink several times or application of preservative free artificial tears prior to capturing corneal images may be helpful. If the mires remain irregular after these precautions, there probably is corneal pathology and consideration should be given to such condition.

## NORMAL CORNEAL TOPOGRAPHIC PARAMETERS AND DEVIATION FROM THE NORMAL

In order to recognize abnormal topography, it is necessary to be able to interpret what is normal. The best way to develop expertise is to routinely examine topographic maps of normal patients with the universal standard scale.[13] Normal corneas will have relatively uniform central power with flattening toward the periphery—particularly toward the nasal side—and smooth contours between contour intervals (Fig. 2). SimK readings should be ~42.75 +/–1.6 D (standard deviation); a good rule of thumb would be to consider K readings less than 38 or greater than 47.5 D abnormal (+/–3 standard deviations from the mean), while those less than 39.5 or greater than 46 D (+/–2 standard deviations) should be regarded with caution. These guidelines have been incorporated into several corneal topographers such that normal values are colored green, cautionary values are yellow and abnormal values are red (Figs 7A to C). This strategy is essential for ease of clinical interpretation.

Parameters outside these ranges do not necessarily indicate that the cornea has pathology. It is not uncommon to see patients with steeper or flatter corneas that are otherwise quite normal by absence of any clinical signs of disease by slit-lamp examination and pachymetry profiles. The finding of otherwise normal corneas with relatively steep or flat curvature parameters can be a familial pattern and topographic evaluation of relatives could be considered for verification. Variations in topography are noted in normal human corneas as described by previous authors.[18-20] Knoll[18] was the first to propose a classification system for normal corneal topography in emmetropic subjects. He classified corneas into four groups based on central asymmetry and amount of peripheral flattening along the horizontal meridian. Bogan et al. described four common topographic patterns in normal corneas—round, oval, symmetric bow tie, asymmetric bow tie and a group of corneas with no readily described or irregular pattern (Figs 8A to E).[20] Rabinowitz et al. also reported similar findings in normal corneas.[21] The approximate distribution of topographic patterns described in normal eyes includes the following: round (23%), oval (21%), symmetric bow tie typical for regular astigmatism (18%), asymmetric bow tie (32%) and irregular (7%). It is important to note that these variations in normal corneal topography are subtle and are consistent with 20/20 or better visual acuity. It is also important to note that although an asymmetric bow tie is one sign of keratoconus, it is only a sign when the gradient is above a certain threshold described

by the I-S index (discussed below). Figure 8D shows an asymmetric bow tie, but it is minimal and does not signal pathology. It is important to establish thresholds for such irregularities in order to distinguish abnormal topography from normal variations; this can be done as noted above by color coding quantitative indices from topographic metrics.

Marked symmetry about the vertical meridian between both eyes of an individual is a hallmark of normal corneas. The two corneas of a normal patient are typically similar in pattern and mean corneal curvature. Forty-three percent of

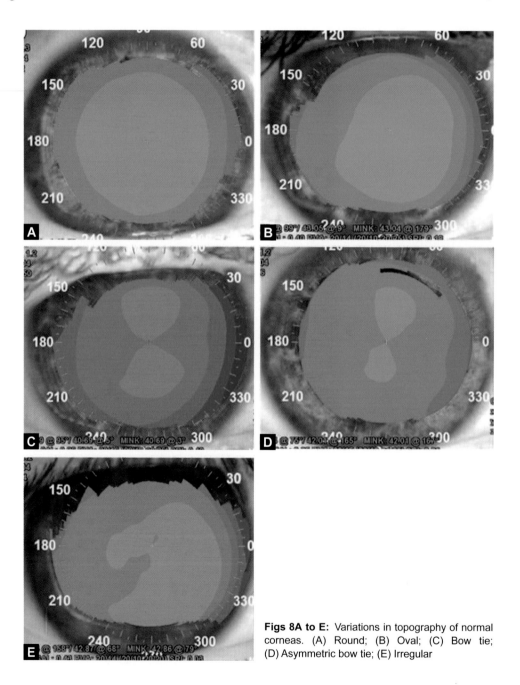

**Figs 8A to E:** Variations in topography of normal corneas. (A) Round; (B) Oval; (C) Bow tie; (D) Asymmetric bow tie; (E) Irregular

right and left eyes were categorized into the same group on pattern recognition and the high correlation of quantitative indices between the two eyes suggests a higher degree of mirror image symmetry as described by Dingeldein.[19] Thus, if astigmatism is present in one cornea, it is also typically present in the contralateral eye. However, if a significant difference is present, the clinician must be more cautious and consider masked corneal pathology, corneal warpage or previous surgery. Deviations from the normal pattern or SimK's discussed above should be a red flag during the screening process, and proper interpretation needs to be completed before proceeding. The most common abnormal corneal topography conditions found in screening, and the known potential sequelae after LASIK are listed in Table 1.

## Contact Lens-Induced Corneal Warpage

Contact lens-induced corneal warpage can be caused by wear of contact lenses, both hard and soft, and can produce a reversible or permanent change in corneal topography not associated with corneal edema. Contact lens-induced warpage is a common topographic abnormality found in refractive screening clinics since a high proportion of patients in these clinics wear contact lenses. The warpage is

**Table 1:** Topographic patterns and their sequelae

| Topographic Abnormality | Cause | Potential Consequence after Refractive Surgery |
|---|---|---|
| Irregular mires with mistracking | Dry eyes, medicamentosa | Poor predictability |
| Irregular contours | Anterior basement membrane dystrophy | Keratectasia |
| Inferior or superior steepening | Corneal warpage | Poor predictability |
| Inferior steepening | Keratoconus, Pellucid marginal degeneration | Keratectasia |
| 'Negative' bow tie, 'C' shaped steepening | Pellucid marginal degeneration | Keratectasia |
| Truncated bow tie | Keratoconus | Keratectasia |
| Asymmetric bow tie | Keratoconus | Keratectasia |
| Lazy 8 or skewed bow tie | Keratoconus | Keratectasia |
| Central or superior steepening | Keratoconus | Keratectasia |

due to contact lens induced corneal molding and is the basis for orthokeratology, a nonsurgical option for the correction of myopia. In orthokeratology, a flatter, looser and large reverse geometry rigid lens is used to mechanically flatten the central corneal contour over time. Swarbrick et al. reported that the initial use of a polymethyl methacrylate (PMMA) lens caused a trend toward central epithelial thinning and mid-peripheral corneal thickening that suggested redistribution of corneal tissue, rather than an overall bending of the cornea.[22]

Corneal warpage manifests with shifts in refraction, changes in keratometry and topographic maps, distortion of keratometer or keratoscopic mires, and a decrease in best-spectacle-corrected visual acuity. Contact lens warpage can masquerade as keratoconus with inferior or superior steepening caused by low or high riding contact lenses, but the induced topographic changes are variable. Superior corneal flattening associated with inferior corneal steepening is the most common topography pattern in keratoconus and contact lens induced warpage. This topographic pattern is secondary to flattening adjacent to the point where the contact lens rests against the cornea. Displacement of epithelial cells from the center to the paracentral zone is believed to cause part of the topographic changes. Corneal warpage is more common with PMMA lenses but can occur with rigid gas permeable and soft contact lenses and is also dependent on the duration of contact lens use.[23,24]

A patient with a history of contact lens wear, needs follow-up exams to ensure refractive stability after discontinuing contact lens use. Discontinuation of contact lens wear for 1 week for soft lenses users and 3 weeks for rigid permeable lenses prior to screening is advocated by some authors. If corneal warpage is suspected during a screening evaluation, re-examination of corneal topography 2–3 weeks later will allow the clinician to test for refractive stability in order to differentiate between true keratoconus and contact lens warpage (pseudokeratoconus). With keratoconus, the area of steepening will generally increase after discontinuing wear as the lens tends to press on the cone; with contact lens warpage, a symmetrical bow tie pattern will often re-emerge. Caveat: topographic and refractive stability may take months to achieve and depends on the type of contact lens used. The mean time with gas-permeable and rigid PMMA lenses was found in one study to be approximately 3 months, with a range from a few weeks to over a year.[23] Examples of topography displaying contact lens warpage producing inferior or superior steepening are shown in Figure 9.

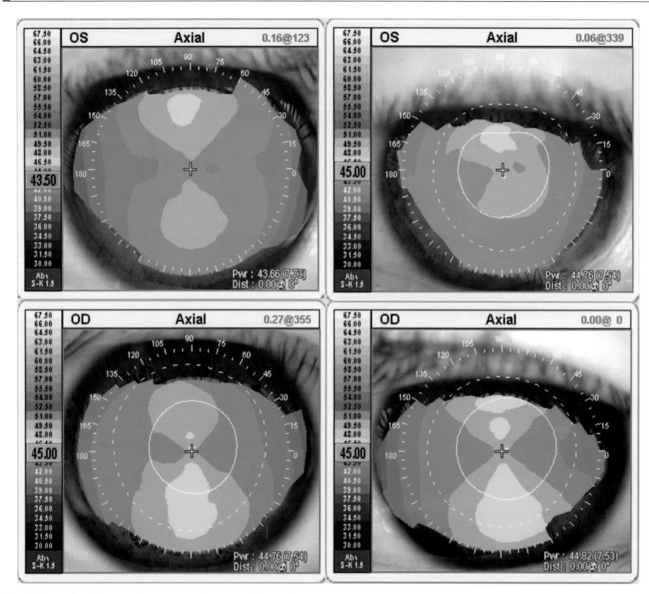

**Fig. 9:** Examples of contact lens warpage. Upper panels result from low riding lenses and lower panels from high riding lenses. None of these are keratoconus as removing the lenses and re-examination several weeks later normalized the topographies

## Topographic Findings in Ectatic Disorders and Refractive Surgery Screening

Keratoconus and PMD are noninflammatory ectatic disorders characterized by progressive stromal thinning, steepening and protrusion of the cornea. Both conditions are normally asymmetrically progressive, with one eye often being more advanced than the other. Less than 2% of cases have been reported as 'unilateral' ectatic disease where one cornea appears completely normal on corneal topography and the fellow eye has mild to advanced signs of keratoconus (Fig. 10).[25] However, since these conditions appear to have a genetic basis that weakens the integrity of

the cornea, it is always recommended to perform corneal topography on both eyes so that the condition will not be overlooked in the unilaterally expressed cases.

### Keratoconus

Screening for early keratoconus is essential because the presence of ectatic degenerative disease is a contraindication for refractive surgery. The most important factor in the preoperative evaluation of a refractive surgery candidate is to rule out the presence of ectatic corneal disorders. Laser ablation procedures in eyes with an overlooked corneal preexisting ectatic disease, may result

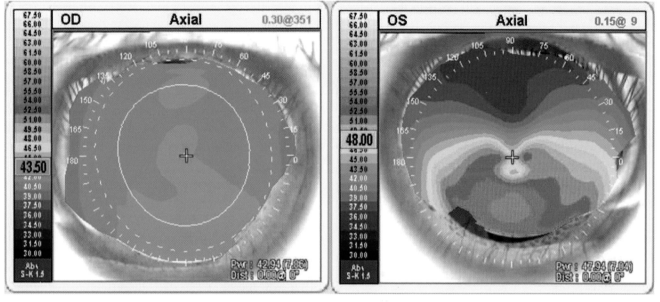

**Fig. 10:** 'Unilateral' keratoconus. There is some inferior steepening in OD, but less than would be consistent with keratoconus suspect (I-S < 1.4 D)

in ectasia progression and deterioration of vision. These patients require close medical and surgical management and may need the riboflavin crosslinking procedure or a corneal transplant. Postrefractive surgery keratectasia is a common cause of litigation.

Refractive surgeons are continuously challenged with the presence of masked corneal ectasia in the preoperative evaluation of refractive candidates. A refractive surgery practice will see far more patients with keratoconus and other topographic abnormalities than would be expected in the general population. The incidence of keratoconus in the general population is very small, perhaps 0.01% or less, but among refractive surgical candidates it can rise to 8% or more.[26] Subsequent work has shown that, as refractive surgery has gained widespread use, the incidence of keratoconus in candidates is reduced significantly, around 1%.[27] Still this is a much higher percentage than in the general population. It is thought that the patients with mild keratoconus who experience spectacle blur owing to corneal aberrations are more apt to seek advanced refractive corrective procedures to achieve acceptable levels of vision.

Corneal topography is a very sensitive method to detect the subtle corneal topographic changes that occur with mild keratoconus. It is also useful to document ectasia after refractive surgery by following serial changes in corneal curvature over time. One problem in making a diagnosis of mild keratoconus or keratoconus suspect is that criteria for these determinations are not well understood. Changes in

corneal topography are generally the earliest and only sign available to the clinician for the detection of keratoconus. In these cases, the accepted terminology for the presence of abnormal corneal topography with signs of keratoconus includes 'keratoconus suspect' and 'forme fruste keratoconus'. Unless the diagnosis is post hoc or the contralateral eye has the diagnosis of keratoconus, such cases should be labeled keratoconus suspect. Retrospectively, after a patient who is suspect of keratoconus develops the disease, the earlier state of the cornea can appropriately be called forme fruste keratoconus. However, in these challenging cases, an advantage of corneal topography is the accuracy of this device to monitor and document serial changes in corneal curvature over time. Increased steepening over a period of time, even in the absence of corneal thinning, is highly suggestive of true clinical keratoconus.

Several keratoconus indices are available on corneal topographers to assist in differentiating keratoconus suspect from normal variations in corneal topography. Rabinowitz and McDonnell[28] were the first to develop numerical indices that were helpful for early detection of keratoconus. These indices measure the power differences between the superior and inferior paracentral corneal regions (designated I-S values) to detect paracentral cones, the central corneal power (Max K) to detect central cones, and the power differences between the left and right eyes to detect the asymmetry between eyes which is characteristic of keratoconus. The I-S value is calculated by taking the difference of the average of 5 superior values at 30° intervals 3 mm above the corneal vertex (optical axis of the topographer) and the average of 5 inferior values at 30° intervals 3 mm below the corneal vertex as shown in Figure 11. Their data suggest that a central corneal power greater than 47.2 D (detects central keratoconus) or an I-S value greater than 1.4 D is consistent with keratoconus suspect, whereas central corneal powers greater than 48.7 D or I-S values greater than 1.9 D are consistent with clinical keratoconus. The latter test is useful with any topographer since in the absence of an automatic calculation of I-S, the display cursor can be moved within a topographic map to collect the needed values manually. The authors recommend this manual calculation when scrutinizing an I-S ratio.

Rabinowitz and Rasheed[29] also developed the KISA% formula as a next step to improve diagnostic evaluation of keratoconus:

$$\text{KISA\%} = (K(I\text{-}S) \times AST \times SRAX)/3$$

in which K = central corneal keratometry power in diopters, I-S = asymmetric dioptric difference between superior and inferior parts of cornea (6 mm apart), AST = difference between steep and flat on SimK meridians, and SRAX = smallest angle between two steep radii subtracted from 180°.

Maeda et al. developed the Klyce/Maeda Keratoconus Prediction Index (KPI), available in some topography devices that helps to differentiate keratoconus from other corneal abnormalities.[30] The KPI value is derived from topographic indices that include the Differential Sector Index (DSI), the Opposite Sector Index (OSI), the Center/ Surround Index (CSI), the Surface Asymmetry Index (SAI), the Irregular Astigmatism Index (IAI) and the percent Analyzed Area (AA). An important aspect of the latter work is that the discriminant analysis-based system was trained to specifically recognize keratoconus from a host of other corneal conditions. While many other keratoconus detection schemes were developed to differentiate keratoconus from normal corneas, the work of Maeda et al. was trained on sets of topographies that included normal, keratoconus, keratoplasty, epikeratophakia, excimer laser photorefractive keratectomy, radial keratotomy, contact lens-induced warpage and other unclassifiable topographies. Inclusion of more classes of corneal pathology than just normal and keratoconus ensures better specificity in clinical screening.

This early work was extended and enhanced by Smolek et al.[31] using a neural network approach, multiple classes of corneal topographies and, importantly, including a classification of keratoconus suspect and PMD (Fig. 12).

## Pellucid Marginal Degeneration

Classic pellucid marginal degeneration is a bilateral peripheral usually inferior corneal thinning disorder characterized by a narrow band of corneal thinning (often approaching 20% normal thickness) separated from the limbus by a relatively uninvolved area 1–2 mm in width. The cornea protrudes above the area of thinning, resulting in high and irregular astigmatism. The cornea above the band of thinning is of normal thickness. The corneal protrusion is most marked central to the area of thinning, and the thickness of the central cornea is usually normal.[32] Similar to keratoconus, PMD is a progressive disorder affecting both eyes, although eyes may progress asymmetrically. In moderate to advanced cases, PMD can easily be differentiated from keratoconus by slit-lamp evaluation because of the classical perilimbal location of the thinning. In early cases, the cornea may appear relatively normal on slit-lamp examination and in advanced cases, it may be difficult to distinguish from keratoconus because the thinning may involve most of the inferior cornea. The topographic pattern of PMD has been described with a 'butterfly' appearance, a 'C' shape rotated 90°, a 'fish mouth' or a 'crab claw'. Other signs include against-the-rule astigmatism and a topographic 'negative blue bow tie' (Fig. 13). When compared to keratoconus, corneal steepening in PMD usually occurs more peripherally in the cornea and is located adjacent to the limbus. Although the topographic patterns of keratoconus and PMD have traditionally been distinguished and this difference may

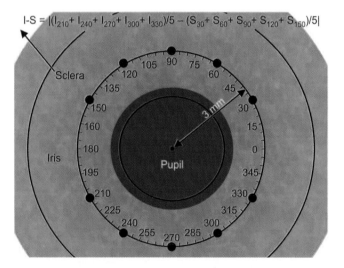

**Fig. 11:** Method for calculating the I-S value used in evaluating asymmetry in corneas for keratoconus

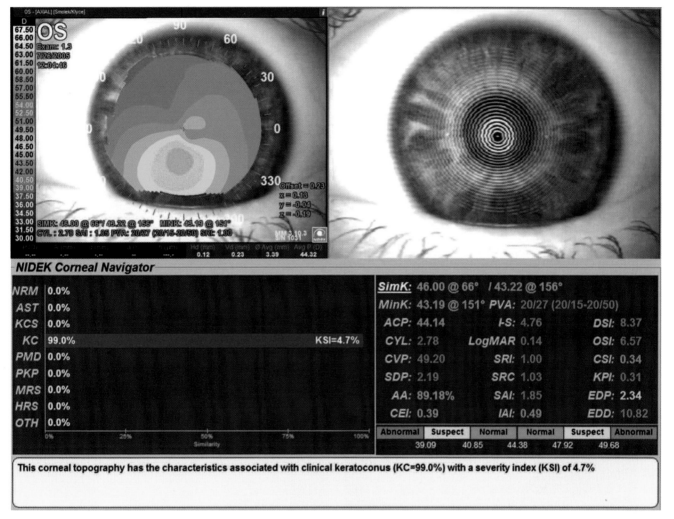

**Fig. 12:** Corneal Navigator used to screen refractive surgical candidates. Color-coding is used to indicate which of the indices is marginal (yellow) or clearly an outlier (red)

be relevant to planning for surgical therapy, it is unclear whether they have different etiologies or if they represent a clinical spectrum of the same underlying pathology. Keratoconus can masquerade as PMD on topography and there have been reports of patients with the keratoconus pattern in one eye and the PMD pattern in the other. The differential diagnosis between these two conditions lies in the pattern of thinning which may only be apparent as the condition progresses from the mildest stages. Keratoconus is associated with a localized area of corneal thinning, whereas the hallmark of PMD is the arcuate band of perilimbal thinning noted above (Fig. 14). In any case, both entities are contraindications for management with keratorefractive surgery because of the elevated risk for iatrogenic ectasia (Fig. 15).

## ADJUNCT SCREENING TOOLS

Corneal topography is a major screening tool to rule out patients who may not be candidates for traditional refractive surgery. Corneal pachymetry measurements are an essential screening tool for complete candidacy evaluation. In certain situations, pupil diameter measurement can be helpful.

### Pachymetry

The measurement of corneal thickness is an invaluable tool during refractive surgical screening. While not an independent risk factor for the development of iatrogenic ectasia by itself, corneal thickness was found to be a statistically significant risk factor for the development

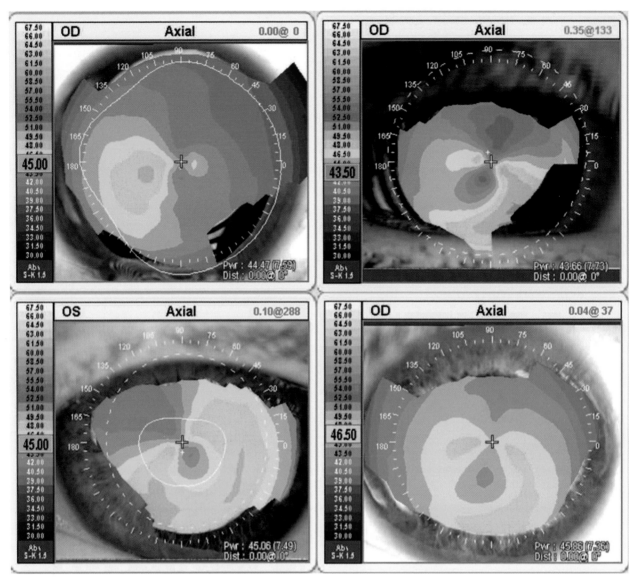

**Fig. 13:** Several instances of topographic pellucid marginal degeneration. Note the 'C' shape and often the 'negative' bow tie with flat area just inferior to the apex. Differentiation will rely on the pattern of associated thinning—focal for keratoconus and perilimbal arcuate thinning for pellucid

of ectasia.[10] With this said, a thin cornea in the face of normal topography and no other risk factors does not mean a patient will develop ectasia with refractive surgery as thin, biomechanically sound corneas likely exist. In addition, corneal thickness must be taken into account when planning surgery to be certain that sufficient residual stromal bed thickness maintains after flap production and tissue ablation. It has been traditional to assure that at least 250 μm of residual stromal bed will be left behind after surgery. The scientific basis for this rule of thumb is weak, but insufficient residual stromal bed thickness is also a risk factor.[10] While the ultrasonic pachymeters have been the standard for assessing corneal thickness on a point-wise basis (usually several central readings followed by four peripheral readings along the horizontal and vertical meridian). Scanning-slit tomographers give a more complete analysis of pachymetry over a large area and allow for evaluation of the overall symmetry and pattern of thinning relative to both corneas. Regional thinning, such as displacement of the thinnest point on the cornea from the corneal apex, should alert the clinician to inspect for additional topographic correlates. If the thinnest point is markedly decentered, this may be associated with pathology and surgery may not be advisable.

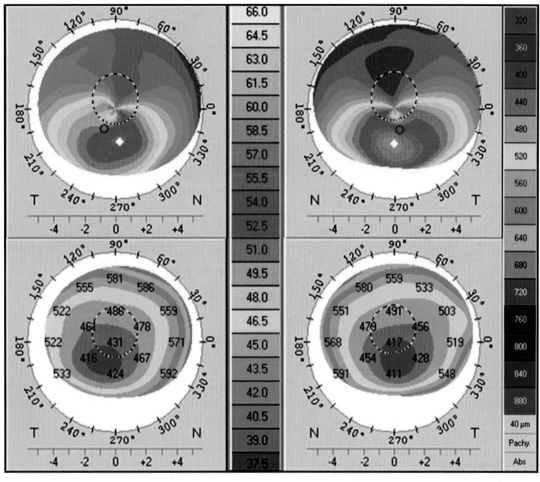

**Fig. 14:** The topography (upper panels) of this case has subtle features suggestive of pellucid marginal degeneration with the 'C' shape in both eyes. However, the focal inferiorly displaced thinnest areas (lower panels) are characteristic of keratoconus. (Center scale: topography, D; right hand scale, pachymetry)

## Pupil Diameter

When excimer laser ablation surgery was first introduced, it was thought that a 5 mm optical zone would be adequate for good vision. In fact, as we know today, small optical zones can interfere with vision when the pupil aperture is not totally within the functional optical zone (the zone where the treatment produces a uniform refractive power).[33] Fortunately, expanded optical zones surrounded by smoothing transitional zones with aspheric treatment algorithms minimize these issues. Although little evidence exists correlating pupil size and outcomes of refractive surgery, incomplete coverage of the pupil can lead to monocular diplopia, ghosting, glare and/or reduced contrast acuity. With this said, it is prudent for the clinician to evaluate both photopic and, in particular, the mesopic pupil sizes in relation to the optical and transition zone diameters. In general, the optical zone of the treatment should be at least 1 mm greater than the mesopic pupil size to allow for intended and unintentional decentration of the treatment area. The clinician should consider additional informed consent when faced with patients with large pupil sizes that are marginally covered with large treatment zones, or avoid using the keratorefractive modality altogether. Virtually all corneal topographers and corneal tomographers image and report pupil diameter, although the Colvard pupillometer type of instrument may more accurately report pupil diameter under a standard lighting condition. The OPD-Scan III (Nidek, Inc., Gamagori, Japan) is a Placido topographer and an ocular aberrometer and reports both photopic and mesopic pupil diameters (Fig. 16).

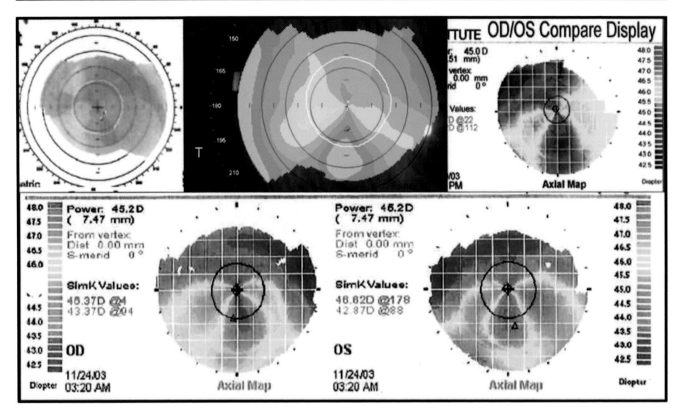

**Fig. 15:** Corneas interpreted as topographic pellucid marginal degeneration suspect. Each of these underwent LASIK and each developed ectasia postoperative. It is helpful to increase the sensitivity of the topographer scale to see these patterns clearly. Note the topography in the upper left is hard to discern because of patient squint and noncontrasting colors

## ▸ CORNEAL TOPOGRAPHERS AND CORNEAL TOMOGRAPHERS

There are a variety of corneal topography models to choose among, many of which offer similar features and presentation formats. For screening applications, Placido-based topographers are preferred over slit-based tomographers as the latter are less sensitive in measuring corneal curvature.

The Orbscan IIz corneal topography system (Bausch & Lomb Surgical, Inc.) is a hybrid system that uses a scanning slit and Placido-based system. The anterior and posterior edges of the slits are captured and analyzed. The slit data provide pachymetric maps as well as anterior and posterior curvature maps while the Placido data provide the topographic maps.

The Pentacam (Oculus, Lynnwood, Wash) uses Scheimpflug optics with its improved depth of field to image the anterior segment from the corneal surface to the lens surface. The rotating camera acquires 100 images from which it extracts 500 data points on the anterior and posterior corneal surfaces. The elevation data from all these images are combined to form a three-dimensional rendering of the cornea and other anterior segment structures. Lacking a

Placido target, the Pentacam slit data are used to generate anterior and posterior corneal surface tomography, including curvature, tangential power and axial power maps.

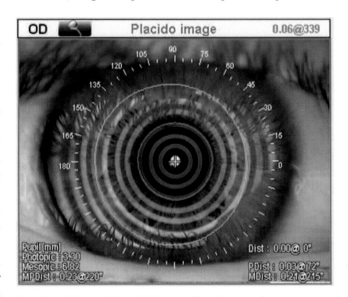

**Fig. 16:** With the Nidek OPD-Scan III both photopic and mesopic pupil diameters are determined for consideration of the size of the functional optical zone prior to laser ablative surgery

Advantages of the Pentacam include the following: high-resolution imaging of the cornea, ability to measure corneas with severe irregularities that may not be amenable to Placido imaging and the ability to calculate pachymetry over a broad corneal area. However, the Pentacam has no Placido-based topographer incorporated in the device. Studies have shown[34-36] that the data obtained with the Pentacam should be interpreted with caution, including corneal astigmatic axes, pupil center, pachymetry, front meridional and axial maps, refractive power maps, pupillometry and equivalent K-readings.

The Galilei (Ziemer, Switzerland) utilizes a rotating dual-Scheimpflug optical system and an integrated Placido topographer. The device analyzes corneal topography, pachymetry over the bulk of the corneal surface and anterior chamber (size and volume). Two cameras in the device scan 180° circumferentially compared to a 360° scan with the single camera in the Pentacam system. This has the potential for reducing data capture time to reduce errors associated with fixation nystagmus and head movement.

The Sirius (Schwind, Kleinostheim, Germany) and the TMS-5 (Tomey, Nagoya, Japan) are new commercially available devices that also measure posterior curvature and elevation maps integrating the data with anterior curvature obtained by Placido-based traditional topography for analysis. Further studies are needed to evaluate the accuracy and reproducibility of these new devices.

## ▶ TOMOGRAPHY ELEVATION MAPS

When screening patients, the Placido-based axial power map has been found to be most clinically useful.[12] The greatest limitation of the Placido corneal topographer is its inability to analyze posterior corneal shape and to provide pachymetry data; these features are available with the corneal tomographers. Direct viewing of corneal shape from elevation data has not been found to be a useful clinical adjunct because, unlike curvature maps, clinically relevant distortions cannot be visualized directly. Therefore, these distortions are enhanced by subtracting a best fit reference surface (usually a sphere or an ellipsoid). It has been suggested that the anterior cornea is more biomechanically sound than the posterior cornea, and posterior elevation changes may be one of the earliest manifestations of keratoconus. Tomidokoro et al.[37] using Orbscan technology, found that both anterior and posterior curvatures were affected in eyes with keratoconus and fellow eyes of patients with diagnosed unilateral keratoconus, which were designated as keratoconus suspect. However, the latter group had an average asymmetry index (I-S) of 4.3 +/–2.8 D confirming that most corneas in this group would be better characterized as mild keratoconus (I-S > 1.9 D as noted above). Fam and Lin found a posterior elevation of 40 μm or more had a sensitivity of 57.7% and a specificity of 89.8% in differentiating keratoconus and at differentiating topographically normal contralateral eyes of keratoconus patients from normals.[38] However, these increased to 99.0% and 92.8% when comparing only keratoconus and normal eyes. Fam and Lin concluded that posterior elevation was of limited use for detection compared to the anterior corneal indices. Thus, manifestations of mild keratoconus do not occur at the posterior corneal surface as promoted by some. The sensitivity and specificity of methods developed to detect keratoconus suspect corneas are not scientifically valid when using the undeveloped fellow eye in 'unilateral keratoconus' patients. In such cases, a more accurate term for undeveloped keratoconus ectasia would be *forme fruste* keratoconus. 'Keratoconus suspect' applies to corneas with very subtle signs on corneal topography such as inferior steepening within the range specified by Rabinowitz and McDonnell,[28] that is with an I-S value from 1.4 D to 1.9 D and no other signs. In this category, the earliest reliable sign of keratoconus are abnormalities seen in corneal topography well before there are detectable changes in pachymetry. Claims contrary to this conclusion generally include mild clinical keratoconus within the keratoconus suspect cohort.

## ▶ CONCLUSION

Placido-based corneal topography is a mature diagnostic tool and continues to be the gold standard to evaluate the anterior corneal surface and to detect abnormal corneal topography such as keratoconus. Corneal tomographers offer extensive pachymetry maps not available on the Placido devices and are able to provide curvature maps of very irregular corneas not amenable to Placido analysis. Educated use of corneal topography and tomography is essential to meet the standard of care in screening refractive surgical candidates and to continue providing safe and effective treatment to our patients.

## ▶ REFERENCES

1. Troutman RC. Surgical keratometer in the management of astigmatism in keratoplasty. Ann Ophthalmol. 1987;19(12):473-4.
2. Rowsey JJ, Reynolds AE, Brown R. Corneal topography. Corneascope. Arch Ophthalmol. 1981;99(6):1093-1100.
3. Doss JD, Hutson RL, Rowsey JJ, et al. Method for calculation of corneal profile and power distribution. Arch Ophthalmol. 1981;99(7):1261-5.

4. Klyce SD. Computer-assisted corneal topography. High-resolution graphic presentation and analysis of keratoscopy. Invest Ophthalmol Vis Sci. 1984;25(12):1426-35.

5. Maguire LJ, Singer DE, Klyce SD. Graphic presentation of computer-analyzed keratoscope photographs. Arch Ophthalmol. 1987;105(2):223-30.

6. Seiler T, Quurke AW. Iatrogenic keratectasia after LASIK in a case of forme fruste keratoconus. J Cataract Refract Surg. 1998;24:1007-9.

7. Lovisolo CF, Fleming JF. Intracorneal ring segments for iatrogenic keratectasia after laser in situ keratomileusis or photorefractive keratectomy. J Refract Surg. 2002;18:535-41.

8. Hardten DR, Gosavi VV. Photorefractive keratectomy in eyes with atypical topography. J Cataract Refract Surg. 2009;35:1437-44.

9. Smolek MK, Klyce SD, Maeda N. Keratoconus and corneal warpage analysis using the keratomorphic diagram. Invest Ophthalmol Vis Sci. 1994;35:4192-4204.

10. Randleman JB, Russell B, Ward MA, et al. Risk factors and prognosis for corneal ectasia after LASIK. Ophthalmology. 2003;110:267-75.

11. American National Standard for Ophthalmics—Corneal Topography Systems—Standard Terminology. Requirements. ANSI Z80.23–1999. Optical Laboratories Association, American National Standards Institute, Inc, 1999.

12. Wilson SE, Klyce SD, Husseini ZM. Standardized color coded maps for corneal topography. Ophthalmology. 1993;13:1723-7.

13. Smolek MK, Klyce SD, Hovis JK. The universal standard scale: proposed improvements to the American National Standards Institute (ANSI) scale for corneal topography. Ophthalmology 2002;109:361-9.

14. American National Standard for Ophthalmics—Corneal Topography Systems—Standard Terminology, Requirements. ANSI Z80.23–2008. Optical Laboratories Association. American National Standards Institute, Inc, 2008.

15. Wilson SE, Klyce SD. Quantitative descriptors of corneal topography. A clinical study. Arch Ophthalmol. 1991;109(3):349-53.

16. Maeda N, Klyce SD, Hamano H. Alteration of corneal asphericity in rigid gas permeable contact lens induced warpage. CLAO J. 1994;20(1):27-31.

17. Hersh PS, Fry K, Blaker JW. Spherical aberration after laser in situ keratomileusis and photorefractive keratectomy. Clinical results and theoretical models of etiology. J Cataract Refract Surg. 2003;29(11):2096-104.

18. Knoll HA. Corneal contours in the general population as revealed by the photokeratoscope. Am J Optom Physiol Opt. 1961;38:389-95.

19. Dingeldein SA, Klyce SD. The topography of normal corneas. Arch Ophthalmol. 1989;107(4):512-8.

20. Bogan SJ, Waring GO 3rd, Ibrahim O, et al. Classification of normal corneal topography based on computer-assisted videokeratography. Arch Ophthalmol. 1990;108(7):945-9.

21. Rabinowitz YS, Yang H, Brickman Y, et al. Videokeratography database of normal human corneas. Br J Ophthalmol. 1996;80(7):610-6.

22. Swarbrick HA, Wong G, O'Leary DJ. Corneal response to orthokeratology. Optom Vis Sci. 1998;75(11):791-9.

23. Ruiz-Montenegro J, Mafra CH, Wilson SE, et al. Corneal topographic alterations in normal contact lens wearers. Ophthalmology. 1993;100(1):128-34.

24. Wang X, McCulley JP, Bowman RW, et al. Time to Resolution of Contact Lens-Induced Corneal Warpage Prior to Refractive Surgery. CLAO J. 2002;28(4):169-71.

25. Holland DR, Maeda N, Hannush SB, et al. Unilateral keratoconus. Incidence and quantitative topographic analysis. Ophthalmology. 1997;104(9):1409-13.

26. Wilson SE, Klyce SD. Screening for corneal topographic abnormalities before refractive surgery. Ophthalmology. 1994;101(1):147-52.

27. Ambrósio R Jr, Klyce SD, Wilson SE. Corneal topographic and pachymetric screening of keratorefractive patients. J Refract Surg. 2003;19(1):24-9.

28. Rabinowitz YS, McDonnell PJ. Computer-assisted corneal topography in keratoconus. Refract Corneal Surg. 1989;5(6):400-8.

29. Rabinowitz YS, Rasheed K. KISA% index: a quantitative videokeratography algorithm embodying minimal topographic criteria for diagnosing keratoconus. J Cataract Refract Surg. 1999;25(10):1327-35.

30. Maeda N, Klyce SD, Smolek MK. Comparison of methods for detecting keratoconus using videokeratography. Arch Ophthalmol. 1995;113(7):870-4.

31. Smolek MK, Klyce SD. Current keratoconus detection methods compared with a neural network approach. Invest Ophthalmol Vis Sci. 1997;38:2290-99.

32. Krachmer JH, Feder RS, Belin MW. Keratoconus and related noninflammatory corneal thinning disorders. Surv Ophthalmol. 1984;28(4):293-322.

33. Tabernero J, Klyce SD, Sarver EJ, et al. Functional optical zone of the cornea. Invest Ophthalmol Vis Sci. 2007;48(3):1053-60.

34. Shankar H, Taranath D, Santhirathelagan CT, et al. Anterior segment biometry with the Pentacam: comprehensive assessment of repeatability of automated measurements. J Cataract Refract Surg. 2008;34(1):103-13.

35. Shankar H, Taranath D, Santhirathelagan CT, et al. Repeatability of corneal first-surface wavefront aberrations measured with Pentacam corneal topography. J Cataract Refract Surg. 2008;34(5):727-34.

36. McAlinden C, Khadka J, Pesudovs K. A comprehensive evaluation of the precision (repeatability and reproducibility) of the Oculus Pentacam HR. Invest Ophthalmol Vis Sci. 2011;52 (10):7731-7.

37. Tomidokoro A, Oshika T, Amano S, et al. Changes in anterior and posterior corneal curvatures in keratoconus. Ophthalmology 2000;107:1328-32.

38. Fam HB, Lim KL. Corneal elevation indices in normal and keratoconic eyes. J Cataract Refract Surg. 2006;32:1281-7.

16 SECTION

# Radial Keratotomy

*John B Cason, Kerry Assil*

## INTRODUCTION

Once the most common elective refractive procedure in the world, radial keratotomy has been replaced by more modern methods of corneal refractive surgery. Historically this procedure has become noted for its lack of acceptable refractive predictability and safety. Yet, the procedure still interests many today because of the lessons learned from its evolution, the large multicenter trial that elucidated its shortcomings, and the many offshoot procedures that developed afterwards that share many of its characteristics that we perform today, like astigmatic keratotomy and limbal relaxing incisions.

One of the largest refractive procedure studies, the Prospective Evaluation of Radial Keratotomy (PERK), proved to be a standard by which many current refractive studies are compared. Prior to this study there was much public demand for the elimination of spectacles while a new capability was developing in Russia that did not require new equipment. Rather it utilized tools already available and thereby bypassed many of the regulatory requirements that typically accompany procedures today. The PERK study served to evaluate the procedure's impact to cornea topography, cornea healing, and refractive stability that directly influenced the development of today's primary refractive procedures, laser *in situ* keratomileusis and photorefractive keratotomy.

Today, radial keratotomy still presents challenges to the ocular surgeon. Residual refractive error still troubles some patients and can be difficult to treat with spectacles. Many patients require hard contact lens correction to alleviate the higher order aberrations that cause some

of their vision disturbances. Some patients desire repeat cornea refractive surgery. Furthermore, some patients are not good candidates for refractive surgery or have unstable corneas that require penetrating keratoplasty. Even in cases where the patient does not need or desire cornea surgery the cataracts that are now developing in this age cohort require special care in regards to intraocular lens calculations and intraoperative care because the near full-thickness wounds can dehisce during surgery and require immediate attention.

## HISTORY

The idea of using cornea incisions to induce changes in cornea shape have roots in early ophthalmology. Snellen first postulated in 1869 that tangential incisions in the cornea would result in flattening in that meridian.[1] This was later confirmed by reports from Schiotz when he reported flattening in the meridian of cataract surgery and by Lans in his rabbit study showing flattening in the incisional meridian and steepening in the meridian 90° away.[2,3]

Nearly fifty years later, Sato created endothelial incisions in the cornea in a radial fashion to flatten the cornea. He derived this technique after observations of keratoconus patients and how their corneas exhibited flattening after the development of hydrops.[4,5] This technique later fell out of favor as the advent of contact lenses provided a simpler and safer solution to ammetropia. However, the notion of creating cuts in the cornea to induce topography changes resurfaced with Beliaev in Russia by making radial cuts in the anterior surface of the cornea at almost full-thickness and then further refined by Fyodorov when he demonstrated titration of effect with the size of the central optical zone.[6] Leo Bores then adopted the procedure in the United States in 1978 changing the centripetal direction cut from the Russians to a centrifugal cut which predominated most of the surgical technique in the US.[7]

Radial Keratotomy remained commonplace worldwide until the mid 1990s when results of the PERK study showed that there was a significant amount of myopic regression. Many patients also became progressively more hyperopic and many further had problems with diurnal variations and other vision disturbances such as glare and halos. During the same time period, the excimer laser was rising in popularity to make way for the adoption of photorefractive keratectomy (PRK) and laser *in situ* keratomileusis (LASIK).

## ➤ TECHNIQUE

The preoperative workup for radial keratotomy was very similar to modern cornea refractive surgery. A full ocular examination was performed with manifest and cycloplegic refractions. Cornea ultrasound pachymetry was also performed in multiple locations to create a pachymetry map (Fig. 1), which was used for the surgery. Sometimes these measurements were repeated in the operating suite or delayed until the procedure itself. Cornea topography was obtained to measure the curvature of the cornea. All of this data along with the age of the patient was used to determine the number of cuts and the size of the optical zone, which titrated the effect of cornea flattening to induce the myopic correction.

During the procedure itself the patient was laid in the supine position and topical anesthetic was instilled in the

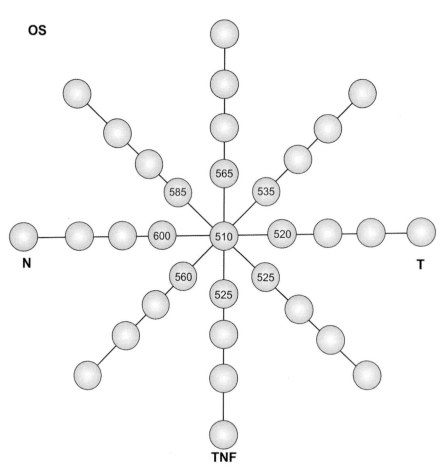

**Fig. 1:** Sample screening pachymetry worksheet demonstrating both central and paracentral values

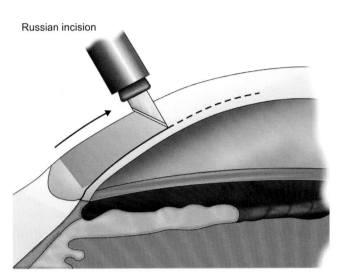

**Fig. 2:** Russian technique: Incisions are made in a radial fashion from the limbus towards the optical clear zone (centripetal)

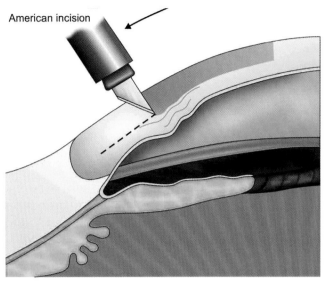

**Fig. 3:** American technique: Incisions are made in a radial fashion from the optical clear zone to the limbus (centrifugal)

operative eye(s). The center of the cornea was marked with a Sinskey hook or other similar instrument followed by marking the optical clear zone with a circular marker. The cornea thickness was then measured with a solid tip ultrasound pachymeter and the depth of the surgical blade was then set at or near the depth of the thinnest pachymetric measurement. The incisions were marked with an inked radial marker and then the incisions were made into the anterior cornea. The manner in which the cuts were made varied some according to the direction of the cuts. Furthermore, the nomograms used varied based on population data or age based cohort adjustments.

The typical Russian technique involved centripetal incisions made from the peripheral limbus towards the optical central clear zone (Fig. 2). The advantage of this technique was better control of depth throughout the incision. However, there was a danger of violating the central clear zone. The American technique consisted of centrifugal cuts made from the central clear zone to the limbus (Fig. 3). This technique had an increased safety profile from a perforation and clear zone standpoint. However, due to bunching of the tissue in the periphery of the cut, the depth was sometimes not sufficient and there was a subsequent lessening of the surgical effect. The combination, or Genesis technique, utilized both of these techniques by starting with a centrifugal partial thickness cut that was followed by a centripetal cut to the optical zone (Figs 4A to C). Using a specially-designed diamond blade, the surgeon was able to utilize a cutting surface on both sides of the blade (Fig. 5). This technique had the advantages of both safety and control of depth to get a more consistent result.[6,8]

## ▶ RESULTS

One aspect of RK vision results was the variability. In comparison to the success of modern cornea refractive surgery the technique resulted in poor predictability, stability, and safety. Lower order aberrations such as sphere and cylinder were sometimes exchanged for higher order aberrations induced by an irregular shaped cornea after the procedure. Enlarging the optical clear zone lessened this effect.[9]

One year after RK surgery, 82% of patients were very or moderately satisfied and 10% were dissatisfied. Fluctuating vision was a complaint in 34% of patients postoperatively compared to 12% prior to the surgery. Ultimately, factors predictive of dissatisfaction were uncorrected visual acuity, residual refractive error and fluctuating vision.[10]

## ▶ PREDICTABILITY

Diameter of the central clear zone, patient age, and depth of incisions were determined to be key factors in predictability.[11] The 90% confidence interval for the optical zone (OZ) was directly correlated to its size and was a sizeable 4.12D at an OZ of 3 mm. At one year, a surgeon could have a 90% confidence interval of 3.5D which meant that the surgical result was within 1.75D of myopia, hyperopia, or somewhere in between.

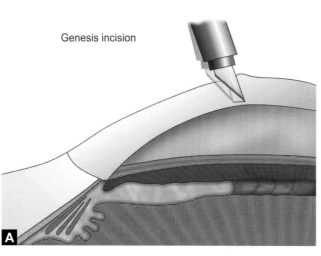

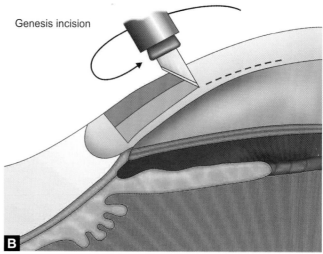

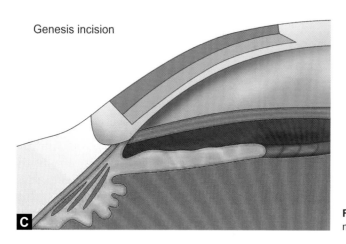

**Figs 4A to C:** Genesis Technique: Centrifugal incisions are first made, followed by centripetal incisions ending at the optical clear zone

The effect of the treatments were directly affected by the healing response of the cornea, which varied by age. Older patients had an exaggerated effect by as much as 1 D per decade. Depth and number of incisions directly affected the predictability as well. A larger number of incisions created more flattening as well as the greater depth of the radial incisions.

## PERK STUDY

The PERK study, led by Dr George Waring III, became the first multicenter clinical trial to evaluate the safety and efficacy and long-term predictability of RK by evaluating 435 patients at 9 centers between March 1982 and October 1983. All surgeries were performed with 45-degree blades and 8 incisions were made with 3.0 and 4.0 optical zones. All patients were within –2 to –8 diopters of myopia. No enhancements were conducted in this prospective trial.[12]

At one year 60% were within 1 D of emmetropia. Thirty percent were undercorrected and 10% were overcorrected by a diopter and for 19% of patients between postoperative month 6 and 12 their refraction changed more than 0.5D.[12] After 3 years, a similar number of patients were under and overcorrected and 76% had 20/40 or better uncorrected vision. However, 12% of patients at this point had refractive shifts more than 1 diopter indicating refractive instability.[13]

At the 4-year point, 23% of patients were more than 1D myopic and the 90% CI was 4.42 D.[14]

The ten-year data began to show another trend in the refractive results, progressive hyperopia. At this point 43% of patients had more than 1D of hyperopia, which was statistically correlated to the size of the optical zone. Sixty percent were within 1D and 38% were within 0.5D.[15]

Ten years after RK, patients were noted to have significant diurnal fluctuation that presumably varied with

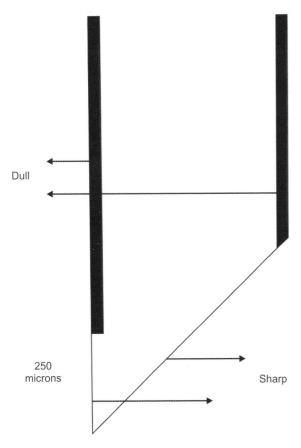

**Fig. 5:** Diamond knife blade design for combined (Genesis) radial incision technique. The sharpened cutting edge extends only 250 microns along the vertical edge from the pointed tip, with the remainder of the vertical margin remaining blunt. The angled margin of the knife is sharpened to provide a cutting edge along its entire length

intraocular pressure variations from morning to night. Symptomatic patients exhibited 0.36D average shifts in their myopia and a concurrent 0.52D shift in keratometry.[16] At 11 years, a shift from minus refraction from 0.50 to 1.62D was seen as well as 31% change in refractive cylinder from morning to day.[17]

## ❧ OTHER RK STUDIES

The Casebeers study consisted of 241 consecutive RK/AK procedures by 1 surgeon. Noticeably different from the PERK study was the use of enhancement procedures for residual and consecutive refractive error. Three years after the procedure there was a 0.6D hyperopic shift that was more prevalent in myopic corrections greater than 6D. Enhancement procedures were needed in 36% of the patients and the hyperopic progression prompted the authors to recommend undertreatment adjustments in the

nomograms. Overall, the postoperative results with enhancements were better than the PERK study. However, 68% of patients had mild to severe vision problems compared with 28% of the control group.[18]

Waring et al. conducted another multicenter trial utilizing the Russian technique and combining RK with AK in order to study the effect of combined astigmatism treatment. Enhancement procedures were utilized during this study compared to the lack of use in the PERK study. Enhancements were performed in 39% of patients. One year results were much more favorable with 89% within 1D and 93% 20/40 or better uncorrected vision. Ninety percent were satisfied with the procedure showing that early results were much more favorable with better management of the astigmatism and overall residual refractive error.[19]

## ❧ RETREATMENTS

Today, RK patients continue to visit their refractive surgeons requesting retreatments for the residual refractive error or the progressive hyperopic shift that developed since the procedure. Care must be taken to avoid performing repeat corneal refractive surgery when there is visually significant cataract contributing more to the deteriorating vision. Furthermore, these patients have irregular corneas and higher order aberrations, which are difficult to treat in native corneas, much less in weakened corneas after RK.

Early retreatments of RK with photorefractive keratectomy (PRK) after the approval of the excimer laser by the FDA were mostly favorable with the exception of the development of stromal haze.[19, 20] This haze in many patients was visually significant and contributed to the shift to LASIK retreatments. However, LASIK had its own problems with pie-wedge dehiscence of the flaps, RK wound dehiscence, epithelial ingrowth, and diffuse lamellar keratitis.[21-27] With the advent of wavefront guided ablation profiles and mitomycin-C to reduce stroma haze, PRK became much more commonplace to treat RK refractive error.[28-31]

The literature data supporting the retreatment of RK refractive error is dispersed over two decades and multiple techniques. There were no published series of patients comparing PRK to LASIK but many that evaluated each individual technique. In general the techniques are equivalent in outcomes and safety but more reported cases of postoperative ectasia have been found after LASIK retreatments showing evidence of further destabilizing the cornea with a lamellar cut after the transverse and radial RK cuts.[22,32]

The RK Retreatment Study Group, led by Dr John Cason, released retrospective multicenter and multisurgeon data comparing PRK to LASIK at the American Society of Cataract and Refractive Surgery 2011 meeting supporting the equal efficacy of wavefront-guided PRK to conventional LASIK with a microkeratome, but a slightly more favorable safety profile in the PRK group. In their evaluation of 112 PRK retreatments and 109 LASIK retreatments, there were 4% total complications in the PRK group consisting exclusively of postoperative haze that was treated successfully with phototherapeutic keratectomy. However, in the LASIK group, there were 12% total complications including 2 cases of ectasia.

## ⯈ CONCLUSION

Overall, RK has successfully treated the ammetropia of many patients and most of the patients were satisfied with the results. In comparison to modern corneal refractive surgery the results did not compare well with PRK and LASIK. However, the lessons learned from RK enabled a greater understanding of cornea healing and response to refractive procedures for corneal refractive surgeons. The evaluation of its safety and efficacy in the PERK study and other observational trials set a standard by which refractive surgery continues to be evaluated.

Furthermore, it is important to note that although radial keratotomy fell out of favor in the refractive surgery community, the surgical principles utilized for this technique are still employed today. Limbal relaxing incisions and astigmatic keratotomies use very similar surgical blades and are used in a similar fashion as their predecessor. The use of these techniques expands the options for refractive and cataract surgeons today.

## ⯈ REFERENCES

1. Snellen H. Die Richtung der hauptmeridiane des astigmatischen Auges. Graefes Arch Ophthalmol. 1869;15:199-207.
2. Schiotz HA. Ein Fall von hochgradigem Hornhautastigmatismus nach Staarextraction. Besserung auf operative Wege. Arch Augenheilk. 1885;15:178-81.
3. Lans LJ. Experimentelle Untersuch ungen uber Entstehung von Astigmatismus durch nicht-perforirende Corneawunden. Graefes Arch Ophthalmol. 1898;45:117-52.
4. Sato T. Treatment of conical cornea (incision of Descemet's membrane). Nippon Ganka Gakkai Zasshi. 1939;43:544-55.
5. Sato T, Akiyama K, Shibata H. A new surgical approach to myopia. Am J Ophthalmol. 1953;36:823-9.
6. Assil KK. Radial Keratotomy: The combined technique. Int Ophthalmol Clin. 1994;34(4):55-77.
7. Bores LD, Myers W, Cowden J. Radial keratotomy: an analysis of the American experience. Ann Ophthalmol. 1981;13:941-8.
8. Verity SM, et al. The combined (Genesis) technique of radial keratotomy. A prospective multicenter study. Refractive Keratoplasty Study Group. Ophthalmology. 1995;102(12):1908-16.
9. Applegate RA, et al. Corneal aberrations and visual performance after radial keratotomy. J Refract Surg. 1998;14(4): 397-407.
10. Bourque LB, et al. Reported satisfaction, fluctuation of vision, and glare among patients one year after surgery in the prospective evaluation of radial keratotomy (PERK) study. Arch Ophthalmol. 1986;104:356-63.
11. Lynn MJ, Waring GO, Sperduto RD. Factors affecting outcome and predictability of radial keratotomy in the PERK study. Arch Ophthalmol. 1987;105:42-51.
12. Waring GO, et al. Results of the prospective evaluation of radial keratotomy (PERK) study one year after surgery. Ophthalmology. 1985;92(2):177-98.
13. Waring GO, et al. Three-year results of the prospective evaluation of radial keratotomy (PERK) study. Ophthalmology. 1987;94(10):1339-54.
14. Waring GO, et al. Results of the prospective evaluation of radial keratotomy (PERK) study 4 years after surgery for myopia. PERK study group. JAMA. 1990;263(8):1083-91.
15. Waring GO, Lynn MJ, McDonnell PJ. Results of the prospective evaluation of radial keratotomy (PERK) study 10 years after surgery. Arch Ophthalmol. 1994;112:1298-308.
16. McDonnell PJ, et al. Morning to evening change in refraction, corneal curvature, and visual acuity 11 years after radial keratotomy in the prospective evaluation of radial keratotomy. The PERK study group. Ophthalmology. 1996;103(2):233-9.
17. Werblin TP, Krider DW, Stafford GM. Casebeer system for refractive keratotomy: patient satisfaction. J Cataract Refract Surg. 1997;23(3):407-12.
18. Waring GO 3rd, Casebeer JC, Dru RM. One-year results of a prospective multicenter study of the Casebeer system of refractive keratotomy: Casebeer Chiron Study Group. Ophthalmology. 1996;103(9):1337-47.
19. McDonnell PJ, et al. Excimer laser myopic photorefractive keratectomy after undercorrected radial keratotomy. J Refract Corneal Surg. 1991;7:146-50.
20. Hahn TW, et al. Excimer laser photorefractive keratectomy to correct residual myopia after radial keratotomy. J Refract Corneal Surg. 1993;9(suppl):S25-S29.
21. Yong L, Chen G, Li W, et al. Laser in situ keratomileusis enhancement after radial keratotomy. J Refract Surg. 2000;16(2):187-90.
22. Lyle AW, Jin GJC. Laser in situ keratomileusis for consecutive hyperopia after myopic LASIK and radial keratotomy. J Cataract Refract Surg. 2003;29:879-88.
23. Oral D, Awwad ST, Seward MS, et al. Hyperopic laser in situ keratomileusis in eyes with previous radial keratotomy. J Cataract Refract Surg. 2005;31:1561-8.
24. Afshari NA, Schirra F, Rapoza PA, et al. Laser in situ keratomileusis outcomes following radial keratotomy, astigmatic keraztotomy, photorefractive keratectomy, and penetrating keratoplasty. J Cataract Refract Surg. 2005;31:2093-100.

25. Munoz G, et al. Femtosecond laser in situ keratomileusis for consecutive hyperopia after radial keratotomy. J Cataract Refract Surg. 2007;33:1183-9.

26. Portellinha et al. Laser in situ keratomileusis for overcorrection after radial keratotomy. J Refract Surg. 2000;16(suppl): S253-6.

27. Francesconi CM, et al. Hyperopic laser-assisted in situ keratomileusis for radial keratotomy induced hyperopia. Ophthalmology. 2002;109:602-5.

28. Nassaralla BA, et al. Prophylactic mitomycin C to inhibit corneal haze after photorefractive keratectomy for residual myopia following radial keratotomy. J Refract Surg. 2007;23:226-32.

29. Ghanem RC et al. Customized topography-guided photorefractive keratectomy with the MEL-70 platform and mitomycin C to correct hyperopia after radial keratotomy. J Refract Surg. 2008;24:911-22.

30. Myrowitz EH, Kurwa A, Parker J, Chuck RS. Wavefront-guided photorefractive keratectomy after radial keratotomy in nine eyes. J Refract Surg; 2009.

31. Koch DD, et al. Wavefront-guided photorefractive keratectomy in eyes with prior radial keratotomy. Ophthalmology 2009; 116:1688-96.

32. Munoz G, et al. Keratectasia after bilateral laser in situ keratomileusis in a patient with previous radial and astigmatic keratotomy. J Cataract Refract Surg. 2005;31:441-45.

# Conductive Keratoplasty

*George O Waring IV, Carolyn A Bates, Jason E Stahl*

## ▶ INTRODUCTION

The theory behind thermokeratoplasty dates back to 1889 when Lans first noted refractive changes in rabbit cornea after application of heat to the peripheral cornea.[1] Heat caused a shrinkage of the cornea in the area of application, reshaping the cornea's curvature. Later attempts to use heat application to flatten keratoconic eyes were unsuccessful, resulting in corneal cell damage, opacities and scarring. Following years of refinement of temperature ranges, investigators began to use heat application in a ring pattern around the peripheral cornea to treat hyperopia and astigmatism. Corneal shrinkage at each spot of heat application along the ring resulted in a band of constriction steepening the central cornea. Over the years, a variety of methods have been used to induce refractive change by selective heating of the cornea, including radial thermal keratoplasty, holmium-YAG laser thermokeratoplasty, $CO_2$ laser thermokeratoplasty and diode laser thermokeratoplasty. Varying degrees of predictability and regression of effect have been reported in the aforementioned techniques.[2]

## ▶ CONDUCTIVE KERATOPLASTY

The most recent incarnation of thermokeratoplasty developed by Mendez et al. is conductive keratoplasty (CK).[3] Conductive keratoplasty is the application of low frequency radio waves to 'shrink' collagen fibrils within the cornea. The low frequency radio waves are delivered through a fine tipped probe applied to the corneal stroma. The tip itself is not a heat source, rather the emitted radio waves cause ionic agitation that increases the temperature of soft tissues, especially connective tissue. In the cornea, the electrical impedance of the stromal collagen results in heat that denatures and 'shrinks' the collagen. Corneal refractive change is produced by localizing the energy delivery to spots along a circumferential band in peripheral cornea. As the collagen shrinks, the band constricts and there is a steepening of the corneal curvature central to the band. The amount of corneal steepening is controlled by treatment placement, intensity and duration. In theory, the energy delivery is self-limiting as denaturation of collagen increases resistance to the current flow.[4]

The advantages of CK over laser reshaping of the central cornea are that it preserves the optical clarity of the visual axis and does not involve any tissue removal. It is used to correct low to moderate levels of hyperopia and astigmatism in ammetropes as well as eyes made ammetropic due to LASIK or cataract surgery. More recently, it is also used to induce monovision in presbyopes.

## ▶ HISTOLOGY

Naoumidi et al.[5] followed the morphological changes of human cornea after CK. Six eyes of six patients with peripheral keratoconus underwent CK treatment followed by penetrating keratoplasty. Changes in corneal structure were assessed with light and electron microscopy of corneal buttons. One day after treatment, the epithelial layer was slightly disrupted where the CK tip had penetrated and an accumulation of fluid perforated Bowman's layer in the treatment area. Overall, the corneal epithelium was only mildly affected by the CK treatment.

The stroma at 1-day post-CK showed extensive changes in morphology. The normally smooth, parallel layers of collagen became disorganized in the treatment area (Fig. 1). Keratocytes underwent cytoplasmic fragmentation, vacuolization and picnotic nuclear changes. Microfibrillar aggregations two to three times the diameter of intact collagen fibers were noted under transmission electron microscopy. Stromal morphology remained normal outside the treatment site, making it possible to identify the affected area as a cylinder of about 120 μm in diameter extending through about 80% of the corneal thickness. Descemet's membrane and the corneal endothelium remained relatively normal in the CK treatment zone.

At 6 months post-CK, the corneal epithelial layer was slightly thickened and Bowman layer in the treatment zone was replaced by irregular connective tissue containing what appeared to be activated fibroblasts. This same loose connective tissue was also present in the stroma within the treatment zone as were cells similar to activated fibroblasts (Fig. 2). Again, the endothelium in the treatment zone appeared normal, except for a slight increase in the amount of structures with vacuoles.[5]

## ▶ CONDUCTIVE KERATOPLASTY TREATMENT

The CK system consists of a radiofrequency energy-generating console, reusable corneal marker, reusable lid speculum, reusable handpiece, disposable keratoplasty tip, and a footpedal controller (Fig. 3). Radiofrequency energy is set to 60% (0.6 W) with a 0.6 second treatment time. The lid speculum acts as the return electrode, so it is important to ensure it has direct contact with the eyelids. The keratoplasty tip has a 45° bend proximally to allow access to the eye over the brow or nasal region and a 90° bend distally to position the tip perpendicular to the corneal surface. A stop at 500 μm from the distal tip indicates the appropriate depth of tip penetration into the cornea.

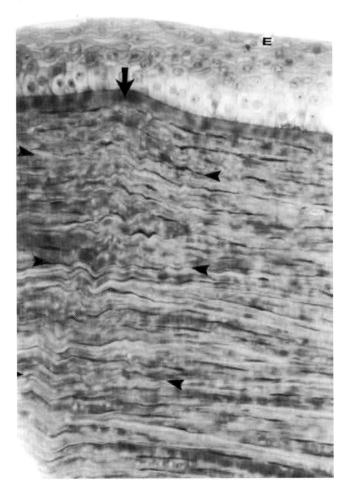

**Fig. 1:** Twenty-four hours after the conductive keratoplasty (CK) treatment (human cornea): crumpled collagen layers (between arrowheads) within the central part of the CK-treated area (thick arrows). E: epithelium. Light microscopy, X 200
*Source:* Reprinted with permission from Naoumidi TL, et al.[5] Conductive keratoplasty: histological study of human corneas. Am J Ophthalmol. 2005;140:984-92. © Elsevier

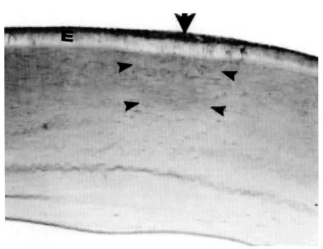

**Fig. 2:** Six months after conductive keratoplasty (CK) treatment (human cornea): the foci of the Bowman's layer as well as the affected corneal stroma, are substituted with fibrous connective tissue along with a large amount of cells resembling fibroblast cells (between small arrowheads). E: epithelial layer. The center of CK-treated area: thick arrows. Light microscopy, X 40
*Source:* Reprinted with permission from Naoumidi TL, et al.[5] Conductive keratoplasty: histological study of human corneas. Am J Ophthalmol. 2005;140:984-92. © Elsevier

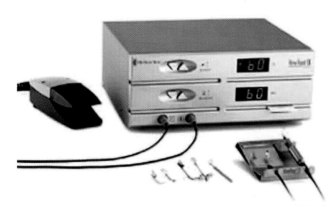

**Fig. 3:** The ViewPoint CK System (Refractec, Inc. Bloomington, MN) consists of a radiofrequency energy-generating console, reusable corneal marker, reusable lid speculum, reusable handpiece, disposable keratoplasty tip, and a footpedal controller
*Source*: Photo courtesy of Refractec, Inc. Bloomington, MN

| Number of Treatment Spots | Treatment Zone Diameter | Correction |
|---|---|---|
| 8 | 7 mm | 0.75 D to 0.875 D |
| 16 | 6 and 7 mm | 1.00 D to 1.0625 D |
| 24 | 6, 7, and 8 mm | 1.75 D to 2.25 D |
| 32 | 6, 7, 8 mm, and in between at 7 mm | 2.375 D to 3.0 D |

**Table 1:** Nomogram for number and placement of treatment spots to achieve desired correction

Appropriate hyperopic patients for CK are over 40, have stable sphere between +0.75 D and +3.25 D with less than 0.75 D of astigmatism, and have a corneal thickness of at least 560 μm at the 6 mm optical zone. Conductive keratoplasty can also be used for the induction of −1.00 D to −2.00 D myopia to improve near vision in the nondominant eye of presbyopic hyperopes or emmetropes. Such patients should have eye dominance assessed with motor and optical techniques and near dominance should be considered.

Conductive keratoplasty treatment spots are evenly spaced in a ring pattern of 6, 7, and/or 8 mm in diameter (Fig. 4). The number of treatment spots is determined by the desired correction (Table 1).[6] Originally, the recommendation for surgeons was to depress the corneal surface

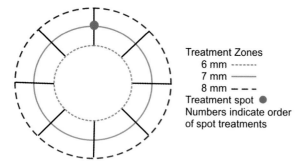

Treatment Zones
6 mm -------
7 mm ———
8 mm – – –
Treatment spot ●
Numbers indicate order of spot treatments

**Fig. 4:** Diagram of radiofrequency spot placements and the order in which the spots are to be applied. Treatment spots are placed at the intersection of the straight lines with each ring. For 16, 24, and 32 spot treatments, spots should be placed around the 6 mm ring first, followed by the 7 mm ring, and finally the 8 mm ring when necessary. The numbers indicate the order in which the treatment spots should be placed

5–7 mm while applying radiofrequency energy. Preliminary information suggests that using the LightTouch, technique, which is application of neutral pressure, improves the effect of CK compared to the FDA studies of standard CK. In standard CK, the probe tip depresses the corneal surface 5–7 mm while applying radiofrequency energy. This causes a mechanical stretching effect on the corneal fibers that resists the natural tendency of the tissue being drawn toward the pulse of RF energy. In LightTouch CK, pressure of the probe on the cornea is neutral, or about 2 mm. This low-compression technique may produce more robust results by minimizing the corneal stretching associated with the standard CK technique (Fig. 5).[7]

A template (OptiPoint Corneal Template, Refractec, Inc. Bloomington, MN) has also been developed to help standardize the CK technique. The template is a light-vacuum suction ring with holes for insertion of the radiofrequency tip. The template is centered on the estimated line of sight allowing accurate placement and depth of the probe tip. Thus compression is limited as with the LightTouch technique, but the tip is still able to penetrate the stroma as in standard CK. In addition, template use allows for more predictable spot placement which reduces induced astigmatism.[8]

## Patient Selection

As mentioned, patients seeking CK treatment for hyperopia should be at least 40 years of age with +0.75 D to +3.25 D of hyperopia. For patients seeking CK monovision as a treatment for presbyopia, they should be hyperopes between +1.00 D and +2.25 D or emmetropes. Peripheral pachymetry reading at the 6 mm optical zone should be less than 560 μm. Excellent uncorrected distance visual acuity (UCDVA) is paramount in the distance eye. Like all refractive procedures, contact lens wearers should discontinue use of their lenses 1–3 weeks prior to the procedure (soft lenses 1 week, hard/rigid lenses 3 weeks).

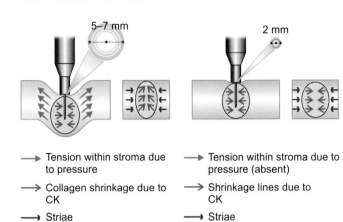

Tension within stroma due to pressure → Tension within stroma due to pressure (absent)

Collagen shrinkage due to CK → Shrinkage lines due to CK

Striae → Striae

**Fig. 5:** In standard CK, the probe tip depresses the corneal surface 5–7 mm while applying radiofrequency energy (Left). This causes a mechanical stretching effect on the corneal fibers that resists the natural tendency of the tissue being drawn toward the pulse of RF energy. In LightTouch CK, pressure of the probe on the cornea is neutral, or about 2 mm. This low-compression technique may produce more robust results by minimizing the corneal stretching associated with the standard CK technique
*Source*: Photo courtesy of Refractec, Inc. Bloomington, MN

For presbyopic patients, eye dominance should be established as previously described to determine the nondominant eye for treatment. Patient education is also critical for this group. They must understand that they will have a good range of functional vision, but may need to use reading glasses for small print or in dim light.

All patients should be counseled that there will be an initial period of myopic overcorrection until 3 to 6 months postoperative which may require temporary spectacles for tasks such as driving. In addition, they must understand that presbyopia is a progressive condition and that retreatment may be necessary in the future.

## Procedure

The CK procedure can be performed under topical anesthesia. Once the desired correction has been determined and the treatment nomogram determined, the patient is placed supine under the operating microscope and the lid speculum inserted. With the patient fixating on a coaxial microscope light, the corneal surface is dried. The CK marker is dampened with gentian violet and centered over the cornea to mark the 6 mm, 7 mm, and 8 mm optical zones and the hash marks designating the positions for CK spot treatments. Centration of the marker on the estimated line of sight is crucial for effective CK treatment.

Treatment spots are applied according to the surgical plan with special care taken to ensure appropriate pressure, tip placement and tip orientation—normal to the corneal

surface. After application of radiofrequency energy, remove the probe. Treatment spots should be placed with a regular cadence in the indicated order. The procedure should be efficient to avoid excessive corneal drying; aiming for one minute or less per series eight spots.

## Efficacy

The US FDA clinical trial was carried out with 20 surgeons at 13 centers. Patients were at least 40 years of age. Study eyes had +0.75 D to +3.00 D hyperopia and 0.76 D or less of cylinder preoperatively and were targeted for plano postoperatively. At 1 year postoperatively, 56% (178/318) of eyes achieved UCDVA of 20/20 or better and 92% (294/318) of eyes achieved 20/40 or better (Fig. 6).[9] Mean manifest refractive spherical equivalent was initially slightly myopic (−0.52 D) and stabilized at 6 months near emmetropia (+0.22 D).[9]

Smaller studies of CK for hyperopia showed similar efficacy results. At 1 year, an UCDVA of 20/20 or better was achieved by 41% (13 of 32) eyes, 59% (19/32) achieved 20/25 or better and 91% (29 of 32) eyes achieved 20/40 or better in a study by Kymionis et al.[10] Pallikaris et al. followed 38 eyes for 30 months after CK for hyperopia. Mean UCDVA went from 0.42(20/40) ± 0.22 preoperative to 0.9(20/25) ± 0.29 at 30 months.[11] Results from Lin and Manche demonstrated improved UCDVA from preop, at which time 35% (8/23) of eyes achieved 20/40 UCDVA or better. Two years postoperatively, 64% (14/21) of eyes had a UCDVA of 20/20 or better, 82% (18/21) had 20/25 or better, and 95% (2122) had 20/40 or better.[12]

One year results from the FDA clinical trial for the use of CK to induce monovision as a treatment for presbyopia demonstrated J1 or better uncorrected near visual acuity (UCNVA) for 38% (20/53) of eyes and J3 or better for 81% (43/53) of eyes treated for near vision. Binocular UCNVA of J1 or better was achieved by 47% (25/53) of patients and J3 or better by 89% (47/53) of patients. Binocular UCDVA was 20/20 or better for 97% (60/62) of patients and 20/40 or better for all patients (62/62). Combined binocular uncorrected near and distance visual acuities are shown in Figure 7.[13]

Ye et al. followed 27 patients who underwent CK for monovision as a correction of presbyopia. Mean UCNVA of the CK eye went from 0.92(20/166) ± 0.16 before treatment to 0.30(20/40) ± 0.13 12 months after treatment (P < 0.05).[14]

Stahl et al. reported longer term data on 10 eyes of 10 patients who underwent CK in the nondominant eye to

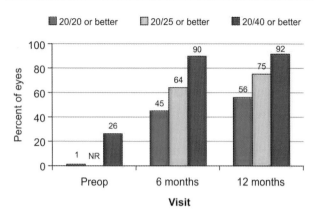

**Fig. 6:** Postoperative Snellen uncorrected distance visual acuities *Source*: McDonald MB, Hersh PS, Manche EE, et al. Conductive Keratoplasty for the Correction of Low to moderate Hyperopia: US Clinical Trial 1-Year Results on 355 Eyes. Ophthalmology. 2002;109(11):1978-89. NR: Not Reported

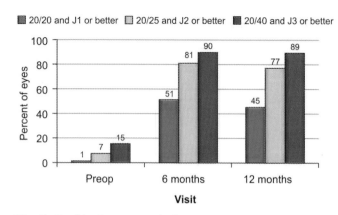

**Fig. 7:** Combined uncorrected distance and near visual acuities. Snellen score indicates minimum distance vision for group and Jaeger score indicates minimum near vision for each group
*Source*: US FDA Refracted ViewPoint™ CK® System - P010018/S005 March 16, 2004. http://www.accessdata.fda.gov/scripts/cdrh/cfdocs/cfTopic/pma/pma.cfm?num=P010018S005. Accessed May 12, 2011

treat presbyopia. Preoperatively, one patient had binocular UCDVA of 20/30 or better and UCNVA of J5 or better. This improved at 1-year post-CK (n = 10) to eight patients with binocular UCDVA of 20/20 or better and J1 or better UCNVA. All patients had UCDVA 20/40 and UCNVA J3. At 3 years postoperative (n = 9), two patients achieved 20/20 UCDVA and J1 UCNVA or better and 7 achieved 20/40 UCDVA and J3 UCNVA or better.[15,16]

Conductive Keratoplasty has also been used to correct hyperopic refractive error after cataract or refractive surgery.[17-19] Claramonte reported that after cataract surgery, only 25% of a group of 16 eyes achieved a UCDVA of 20/40 or better due to residual hyperopia. After refractive adjustment with CK, 62.5% of eyes had a UCDVA of 20/40 or better at 12 months postoperative.[17]

Conductive Keratoplasty in 39 eyes of 38 patients for the treatment of presbyopia with monovision demonstrated good refractive stability and predictability in eyes that had previously had LASIK surgery and eyes that had no previous surgery. The binocular outcomes at 1 year postoperative were similar for the post-LASIK and non-LASIK groups. After CK treatment in the nondominant eye, binocular mean UCDVA was −0.18 ± 0.00(20/13) in the post-LASIK group and −0.09 ± 0.12(20/16) in the non-LASIK group and mean UCNVA was 0.22 ± 0.25(20/33) and 0.20 ± 0.17(20/31) respectively.[19]

## Safety

One of the advantages of CK is the safety of the procedure. Unlike LASIK, corneal manipulations with CK are peripheral. They do not directly affect the visual axis or

ablate corneal tissue. Across 11 studies that reported safety as lines of BCVA lost, 7 of a total of 770 eyes (1%) lost 2 lines of BCDVA.[2,9-14,16-18,17,18] All seven patients with a 2 line loss of BCDVA were part of the initial FDA clinical trial treating hyperopia,[9] exceeding FDA safety standards.

Effects of the radiofrequency waves do not damage the corneal endothelium. Histological changes are minimal in the endothelial layer[5,9] and endothelial cell counts at the corneal periphery, mid-periphery and centrally showed no significant change from preoperative values after 1 year of follow-up.[9]

Contrast sensitivity is also spared with CK. Because the treatment zones are at the periphery of the cornea, post-operative contrast sensitivity measurements remain within normal limits.[9,11,14]

## Predictability

Predictability of hyperopic corrections by reshaping the corneal curvature is more variable than myopic corrections due to the increased difficulty of precisely steepening the corneal curvature to decrease hyperopia. Variability in centration of optical zone, angle of treatment tip, and depth of tip in the stroma can all affect the refractive correction achieved. Predictability in most published studies of CK for hyperopia is acceptable (Table 2)[21] and within the range reported for LASIK treatment for hyperopia.[19-20]

## Stability

One of the main issues with all corneal treatments for hyperopia is regression over time. Most CK treated eyes show

**Table 2:** Difference between targeted and achieved MRSE in eyes treated with conductive keratoplasty

| Study | n | Follow-up (Months) | MRSE within ± 0.5 D of Target | MRSE within ±1.0 D of Target |
|---|---|---|---|---|
| Tomita[19] | 5 | 12 | 50.0% | 100.0% |
| Claramonte[17] | 16 | 12 | 56.3% | 81.3% |
| Ayoubi[21] | 32 | 12 | 46.9% | 75.0% |
| McDonald[9] | 318 | 12 | 63.0% | 89.0% |
| Ye[14] | 38 | 12 | 68.0% | 92.0% |
| P010018/S005[13] | 63 | 12 | 0.0% | 0.0% |
| Lin[12] | 22 | 24 | 64.0% | 91.0% |
| Naoumibi[20] | 47 | 24 | 61.0% | 83.0% |
| Pallikaris[11] | 30 | 30 | 68.0% | 92.0% |
| Stahl[16] | 10 | 36 | 44.0% | 100.0% |
| Chang[18] | 7 | 3–24 | 71.4% | 85.7% |
| Kymionis[10] | 32 | 8–18 | 21.0% | 26.0% |
| Ehrlich[26] | 16 | 44–90 | 6.3% | 43.7% |

a slight myopic overcorrection initially after treatment that resolves and stabilizes at 3–6 months postoperative.[9,11,13,26] There are few studies of CK that report results beyond 1-year postoperative.

Two studies with 24 months of follow-up report showed decreasing changes in MRSE between visits over time. Mean MRSE changed −0.05 D between 3 and 6 months, −0.16 D between 6 and 12 months, and +0.02 D between 12 and 24 months post CK in a study of 47 eyes treated for hyperopic astigmatism.[21] Eighteen eyes treated for low to moderate myopia showed a similar pattern of change in MRSE between visits. The mean change in MRSE was +0.057 D per month between 3 and 6 months, +0.033 D per month between 6 and 9 months, +0.027 D per month between 9 and 12 months, and +0.024 D per month between 12 and 24 months.[12]

With a 30 month follow-up, Pallikaris et al. reported a mean change in MRSE of +0.06 D between 3 and 6 months after surgery, +0.01 D between 6 and 12 months, and +0.04 D between 12 and 24 months postoperatively.[11]

A small study (16 eyes of 9 patients) with a mean follow-up of 73.1 months (range 44 to 90 months) showed mean SE regressed from +0.295 ± 0.31 D at 12 months to +1.00 ± 0.35 at 4 years and +1.39 ± 0.31 at the final visit, which was similar to the preoperative SE of 1.45 ± 0.29 D. Using linear regression, the authors suggest a rate of regression of

+0.0184 D per month after 6 months postoperative. This difference in SE between visits was statistically significant.[21]

Pallikaris et al. noted their 30 month CK results demonstrated greater postoperative stability than stability reported for eyes treated with LASIK or PRK for low to moderate hyperopia.[11] Conversely, Ayoubi et al. have recently reported that femtosecond LASIK provides more stable correction in emmetropic presbyopes undergoing monovision than light-touch CK, with 50% of CK patients requiring retreatment.[21]

Confounding the estimation of the refractive stability of CK is the natural progression of hyperopia over time. Ehrlich et al. estimated the rate of refractive regression after CK as +0.0184 D per month after 6 months postoperatively. From that series they also report one untreated fellow eye with a change of +0.50 D 3 months after treatment.[26] Stahl et al. reported data on 9 of 10 eyes treated with CK for presbyopic monovision with a 3-year follow-up. There was no significant change in keratometry between 1 and 3 years postoperative. During this 2-year period, the MRSE of the treated eyes showed a mean change in MRSE of +0.25 D. In this same study, there was a mean change in MRSE of +0.18 D-year over the study period for untreated fellow eyes, an amount similar to the 'regression' of effect in the CK treated eyes.[16]

## ▶ SURGICALLY-INDUCED ASTIGMATISM

Hersh has reported that the amount of surgically induced astigmatism (SIA) increases as the number of treatment spots increases. Mean magnitude of SIA in 203 eyes treated for hyperopia was 0.64 ± 0.40 D in eyes treated with eight spots, 0.61 ± 0.46 D with 16 spots, 0.69 ± 0.42 D with 24 spots and 0.74 ± 0.38 D in eyes with 32 treatment spots. The increase in absolute cylinder decrease over time postoperatively.[2] In the FDA clinical trial for hyperopia, an increase in cylinder greater than or equal to 1.0 D was reported in 21% of patients at 1 month, 14% at 6 months, and 6% at 12 months postoperative.[9] Results from the clinical trial for presbyopia were similar: 28% at 1 month, 9.6% at 6 months, and 8% at 12 months.[13] Smaller studies reported no eyes with over 1.0 D of SIA at their final visit.[12,14,16,19] One exception was one eye in the study by Tomita that had a greater than 1.0 D increase in SIA, but maintained a BCDVA of 20/13.[19]

## Complications

Intraoperative complications or adverse events are rare in published reports of CK.[2,9,11-14,16,21] Most common symptoms are those reported for all refractive procedures, glare, halos, variable vision in dim light, and light sensitivity, none of which are rated as severe.

## Patient Evaluation

Data reported on subjective patient satisfaction after CK suggests patient satisfaction was high. Seventy-nine to ninety-two percent of patients were satisfied or extremely satisfied with their outcomes.[9,11-14] At 2 years postoperative, 92% of patients reported improved quality of vision after the CK procedure.[12] Patients treated for presbyopia also reported high levels of spectacle independence for all distances.[14] An exception is a study by Ayoubi comparing LASIK to CK which found lower levels of satisfaction (34.4% of 32 patients) for the CK group compared to the LASIK group.[21]

## ▶ CONCLUSION

Conductive keratoplasty for the treatment of hyperopia and induction of myopia in presbyopic monovision is effective, predictable and safe. The procedure does not involve tissue removal and spares the visual axis. The procedure avoids flap complications in theory preserves the biomechanical properties and corneal sensitivity properties of the cornea. Contrast sensitivity is not impaired, and patient satisfaction is high at 3 years postoperatively. The system is easily portable and the procedure can be done in an office setting under topical anesthesia. Drawbacks include the initial myopic shift after treatment and the lack of consensus as to the long-term stability of the results. Hopefully, continued standardization of the procedure and consistent studies of long-term stability will improve both our understanding and implementation of the CK procedure.

*Note*: The authors have no financial interest in any devices mentioned herein.

## ▶ REFERENCES

1. Lans LJ. Experimentelle Untersuchungen uber Entstehung von Astigmatismus durch nicht-perforirende Corneawunden. Graefes. Arch Ophthalmol. 1889;44:117-52.
2. Hersh PS. Optics of conductive keratoplasty: implications for presbyopia management. Trans Am Ophthalmol Soc. 2005;103:412-56.
3. Mendez A, Mendez Noble A. Conductive keratoplasty for the correction of hyperopia. In: Sher NA (ed). Surgery for Hyperopia and Presbyopia. Baltimore: Williams & Wilkens; 1997. pp. 163-71.
4. Choi B, Kim J, Welch AJ, et al. Dynamic impedance measurements during radio-frequency heating of cornea. IEEE Trans Biomed Eng. 2002;49:1610-6.
5. Naoumidi TL, Pallikaris IG, Naoumidi II, et al. Conductive keratoplasty: histological study of human corneas. Am J Ophthalmol. 2005;140:984-92.
6. US FDA Refractec ViewPoint CK System P010018. April 20, 2002. http://www.accessdata.fda.gov/scripts/cdrh/cfdocs/cfPMA/pma.cfm?id=15339. Accessed May 12, 2011.
7. Asbell PA, Tinio B, Ahdoot M, et al. Effect of neutral pressure conductive keratoplasty over six months in the treatment of hyperopia and presbyopia. Invest Ophthalmol Vis Sci. 2006;47(Suppl):S5864.
8. Stahl ED, Durrie DS. Template-Guided Conductive Keratoplasty Using the ViewPoint CK System for Optimizing Near Vision. Presented at the Annual Meeting of the ASCRS April 27-May, 22007, San Diego, CA. Abstract # 299724.
9. McDonald MB, Hersh PS, Manche EE, et al. Conductive Keratoplasty for the Correction of Low to Moderate Hyperopia: US Clinical Trial 1-Year Results on 355 Eyes. Ophthalmology. 2002;109(11):1978-89.
10. Kymionis GD, Naoumidi TL, Aslanides IM, et al. Intraocular pressure measurements after conductive keratoplasty. J Refract Surg. 2005;21(2):171-5.
11. Pallikaris IG, Naoumidi TL, Astyrakakis NI. Long-term results of conductive keratoplasty for low to moderate hyperopia. J Cataract Refract Surg. 2005;31(8):1520-9.
12. Lin DY, Manche EE. Two-year results of conductive keratoplasty for the correction of low to moderate hyperopia. J Cataract Refract Surg. 2003;29(12):2339-50.
13. US FDA Refracted ViewPoint™ CK® System - P010018/S005 March 16, 2004. http://www.accessdata.fda.gov/scripts/cdrh/cfdocs/cfTopic/pma/pma.cfm?num=P010018S005. Accessed May 12, 2011.
14. Ye P, Xu W, Tang X, et al. Conductive keratoplasty for symptomatic presbyopia following monofocal intraocular lens implantation. Clin Experiment Ophthalmol. 2010;39(5):404-11.doi: 10.1111/j.1442-9071.2010.02464.x.
15. Stahl JE. Conductive Keratoplasty for Presbyopia: 1-year Results. J Refract Surg. 2006;22(2):137-44.
16. Stahl JE. Conductive Keratoplasty for Presbyopia: 3-year Results. J Refract Surg. 2007;23(9):905-10.
17. Claramonte PJ, Alio′ JL, Ramzy MI. Conductive keratoplasty to correct residual hyperopia after cataract surgery. J Cataract Refract Surg. 2006;32:1445-51.
18. Chang JSM, Lau SYF. Conductive Keratoplasty to Treat Hyperopic Overcorrection After LASIK for Myopia. J Refract Surg. 2011;27:49-55.
19. Tomita M, Watabe M, Ito M, et al. Conductive keratoplasty for the treatment of presbyopia: comparative study between post- and non-LASIK eyes. Clin Ophthalmol. 2011;5:231-7.
20. Naoumidi TL, Kounis GA, Astyrakakis NI, et al. Two-year follow-up of conductive keratoplasty for the treatment of hyperopic astigmatism. J Cataract Refract Surg. 2006;32(5):732-41.

21. Ayoubi MG, Leccisotti A, Goodall EA, et al. Femtosecond laser in situ keratomileusis versus conductive keratoplasty to obtain monovision in patients with emmetropic presbyopia. J Cataract Refract Surg. 2010;36(6):997-1002.

22. US FDA. Technolas 217A Excimer Laser System. P990027/S004. February 25,2003. http://www.fda.gov/cdrh/pdf/p990027S004. html. Accessed June 3, 2011.

23. US FDA. Visx Star S2 and S3 Excimer Laser Systems. P930016/S012. April 27, 2001. http://www.fda.gov/cdrh/pdf/ p930016s012.html. Accessed June 3, 2011.

24. US FDA, WaveLight ALLEGRETTO WAVE™ Excimer Laser System. P030008. October 10, 2003. http://www.fda.gov/cdrh/ PDF3/p030008.html. Accessed June 3, 2011.

25. Autrata R, Rehurek J. Laser-assisted subepithelial keratectomy and photorefractive keratectomy for the correction of hyperopia: Results of a 2-year follow-up. J Cataract Refract Surg. 2003;29(11):2105-14.

26. Ehrlich JS, Manche EE. Regression of effect over long-term follow-up of conductive keratoplasty to correct mild to moderate hyperopia. J Cataract Refract Surg. 2009;35(9):1591-6.

# CHAPTER 97

# Incisional Surgery for Natural and Surgically-Induced Astigmatism

*Matthew D Council*

## ❧ INTRODUCTION

As patients' expectations regarding visual outcomes after cataract surgery increase and as modern presbyopia-correcting lenses become more common, management of pre-existing and surgically-induced astigmatism becomes increasingly important. The surgical correction of astigmatism has thus become an important component of modern eye surgery.

Currently, multiple methods of correcting corneal astigmatism exist. These include placement of the main corneal incision on the steep axis or the use of paired corneal incisions[1], the use of a toric intraocular lens (IOL), limbal relaxing incisions (LRIs), and refractive laser surgery. Excellent visual outcomes can be obtained with the use of later generation toric IOLs and modern refractive laser surgery. However, not all patients may be candidates for these techniques secondary to the cost of the treatment or the amount of corneal astigmatism. In these cases, LRIs represent an excellent alternative or adjunctive technique. The discussion of toric lenses and refractive laser surgery is outside the scope of this chapter. This chapter will focus on the use of LRIs for the correction of corneal astigmatism.

Astigmatic keratotomy has been used since 1980s. Over the past decade and a half, the use of LRIs has become increasingly common. The availability of several established nomograms and an online calculator has facilitated the acceptance of this technique. Compared to astigmatic keratotomy, LRIs are more forgiving and less likely to induce irregular astigmatism. In a recent survey, one third of cataract surgeons chose LRIs as their preferred method of correcting pre-existing astigmatism.[2] Numerous studies have shown this technique to be safe and effective.[3-9] This chapter will provide an overview of the necessary steps to utilize this important technique.

## ❧ PATIENT SELECTION

Careful assessment of a patient's corneal astigmatism is an essential component of any preoperative exam. Even if it is not the intent of the patient or surgeon to address this issue at the time of cataract surgery, the patient should be advised of their likely need for spectacles postoperatively if they have a significant amount of pre-existing astigmatism. When correction of astigmatism is planned, a goal of less than one diopter of residual astigmatism is desired when using traditional monofocal lenses. For modern presbyopia-correcting surgery, less than 0.5 diopters of postoperative cylinder should be the goal. There are few patient contraindications to this technique. However, this technique should not be used in patients with pre-existing corneal disorders, such as keratoconus or a neurotrophic cornea.

## ❧ PREOPERATIVE MEASUREMENTS

Care should be taken preoperatively to correctly identify the amount and axis of the patient's corneal astigmatism. The patient's pre-existing spectacle correction or a recent manifest refraction may indicate prior astigmatic correction. The astigmatism may also be identified when taking keratometry measurements as part of preoperative biometry.

It is recommended to verify the patient's astigmatism using several different methods. Manual keratometry can be used to quantify the amount and axis of the astigmatism. Corneal topography is useful for several reasons (Fig. 1).

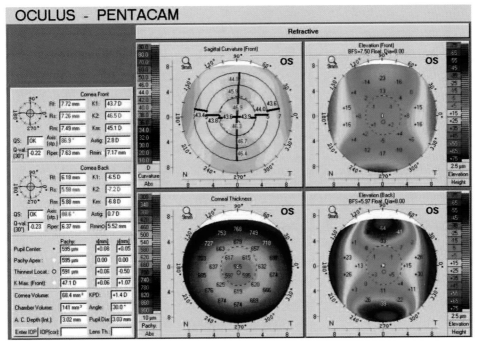

**Fig. 1:** Corneal topography showing with-the-rule astigmatism suitable for correction by LRIs

Topography can show irregular astigmatism, such as that from anterior basement membrane dystrophy that may not be correctable by surgical management alone. It can also alert the physician to forme fruste keratoconus or other ectatic disease. Limbal relaxing incisions are not recommended in the setting of abnormal topography as they may lead to worsening of ectasia.[10,11] Finally, the preoperative K's can further be documented with an autokeratometer or with the K readings from the IOL master.

As a general rule, the K values from these different modalities should all agree. Sometimes, the astigmatic correction in the manifest refraction or old spectacle correction may not agree with the other measurements. This can be due to lenticular astigmatism, which will be eliminated at the time of cataract surgery. In this setting, however, the measurements from the other modalities should agree. If there is conflicting data, it may be wise to defer surgical correction of astigmatism at the time of cataract removal. The astigmatism can always be corrected at a later date when measurements have stabilized. This can be accomplished with the use of LRIs done in the operating room or the office or with refractive laser surgery. One advantage of refractive laser surgery is that any residual refractive error may then also be corrected at the same time.

In author's practice, corneal topography is used to identify the main axis of the astigmatism. Manual keratometry is used to quantify the amount of cylinder to be corrected. The K readings from the IOL master are used to determine the average K value for IOL calculations.

## NOMOGRAMS

Numerous nomograms for LRIs exist. Two of the most commonly used are the DONO or Donnenfeld nomogram (designed by Eric Donnenfeld) and the Nichamin Age and Pachymetry Adjusted (NAPA) nomogram (designed by Louis Nichamin). Knowing the age of the patient and the amount of astigmatism to be corrected, the following tables can be consulted to determine the number and length of the LRIs (Tables 1 to 3). More precise results can be obtained through the use of computer software which takes into account the placement and astigmatic effect of the main phacoemulsification incision. Through the use of vector analysis, this software can model these different effects and produce a surgical plan which includes an estimate of the expected residual astigmatism.[12] When using vector analysis in this way, it is helpful for the surgeon to be aware of the average amount of astigmatism induced by their surgical technique. Software is available for a surgeon to track their surgical outcomes and to obtain this information.[13] Similarly, software is available for surgical planning when some toric IOLs are utilized.[14] Regardless of the nomogram

CHAPTER **97**

**Table 1:** The Donnenfeld nomogram for LRIs[20]

| Preoperative Astigmatism | Number of Incisions | Length of Incisions (Clock Hours) |
|---|---|---|
| 0.50 D | 1 | 1.5 |
| 0.75 D | 2 | 1 |
| 1.50 D | 2 | 2 |
| 3.00 D | 2 | 3 |

*All incisions are placed 0.5 mm from the limbus in the correct axis.*

*Patients who have against-the-rule astigmatism or who are less than 45 years old may benefit from slightly longer incisions. Shorter incisions may be indicated for patients older than 65 years.*

used, the surgical plan should be physically documented for use at the time of surgery. Clear documentation of the plan will lessen the risk of off-axis or wrong-axis surgery, which could worsen the patient's pre-existing astigmatism.

## ❧ TECHNIQUE

Limbal relaxing incisions may be performed at the time of cataract surgery or as a standalone procedure performed in the operating suite or the office procedure room. The technique is similar in both cases. The eye must be marked preoperatively as a reference for axis determination. This is best done with the patient in an upright position in primary gaze before they have received sedation. When a patient reclines, the eye may cyclotort in an unpredictable fashion, making upright marking essential.[15] Several different methods exist for marking the cornea preoperatively. All involve placing reference marks to aid in later alignment with an axis marker in surgery (Fig. 2). Marks are frequently placed at 3, 6 and 9 o'clock.

After the eye is marked, the patient is prepared for surgery in the usual fashion. The LRIs are usually performed before the removal of the cataract at the start of the case. Pachymetry measurements can be taken over the peripheral cornea before the prep if using the pachymetry-adjusted NAPA nomogram. Following the prep, an axis marker is aligned with the previously placed corneal marks. The beginning and end point of each LRI is then identified and/or marked. An additional mark may be made for placement of the main phaco incision. Viscoelastic is then placed over

**Table 2:** Nichamin nomogram with empiric 600-micron blade depth setting[21,22]

Intralimbal relaxing incision nomogram for modern phaco surgery: empiric blade-depth setting of 600 μm

Spherical (up to + 0.75 × 90 or + 0.50 × 180)

*Incision design*: 'Neutral' temporal clear corneal incision (i.e., 3.5 mm or less, single plane, just anterior to vascular arcade)

Against-the-rule, (Steep axis 0–44°/136–180°)

Paired incisions in degrees of arc

| Preoperative cylinder | 30–40 y | 41–50 y | 51–60 y | 61–70 y | 71–80 y | 81–90 y | 90+y |
|---|---|---|---|---|---|---|---|
| | Nasal limbal arc only | | | | | 35° | |
| + 0.75 to + 1.25 | 55° | 50° | 45° | 40° | 35° | | |
| + 1.50 to + 2.00 | 70° | 65° | 60° | 55° | 45° | 40° | 35° |
| + 2.25 to + 2.75 | 90° | 80° | 70° | 60° | 50° | 45° | 40° |
| + 3.00 to + 3.75 | 70° | 90° | 85° | 70° | 60° | 50° | 45° |
| | o.z = 5 mm | o.z = 9 mm | | | | | |

*Incision design*: The temporal incision, if greater than 40° of arc, is made by first creating a two-plane, grooved phaco incision (600 μ depth), which is then extended to the appropriate arc length at the conclusion of surgery.

With-the-rule, (Steep axis 45°–135°)

| + 1.00 to + 1.50 | 50° | 45° | 40° | 35° | 30° | | |
| + 1.75 to + 2.25 | 60° | 55° | 50° | 45° | 40° | 35° | 30° |
| + 2.50 to + 3.00 | 70° | 65° | 60° | 55° | 50° | 45° | 40° |
| + 3.25 to + 3.75 | 80° | 75° | 70° | 65° | 60° | 55° | 45° |

*Incision design*: 'Neutral' temporal clear corneal along with the following peripheral accurate incisions.

When placing intralimbal relaxing incisions following or concomitant with radial relaxing incisions, total arc length is decreased by 50%

**Table 3:** Nichamin nomogram with adjustable blade depth[21,22]

Intralimbal arcuate astigmatic nomogram

With-the-rule (Steep axis 45°–135°)

| Preoperative cylinder (Diopters) | Paired incisions in degrees of arc | | | | | |
|---|---|---|---|---|---|---|
| | 20–30 yrs old | 30–40 yrs old | 41–50 yrs old | 51–60 yrs old | 61–70 yrs old | 71–80 yrs old |
| 0.75 | 40 | 35 | 35 | 30 | 30 | |
| 1.00 | 45 | 40 | 40 | 35 | 35 | 30 |
| 1.25 | 55 | 50 | 45 | 40 | 35 | 35 |
| 1.50 | 60 | 55 | 50 | 45 | 40 | 40 |
| 1.75 | 65 | 60 | 55 | 50 | 45 | 45 |
| 2.00 | 70 | 65 | 60 | 55 | 50 | 45 |
| 2.25 | 75 | 70 | 65 | 60 | 55 | 50 |
| 2.50 | 80 | 75 | 70 | 65 | 60 | 55 |
| 2.75 | 85 | 80 | 75 | 70 | 65 | 60 |
| 3.00 | 90 | 90 | 85 | 80 | 70 | 65 |

Against-the-rule (Steep axis 0–44°/136–180°)

| | 20–30 yrs old | 30–40 yrs old | 41–50 yrs old | 51–60 yrs old | 61–70 yrs old | 71–80 yrs old |
|---|---|---|---|---|---|---|
| 0.75 | 45 | 40 | 40 | 35 | 35 | 30 |
| 1.00 | 50 | 45 | 45 | 40 | 40 | 35 |
| 1.25 | 55 | 55 | 50 | 45 | 40 | 35 |
| 1.50 | 60 | 60 | 55 | 50 | 45 | 40 |
| 1.75 | 65 | 65 | 60 | 55 | 50 | 45 |
| 2.00 | 70 | 70 | 65 | 60 | 55 | 50 |
| 2.25 | 75 | 75 | 70 | 65 | 60 | 55 |
| 2.50 | 80 | 80 | 75 | 70 | 65 | 60 |
| 2.75 | 85 | 85 | 80 | 75 | 70 | 65 |
| 3.00 | 90 | 90 | 85 | 80 | 75 | 70 |

Blade depth setting is at 90% of the thinnest pachymetry

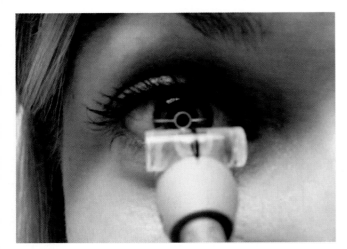

**Fig. 2:** Reference marks are placed at 3 and 9 o'clock with the patient in the upright position

the surface of the cornea overlying the planned incision. A diamond knife or other suitable instrument is then used to make the incision (Fig. 3). One may use a blade preset to 600 microns depth for the DONO nomogram or an adjustable blade, if using the NAPA nomogram (where the blade depth is set to 90% of the thinnest pachymetry reading). The incision is placed in the peripheral cornea just inside the limbus. The blade is fully inserted perpendicular to the corneal surface at one end of the planned LRI. The blade is then drawn back towards the surgeon in a curvilinear fashion to complete the incision. A blunt tip cannula is then swept through the LRI, and balanced salt solution is irrigated through the incision. This ensures that the LRI is complete and not full thickness. The surgeon then proceeds with the remainder of the cataract surgery.

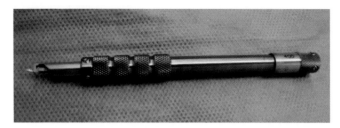

**Fig. 3:** A surgical blade with adjustable depth is used to make the partial thickness incisions

It is possible to overlap the phaco incision with a LRI when necessary in cases of significant against-the-rule astigmatism. If the complete LRI is created before the phaco incision is made, one will often encounter wound gape and leakage around the phaco handpiece, creating a suboptimal surgical environment. To avoid this situation, the surgeon first creates a partial LRI corresponding to the width of the planned phacoemulsification incision. The eye is then entered with the keratome through the previously created LRI. At the end of the case, prior to removal of viscoelastic, the LRI is then extended to its full width.

Postoperative care is the same as with standard cataract surgery, though it is advisable to continue the topical antibiotic until the epithelium over the incision has healed.

## ⯈ COMPLICATIONS

### Infection

As with any incision, infection is possible. Postoperatively, the incision site is monitored closely for signs of infection, and prompt treatment is instituted as needed.

### Bleeding

If there is any pannus, bleeding is sometimes encountered during surgery. This is usually minor and self-limited.

### Full-thickness Perforation

If the cornea is abnormally thin or pachymetry is inaccurate, full-thickness perforation may rarely occur. Based on the incision geometry, these incisions are not self-sealing and cannot be closed with stromal hydration alone. In the case of perforation, the incision is closed with suture. The surgeon may then decide whether to proceed with removal of the cataract or wait until the incision is healed and proceed with cataract surgery at a later date.

### Ectasia

The LRIs weaken the corneal stroma and thus could theoretically lead to postoperative ectasia.[10,11] For this reason, preoperative topography is recommended. If abnormal topography, such as forme fruste keratoconus is identified, LRIs should be avoided.

### Weakening of the Globe

Rupture at the site of prior radial and astigmatic keratotomy sites is possible following trauma.[16]

### Decreased Corneal Sensation

Severing of corneal nerves with the incision may lead to worsening corneal hypesthesia in susceptible individuals. Caution should be advised in patients with decreased corneal sensation.[17]

### Misalignment or Wrong Axis Surgery

Care should be taken when marking the eye preoperatively and when making the incisions. A small alignment error can exist with current marking techniques, which may lessen their effect.[18] If care is not taken, it is possible to place the LRIs on the flat meridian, leading to a worsening or even doubling of the astigmatic error. To prevent these errors, a written surgical plan should be available in the operating suite and should be consulted before the incisions are made.

## ⯈ FUTURE DIRECTIONS

Several different femtosecond lasers have been recently approved or are seeking approval by the US Food and Drug Administration (FDA) for use in cataract surgery.[19] An exciting new application of these lasers is their use for making relaxing incisions to precisely treat corneal astigmatism. As these lasers enter the clinical realm, their accuracy will likely to lead the refinement of existing nomograms, leading to more reproducible and predictable correction of astigmatism at the time of cataract surgery.

## ⯈ CONCLUSION

The identification and management of corneal astigmatism is an essential component of modern cataract surgery. To obtain the best refractive results, astigmatic error must be minimized. Significant advances have been made with newer toric IOLs and with refractive laser surgery. Limbal relaxing incisions are an excellent alternative or adjunctive technique and should be included in the armamentarium of the eye surgeon.

## ✷ REFERENCES

1. Qammar A, Mullaney P. Paired opposite clear corneal incisions to correct preexisting astigmatism in cataract patients. J Cataract Refract Surg. 2005;31(6):1167-70.
2. Bethke W. Toric IOLs are gaining fans. Re Ophthalmol. 2011.
3. Ouchi M, Kinoshita S. Prospective randomized trial of limbal relaxing incisions combined with microincision cataract surgery. J Refract Surg. 2010;26(8):594-9.
4. Cristóbal JA, Del Buey MA, Ascaso FJ, et al. Effect of limbal relaxing incisions during phacoemulsification surgery based on nomogram review and numerical simulation. Cornea. 2009;28(9):1042-9.
5. Carvalho MJ, Suzuki SH, Freitas LL, et al. Limbal relaxing incisions to correct corneal astigmatism during phacoemulsification. J Refract Surg. 2007;23(5):499-504.
6. Kaufmann C, Peter J, Ooi K, et al. Queen Elizabeth Astigmatism Study Group. Limbal relaxing incisions versus on-axis incisions to reduce corneal astigmatism at the time of cataract surgery. J Cataract Refract Surg. 2005;31(12):2261-5.
7. Bayramlar HH, Dağlıoğlu MC, Borazan M. Limbal relaxing incisions for primary mixed astigmatism and mixed astigmatism after cataract surgery. J Cataract Refract Surg. 2003;29(4):723-8.
8. Müller-Jensen K, Fischer P, Siepe U. Limbal relaxing incisions to correct astigmatism in clear corneal cataract surgery. J Refract Surg. 1999;15(5):586-9.
9. Budak K, Friedman NJ, Koch DD. Limbal relaxing incisions with cataract surgery. J Cataract Refract Surg. 1998;24(4):503-8.
10. Shaikh S, Shaikh NM, Manche E. Iatrogenic keratoconus as a complication of radial keratotomy. J Cataract Refract Surg. 2002;28(3):553-5.
11. Wellish KL, Glasgow BJ, Beltran F, et al. Corneal ectasia as a complication of repeated keratotomy surgery. J Refract Corneal Surg. 1994;10(3):360-4.
12. http://www.lricalculator.com/ [Accessed January 2012].
13. http://www.doctor-hill.com/physicians/download.htm [Accessed January 2012].
14. http://www.acrysoftoriccalculator.com/ [Accessed January 2012].
15. Chernyak DA. Cyclotorsional eye motion occurring between wavefront measurement and refractive surgery. J Cataract Refract Surg. 2004;30(3):633-8.
16. Lee BL, Manche EE, Glasgow BJ. Rupture of radial and arcuate keratotomy scars by blunt trauma 91 months after incisional keratotomy. Am J Ophthalmol. 1995;120(1):108-10.
17. Moon SW, Yeom DJ, Chung SH. Neurotrophic corneal ulcer development following cataract surgery with a limbal relaxing incision. Korean J Ophthalmol. 2011;25(3):210-3.
18. Visser N, Berendschot TT, Bauer NJ, et al. Accuracy of toric intraocular lens implantation in cataract and refractive surgery. J Cataract Refract Surg. 2011;37(8):1394-402.
19. Palanker DV, Blumenkranz MS, Andersen D, et al. Femtosecond laser-assisted cataract surgery with integrated optical coherence tomography. Sci Transl Med. 2010;2(58):58-85.
20. Donnenfeld ED. Redeeming the reputation of LRIs. Cataract and Refractive Surgery Today. 2007:48-9.
21. Nichamin LD. Nomogram for limbal relaxing incisions. J Cataract Refract Surg. 2006;32(9):1408.
22. Nichamin LD. Astigmatism control. Ophthalmol Clin North Am. 2006;19(4):485-93.

# CHAPTER 98

# Shaping the Future and Reshaping the Past: The Art of Vision Surgery

*Arun C Gulani*

In our ongoing quest towards achieving a goal of 'Super Vision', we continue to raise the bar on safety and predictability in effort to enable each and every patient to become a candidate for visual freedom!

In order to achieve such high aspirations, we must first believe that there are no limits to refractive surgery options, combinations and stages if we are dedicated to reaching emmetropia in each and every case.

As we shape this future, it is very important that we first understand the past; thus, we shall briefly review the origin of two of the most fundamental refractive surgical procedures (keratomileusis and lamellar keratoplasty), the underlying concepts of which to date remain unchanged, though technology has continued to evolve by leaps and bounds.

## ⯈ HISTORY OF LAMELLAR REFRACTIVE SURGERY (KERATOMILEUSIS AND AUTOMATED LAMELLAR KERATOPLASTY)

Lamellar refractive keratoplasty developed from the original concepts and work of Dr Jose Barraquer at his clinic in Bogota, Columbia. The original myopic keratomileusis technique was a very involved process. A corneal disk of approximately 300 microns thickness was removed in a freehand fashion with a paufique knife or corneal dissector. Dr Barraquer then actually transported this disk of tissue in his car across Bogota to a separate facility, where he glued it onto a contact lens lathe and carved and reshaped the stromal side to thin out the center, creating a concave lens. This lens (no longer a lamellar disk) was then transported back across Bogota to the operating room, where it was repositioned upon the patient's eye. Two interrupted sutures were placed, and a conjunctival flap was raised, inverted and laid over the keratomileusis. The patient's eye was then sewn shut to allow healing.

Overall, the initial patients experienced good results, with 80 percent manifesting a visual improvement. Casimir Swinger, Lee Nordan and Richard Troutman later introduced these techniques to the United States. These pioneers, motivated by achieving procedurally-oriented goals of automation and precision, attempted to improve classical keratomileusis; however, their efforts were largely overcome by the technical difficulties and steep learning curves associated with this new procedure.

Keratomileusis *in situ*, in which a shaping, second resection is made upon the bed after a primary cap is resected, was also developed in Bogota and pioneered by Barraquer and Dr Luiz Ruiz. Their patients experienced both a more rapid recovery of vision and a more comfortable postoperative course. Leo Bores performed the first cases of keratomileusis *in situ* in the United States in November 1987, where he furthered advancement of this technique. Lamellar keratoplasty then later became known as automated lamellar keratoplasty (ALK) when, in the late 1980s, Luis Ruiz developed an automated geared keratome that controlled the speed of the pass across the eye, so that more consistent cuts were possible.

This new keratome and the procedure crafted around it, automated lamellar keratoplasty, have provided ease of technique, rapid recovery and a wide range of potential correction. Early results with this relatively quick and simple technique have been promising. Procedures could be performed safely with topical anesthesia. Moreover, recovery time for the patient improved and there was less suture-induced astigmatism. Disadvantages with this technique, however, included potential irregular astigmatism and loss of caps, which was addressed by returning to Barraquer's original keratomileusis *in situ* procedure using the flap technique. The never-ending quest for higher accuracy eventually incorporated the excimer laser to finally lead to the advent of LASIK (laser-assisted *in situ* keratomileusis) as we know it today.

Keratomileusis and lamellar corneal surgeries can be combined into a modern day concept, in which laser refractive surgery is the keratomileusis and lamellar corneal manipulations become preparatory (to prepare for laser vision surgery) or reparatory (to repair laser vision surgery complications) in leading the patients to emmetropia.

## ❧ GULANI CARDINAL RULES FOR REFRACTIVE SURGEONS

1. For any patient coming to clinic to be evaluated for laser vision surgery, there exists no such query as 'Am I a candidate?' Any patient who has a normal eye, with a normal optic nerve and brain, deserves perfect vision.
2. A 'refractive surgeon' must know how to 'refract', i.e. Garbage In-Garbage Out.
3. I do not believe in differentiating between cornea, LASIK and cataract surgeons. We are all 'vision corrective' surgeons!
4. There is no case that is 'complex'. Every case is 'unique'. By this concept, there is also no case that is 'routine'.

Given these rules, every patient with a normal eye is a candidate for vision corrective surgery, and it is our responsibility to take the time to customize a plan for their individual quest for improved vision.

Towards this endeavor, the author has suggested the 5S system leading to a superspecialty of Corneoplastique™. In this system, a plan is devised to reshape the cornea using the excimer laser appropriately, in keeping with the goals of refractive treatment specific to each case. The goal at all times, for patients and surgeons both, should be unaided 20/20 vision for the patient. The five Ss stand for Shape, Sight, Scar, Site and Strength (Fig. 1). The 5S system addresses the following questions in order to customize a treatment plan that provides optimum visual outcomes for the patient:

*Sight*: Is the patient correctable to 20/20 with glasses and/or gas permeable contact lenses?
*Site*: Is the involvement central or peripheral?
*Scar*: Is the cornea clear or opaque?
*Strength*: Is the cornea thick or thin?
*Shape*: Is the curvature steep, flat, or is there astigmatism (regular/irregular)?

No matter what the etiology, the 5S system can determine the pathology and direct appropriate management.[1,2]

This system can be applied to every refractive patient of myopia, hyperopia, and astigmatism seeking vision beyond 20/20, as well as to those patients who have undergone previous refractive surgery who are seeking 20/20 vision once again. The author's goal is to achieve the very best vision possible for each patient.

This latter population of patients, those who have already undergone refractive surgery, consists of millions of people who constitute, in the author's opinion, an

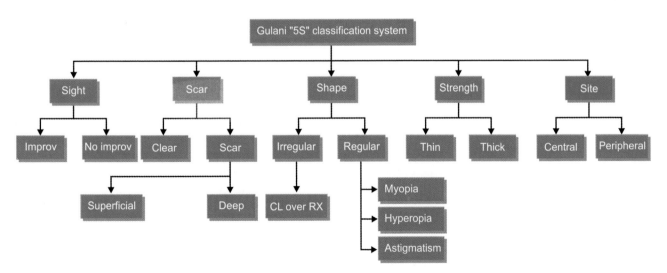

**Fig. 1:** Gulani 5S classification system

emerging epidemic in the world of ophthalmology, for which physicians need to prepare. Most of these patients can be corrected back to enjoy the excellent vision that they had once appreciated using modern technology. In a way, turning back the clock![3,4] One must make their diagnosis based on clinical evaluations along with surgical plan based on a logical approach to excellent vision. In this setting, such patients may be approached using the previously mentioned laser corneoplastique concept, along with the 5S classification system, to allow the author to practically address any previous refractive surgery in turning back the clock and once again aiming for unaided emmetropia with modern technologies.[5,6]

For the case of previous refractive surgeries, a newly-proposed classification system is described below that may be beneficial in clarifying the subjective and objective principles to keep in mind when approaching such patients. This system may be universally applied in studying the surgery, clarifying the visual effects-complaint relationship, and planning steps in rehabilitation of vision for the patient.

The classification system may be divided into primary and secondary visual factors that both aid in the patient evaluation process and simplify a universal approach to diagnosis and surgical planning.[7] Primary visual factors help evaluate the patient's symptoms, along with implied optical and refractive components. Secondary factors allow us to plan combination surgeries in our quest to address the eye for optimal optical performance.

## GULANI CLASSIFICATION FOR PREVIOUS REFRACTIVE SURGERY

### Primary Visual Factors

#### Quantitative

- Decreased visual acuity (Myopia, Hyperopia, Astigmatism).

#### Qualitative

- Irregular astigmatism
- Small optic zone
- Incisions.

### Secondary (Associated) Visual Factors

- Presbyopia
- Cataracts
- Corneal scars
- Corneal instability (thin/ectasia/trampoline effect).

Once the above is determined, the plan simply unfolds in front of your eyes. The seemingly complex eye now provides the cornea as a platform of visual rehabilitation along with, if needed, associated surgeries like cataract & IOL, etc. This is what the author calls refractive surgery to the rescue using the most accurate and elegant way to correct vision components.

These previous refractive surgeries can range from radial keratotomy to epikeratophakia, combinations of various refractive surgeries and even LASIK complications (Fig. 2).

Surface laser ablation in the form of advanced surface ablation (ASA) is a very useful tool for correcting superficial irregularity,[8] reshaping the cornea, as well as simultaneous scar peel with corneal shaping.[9] In many a cases, double ablation ASA/PRK can be used to smooth the surface and achieve refractive outcomes, including widening small optic zones of previous refractive surgeries.

The most important key factor is to determine whether just shaping is required or whether the cornea needs to be rehabilitated prior to this.

Shape correction following most previous refractive surgeries can be achieved with the excimer laser, but architectural correction of the cornea, in the form of clearance (from scars) and strength (thickness) recovery (ectasia/epiKphakia) prior to shaping, can help prepare for the final laser vision surgery.[10]

In a majority of cases, excimer laser surgery in a superficial ablation mode of ASA can be used to address the shape in leading to emmetropia.[11]

In cases of corneal thickness or corneal instability, one needs to prepare the cornea by lamellar techniques (anterior or posterior) or inserts (INTACS, etc.)[12,13] to then present it for reshaping using laser vision surgery.

In cases of surface ocular surface irregularity, we can perform sutureless (glue) amniotic membrane surgery with excellent rehabilitation[14] (Fig. 3).

If lamellar surgery is contemplated to rehabilitate the cornea, then we can plan for sutureless lamellar, anterior sutured (Barraquer Anti-Torque), deep anterior lamellar or sutureless posterior lamellar surgeries[15] and in this way prepare the cornea for future excimer surgery (Fig. 4).

Automated sutureless lamellar surgeries can be performed using microkeratomes, artificial anterior chambers and femtosecond lasers.[16,17]

In case of deep corneal pathologies with severe irregularity, hand lamellar techniques need to be performed manually using a resistance guide technique (Gulani multidirectional dissector) of lamellar separation at the depth

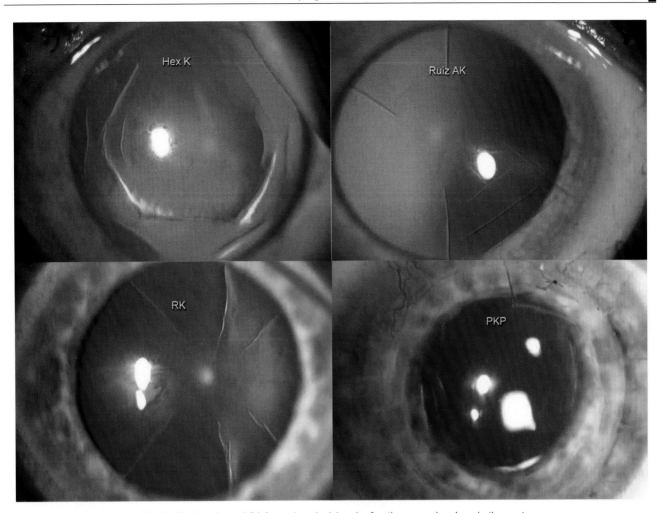

**Fig. 2:** Excimer laser ASA for various incisional refractive surgeries done in the past

of corneal pathology. Using this technique, surgical lights of the microscope may be shut off and a specially-designed side fiberoptic light can be utilized for illumination (Figs 5 and 6).

At this point, two important points need to be emphasized:

1. The donor thickness always decreases due to deturgescence.
2. The size may vary because of the suction in the donor eye.

Hand lamellar surgery gives the surgeon the control to go to whatever corneal depth is required. Also, when automated lamellar keratoplasty fails during surgery, one can convert to the hand lamellar procedure to salvage and proceed successfully.[16]

The femtosecond lasers (Intralase, Zeimer, Carl Zeiss, Femtec, etc.) are being used to perform lamellar corneal sections in the donor and recipient and further design

improvements will make this the future technology for perfecting the art of corneal restoration in clinic.

Suturing techniques vary. A sutureless procedure can be used when a thin optical automated flap lamellar replacement is performed, especially in young patients in whom the endothelium and the rest of the corneal tissue are normal. Various tissue glues are under investigation too.

Use of a superficial suture in the periphery of the cornea will produce a trampoline effect to hold the cornea in place. Another option is the Barraquer 8-bite antitorque stitch to eliminate or decrease astigmatism postoperatively. In deep lamellar procedures, 16-bite stitching must be used to ensure integration of the walls of the lamellar replacement with the cornea.

Lamellar surgery can also be performed on the posterior aspect of the cornea in patients with Fuchs' dystrophy in whom the endothelium must be replaced.[18]

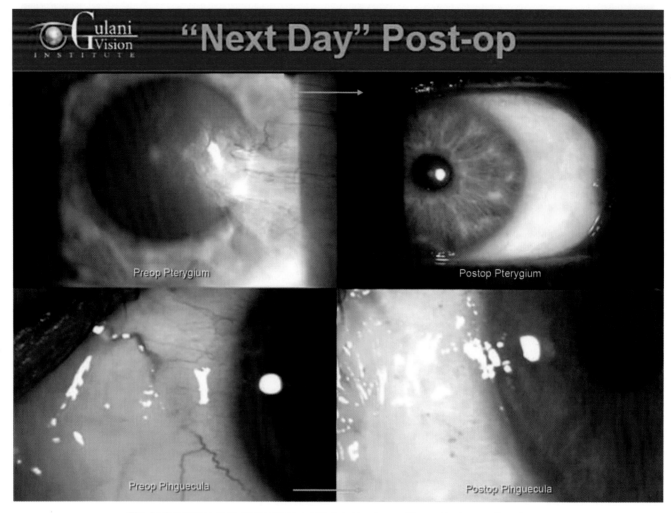

**Fig. 3:** Sutureless amniotic membrane graft for pterygiums with excellent cosmetic outcome

In the author's technique, the author enters through a paracentesis and peel of the descemet's membrane with a single instrument (Gulani KHT dissector/peeler) and also retrieve it with this same instrument. Then using a central self-sealing corneal incision, the graft is placed and floated with air till excellent adherence is achieved (Fig. 7). After good corneal stability is achieved, one may proceed with excimer laser surgery towards the goal of unaided emmetropia.

Thus, lamellar surgery can replace surface contour and/or tissue strength and stabilize the patient's cornea to maximize clarity. The visual endpoint can then be pursued in a staged manner with surface laser ablation, such as photorefractive keratectomy for corneal reshaping.[19]

Lamellar corneal surgery is the original starting point for LASIK and also the end point for any complications arising from LASIK. This is why lamellar surgery is very important. Most complications associated with LASIK are related to the cornea.[20,21]

The cornea can also be rehabilitated with INTACS in cases of post-LASIK ectasia (Fig. 8). In such cases too, one can still have the liberty of performing laser surgery (ASA) on top of the INTACS to address residual astigmatism (Fig. 9).

Let us analyze this concept. The fact that the keratoconus or LASIK ectasia has been stabilized by the INTACS (acting like braces) allows us to shape the cornea just a little more (Fig. 10) (of course contact lenses and glasses are the noninterventional options here), since astigmatism removes the least amount of tissue when ablated with the excimer laser.

This is also the reason why the author does perform excimer laser surgery (ASA) for a population of keratoconus patients who qualify by his criteria and see 20/20 best

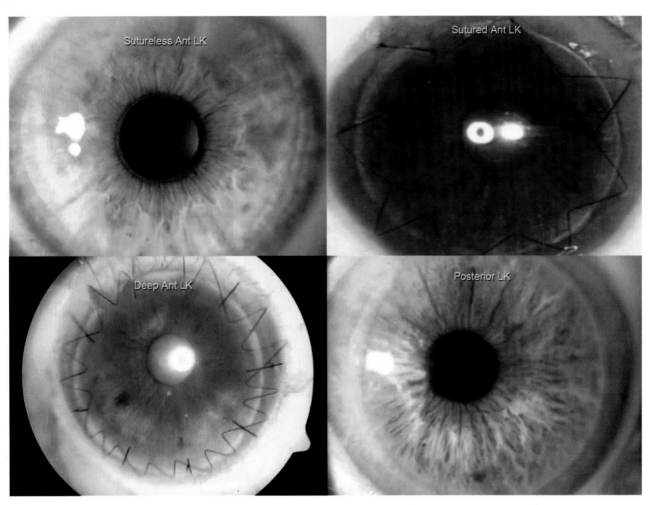

**Fig. 4:** Various lamellar transplant surgeries to rehabilitate the cornea

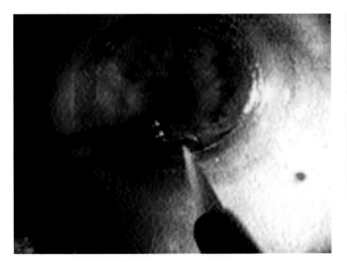

**Fig. 5:** Hand lamellar dissection with special fiber optic accessory lights

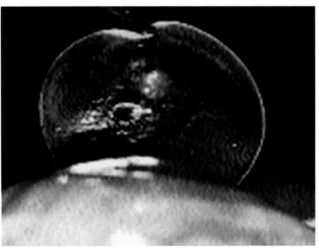

**Fig. 6:** Corneal scar contained in the automated lamellar flap

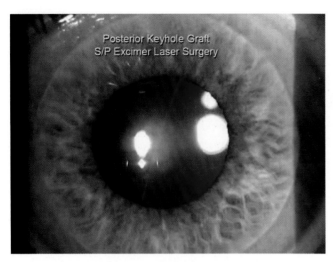

Fig. 7: Postoperative appearance of Gulani keyhole transplant (DSAEK/DSEK)

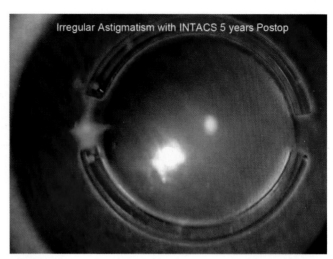

Fig. 8: Excimer ASA after INTACS to correct residual astigmatism

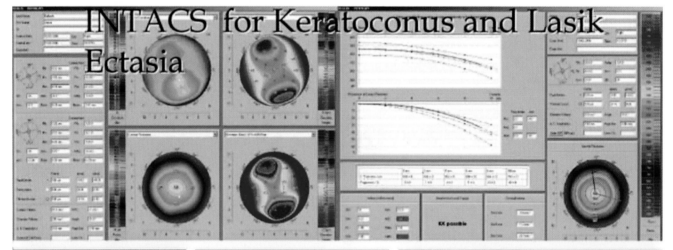

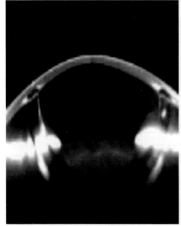

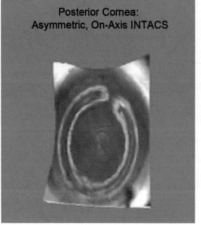

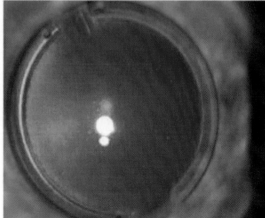

Fig. 9: INTACS for keratoconus and LASIK ectasia

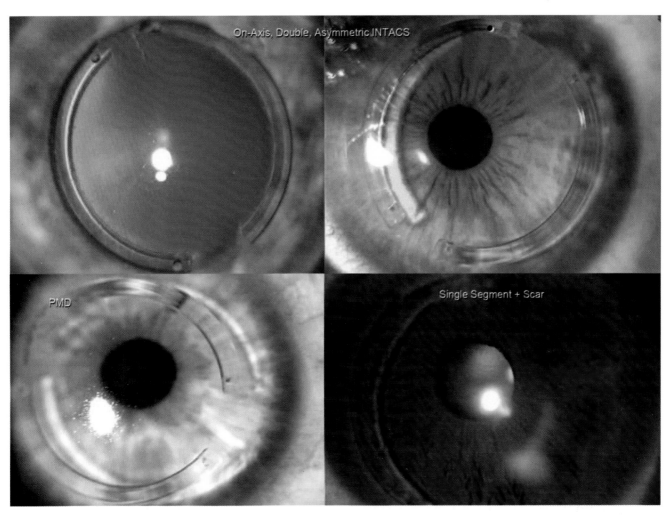

**Fig. 10:** Different inserting approaches, asymmetric heights and segments for INTACS for stabilizing the corneal shape

corrected with hard contact lens trials. He suggests laser vision surgery in a surface ASA mode; however, he does educate them that INTACS is the back up if they do progress in ectasia, either by natural progression or due to the laser surgery (Note: LASIK cannot be allowed on ectatic corneas).

INTACS is an excellent way to correct or minimize their ectasia, but since it is an inaccurate surgery, it should be reserved for patients with keratoconus who are best corrected to 20/40 or less.[22]

When considering intraocular surgery with lens implants, take full advantage of correcting not only the axial opacity (cataract) but also the refractive error with correct lens power calculation.

Additionally, also take care of associated optical concerns with appropriate lens implant choices, i.e. presbyopia correcting lens implants for presbyopia. Similarly, utilize toric lens implants for astigmatism in cases of high astigmatism to compliment future laser astigmatic correction on the cornea.

This could also imply piggyback IOLs or IOL exchanges for appropriate emmetropic goals.

Thus, once again when fixing the eye, first address intraocular concerns followed by laser corneal surgery (ASA) since this laser corneal surgery step can not only correct for final unaided vision, but also address residual refractive errors for less than perfect intraocular calculations.

Each step of surgery in combined stages should prepare for the success of the next step towards final emmetropia.

Various modalities like collagen crosslinking,[23,24] conductive keratoplasty,[25] intracorneal implants and glues can be used as adjuncts to a staged approach in reversing vision. This wide spectrum of applications is only limited by our logic and imagination; that is, responsible thinking and knowledge of anatomy, optics and physiology, as they apply to selecting the most appropriate surgery or surgeries, should be kept in mind and effectively utilized synergistically to achieve an optimal visual outcome for the patient.

For example:

- Conductive keratoplasty (CK) in RK surgery (think about destabilizing the already unstable RK incisions and even causing an incisional gape). Do not combine a contractive (CK) procedure with a relaxing (incisional) procedure.

The following self-reflecting principles may be followed by any surgeon correcting past surgeries:

- Am I performing the most effective surgery for this patient, with the least amount of intervention possible?
- This patient has undergone surgery already in the past. I should not perform any surgery without it leading to a better vision.
- This patient will, in the future, most likely need surgery. Am I preparing this patient for the future for a logical next step or future technology?
- The surgeon who operated on this patient obviously did the best they could, taking to heart the patient's hopes of improving his/her vision. How am I continuing with that concept in turning back the clock?
- Am I in anyway causing this patient to head towards an endpoint of irreversible blindness?
- Am I utilizing the most current technology and advanced surgical techniques to give this patient the best vision his or her eye is capable of achieving?
- Is this patient best helped by nonsurgical methods of advanced contact lenses or glasses?
- Am I doing what is the best for this patient or doing only what I am limited to by my knowledge or training, ie. PKP compared to lamellar surgery?

The questions above, along with the classification systems previously described, can outline a plan that will direct you towards achieving excellent vision for your patients.

These very principles follow the concepts that have been integrated under the new system of Corneoplastique™, wherein topical, brief, elegant, esthetically pleasing, minimally interventional surgeries are used singly, or in stages, to reach an ultimate goal of unaided emmetropia. Final fine tuning is performed using the excimer laser to further facilitate early rehabilitation and esthetically pleasing outcomes, in association with improved, uncorrected visual acuity.[26-28]

This is in contrast to the more extensive standard surgical techniques like penetrating keratoplasties (PK), etc., where in most cases, the final unaided visual outcome, despite a long rehabilitation period, is less than optimal.[29] Synergistically though, these standard surgeries, due to their proven track record, can always serve as a backup plan in selection of any of the above mentioned techniques.

Now that we understand the concept of thinking and approach, we know that where the patient had their surgery, what technology was used and who did it is irrelevant. What is important is the presentation of the patient and their complaints.

Listen to the patient and enumerate their concerns related to lifestyle limitations, occupations or hobbies and direct your surgical approach with that goal. You will be amazed how well your patients will grasp these concepts and become a part of the team, dedicated to improvement of their vision.

Let us therefore understand the principles of fixing the eye like a camera, first from within, when applicable, and then finally correcting for unaided vision using the cornea and excimer laser, as we go through some case scenarios.

Let us first look at patients with radial keratotomy:

Patients with RK may present with a variety of RK incisions. They can have 4, 8, 16 or 32 incision surgeries and all kinds of patterns and linearity based on their refractive errors, surgeon's style or training, and when the RIK was initially performed. They may also include additional incisional surgeries like astigmatic keratotomy (AK), enhancement RK and even hexagonal keratotomy (Fig. 11A). Additionally, they may present with intraocular surgeries like pseudophakia or phakic implants. Most of the presentations of radial keratotomy can be addressed with laser vision surgery in reshaping the cornea.[30]

In some cases, there may be associated factors, like Lasso sutures, in place (Fig. 11B). They are not as big a problem as they might appear. If the purse-string sutures are deep enough and the cornea is stable, there is no need to dig after them. Once that is established, you approach the patient similar to other post-PK patients, determining their vision, what the suture is doing to the vision, if anything, such as astigmatism and surface irregularity. If it is not doing anything, then proceed with straight laser on these cases. However, if the purse-string suture is inducing a lot of change, to the point you can see the traction from it, or if it is recent, superficial or broken, then remove it and wait a month (or more based on topographic stability) before doing your laser for final reshaping.

In many cases (since patients with RK are now in their cataractous ages), they will likely also need cataract surgery. Here too, plan to maximally improve all optical imperfections so you always plan for the most effective vision by performing the least amount of intervention for the patient and help them gain maximum advantage for their vision.

You can plan for cataract surgery in such a way that you can address not only their hazy vision due to the cataract but also their refractive errors, i.e. hyperopia with appropriate

IOL power calculations. For their associated problems, such as presbyopia and or astigmatism, you may select premium IOLs including accommodative, multifocal lens implants, toric lens implants, etc.

The author has had good success with ReStor Lens implants in such patients (Fig. 11C) by optimizing their eye from within the eye first and then getting ready for laser vision surgery to address three more aspects:

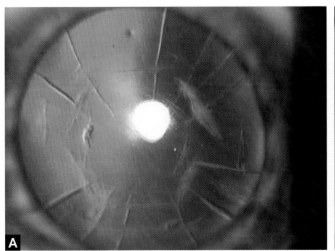
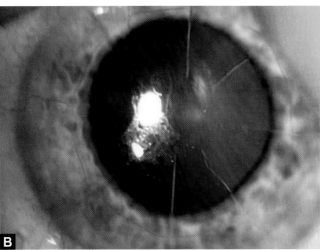

## Hyperopia S/P RK & CAT

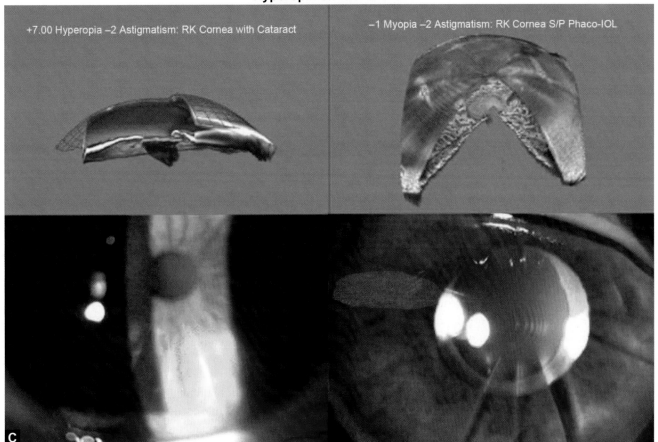

**Figs 11A to C:** (A) RK with hexagonal keratotomy; (B) RK with Greene's Lasso suture; (C) ReStor IOL implant post RK with cataract

1. Residual refractive error
2. Astigmatism
3. Increasing the optical zone to excellent visual outcomes without glasses (remember most RK surgeries were done with small optical zones).

Do not get too anxious about having to perform cataract surgery on a post-RK eye. Here are some helpful tips:

• Select the site of entry based on astigmatism axis and available space between two radial incisions.

• Author's phaco-feed technique: Use low flow phaco-emulsification, aqualase or phacochop techniques to keep the pressure in the eye down as you work. Also keep the phaco probe stationary in the incision (so as not to torque or cause stress on the adjacent RK incisions) and feed the cataract with your second hand /instrument into it.

• Always remember that these patients were once myopic in refraction (even though today they are presenting with hyperopia) and still have the myope's ocular anatomy, so all the risks of cataract surgery in myopia (namely retinal issues) still apply.

You may see patients who have had multiple surgeries in attempt to address induced complications or inadequate outcomes of previous ones, thus leading to bizarre combinations of surgeries. For example, a patient had undergone RK, AK, LASIK and cataract surgery in her right eye. When the patient presented to me, she was status post RK/AK/LASIK/piggyback IOL OD with 20/400 uncorrected, best corrected to 20/40. In this case, first analyze the primary and secondary factors mentioned above, irrespective of the number of surgeries already performed and then determine her corneal platform for laser reshaping. In this case, despite all of the patient's previous surgeries, it was concluded that her refractive error and irregular astigmatism were the cause of visual deterioration; thus, a combined excimer laser ASA/PRK treatment with mitomycin was performed, and the patient reached 20/20 uncorrected for distance and 20/25 for near (Fig. 12).

Patients with corneal scarring are repeatedly told they are not candidates for laser vision surgery; this new technique, however, could change that. The patient sees 20/20 despite a remaining residual scar. So in this case, don't chase the scar, you chase the shape.

Corneal scars, in particular, can be easily salvaged unless they are full thickness into the cornea (which will require PK). Even then we can surely come back with the excimer PRK for dealing successfully with the postoperative astigmatism (Figs 13A and B).[8]

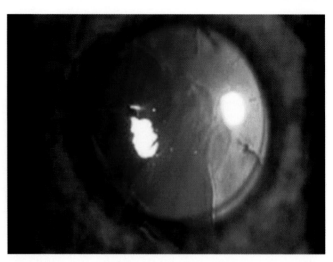

**Fig. 12:** Combined excimer laser ASA/PRK treatment in a post RK/AK/LASIK/Piggyback IOL case

For scars which are anterior (and most of them are), we need to determine depth (plan for corneal build up as needed if thin/thick/irregular, etc).

Supra-Bowman scars can be peeled off under the excimer laser and PRK continued to full refractive correction (Fig. 14).

If the scar looks like it is not a sheet of tissue, but actually has become part of the corneal stroma (i.e. herpetic scars which are usually gelatinous on touching), then use that scar as a masking agent to perform the refractive PRK without lifting or removing it (Fig. 15).

It is important to keep in mind that a great deal can be revealed on removing the epithelium.

Let us now take cases of patients with corneal scars following LASIK surgery. This patient was referred with best corrected 20/100 vision and an obvious corneal scar after LASIK surgery. Using the 5S system, he had central involvement and a scar, the cornea had good thickness, while the shape was affected because of irregular astigmatism. With a rigid contact lens and a subjective analysis, his vision improved to 20/25.

In this case, the central scar and shape (the only three affected Ss) were addressed by performing an excimer laser ASA with mitomycin C on his LASIK flap. The patient subsequently achieved an uncorrected vision of 20/15 in this eye (Fig. 16).

In a different example, another LASIK complication patient had a similar corneal scar but also thin residual cornea. To treat this patient, the previous LASIK flap was replaced with a thicker sutureless lamellar corneal transplant (If more than 180 microns, perform a Barraquer anti-torque,

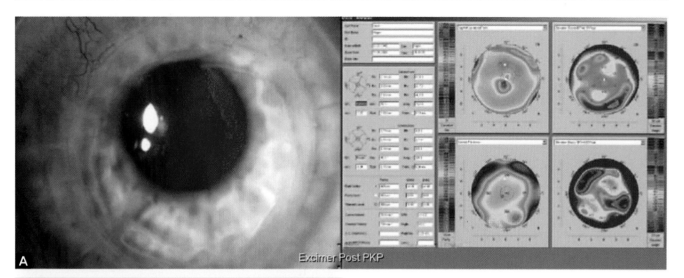

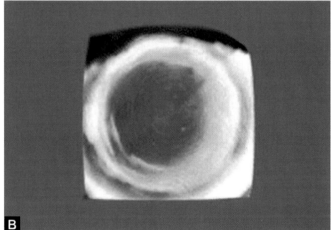

**Figs 13A and B:** Excimer ASA postpenetrating keratoplasty to correct high astigmatism

8-bite, continuous suture. Also, remember the donor corneal lamella and the 10% rule of resoluted thickness), thus addressing the central site, clarity and corneal thickness. Three months later, with potential vision on test showing possibility of 20/25, the excimer laser was used to address the final 'S' shape, resulting in uncorrected vision of 20/20 in this eye (Figs 17A and B).

Now let us take a patient with an opposite problem: aphakic epikeratophakia with decentered, scarred epilenticle. Here the cornea has a problem with all 5 Ss [It is thicker (Strength), Scarred, central Site affected with poor Shape and Sight]. A general approach is outlined below.

*Stage I:* Remove the epilenticle (Scar and Strength are addressed).

*Stage II:* Secondary IOL (Sight is addressed).

*Stage III:* If needed, further use of excimer laser to fine tune the Shape and further improve Sight.

Corneal transplants have been shown to be effective in these patients, but we need to ask whether a less invasive treatment approach would benefit a specific epikeratophakia patient. This is where we can apply the 5S classification; to illustrate, let us again look at this aforementioned patient who underwent aphakic epikeratophakia nearly two decades earlier and presented with decentered, scarred epilenticle with poor vision best corrected to 20/200.

First let us determine the first S—sight. By using a hard contact lens, the patient was able to achieve 20/25 vision. Turning to the site, (second S), it was determined that the epilenticle was decentered, and there was an opaque scar (third S). The cornea was thick since this was added tissue (fourth S), and the patient had irregular astigmatism with hyperopia (fifth S).

Using this classification system, the plan was Step1: Remove the epilenticle (the scar, site and increased thickness were thus addressed). On removing the epilenticle disk from

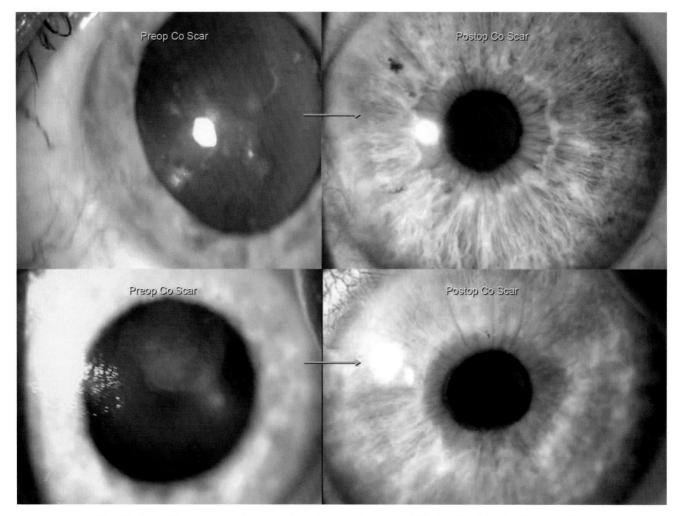

**Fig. 14:** Supra-Bowman corneal scars peeled prior to excimer laser ASA aimed for full refractive correction

the patient's cornea, the underlying cornea was pristine. By removing the disk, we had removed the scar, corrected the center and the new cornea had normal thickness. The surgery also addressed the shape of the cornea. The only thing remaining was sight (S1) so we proceeded with high-speed vitrectomy and secondary IOL placement to correct her aphakia. This resulted in uncorrected vision of 20/25 in this woman's eye (Fig. 18).

Just to reiterate the application and thought process, another epikeratophakia patient had a scarred myopic lenticle with pseudophakia (20/400 vision). There the previous 4Ss were addressed in the above fashion and instead of performing an intraocular IOL placement (since she was already pseudophakic), excimer surface ablation was performed to address the S5 for shape (irregular astigmatism and residual ammetropia), resulting in uncorrected vision of 20/30, in this eye.

In a third case of myopic epikeratophakia, a young individual presented with central scarring (uncorrected vision 20/400, best corrected 20/70 distorted). It was determined that the scar was superficial, and that the patient had thin cornea underneath that would not allow for any excimer ASA shaping if his epilenticle were removed. Also, being young, he did not want any intraocular surgery.

Correction of his ammetropia was calculated at −5.00 D with Grade I irregular astigmatism. In this instance, just enough tissue could be removed to leave him with good thickness, relative central clarity and corrected shape and irregularity (The backup plan being that if this approach of least intervention does not work then we shall remove his epilenticle and plan for a phakic implant). So, a central myopic ablation was performed with superficial scar removal as Stage I. The patient already is seeing uncorrected 20/40, and has been ecstatic with his recovery (Fig. 19).

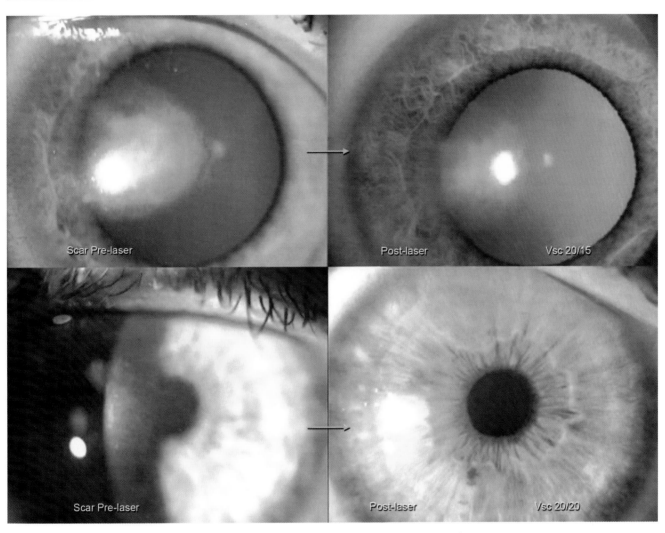

**Fig. 15:** Scar as a masking agent to perform the refractive ASA without lifting or removing it

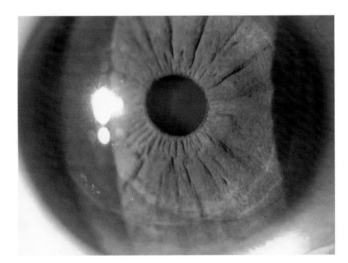

**Fig. 16:** Excimer laser ASA application for corneal scar post-LASIK surgery

These examples illustrate that the 5S system can be effectively utilized to first achieve a clear and stable cornea; then, all that needs to be done is to derive the optimum shape (as long as there is no progressive or irreversible intraocular pathology) for unaided emmetropia.

A complete and thorough evaluation of the optical system of the eye from the cornea to the retina is necessary. This complete information is important when using the Corneoplastique™ because it uses the complete anterior segment and finally the cornea as a platform for visual rehabilitation.

In another case, a patient was referred with resultant legal blindness in his left eye. He had a history of PRK and pseudophakia (barely visible through the opaque anterior cornea) and had just had a traumatic accident. He presented with extensive conjunctival scarring, central diffuse corneal scar and corneal pannus in two quadrants. Again, applying our 5S system, as Stage 1 the ocular surface and corneal pannus, including superficial corneal scar, was cleared using an amniotic membrane graft with glue. The patient was thrilled with the esthetic appearance and also better

vision of 20/80. Stage 2 (following potential vision testing with a contact lens trial) was implemented. Three months later, the residual corneal scar and irregular corneal surface was addressed with the excimer laser resulting in a clear anterior cornea and expected shape to uncorrected 20/40 vision. At this point with newly-achieved visible clarity, an opaque posterior capsule was identified, and a YAG laser capsulotomy was performed. The patient sees uncorrected 20/15 in this eye (Figs 20A to D).

Let us examine another example to reiterate the symbiosis of intraocular planning with corneal rehabilitation.

This patient was referred after she had phacoemulsification and multifocal ReSTOR IOL implantation (ReStor SN60D3) in her left eye, followed by YAG capsulotomy. She was frustrated with her vision as the surgery left her with debilitating glare and reduced vision in this left eye. Due to residual spectacle blur following cataract surgery, her eye surgeon performed a laser PRK procedure after 9 months of her IOL surgery. This was followed by development of corneal scar and astigmatism with the refraction of +5.25, −1.25 × 180.

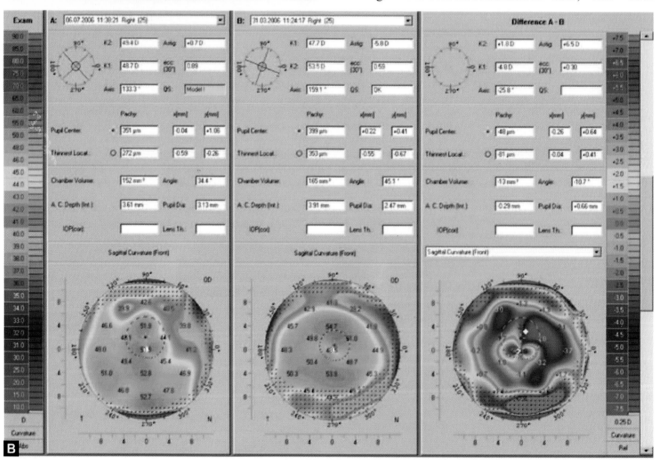

**Figs 17A and B:** (A) Sutureless lamellar corneal transplant followed by excimer ASA for corneal scar post-LASIK with thin residual cornea; (B) Pentacam evaluation of significantly improved keratometry following lamellar keratoplasty

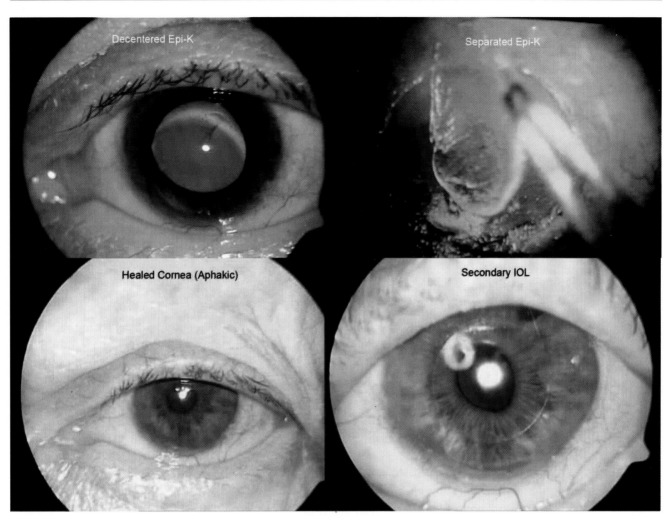

**Fig. 18:** Decentered epikeratophakia with aphakia managed with application of 5S classification system

Her eye surgeon then performed another PRK for the same. This patient slipped into depression convinced she had no recourse after the postoperative results of second PRK with vision 20/200 in her left eye. She presented to us after 7 months of her last PRK with complaints of poor visual status despite best corrected glasses and contact lenses, and she wished to seek surgical correction for the same.

Applying the same 5S system, we proceeded with our plan. First, her scar was cleared using laser ASA technique, inducing a finite refractive error. Once her cornea was cleared, her vision improved to 20/25 with a contact lens trial of +6.00 D of hyperopia. Given that she had ND YAG laser capsulotomy, exchanging her IOL would lead to vitreous disturbance and decrease her chance of perfecting vision. Having corrected her Site, Scar and Strength, her refraction needed to be corrected (The author does not recommend corneal surgery for 6 D hyperopia). After an indepth clinical

exam including optical path difference scanning system (OPD) and Pentacam evaluation, a piggyback IOL with iridectomy was performed. She now sees 20/20 at distance and 20/20 at near without glasses (Fig. 21).

Let us see if these surgeries were in sync with our Corneo- plastique principles:

Both stages of surgeries were topical, brief, esthetically pleasing and aimed for unaided emmetropia.

What was the thought process during the entire procedure planning:

All cardinal rules were followed and approach was aimed not only to salvage but to actually perfect her vision.

What does the patient remember about her surgical experience:

She felt she was an integral team player in her own quest for perfect vision who recollected pleasant, no-injection, no-patch procedures that lasted 5–10 minutes each.

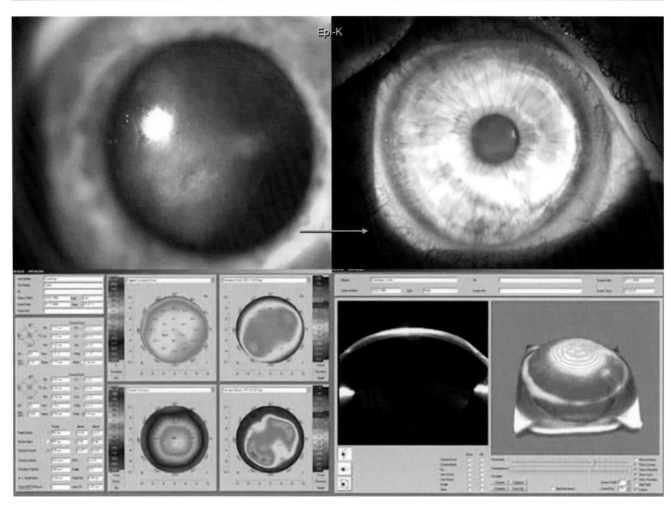

**Fig. 19:** Excimer ASA for scar with epikeratophakia to a refractive outcome

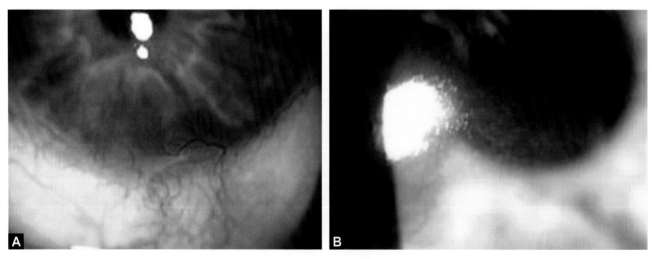

**Figs 20A and B**

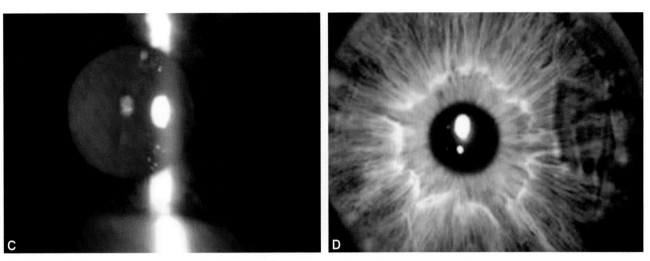

**Figs 20A to D:** Application of staged correction using amniotic clearance followed by YAG excimer laser and YAG laser to unaided emmetropia

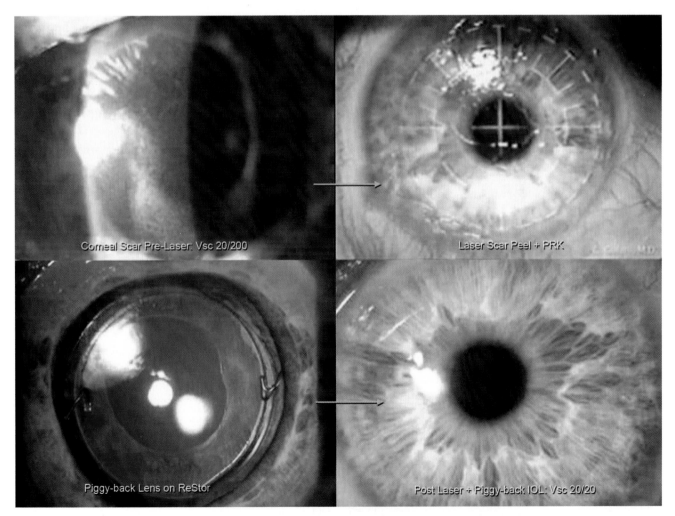

**Fig. 21:** Excimer laser ASA followed by piggy-back IOL implant for management of patient with previous ReStor lens and PRK complication of corneal scar

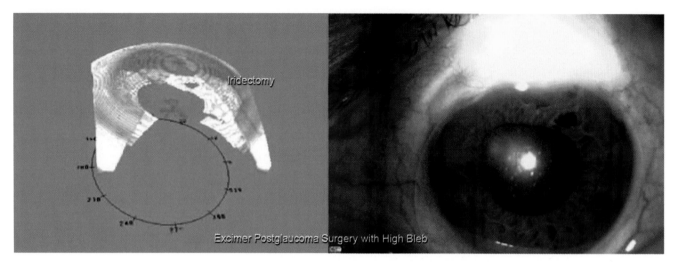

Iridectomy

Excimer Postglaucoma Surgery with High Bleb

**Fig. 22:** Excimer laser surgery for high astigmatism following postglaucoma filtering bleb in a case of controlled glaucoma

So with above examples and many more (Figs 22 and 23), you will be able to design a plan to correct patients' vision by looking at his or her clinical presentation and then adding appropriate diagnostic details in order to arrive at a logical and efficacious plan of care.

As eye surgeons, we must always strive for 20/20 or better for patients, no matter what surgery they may have had in the past. In every case, caution must be exercised in patient selection and technique selection, as in all LASIK/ Refractive surgery cases. We have an obligation to do the best we can with the patient's safety and outcome as our primary goal.

As for choice of technology, the author uses the VISX Star S4 laser (AMO, Irvine, California) and is involved in trials internationally for femtosecond laser advances in

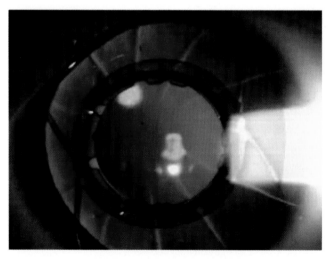

**Fig. 23:** RK with phakic implant

cornea and cataract surgery. In author's practice, he uses the newly-released Marco 3D Wave (OPD-III, Nidek Inc, Japan) which enables him to review not only the topography and wavefront aberrations but also detailed internal and corneal OPD along with SA values. This is beneficial in correcting previous refractive surgery cases, as well as in understanding and correcting refractive complications. For example, in a case of LASIK ectasia followed by placement of INTAC ring segment, which the patient's surgeon performed resulting in distorted vision of 20/400, the same surgeon decided that the and only option for improving vision was a corneal transplant. After detailed OPD testing and planning, author determined a laser ASA technique and resulted in 20/40 uncorrected vision (Fig. 24).

When we are aiming for vision beyond 20/20 in every case, we must be sensitive to and address every aspect of vision therein. So, in such cases, we can use spherical aberration-correcting implants to improve contrast sensitivity and vision quality. Since the cataractous lens will be removed anyways, we must try and counter the corneal spherical aberration by selecting the appropriate premium lens implant. This is also applicable to previous refractive surgery cases like postmyopic refractive surgery (SA is usually high positive) where we can use the Tecnis multifocal IOL (which corrects 0.27 microns of SA) and posthyperopic refractive surgery cases (SA is usually high negative) where we can use a standard monofocal lens implant (which usually induce positive SA). For example, in this case of previous RK and LASIK with cataract, we were able to use a ReStor multifocal lens implant combined with Laser ASA and result in uncorrected vision of 20/20 and near (Fig. 25).

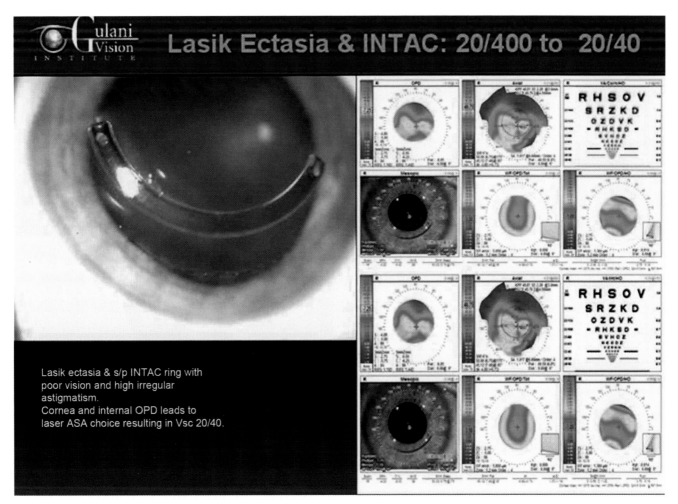

**Fig. 24:** LASIK ectasia case with INTAC ring with internal and corneal OPD underwent laser ASA to excellent vision outcome

The author uses the Pentacam (Oculus) as an adjunct to his thought process during clinic[31-35] and high definition imaging systems[36,37] both to document his outcomes and also to translate his thought process for the patients and their families.

This also further bolsters the confidence that they gain from you since they know you have thought through the whole process before embarking on the stages of improving one's vision rather than performing surgery and then piecing plans together as you go.

These patients also understand that their 20/20 will not be as good as a virgin refractive case, but given where they are coming from, and given what minimal trauma they will be going through with these techniques, it is a win-win for the team (patient & doctor).

Also, if the patient is already very happy at any intermediary stage (if you were planning combined stages), stop! The patient and their satisfaction is what we are addressing, not a topography chart.

This will open up the doors to millions of patients of previous refractive surgeries who have been told that they cannot be helped. This will also open up the flood gates to patients with inadequate and complicated outcomes of laser vision surgery for a second chance at enjoying terrific vision.

Our ability to understand the past will help us lead into the future and also navigate the waters of innovation so that not only can we endeavor to achieve supervision for our refractive patients of today, but we can also reshape the future of refractive patients from the past.

## ⋗ ACKNOWLEDGMENT

I would like to acknowledge Dr Lee Nordan and the Late Dr Ignacio Barraquer for fueling my endeavor in this direction (Figs 26 and 27).

I also want to acknowledge my Visiting Research Intern: Ms Melisa Kulaozovic, BS (Munich, Germany).

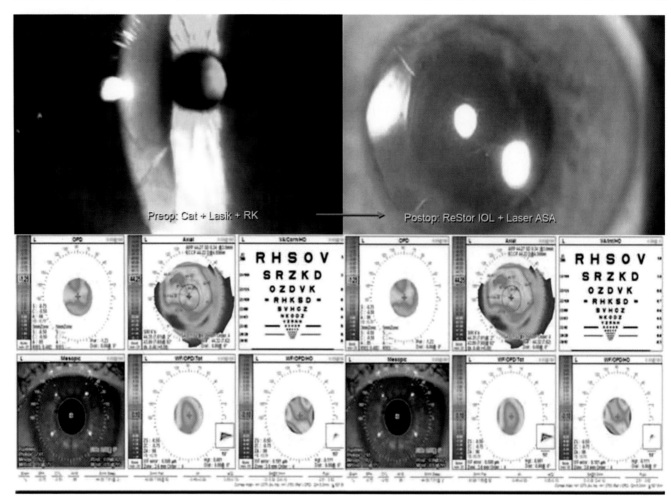

**Fig. 25:** RK case with LASIK and cataract with postoperative corneal and internal OPD evaluating
20/20 vision with ReStor lens implant and laser ASA combination

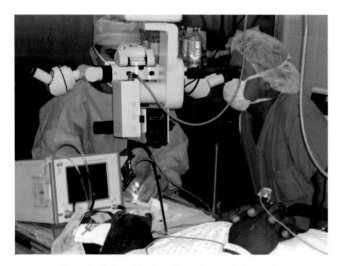

**Fig. 26:** Dr Lee Nordan observing Dr Gulani raise
lamellar keratoplasty to Corneoplastique™

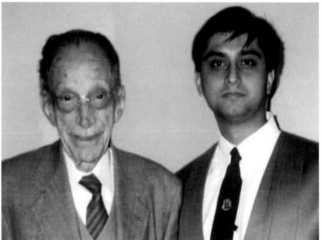

**Fig. 27:** Dr Barraquer with Dr Gulani

# ❖ REFERENCES

1. Gulani AC. Gulani 5S classification system. Tips & Tricks in LASIK Surgery. New Delhi: JP Publishers; 2007. pp. 91-100.
2. Gulani AC. 5S Classification System. California: ASCRS; 2006.
3. Gulani AC, Holladay J, Belin M, et al. Future technologies in LASIK—Pentacam advanced diagnostic for laser vision surgery. Expert Rev Ophthalmol. 2012 (in Press).
4. Gulani AC. 'Future Directions in Lasik'. Corneal Refractive Surgery in Video Atlas of Ophthalmic Surgery. XLV. 2008.
5. Gulani AC. Corneoplastique™. Tech Ophthalmol. 2007;5(1): 11-20.
6. Gulani AC. Corneoplastique: art of vision surgery (Abstract). J Am Soc Laser Med Surg. 2007;19:40.
7. Gulani AC. A new concept for refractive surgery. Ophthalmology Management. 2006;10(4):57-63.
8. Knrz MC, Jendritza B. Topographically-guided laser in situ keratomileusis to treat corneal irregularities. Ophthalmology. 2000;107:1138-43.
9. Gulani AC. Excimer laser PRK and corneal scars: refractive surgery to the rescue. Mastering Advanced Surface Ablation Techniques. New Delhi: JP Publishers; 2007. pp. 246-8.
10. Gulani AC. Corneoplastique system repairs cornea before or after laser refractive surgery. Ocular Surgery News. 2007;25 (21):124-5.
11. Gulani AC. "Future of laser vision surgery" video DVD rom. Advanced Surface Ablation Techniques; 2007.
12. Kymionis GD, Aslanides IM, Siganos CS, et al. INTACS for early pellucid marginal degeneration. J Cataract Refract Surg. 2004;30:230-3.
13. Colin J, Cochner B, Savary G, et al. INTACS inserts for treating keratoconus: one year results. Ophthalmology. 2001;108: 1409-14.
14. Gulani AC. Sutureless amniotic surgery for pterygium: cosmetic outcomes for ocular surface surgery. Techniques in Ophthalmology. 2008;6(2):41-4.
15. Gulani AC. Gulani Keyhole Transplant. Corneal Refractive Surgery in Video Atlas of Ophthalmic Surgery. XXXVII. (2) 2008.
16. Gulani AC. Principles of surgical treatment of irregular astigmatism in unstable corneas. Textbook of Irregular Astigmatism. Diagnosis and Treatment. Thorofare, NJ: SLACK Incorporated; 2007. pp. 251-61.
17. Gulani AC. Lamellar corneal procedure useful for reparative surgery. Ophthalmology Times; 2003.
18. Melles G, Kamminga N. Posterior lamellar keratoplasty can be an effective surgical technique to manage corneal endothelial disorders. Ophthalmologe. 2003;100(9):689-95.
19. Pedrotti E, Sbabo A, Marchini G. Customized transepithelial photorefractive keratectomy for iatrogenic ametropia after penetrating or deep lamellar keratoplasty. J Cataract Refract Surg. 2006;32(8):1288-91.
20. Neumann AC, Gulani AC. Lamellar surgery: counterpoints and complications. In: Elander, Rich, Robin (Eds). Textbook of Refractive Surgery. Saunders Inc. 1996;24:291-7.
21. Gulani AC. How to put logic into action after Lasik. Rev Ophthalmol. 2006;XIII (9):60-4.
22. Gulani AC. INTACS: a refractive surgery to prepare and repair. INTACS Round Table. Chicago: ASCRS; 2007.
23. Kohlhaas M, Spoerl E, Spck A, et al. A new treatment of keratectasia after LASIK with riboflavin/UVA light cross-linking. Klin Monatsbl Augenheilkd. 2005;222(5):430-6.
24. Schnitzler E, Sporl E, Seiler T. Irradiation of cornea with ultraviolet light and riboflavin administration as a new treatment for erosive corneal processes, preliminary results in four patients. Klin Monatsbl Augenheilkd. 2000;217(3):190-3.
25. Hesrh PS, Fry KL, Chandrashekhar R, et al. Conductive keratoplasty to treat complications of LASIK. J Refract Surg. 2003;19: 425-32.
26. Gulani AC. Corneoplastique: art of laser vision surgery. Corneal Refractive Surgery in Video Atlas of Ophthalmic Surgery. 2008;XXXVIII(2).
27. Gulani AC. "Corneoplastique" Video Journal of Ophthalmology, MO: Media Mill. 2007;II(4).
28. Gulani AC. Corneoplastique™: Art of Vision Surgery (Abstract). Berlin, Germany: ISOPT; 2006.
29. Muraine M, Sanchez C, Watt L, et al. Long-term results of penetrating keratoplasty. A 10 year plus retrospective study. Graefes Arch Clin Exp Ophthalmol. 2003;241(7):571-6.
30. Gulani AC, McDonald M, Majmudar P, et al. Meeting the challenge of Post-RK patients. Rev Ophthalmol. 2007; IV(10): 49-54.
31. Gulani AC. Pentacam technology in LASIK: the shape of vision. LASIK Surgery. New Delhi: JP Publishers; 2007. pp. 51-61.
32. Gulani AC. Pentacam technology in customized refractive surgery. Mastering the Techniques of Customized Lasik. New Delhi: JP Publishers; 2007. pp. 156-64.
33. Bansal J, Gulani AC. Excimer laser enhancements after multifocal IOLs. In: Textbook of Premium Cataract Surgery: A Step by Step Guide. Hovanesian J Slack (Ed) Inc, Thoroghfare, NJ; 2012.pp.135-45,15.
34. Donnenfeld E, Gulani AC. Femtosecond laser for astigmatism correction during cataract surgery. JP Publishers. 2012;21: 155-61.
35. Maus M, et al. Pentacam. Textbook of Corneal Topography in the Wavefront Era. NJ: SLACK Incorporated; 2006.pp. 281-93.
36. Gulani AC. 'Future directions in lasik'. Corneal Refractive Surgery in Video Atlas of Ophthalmic Surgery. XLV. 2008.
37. Gulani AC, et al. 'Innovative real-time illumination system for LASIK surgery'. Clinical & Surgical Ophthalmology. Journal of Canadian Society of Cataract & Refractive Surgery. 2003;6: 244-6.

# CHAPTER 99

# Intrastromal Corneal Implants for the Treatment of Presbyopia

*George O Waring, Stephen D Klyce*

## ❧ INTRODUCTION

Presbyopia, the progressive loss of the eye's ability to accommodate, affects more than 80 million emmetropic presbyopes in the United States. Corneal surgery to treat presbyopia, such as presbyopic laser-assisted *in situ* keratomileusis (LASIK), monovision LASIK or monovision conductive keratoplasty (CK), requires permanent changes in corneal structure. Multifocal and accommodating intraocular lenses treat presbyopia, but the procedure is intraocular with a slightly higher risk profile. As a result, corneal inlays are gaining attention as a promising new paradigm for the surgical treatment of presbyopia. Inlays currently in development or clinical trials are the KAMRA™ (AcuFocus™, Irvine, CA), Vue+™ (ReVision Optics™, Lake Forest, CA) and Flexivue™ microlens (Presbia™, Amsterdam, Netherlands). Each is distinctive in size, material and mechanism of action (Fig. 1).

Corneal inlays are removable, repositionable and reversible. These additive technologies do not require removal of corneal tissue and can be combined with other refractive techniques in order to treat both presbyopia and ametropia. These features make corneal inlays an attractive treatment for the burgeoning presbyopic population.

## ❧ BACKGROUND

Corneal inlays have been around for decades. Jose Barraquer proposed treating aphakia and high myopia by implanting a flint glass or plexiglass synthetic lenticule into the cornea (synthetic keratophakia) in 1949.[1] Inlays of high index polymers, such as polymethyl methacrylate (PMMA) and polysulfone, were developed by Peter Choyce to treat Fuch's dystrophy and high myopia.[2] However, all these materials were relatively impermeable, depriving the cornea of fluids and nutrients while retaining metabolic by-products. The results were thinning of the anterior stroma and keratolysis. Claes Dohlman's team developed a permeable hydrogel lenticule in 1967.[3] Hydrogel inlays produced with high water content do not markedly impede metabolic gradients across the stroma, allowing nutrient flow to the anterior cornea. Unfortunately, the hydrogel polymers had a low index of refraction and thus, by themselves, had a relatively limited optical power without becoming bulky enough to change the corneal surface curvature.

The use of animal models, as well as micromolecular gradient and stromal hydration computations by McCarey, Klyce and others led to the understanding that corneal inlays needed to be thin, small diameter, highly permeable and implantable relatively deep in corneal stroma (Fig. 2).[4-7] The nutrient permeable corneal endothelium and the gas permeable corneal epithelium synergistically transport

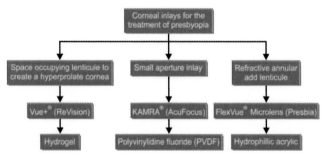

**Fig. 1:** Flow chart depicting classification of corneal inlays based on mechanism of action

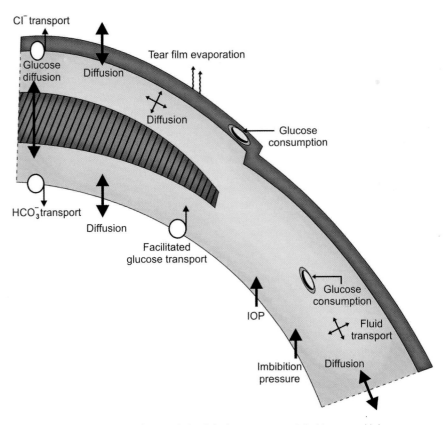

**Fig. 2:** Schematic of corneal physiologic processes related to corneal inlays

ions out of the stroma. Such a design allows oxygen from tear film and glucose from aqueous humor to nourish corneal cells while catabolic waste products flow out to the aqueous humor with minimal restriction.[8] This allows the cornea to maintain its osmotic balance and thickness in order to provide a healthy environment for corneal cells and to remain transparent.

This knowledge has led to an evolution of material and design culminating in the corneal inlays in clinical trials today. The early inlay designs have included the kerato-gel™ (Allergan, Inc., Irvine CA). Designed for aphakia, this inlay was composed of lidofilcon A (Fig. 3). The chiron™ inlay (Bausch and Lomb, Rochester NY) was a meniscus hydrogel optical lens that ranged from +1.50 to +3.50 D in add power with a diameter ranging from 1.80–2.20 mm. This permeable lenticule was well-tolerated, and a slit lamp image from a 16-year postoperative patient is displayed in Figure 4.

The PermaVision™ intracorneal lens (Anamed™, Lake Forest, CA) was composed of a hydrogel-based material called Nutrapore™ with water content of 78%. This lens, measuring 5.0–5.5 mm in diameter with central thickness

of 30–60 μm, was designed to alter the surface curvature of the cornea. This was followed by the IntraLens™ that altered surface curvature to create a multifocal cornea for the treatment of hyperopia and presbyopia. This line of inlays culminated in the current Vue+ inlay. The intracorneal

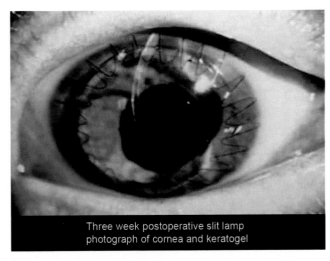

Three week postoperative slit lamp photograph of cornea and keratogel

**Fig. 3:** Slit lamp photograph of an original kerato-gel™ for aphakia 3 weeks postoperative

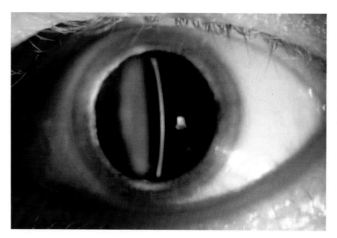

**Fig. 4:** Slit lamp photograph of a chiron corneal inlay 16 years post-operative
*Source*: GO Waring IV and DS Durrie

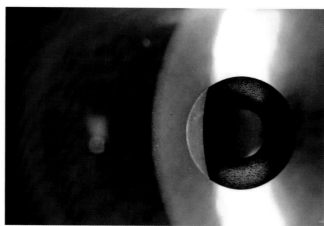

**Fig. 5:** Postoperative slit lamp photo of a KAMRA™ small aperture inlay
*Source*: AcuFocus™, Inc

microlens™ (BioVision™ AG, Brüggs, Switzerland) was a 3.0 mm diameter, 20 μm thick hydrogel annular add inlay with a central opening free of optical power that also allowed nutrient flow to the anterior central cornea. This inlay was designed to be placed into a stromal pocket with a mechanical microkeratome pocket maker. The microlens™ went on to be known as the InVue, the precursor to the Flexivue microlens inlay.

Three corneal inlays are currently available outside the United States and are at various stages in the US Food and Drug Administration (FDA) approval process for the United States.

## ▶ KAMRA™ SMALL APERTURE INLAY

The KAMRA™ corneal inlay is a 3.8 mm diameter annulus with a central 1.6 mm aperture. The inlay utilizes the properties of the small aperture to increase depth of field by reducing the angle of light that reaches the lens from objects outside of the plane of focus. This decreases the zone of confusion at the retina, improving the quality of images outside of the plane of focus. A slit lamp photograph of the KAMRA™ inlay is shown in Figure 5. The inlay is 5 μm thick and made of biocompatible polyvinylidine fluoride (PVDF). Eight thousand four hundred laser-etched openings of 5.5–11.5 μm maintain the metabolic flow to the anterior cornea and are distributed in a pseudo-random pattern to prevent diffraction issues at night.

The KAMRA™ corneal inlay has completed enrollment in its clinical trial as part of the FDA approval process in the United States. Studies have been completed outside the

United States where the inlay is commercially available. Seyeddain et al. reported 2 years data on the KAMRA™ inlay implanted in 32 eyes and found 96.9% of patients read J3 or better in the implanted eye with mean binocular uncorrected near visual acuity (UCNVA) improvement from J6 preoperatively to J1 after 24 months. Mean binocular uncorrected intermediate visual acuity (UCIVA) was 20/20 at 1 month and remained 20/20 throughout the 24-month follow-up. Mean uncorrected distance visual acuity (UCDVA) was 20/20 in the implanted eye and 20/16 binocularly.[9] Yilmaz et al. reported 1 year data on 39 presbyopic patients; 12 were naturally emmetropic and 27 had emmetropia resulting from previous hyperopic LASIK. Of the 39 inlays implanted, three were explanted during the study. At 1 year, the mean UCNVA improved from J6 (preoperatively) to J1+. All implanted eyes had an UCNVA of J3 or better and 85.3% were J1 or better. Binocularly, the mean UNCVA remained J1 or better throughout the study. The mean UCDVA in eyes with an inlay did not change significantly from preoperative and remained 20/20 throughout the study period. All three eyes with inlay explantation returned to within ±1.00 D of the preoperative refraction for both near and distance acuity, with no loss of best corrected distance visual acuity.[10] A contralateral comparison of the Optical Quality Analysis System™ (OQAS, Visiometrics™, Spain) demonstrates a broadened defocus curve and reduced simulated retinal blur in the implanted eye (Fig. 6).

Currently, a combined LASIK and KAMRA™ implant procedure is being used outside the United States to correct ametropia and presbyopia. After laser ablation, the

## Optical Quality Analysis System

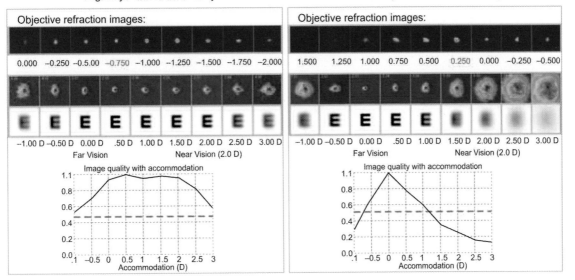

**Fig. 6:** Contralateral comparison of the ocular quality assessment system after KAMRA™ small aperture inlay implantation in the right eye, demonstrates a broadened defocus curve, as well as an improved point spread function and improved simulated retinal image at near
*Source*: AcuFocus™, Inc

KAMRA™ inlay can easily be placed beneath the LASIK flap. This procedure allows surgeons to set the postoperative refractive target, thereby optimizing a patient's refractive status and outcomes.

### ▶ VUE+ SPACE OCCUPYING INLAY

The Vue+ corneal inlay, (formerly the Presbylens™), was developed in 2007 for the treatment of emmetropic presbyopes. Made of a proprietary hydrogel based material, the inlay has water content and refractive index similar to the human cornea. The material is highly permeable allowing sufficient fluid and nutrient transmission flow to maintain a healthy cornea.

The inlay is 2 mm in diameter, 10 μm thick at the periphery and 24–40 μm thick centrally. A slit lamp biomicroscopic photograph of the Vue+ inlay is shown in Figures 7A and B. The differential thickness across the inlay changes the surface curvature of the cornea, creating a multifocal surface. This improves near and intermediate visual acuities. The effect on distance acuity is minimal as light rays outside the 2 mm inlay area remain focused on the retina, especially with pupil dilation. In bright light, pupil constriction creates a pseudoaccommodative state utilizing the steepened central cornea.

At this time, the Vue+ inlay is commercially available in the European Union and the first phase of the FDA clinical trials for approval in the United States has been completed. Preliminary data on eight presbyopic emmetropes implanted with the earlier 1.5 mm version of the inlay have been reported. The inlay was placed under a lamellar flap. All eight implanted eyes achieved 20/32 or better UCNVA at 2 years postoperative. The mean gain in UCNVA was 3.6 lines with a binocular mesopic UCDVA of 20/25 or better for all patients. All subjects reported that they were satisfied with the surgery and able to perform typical near tasks without glasses. In a concomitant animal study, the implanted corneas remained clear and tolerated the inlays well (GD Sharma et al. 2010;ARVO Abstract 813).

### ▶ FLEXIVUE MICROLENS ANNULAR ADD LENTICULE

Of the three corneal inlays discussed here, only the Flexivue microlens has a refractive optic with separate distance and near focal points. The inlay is 3 mm in diameter with an edge thickness of 20 μm. The inlay is composed of a hydrophilic acrylic polymer that allows fluid and nutrient flow to the cornea. The central zone of the inlay has no

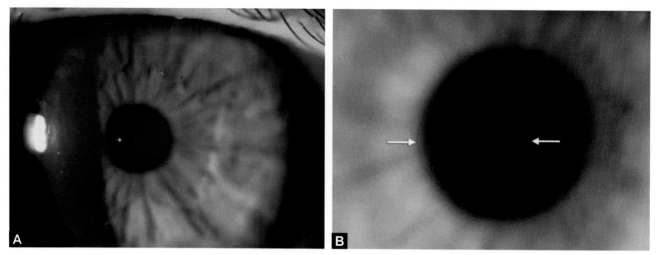

**Figs 7A and B:** Slit lamp photograph of the ReVision Vue™ inlay placed on stromal bed
*Source*: ReVision Optics™, Inc. White arrows indicate perimeter of inlay.

refractive power. The periphery has a refractive index higher than that of the cornea for a total of +1.25 to +3.00 D of add power.

The Flexivue microlens inlay is available in Europe where initial data are promising. In a study of 43 patients (average age, 52 years) with a mean preoperative UCDVA of 20/20 and mean UCNVA of 20/50, all patients had an increase in the uncorrected near VA after 1 week. By 1 year, 93% of patients had an UCNVA of J2 or better (Pallikaris et al. unpublished data, 2009).

### ᐅ IMPLANTING CORNEAL INLAYS

The implantation procedure is similar for all three corneal inlays. The main difference is the depth of placement. The curvature changing Vue+ inlay is placed superficially at a depth of 120–130 µm. The small aperture KAMRA™ and refractive Flexivue microlens are placed deeper, at about 200 µm, to avoid changing the curvature of the cornea. The inlay is placed in the nondominant eye, although patients who are near dominant may prefer to have the implant placed in their distance-dominant eye. Eye dominance should be assessed by both sensory and motor dominance assessment techniques.

Corneal inlays may be placed under a lamellar flap or within a corneal pocket. Ziemer Femto LDV™ (Ziemer Group AG, Port, Switzerland) offers pocket software. A pocket can be created by placing a keyhole shaped plastic shield in the cone of the laser to block pulses, resulting in a pocket instead of a flap (PS Binder et al., 2010; ARVO Abstract 2868). New femtosecond pocket software is currently in development for the IntraLase™ (Abbott Medical Optics, Santa Ana, CA). Each technique has its advantages. Relative to a lamellar flap, creation of a corneal pocket preserves the majority of peripheral corneal nerves maintaining corneal sensitivity and potentially allowing quicker visual recovery. In addition, the peripheral biomechanical properties of the cornea are maintained and flap-related complications are avoided. Creation of a lamellar flap, however, can be an attractive alternative as it offers access to the stromal bed for excimer ablation, allowing for refractive target control and the ability to treat ametropia. In addition, a lamellar flap allows easy access to the inlay in the event repositioning or removal is warranted. The primary difference between a standard LASIK flap is that the technique is relatively dry and thicker flaps may be used to avoid surface curvature changes.

The Flexivue microlens inlay has an insertion device to place the lens into a corneal pocket. Otherwise, corneal inlays are positioned beneath a flap or within a pocket at the desired depth and centered. Inlay centration is critical for optimum performance for all of the corneal inlays.[10] The basis for proper centration is using a coaxially fixated light source on a surgical microscope with patient-assisted fixation. A surgical marker is often useful to clearly identify the target position once it is established by taking into account the first Purkinje image and center of the entrance pupil as landmarks, accounting for the degree of angle kappa. New devices, such as the AcuTarget™ (SMI, Berlin, Germany) are also in development to aid in identifying the proper inlay position.

## ❧ POTENTIAL COMPLICATIONS AND MANAGEMENT

As doctors' understanding of corneal physiology and wound healing have improved, early generation implant adverse events, such as corneal stromal opacity, haze variants, para-inlay epithelial or extracellular matrix deposits, infiltration and keratolysis,[11-14] have decreased significantly. Modifications in postoperative medical regimens and ocular surface optimization, including the correct use of postoperative steroid and perioperative cyclosporine, may also play a role in the improved tolerance and refractive stability of current inlay designs. In addition, a new generation of femtosecond lasers with increased repetition rates, as well as tighter spot and line separation are allowing surgeons to better modulate wound healing responses and decrease forward light scatter. Recognizing focal surface irregularities in the form of epitheliopathy or paracentral irregular 'dellen' like curvature changes associated with the inlay location indicate the use of aggressive treatment of the ocular surface with preservative-free lubricants, cyclosporine, omega-3 fatty acids and antikeratolytic agents such as doxycyline. In the very rare case of progression, extraction is advised with close follow-up. In such cases, the cornea typically heals without further sequelae. Visually significant epithelial ingrowth or deep lamellar keratitis should be managed in the usual fashion, removing the inlay as warranted in severe cases. In the case of decentration, inlays may be easily repositioned concentric with the estimated line of sight to dramatically improve distance and near acuities.[9]

## ❧ CONCLUSION

Half a century after the development of the first corneal implant, materials, designs and techniques are now available, allowing for successful corneal inlay implantation for the treatment of presbyopia. The mechanisms of action for current inlays differ, but all are implanted monocularly, typically in the nondominant eye beneath a LASIK flap or within a laser-created pocket. The inlays are biocompatible and allow adequate molecular flow across the cornea. The procedure is minimally invasive and reversible, making this a viable treatment for presbyopia. Surgeons are currently looking to expand the range of procedures to include implantation in postrefractive patients, including pseudophakic, postlaser vision correction and post-thermal keratoplastic presbyopes.

## ❧ REFERENCES

1. Barraquer JI. Queratoplatica Refractiva. Estudios e informaciones. Oftalnologicas. 1949;2:10.
2. Choyce P. The present status of intracorneal implants. J. Cataract Ophth. 1968;3:295.
3. Dohlman CH, Refojo MF, Rose J. Synthetic polymers in corneal surgery: glyceryl methacylate. Arch Ophthalmol. 1967;177:52-8.
4. Klyce SD, Dingeldein SA, Bonanno JA, et al. Hydrogel implants: Evaluation of first human trial. Invest Ophthalmol Vis Sci Suppl. 1988;29:393.
5. McCarey BE. Alloplastic Refractive Keratoplasty. In: Sanders DR, Hofmann RF, Salz JJ (Eds). Refractive Corneal Surgery. SLACK Inc; 1986. pp. 531-48.
6. Klyce SD, Russell SR. Numerical solution of coupled transport equations applied to corneal hydration dynamics. J Physiol. 1979;292:107-34.
7. Larrea X, De Courten C, Feingold V, et al. Oxygen and glucose distribution after intracorneal lens implantation. Optom Vis Sci. 2007;84(12):1074-81.
8. Klyce SD. Stromal lactate accumulation can account for corneal edema osmotically following epithelial hypoxia in the rabbit. J Physiol.1981;321:49-64.
9. Seyeddain O, Riha W, Hohensinn M, et al. Refractive surgical correction of presbyopia with the acufocus small aperture corneal inlay: two-year follow-up. J Refract Surg. 2010;26:1-9.
10. Yilmaz OF, Bayraktar S, Agca A, et al. Intracorneal inlay for the surgical correction of presbyopia. J Cataract Refract Surg. 2008;34(11):1921-7.
11. Barraquer JI. Modification of refraction by means of intracorneal inclusions. Int Ophthalmol Clin. 1966;6:53-78.
12. Werblin TP, Patel AS, Barraquer JI. Initial human experience with Permalens myopic hydrogel intracorneal lens implants. Refract Corneal Surg. 1992;8:23-6.
13. Mulet ME, Alio JL, Knorz MC. Hydrogel intracorneal inlays for the correction of hyperopia: outcomes and complications after 5 years of follow-up. Ophthalmology. 2009;116(8):1455-60.
14. Alió JL, Mulet ME, Zapata LF, et al. Intracorneal inlay complicated by intrastromal epithelial opacification. Arch Ophthalmol. 2004;122(10):1441-6.

CHAPTER 99

# CHAPTER 100

# Excimer Laser Surface Ablation: Photorefractive Keratectomy and Laser Subepithelial Keratomileusis

*Gitane Patel*

## HISTORY

The first experimental use of the excimer laser on human tissue occurred in 1981, amongst three IBM researchers who used the laser to cleanly etch designs in their day-old Thanksgiving turkey.[1] By 1983, Rangaswamy Srinivasan, one of the original IBM researchers, and Steven Trokel presented findings showing that the excimer laser could have practical applications in corneal surgery.[2] By the early 1990s, it became evident that photorefractive keratectomy (PRK) had the potential to become a cornerstone of refractive corrective eye surgery.[3] An alternative procedure, laser-assisted subepithelial keratomileusis (LASEK), was developed in 1999 by Massimo Camellin in order to address some of the complications associated with PRK.[4]

## EXCIMER LASER

The realm of laser vision corrective surgery was brought into existence by the advent of the 193 nm excimer laser. The term 'excimer' stems from the words 'excited dimer'. The laser emits light of ultraviolet intensity of 193 nm, which is produced by the excitation of argon, which then binds with a fluorine atom. This light causes a photo-disruptive effect on corneal stromal tissue, vaporizing the tissue with minimal heat production. This unique effect allows molding of the corneal stroma by the laser without significant effect on surrounding tissues.[2]

## PRK, LASIK AND LASEK

Photorefractive keratectomy and LASEK, in effect, are the same procedure. In PRK, the epithelium is completely removed, either by using manual scraping, the excimer laser,[5] or using alcohol (which may lead to a smoother Bowman's surface and better overall results).[6] In LASEK, the epithelium is loosened using alcohol, but left on a hinge, to be repositioned into place at the end of the procedure.[4] The hope here is to reduce postoperative pain by covering the bare stroma with the epithelium. In laser-assisted *in situ* keratomileusis (LASIK), a hinged lenticule of corneal stroma is created, using either the microkeratome or the femtosecond laser, the lenticule is retracted during the ablation, and it is repositioned at the end of the procedure.[7]

In PRK, the epithelium within the ablation zone is completely removed before the ablation. If using a blade to remove the epithelium, care must be taken not to cause aberrations in Bowman's layer. Additionally, all epithelium within the ablation zone must be completely removed to avoid undertreated islands, which may lead to irregular astigmatism and decreased vision postprocedure. Alternatively, 20% alcohol can be applied over the epithelium to loosen it. The epithelium can then be gently swept or scraped away using a methylcellulose sponge or blade. Finally, the excimer laser itself can be used to ablate the epithelium just prior to performing the refractive ablation. Generally, a bandage contact lens is placed at the end of the procedure to aid in pain control and re-epithelialization.

In LASEK, a trephine or sharp instrument is used to demarcate an epithelial hinge. Then, 20% alcohol solution is used to loosen the epithelium, which is then retracted back for the ablation. This flap is then repositioned after the laser ablation has completed. A bandage contact lens is then placed.

Laser-assisted in situ keratomileusis is significantly different from other procedures because a thin stromal flap is created, retracted and replaced after the procedure. This flap, generally 120–160 μm in thickness, may be created either by a microkeratome or a femtosecond laser. Afterward, a contact lens is not generally necessary, and visual rehabilitation is almost immediate and painless.

## ▶ PREOPERATIVE MANAGEMENT

An unmistakably important aspect of preoperative management for laser surface refractive surgery is patient selection. Patients should understand first and foremost that their visual acuity after laser refractive surgery will be no better than with glasses or contact lenses. In particular, the myopic prepresbyope should be thoroughly counseled on the decrease in near visual acuity after the procedure. The patient should be instructed to stay out of soft contact lenses for at least 1 week, and rigid contact lenses for at least 3 weeks, prior to presurgical evaluation, in order to gain the highest accuracy in preoperative refractive and wavefront measurements. Corneal pachymetry, topography, and wavefront measurements should be made before the procedure.

A thorough medical history should be taken, including general medical history and history of any eye disease, including collagen vascular disease, inflammatory eye disease, dry eye syndrome, and/or prior eye surgeries. Retinoic acid derivative medications, such as isotretoin, should be stopped, as these may have a negative effect on healing.[8] Amiodarone use is a contraindication for refractive laser eye surgery. A complete ophthalmic examination, including manifest and cycloplegic refraction, pupil size measurements, and careful corneal examination should be performed. Any signs of ocular disease, including glaucoma, macular degeneration, or macular epiretinal membrane, among others, should be carefully searched for, as these may affect the postoperative vision. Patients with incipient cataracts may be better considered for future cataract surgery, since the cataract will not only decrease the best spectacle-corrected visual acuity (BSCVA), but also cause a refractive change with time. Special attention should be paid to any evidence of corneal disease or opacities, as these may negatively affect the laser ablation, as well as the action of the femtosecond laser during flap creation. The corneal topography should be carefully reviewed in every patient for signs of corneal ectasia or risk thereof. Signs of latent or intermittent strabismus should be searched for, as fusion may be affected by monovision treatments.[9] Patients with anterior basement membrane dystrophy may fare better with PRK than with LASIK because the former may help both reduce the signs of such and avoid the occurrence of epithelial sloughing.[10]

Also, patients whose residual stromal bed thickness may be less than 250 μm with LASIK may still be refractive surgical candidates with PRK or LASEK.[11] A patient with a deep orbit may present a challenge with placing the keratome or femtosecond laser suction ring. Excessively steep (48D) or flat (40D) eyes may suffer from buttonholes or free caps, respectively, and may also be better managed with PRK or LASEK.

## ▶ TECHNIQUE

Laser-assisted in situ keratomileusis technique is covered in Chapter 95. After epithelial removal/flap formation, PRK and LASEK techniques are identical. Before beginning the procedure, a reference mark may be placed in the eye at 180°. The patient is then laid flat under the laser. A small dose of anxiolytic such as diazepam may be given preoperatively for patient comfort. A topical anesthetic, such as tetracaine, should be used. Iris registration may be used to reduce error from cyclotorsion,[12] while pupil tracking may help account for eye movement. It is still important, however, to encourage the patient to stare at the fixation target. The foot pedal is depressed to engage the laser. In eyes with high myopia or after previous corneal surgery, mitomycin C (MMC) 0.02% may be used to help prevent the complication of corneal haze.[13] At the conclusion of the treatment, the cornea is irrigated with a 30-guage cannula and (in LASEK) the epithelial flap repositioned. A drop of a topical steroid, NSAID and antibiotic are usually given. A bandage contact lens is then placed, and a clear eye shield is positioned over the eye. If bilateral treatment is planned, this is normally performed concurrently.

## ▶ POSTOPERATIVE MANAGEMENT

Generally, a topical fourth generation fluoroquinolone, such as moxifloxacin or gatifloxacin, administered four times a day, a topical steroid, such as loteprednol 0.5% administered four times a day, and a topical NSAID, such as bromfenac 0.09%, administered once a day are prescribed. The topical NSAID and antibiotic are normally continued until the epithelial defect has healed and the contact lens has been removed. The steroid is continued on a taper for up to 6 months depending on refractive stability and haze formation.[14] High dose vitamin C may be used to help in wound healing and haze prevention.[15]

CHAPTER 100

## ⋟ OUTCOMES

Despite the promise of less postoperative pain, LASEK has not shown any benefit with regards to postoperative pain, re-epithelialization, or final outcomes when compared to PRK, although there may be less postoperative haze with LASEK.[16]

A 14-year follow-up study of myopic PRK showed that refractive stability is long standing—the average uncorrected visual acuity was close to 20/20 amongst those with low to moderate myopia and about 20/25 amongst those with high myopia.[17] At 6 months after wavefront-guided ablation, 75% of eyes reach 20/20 or better,[18] with almost all reaching better than 20/40. There can, however, be some decreased contrast sensitivity, which affect low-light visual acuity.[19]

In hyperopic PRK, the ablation occurs in the periphery of the ablation zone, steepening the cornea. There is normally an early overcorrection, which, due to epithelial molding, regresses to the desired target refraction over 3–6 months.

At 1 year, 93% of patients with low to moderate hyperopia may reach an uncorrected visual acuity of 20/40, while 70% reach 20/20.[20] Patients with higher hyperopia, greater than +3.75 D, 48% reach 20/40 uncorrected, while 34% reach 20/20. Up to 19% may lose two or more lines of best corrected vision. Hyperopic LASIK, combined with MMC, has shown similar results, with 94% reaching better than 20/40 uncorrected, but with less haze occurrence.[21]

## ⋟ MITOMYCIN C

Mitomycin C was first used to treat postcorneal haze resulting from PRK treatment.[22] Since then, it has become commonplace to prophylactically treat patients with higher treatments (−6.00 D and greater) to prevent haze formation.[23] Mitomycin C 0.02% is placed over the cornea at the end of the treatment for 2 minutes using a methylcellulose sponge, and then the eye is rinsed. It has also been utilized to successfully reduce haze formation in hyperopic treatments.[19]

## ⋟ MONOVISION

If the presbyope or prepresbyope desires to retain some functional near vision, one eye may be targeted for slight myopia (generally anywhere from −0.5 D to −2 D). The vast majority of patients tend to retain both excellent distance vision as well as functional intermediate vision,

with up to 88% patient satisfaction.[24] Generally, the dominant eye is set for distance and the nondominant eye for intermediate, but crossed-monovision may also be employed successfully.

## ⋟ PHOTOREFRACTIVE KERATECTOMY AFTER PREVIOUS CORNEAL SURGERY

Photorefractive keratectomy has been performed following previous PRK, LASIK, radial keratotomy (RK), conductive keratoplasty (CK) and penetrating keratoplasty (PKP).

Following PRK for errors greater than −6 D, the rates of regression may be up to 2 D 10 years following the procedure.[25] Retreatment may be an option to correct the error. Haze with PRK retreatment may be moderate to severe in up to 8% of eyes[26] without the use of MMC. As a result, many centers routinely use MMC for any PRK retreatment.

Photorefractive keratectomy may be performed after LASIK, if for example, there is a complication with flap creation, such as a buttonhole or doughnut-shaped flap.[27] If the surgeon does not feel that recutting the flap at a future date is a good option, or if there are limitations due to residual stromal bed thickness, PRK may be an option.

Radial keratotomy hyperopic shifts may be treated effectively with a PRK treatment.[28] Once again, due to the risk of corneal haze, MMC is routinely used.[29] Wavefront-guided treatments may aid in improving visual outcomes.[30]

Good results have been obtained with PRK in patients who have already undergone successful PKP.[31] It offers a solution for patients who may not be able to tolerate contact lenses and in whom the anisometropia is too great for glasses. The use of MMC has improved the outcomes of PRK postkeratoplasty.[32] However, the chance of postoperative haze and graft failure may still be increased in these patients.

Residual refractive error after cataract surgery is also effectively treated with PRK.[33]

## ⋟ COMPLICATIONS

### Haze

Corneal haze is a complication of LASEK and PRK, with higher treatments being more prone to visually significant corneal hazing.[34] It is thought to occur secondary to deposition of extracellular matrix materials secreted by fibroblasts in the area of hazing.[35] This hazing, if significant enough, may lead to glare or regression.

A mild, reticular pattern of anterior corneal stromal hazing is common early after treatment, but in most patients, this clears over time without visual sequelae.[36] Moreover, the use of MMC for higher treatments has reduced the occurrence of visually significant haze even further.[37] Patients with deeper ablation depth,[38] smaller treatment diameters,[39] and ultraviolet light exposure are at higher risk for corneal haze. The use of steroids postoperatively helps to reduce the formation of late onset haze.[40] Use of ascorbate may also reduce the postoperative haze.[41]

If a patient develops significant haze or the related regression of correction, it is important to institute topical steroids frequently for weeks to stop the regression and/or haze. If this is unsuccessful, then other viable interventional strategies, including phototherapeutic keratectomy with MMC[42] or corneal scraping with MMC, may be indicated.[43]

## Infectious Keratitis

Corneal infiltrates may occur in up to 0.8% of PRK patients, with a handful of these possessing confirmed infectious etiologies.[44] Generally, the bandage contact lens is discontinued, and dosages of steroids and antibiotics are increased, with close follow-up, in the case of an infiltrate with low infectious suspicion.[45] The most likely cases are gram positive bacteria, including *Staphylococcus aureus* (as well as methicillin resistant variants), *Staphylococcus epidermis, Streptococcus viridans and Streptococcus pneumoniae*.[46] Case reports of atypical Mycobacterium,[47] fungus,[48] and herpetic keratitis[49] have also been documented. Urgent treatment with fourth generation flouroquinolones and/or fortified antibiotics may be necessary. If permanent corneal scarring ensues, therapeutic PRK[50] or PKP may be required.

## Decentered Ablation

A decentered ablation occurs when the center of the ablation is eccentric to the center of the pupil or visual axis. It is important to ensure that the patient's head is positioned correctly, that the eye tracker is functional, and that the surgeon's eyepiece is aligned correctly with the laser. Decentration may cause comma-shaped aberration, astigmatism, and loss of focus,[51] which may decrease the visual outcome. Topography-guided laser treatment may be effective in treating this condition.[52,53]

## Dry Eyes

Dry eyes, as in LASIK, are common in the months ensuing PRK or LASEK surgery. Although this normally resolves by 6 months' time,[54] some long-term symptoms may remain. However, duration of symptoms is less than after LASIK.[55] Nerve growth factor and corneal sensation may play a role in this process.[54]

It is prudent to assess and treat tear film abnormalities or deficiencies before performing refractive surgery. Methods may include frequent use of preserved or nonpreserved artificial tears and gels, placement of punctal plugs, and treatment of blepharitis. For patients with more severe dry eyes, starting cyclosporine (Restasis, Allergan) eye drops before surgery may be required.

In summary, both PRK and LASEK are safe and effective refractive procedures for the correction of myopia, hyperopia and astigmatism. Photorefractive keratectomy and LASEK, as compared to LASIK, provides the advantages of a flap-free procedure, which can reduce the potential for ectasia and flap complications, at the cost of a slower, more uncomfortable visual recovery, but with the same end results. Proper patient selection, safe and consistent surgical technique, and adequate perioperative care are important aspects to obtain positive results with the use of PRK and LASEK in the management of patients with refractive errors.

## ❧ REFERENCES

1. Wynn JJ. Excimer Laser Surgery. http://www.ibm.com/ibm100/us/en/icons/excimer/.
2. Trokel SL, Srinivasan R, Braren B. Excimer laser surgery of the cornea. Am J Ophthalmol. 1983;96(6):710-5.
3. Lindstrom RL, Sher NA, Chen V, et al. Use of the 193-NM excimer laser for myopic photorefractive keratectomy in sighted eyes: a multicenter study. Trans Am Ophthalmol Soc. 1991;89:155-72; discussion 172-82.
4. Camellin M. LASEK may offer advantages of both LASIK and PRK. Ocular Surgery News. 1999:28.
5. Lee YG, Chen WY, Petroll WM, et al. Corneal haze after photorefractive keratectomy using different epithelial removal techniques: mechanical debridement versus laser scrape. Ophthalmology. 2001;108(1):112-20.
6. Carones F, Fiore T, Brancato R. Mechanical vs. alcohol epithelial removal during photorefractive keratectomy. J Refract Surg. 1999;15(5):556-62.
7. Pallikaris IG, Papatzanaki ME, Siganos DS, et al. A corneal flap technique for laser in situ keratomileusis. Human studies. Arch Ophthalmol. 1991;109(12):1699-702.
8. Fraunfelder FT, LaBraico JM, Meyer SM. Adverse ocular reactions possibly associated with isotretinoin. Am J Ophthalmol. 1985;100(4):534-7.
9. Godts D, Trau R, Tassignon MJ. Effect of refractive surgery on binocular vision and ocular alignment in patients with manifest or intermittent strabismus. Br J Ophthalmol. 2006;90(11):1410-3.

10. Zaidman GW, Hong A. Visual and refractive results of combined PTK/PRK in patients with corneal surface disease and refractive errors. J Cataract Refract Surg. 2006;32(6):958-61.

11. Melki SA, Azar DT. LASIK complications: etiology, management, and prevention. Surv Ophthalmol. 2001;46:95-116.

12. Chernyak DA. Iris-based cyclotorsional image alignment method for wavefront registration. IEEE Trans Biomed Eng. 2005;52(12):2032-40.

13. Shalaby A, Kaye GB, Gimbel HV. Mitomycin C in photorefractive keratectomy. J Refract Surg. 2009;25(1 Suppl):S93-7.

14. Vetrugno M, Maino A, Quaranta GM, et al. The effect of early steroid treatment after PRK on clinical and refractive outcomes. Acta Ophthalmol Scand. 2001;79(1):23-7.

15. Stojanovic A, Ringvold A, Nitter T. Ascorbate prophylaxis for corneal haze after photorefractive keratectomy. J Refract Surg. 2003;19(3):338-43.

16. Zhao LQ, Wei RL, Cheng JW, et al. Meta-analysis: clinical outcomes of laser-assisted subepithelial keratectomy and photorefractive keratectomy in myopia. Ophthalmology. 2010;117(10):1912-22. Epub 2010 Aug 14.

17. Bricola G, Scotto R, Mete M, et al. A 14-year follow-up of photorefractive keratectomy. J Refract Surg. 2009;25(6):545-52.

18. Moshirfar M, Schliesser JA, Chang JC, et al. Visual outcomes after wavefront-guided photorefractive keratectomy and wavefront-guided laser in situ keratomileusis: Prospective comparison. J Cataract Refract Surg. 2010;36(8):1336-43.

19. Tanabe T, Miyata K, Samejima T, et al. Influence of wavefront aberration and corneal subepithelial haze on low-contrast visual acuity after photorefractive keratectomy. Am J Ophthalmol. 2004;138(4):620-4.

20. Stevens J, Giubilei M, Ficker L, et al. Prospective study of photorefractive keratectomy for myopia using the VISX StarS2 excimer laser system. J Refract Surg. 2002;18(5):502-8.

21. Leccisotti A. Mitomycin-C in hyperopic photorefractive keratectomy. J Cataract Refract Surg. 2009;35(4):682-7.

22. Raviv T, Majmudar PA, Dennis RF, et al. Mitomycin-C for post-PRK corneal haze. J Cataract Refract Surg. 2000;26(8):1105-6.

23. Carones F, Vigo L, Scandola E, et al. Evaluation of the prophylactic use of mitomycin-C to inhibit haze formation after photorefractive keratectomy. J Cataract Refract Surg. 2002;28(12):2088-95.

24. Jain S, Ou R, Azar DT. Monovision outcomes in presbyopic individuals after refractive surgery. Ophthalmology. 2001;108(8):1430-3.

25. Alió JL, Muftuoglu O, Ortiz D, et al. Ten-year follow-up of photorefractive keratectomy for myopia of more than -6 diopters. Am J Ophthalmol. 2008;145(1):37-45.

26. Maloney RK, Chan WK, Steinert R, et al. A multicenter trial of photorefractive keratectomy for residual myopia after previous ocular surgery. Summit Therapeutic Refractive Study Group. Ophthalmology. 1995;102(7):1042-52; discussion 1052-3.

27. Kapadia MS, Wilson SE. Transepithelial photorefractive keratectomy for treatment of thin flaps or caps after complicated laser in situ keratomileusis. Am J Ophthalmol. 1998;126(6):827-9.

28. Myrowitz EH, Kurwa A, Parker J, et al. Wavefront-guided photorefractive keratectomy after radial keratotomy in nine eyes. J Refract Surg. 2009;25(5):470-2.

29. Anbar R, Malta JB, Barbosa JB, et al. Photorefractive keratectomy with mitomycin-C for consecutive hyperopia after radial keratotomy. Cornea. 2009;28(4):371-4.

30. Koch DD, Maloney R, Hardten DR, et al. Wavefront-guided photorefractive keratectomy in eyes with prior radial keratotomy: a multicenter study. Ophthalmology 2009:116(9):1688-96.

31. Huang PY, Huang PT, Astle WF, et al. Laser-assisted subepithelial keratectomy and photorefractive keratectomy for post-penetrating keratoplasty myopia and astigmatism in adults. J Cataract Refract Surg. 2011;37(2):335-40.

32. Forseto Ados S, Marques JC, Nosé W. Photorefractive keratectomy with mitomycin C after penetrating and lamellar keratoplasty. Cornea. 2010;29(10):1103-8.

33. Artola A, Ayala MJ, Claramonte P, et al. Photorefractive keratectomy for residual myopia after cataract surgery. J Cataract Refract Surg. 1999;25(11):1456-60.

34. Caubet E. Course of subepithelial corneal haze over 18 months after photorefractive keratectomy for myopia [corrected]. Refract Corneal Surg. 1993;9(2 Suppl):S65-70.

35. Lee YC, Wang IJ, Hu FR, et al. Immunohistochemical study of subepithelial haze after phototherapeutic keratectomy. J Refract Surg. 2001;17(3):334-41.

36. Honda N, Hamada N, Amano S, et al. Five-year follow-up of photorefractive keratectomy for myopia. J Refract Surg. 2004;20(2):116-20.

37. Bedei A, Marabotti A, Giannecchini I, et al. Photorefractive keratectomy in high myopic defects with or without intraoperative mitomycin C: 1-year results. Eur J Ophthalmol. 2006;16(2):229-34.

38. Møller-Pedersen T, Cavanagh HD, Petroll WM, et al. Corneal haze development after PRK is regulated by volume of stromal tissue removal. Cornea. 1998;17(6):627-39.

39. O'Brart DP, Corbett MC, Verma S, et al. Effects of ablation diameter, depth, and edge contour on the outcome of photorefractive keratectomy. J Refract Surg. 1996;12(1):50-60.

40. Vetrugno M, Maino A, Quaranta GM, et al. The effect of early steroid treatment after PRK on clinical and refractive outcomes. Acta Ophthalmol Scand. 2001;79(1):23-7.

41. Stojanovic A, Ringvold A, Nitter T. Ascorbate prophylaxis for corneal haze after photorefractive keratectomy. J Refract Surg. 2003;19(3):338-43.

42. Porges Y, Ben-Haim O, Hirsh A, et al. Phototherapeutic keratectomy with mitomycin C for corneal haze following photorefractive keratectomy for myopia. J Refract Surg. 2003;19(1):40-3.

43. Vigo L, Scandola E, Carones F. Scraping and mitomycin C to treat haze and regression after photorefractive keratectomy for myopia. J Refract Surg. 2003;19(4):449-54.

44. de Oliveira GC, Solari HP, Ciola FB, et al. Corneal infiltrates after excimer laser photorefractive keratectomy and LASIK. J Refract Surg. 2006;22(2):159-65.

45. Rao SK, Fogla R, Rajagopal R, et al. Bilateral corneal infiltrates after excimer laser photorefractive keratectomy. J Cataract Refract Surg. 2000;26(3):456-9.

46. Donnenfeld ED, O'Brien TP, Solomon R, et al. Infectious keratitis after photorefractive keratectomy. Ophthalmology. 2003;110(4):743-7.

47. Kouyoumdjian GA, Forstot SL, Durairaj VD, et al. Infectious keratitis after laser refractive surgery. Ophthalmology. 2001;108 (7):1266-8.

48. Periman LM, Harrison DA, Kim J. Fungal keratitis after photorefractive keratectomy: delayed diagnosis and treatment in a co-managed setting. J Refract Surg. 2003;19(3):364-6.

49. Lu CK, Chen KH, Lee SM, et al. Herpes simplex keratitis following excimer laser application. J Refract Surg. 2006;22(5): 509-11.

50. Faschinger CW. Phototherapeutic keratectomy of a corneal scar due to presumed infection after photorefractive keratectomy. J Cataract Refract Surg. 2000;26(2):296-300.

51. Bühren J, Yoon G, Kenner S, et al. The effect of optical zone decentration on lower- and higher-order aberrations after photorefractive keratectomy in a cat model. Invest Ophthalmol Vis Sci. 2007;48(12):5806-14.

52. Lin DY, Manche EE. Custom-contoured ablation pattern method for the treatment of decentered laser ablations. J Cataract Refract Surg. 2004;30(8):1675-84.

53. Toda I, Yamamoto T, Ito M, et al. Topography-guided ablation for treatment of patients with irregular astigmatism. J Refract Surg. 2007;23(2):118-25.

54. Kanellopoulos AJ, Pallikaris IG, Donnenfeld ED, et al. Comparison of corneal sensation following photorefractive keratectomy and laser in situ keratomileusis. J Cataract Refract Surg. 1997;23:34-8.

55. Hovanesian JA, Shah SS, Maloney RK. Symptoms of dry eye and recurrent erosion syndrome after refractive surgery. J Cataract Refract Surg. 2001;27(4):577-84.

# LASIK Instrumentation: Microkeratomes, Excimer Lasers and Wavefront Analyzers

*Fasika Woreta, Yassine J Daoud, Kraig S Bower*

## ❧ INTRODUCTION

Laser *in situ* keratomileusis (LASIK) is the most common refractive surgery performed today.[1] Over the past two decades, advances in microkeratome design, laser technology, and wavefront-guided technology have led to substantial improvements in the safety, efficacy and predictability of surgical outcomes. This chapter will provide an overview of the principles of the mechanical microkeratome, as well as review the most commonly used microkeratomes and femtosecond lasers. The principles of the excimer laser and commonly used excimer lasers will also be discussed. Finally, the theories of wavefront analysis and specific FDA-approved wavefront-guided systems will be reviewed.

## ❧ MICROKERATOMES

### Historical Background

In the 1958 in Bogota, Columbia, Dr Jose I Barraquer developed the first manual microkeratome with a cutting angle of 0°. In 1962, he designed an improved keratome with a cutting angle of 26° and a suction ring. In 1991, based on Barraquer's work, Dr Ioannis Pallikaris introduced the concept of the creation of a corneal hinge and performed the first photoablation under a nasal corneal flap.[2] This was a significant advancement in the field of refractive surgery and today the creation of a hinged corneal flap of optimal thickness is a critical part of the LASIK operation. The rate of micokeratome-related flap complications such as incomplete caps, thin or irregular caps, decentered caps, and button-holes have been reported to range from 0.3 to 1.9%.[3,4] Thick flaps decrease residual stromal bed thickness and can be associated with corneal ectasia.[5] Postoperative flap related complications include flap striae, flap displacement, diffuse lamelllar keratitis (DLK), epithelial effects, and epithelial ingrowth.[6,7] The main criteria for a microkeratome are safety, reliability and reproducibility of flap diameter and thickness

The Bausch & Lomb automated corneal shaper (ACS), introduced in 1994, was the most popular and frequently used keratome for many years. Based on the automated lamellar keratotomy (ALK) technique designed by A Ruiz, it was one of the earliest microkeratomes and served as a model for modern keratomes. This keratome could be advanced automatically with the theoretical advantage of an improved consistency of cut.[8] It created a nasal hinge with depth settings of 160–200 microns.[8,9] Since then, many models of microkeratomes have been introduced, with safer and more reliable designs. This section will review the basic components of a microkeratome and commonly used microkeratomes.

### Components of the Microkeratome

The basic components of a microkeratome consist of control console, body or motor, head, blade and suction ring.[8,10-12]

- The control console contains the power supply and vacuum pump, which transmit vacuum to the suction ring through disposable suction tubing. The console contains a front panel display and two foot-pedals, which control the motor (forward/backward) and suction pump (activate/deactivate).

- The motor is housed in a cylindrical handpiece attaching to the console by the power supply cord. On the other side, it is screwed vertically onto the head and attaches to the blade holder, transmitting oscillation to the blade. The blade can be moved forward manually or through an automated gear mechanism.

- The head is composed of gears, a blade holder, a stopping plate, and a depth plate to set flap thickness. The motor activates the gear mechanism, allowing automated movement. The stop mechanism allows for the creation of a hinge and can be adjusted. Newer keratomes have fixed plate depths, as replaceable depth plates can lead to a deeper than intended cut if incorrectly inserted.

- The microkeratome blade is shaped on both sides. It is disposable and inserted manually or with a blade insertion system into the microkeratome head. If moved forward manually, the surgeon can modify flap thickness by using a faster pass to create a thinner flap and a slower pass for a thicker flap. Automated microkeratomes have a fixed passed speed with horizontal blade oscillations varying from 12,000 to 18,000 oscillations per second. The blade entry angles vary from 25° to 30° in the majority of microkeratomes.

- The suction ring consists of a handle and circular ring with an inner diameter of 8–8.5 mm on average, which has a vacuum outlet from below to hold the globe. Suction rings with different inner ring diameters are available with some models and flap diameter depends on both the inner ring diameter and steepness of the cornea, with larger rings and steeper corneas resulting in larger flaps. Before each procedure, the suction should be checked carefully. Newer microkeratomes stop blade oscillation if there is loss of suction.

The next section will review specific models of mechanical microkeratomes including the Hansatome (Bausch & Lomb), Zyoptix XP (Technolas Perfect Vision), the Summit Krumeich-Barraquer Microkeratome (SKBM, Alcon), the Amadeus II Microkeratome (Abott Medical Optics), MK-2000 (Nidek), the Carriazo-Barraquer Microkeratome (Moria), and the Carriazo-Pendular Microkeratome (SCHWIND eye-tech-solutions). A comparison of these microkeratomes is displayed in Table 1, with selected microkeratome models displayed in Figures 1A to E. With the exception of the Amadeus microkeratome, flaps created with microkeratomes are generally thinner than the specified plate depth.

## Hansatome (Bausch & Lomb)

The Hansatome, by Bausch & Lomb Surgical, is the most commonly used instrument for creating a flap, utilized by 45% of surgeons in a 2004 survey by the US Members of the International Society of Refractive Surgery of the American Academy of Ophthalmology.[1] The Hansatome is a two-piece mechanical microkeratome, consisting of a handpiece with an electric motor connected to the head of the microkeratome and an oscillating stainless steel blade oriented at an angle of 25°. The blade oscillates within the microkeratome head at 7,500 oscillations per minute. There is a curved elevated gear track, which should be nasally positioned to create a superior hinge. Both the handpiece and motor are placed vertically on the suction ring, providing stability and traction during the cut. The standard suction ring has an outer diameter of 20 mm and the inner diameters are available in 8.5 mm or 9.5 mm. For patients with narrow palpebral fissures, tight lids, or deep-set orbits, microrings are available with an outer diameter of 19 mm and the same available inner diameters. The keratome head has a secure, nonremovable depth plate intended to create a flap of a specific thickness. Plates of different thicknesses (160, 180 and 200 µM) are available, with the most commonly used plates being the 160 and 180 µM plates.[9,11-13] The actual flap thickness is usually less than the predicted flap thickness.[11,14,15] In a prospective multicenter study, the mean flap thickness for the 160 and 180 µM plates were 129 ± 21 µM and 136 ± 25 µM, respectively.[12,15]

In the past, epithelial defects were common with the Hansatome, reported to range from 3.3% to 15%.[3,15-17] Epithelial defects after LASIK have been associated with diffuse lamellar keratitis, epithelial ingrowth and delayed visual recovery[18-20] With the advent of zero compression heads, designed to reduce the incidence of epithelial defects by eliminating compression of the flap and shearing forces on the epithelium, the incidence of epithelial defects has been reduced significantly, now reported to be about 0.4%.[20]

## Zyoptix XP Microkeratome (Technolas Perfect Vision)

The Zyoptix XP is the most recent mechanical microkeratome released by Bausch & Lomb, with several advantages over the Hansatome. These improvements include the absence of external gears and an elevated suction ring,

101
CHAPTER

**Table 1:** Comparison of microkeratome models

| Microkeratome | Manufacturer | Oscillation Speed (rpm) | Translational Speed (mm/sec) | Flap Thicknesses (μM) | Flap Diameters (mm) | Hinge Position |
|---|---|---|---|---|---|---|
| Hansatome | Bausch & Lomb | 7,500 | Preset (~ 6 seconds to cut flap) | 160 180 200 | 8.5 9.5 | Superior |
| Zyoptix XP | Technolas perfect vision | 61,000 | 12.0 | 120 140 160 | 8.5 9.5 | 360° hinge placement |
| Summit Kruemeich-Barraquer | Alcon | 5,000–20,000 | Up to 3 | 130 160 | 8.0–10.0 | Nasal |
| Amadeus II | Abott medical optics | 4,000–20,000 | 1.5–4.0 | 110 120 140 160 | 8.5 9.0 9.5 10.0 | Nasal |
| Nidek MK-2000 | Nidek | 9,000 | 2.0 | 130 160 180 | 9 10 | Typically nasal, other positions possible |
| Carriazo-Barraquer | Moria | 15,000 | Manual control (most common 2.5–4.0) | 130 160 180 | 7–10.5 | 360° hinge placement |
| Moria M2 | Moria | 15,000 | 2.1 or 3.1 available | 130 160 | 7–10.5 | 360° hinge placement |
| Carriazo-Pendular | SCHWIND eye-tech solutions | Up to 15,000 | Up to 6 | 90 110 130 150 170 | 9 10 | 360° hinge placement |

minimizing the potential for physical obstruction of the microkeratome as it moves forward and interference with drapes and eyelashes. The hinge position can be varied 360° as desired by the surgeon. The motor sleeve is autoclavable, allowing for easier sterilization. The right eye/ left eye selector switch facilitates transition between eyes without total disassembly, as is required for the Hansatome. This eliminates risk of improper reassembly, resulting in improved safety. All parts are 100% interchangeable unlike the Hansatome, preventing the need to return the entire

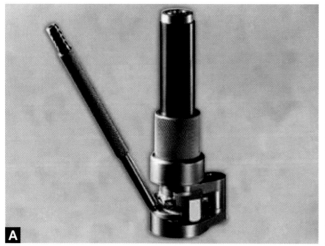
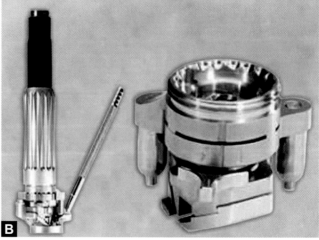

**Figs 1A and B**

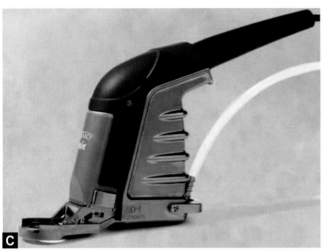

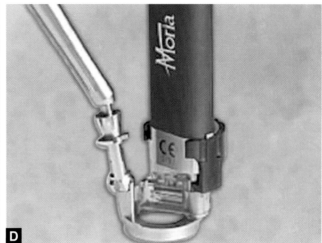

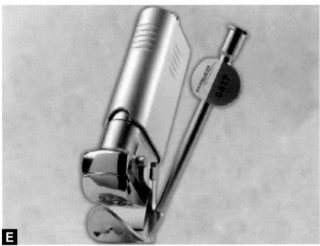

**Figs 1A to E:** Depiction of microkeratomes used for LASIK flap creation. (A) Hansatome (Bausch & Lomb); (B) Zyoptix XP Microkeratome (Technolas Perfect Vision); (C) Amadeus II (Abott Medical Optics); (D) Moria M2 (Moria); (E) Carriazo-Pendular Microkeratome (SCHWIND eye-tech-solutions). Note pendular cutting head

unit to the manufacturer for repair of only one component. The XP blades are also manufactured with tighter blade tolerance than the blades used with Hansatome. Finally, the Zyoptix XP allows for less variation in flap thickness than the Hansatome, reducing the standard deviation in flap thickness from 20.7µM to 14.8 µM.[12,21]

## Summit-Krumeich-Barraquer Microkeratome (Alcon)

The Summit-Krumeich-Barraquer microkeratome was a microkeratome in which the blade could be passed either manually or automatically. It had a dual motor system, which regulated translational speed and blade oscillation rate independently. Both of these parameters could be adjusted by the surgeon, with the blade advancement rate ranging from 0.5 to 4.0 mm/second and the blade oscillation rate ranging from 4,000 to 20,000 oscillations per minute. This dual motor design provided a safety advantage,

allowing the blade to reach full oscillating speed before forward movement and the blade oscillation to be turned off during backward movement.[22,23] The microkeratome had four suction rings to create flaps ranging from 8.0 mm to 9.5 mm in diameter. One advantage was that the applanation plate was transparent, allowing visualization of the cornea during the creation of the flap.[24] However, this microkeratome was recalled by Alcon in 2003, as the adhesive holding applanation plate in place was found to deteriorate over time, leading to misalignment of the window and deeper than intended flaps. It is no longer available on the market.

## Amadeus II (Abott Medical Optics)

The Amadeus microkeratome is a one-piece microkeratome designed with emphasis on safety and efficiency. Initially manufactured by Abbot Medical Optics (AMO), it is now marketed by Zeimer Ophthalmic Systems. It can be operated with a single hand and consists of only three pieces to assemble. In addition, each piece can be assembled in only one way, eliminating the possibility of improper assembly. It is fully assembled when handed to the surgeon, avoiding the need for on the eye assembly and therefore reducing required suction time. It has a dual motor system with separate motors for both translation of the microkeratome and oscillation of the blade. The blade oscillation rate is customizable from 4,000 to 20,000 rpm and translation speed from 1.5 to 4.0 mm/seconds. It is gearless, avoiding the risk of gear jams. Four suction ring sizes, 8.5 mm, 9.0 mm, 9.5, and 10.0 mm are available. Only a nasal hinge can be created. Depth plates are available to create 140, 160 and 180 µM flaps. In the multicenter trial by Solomon and colleagues using an earlier version of the Amadeus, the mean flap thickness for the 130, 140 and 160 µM plates were 147 ± 24 µM, 134 ± 15 µM, and 180 ± 34 µM, respectively.[15] There are multiple computer-controlled safety checks at every step of the procedure, including assembly, suction, and advancement.[25] Visualization of the cornea is possible during flap creation through the applanation plate. Another major advantage is that is the only microkeratome system that has a multipurpose platform for use in anterior and posterior keratoplasty.

## MK-2000 (Nidek)

The MK-2000, like the Amadeus microkeratome, is a one-piece microkeratome with several advantages: automated drive, no external gears, independent translational and blade oscillation movement, the ability for one-handed operation, assembly prior to placement on the eye, and visible flap formation during forward movement of the head. The blade oscillates at a fixed rate of 9,000 rpm with a cut angle of 25° and the translational movement of the blade holder forward and backward is fixed at a rate of 2 mm per second. The MK-2000 microkeratome is easier to use in patients with narrow palpebral fissures, tight lids, or deep orbits than the two-piece Hansatome, as it is a smaller size for suction rings of the same diameter. The suction ring has dual suction ports with a feedback sensor, with an alarm to indicate when suction is not sufficient. In addition, the blade cannot be moved forward with the alarm active, providing a safety mechanism.[12,23,26,27] Two suction rings of sizes 8.5 mm and 9.5 mm and three microkeratome plate holders with depths of 130 µM, 160 µM or 180 µM are available. A nasal hinge is typically created, but other positions are possible. In the multicenter trial by Solomon, the actual mean flap thickness created was

less than the predicted, with the 130 µM plate thickness producing a mean flap thickness of 111 ± 19 µM and the 160 µM producing a mean flap thickness of 121 ± 12 µM.[15]

## Corriazo-Barraquer Microkeratome (Moria)

The Moria CB microkeratome was one of the first pivoting microkeratomes, allowing the position of the flap hinge to be varied by 360°. The microkeratome head fits into a dovetail groove and thus no gears are exposed. There is only one way to insert the preassembled blade, avoiding improper insertion. The blade oscillates at 15,000 rpm with a cutting angle of 26°. It is a manual keratome and thus and the translational speed can be varied by the surgeon, with faster passes creating thinner flaps. The microkeratome has a dual-vacuum setting (20 mm Hg and 65 mm Hg), allowing the suction ring to remain attached to the cornea at a lower intraocular pressure. Suction rings of five different sizes are available, ranging from 7 mm to 10.5 mm, and thus can accommodate those with small palpebral fissures. There are three depth settings labeled 110 µM, 130 µM or 150 µM, but in actuality the flaps created are thicker by at least 30 µM.[12,15]

The Moria M2 automated microkeratome has many of the same features of the Moria CB, with the advantage of a dual motor system with automated translation to improve the consistency of flap creation.[12,22,28] Single-use Moria M2 microkeratomes are now available, with the advantages of decreasing complications related to improper sterilization such as DLK and infectious keratitis, and errors in assembly, as the blade is preassembled within the disposable head.[29-31]

## Corriazo-Pendular Microkeratome (SCHWIND eye-tech-solutions)

The Carriazo-Pendular microkeratome is one of the newest generations of microkeratomes, utilizing a novel ball-shaped blade and cutting head. It is the only microkeratome with a convex application during the cut, thus producing a flap of uniform thickness and reducing the risk of a central buttonhole. The sterile curved blade is provided in a unique blade box, which allows for blade assembly without contact. The flap hinge can be freely selected (360°). The system contains dual motors for blade oscillation and advancement. Translation can be controlled manually or by a motor with speeds up to 6 mm/second. Blade oscillation can be increased to up to 15,000 rpm. Four suction rings are available for flap diameters of 9 and 10 mm and for right and left eye applications. The cutting heads are available for 90, 110, 130, 150 and 170 µM flap thicknesses. Using the 90 µM head, Kymionis and colleagues found a mean flap thickness of 79.88 ± 6.94 µM.[32]

## FEMTOSECOND LASER

In 1999, the method of creating a LASIK flap by using the femtosecond laser instead of a blade was described. The femtosecond laser is a focusable near infrared laser with a wavelength of 1053 nm, consisting of a solid state neodymium (Nd): Glass laser source. It uses ultrafast pulses in the femtosecond ($100 \times 10^{-15}$ second) duration range, which are amplified and delivered by a beam focused to 3–5 µM in size to the corneal stroma. The laser vaporizes the tissue by the process of photodisruption, creating small cavitation bubbles with minimal damage to the surrounding tissues. The pulses are repeated at a rate of 3–5 kHz with many pulses applied in the same area to create a dissection plane within the corneal stroma.[12,33,34] The computer-controlled delivery system can be programmed to create a lamellar flap using a contiguous spiral or more commonly, the raster pattern, requiring 500,000–800,000 spots.[34]

Advantages to the femtosecond laser over a mechanical keratome include increased consistency of flap thickness and diameter, a more planar instead of meniscus-shaped flap, which may have optical advantages, less flap-related complications such as free caps and buttonholes, and a reduction in suction pressure required.[33,35,36] There also may be less higher order optical aberrations, less induced astigmatism, improved contrast sensitivity, faster visual recovery times, and better uncorrected distance visual acuity.[35,37] Major disadvantages over the mechanical microkeratomes are the increased cost and physical size of femtosecond lasers. In addition, rare side effects unique to high energy femtosecond lasers include transient-light sensitivity syndrome and anterior chamber gas bubble formation.[38,39] The production of an opaque bubble layer (OBL) is also related to excessive energy and can interfere with treatment if it migrates into the superficial stroma.[40-42]

The first femtosecond laser, the IntraLase (Abott Medical Optics, California), gained FDA approval in 2001. There has been a dramatic increase in the market share of femtosecond lasers purchased for LASIK flap creation, increasing from 0% in 2011 to over 50% in 2010. Other commercially available femtosecond lasers besides the IntraLase include the Technolas 520F (Technolas Perfect Vision, Germany), VisuMax femtosecond laser (Carl Zeiss Meditec, Germany), Femto LDV femtosecond laser (Ziemer Ophthalmic Systems Group, Switzerland), and the WaveLight FS200 femtosecond laser (Alcon Laboratories, Inc., Fort Worth, Texas) (Figs 2A to E).[35,43] A comparison of the different femtosecond lasers is shown in Table 2. In addition to flap creation for LASIK, the FDA has approved several femtosecond devices for other uses, including intrastromal corneal ring segment placement and corneal transplant applications.

### IntraLase (Abott Medical Optics)

The IntraLase system has undergone progressive refinements since it was introduced in 2001. The current fifth-generation IntraLase (iFS Intralase) has increased laser pulse rates (from 10 kHz in earlier designs to 150 kHz), allowing for shorter flap-cutting times (< 20 seconds) and less energy to cut the flap. It also allows for enhanced flap customization capabilities such as inverted bevel-in

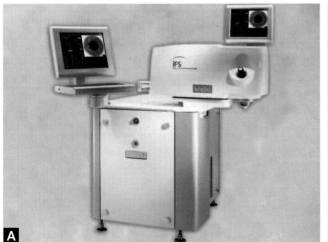
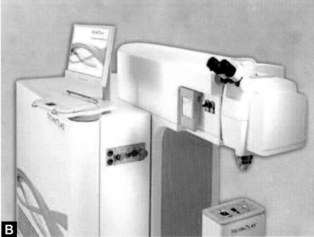

**Figs 2A and B**

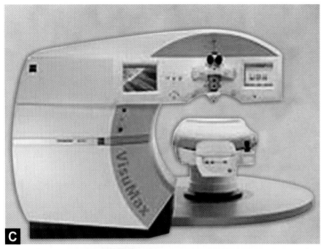

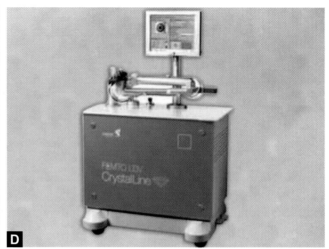

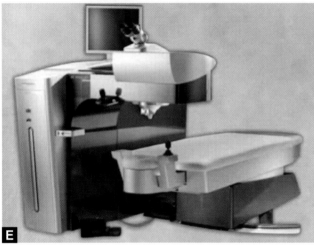

**Figs 2A to E:** Commercially available femtosecond lasers for LASIK flap creation. (A) IntraLase iFS laser (Abott Medical Optics); (B) TECHNOLAS 520F (Technolas Perfect Vision); (C) VisuMax (Carl Zeiss Meditec); (D) Femto LDV (Ziemer); (E) Wavelight UltraFlap (Alcon)

side cuts with angles up to 150°, providing greater optical wound healing and flap stability. A flat applanation glass is docked with high vacuum connected to a syringe, allowing for the creation of uniformly thin, planar flaps. The flat applanation glass plate requires intraocular pressure elevations from 60–100 mm Hg. Suction is extremely reliable and suction breaks are rare. A raster cut pattern is used to create the flap. It has a high-precision computer based delivery system, allowing for variation in flap shape, depth, and diameter.[42] The video microscope provides excellent visualization of centration, and centering software allows the surgeon to compensate for decentration that occurs during suction ring placement. These parameters have led to the IntraLase being the most popular femtosecond laser in the United States, with over 3.5 million cases performed with it. Disadvantages include its sensitivity to changes in the environment, requiring a constant temperature and humidity, and its large physical size.[44]

## Technolas 520F (Technolas Perfect Vision)

The original Technolas laser, the FEMTEC laser, was introduced to the market in 2006. Similar to the earlier generations of the IntraLase, the original pulse rate was 10 kHz. The newest version, the TECHNOLAS 520F, operates with a frequency of 80 kHz, allowing for flap creation in about 20 seconds. One major advantage is that it uses a curved patient interface, requiring less suction pressure during treatment. This increases patient comfort and enables the patient to maintain fixation throughout treatment. However, the low vacuum allows for an easier break in suction if the patient is not cooperative. Corneal lamellar cuts are made parallel to the curved applanating lens in a spiral pattern, allowing the OBL to stay in the periphery.[42] Centration software allows recentering under the curved interace. The CustomFlap software allows for customization of flap diameter, thickness, hinge position

**Table 2:** Comparison of commercially available femtosecond lasers

|  | IntraLase iFS | Technolas 520F | VisuMax | Femto LDV | WaveLight FS 2000 |
|---|---|---|---|---|---|
| Manufacturer | Abott Medical Optics | Technolas Perfect Vision | Carl Zeiss, Meditec | Zeimer Ophthalmic Systems Group | Alcon |
| Laser concept | Amplifier | Amplifier | Fiber-optic amplifier | Oscillator | Amplifier |
| Repetition rate (kHz) | 150 | 80 | 200 | > 20 MHz | 200 |
| Pulse duration (fs) | 600–800 | 500–700 | 220–580 | 200–350 | 200–300 |
| Pulse energy (nJ) | 500–1300 | > 500 | < 300 | < 100 | 300–1500 |
| Spot size (µM) | < 3 | 1 | 1 | 2 | 5 |
| Operation speed (sec) | < 20 | 25 | 20–40 | 15–20 | < 10 |
| Docking patient interface | Flat | Curved | Curved | Flat | Flat |
| Size/mobility | Bulky, fixed | Bulky, fixed | Very bulky, fixed | Very small, mobile | Bulky, fixed |
| Customizable features | High | High | Very high | Limited | High |
| Sensitive to temperature and humidity | Yes | Yes | No | No | No |

and geometry. A refractive procedure for presbyopia, known as the Intracor, is being investigated as a minimally nvasive treatment for presbyopia as part of this platform. Results in Europe have shown promising results.[45]

## VisuMax Femtosecond Laser (Carl Zeiss Meditec)

The VisuMax was also introduced in 2006. Like the Technolas 520F, it uses a curved docking interface, allowing for lower suction pressures. Its laser has been upgraded to operate at a pulse rate of 500 kHz, using a low pulse energy profile (< 1 µJ) and a spiral pattern. A computer controlled vacuum system controls the suction, which is applied at the corneal limbus. This allows for more precise tissue removal, but limits flap diameters. Unlike the IntraLase and FEMTEC, it is an industrial laser that is not sensitive to changes in the environment. Of all the femtosecond lasers, it has the largest physical size and is the most expensive.[42-44]

Femtosecond-only vision correction using this system is available outside the US. (RelEx, Carol Zeiss Meditech), which comprises both the femtosecond lamellar extraction (FLEx) and small-incision lamellar extraction (SMILE). With SMILE, a small incision less than 4 mm is used to remove the refractive lenticule, eliminating the need for flap creating or excimer ablation.

## Femto LDV Femtosecond Laser (Ziemer Ophthalmic Systems)

The Femto Leonardo Da Vinci system (Femto LDV) was FDA-approved in 2006 and is the smallest and only

mobile femtosecond laser available. It has a handheld laser delivery system, which fits under all excimer lasers and thus does not require any movement of the patient. It is the only femtosecond laser to use an oscillator as a laser source, allowing for a less bulky laser system and faster start-up time. The other femtosecond lasers use an amplifier to reach sufficient energy density. The Femto LDV operates with a pulse rate 1,000 times higher than other femtosecond lasers (in the MHz range), allowing for flap creation in about 15–20 seconds. Low pulse energy, in the nanojoule range is achieved, resulting in reduced OBL formation and improved precision. It uses a computer-controlled vacuum to maintain suction system. Like the VisuMax, it is an industrial laser that is not sensitive to changes in the environment.[42-44]

In contrast to the other femtosecond lasers, which use highly flexible computer-controlled flap diameters and cutting depths, the FemtoLDV uses suction rings of different diameters (8.5, 9.0, 9.5 and 10.0 mm) to determine flap diameter and a distance foil to determine cutting depth. Thus the flap-making approach is more similar to making a cut with a microkeratome. Similar to the IntraLase, the Femto LDV has a flat instead of curved applanating surface, requiring higher suction pressures. Another disadvantage is that unlike the other femtosecond lasers, there is no direct visualization during the cutting process.

## Wavelight FS 2000 Laser (Alcon)

The Wavelight is the newest available femtosecond laser, released onto the market in 2011. It has a pulse repetition rate of 200 kHz, allowing for the creation of LASIK flaps

CHAPTER 101

in about 6 seconds. It uses pulse energies in the range of 0.3–1.5 µJ, applying laser spots in a raster pattern on the cornea. The surgeon is able to customize the diameter, depth, angle and location of the corneal flaps. Like the IntraLase, it has a flat applanation docking device interface. The main advantage of the WaveLight is that it minimizes OBL formation through the creation of specific venting channels during flap formation.[41,43]

## ▸ EXCIMER LASER

The excimer laser is an ultraviolet laser, with its name derived from the terms excited and dimer. When a reactive gas such as fluorine is mixed with an inert gas such as argon and electrically stimulated, light of wavelength 193 nm is emitted. This produces energy levels high enough to break covalent carbon-carbon bonds, a process known as photoablation.[34]

Excimer laser delivery systems can be classified into one of three types: broad-beam, scanning-slit and flying-spot systems. A broad-beam laser uses a large beam diameter (6–8 mm) with the main disadvantage of beam inhomogeneity causing irregular ablation. Slit-scanning lasers use small beam diameters with slit holes that can be varied to perform smoother ablations. Flying-spot lasers (also known as scanning spot lasers) have the smallest beam diameters (0.8–2 mm) and can produce the smoothest ablations. The scanning-slit and flying-spot lasers require eye-tracking technology to avoid decentration during treatment.[7] There have been many improvements in the excimer laser in refractive surgery, including flying-spot lasers, eye-tracking technology, and the ability for customization.[46] Different excimer lasers are summarized below and compared in Table 3.

## Zytopix Technolas Platform (Technolas Perfect Vision)

This system utilizes the 217 Zyoptix excimer laser by Technolas Perfect Vision, which is a flying-spot laser. The laser beam has an ablation diameter of 2 mm, which a laser pulse duration of 18 nanoseconds and an ultrafast repetition rate of 50 Hz. The ablation software used for conventional treatment, called PlanoScan, produces a multizone treatment with a smooth ablated surface, minimizing symptoms of nighttime glare. The system also contains an eye-tracker system and blocks treatment if it detects movements greater than 3 mm. The newest version includes advanced rotational eye tracking and iris registration. Wavefront integration incorporates a multidimensional Orbscan II software and Zywave Schack-Hartman aberrometer, allowing for wavefront-guided ablation.[46] It is FDA-approved for LASIK treatments for myopia up to −12.0 D with or without astigmatism up to −3.0 D and for hyperopia up to +4.0 D with or without up to +2.0 D of astigmatism. For the wavefront-guided platform, it is approved for myopia up to −7.0 with or without astigmatism up to −3.0 D.

| **Table 3:** Comparison of FDA-approved excimer lasers | | | | | | |
|---|---|---|---|---|---|---|
| | VISX Star S4 IR | WaveLight Allegretto Wave | TECHNOLAS T217P | MEL 80 | LADARVision 4000 | EC-5000 |
| Manufacturer | Abott Medical Optics | Alcon | Technolas Perfect Vision | Carl Zeiss, Meditec | Alcon | Nidek |
| Ablation Type | Broad beam<br><br>Variable spot scanning | Flying-spot | Flying-spot | Flying-spot | Flying-spot | Scanning-slit |
| Beam size (mm) | 0.65–6.5 | 0.95 | 1/2 (alternates) | 0.7 | 0.8 | 2 × 9 |
| Beam Profile | Top Hat | Gaussian | Truncated Gaussian | Gaussian | Gaussian | Gaussian |
| Pulse Frequency (Hz) | 10–20 | 200–400 | 100 | 250 | 60 | 100 |
| Eye Tracker Sampling Rate (Hz) | 60 | 4000 | 240 | 250 | 4000 | 200 |
| Iris registration | Yes | No | Yes | No | No | No |
| FDA-approved custom wavefront | Yes (CustomVue™) | Yes | Yes | No | Yes (Custom Cornea™) | No |

## LADARVision 4000 System (Alcon)

The LADARVision 4000 excimer laser was approved by the FDA in 1999 for clinical use in the United States. It utilizes flying-spot technology, consisting of a laser beam with a Gaussian energy distribution profile and a small diameter of 0.8 mm. The system consists of a sophisticated eye-tracker system, the LADARTracker, which is able to track movements of the eye 4,000 times per second, faster than any other excimer systems used today. This allows each laser spot to hit its target with great precision, with a mean error of 37 microns.[46] It is FDA-approved for LASIK treatment of myopia up to –9.0 D with or without astigmatism from –0.5 to –3.0 D and for hyperopia less than 6.0 D with or without astigmatism up to 6D. CustomCornea™ with the LADARVision system allows for wavefront-guided surgery and is FDA-approved for myopia up to –7.0 D with or without astigmatism less than 0.5 D.

## EC-5000 Excimer Laser (Nidek)

The Nidek EC-5000 excimer laser is FDA-approved for the treatment of myopia and astigmatism. It utilizes a scanning-slit delivery system and advantages include an eye-tracking system, the ability to vary the optical and transition zone size, and the potential for future wavefront customization.[12] In the US, it is FDA-approved for myopia up to −14.0 D with or without astigmatism up to −4.00 D and for the correction of hyperopia ranging from +0.5 D to +5.0 D sphere and astigmatism up to 2.0 D cylinder.

## VISX STAR S4 Excimer Laser (AMO)

The VISX STAR S4 laser is one of the most widely used excimer lasers in United States. Its advantages include the following features: variable spot scanning, Active Trak 3-D eye tracking, autocentering and iris registration.[12] The variable spot scanning allows the beam size to vary from 2 to 6 mm, allowing for smoother treatment. The autocentering feature automatically finds the geometric center of the undilated pupil. Iris registration allows for the control of intraoperative rotational eye movements and allows for proper centration of laser ablation. It can be performed even with an eccentric pupil. It is FDA-approved for LASIK for myopia up to –14.0 D with or without –0.50 to –5.0 D of astigmatism and for hyperopia between +0.5 D and +5.0 D with or without astigmatism up to +3.0 D. The VISK Star S4 laser with CustomVue™ allows for wavefront-guided LASIK and is approved for myopia up to –6.0 D with or without astigmatism up to –3.0 D.

## Mel 80 Excimer Laser System (Carl Zeiss Meditec)

In 2006, the FDA approved the Mel 80 excimer laser system for LASIK treatment of myopia up to –7.0 diopters, with or without astigmatism of up to –3.0 D. The Mel 80 excimer laser is a flying-spot laser that operates with a Gaussian beam profile and a spot size of 0.7 mm. It emits a 4–6 nanosecond pulse at a frequency of 250 Hz. It has an infrared pupil tracking system processed at the same frequency of 250 Hz.[47] This platform is wavefront-optimized with a prolate optimization function, designed to reduce the induction of higher-order aberrations.[48]

## WaveLight Allegretto Wave System

The WaveLight ALLEGRETTO WAVE™ excimer laser is a flying-spot laser with a pulse repetition rate of 200–400 Hz and an ablation spot diameter of 0.10 mm. It is the fastest excimer laser available in the US and includes a sophisticated eye-tracking system with a frequency of 250 or 400 Hz to match the frequency of the laser. It is FDA-approved for LASIK to treat myopia up to –12.0 D with or without astigmatism up to –6.0 D and hyperopia up to +6.0 D with and without astigmatism up to 5.0 D. The standard treatment is wavefront-optimized, with algorithms designed to maintain the normal prolate shape of the cornea and avoid the induction of higher-order aberrations.[48-51] The ALLEGRETTO analyzer (a Tscherning aberrometer) is available for use with this excimer laser system for wavefront-guided LASIK and approved to treat myopia up to –8.0 D with astigmatism up to –3.0 D and hyperopia up to +5.0 with astigmatism up to +6.0 D. In a prospective study by the US Food and Drug Administration, no statistically significant differences between wavefront-guided and wavefront-optimized treatments were found in the majority of eyes, suggesting that wavefront-guided treatments are not required in the majority of cases with this laser.[51]

## SCHWIND AMARIS Excimer Laser (SCHWIND eye-tech-solutions)

Although not yet FDA-approved in the US, the SCHWIND AMARIS is a commercially available flying-spot excimer laser that utilizes a 500 Hz repetition rate with a super-Gaussian ablation profile. Spot placement is randomized to minimize heat buildup between laser pulses. A high-speed 6D eye tracking system with a frequency of 1050 Hz is available. Both aspheric-based and wavefront-guided ablations are available with this system.[52,53]

101 CHAPTER

## Wavefront Analyzers

The ability to measure wavefront aberration in the human eye introduced a new era in refractive surgery.[54,55] As ocular wavefront aberrations were linked to contrast sensitivity and visual symptoms, custom LASIK was created to correct these wavefront aberrations in addition to standard correction of myopia, hyperopia and astigmatism.[55] Custom LASIK was approved for the correction of myopia and myopic astigmatism in the US in 2002.

Wavefront aberrations can be expressed mathematically in polynomial expansions known as Zernike polynomials and are classified into lower and higher-order aberrations. Lower-order aberrations can be corrected with conventional LASIK surgery. Higher-order aberrations, which represent 17% of the total optical error in humans,[56] include the following:

- Third order: coma and trefoil
- Fourth order: spherical aberration and secondary astigmatism
- Fifth order: secondary coma
- Sixth order: secondary spherical aberration

Wavefront aberrometers are used to measure to the total aberrations of the eye. In the Hartman-Shack aberrometer, a small ray of infrared light is projected onto a small spot on the retina. The reflected light from the fovea is imaged onto a lenslet array and collected by a charge-coupled device camera. The deviation of each spot from its corresponding lenslet axis is used to calculate the aberrations.[55,56] In Tscherning aberrometry, a collimated laser beam (a frequency doubled Nd:YAG) is used to illuminate a grid mask to produce parallel beams entering the eye. A lens is used to focus the beams on the retina. The grid pattern of the retina is then captured and aberrations are calculated based on deviations from the ideal wavefront.[55,56]

Fourier analysis is an alternative to Zernike polynomials for describing optical wavefronts. This method reconstructs wavefront data by decomposing the image into spatial frequency components and may be more accurate in eyes with higher aberration.[57-60]

Wavefront-guided lasers currently FDA-approved in the United States include the Zyoptix Technolas, LADAR CustomCornea™, VISX CustomVue™, and the Allegretto Wavelight. The Zyoptix, LADAR CustomCornea, and VISX CustomVue utilize Hartman-Shack technology and the Allegretto Wavelight utilizes Tscherning aberrometry. The WaveScan aberrometer, which is linked to the VISX CustomVue™ system, is the first aberrometer to use Fourier analysis.[55]

## ⊁ REFERENCES

1. Duffey RJ, Leaming D. US trends in refractive surgery: 2004 ISRS/AAO Survey. J refract surg. 2005;21(6):742-8.
2. Buratto L BS. From keratomileusis to LASIK. In: Buratto L BS (Ed.). Custom LASIK: surgical techniques and complications. NJ: SLACK Incorporated; 2003. pp. 3-8.
3. Gimbel HV, Penno EE, van Westenbrugge JA, et al. Incidence and management of intraoperative and early postoperative complications in 1000 consecutive laser in situ keratomileusis cases. Ophthalmology. 1998;105(10):1839-47.
4. Jacobs JM, Taravella MJ. Incidence of intraoperative flap complications in laser in situ keratomileusis. J Cataract Refract Surg. 2002;28(1):23-8.
5. Haw WW, Manche EE. Iatrogenic keratectasia after a deep primary keratotomy during laser in situ keratomileusis. Am J Ophthalmol. 2001;132(6):920-1.
6. Sutton GL, Kim P. Laser in situ keratomileusis in 2010—a review. Clin Experiment Ophthalmol. 2010;38(2):192-210.
7. Maldonado MJ, Nieto JC, Pinero DP. Advances in technologies for laser-assisted in situ keratomileusis (LASIK) surgery. Expert Rev Med Devices. 2008;5(2):209-29.
8. Buratto L BS, Salib G. LASIK with a nasal hinge. In: Buratto L BS (Ed). Custom Lasik: surgical techniques and complications. NJ: SLACK Incorporated; 2003. pp.93-117.
9. Probst LE. Lasik: a color atlas and surgical synopsis. Thorofare, NJ: Slack Inc. 2001;7:. 371.
10. Alwan YM. Understanding microkeratomes. Technical Communique Surgicals Division, Medicals International SARL, 2002; 5:2011.
11. Behrens A, Langenbucher A, Kus MM, et al. Experimental evaluation of two current-generation automated microkeratomes: the Hansatome and the Supratome. Am J Ophthalmol. 2000;129(1):59-67.
12. Feder RS, Rapuano CJ. The LASIK handbook: a case-based approach. Volume 10. Philadelphia: Lippincott Williams & Wilkins. 2007. p. 277.
13. Buratto L. Down-up LASIK with the Hansatome In: Buratto L, Brint SF (Eds). CUSTOM LASIK: surgical techniques and complications, 3rd edition. Thorofare, NJ: Slack; 2003. pp.119-50.
14. Giledi O, Mulhern MG, Espinosa M, et al. Reproducibility of LASIK flap thickness using the Hansatome microkeratome. J Cataract Refract Surg. 2004;30(5):1031-7.
15. Solomon KD, Donnenfeld E, Sandoval HP, et al. Flap thickness accuracy: comparison of 6 microkeratome models. J Cataract Refract Surg. 2004;30(5):964-77.
16. Lindstrom RL, Linebarger EJ, Hardten DR, et al. Early results of hyperopic and astigmatic laser in situ keratomileusis in eyes with secondary hyperopia. Ophthalmol. 2000;107(10):1858-63; discussion 63.
17. Bashour M. Risk factors for epithelial erosions in laser in situ keratomileusis. J Cataract Refract Surg. 2002;28(10):1780-8.
18. Shah MN, Misra M, Wihelmus KR, et al. Diffuse lamellar keratitis associated with epithelial defects after laser in situ keratomileusis. J Cataract Refract Surg. 2000;26(9):1312-8.
19. Sachdev N, McGhee CN, Craig JP, et al. Epithelial defect, diffuse lamellar keratitis, and epithelial ingrowth following post-LASIK epithelial toxicity. J Cataract Refract Surg. 2002;28(8):1463-6.

16 SECTION

20. Taneri S. Laser in situ keratomileusis flap thickness using the Hansatome microkeratome with zero compression heads. J Cataract Refract Surg. 2006;32(1):72-7.

21. Pepose JS, Feigenbaum SK, Qazi MA, et al. Comparative performance of the Zyoptix XP and Hansatome zero-compression microkeratomes. J Cataract Refract Surg. 2007;33(8):1386-91.

22. Miranda D, Smith SD, Krueger RR. Comparison of flap thickness reproducibility using microkeratomes with a second motor for advancement. Ophthalmol. 2003;110(10):1931-4.

23. Naripthaphan P, Vongthongsri A. Evaluation of the reliability of the Nidek MK-2000 microkeratome for laser in situ keratomileusis. J Refract Surg. 2001;17(2 Suppl):S255-8.

24. Ucakhan OO. Corneal flap thickness in laser in situ keratomileusis using the summit Krumeich-Barraquer microkeratome. J Cataract Refract Surg. 2002;28(5):798-804.

25. Solomon KDS, Helga P. Amadeus Microkeratome In: Buratto L, Brint SF (Eds). CUSTOM LASIK: surgical techniques and complications, 3rd edition. Thorofare, NJ: Slack, 2003.

26. Sarkisian KA, Petrov AA. Experience with the Nidek MK-2000 microkeratome in 1,220 cases. J Refract Surg. 2001;17(2 Suppl): S252-4.

27. Schumer DJ, Bains HS. The Nidek MK-2000 microkeratome system. J Refract Surg. 2001;17(2 Suppl):S250-1.

28. Muallem MS, Yoo SY, Romano AC, et al. Corneal flap thickness in laser in situ keratomileusis using the Moria M2 microkeratome. J Cataract Refract Surg. 2004;30(9):1902-8.

29. Kanellopoulos AJ, Pe LH, Kleiman L. Moria M2 single use microkeratome head in 100 consecutive LASIK procedures. J Refract Surg. 2005;21(5):476-9.

30. Huhtala A, Pietila J, Makinen P, et al. Corneal flap thickness with the Moria M2 single-use head 90 microkeratome. Acta ophthalmologica Scandinavica. 2007;85(4):401-6.

31. Du S, Lian J, Zhang L, et al. Flap thickness variation with 3 types of microkeratome heads. J Cataract Refract Surg. 2011;37(1):144-8.

32. Kymionis GD, Portaliou DM, Tsiklis NS, et al. Thin LASIK flap creation using the SCHWIND Carriazo-Pendular microkeratome. J Refract Surg. 2009;25(1):33-6.

33. Traub I, Kurtz R, Juhasz T, et al. LASIK flaps with the femtosecond laser In: L B, S B (Eds). CUSTOM LASIK: surgical techniques and complications, 3rd edition. Thorofare, NJ: Slack, 2003.

34. Loh RSH DR. LASIK instrumentation: microkeratomes, excimer lasers, and wavefront analyzers. In: Smolin G, Foster CS, Azar DT, Dohlman CH (Eds). Smolin and Thoft's the cornea: scientific foundations and clinical practice, 4th edition. Philadelphia: Lippincott Williams & Wilkins, 2005.

35. Gil-Cazorla R, Teus MA, de Benito-Llopis L, et al. Femtosecond Laser vs Mechanical Microkeratome for Hyperopic Laser In Situ Keratomileusis. Am J Ophthalmol. 2011;152(1):16-21 e2.

36. Ahn H, Kim JK, Kim CK, et al. Comparison of laser in situ keratomileusis flaps created by 3 femtosecond lasers and a microkeratome. J Cataract Refract Surg. 2011;37(2):349-57.

37. Montes-Mico R, Rodriguez-Galietero A, Alio JL. Femtosecond laser versus mechanical keratome LASIK for myopia. Ophthalmology. 2007;114(1):62-8.

38. Haft P, Yoo SH, Kymionis GD, et al. Complications of LASIK flaps made by the IntraLase 15- and 30-kHz femtosecond lasers. J Refract Surg. 2009;25(11):979-84.

39. Srinivasan S, Rootman DS. Anterior chamber gas bubble formation during femtosecond laser flap creation for LASIK. J Refract Surg. 2007;23(8):828-30.

40. Moshirfar M, Gardiner JP, Schliesser JA, et al. Laser in situ keratomileusis flap complications using mechanical microkeratome versus femtosecond laser: retrospective comparison. J Cataract Refract Surg. 2010;36(11):1925-33.

41. Mrochen M, Wullner C, Krause J, et al. Technical aspects of the WaveLight FS200 femtosecond laser. J Refract Surg. 2010;26 (10):S833-40.

42. Soong HK, Malta JB. Femtosecond lasers in ophthalmology. Am J Ophthalmol. 2009;147(2):189-97 e2.

43. Reggiani-Mello G, Krueger RR. Comparison of commercially available femtosecond lasers in refractive surgery. Expert Rev Ophthalmol. 2011;6(1):55-65.

44. Lubatschowski H. Overview of commercially available femtosecond lasers in refractive surgery. J Refract Surg. 2008;24 (1):S102-7.

45. Holzer MP, Mannsfeld A, Ehmer A, et al. Early outcomes of INTRACOR femtosecond laser treatment for presbyopia. J Refract Surg. 2009;25(10):855-61.

46. Buratto L, Brint SF. The excimer laser. In: Buratto L, Brint SF (Eds). Custom LASIK: surgical techniques and complications, 3rd edition. Thorofare, NJ: Slack; 2003. pp.391-434.

47. Goes FJ. LASIK for myopia with the Zeiss meditec MEL 80. J Refract Surg. 2005;21(6):691-7.

48. Myrowitz EH, Chuck RS. A comparison of wavefront-optimized and wavefront-guided ablations. Curr Opin Ophthalmol. 2009; 20(4):247-50.

49. Kim A, Chuck RS. Wavefront-guided customized corneal ablation. Curr Opin Ophthalmol. 2008;19(4):314-20.

50. George MR, Shah RA, Hood C, et al. Transitioning to optimized correction with the WaveLight ALLEGRETTO WAVE: case distribution, visual outcomes, and wavefront aberrations. J Refract Surg. 2010;26(10):S806-13.

51. Stonecipher KG, Kezirian GM. Wavefront-optimized versus wavefront-guided LASIK for myopic astigmatism with the ALLEGRETTO WAVE: three-month results of a prospective FDA trial. J Refract Surg. 2008;24(4):S424-30.

52. Arbelaez MC, Aslanides IM, Barraquer C, et al. LASIK for myopia and astigmatism using the SCHWIND AMARIS excimer laser: an international multicenter trial. J Refract Surg. 2010;26(2):88-98.

53. Arbelaez MC, Arba Mosquera S. The SCHWIND AMARIS Total-Tech Laser as An All-Rounder in Refractive Surgery. Middle East Afr J Ophthalmol. 2009;16(1):46-53.

54. Liang J, Grimm B, Goelz S, et al. Objective measurement of wave aberrations of the human eye with the use of a Hartmann-Shack wave-front sensor. J Opt Soc Am A Opt Image Sci Vis. 1994;11(7):1949-57.

55. Awwad ST, McCulley JP. Wavefront-guided LASIK: recent developments and results. Int Ophthalmol Clin. 2006;46(3): 27-38.

56. Yeh PC, Azar DT. Smolin and Thoft's The cornea: scientific foundations and clinical practice. In: Smolin G, Foster CS, Azar DT, Dohlman CH (Eds). Wavefront-guided custom LASIK and LASEK: techniques and outcomes, 4th edition. Philadelphia: Lippincott Williams & Wilkins; 2005.

57. Klyce SD, Karon MD, Smolek MK. Advantages and disadvantages of the Zernike expansion for representing wave aberration of the normal and aberrated eye. J Refract Surg. 2004;20 (5):S537-41.

58. Wang L, Chernyak D, Yeh D, et al. Fitting behaviors of Fourier transform and Zernike polynomials. J Cataract Refract Surg. 2007;33(6):999-1004.

59. Smolek MK, Klyce SD. Goodness-of-prediction of Zernike polynomial fitting to corneal surfaces. J Cataract Refract Surg. 2005;31(12):2350-5.

60. Dai GM. Comparison of wavefront reconstructions with Zernike polynomials and Fourier transforms. J Refract Surg. 2006;22(9):943-8.

# LASIK Techniques and Outcomes

*Andrea Cruzat, Roberto Pineda*

## ▶ ABSTRACT

Laser *in situ* keratomileusis (LASIK) has become one of the most popular surgeries in the world to correct refractive error due to minimal postoperative pain, quick visual recovery, refractive accuracy and safety. The creation of a corneal flap is the most important step and is essential for a successful procedure. Predictable flap thickness is critical to perform LASIK safely. At present, a LASIK flap can be created with a mechanical microkeratome or a femtosecond laser. In this chapter, we will review the technique of both systems and compare their outcomes. There are many studies comparing these two LASIK techniques showing variable results. Some studies have shown equivalency between femtosecond laser and the mechanical microkeratome, while others have shown better outcomes with the femtosecond laser. Although further studies are needed to compare these techniques, current literature favors LASIK flaps created with a femtosecond laser as this approach appears to provide better visual outcomes, improved astigmatic neutrality, induction of fewer higher order aberrations (HOAs), decreased epithelial injury, and creates less dry eye compared to traditional mechanical microkeratomes. Laser LASIK flaps are more reproducible and uniform with greater predictable flap thickness and diameters, smoother stromal beds and lower rates of flap complications. Nevertheless, mechanical microkeratomes have a longer track record of safety and cost significantly less than femtosecond lasers.

## ▶ INTRODUCTION: HISTORY

In 1963, at the Barraquer ophthalmologic clinic (Bogotá, Colombia), Ignacio Barraquer developed a refractive surgery technique called keratomileusis (corneal reshaping), introducing the concept of corneal lamellar surgery for correction of refractive errors.[1]

In 1980, R Srinivasan, a scientist, who was using the excimer laser to make microscopic circuits in microchips for informatics equipment, discovered that the excimer laser could also be used to cut organic tissues with high accuracy without significant thermal damage. Later, in 1983, Srinivasan in collaboration with Stephen Trokel, performed the first photorefractive keratectomy (PRK) or keratomileusis *in situ* (without separation of corneal layer) in Germany.

In 1989, the first patent for LASIK was granted (by the US Patent Office) to Gholam Ali. Peyman, MD called 'Method for Modifying Corneal Curvature', describing the surgical procedure in which a flap is cut in the cornea and pulled back to expose the corneal bed. This exposed surface is then ablated to the desired shape with an excimer laser, following which the flap is replaced. In 1990, Pallikaris et al.[2,3] and Buratto et al.[4] introduced the techniques combining lamellar procedures with excimer laser ablation. These advances led to the development of modern LASIK procedures.

LASIK technique consists of basically three steps: (1) construction of an anterior lamellar corneal flap;

(2) application of a UV laser to ablate the posterior corneal stroma under the lifted flap and (3) replacement of the reflected corneal flap.[5] Considerable technological advancement has been made over the last 20 years in the first two steps, making LASIK the most popular corneal refractive surgery procedure.

The UV laser, (excimer or solid-state lasers) used to ablate the corneal stroma, has developed significantly since the first ArF excimer laser was used for ablation of organic tissue in the early 1980s. Several beam delivery systems have been used by both excimer and nonexcimer lasers, including: circle/linear scanning, slit scanning, expanding diaphragm, rotating disk, erodible mask, absorbing cell and fiber coupling. The first generation (1986) broad beam laser technology consisted of a large beam size of 5–6 mm at a low repetition rate (20 Hz) and high beam energy (30 mJ on the corneal surface), while the newer generation (1996) scanning laser systems (flying spot) utilize a smaller beam spot size of 0.5–1.5 mm at a high repetition rate excimer laser (200–500 Hz) with lower beam energy (0.8–2.0 mJ) providing more accuracy, smoother surface and flexibility of the ablation profiles (Fig. 1).

Eventually, the single-zone method used at the early stages was improved to a multi-zone to reduce the amount of tissue removed. The invention of eye-tracking systems to minimize off-center ablation caused by eye movement and the development of computer-programmed algorithms

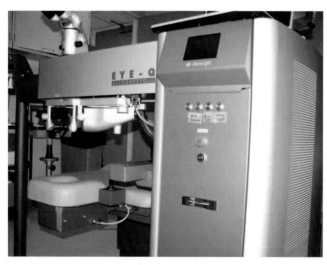

**Fig. 1:** Excimer laser system to perform LASIK. The newer generation of excimer lasers have scanning laser systems (flying spot) utilizing a smaller beam spot size of 0.5–1.5 mm at a high repetition rate (200–500 Hz) with lower beam energy (0.8–2.0 mJ) providing more accuracy, smoother surface and flexibility of the ablation profiles. The model shown in the figure is a WaveLight® Allegretto Wave® Eye-Q (Erlangen, Germany) approved by the FDA on 2006.

improved the consistency of the excimer lasers. Empirical correction factors based on the population patient data were introduced by laser manufacturers to compensate for the increase of surface aberrations after LASIK. The software-driven scanning technology permit a personalized treatment with the use of wavefront-guided ablations to treat high order aberrations and advanced topography with elevation maps to guide the laser to perform customized LASIK for the treatment of irregular corneal surfaces, off-centered cornea after refractive surgery or regional correction for astigmatism, so-called topography-guided LASIK (reviewed Lin JT[5]).

As LASIK flap creation is the critical step in successful LASIK surgery, substantial effort has been put into producing safer instruments for the flap construction. During the first 10 years of the procedure, the LASIK flap was created with mechanical microkeratomes and complications such as incomplete or partial flaps, free flaps, buttonholes, and small irregular flaps, were a menace particularly in steep or flat corneas, limiting the number of eyes that could safely have LASIK. Fortunately, safer models of mechanical microkeratomes were developed and the femtosecond laser became available for LASIK flap formation. Since the introduction of femtosecond laser models, considerable progress has been made in improving flap geometry and limiting LASIK flap complications.

Currently, there are a variety of microkeratomes as well as femtosecond lasers that have been developed for LASIK flap creation and are in clinical use. The IntraLase femtosecond laser and the mechanical microkeratome platforms have different mechanisms of action to create the corneal flap. Previous studies report the advantages and disadvantages of mechanical microkeratome and the IntraLase femtosecond laser. The purpose of this chapter is to describe the different LASIK techniques and review and summarize the outcomes for both the microkeratome and the femtosecond laser.

## TECHNIQUES: MECHANICAL MICROKERATOME VERSUS LASER KERATOME

### Mechanical Microkeratome

The LASIK mechanical microkeratome creates an anterior lamellar circular corneal flap in the cornea, leaving an uncut portion called the 'hinge', as an attachment point between the flap and the corneal bed. It uses shear force through the use of an oscillating blade, traveling across the cornea in a torsional or translational path. It is necessary to provide a stable platform for the microkeratome cutting head, so a suction ring, connected to a vacuum pump, is applied to adhere to the globe and raises the intraocular pressure (IOP) to a level that immobilizes and increases sectility of the cornea so it cannot move away from the microkeratome blade when the flap is cut. The size of the suction ring, the vertical dimension of the ring and the diameter of the opening are major factors in how the cornea protrudes and is exposed to the cutting blade, determining the flap thickness, the diameter of the flap and the size of the LASIK flap hinge.

The mechanical microkeratome has several important components (Figs 2A and B): a very sharp disposable cutting blade, the applanation head or plate that flattens the cornea in advance of the cutting blade. The motor, either electrical or gas-driven turbine, oscillates the blade rapidly, typically between 6,000 and 15,000 cycles per minute. The same motor or a second motor is used to mechanically advance the cutting head, which is attached to the suction ring, across the cornea, although in several models the surgeon manually controls the advance of the cutting head.[6] The theoretical flap thickness is determined by the distance between the blade and the fixed microkeratome plate.[7] Other important variables that determines the flap thickness are the quality and the entry angle of the blade, the translation speed and oscillation rate, the consistency across the cornea, the suction ring pressure setting and suction duration, the mechanism of the cut, room humidity, the preoperative corneal thickness, keratometry, astigmatism and the corneal diameter.[8]

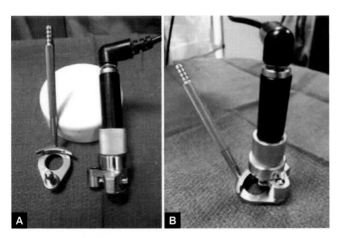

**Figs 2A and B:** Mechanical microkeratome. The Bausch & Lomb Hansatome corneal microkeratome for LASIK. Nondisposable vertical microkeratome model. (A) Separated microkeratome and suction ring, note the geared outer track of the suction ring; (B) An assembled microkeratome, note the motor is directly above the operating surface.

Microkeratome complications are often related to faulty blade, improper placement, motor jam or suction loss, translating clinically as incomplete flap creation, flap buttonhole, severe flap deformation, irregular flap cuts or free cap.

In the 1950s, Barraquer designed the first microkeratome to create a corneal flap. With the increasing popularity of LASIK, many ophthalmic companies have developed different versions of microkeratomes, starting with manual and evolving to newer automated microkeratomes. Today a wide number of choices are available with different variables. A summary of the different mechanical microkeratomes and their characteristics is presented in Table 1.

## Laser Keratome

The femtosecond laser is a solid-state laser that creates the corneal flap by generating ultrashort (femtosecond $10^{-15}$ seconds) pulses of laser at a near-infrared (1,053 nm) wavelength as closely spaced spots, at a predetermined depth in the cornea producing corneal tissue cutting by microphotodisruption. These pulses reach a high peak power, generating hot plasma, initiating a process of tissue ionization, commonly called 'laser-induced optical breakdown'. This hot plasma expands as shock waves and creates an intrastromal cavitation bubble composed primarily of water and carbon dioxide. Multiple high-pressure cavitation bubbles coalesce expanding along the path of least resistance resulting in an intrastromal cleavage plane. The femtosecond laser delivers a series of pulses in a specified spiral or raster pattern to create the corneal lamellar intrastromal cut and then extends the laser cut vertically toward the surface creating a side cut to complete the LASIK flap.[9,10] A predefined arc along a portion of the LASIK flap edge is left uncut to create the hinge. The entire process takes place through a glass applanation plate that is fixed to the eye with low-pressure suction ring.

The first commercially available femtosecond laser, IntraLase, was approved in the United States in 2000 with a speed of 6 kHz, which increased in rate to 10 kHz, 15 kHz, 30 kHz, 60 kHz, 150 kHz, 200 kHz lasers and currently up to MHz (Fig. 3). The different femtosecond lasers differ in energy parameters and pulse rates, key determinants in the efficacy and safety of flap formation, the slower the pulse rate, the more energy required to generate the flap. The femtosecond lasers systems can be classified into two groups. Group one is characterized by high pulse energy and low pulse frequency (including the IntraLase and the Femtec), while group two is characterized by low pulse energy and

**Table 1:** Types of microkeratomes and their characteristics

| Mechanical Microkeratomes Manufacturer/ Model Name | Oscillation Speed (rpm) | Flap Diameter (mm) | Depth (flap thickness) (µm) | Mechanism/Motor | Advance Rate (mm/s) | Hinge Position/Horizontal vs Vertical Microkeratome | Automatic vs Manual/ Disposable vs Non-disposable |
|---|---|---|---|---|---|---|---|
| Automated Corneal Shaper (ACS)/Bausch & Lomb—Chiron (Rochester, NY) | 7,500 | ≥ 9.0 | 130, 160, 180, 200 | Gear driven/Electric motor | 3.7 | Nasal hinge/Horizontal | Automatic/Nondisposable. No longer available |
| Carriazo-Barraquer (CB)/Moria and Schwind (Doylestown, PA) | 15,000 | 7.0–10.5 | 130, 160, 180 | Inner drive mechanism/Motor: gas turbine or electric | 3.7 | Variable hinge, nasal and superior/ Vertical | Manual (turbine) or Automatic (electric)/ Nondisposable, single use available |
| M2/Moria (Doylestown, PA) | 15,000 | Up to 10.5 | 130, 160 | Sliding, no gears/ Dual electric motor | 2 or 3 | Variable hinge position | Automatic/Nondisposable, single use available |
| One Use-Plus (SBK) M2/Moria (Doylestown, PA) | 15,000 | Up to 10.5 | 100, 120 | Linear system/Dual gas turbine motor | 2 or 3 | Nasal hinge | Automatic/Disposable |
| Hansatome/Bausch & Lomb—Chiron (Rochester, NY) | 14,000 | 8.5, 9.5 | 160, 180, 200 | One outer gear/ Electric motor | 6.0 | Superior hinge/ Vertical | Automatic/Nondisposable |
| MK-2000/Nidek | 9,000 | 8.5, 9.0, 9.5, 10.0 | 130, 160, 180 | Geared, but no exposed/Dual electric motors | 2.0 | Variable hinge, nasal/Horizontal | Automatic/Nondisposable |
| Amadeus/Allergan (Ziemer Group) | 4,000–20,000 | 8.5, 9.0, 9.5, 10.0 | 140, 160, 180, 220, 300 | Linear, no external gear/Electric motor | 1.5–4.0 | Variable hinge, nasal or superior/ Horizontal | Automatic/Nondisposable |
| Summit Krumeich-Barraquer (SKBM)/ Alcon (Fort Worth, TX) | 4,000–20,000 | 9.5, 10.0 | 130, 160, 180 | Sliding, no gear/ Dual electric motors | 0.1–3.0 | Horizontal | Automatic/Nondisposable |
| Rondo microkeratome/Wavelight AG (Erlangen, Germany) | 9,000 | 8.0, 8.5, 9.0, 9.5, 10.0 | 100, 130, 150 | Electric motor | 2.8 | Variable hinge position | Automatic/Nondisposable |
| Med-Logics/Med-Logics | 8–13,000 | 8.0–10.0 | 160, 180 | Design: sliding/ Electric motor | 3.5 | Horizontal | Automatic/Nondisposable |
| Carriazo-Pendular/ SCHWIND (Kleinostheim, Germany) | 9–15,000 | 8, 9, 10 | 90, 110, 130, 150, 170 | Geared, but not exposed/Dual electric motor or nitrogen turbine | 3 (range 2–5) | Variable hinge position | Automatic (electric) or Manual (turbine)/ Nondisposable |
| BD K-3000/Becton | 12,000 | 8.5, 9.0, 9.5, 10 | 130, 160, 180 | Design: track & reel/Dual electric motor | 4.4 | Nasal hinge/Horizontal | Automatic/Nondisposable |
| Ultrashaper/Laser-Sight Technologies (with Becton-Dickinson) | 7,200 | ≥ 7.2 | 130, 160 | Design: sliding, no external gears/ Electric motor | N/A | Horizontal | Automatic/Nondisposable |
| Unishaper Automated Disposable Keratome (ADK)/LaserSight Technologies (with Becton-Dickinson) | 7,500 | ≥ 8.5 | 130, 160 | Design: gear driven, but not exposed/Dual electric motor | 4.5 | Variable hinge position | Automatic/Disposable |

*Contd...*

| Mechanical Microker-atomes Manufacturer/ Model Name | Oscil-lation Speed (rpm) | Flap Di-ameter (mm) | Depth (flap thickness) (μm) | Mechanism/Motor | Advance Rate (mm/s) | Hinge Position/Hori-zontal vs Vertical Microkeratome | Automatic vs Manual/ Disposable vs Non-disposable |
|---|---|---|---|---|---|---|---|
| Flapmaker/Refractive Technologies (Cleve-land, Ohio) | 12,500 | 8.0, 8.5, 9.5,10.5 | 130, 160, 180, 200, 220 | Design: sliding/ Electric motor | 6.8 | Variable hinge position | Automatic/Disposable |
| LSK-1/Moria (Doyles-town, PA) | 15,000 | 7.5 to ≤ 10 | 130, 160, 180 | Design: sliding/ Motor: gas turbine | Variable | Nasal hinge/Hori-zontal | Manual/Disposable and nondisposable available |

mm/s: millimeters per second; rpm: revolutions per minute; μm: micrometers; mm: millimeters

high pulse frequency (including the Femto LDV).[11] For example, the higher energy used with the 6 kHz, 10 kHz and 15 kHz IntraLase models, produce larger shock waves that result in more tissue damage and in larger cavitation bubbles that can block subsequent pulses and interfere with the cutting process. With higher pulse repetition rate models (60 kHz,150 kHz and MHz IntraLase models) lower energy settings and closer spot and line separation enhances the quality of the cleavage plane, making it easier to lift the flap, reducing the level of inflammation, increasing the speed of the procedure and creating smoother corneal stromal beds[12] (Figs 4A and B).

Discussed in another chapter in more depth, complications unique to the femtosecond laser include: opaque bubble layer (OBL), vertical gas/bubble break, bubbles in the anterior chamber, rainbow glare and transient light sensitivity

syndrome (TLSS). In TLSS, the patient presents with delayed onset (2–6 weeks) of photophobia after uneventful LASIK surgery with an unremarkable slit lamp examination. It is a side effect attributed to the femtosecond laser associated with the energy of the device.[13,14] Treatment with intensive topical corticosteroid improve symptoms and support an inflammatory theory.[15] The incidence of TLSS significantly decreased when newer femtosecond lasers were introduced with faster rates of flap creation and lower raster bed energies.[14] A summary of the different femtosecond lasers and their characteristics is presented in Table 2.

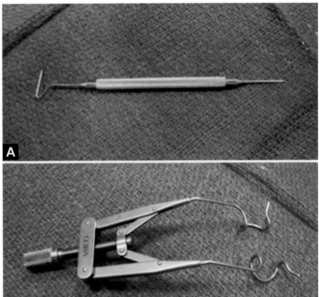

**Figs 4A and B:** Femtosecond LASIK instruments. (A) Seibel-Intra-LASIK Flap lifter (Rhein Medical Tampa, Florida) for separation and lifting a femtosecond created flap. Although dissection of the flap is easier with the newer femtosecond laser models, a special instrument is required to lift the flap; (B) Lieberman-style speculum is recom-mended for good exposure during the LASIK procedure.

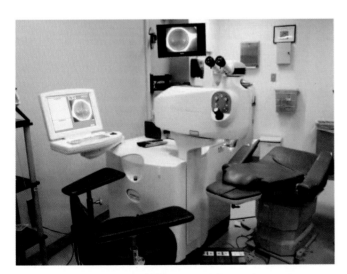

**Fig. 3:** Femtosecond laser. Different models vary in energy param-eters and pulse rates, key determinants in the efficacy, safety and time of flap formation. The slower the pulse rate, the more energy required to generate the flap. Pictured is the IntraLase femtosecond laser (FS 60Hz)/IntraLase Corp., Abbot Medical Optics Inc (Santa Ana, CA).

**Table 2:** Types of femtosecond lasers and their characteristics

| Femtosecond Lasers | Repetition Rate/ Wavelength | Pulse Width (fs)/ Spot Size (nm)/ Pulse Energy (µJ) | Clinical Aspects/Corneal Flap (operation speed at 9.0–9.5 mm) /Environmental requirements | Additional Features |
|---|---|---|---|---|
| 10 kHz Pulsion femto-second laser/IntraLase Corporation (Irvine, CA) | 10 kHz/1,040 nm | | Planar applanation/Manual suction/ Speed: 120 seconds/Constant temperature and humidity required | 1st generation/High pulse energy (µJ) and low pulse frequency (kHz) |
| IntraLase 15 kHz femtosecond laser | 15 kHz/1,040 nm | /2.7 µJ | Planar applanation/Manual suction/ Speed: 90 seconds/Constant temperature and humidity required | 2nd generation (2003)/High pulse energy (µJ) and low pulse frequency (kHz) |
| IntraLase 30 kHz femtosecond laser | 30 kHz/1,040 nm | /1.9 µJ | Planar applanation/Manual suction/ Speed: 40 seconds/Constant temperature and humidity required | 3rd generation (2005)/High pulse energy (µJ) and low pulse frequency (kHz) |
| IntraLase femtosecond laser/IntraLase Corp., Abbot Medical Optics Inc. (Santa Ana, CA) | 60–150 kHz/1,040 nm | > 500 fs/ spot size: > 1 µm/0.45–1.0 µJ | Planar applanation/Manual suction/ Speed: 8–30 seconds/Constant temperature and humidity required | 4th generation (60 kHz—2006). 5th generation (150 kHz) got FDA approval 2008. Advanced incision capabilities. High pulse energy (µJ) and low pulse frequency (kHz) |
| Femtec/20/10 Perfect Vision AG (Heidelberg, Germany) | 10–80 kHz/1,040 nm | > 500 fs/spot size: > 1 µm/> 1.0 µJ | Curved applanation cone: less corneal distortion, eye compression and elevation of IOP. Computer-controlled suction/Speed: 36 seconds to 1 minute/Constant temperature and humidity required | FDA approval 2004. High pulse energy (µJ) and low pulse frequency (kHz). Potential for IntraCor: changes the shape of the cornea from within, without cutting a flap. Very small and mobile compared to the others bulky and fixed |
| VisuMax FS Laser/ Carl Zeiss Meditec, Inc. (Dublin, California) | 200 kHz/ 1,040 nm | 220–580 fs/spot size: 1 µm/< 1.0 µJ | Curved applanation cone: less corneal distortion, eye compression and elevation of IOP. Computer-controlled suction/Speed: between 20 and 60 seconds/Room temperature, humidity can vary | FDA approval 2007. Potential for ReLEx (refractive lenticule extraction): A lenticule of intrastromal corneal tissue and a flap-like access cut are created with the laser, the lenticule is then manually removed and the flap repositioned |
| Femto LDV/Ziemer Ophthalmic Systems Group (Port, Switzerland) (formerly called Da Vinci or Ziemer femtosecond laser) | 1MHz/1,040 nm | 250 fs/spot size: < 1 µm/some µJ | Applanation with glass. Better cleavage plane (easier to lift the flap), less inflammation, faster speed of the procedure, smoother corneal stromal beds, does not create an opaque bubble layer. Computer-controlled suction/speed: 30–40 seconds/Room temperature, humidity can vary | FDA approval 2006. Low pulse energy (nanoJ) and high pulse frequency (MHz). Ultrashort pulses of lower energy with a very high repetition rate (> 1 MHz). Less programmable features (flap's diameter, centration, hinge, side-cut angle) |
| FS 200 femtosecond laser/Wavelight GmbH (Erlangen, Germany) | 200 kHz/ 1,050 nm | 350 fs/spot size: 5µm/ 0.3–1.5 µJ | | Three dimensional tissue cutting, broad-spectrum applications in corneal surgery |
| TPV femtosecond laser/Technolas Perfect Vision GmbH (Munich, Germany) | In development | | | Will combine cataract and refractive capabilities |

kHz: kiloHertz; MHz: MegaHertz; fs: femtosecond; µJ: microJoules; nanoJ: nanoJoules; µm: micrometer; nm: nanometers

## ▶ OUTCOMES

### Flap Thickness and Flap Diameter

The importance of flap thickness and its predictability is a key factor in LASIK safety. Flaps that are too thin increase the risk for a flap tear, striae and folds, or even a buttonhole, free flap, irregular, incomplete, or intraepithelial flap that are associated with greater risk of subepithelial haze due to epithelium and basement membrane damage.[16,17] Conversely, thick flaps may reduce the biomechanical stability of the cornea and limit the amount of stromal ablation thereby increasing the risk of iatrogenic corneal ectasia when insufficient posterior stromal bed remains.[7,18,19] Some studies have shown by mathematical analysis that the mean, the standard deviation and the range of flap thickness performed with various devices are risk factors for the development of ectasia.[7,20-22] Hence, it is important to create a regular flap with a narrow standard deviation from the predicted flap thickness.

With the microkeratome, multiple factors determine the corneal thickness profile, such as the quality of the blade's edge, speed of the microkeratome pass, speed of blade oscillation, ease of corneal pass, and advancement of the microkeratome along the track of the suction ring.[14] Previous clinical studies have shown the inaccuracies of different microkeratomes with low predictability and high variability in flap thickness, in the range of ±20 to ±40 μm.[23-29] Solomon et al. compared 6 microkeratomes models evidencing the large variability in the flap thickness.[30] In general, mechanical microkeratome flaps are meniscus shaped, being thicker in the periphery and thinner in the center, increasing the risk for buttonhole perforation.[12,31,32] Additionally, the flap diameter also has poor predictability with the mechanical microkeratome with a positive correlation between mean corneal curvature and LASIK flap diameter (steeper corneas have wider diameter flaps that may impinge on the limbus and flatter corneas have smaller diameter flaps that may not allow the full laser ablation to be delivered, predisposing to halos, glare, and other visual disturbances in eyes with larger pupils).[33,34]

Femtosecond lasers create thinner LASIK flaps with higher predictability and less deviation from the intended thickness. According to several studies, the variability is within ±20 μm of the intended flap thickness.[14,27,33,35-39] Femtosecond laser flaps also tend to be more uniform in thickness than microkeratome flaps, producing a planar-shaped flap.[12,31,32] The femtosecond flaps are also more predictable in their diameter, with smaller variability in flap diameter and is independent of corneal curvature.[33,34] Studies have shown that the faster femtosecond lasers have better predictability compared to the earlier femtosecond models.[40] This better flap thickness predictability with the femtosecond laser should be expected to reduce the incidence of ectasia compared to eyes operated with a mechanical microkeratome. It may also assure greater residual stroma in patients requiring enhancements.[20] Stonecipher et al. showed in a prospective study (n = 18,471 eyes) that the enhancement rates seen in mechanical microkeratome LASIK was 4.2% compared to 1.6% with femtosecond LASIK, demonstrating that better predictability also results in better refractive outcomes, which means fewer enhancements.[14]

### Epithelial Preservation

Epithelial preservation is an important factor in the healing process and for visual recovery. Epithelial defects cause postoperative pain, photophobia and a higher incidence of postoperative complications such as epithelial ingrowth, slower visual recovery, flaps complications, increased re-treatment rates and greater inflammation [diffuse lamellar keratitis (DLK)].[20,41-44]

Reports have favored the femtosecond laser with regard to loose epithelium or epithelial slides and epithelial defects during flap creation.[20,33] Although the development of newer mechanical keratome designs have reduced the incidence of these epithelial-related issues the rate still remains significant with newer design mechanical microkeratomes reporting epithelial slides in as many as 2.6% of these flaps.[45] This is in contrast to the femtosecond laser which requires no moving instrumentation during the procedure while mechanical keratomes pivot the keratome head across the corneal epithelium under high pressure, making the development of an epithelial defect more likely.[20] When LASIK is performed with a femtosecond laser, it is uncommon to generate epithelial defects, even in eyes with anterior basement dystrophy; however, in some cases epithelial damage can occur in the area overlying the stromal pocket produced by the laser.[9]

### Stromal Wound Healing and Inflammation

In 1997, Wilson et al.[46] showed a significant difference in the wound healing response between the femtosecond laser and microkeratomes. According to different studies investigating wound healing and inflammation and when comparing mechanical microkeratomes and femtosecond laser flaps, there is a correlation between the energy delivered to the cornea and stromal cell death and corneal inflammation.[9,12,47-50] In a study performed by Netto et al.[12], flaps created with higher energy lasers (IntraLase 15 kHz), induced more cell death, stromal cell proliferation and inflammatory cell infiltration than flaps created with the 30 kHz or 60 kHz laser or the Hansatome microkeratome (Bausch & Lomb). Also, the type of stromal cell death triggered by the femtosecond laser was necrosis, a more potent promoter of inflammation, versus apoptosis with the microkeratome.[12]

Consistent with this study, earlier models of femtosecond lasers with higher energy (6 kHz and 15 kHz models), produced an increased incidence of DLK and slower visual recovery, while models with lower energy (60 kHz), induced a small inflammatory response similar to that of microkeratomes.[12,48,49] Another important distinction of the femtosecond laser versus the microkeratome for LASIK is the stronger healing and adhesion strength of the flap edge and flap interface which likely reduces the risk for flap dislocation associated with trauma.[51,52] However, this difference was small when comparing lower energy femtosecond laser (60 kHz) with conventional microkeratome.[12]

## Aberrations

Higher order aberrations commonly increase after LASIK procedures.[53] Some studies have shown that flap formation itself can induce optical aberrations prior to the laser ablation, although some increase in total HOAs is attributable to laser ablation as well.[54-57] Regardless of the device used to create a LASIK flap, it is important that the ablation surface be smooth to limit the generation of HOAs.[57,58] Several recent studies have shown that mechanical microkeratome flaps increase lower order[59,60] as well as high order aberrations.[54,61] Furthermore, studies comparing both systems have demonstrated less induction of HOAs when creating the LASIK flap with the femtosecond laser than with a mechanical microkeratome.[62-66] Tran et al. found a statistically significant increase in HOAs with the Hansatome microkeratome (Bausch & Lomb) group but not in the femtosecond laser group.[66] Kezirian et al. performed a study comparing surgically induced astigmatism, showing that femtosecond laser induced less astigmatism than the mechanical microkeratome.[20] The authors explained the smaller induction of astigmatism in the IntraLase group as the result of flap morphology as laser flaps are circular rather than truncated, extending beneath the hinge. The study also attributed a role to the programmed edge angle

of the flap and constant flap thickness.[20] Moreover, a study by Durrie et al. showed significantly less astigmatism and trefoil in the femtosecond laser group after surgery versus the mechanical microkeratome.[65]

## Refraction Predictability and Visual Acuity

Several studies have compared the refractive, visual and best corrected acuity outcomes of the mechanical keratomes and femtosecond lasers. Some studies, such as Patel et al.[67] (n = 42 eyes) found no difference in visual outcomes between femtosecond and microkeratome LASIK. Similarly, Lim et al.[68] (n = 55 eyes) and Kezirian et al.[20] (n = 375 eyes) concluded that the method of flap creation did not affect postoperative uncorrected visual acuity (UCVA). Alternatively, Tanna et al. (n = 2,000 eyes), showed that the femtosecond laser improves both the speed of visual recovery as well as UCVA through 3 months postoperative when compared to mechanical microkeratome.[69] The study explained that the improvement occurred despite similar refractive predictability in both the femtosecond and the mechanical microkeratome group. Thus, the improved UCVA was not due to residual refractive error in the microkeratome group.[69] Furthermore, Durrie et al.[65] (n = 102 eyes) and others have shown that the femtosecond laser produces statistically better visual outcomes and contrast sensitivity.[47] Some studies have shown better predictability of the manifest refraction spherical equivalent and a less surgically induced refractive change with the femtosecond laser versus the mechanical keratome.[14,20,65] Some of the factors used to explain this phenomenon is that femtosecond LASIK has better regularity, planar-shaped flaps, better predictable flap thickness, more accurate repositioning of the flap at the end of the procedure and improved smoothness of the stromal bed compared to the mechanical flaps. Also, the creation of the femtosecond flap is a relatively dry procedure resulting in more standardized tissue hydration, unlike the microkeratome where the cornea is regularly irrigated.[14]

## Biomechanics

The importance of corneal biomechanics has been acknowledged as a fundamental part of LASIK outcomes. The geometry of the flap in terms of planarity (uniform thickness throughout) is important since a meniscus-shaped flap (microkeratome) cut deeper in the periphery and may damage more of the strong corneal collagen fibers to achieve a similar central thickness compared to a planar flap (femtosecond).[36]

LASIK produces a reduction in corneal biomechanical stability because a significant number of collagen fibers are severed and there is minimal biomechanical loading distributed in the flap.[14,70] Some studies propose that the human corneal stroma heals in an incomplete fashion after LASIK resulting in a weak stromal scar (explaining why flaps can be relifted many years after surgery), but femtosecond laser flaps have shown to heal stronger peripherally than conventional microkeratome flaps, however, well below the tensile strength of normal corneal tissue.[14,71]

Studies have suggested that flaps around 100–110 μm thickness are the optimum flaps, providing the greatest biomechanical stability and the lowest complication rate, while thick flaps alter the corneal lamellae and weakened the cornea.[37,49,72] Further research is needed focused on the effect of flap thickness and flap morphology on corneal biomechanics comparing microkeratomes and femtosecond laser.

## Dry Eye

Dry eye is reported as the most common complication after LASIK and a major cause of patient and surgeon dissatisfaction.[73-79] Although dry eye after LASIK is usually a temporary complication and ameliorates over time, it is most noted in the 1st month and improves after 3–6 months.[80,81] The incidence of this complication ranges from 0.25% to more than 50% of patients that have had LASIK.[74-77,82-84] Although multifactorial, one of the main mechanisms may be the damage to the afferent sensory nerves producing a neurotrophic cornea.[76,85-87] Central sub-basal and stromal nerve fiber bundles are absent immediately after LASIK due to the transection of nerves during the flap creation and subsequent stromal photoablation.[88] Other possible mechanisms of LASIK-associated dry eye are the reduction of blinking reflex and tear production, increased tear evaporation, altered tear-film stability due to altered corneal curvature, inflammation, injury to goblet cells at the limbus with the suction ring or the effects of medication.[76,85] Altering the flap characteristics and how the flap is created in LASIK may also affect postoperative LASIK dry eye.

The prolonged reduction in corneal sensation after refractive surgery is due to the interruption of the normal organization and regeneration of the corneal nerves. The recovery of corneal sensation after LASIK to preoperative values has been estimated to be between 3 and 16 months, with an average approximately of 6 months.[78,87,89-94] Stachs et al. showed that corneal sensation plateaus at 12 months postoperatively when it reaches 90–100% of esthesiometry values measured in normal corneas, although at earlier time points corneal sensation is markedly lower.[95]

Regarding nerve regeneration, 1 month after LASIK, very thin nerves of the sub-basal nerve plexus fibers can be visualized[95] but the number of sub-basal and stromal nerve fiber bundles are decreased by 90% as compared to the preoperative values.[95,96] In one study by Slowik et al., they did not observe sub-basal nerves in the central cornea during the first 4 months after LASIK.[97] During the 1st year after LASIK, reinnervation occurs, with corneal nerves being detected in the central cornea by 6 months.[88,98] However, the nerve density after LASIK remains less than a half of the preoperative values even at 12 months.[95,96,99] In addition, decreased sub-basal nerve density is observed at 2–3 years after LASIK.[88] Stachs et al. showed that at 2 years after LASIK, the whorl-shaped configuration of the sub-basal nerve plexus was not visualized and that the nerve fibers recovered to a near-normal state but were abnormally curved, thin and nonbranching.[95] Studies quantifying the sub-basal nerve density have shown to be reduced by 51%, 35% and 34% at 1, 2 and 3 years respectively.[100] At 5 years following surgery, nerve regeneration appears to be complete.[100] A strong correlation has been observed between corneal sensation and sub-basal nerve morphology and density after LASIK, showing that corneal sensitivity improves as the sub-basal nerves regenerate so that both function and nerve morphology seem to approach normal levels in about 6 months.[90,91,99,101] Interestingly, a study comparing corneal wound healing and nerve regeneration showed no difference between flaps created with femtosecond laser as compared to mechanical microkeratome.[102] This was confirmed by Patel et al. in a study where the patients were followed until 36 months after LASIK and the sub-basal nerve density and corneal sensitivity did not differ between methods of flap creation; however, the study had a large standard deviation of nerve density, the sample size was small and examined through a confocal microscope whose optical design is not the best to evaluate corneal nerves.[103] Conversely, in a small series of eyes, Lim et al. suggested that corneal sensitivity recovers faster after femtosecond laser flap creation compared with microkeratome.[68] Regarding corneal sensation and hinge position, initial studies have shown that postoperative corneal sensation may be higher and recover faster in eyes with nasally hinged flaps than in eyes with superiorly hinged flaps, inducing less neurotrophic dry eye.[82,104] However, later studies did not find an association between corneal sensation and hinge position with a microkeratome or a femtosecond laser.[82,93,105]

There are controversial results regarding the incidence of dry eye after femtosecond versus mechanical microkeratome LASIK. Golas et al. showed that there is no significant difference in self-reported dry eye symptoms between the mechanical keratome and the femtosecond laser.[80] By the other hand, other studies have shown a decrease in the incidence of LASIK induced dry eye when the flap is created with a femtosecond laser. For example, Salomao et al. found a 9% incidence of LASIK induced dry eye with a femtosecond laser compared with 46% with a microkeratome.[27]

Possible explanations for the decreased dry eye incidence with the femtosecond laser could be that this technique creates planar flaps with a defined side-cut angle, allowing a more precise realignment of the flap compared with microkeratome flaps (tapered edges), possibly producing less damage to corneal nerves.[103] Other explanations as to why there is less induction of dry eye are attributable to thinner flaps, reducing the amount of tissue for nerve regeneration, speeding up the recovery of corneal sensation,[106] as well as, less damage to limbal cells, including goblet cells, produced by the femtosecond fixation ring.

Further studies are required to assess flap configuration, hinge position or other factors accountable for the lower incidence of LASIK induced dry eye with the use of the femtosecond laser.

Comparison of outcomes of femtosecond laser versus microkeratome is given in Table 3.

**Table 3:** Comparison of outcomes of femtosecond laser versus microkeratome

| Outcome | Mechanical Microkeratome | Femtosecond Laser |
| --- | --- | --- |
| Flap thickness | Meniscus-shaped flap: thinner in the center, thicker in the periphery.[12,31,32] | Planar-shaped flap: even thickness across the flap.[12,31,32] |
| | High variability in flap thickness.[30] Thickness ±20 to ±40 μm.[23-29] | Higher predictability and less deviation from the intended thickness compared to microkeratome.[34,35,107] Variability is within ±20 μm of the intended flap thickness.[14,27,33,35-39] |
| Flap diameter | Diameter is function of corneal power: steeper corneas have wider diameter flaps; flatter corneas have smaller diameter flaps.[33,34] | More accurate in flap diameter, small variability in flap diameter independent of corneal curvature.[33,34] |
| Flap hinge | Hinge is nasal or superior, depending on the microkeratome | Surgeon can select the position and diameter of the hinge (superior, horizontal or oblique-hinged flap) |
| Visual outcome | No difference in visual outcomes between femtosecond and microkeratome LASIK.[20,67,68,108] No difference in postoperative un-corrected visual acuity.[20,68] | Faster visual recovery and improved un-corrected visual acuity.[65,69] Better visual outcomes and contrast sensitivity.[47] Better predictability of the manifest refraction spherical equivalent and a less surgically induced refractive change.[14,20,65] |
| Epithelial preservation | Incidence of epithelial defects 2.6%.[45] | Less epithelial defects.[20,33] Only some cases of epithelial damage overlying the stromal pocket produced by the laser.[9] |
| Enhancement rate | Enhancement rate 4.2% (n = 18,471 eyes).[14] | Enhancement rate 1.6% with IntraLase.[14] |
| Stromal wound healing and inflammation | No difference in cell death and corneal inflammation between microkeratome and 60 kHz femtosecond laser.[12,47] | The higher the energy of the laser (15 kHz vs 30 and 60 kHz), triggers more cell death, stromal cell proliferation and inflammation.[9,12,47-50] |
| | Cell death induced by microkeratomes is apoptosis, while with FS lasers is necrosis.[12] | Cell death induced is necrosis, promoting more inflammation than apoptosis.[12] |
| | Weaker healing of the flap compared to FS laser flaps.[12,51] | Stronger healing at the flap edge and in the flap interface.[12,51] |
| Diffuse lamellar keratitis (DLK) | Lower incidence of DLK, comparable to lower energy (≥60 kHz) femtosecond laser.[12,48,49] | Higher energy lasers (earlier models: 6 kHz and 15 kHz) have increased incidence of DLK and slower visual recovery.[48] Lower energy models (60 kHz) are comparable to microkeratomes.[12,48,49] |

*Contd...*

| Outcome | Mechanical Microkeratome | Femtosecond Laser |
| --- | --- | --- |
| High order aberrations and surgically induced astigmatism | Increased lower order[59,60] and high order aberrations.[54,61] More induction of HOAs as compared to femtosecond laser.[62-66] | Less induction of HOAs.[62-66] |
| | More induction of astigmatism.[20,65] | Less induction of astigmatism.[20,65] |
| Biomechanics | Meniscus-shaped flap damage more the peripheral fibers.[36] Weaker stromal scar, especially in the periphery when compared to femtosecond LASIK.[14,71] | Planar-shaped flaps may damage less peripheral fibers.[36] Stronger stromal peripheral scar than conventional mechanical microkeratome.[14,71] |
| Dry eye, corneal sub-basal nerve density and corneal sensitivity | Sub-basal nerve density and corneal sensitivity did not differ between methods (36 months of follow-up).[103] | Flap creation by FS did not show a difference in the stromal bed morphology or nerve regeneration when compared with the microkeratome.[102] Corneal sensitivity recovers faster after FS laser compared with microkeratome.[68] |
| | Controversial results of incidence of dry eye after LASIK. Golas et al. showed no significant difference in dry eye symptoms between the mechanical keratome and the femtosecond laser.[80] | Decrease in the incidence of LASIK-induced dry eye when the flap is created with a femtosecond laser, 9% vs 46% with a microkeratome.[27] |
| | Controversial results. Corneal sensation higher and recover faster in nasally hinged flaps than in superiorly hinged flaps, inducing less neurotrophic dry eye.[82,104] Later studies show no effect on hinge position in dry eye and/or corneal sensation with a mechanical microkeratome.[80,91] | No effect on hinge position in dry eye and/or corneal sensation with a femtosecond laser.[82,93,105] |

## CONCLUSION

LASIK technology has progressed rapidly over the past decade. After reviewing the techniques and outcomes of both mechanical and laser keratomes, the latter appears to significantly reduce flap-related complications and improve visual outcomes over mechanical microkeratome technology. In the most recent ASCRS 2011 survey, over 50% of the LASIK flaps created in the USA are made with a femtosecond laser. The safety and advantages of the femtosecond laser over mechanical microkeratomes includes improved uniformity of the flap, better predictability and reproducibility of flap thickness, lower incidence of flap-related complications, reduction of induced surgical astigmatism and HOA, better stromal bed quality as well as biomechanical outcomes.

It seems likely that femtosecond LASIK will become more common throughout the world with the introduction of several new models of femtosecond laser. Another important consideration is financial, as femtosecond lasers are a more expensive alternative, not all refractive centers will be able to offer this technology. Although some complications such as TLSS and vertical gas/bubble break are specific to femtosecond lasers, they are infrequent with the most recent models of femtosecond lasers. Several new femtosecond laser models have been recently introduced, and they offer additional functions other than flap creation for keratoplasty and cataract surgery. Further experience is needed to evaluate the efficacy and safety of these new laser platforms.

## REFERENCES

1. Barraquer JI. Basis of refractive keratoplasty—1967. Refract Corneal Surg. 1989;5(3):179-93.
2. Pallikaris IG, Papatzanaki ME, Siganos DS, et al. A corneal flap technique for laser in situ keratomileusis. Human studies. Arch Ophthalmol. 1991;109(12):1699-702.
3. Pallikaris IG, Papatzanaki ME, Stathi EZ, et al. Laser in situ keratomileusis. Lasers Surg Med. 1990;10(5):463-8.
4. Buratto L, Ferrari M, Rama P. Excimer laser intrastromal keratomileusis. Am J Ophthalmol. 1992;113(3):291-5.
5. Lin JT. Principles of scanning lasers for customized LASIK. In: Garg A, Alió JL, Pajic B, Mehta CK (Eds). Mastering the Techniques of LASIK, EPILASIK, and LASEK (Techniques and Technology). New Delhi, India: Jaypee Brothers Medical Publishers; 2007. pp. 27-47.
6. Rapuano CJ, Belin MW, Boxer-Walcher BS, et al. Refractive surgery. In: Rapuano CJ (Ed). Basic and Clinical Science Course. San Francisco, CA: American Academy of Ophthalmology; 2010-2011.
7. Seiler T, Koufala K, Richter G. Iatrogenic keratectasia after laser in situ keratomileusis. J Refract Surg. 1998;14(3):312-7.
8. Paschalis EI, Aristeidou AP, Foudoulakis NC, et al. Corneal flap assessment with Rondo microkeratome in laser in situ keratomileusis. Graefes Arch Clin Exp Ophthalmol. 2011;249(2):289-95.

9. Salomao MQ, Wilson SE. Femtosecond laser in laser in situ keratomileusis. J Cataract Refract Surg. 2010;36(6):1024-32.

10. Kurtz RM, Liu X, Elner VM, et al. Photodisruption in the human cornea as a function of laser pulse width. J Refract Surg. 1997;13(7):653-8.

11. Lubatschowski H. Overview of commercially available femtosecond lasers in refractive surgery. J Refract Surg. 2008;24(1):S102-7.

12. Netto MV, Mohan RR, Medeiros FW, et al. Femtosecond laser and microkeratome corneal flaps: comparison of stromal wound healing and inflammation. J Refract Surg. 2007;23(7):667-76.

13. Stonecipher KG, Dishler JG, Ignacio TS, et al. Transient light sensitivity after femtosecond laser flap creation: clinical findings and management. J Cataract Refract Surg. 2006;32(1):91-4.

14. Stonecipher K, Ignacio TS, Stonecipher M. Advances in refractive surgery: microkeratome and femtosecond laser flap creation in relation to safety, efficacy, predictability, and biomechanical stability. Curr Opin Ophthalmol. 2006;17(4):368-72.

15. Munoz G, Albarran-Diego C, Sakla HF, et al. Transient light-sensitivity syndrome after laser in situ keratomileusis with the femtosecond laser Incidence and prevention. J Cataract Refract Surg. 2006;32(12):2075-9.

16. Rocha KM, Kagan R, Smith SD, et al. Thresholds for interface haze formation after thin-flap femtosecond laser in situ keratomileusis for myopia. Am J Ophthalmol. 2009;147(6):966-72.

17. Biser SA, Bloom AH, Donnenfeld ED, et al. Flap folds after femtosecond LASIK. Eye Contact Lens. 2003;29(4):252-4.

18. Randleman JB, Woodward M, Lynn MJ, et al. Risk assessment for ectasia after corneal refractive surgery. Ophthalmology. 2008;115(1):37-50.

19. Randleman JB, Dawson DG, Grossniklaus HE, et al. Depth-dependent cohesive tensile strength in human donor corneas: implications for refractive surgery. J Refract Surg. 2008;24(1):S85-9.

20. Kezirian GM, Stonecipher KG. Comparison of the IntraLase femtosecond laser and mechanical keratomes for laser in situ keratomileusis. J Cataract Refract Surg. 2004;30(4):804-11.

21. Probst LE, Machat JJ. Mathematics of laser in situ keratomileusis for high myopia. J Cataract Refract Surg. 1998;24(2):190-5.

22. Genth U, Mrochen M, Walti R, et al. Optical low coherence reflectometry for noncontact measurements of flap thickness during laser in situ keratomileusis. Ophthalmology. 2002;109(5):973-8.

23. Pietila J, Makinen P, Suominen S, et al. Corneal flap measurements in laser in situ keratomileusis using the Moria M2 automated microkeratome. J Refract Surg. 2005;21(4):377-85.

24. Arbelaez MC. Nidek MK 2000 microkeratome clinical evaluation. J Refract Surg. 2002;18(3 Suppl):S357-60.

25. Ucakhan OO. Corneal flap thickness in laser in situ keratomileusis using the summit Krumeich-Barraquer microkeratome. J Cataract Refract Surg. 2002;28(5):798-804.

26. Shemesh G, Dotan G, Lipshitz I. Predictability of corneal flap thickness in laser in situ keratomileusis using three different microkeratomes. J Refract Surg. 2002;18(3 Suppl):S347-51.

27. Salomao MQ, Ambrosio R, Wilson SE. Dry eye associated with laser in situ keratomileusis: mechanical microkeratome versus femtosecond laser. J Cataract Refract Surg. 2009;35(10):1756-60.

28. Taneri S. Laser in situ keratomileusis flap thickness using the Hansatome microkeratome with zero compression heads. J Cataract Refract Surg. 2006;32(1):72-7.

29. Pepose JS, Feigenbaum SK, Qazi MA, et al. Comparative performance of the Zyoptix XP and Hansatome zero-compression microkeratomes. J Cataract Refract Surg. 2007;33(8):1386-91.

30. Solomon KD, Donnenfeld E, Sandoval HP, et al. Flap thickness accuracy: comparison of 6 microkeratome models. J Cataract Refract Surg. 2004;30(5):964-77.

31. von Jagow B, Kohnen T. Corneal architecture of femtosecond laser and microkeratome flaps imaged by anterior segment optical coherence tomography. J Cataract Refract Surg. 2009;35(1):35-41.

32. Talamo JH, Meltzer J, Gardner J. Reproducibility of flap thickness with IntraLase FS and Moria LSK-1 and M2 microkeratomes. J Refract Surg. 2006;22(6):556-61.

33. Binder PS. Flap dimensions created with the IntraLase FS laser. J Cataract Refract Surg. 2004;30(1):26-32.

34. Binder PS. One thousand consecutive IntraLase laser in situ keratomileusis flaps. J Cataract Refract Surg. 2006;32(6):962-9.

35. Kim JH, Lee D, Rhee KI. Flap thickness reproducibility in laser in situ keratomileusis with a femtosecond laser: optical coherence tomography measurement. J Cataract Refract Surg. 2008;34(1):132-6.

36. Stahl JE, Durrie DS, Schwendeman FJ, et al. Anterior segment OCT analysis of thin IntraLase femtosecond flaps. J Refract Surg. 2007;23(6):555-8.

37. Slade SG. The use of the femtosecond laser in the customization of corneal flaps in laser in situ keratomileusis. Curr Opin Ophthalmol. 2007;18(4):314-7.

38. Dupps WJ, Wilson SE. Biomechanics and wound healing in the cornea. Exp Eye Res. 2006;83(4):709-20.

39. Chan A, Ou J, Manche EE. Comparison of the femtosecond laser and mechanical keratome for laser in situ keratomileusis. Arch Ophthalmol. 2008;126(11):1484-90.

40. Pfaeffl WA, Kunze M, Zenk U, et al. Predictive factors of femtosecond laser flap thickness measured by online optical coherence pachymetry subtraction in sub-Bowman keratomileusis. J Cataract Refract Surg. 2008;34(11):1872-80.

41. Shah MN, Misra M, Wihelmus KR, et al. Diffuse lamellar keratitis associated with epithelial defects after laser in situ keratomileusis. J Cataract Refract Surg. 2000;26(9):1312-8.

42. Mulhern MG, Naor J, Rootman DS. The role of epithelial defects in intralamellar inflammation after laser in situ keratomileusis. Can J Ophthalmol. 2002;37(7):409-15.

43. Wang MY, Maloney RK. Epithelial ingrowth after laser in situ keratomileusis. Am J Ophthalmol. 2000;129(6):746-51.

44. Dastgheib KA, Clinch TE, Manche EE, et al. Sloughing of corneal epithelium and wound healing complications associated with laser in situ keratomileusis in patients with epithelial basement membrane dystrophy. Am J Ophthalmol. 2000;130(3):297-303.

45. Duffey RJ. Thin flap laser in situ keratomileusis: flap dimensions with the Moria LSK-One manual microkeratome using the 100-microm head. J Cataract Refract Surg. 2005;31(6):1159-62.

46. Wilson SE. Molecular cell biology for the refractive corneal surgeon: programmed cell death and wound healing. J Refract Surg. 1997;13(2):171-5.

47. de Medeiros FW, Kaur H, Agrawal V, et al. Effect of femtosecond laser energy level on corneal stromal cell death and inflammation. J Refract Surg. 2009;25(10):869-74.

48. Javaloy J, Vidal MT, Abdelrahman AM, et al. Confocal microscopy comparison of intralase femtosecond laser and Moria M2 microkeratome in LASIK. J Refract Surg. 2007;23(2):178-87.

49. Chang JS. Complications of sub-Bowman's keratomileusis with a femtosecond laser in 3009 eyes. J Refract Surg. 2008;24(1):S97-101.

50. Krueger RR, Dupps WJ. Biomechanical effects of femtosecond and microkeratome-based flap creation: prospective contralateral examination of two patients. J Refract Surg. 2007;23(8):800-7.

51. Kim JY, Kim MJ, Kim TI, et al. A femtosecond laser creates a stronger flap than a mechanical microkeratome. Invest Ophthalmol Vis Sci. 2006;47(2):599-604.

52. Knorz MC, Vossmerbaeumer U. Comparison of flap adhesion strength using the Amadeus microkeratome and the IntraLase iFS femtosecond laser in rabbits. J Refract Surg. 2008;24(9):875-8.

53. Subbaram MV, MacRae S, Slade SG, et al. Customized LASIK treatment for myopia: relationship between preoperative higher order aberrations and refractive outcome. J Refract Surg. 2006;22(8):746-53.

54. Pallikaris IG, Kymionis GD, Panagopoulou SI, et al. Induced optical aberrations following formation of a laser in situ keratomileusis flap. J Cataract Refract Surg. 2002;28(10):1737-41.

55. Waheed S, Chalita MR, Xu M, et al. Flap-induced and laser-induced ocular aberrations in a two-step LASIK procedure. J Refract Surg. 2005;21(4):346-52.

56. Huang D, Arif M. Spot size and quality of scanning laser correction of higher order wavefront aberrations. J Refract Surg. 2001;17(5):S588-91.

57. Porter J, MacRae S, Yoon G, et al. Separate effects of the microkeratome incision and laser ablation on the eye's wave aberration. Am J Ophthalmol. 2003;136(2):327-37.

58. Vinciguerra P, Azzolini M, Airaghi P, et al. Effect of decreasing surface and interface irregularities after photorefractive keratectomy and laser in situ keratomileusis on optical and functional outcomes. J Refract Surg. 1998;14(2 Suppl):S199-203.

59. Wilson SE, Mohan RR, Hong JW, et al. The wound healing response after laser in situ keratomileusis and photorefractive keratectomy: elusive control of biological variability and effect on custom laser vision correction. Arch Ophthalmol. 2001;119(6):889-96.

60. Oshika T, Klyce SD, Applegate RA, et al. Comparison of corneal wavefront aberrations after photorefractive keratectomy and laser in situ keratomileusis. Am J Ophthalmol. 1999;127(1):1-7.

61. Hersh PS, Fry K, Blaker JW. Spherical aberration after laser in situ keratomileusis and photorefractive keratectomy. Clinical results and theoretical models of etiology. J Cataract Refract Surg. 2003;29(11):2096-104.

62. Sarayba MA, Ignacio TS, Binder PS, et al. Comparative study of stromal bed quality by using mechanical, IntraLase femtosecond laser 15- and 30-kHz microkeratomes. Cornea. 2007;26(4):446-51.

63. Medeiros FW, Stapleton WM, Hammel J, et al. Wavefront analysis comparison of LASIK outcomes with the femtosecond laser and mechanical microkeratomes. J Refract Surg. 2007;23(9):880-7.

64. Buzzonetti L, Petrocelli G, Valente P, et al. Comparison of corneal aberration changes after laser in situ keratomileusis performed with mechanical microkeratome and IntraLase femtosecond laser: One-year follow-up. Cornea. 2008;27(2):174-9.

65. Durrie DS, Kezirian GM. Femtosecond laser versus mechanical keratome flaps in wavefront-guided laser in situ keratomileusis: prospective contralateral eye study. J Cataract Refract Surg. 2005;31(1):120-6.

66. Tran DB, Sarayba MA, Bor Z, et al. Randomized prospective clinical study comparing induced aberrations with IntraLase and Hansatome flap creation in fellow eyes: potential impact on wavefront-guided laser in situ keratomileusis. J Cataract Refract Surg. 2005;31(1):97-105.

67. Patel SV, Maguire LJ, McLaren JW, et al. Femtosecond laser versus mechanical microkeratome for LASIK: a randomized controlled study. Ophthalmology. 2007;114(8):1482-90.

68. Lim T, Yang S, Kim M, et al. Comparison of the IntraLase femtosecond laser and mechanical microkeratome for laser in situ keratomileusis. Am J Ophthalmol. 2006;141(5):833-9.

69. Tanna M, Schallhorn SC, Hettinger KA. Femtosecond laser versus mechanical microkeratome: a retrospective comparison of visual outcomes at 3 months. J Refract Surg. 2009;25(7 Suppl):S668-71.

70. Qazi MA, Roberts CJ, Mahmoud AM, et al. Topographic and biomechanical differences between hyperopic and myopic laser in situ keratomileusis. J Cataract Refract Surg. 2005;31(1):48-60.

71. Schmack I, Dawson DG, McCarey BE, et al. Cohesive tensile strength of human LASIK wounds with histologic, ultrastructural, and clinical correlations. J Refract Surg. 2005;21(5):433-45.

72. Durrie DS, Slade SG, Marshall J. Wavefront-guided excimer laser ablation using photorefractive keratectomy and sub-Bowman's keratomileusis: a contralateral eye study. J Refract Surg. 2008;24(1):S77-84.

73. Hovanesian JA, Shah SS, Maloney RK. Symptoms of dry eye and recurrent erosion syndrome after refractive surgery. J Cataract Refract Surg. 2001;27(4):577-84.

74. Jabbur NS, Sakatani K, O'Brien TP. Survey of complications and recommendations for management in dissatisfied patients seeking a consultation after refractive surgery. J Cataract Refract Surg. 2004;30(9):1867-74.

75. Levinson BA, Rapuano CJ, Cohen EJ, et al. Referrals to the Wills Eye Institute Cornea Service after laser in situ keratomileusis: reasons for patient dissatisfaction. J Cataract Refract Surg. 2008;34(1):32-9.

76. Ambrosio R, Tervo T, Wilson SE. LASIK-associated dry eye and neurotrophic epitheliopathy: pathophysiology and strategies for prevention and treatment. J Refract Surg. 2008;24(4):396-407.

77. Ang RT, Dartt DA, Tsubota K. Dry eye after refractive surgery. Curr Opin Ophthalmol. 2001;12(4):318-22.

78. Toda I, Asano-Kato N, Komai-Hori Y, et al. Dry eye after laser in situ keratomileusis. Am J Ophthalmol. 2001;132(1):1-7.

79. Toda I. LASIK and the ocular surface. Cornea. 2008;27(Suppl 1):S70-6.

80. Golas L, Manche EE. Dry eye after laser in situ keratomileusis with femtosecond laser and mechanical keratome. J Cataract Refract Surg. 2011; 37(8):1476-80.

81. Mian SI, Li AY, Dutta S, et al. Dry eyes and corneal sensation after laser in situ keratomileusis with femtosecond laser flap creation effect of hinge position, hinge angle, and flap thickness. J Cataract Refract Surg. 2009;35(12):2092-8.

82. Vroman DT, Sandoval HP, Fernandez de Castro LE, et al. Effect of hinge location on corneal sensation and dry eye after laser in situ keratomileusis for myopia. J Cataract Refract Surg. 2005;31(10):1881-7.

83. Hammond MD, Madigan WP, Bower KS. Refractive surgery in the United States Army, 2000-2003. Ophthalmology. 2005;112(2):184-90.

84. Yu EY, Leung A, Rao S, et al. Effect of laser in situ keratomileusis on tear stability. Ophthalmology. 2000;107(12):2131-5.

85. Wilson SE, Ambrosio R. Laser in situ keratomileusisinduced neurotrophic epitheliopathy. Am J Ophthalmol. 2001; 132(3): 405-6.

86. Wilson SE. Laser in situ keratomileusis-induced (presumed) neurotrophic epitheliopathy. Ophthalmology. 2001;108(6): 1082-7.

87. Battat L, Macri A, Dursun D, et al. Effects of laser in situ keratomileusis on tear production, clearance, and the ocular surface. Ophthalmology. 2001;108(7):1230-5.

88. Calvillo MP, McLaren JW, Hodge DO, et al. Corneal reinnervation after LASIK: prospective 3-year longitudinal study. Invest Ophthalmol Vis Sci. 2004;45(11):3991-6.

89. Matsui H, Kumano Y, Zushi I, et al. Corneal sensation after correction of myopia by photorefractive keratectomy and laser in situ keratomileusis. J Cataract Refract Surg. 2001;27(3):370-3.

90. Perez-Gomez I, Efron N. Change to corneal morphology after refractive surgery (myopic laser in situ keratomilesis) as viewed with a confocal microscope. Optom Vis Sci. 2003;80(10):690-7.

91. Bragheeth MA, Dua HS. Corneal sensation after myopic and hyperopic LASIK: clinical and confocal microscopic study. Br J Ophthalmol. 2005;89(5):580-5.

92. Chuck RS, Quiros PA, Perez AC, et al. Corneal sensation after laser in situ keratomileusis. J Cataract Refract Surg. 2000;26(3):337-9.

93. Kumano Y, Matsui H, Zushi I, et al. Recovery of corneal sensation after myopic correction by laser in situ keratomileusis with a nasal or superior hinge. J Cataract Refract Surg. 2003;29(4):757-61.

94. Kanellopoulos AJ, Pallikaris IG, Donnenfeld ED, et al. Comparison of corneal sensation following photorefractive keratectomy and laser in situ keratomileusis. J Cataract Refract Surg. 1997;23(1):34-8.

95. Stachs O, Zhivov A, Kraak R, et al. Structural-functional correlations of corneal innervation after LASIK and penetrating keratoplasty. J Refract Surg. 2010;26(3):159-67.

96. Lee BH, McLaren JW, Erie JC, et al. Reinnervation in the cornea after LASIK. Invest Ophthalmol Vis Sci. 2002;43(12):3660-4.

97. Slowik C, Somodi S, Richter A, et al. Assessment of corneal alterations following laser in situ keratomileusis by confocal slit scanning microscopy. Ger J Ophthalmol. 1996;5(6):526-31.

98. Lee SJ, Kim JK, Seo KY, et al. Comparison of corneal nerve regeneration and sensitivity between LASIK and laser epithelial keratomileusis (LASEK). Am J Ophthalmol. 2006;141(6):1009-15.

99. Linna TU, Vesaluoma MH, Perez-Santonja JJ, et al. Effect of myopic LASIK on corneal sensitivity and morphology of subbasal nerves. Invest Ophthalmol Vis Sci. 2000;41(2):393-7.

100. Erie JC, McLaren JW, Hodge DO, et al. Recovery of corneal subbasal nerve density after PRK and LASIK. Am J Ophthalmol. 2005;140(6):1059-64.

101. Cruzat A, Pavan-Langston D, Hamrah P. In vivo confocal microscopy of corneal nerves: analysis and clinical correlation. Semin Ophthalmol. 2010;25(5-6):171-7.

102. Sonigo B, Iordanidou V, Chong-Sit D, et al. In vivo corneal confocal microscopy comparison of intralase femtosecond laser and mechanical microkeratome for laser in situ keratomileusis. Invest Ophthalmol Vis Sci. 2006;47(7):2803-11.

103. Patel SV, McLaren JW, Kittleson KM, et al. Subbasal nerve density and corneal sensitivity after laser in situ keratomileusis: femtosecond laser vs mechanical microkeratome. Arch Ophthalmol. 2010;128(11):1413-9.

104. Donnenfeld ED, Solomon K, Perry HD, et al. The effect of hinge position on corneal sensation and dry eye after LASIK. Ophthalmology. 2003;110(5):1023-9.

105. Mian SI, Shtein RM, Nelson A, et al. Effect of hinge position on corneal sensation and dry eye after laser in situ keratomileusis using a femtosecond laser. J Cataract Refract Surg. 2007;33(7):1190-4.

106. Nassaralla BA, McLeod SD, Boteon JE, et al. The effect of hinge position and depth plate on the rate of recovery of corneal sensation following LASIK. Am J Ophthalmol. 2005;139(1):118-24.

107. Sutton G, Hodge C. Accuracy and precision of LASIK flap thickness using the IntraLase femtosecond laser in 1000 consecutive cases. J Refract Surg. 2008;24(8):802-6.

108. Azar DT, Ghanem RC, de la Cruz J, et al. Thin-flap (sub-Bowman keratomileusis) versus thick-flap laser in situ keratomileusis for moderate to high myopia: case-control analysis. J Cataract Refract Surg. 2008;34(12):2073-8.

# LASIK Outcomes in Astigmatism

*John J DeStafeno, John P Berdahl*

## ❧ INTRODUCTION

Astigmatism is a common form of refractive error, due to corneal or lenticular curvature meridional differences, in which light rays entering the eye do not focus into a single point resulting in a blurred visual image. First described by Thomas Young in 1801, astigmatism is currently present in more than 90% of adult eyes. Additionally, as much as 44% of the general population has more than 0.50 diopter (D) of astigmatism, and 8% of the population has 1.50 D or more.[1] In this modern era of ophthalmic surgery, uncorrected astigmatism can have a significant impact on visual outcomes, emphasizing the importance of detection and management of this condition.

Over the course of the past century, the evolution of medical and surgical correction of astigmatism has continued to evolve. Currently, astigmatism is managed with several modalities including spectacles, contact lenses, compression sutures, keratotomy procedures, toric and phakic intraocular lenses, and varying forms of excimer laser ablation. In this chapter, we will focus on excimer laser corrective surgery, specifically laser *in situ* keratomileusis (LASIK), for the treatment of astigmatism, exploring the varying techniques, visual outcomes, and comparisons to other currently used technologies.

## ❧ DEFINITIONS

The term astigmatism is derived from the Greek a-, meaning 'not' and stigma-, meaning 'point or mark'. Astigmatism is typically categorized into regular or irregular astigmatism. Regular astigmatism occurs when the meridian of the maximum and minimum curvature are at right angles.

Regular astigmatism is generally categorized as with-the-rule (meridian of maximum curvature with 30° of vertical) or against-the-rule (meridian of maximum curvature within 30° of horizontal). With-the-rule astigmatism is more prevalent in the younger population, transitioning to against-the-rule astigmatism with aging, due to possible changes in corneal curvature. Regular astigmatism is commonly corrected through the use of spherocylindrical lenses (Fig. 1).

Irregular astigmatism presents when the two principal meridians of the eye are not at right angles to each other. Furthermore, there may be variations in refraction in a single meridian of the eye.[2] Unlike regular astigmatism, irregular astigmatism is often encountered due to trauma, scarring, corneal surgery and corneal diseases (keratoconus). Irregular astigmatism can be classified into two distinct types: (1) regularly irregular and (2) irregularly irregular astigmatism. Loosely defined, regularly irregular astigmatism has an identifiable pattern (the asymmetric bowtie) while irregularly irregular astigmatism has no recognizable pattern on corneal topography.[3] Irregular astigmatism cannot be corrected with spherocylindrical lenses and is often difficult to measure and treat. Correction may be obtained through the use of rigid contact lenses and surgery (Fig. 2).

## ❧ HISTORY

The use of the excimer laser to ablate precise corneal shapes in animal models was first described by Trokel et al. in 1983.[4] Further progress was made in the early 1990s with the use of toric ablation patterns for the treatment of astigmatism. Early work by McDonnell and colleagues

16
SECTION

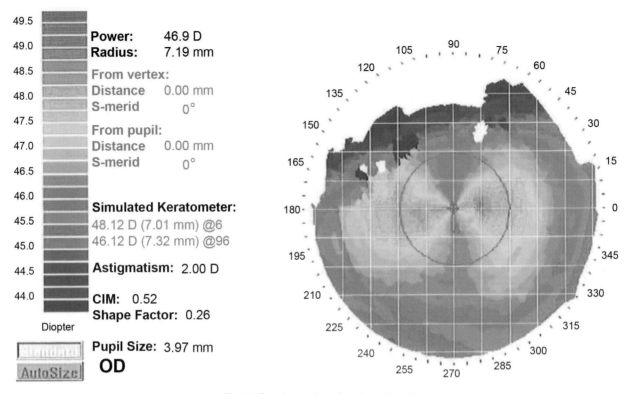

49.5
49.0
48.5
48.0
47.5
47.0
46.5
46.0
45.5
45.0
44.5
44.0

Diopter

**Power:** 46.9 D
**Radius:** 7.19 mm

**From vertex:**
**Distance** 0.00 mm
**S-merid** 0°

**From pupil:**
**Distance** 0.00 mm
**S-merid** 0°

**Simulated Keratometer:**
48.12 D (7.01 mm) @6
46.12 D (7.32 mm) @96

**Astigmatism:** 2.00 D

**CIM:** 0.52
**Shape Factor:** 0.26

**Pupil Size:** 3.97 mm
**OD**

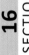

**Fig. 1:** Regular against-the-rule astigmatism

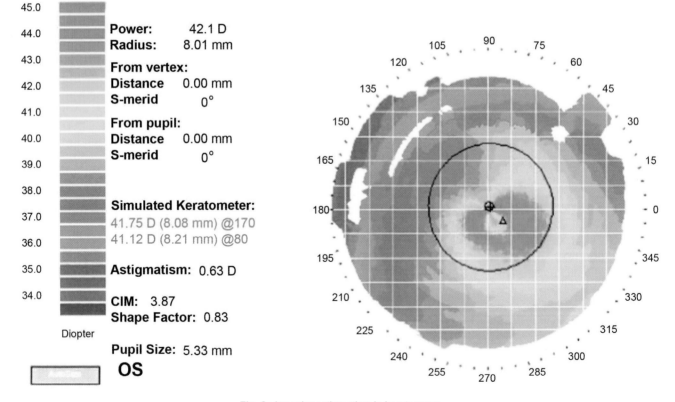

45.0
44.0
43.0
42.0
41.0
40.0
39.0
38.0
37.0
36.0
35.0
34.0

Diopter

**Power:** 42.1 D
**Radius:** 8.01 mm

**From vertex:**
**Distance** 0.00 mm
**S-merid** 0°

**From pupil:**
**Distance** 0.00 mm
**S-merid** 0°

**Simulated Keratometer:**
41.75 D (8.08 mm) @170
41.12 D (8.21 mm) @80

**Astigmatism:** 0.63 D

**CIM:** 3.87
**Shape Factor:** 0.83

**Pupil Size:** 5.33 mm
**OS**

**Fig. 2:** Irregular astigmatism in keratoconus

described the use of toric ablation to flatten primarily the steep axis in four patients with cylindrical errors.[5] The authors found an unintentional hyperopic shift that occurred as the flat meridian, in addition to the steep meridian, was flattened as well. These results led others to address the issues with toric ablations. In 1995, Alio et al. reported results of 46 patients who underwent an updated cylindrical ablation profile to correct simple myopic astigmatism. The mean preoperative cylinder was −2.50 D with 1 year results displaying mean residual cylinder of −0.50 D and 20/25 Snellen visual acuity.[6]

The first early work with hyperopic excimer ablation was reported by Dausch and colleagues in 1993.[7] Hyperopic astigmatic correction is achieved by preferentially steepening the flat meridian. This ablation technique induces little effect on the spherical portion of the refraction. Argento et al. provided one of the earlier reports on correction of simple hyperopic astigmatism and found a 2.86 D decrease in cylindrical correction with 20/25 Snellen visual acuity.[8] Further early reports of treatment for primary or secondary hyperopia are limited as most did not treat astigmatism or there were combined results of the spherical and astigmatic cohorts. In addition, vector analysis of astigmatism results was not routinely performed, leading to difficulty determining the true efficacy of treatment.[9]

## LASIK TREATMENT OF ASTIGMATISM

In 1997, the Food and Drug Administration (FDA) approved the use of excimer LASIK for the treatment of astigmatism. The excimer laser operates at a wavelength of 193 nm and ablates approximately 0.25 μm of stromal tissue with each pulse.[10] Myopic astigmatic corrections apply pulses along the central part of the flat meridian in an elliptical pattern, flattening the steep meridian. In contrast, hyperopic astigmatic corrections apply pulses predominantly in the periphery, steepening the flat meridian.

Traditionally, excimer lasers correct spherocylindrical error using an ablation profile based solely on the manifest refraction, commonly referred to as conventional LASIK. Conventional treatments do not address spherical and coma aberrations (higher order aberrations, HOAs). The introduction of Wavefront-guided laser platforms can help identify and correct coma, trefoil, quadrafoil, and higher order spherical aberration in addition to astigmatism. Zernike polynomials are used to outline a convenient mathematical identification of the aberration content in the optical wavefront, which results in a more precise and customized treatment profile than conventional treatments. From these measurements, an ablation profile is created that is applied using variable beam or scanning spot technology.

Wavefront-guided treatments have been shown to improve visual quality such as decreased halos, glare and other symptoms, along with increased visual acuity in low-contrast conditions. A recent review of the literature by the American Academy of Ophthalmology in 2008, supported the visual benefits of wavefront-guided LASIK for myopia and astigmatism.[11]

Recently, the approval of the WaveLight laser combined with wavefront analysis, now gives surgeons a choice between a wavefront-optimized surgery and a wavefront-guided surgery. The wavefront-optimized surgery uses data derived from the laboratory to determine the optimal tissue ablation plan, while the wavefront-guided surgery uses data derived from a custom evaluation of each eye to determine an optimized treatment plan for the individual patient. Several groups have compared wavefront-optimized to wavefront-guided LASIK for the correction of myopic astigmatism and have shown excellent uncorrected Snellen visual acuity and appear to be equally effective options in correcting astigmatism.[12,13]

Topography-guided treatments have been used most predominantly to correct irregular corneas with excellent results.[14,15] They have the advantage of delivering treatment based on the shape of the corneal surface, can treat a wider area on the cornea than wavefront-based ablations, are not affected by lenticular opacities, and may be more stable due to treating the cornea rather than aberrometry measurements alone. However, a major disadvantage of topography-guided treatments is that they do not account for all the refractive elements of the eye and, therefore, do not treat lenticular aberrations. This uncoupling of corneal and lenticular aberrations may lead to reduced quality of vision.[16]

Due to limitations in both wavefront-based and topography-guided ablations, the combination of these two treatments to provide a higher level of visual correction has been suggested by some. Alpins et al. compared patients treated with wavefront-guided treatment alone versus those treated with both wavefront and topography-guided treatments for the correction of myopic astigmatism. The combination group had a greater reduction in astigmatism and better visual outcomes.[17] Further studies are needed to establish the possible benefit of these treatment profiles and the effect on overall visual quality.

## ASTIGMATIC AXIS OF CORRECTION

The outcome of LASIK for astigmatism is dependent on both the magnitude and orientation of the axis of correction. In regular astigmatism, magnitude can be measured relatively accurately through the use of manifest refraction, topographers, etc. Small errors in magnitude may lead to under- or overcorrections that have less of an effect of the visual outcome than axis misalignment. Axis misalignment is important not only in the treatment of astigmatism but also in wavefront-guided surgery due to treatment profiles not being radially symmetric. Small degrees of error in axis alignment lead to significant reduction in astigmatic correction[18] (Table 1).

Cyclotorsion is a well-known factor leading to axis misalignment. Patients transitioning from seated to supine positioning can lead to astigmatic changes on the magnitude of 0–14 degrees.[19] Fortunately, proper alignment has been aided by the introduction of iris registration and dynamic tracking technologies (Fig. 3). In 2005, Chernyak initially reported the use or iris registration for enhanced alignment of laser treatments.[20] Khalifa and colleagues reported on a double-blind study with three patient groups: (1) Conventional LASIK and manual marking, (2) Wavefront-guided LASIK and manual marking and (3) Wavefront-guided LASIK with iris registration (LASIK+IR). The LASIK+IR group had better postoperative UCVA (100% 20/30 or better; 90% 20/20 or better; 20% 20/16 or better) than the other groups. The LASIK+IR group had the highest predictability of spherical refraction and the highest predictability of cylinder refraction. They also had a significantly smaller increase postoperatively in coma, trefoil and secondary astigmatism.[21]

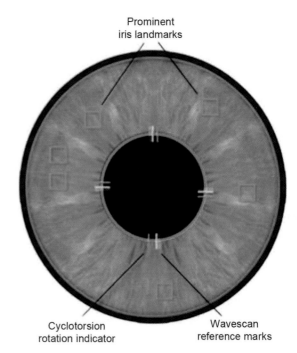

**Fig. 3:** Iris registration VISX CustomVue
*Source:* Photograph courtesy of Abbott Medical Optics, Santa Ana, CA

Iris registration does not actively track the iris during excimer laser treatment; rather the treatment is aligned only at the time of registration. This limitation may lead to a dynamic misalignment between the laser and the ablation bed due to the intraoperative rotational activity of the eye (Fig. 4). Therefore, dynamic iris tracking programs have been developed to account for this dynamic misalignment. A 2011 study by Prakash and colleagues performed a comparative study looking at outcomes for myopic astigmatism using LASIK without iris registration, with iris registration and with iris registration-assisted dynamic rotational eye tracking. The authors concluded

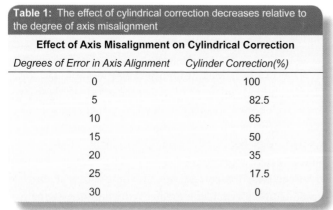

**Table 1:** The effect of cylindrical correction decreases relative to the degree of axis misalignment

| Effect of Axis Misalignment on Cylindrical Correction | |
|---|---|
| *Degrees of Error in Axis Alignment* | *Cylinder Correction(%)* |
| 0 | 100 |
| 5 | 82.5 |
| 10 | 65 |
| 15 | 50 |
| 20 | 35 |
| 25 | 17.5 |
| 30 | 0 |

*Source:* Adapted from Kim YJ, Sohn J, Tchah H, Lee CO. Photo-astigmatic refractive keratectomy in 168 eyes: six-month results. J Cataract Refract Surg. 1994; 20:387-91.

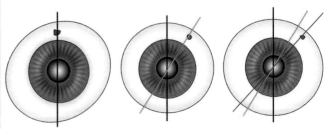

**Fig. 4:** Dynamic misalignment. The black mark represents an iris landmark. Left: Preablation reference, upright position. Middle: Preablation supine position displaying cyclotorsion. Right: Active cyclotorsion during excimer ablation. Note the change in degree of cyclotorsion from the start of ablation (middle) to the intraoperative ablation (right)
*Source:* Courtesy of A Agarwal

the mean postoperative refractive error and cylindrical values were significantly lower in the cases that underwent iris recognition and dynamic tracking. In addition, using Alpins analysis, difference vector, error angle, correction index, success index and flattening index were best in the iris recognition and dynamic tracking group.[22]

## LASIK IN IRREGULAR ASTIGMATISM

Irregular astigmatism, optical distortions that cannot be corrected with spherocylindrical lenses, can be caused by ocular disease, trauma and postsurgical forms. Prior to the advent of excimer lasers, limited surgical treatments including selective incisions, sutures, lamellar and full thickness keratoplasty were used with limited success. The majority of the work with excimer laser for the correction of irregular astigmatism has been conducted using surface ablation yet we felt this to be a relevant discussion in astigmatism outcomes.

Although refractive corneal surgery with the excimer laser can result in irregular astigmatism, it is currently the most promising technology available to correct this unwanted outcome. Both topography and wavefront-guided ablations have been used for corneal irregularities including decentered ablations and corneal islands.[23-25] Various laser platforms are combined with elevation-based corneal topography to correct irregular astigmatism. One such model, the Corneal Interactive Programmed Topographic Ablation (CIPTA), was studied by Allesio and colleagues whom treated 42 eyes with decentered photorefractive keratectomy (PRK) ablations and reported a decrease in decentration from 1.19 mm to 0.15 mm and improved mean visual acuity to 20/26 in all patients.[26]

Masking agents (e.g. sodium hyaluronate) are another option employed to treat irregular astigmatism. Excimer laser assisted by sodium hyaluronate (ELASHY) is a technique used to create a smooth ablation bed, essentially treating the 'peaks' and protecting the 'valleys' in the corneal profile.[27] In a similar fashion, Biomask, a porcine Type I collagen material, has been used in conjunction with phototherapeutic keratectomy (PTK) for surface irregularities. Corneal surface and mean visual acuity have been reported to improve using these techniques.[28]

## LASIK AFTER PENETRATING KERATOPLASTY

Despite the advances in graft selection and surgical techniques, residual refractive error remains a major cause of decreased visual acuity after penetrating keratoplasty (PK). Astigmatism after PK for keratoconus is typically 2–6 D, with approximately 15% greater than 5.00 D.[29] Wound suturing, corneal relaxing incisions and wedge resections are some techniques that have been used to correct astigmatic error after PK. With the advent of laser surgical correction after PK, several studies have reported the benefit of LASIK of other refractive procedures for the correction of refractive error after PK.

The use of LASIK for the correction of myopia is more effective and predictable than the correction of myopic astigmatism. This is not to state that use of the LASIK for astigmatic correction has been unsuccessful. Lee and Kim reported a 3.80 D and near 54% mean reduction in astigmatism after LASIK post-PK.[30] The authors also found an increase in corrected visual acuity and greater tolerance to spectacles/contact lenses. Furthermore, a greater understanding of the biomechanical changes of the cornea after lamellar keratectomy (flap creation) and the development of femtosecond lasers has improved astigmatism outcomes. For example, some surgeons advocate two-step LASIK (creation of lamellar flap, followed by LASIK at a later date) due to biomechanical changes of the cornea. Studies have shown a decrease in astigmatic error after lamellar flap creation, possibly leading to inaccurate correction if performed in a one-stage procedure.[31,32] Femtosecond thin-flap LASIK may allow for the advantage of treatment within the corneal graft limits and greater customization of flap parameters. Baraquet et al. performed consecutive femtosecond thin-flap LASIK on 11 consecutive eyes and found a mean preoperative astigmatism decrease from $-6.60 \pm 3.60$ D to $-2.90 \pm 2.00$ D 6 months after surgery.[33]

Although, the refractive results for LASIK after PK currently do not approach those in eyes without a history of PK, these promising results and further advances in femtosecond technology and ablation profiles will allow for greater precision and predictability of LASIK astigmatism correction after PK.

## LASIK COMPARED TO PHAKIC TORIC IMPLANTED COLLAMER LENS

As demonstrated throughout this chapter, a full-range of astigmatism can be managed well with LASIK corneal refractive surgery. Alternative treatment options continue to evolve, including phakic implantable and pseudophakic intraocular lenses.

Several studies have reported the benefits of toric lens implantation when compared to corneal refractive surgery.[34-37] In 2007, Schallhorn et al. compared 43 eyes implanted with toric implantable contact lens (toric ICL) and 45 eyes receiving PRK with mitomycin C for moderate to high myopia (−6.00 to −20.00 D) with moderate astigmatism (1.00 to 4.00 D). The authors concluded toric ICL had better performance for safety, efficacy, predictability and stability when compared to the PRK eyes.[36] Quality of vision has also been investigated after lens implantation compared to laser refractive surgery. Night driving (via a night driving stimulator) was found to be superior in toric ICL patients when compared to PRK patients with and without glare present.[37]

Toric lens implantation can also be used for eyes with irregular astigmatism with some success. Although there are currently no direct comparative studies between toric ICL and LASIK for treatment of irregular astigmatism, improvements in best-corrected and uncorrected visual acuity after toric ICL implantation have been reported in patients with dystrophic disease (pellucid marginal degeneration) and postkeratoplasty anisometropia and astigmatism.[38,39] These studies suggest toric lens implantation may become a viable option for the correction of a full-range of astigmatism as well.

## ❧ EXCIMER LASER OUTCOMES IN CORRECTION OF ASTIGMATISM

This chapter has outlined the advancements and outcomes of astigmatism correction using laser based refractive surgery, specifically LASIK. Outcomes of any surgical procedure rely on many factors including proper patient selection, preoperative testing accuracy, surgical technique and postoperative management. With regards to LASIK, preoperative parameters such as accurate manifest refractions, topographic imaging and wavefront testing are essential in correcting the full amount of refractive error. Special attention to flap/hinge creation, hydration of the stromal bed, centration of the ablation and avoidance of striae are paramount. Postoperative management of ocular surface disease, diffuse lamellar keratitis, epithelial in growth and flap irregularities further enhance outcomes.

When analyzing overall outcomes of excimer laser surgery for astigmatism correction, the United States FDA trials provide useful data in evaluating the current level of effectiveness. The FDA Ophthalmic Devices Panel targeted a goal of an effective mean reduction of absolute cylinder as 64% at a 1997 meeting.[40] For comparison purposes, aggregate data from the FDA trials using newer laser technologies (WaveLight Allegreto, LADARVision 4000, VISX Star S4, Technolas 217z Zyoptix) were compiled for the correction of myopic, hyperopic and mixed astigmatism. A reduction in 66% of absolute cylinder was achieved with these newer laser platforms (Table 2).

As reported in aforementioned studies, higher levels of preoperative astigmatism resulted in a greater percentage reduction. Using vector analysis methods, the FDA studies demonstrate higher levels of astigmatism (> 3.0 D) are typically slightly undercorrected while the converse is true for lower levels of astigmatism (< 1.0 D); they are typically slightly overcorrected. Further analysis confirms the excellent accuracy of astigmatism correction. In a limited subset of patients (n = 411), over 92% of patients were within 1.00 D and over 67% were within 0.50 D of the targeted refractive goal.[40]

## ❧ CONCLUSION

Astigmatism is a common refractive error that can be a significant cause of decreased visual acuity and quality. LASIK refractive surgery is a well-established and proven technology for astigmatism correction. Further advances in excimer lasers, eye tracking technology, and wavefront and topographic-guided ablations are likely to enhance outcomes in the future.

**Table 2:** Effectiveness of excimer laser on cylindrical correction. Higher levels of preoperative cylinder resulted in a greater reduction of absolute cylinder

| Excimer Laser Reduction of Absolute Cylinder | |
| --- | --- |
| *Preoperative Cylinder* | *Percent Reduction* |
| All | 66.34756 |
| < 0.50 D | 53.3 |
| < 0.50 to < 1.00 D | 52.47365 |
| 1.00 to < 2.00 D | 69.61911 |
| 2.00 to < 3.00 D | 78.92474 |
| ≥ 3.00 D | 83.90645 |

# ❖ REFERENCES

1. Fledelius HC, Stubgaard M. Changes in refraction and corneal curvature during growth and adult life. A cross sectional study. Acta Ophthalmol (Copenh). 1986;64:487-91.

2. Cline D, Hofstetter HW, Griffin JR. Dictionary of Visual Sciences, 4th edition. Newton, MA: Butterworth-Heinemann; 1997.

3. Goggin M, Alpins N, Schmid L. Management of irregular astigmatism. Curr Opin Ophthalmol. 2000;11:260-6.

4. Trokel SL, Srinivason R, Braren B. Excimer laser surgery of the cornea. Am J Ophthalmol. 1983;96:710-5.

5. McDonnell PJ, Moreira H, Garbus J, et al. Photorefractive keratectomy to create toric ablations for correction of astigmatism. Arch Ophthalmol. 1991;109:1370-3.

6. Alio JL, Artola A, Ayala AJ, et al. Correcting simple myopic astigmatism with the excimer laser. J Cataract Refract Surg. 1995;21:512-5.

7. Dausch D, Klein R, Schroder E. Excimer laser photorefractive keratectomy for hyperopia. Refract Corneal Surg. 1993;9:20-8.

8. Argento CJ, Cosentino MJ, Biondini A. Treatment of Hyperopic Astigmatism. J Cataract Refract Surg. 1997;23:1480-90.

9. Varley GA, Huang D, Rapuano CJ, et al. LASIK for hyperopia, hyperopic astigmatism, and mixed astigmatism: a report by the American Academy of Ophthalmology. Ophthalmology. 2004;111(8):1604-17.

10. Campos M, Wang XW, Hertzog L, et al. Ablation rates and surface ultrastructure of 193 nm excimer laser keratectomies. Invest Ophthalmol Vis Sci. 1993;34(8):2493-500.

11. Schallhorn SC, Farjo AA, Huang D, et al. Wavefront-guided LASIK for the correction of primary myopia and astigmatism: a report by the American Academy of Ophthalmology. Ophthalmology. 2008;115(7):1249-61.

12. Miraftab M, Seyedian MA, Hashemi H. Wavefront-guided vs wavefront-optimized LASIK: a randomized clinical trial comparing contralateral eyes. J Refract Surg. 2011;4:245-50.

13. Stonecipher KG, Kezirian GM. Wavefront-optimized versus wavefront-guided LASIK for myopic astigmatism with the ALLEGRETTO WAVE: three-month results of a prospective FDA trial. J Refract Surg. 2008;4:S424-30.

14. Jankov MR, Panagopoulou SI, Tsiklis NS, et al. Topography-guided treatment of irregular astigmatism with the wavelight excimer laser. J Refract Surg. 2006;22(4):335-44.

15. Yoshida Y, Nakamura T, Hara S, et al. Topography-guided custom ablation for irregular corneal astigmatism using the NIDEK NAVEX Laser System. J Refract Surg. 2008;24(1):24-32.

16. Wang M. Irregular Astigmatism: Diagnosis and Treatment. Thorofare, NJ: Slack Inc.; 2008. pp. 274-5.

17. Alpins N, Stamatelatos G. Clinical outcomes of laser in situ keratomileusis using combined topography and refractive wavefront treatments for myopic astigmatism. J Cataract Refract Surg. 2008;34(8):1250-9.

18. Kim YJ, Sohn J, Tchah H, et al. Photoastigmatic refractive keratectomy in 168 eyes: 6 months results. J Cataract Refract Surg. 1994;20:387-91.

19. Smith EM, Talamo JH, Assil KK, et al. Comparison of astigmatic axis in the seated and supine positions. J Refract Corneal Surg. 1994;10:615-20.

20. Chernyak DA. Iris-based cyclotorsional image alignment method for wavefront registration. IEEE Trans Biomed Eng. 2005;52:2032-40.

21. Khalifa M, El-Kateb M, Shaheen MS. Iris registration in wavefront-guided LASIK to correct mixed astigmatism. J Refract Surg. 2009;35(3):433-7.

22. Prakash G, Agarwal A, Ashok Kumar D, et al. Comparison of laser in situ keratomileusis for myopic astigmatism without iris registration, with iris registration, and with iris registration-assisted dynamic rotational eye tracking. J Cataract Refract Surg. 2011;37(3):574-81.

23. Knorz M, Jendritza B. Topographically-guided laser in-situ keratomileusis to treat corneal irregularities. Ophthalmology. 2001;107:1138-43.

24. Toda I, Yamamoto T, Ito M, et al. Topography-guided ablation for treatment of patients with irregular astigmatism. J Refract Surg. 2007;23:118-25.

25. Reinstein DZ, Archer TJ, Gobbe M. Combined corneal topography and corneal wavefront data in the treatment of corneal irregularity and refractive error in LASIK or PRK using the Carl Zeiss Meditec MEL 80 and CRS-Master. J Refract Surg. 2009;25(6):503-15.

26. Alessio G, La Tegola M, Sborgia C. Topography-driven photorefractive keratectomy: results of corenal interactive programmed topographic ablation software. Ophthalmology. 2000;107:1578-87.

27. Kornmehl E, Steinert R, Puliafito C. A comparative study of masking fluids for excimer laser phototherapeutic keratectomy. Arch Ophthalmol. 1991;109:860-3.

28. Kremer F, Aronsky M, Bowyer B, et al. Treatment of corneal surface irregularities using Biomask as an adjunct to excimer laser phototherapeutic keratectomy. Cornea. 2002;21:28-32.

29. Olson RJ, Pingree M, Ridges R, et al. Penetrating keratoplasty for keratoconus: a long-term review of results and complications. J Cataract Refract Surg. 2000;26(7):987-91.

30. Lee HS, Kim MS. Factors related to the correction of astigmatism by LASIK after penetrating keratoplasty. J Refract Surg. 2010;26(12):960-5.

31. Busin M, Zambianchi L, Garzione F, et al. Two-stage laser in situ keratomileusis to correct refractive errors after penetrating keratoplasty. J Refract Surg. 2003;19(3):301-8.

32. Kollias AN, Schaumberger MM, Kreutzer TC, et al. Two-step LASIK after penetrating keratoplasty. Clin Ophthalmol. 2009;3:581-6.

33. Barequet IS, Hirsh A, Levinger S. Femtosecond thin-flap LASIK for the correction of ametropia after penetrating keratoplasty. J Refract Surg. 2010;26(3):191-6.

34. Kamiya K, Shimizu K, Igarashi A, et al. Comparison of collamer toric implantable [corrected] contact lens implantation and wavefront-guided laser in situ keratomileusis for high myopic astigmatism. J Cataract Refract Surg. 2008;34(10):1687-93.

35. Sanders DR, Sanders ML. Comparison of the toric implantable collamer lens and custom ablation LASIK for myopic astigmatism. J Refract Surg. 2008;24(8):773-8.

36. Schallhorn S, Tanzer D, Sanders DR, et al. Randomized prospective comparison of visian toric implantable collamer lens and conventional photorefractive keratectomy for moderate to high myopic astigmatism. J Refract Surg. 2007; 23(9):853-67.

37. Schallhorn S, Tanzer D, Sanders DR, et al. Night driving simulation in a randomized prospective comparison of visian toric implantable collamer lens and conventional PRK for moderate to high myopic astigmatism. J Refract Surg. 2010;26(5):321-6.

38. Kamiya K, Shimizu K, Hikita F, et al. Posterior chamber toric phakic intraocular lens implantation for high myopic astigmatism in eyes with pellucid marginal degeneration. J Cataract Refract Surg. 2010;36(1):164-6.

39. Akcay L, Kaplan AT, Kandemir B, et al. Toric intraocular collamer lens for high myopic astigmatism after penetrating keratoplasty. J Cataract Refract Surg. 2009;35(12):2161-3.

40. Porter IW, Azar DT. A complete surgical guide for correcting astigmatism. In: Henderson BA, Gills JP (Eds). Thorofare, NJ: Slack Inc.; 2011. pp. 33-5.

# LASIK Combined with Other Procedures

*John B Cason*

## ♣ INTRODUCTION

Laser *in situ* keratomileusis (LASIK) remains today the most common and successful elective refractive procedure in the world. The vast majority of these procedures are performed in both eyes in a single session and without the need for any other combined procedures to achieve the desired refractive result. However, as the success of this procedure has grown, the desire to combine the optical capabilities of LASIK with other surgeries has developed as well.

By staging this procedure or performing it concurrently, synergistic vision results are possible. While vision results might be superior with a combined or sequential procedure there are more frequent complications which should be discussed in the informed consent process. Sometimes an enhancement for a prior refractive surgery is desired yet the original procedure is not desired or practical. LASIK is a great alternative at times due to the quick vision recovery and in some cases a more stable refractive result. Other times the desired result is not possible with one procedure alone and this can be planned from the beginning of the surgical planning process.

The purpose of this chapter is to discuss the combination procedures either by initial design or by necessity after a prior procedure. There are many times that LASIK can be used as a second procedure for enhancement. However, the enhancements for residual or refractive error would be best discussed in detail in its own right.

## ♣ ON-FLAP PHOTOREFRACTIVE KERATECTOMY

Photorefractive keratectomy (PRK) is an alternative refractive procedure during which the epithelium is removed by mechanical or laser and then the refractive treatment is performed. In general, PRK after LASIK is not considered a first line treatment. However, there are circumstances where LASIK has been performed and flap re-lift is not desired. For example, the amount of residual stroma bed may be close to 250 microns, the flap might not be stable, or the risk for epithelial ingrowth might be high with re-lift. Furthermore, this procedure has been performed successfully to treat anterior basement membrane dystrophy after LASIK surgery.[1]

Flap complications during LASIK are very problematic and frequently result in aborting the procedure, waiting for a period of stability, and then returning to the operating room. Buttonholes, incomplete flaps and thin flaps all create difficulties in achieving good vision with LASIK by itself. PRK adds a degree of safety by avoiding manipulation of the subpar flap.

Despite the favorable safety profile of PRK after LASIK, stroma haze prevention with mitomycin-C (MMC) must be considered. Haze is not uncommon after this combined procedure and can cause regression and decrease in best corrected vision.[2,3] Possibly, the stroma keratocytes are already activated by the flap creation and subsequent laser treatment induces an exaggerated healing response especially when the ablation depth is more than 40 microns or approximately two diopters of treatment.[4] It is controversial whether or not Laser assisted subepithelial keratectomy (LASEK) causes less haze than PRK and there have been no studies directly comparing conventional to wavefront-guided treatments.[4,5] However, in a retrospective study, Srinivasan et al. showed that there was very little significant haze during the healing process of on-flap PRK even with contact times of 30 seconds.[6]

One use of on-flap PRK is for the treatment of complications after LASIK. On-flap PRK has been showed to treat buttonhole complications with good uncorrected vision outcomes.[7,8] In cases of flap striae, Steinert et al. used PRK, removing approximately 10 microns without MMC, and did not encounter any significant haze during the postoperative healing period.[9] A published multicenter, multi-surgeon retrospective study showed that flap complications were safely and effectively treated with on-flap PRK with MMC and achieved 20/20 or better uncorrected vision results in 77% of patients. There was one patient that needed a retreatment for visually significant haze. However, that patient did not receive intraoperative MMC. During this study, many different epithelium removal techniques were used, including no-touch laser removal, mechanical scraping and alcohol assisted. There were also variable waiting intervals between the initial LASIK procedure and PRK.[8]

The wait time between LASIK and PRK is very important for the final visual outcome. Waiting a period of 3 months could allow enough time for the activated stromal keratocytes to downregulate and decrease the chances of stroma haze.[10] However, it is also possible in cases of potential visually significant scarring that the PRK procedure should be performed between 2 weeks and 3 months. During this time, the flap would stabilize but the scarring response would not have matured to the point that keratometry changes would occur.[7,8,11-13]

## ▶ PHAKIC INTRAOCULAR LENSES

Bioptics is a surgical technique first described by Zaldivar et al. that was useful in treating large amounts of refractive error that would not safely or adequately treated with phakic intraocular lens (PIOL) alone.[14] The philosophy behind this type of treatment is to treat the largest magnitude of the refractive error with the PIOL procedure. With a smaller amount of residual refractive error, less tissue is removed in the cornea which results in less chance of regression, residual refractive error, glare and halos. With a smaller correction there is more accuracy in the final outcome.

There are different types of phakic IOLs differentiated by where they are placed. Two options exist including in the ciliary sulcus just in front of the crystalline lens and in front of the iris in the anterior chamber and can be fixated in the iris or in the angle. Each has characteristics that are both favorable and problematic and must be considered.

In a retrospective study, LASIK and PRK were performed at least 6 weeks after PIOL insertion for treatment of residual refractive error. In this study, 91% of LASIK and 98% of PRK patients were within 1 diopter of emmetropia. However, LASIK was used to treat larger amounts of refractive error due to the fact MMC was not used.[15] In several other studies, approximately 80% of patients were within 0.5 D and almost all were within 1 D.[14-20]

Another consideration in bioptic treatments is whether or not the flap is created during the PIOL insertion or during the LASIK treatment. By creating the LASIK flap during the PIOL insertion, it is possible to allow keratometry stability prior to the LASIK treatment, especially if there are any aberrations created by the flap itself. In a prospective comparative series, 3–5 months wait time was used prior to LASIK treatment.[16]

Depending on the type of PIOL used, there might be variable amounts of endothelial cell loss. Variable reports show no statistically significant loss versus 4% in myopia and almost 11% in hyperopic treatments and iris-fixated lenses.[16-20] This cell loss is presumably due to the PIOL insertion itself or continued damage from the presence of the lens in such proximity to the endothelium. In one prospective trial, the endothelial cell loss was approximately 4% overall but there was no statistically significant difference in cell loss before and after the LASIK procedure which showed that the LASIK procedure itself is not a likely contributor to this process.[19]

## ▶ POSTERIOR CHAMBER INTRAOCULAR LENS

In combination with clear lens extraction and cataract surgery, LASIK has good success with achieving desirable uncorrected vision. This appears to be the case whether the surgeon plans the combination as a staged primary procedure or to retreat undesirable refractive error after lens extraction and intraocular lens implantation. Of note, most studies using this technique utilized at least a 3 months wait period between intraocular surgery and LASIK in order to achieve complete resolution of postoperative corneal edema and topography changes after the lens removal.

Postoperative uncorrected vision results have been comparable with native cornea LASIK.[21] Approximately 80–90% of patients achieve 20/40 or better vision and almost 50% are 20/20 or better.[21-24] However, many of these studies were conducted with older ablation profiles and these estimates could be conservative. The surgeon should keep in mind the very high vision expectations of elective surgery patients and weigh the desired correction with risks of intraocular surgery, including endophthalmitis, retinal detachment, macula edema and endothelial cell damage. For very high amounts of refractive error, these risks might be tolerable if the patient is highly motivated to achieve good unaided vision results.

When comparing PRK to LASIK after clear lens extraction, there appears to be no significant difference in vision results.[23] However, the data comparing these two modalities has been retrospective in nature and the refractive error between the two groups of patients has not been studied in an equivalent fashion.

Recently, the use of multifocal, zonal refractive, and accommodating intraocular lenses has pioneered the treatment of presbyopia and achieving good near vision for many lens extraction patients. This has extended mostly to cataract patients who have active lifestyles and desire near and distance vision correction simultaneously and do not wish to use spectacles for most if not all vision tasks. To achieve this goal, the reduction of as much of the refractive error as possible is critical considering that many multifocal patients that are not happy with their surgery are not happy with the residual refractive error present.[25-26]

Vision outcomes are very favorable after multifocal intraocular lens implantation and LASIK. Approximately, 90% of these patients are within 0.5 D of emmetropia and are reading J1 or better at near.[27-32] These results are more favorable than the monofocal lens results mentioned above and this is most likely due to the different technologies used in LASIK in the more recent studies performed for multifocal lenses. However, in one study, there was no difference between monofocal and multifocal lens LASIK treatments for myopia but there was a statistically significant difference in treating hyperopia in favor of the monofocal group.[32]

Considering there are multiple ablation profiles, the surgeon must decide which is most favorable for the lens technology and resulting optics. Topography guided, wavefront guided, wavefront optimized and conventional platforms form many of the choices from which to decide. It is not entirely clear which type of technology is best in combination with LASIK. In one prospective study, the zonal refractive and diffractive lens technologies after LASIK had good improvement in vision but higher order aberrations were not significantly changed. The authors postulated that the wavefront analyzers were unable to accurately measure the different optical characteristics of these lenses.[28]

When comparing PRK to LASIK, a retrospective review showed that there is not a statistical difference between outcomes between these two types of surgery.[29] Furthermore, LASIK can achieve a good vision outcome when performed on patients with a history of multifocal IOL implantation and simultaneous limbal relaxing incisions.[31]

## PENETRATING KERATOPLASTY

The most common methods to correct residual irregular astigmatism and refractive error after penetrating keratoplasty (PKP) are spectacles and contact lenses. Most frequently, the residual astigmatism is so irregular that the use of hard contact lens is preferable to soft contact lens. However, in some circumstances the patient is not able to tolerate any of these options due to significant graft-host mismatch, high astigmatism or lifestyle factors, and the use of LASIK can be very helpful in these situations. Most patients cannot tolerate anisometropia of greater than 3 D or astigmatism greater than 4 D.

The goal of refractive surgery in many of these cases is to get the refractive error within this range so that the patient can better tolerate other vision options rather than achieving emmetropia in most elective cases. The consensus opinion is to wait at least until the 12th postoperative month and at least 3 months after final suture removal.[33]

In general, LASIK can achieve very good results after PKP. Most patients are able to achieve refractive errors that are tolerable for glasses and hard contact lenses. In a prospective study performed by Donnenfeld et al. almost all patients had less than 3 D of anisometropia and 4 D of astigmatism.[34]

LASIK in these patients is well-tolerated. However, there is an increase in complications in comparison with LASIK in native corneas. Herpes simplex virus could reactivate as a result of the excimer laser. Most of the problems encountered are from flap creation. There is a high chance of epithelial ingrowth, flap dislocation, PKP wound dehiscence, and a possibility that the patient might need further enhancements or repeat PKP from either rejection or high astigmatism.[35] Some case reports exist showing that flap dislocation can result from corneal edema and that this can be more likely to occur in the first 1–2 years of PKP healing.[36] In cases of endothelial dysfunction, like pseudophakic bullous keratopathy, the presence of edema can cause a similar dislocation from poor adherence of the flap from abnormal hydrostatic forces.[37] Endothelial cell counts appear to be stable after LASIK and it is difficult to show if there is any increase in graft rejection.[34]

Data appears to support doing a two-stage procedure when performing LASIK after PKP. The creation of the flap may create changes in the cornea topography and some studies indicate that one should cut the flap and then wait for topographic stability before performing LASIK.[38-41] One study even reported that in some cases the patient did not require laser keratectomy after the flap creation had been performed. In some cases as much as 50% of the astigmatism was reduced by the flap creation alone.[39]

*Disclaimer*

The views expressed in this chapter are those of the author and do not necessarily reflect the official policy or position of the Department of the Navy, or Department of Defense, nor the US Government.

No financial interests to disclose.

## ▶ REFERENCES

1. Rojas MC, Manche EE. Phototherapeutic keratectomy for anterior basement membrane dystrophy after laser in situ keratomileusis. Arch Ophthalmol. 2002;120:722-7.

2. Carones F, Vigo L, Carones AV, et al. Evaluation of photorefractive keratectomy retreatments after regressed myopic laser in situ keratomileusis. Ophthalmology. 2001;108:1732-7.

3. Beerthuizen JJ, Siebelt E. Surface ablation after laser in situ keratomileusis: retreatment on the flap. J Cataract Refract Surg. 2007;33(8):1376-80.

4. Cagil N, Aydin B, Ozturk S, et al. Effectiveness of laser assisted subepithelial keratectomy to treat residual refractive errors after laser insitu keratomileusis. J Cataract Refract Surg. 2007;33(4):642-7.

5. Saeed A, O'Doherty M, O'Doherty J, et al. Laser assisted subepithelial keratectomy retreatment after laser in situ keratomileusis. J Cataract Refract Surg. 2008;34:1736-41.

6. Srinivasan S, Drake A, Herzig S. Photorefractive keratectomy with 0.02% mitomycin-C for treatment of residual refractive error after LASIK. J Refract Surg. 2008;24(1):S64-7.

7. Lane HA, Swale JA, Majmudar PA. Prophylactic use of mitomycin-C in the management of a buttonholed LASIK flap. J Cataract Refract Surg. 2003;29(2):390-2.

8. Weisenthal RW, Salz J, Sugar A, et al. Photorefractive keratectomy for treatment of flap complications in laser in situ keratomileusis. Cornea. 2003;22(5):399-404.

9. Steinert RF, Ashrafzadeh A, Hersh PS. Results of phototherapeutic keratectomy in the management of flap striae after LASIK. Ophthalmology. 2004;111(4):740-6.

10. Slade SG. LASIK complications. In: Machatt JJ (Ed). Excimer laser refractive surgery. Practice and principles. Thorofare, NJ: Slack, Inc. 1996:360-8.

11. Wilson SE. LASIK: management of common complications. Cornea. 1998;17(5):459-67.

12. Kapadia MS, Wilson SE. Transepithelial photorefractive keratectomy for treatment of thin flaps or caps after complicated laser in situ keratomileusis. Am J Ophthalmol. 1998;126(6):827-9.

13. Wilson SE. Transepithelial PRK/PTK for treatment of donut-shaped flaps in LASIK. Refract Surg Outlook. 2001;1-4.

14. Zaldivar R, Davidorf JM, Oscherow S, et al. Combined posterior chamber phakic intraocular lens and laser in situ keratomileusis: bioptics for extreme myopia. J Refract Surg. 1999;15(3):299-308.

15. Arne JL, Lesueur LC, Hulin HH. Photorefractive keratectomy or laser in situ keratomileusis for residual refractive error after phakic intraocular lens implantation. J Cataract Refract Surg. 2003;29:1167-73.

16. Guell JL, Vazquez M, Gris O. Adjustable refractive surgery: 6 mm artisan lens plus laser in situ keratomileusis for the correction of high myopia. Ophthalmology. 2001;108:945-52.

17. Perez-Santonja JJ, Bueno JL, Zato MA. Surgical correction of high myopia in phakic eyes with Worst-Fechner myopia intraocular lenses. J Refract Surg. 1997;13:268-81.

18. Meltendorf C, Cichocki M, Khonen T. Laser in situ keratomileusis following the implantation of iris-fixated phakic intraocular lenses. Ophtalmologica. 2008;222(2):69-73.

19. Munoz G, Alió JL, Montés-Micó R, et al. Angle supported phakic intraocular lenses followed by laser in situ keratomileusis for the correction of high myopia. Am J Ophthalmol. 2003;136:490-9.

20. Munoz, Alió JL, Montés-Micó R, et al. Artisan iris claw phakic intraocular lens followed by laser in situ keratomileusis for high hyperopia. J Cataract Refract Surg. 2005;31:308-17.

21. Kim P, Briganti EM, Sutton GL, et al. Laser insitu keratomileusis for refractive error after cataract surgery. J Cataract Refract Surg. 2005;31:979-86.

22. Avala MJ, Pérez-Santonja JJ, Artola A, et al. Laser insitu keratomileusis to correct residual myopia after cataract surgery. J Refract Surg. 2001;17(1):12-6.

23. Pop M, Payette Y, Amyot M. Clear lens extraction with intraocular lens followed by photorefractive keratectomy or laser in situ keratomileusis. Ophthalmology. 2001;108:104-11.

24. Velarde JI, Anton PG, deValentin-Gamazo L. Intraocular lens implantation and laser in situ keratomileusis (bioptics) to correct high myopia and hyperopia with astigmatism. J Refract Surg. 2001;17(2):S234-7.

25. Devries NE, Webers CA, Touwslager WR, et al. Dissatisfaction after implantation of multifocal intraocular lenses. J Cataract Refract Surg. 2011;37(5):859-65.

26. Woodward MA, Randleman JB, Stulting RD. Dissatisfaction after multifocal intraocular lens implantation. J Cataract Refract Surg. 2009;35(6):992-7.

27. Alfonso JF, Fernández-Vega L, Montés-Micó R, et al. Femtosecond laser for residual refractive error correction after refractive lens exchange with multifocal intraocular lens implantation. Am J Ophthalmol. 2008;146:244-50.

28. Jendrizza BB, Knorz MC, Morton S. Wave-front guided excimer laser vision correction after multifocal IOL implantation. J Refract Surg. 2008;24(3):274-9.

29. Macsai MS, Fontes BM. Refractive enhancement following presbyopia-correcting intraocular lens implantation. Curr Opinion Ophthalmol. 2008;19(1):18-21.

30. Muftuoglu O, Prasher P, Chu C, et al. Laser in situ keratomileusis for residual refractive errors after apodized diffractive multifocal intraocular lens implantation. J Cataract Refract Surg. 2009;35(6):1063-71.

31. Muftuoglu O, Dao L, Cavanagh HD, et al. Limbal relaxing incisions at the time of apodized diffractive multifocal intraocular lens implantation to reduce astigmatism with or without subsequent laser in situ keratomileusis. J Cataract Refract Surg. 2010;36:456-64.

32. Pinero DR, Avala Espinosa MJ, Alio JL. LASIK outcomes following multifocal and monofocal intraocular lens implantation. J Refract Surg. 2010;26(8):569-77.

33. Kuryan J, Channa P. Refractive surgery after corneal transplant. Curr Opin Ophthalmol. 2010;21(4):259-64.

34. Donnenfeld ED, Kornstein HS, Amin A, et al. Laser in situ keratomileusis for correcting myopia and astigmatism after penetrating keratoplasty. Ophthalmology. 1999;106:1966-75.

35. Hardten DH, Chittcharus A, Lindstrom RL. Long term analysis of LASIK for the correction of refractive errors after penetrating keratoplasty. Cornea. 2004;23(5):479-89.

36. Chan CC, Rootman DS. Corneal lamellar flap retraction after LASIK following penetrating keratoplasty. Cornea. 2004;23(6):643-6.

37. Solomon R, Donnenfeld ED, Perry HD, et al. Post-LASIK corneal flap displacement following penetrating keratoplasty for bullous keratopathy. Cornea. 2005;24:874-8.

38. Busin, Zambianchi L, Garzione F, et al. Two stage laser in situ keratomileusis to correct refractive errors after penetrating keratoplasty. J Refract Surg. 2003;19(3):301-8.

39. Busin M, Arffa RC, Zambianchi L, et al. Effect of hinged lamellar keratotomy on postkeratoplasty eyes. Ophthalmology. 2001;108(10):1845-51.

40. Kollias, Schaumberger MM, Kreutzer TC, et al. Two step LASIK after penetrating keratoplasty. Clinical Ophthalmology. 2009;3:581-6.

41. Lee GA, Pérez-Santonja JJ, Maloof, et al. Effects of lamellar keratotomy on postkeratoplasty astigmatism. Br J Ophthalmol. 2003;87(4):432-5.

# Wavefront-Guided Custom LASIK and LASEK: Techniques and Outcomes

*John P Berdahl*

## ❧ INTRODUCTION

Over the last 20 years, refractive surgery has enjoyed tremendous technological advancements. One of the most exciting advancements has been the application of wavefront technology to guide and optimize refractive surgery treatments.[1-3] The goal of wavefront-guided LASIK and LASEK is to use additional measurements of aberrations within the optical system (beyond sphere and cylinder) to achieve a more optically perfect ablation.

Traditionally, refractive surgery was able to only treat lower order aberrations such as spherical error and astigmatism. By treating only lower order aberrations, conventional treatments have been unable to move us closer toward realizing 'ideal theoretical vision'. However, the ability to produce repeatable measurements of the higher order aberrations (HOAs)[4] has allowed surgeons and optical engineers to develop ablation profiles that are customized or optimized to a patient's individual optical system. These treatment profiles allow us to limit the induced HOAs, limit the visual quality complaints and loss of best-corrected visual acuity (BCVA) resulting from refractive surgery.

In this chapter, we will explore new techniques and surgical outcomes related to wavefront-guided technology.

## ❧ OPTICAL CONSIDERATIONS

### Visual Quality and Visual Acuity

The majority of a patient's 'blur' is dictated by the spherocylindrical refraction; however, a significant portion of image blur can also come from HOAs. Other less important sources of blur include diffraction and opacities.

It has been understood for a long time that the treatment of spherocylindrical refractions may not completely fix a patient's optical system. This is particularly true in cases of irregular astigmatism such as keratoconus. This understanding has brought objectivity to eye surgeons' long-held understanding that visual quality and visual acuity are two different things, and that 20/20 vision does not always equate with visual satisfaction. Even after a patient has a 20/20 correction and a manifest refraction of plano, the patient can experience bothersome issues with visual quality despite an excellent visual acuity. This dissonance between quality and acuity is one of the driving forces behind the rapid technological advancement of wavefront-guided refractive surgery.

### Limits of Vision: The Root Mean Square

The root mean square (RMS) is defined as a 'statistical measure of the magnitude of a varying quantity', and it is important to understand in relation to the theoretical limits of vision. The RMS is the square root of the mean of the square of any number of discrete values. In simplest terms, the RMS is a summation of the eye's aberrations, and it is typically measured at the micron level. Wavefront analysis now allows 0.05 micron measurements of the RMS deviation.

In the 1990s, Andrea Marechal determined that the human eye could measure aberrations to 0.07 microns of RMS. This corresponds to a visual acuity of 20/6. From this theoretical limit of vision, the idea of 'super vision' was born. Surgeons have debated whether or not the theoretical limit of 20/6 vision can actually be achieved clinically.

It has been demonstrated that the retina is actually the limiting factor and can produce a Snellen visual acuity of approximately 20/8. Since surgeons and patients enjoy seeing 20/15 or 20/10, surgeons have continued to push the limits of visual acuity. The visual cortex also contributes to the spatial resolution capable within the human eye, although the potential of the visual cortex has yet to be identified conclusively. Hence, the three factors in image quality are the optics of the eye, the retinal resolution, and the cortical processing that ultimately results in 'seeing' an image. Wavefront technology has begun to address the optical imperfections within the visual system, but cannot improve upon the retinal resolution and cortical processing.

## Basic Optics of Refractive Surgery

In the early days of refractive surgery of myopic photoablation with the excimer laser, wavefront analysis quickly became important. As surgeons flattened the center cornea, a more oblate profile of the cornea was created instead of a more physiologic prolate corneal shape. The oblate cornea induced an increase in HOAs that led to a decrease in the quality of vision for patients. The increase of HOAs led to the quick adoption of wavefront-guided and wavefront-optimized refractive surgery systems to improve visual quality.

Irregularities within the optically important zone of the cornea can lead to HOAs that can create symptomatic ghosting and image blur. The effects of these can be debilitating, even in the setting of fairly good visual acuity. Most HOAs cause a degradation of vision; however,

some HOAs (such as vertical coma) may correlate with better uncorrected visual acuity (UCVA) or can lead to an increased depth of focus in a naturally multifocal cornea. Clinical trials have shown that correction of HOAs at the time of refractive surgery improves visual outcome, decreases the incidence of HOAs, improves visual quality and contrast sensitivity, and decreases night-time glare.[5-9]

## ➤ WAVEFRONT BASICS

### Premeasurement Considerations

In general, preoperative considerations for wavefront-guided treatment are similar to conventional LASIK.[10] The majority of HOAs are generated at the corneal surface. However, other areas (such as the posterior cornea, the lens, the tear film and other defects of the ocular media) can lead to HOAs as well. Therefore, when performing a refractive laser vision correction on the surface of the cornea, one must understand that nearly all of the HOAs from each of the different ocular media are incorporated into the wavefront profile, and ultimately the treatment of the eye.

It is also important to make sure that each patient has an adequate tear film when obtaining this data, since the tear film can be variable from moment to moment. Additionally, wavefront should be centered on the visual axis of the eye. If the patient is not properly looking at the wavefront source, HOAs can be induced.

A 'wavefront' is best understood as a planar wave of monochromatic light moving in a single direction (Figs 1A and B). As the planar wave of light enters the eye, it will be

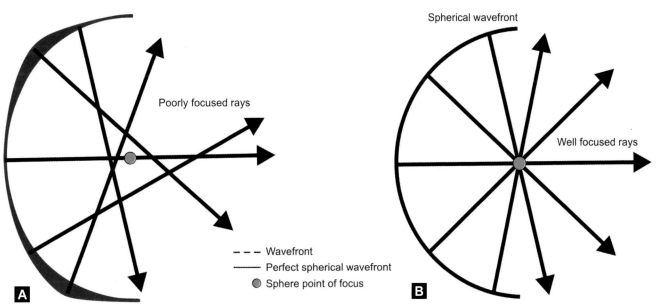

**Figs 1A and B:** Wavefront. (A) Poorly-focused rays; (B) Well-focused rays

curved by the converging power of the cornea and the lens. Any irregularities of the cornea, the lens, the ocular surface or the posterior cornea will cause HOAs to be presented.

As the path of light continues to make its way to the retina, the distance it travels can be determined by the time that it takes to reach the retina and bounce back to the wavefront sensor. Wavefront data can be referenced at the pupil or cornea plane. Regardless of where the data is measured, the surgeon must also consider the role of the pupil in the formation of images. A constricted pupil increases the depth of field of light and decreases the amount of contribution from the peripheral lens and cornea. Conversely, an increased pupil size decreases the depth of field and increases the contribution of the peripheral cornea and lens. A wavefront sensor is then used to detect and report these aberrations in a report called a waveform. Light scatter is not measured by a wavefront sensor, so a clean waveform does not indicate that a cataract or other sources of scatter are not present. It is important to note that pupil size will change the wavefront, which can result in a person having a different visual experience in a scotopic situation compared to a photopic one. With the use of multiple devices (such as topography), the corneal contribution of the wavefront can be determined separately from other portions of the wavefront, which is helpful for planning a treatment.

## Wavefront Acquisition

Typically, a patient is seen in the office and a wavefront measurement is obtained in the setting of an undilated pupil with adequate lubrication. It is important to note that the position of the eyelids, inadequate fixation, tearing, dryness and opacities may prevent an adequate wavefront image from being obtained. Sensors can help to determine the quality of the wavefront image, and it is possible to look directly at this Hartmann-Shack image to ensure there is no dropout of information. Once a satisfactory wavefront is obtained, it should be compared to the manifest reaction and topography of the patient's eye. This will help to ensure that the measurements corroborate and one can be more confident that the appropriate treatment profile has been chosen.

Interestingly, in patients with small amounts of astigmatism, the different wavefront profiles can have widely varying axes of astigmatism. However, when one looks at the actual ablation profile, the profiles look quite similar. This can reinforce that the appropriate wavefront measurement has been chosen.

Patients with very early cataracts or approaching the age where cataracts begin to develop may have significant contributions to their waveform from the cataract. Because of this, wavefront-guided treatments may be preferable in patients who may have an impending cataract.

## Wavefront Aberrometry

Phoropters have traditionally measured at the 0.25 diopter level. Keratometers and topographers measure at the same level. However, excimer lasers can ablate tissue to the level of 0.25 microns. Since our ability to customize the corneal surface exceeded our ability to measure the refractive state of the eye, excimer laser companies had strong motivation to improve the ability to measure the refractive state of the eye more accurately and hence measure the HOAs.

Five types of wavefront analysis were developed, including Hartmann-Shack aberrometers, ray tracing aberrometers, Tscherning aberrometers, dynamic spatial skiascopy and holographic imaging. Each has its own unique nuance, but they all generally produce similar wavefronts of the optical state of the eye.

Patients are usually bothered by 0.4 microns RMS, but can detect a change from their previous refractive state of 0.2 microns RMS. Lou Catania, OD has beautifully outlined this as a clinical awareness threshold of greater than or equal to 0.4 microns RMS and a clinical differential threshold of greater than 0.2 microns RMS. This becomes incredibly important as a patient undergoes laser vision correction, because induced HOAs have a tendency to bother patients more than HOAs that are already present in the optical system.

As the FDA began to approve wavefront-guided custom ablation, it was found that visual acuity and visual quality were improved significantly. Wavefront-guided treatments were not able to consistently correct HOAs, but they were found to induce less HOAs than conventional treatments. This is important because patients are more sensitive to induced HOAs than previously existing HOAs. The underlying reason why HOAs cannot be corrected is because of the dynamic state of the ocular surface. Not only is the tear film constantly changing, but the squamous epithelial cells present on the surface of the cornea change as well. These cells have a minimal size of 5 microns at which they retain their refractive characteristics. Since excimer lasers can ablate to 0.25 microns, but because of the turnover of the tear film and the squamous epithelium the wavefront can change. Epithelial hyperplasia also occurs after refractive surgery, which can change the HOA profile.

## Wavefront Images and Measurements

A Hartmann-Shack image is the most typical way that the wavefront sensor collects images. A wavefront is projected into the eye and goes through the ocular media on the way to the retina. This information bounces off the retina and is observed by a grid of photosensitive microcameras. This is the raw data that generates the actionable waveform. After creating this image, complex mathematical algorithms can be used to separate the image into separate waveform functions.

## ▶ INTERPRETING WAVEFRONTS

### Zernike Coefficients and Other Methods of Analysis

The most common way to analyze this data is with Zernike coefficients. Figure 2 with the Zernike method, each coefficient measures a different optical aberration. Lower order aberrations (like piston tip and tilt) are typically not included. The important lower order aberrations which are measured include sphere and cylinder. HOAs such as vertical coma, horizontal coma, trefoil, quadrafoil and others have much more bearing on the optical quality. The Zernike method essentially deconstructs the complete waveform into multiple individual waveforms which are simpler than the whole waveform and can be more easily identified. In theory, the

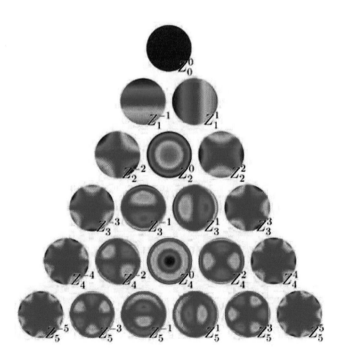

**Fig. 2:** Zernike coefficient tree

HOA profile can be deconstructed into an infinite number of coefficients that can perfectly describe the wavefront. However, Zernike coefficients are not able to fully represent nonradially symmetric irregularities, so the Zernike approach is not ideal in every situation.

### Coma

In cases involving coma (Fig. 3), patients often state that they see double or shadows, or that their vision is just not clear despite being able to see at the 20/15 level or better. Coma can be represented by vertical coma or horizontal coma and in some cases oblique coma. Typically, these patients have more than 0.4 microns RMS. The wavefront of coma typically shows a bimodal pattern of two opposite powers distributed symmetrically in the pupil. Understandably, coma can produce a secondary image because of the two different foci present in the bimodal pattern. Mild coma may represent small aberrations coming from the media or from the cornea or the Crystalens; however, larger amounts of coma typically are caused by abnormalities to the corneal surface.

### Trefoil

Trefoil (Fig. 4) is another common third-order aberration that is typically associated with scotopic vision. Smaller pupils have a tendency to reduce or eliminate trefoil because it often originates in the peripheral cornea. Under mesopic conditions, a peripheral cornea contributes more to the wavefront and the patient often experiences streaking or tails from a point source of light. Trefoil typically manifested shows a radial symmetry of the wavefront with a trimodal distribution showing three distinct areas that typically have a radial symmetry. These three foci of aberration result in streaks of vision. Again, patients with 0.3–0.4 microns RMS can experience more trefoil. Trefoil can be related to the microkeratome path in LASIK, changes in the crystalline lens or corneal distortions, or limbal relaxing incisions.

### Spherical Aberration

Spherical aberrations (Fig. 5) are fourth order HOA and very common. Typically, patients with spherical aberrations see halos around lights at night time. Patients also see halos around letters in the Snellen chart. Spherical aberration always is symmetrical in nature so tails or streaks are typically not present. Spherical aberrations are represented in a wavefront by a very symmetrical increase in the wavefront from central to peripheral. The point spread function looks like concentric rings. Positive spherical aberration can

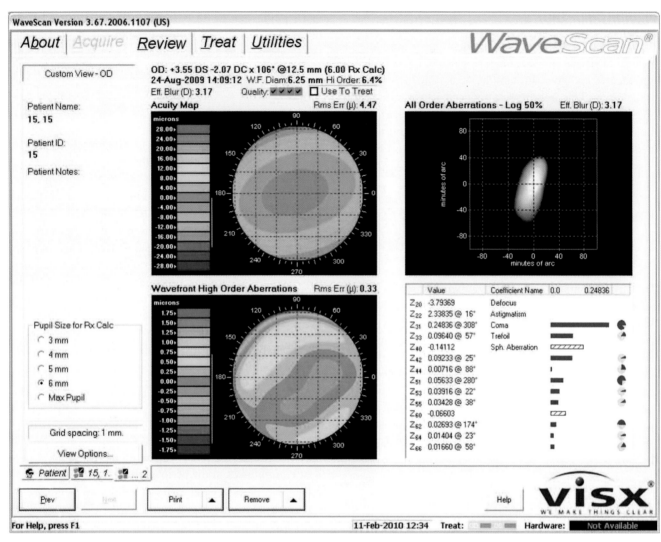

**Fig. 3:** Wavefront of coma
*Source:* Image courtesy of AMO

improve near vision at the expense of distance vision quality. Combining a small pupil with positive spherical aberration can improve peoples' near vision in a quite pleasing way. Spherical aberration is typically caused by changes in the crystalline lens or the peripheral cornea in dilated pupils.

Further work is being performed to investigate whether Fourier analysis using either Fourier transforms or Fourier sequences may provide a way to fully represent a waveform with fully deconstructed individual mathematical models.[11]

Devices such as the Optical Quality Analysis System (OQAS) (Visionmetrics, Terrassa, Spain) and the iTrace Visual Function Analyzer (Tracey Technologies, Houston Texas) can use these waveforms to create point-spread functions that describe the visual effects of these HOAs. They can also produce a Snellen chart that can simulate the blur that a patient experiences.

## Point Spread Function

Zernike polynomials provide the mathematical and theoretical underpinning for wavefront analysis; however, the point spread function gives the surgeon and the patient a visual understanding of the optical aberrations within a system. Often times after showing a patient a point spread function they will say, 'that is exactly what I see!' In an aberration-free system, a point source of light would have no spreading. Once aberrations are induced, that light is

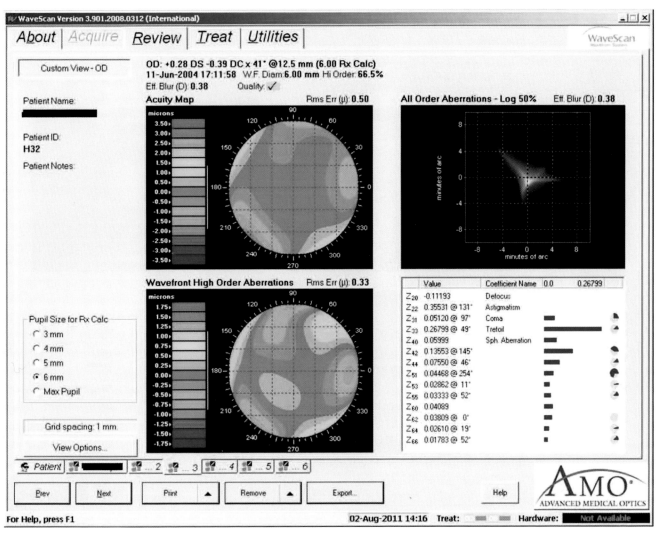

**Fig. 4:** Wavefront of trefoil
*Source:* Image courtesy of AMO

refracted and becomes distorted, creating a new image pattern. The point spread function helps the surgeon visually see what the patient is trying to describe.

## Wavefront with Iris Registration

Iris registration is often used in conjunction with custom wavefront technology in order to ensure that the wavefront is superimposed on the cornea properly. Since the eye can experience torsional rotation of up to 15–20° upon lying supine, iris registration identifies iris landmarks and rotates the treatment accordingly. Studies have shown that iris registration software in conjunction with wavefront-guided technology may help achieve better visual and refractive outcomes in LASIK treatments.[12,13]

## Special Cases

Higher order aberrations such as negative spherical aberration or large amounts of coma may be a sign that underlying irregularities of the cornea should be investigated further. This could be due to conditions such as corneal scarring, keratoconus or prior surgery.

## Flap Creation

Wavefront-guided treatments and measurements can also be affected by the technology used to create the flap during LASIK. The creation of the LASIK flap alone can modify the eye's optical characteristics in lower order aberrations and HOAs. Studies have shown that eyes receiving flaps

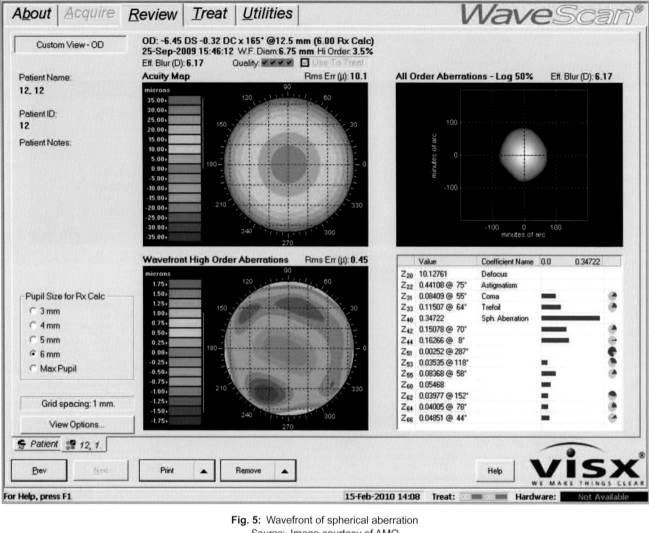

**Fig. 5:** Wavefront of spherical aberration
*Source*: Image courtesy of AMO

made using a microkeratome see an increase in HOAs post-operatively, while eyes with flaps made with a femto laser see less increase.[14,15] Because wavefront-guided LASIK treatments use measurements made preoperatively, flap technology may factor into the efficacy of the wavefront measurements.

Custom wavefront-guided treatment has been in practice now for a number of years and has continued to improve. Data has shown that wavefront-guided and wavefront-optimized treatments produce excellent visual quality, visual acuity and patient satisfaction.

The custom aspect of wavefront treatment takes a wavefront image of the patient's optical system and then creates an individualized laser ablation pattern to compensate for the HOAs that are uniquely present in each eye. These treatments can require more tissue consumption while attempting to offer a more customized outcome.

## Custom Wavefront as Enhancement

Custom wavefront-guided treatments can also be used as enhancements to attempt to improve image quality in patients who have had previous custom treatments or conventional treatments. Enhancements are dependent on discovering any visual difficulty the patient may be experiencing despite their improved visual acuity. Studies have indicated that wavefront-guided LASIK appears to be better than conventional LASIK for treating residual refractive errors.[16] A significant reason for this is that wavefront-guided LASIK does not increase HOAs and does not modify contrast sensitivity.[17] The improvements in optical measurement we receive through wavefront-sensing technology and wavefront-guided treatments have allowed us to identify and treat these problems of optical quality consistently during enhancements.

## ⟩ CONCLUSION

Wavefront analysis is continuing to mature, and has greatly improved in the past 5 years. Zernike polynomials have been very helpful in deconstructing wavefront images and improving our ability to treat HOAs. Future analysis of Fourier transforms may improve our sophistication further.

Wavefront maps need to be interpreted carefully and should fit well with other data, including the manifest reaction, corneal topography and the clinical exam.

As wavefront technology continues to improve, visual outcomes for our patients continue to improve as well. As we progress, the quality of the ablation profile will no longer be the limiting factor in the quality of our patients' vision. Other factors, such as dryness, lenticular changes and retinal resolution, and cortical image processing will ultimately be the factors that limit a patient's vision.

## ⟩ REFERENCES

1. Schallhorn SC, Farjo AA, Huang D, et al. Wavefront-guided LASIK for the correction of primary myopia and astigmatism: a report by the American Academy of Ophthalmology. Ophthalmology. 2008;115(7):1249-61.

2. Nuijts RM, Nabar VA, Hament WJ, et al. Wavefront- guided versus standard laser in situ keratomileusis to correct low to moderate myopia. J Cataract Refract Surg. 2002;28:1907-13.

3. Phusitphoykai N, Tungsiripat T, Siriboonkoom J, et al. Comparison of conventional versus wavefront-guided laser in situ keratomileusis in the same patient. J Refract Surg. 2003;19:S217-20.

4. Liang J, Grimm B, Goelz S, et al. Objective measurement of wave aberrations of the human eye with the use of a Hartmann-Shack wave-front sensor. J Opt Soc Am A Opt Image Sci Vis. 1994;11(7):1949-57.

5. Alio JL, Pinero D, Muftuoglu O. Corneal wavefront-guided retreatments for significant night vision symptoms after myopic laser refractive surgery. Am J Ophthalmol. 2008;145(1):65-74.

6. Durrie DS, Stahl J. Randomized comparison of custom laser in situ keratomileusis with the Alcon CustomCornea and the Bausch & Lomb Zyoptix systems: one-month results. J Refract Surg. 2004;20:S614-8.

7. Kim TI, Yang SJ, Tchah H. Bilateral comparison of wavefront-guided versus conventional laser in situ keratomileusis with Bausch and Lomb Zyoptix. J Refract Surg. 2004;20:432-8.

8. Slade S. Contralateral comparison of Alcon CustomCornea and VISX CustomVue wavefront-guided laser in situ keratomileusis: one-month results. J Refract Surg. 2004;20:S601-5.

9. Pop M, Payette Y. Correlation of wavefront data and corneal asphericity with contrast sensitivity after laser in situ keratomileusis for myopia. J Refract Surg. 2004;20:S678-84.

10. Sugar A, Rapuano CJ, Culbertson WW, et al. Laser in situ keratomileusis for myopia and astigmatism: safety and efficacy: a report by the American Academy of Ophthalmology. Ophthalmology. 2002;109:175-87.

11. Wang L, Chernyak D, Yeh D, et al. Fitting behaviors of Fourier transform and Zernike polynomials. J Cataract Refract Surg. 2007;33:999-1004.

12. Ghosh S, Couper TA, Lamoureux E, et al. Evaluation of iris recognition system for wavefront-guided laser in situ keratomileusis for myopic astigmatism. J Cataract Refract Surg. 2008;34(2):215-21.

13. Kohnen T, Kuhne C, Cichocki M, et al. Cyclorotation of the eye in wavefront-guided LASIK using a static eyetracker with iris recognition. Ophthalmologe. 2007;104(1):60-5.

14. Tran DB, Sarayba MA, Bor Z, et al. Randomized prospective clinical study comparing induced aberrations with IntraLase and Hansatome flap creation in fellow eyes: potential impact on wavefront-guided laser in situ keratomileusis. J Cataract Refract Surg. 2005;31(1):97-105.

15. Durrie DS, Kezirian GM. Femtosecond laser versus mechanical keratome flaps in wavefront-guided laser in situ keratomileusis: prospective contralateral eye study. J Cataract Refract Surg. 2005;31(1):120-6.

16. Alio JL, Montes-Mico R. Wavefront-guided versus standard LASIK enhancement for residual refractive errors. Ophthalomology. 2006;113(2):191-7.

17. Lee HK, Choe CM, Ma KT, et al. Measurement of contrast sensitivity and glare under mesopic and photopic conditions following wavefront-guided and conventional LASIK surgery. J Refract Surg. 2006;22(7):647-55.

# LASIK Complications

*Mark E Whitten*

## ❧ INTRODUCTION

In considering a format for this chapter, the author has called upon his experience in performing more than 100,000 original LASIK procedures and countless LASIK second procedures ('enhancements'). With a normal complication rate of about 1/4,000, he should have statistically gained first hand knowledge regarding most of the complications mentioned herein (and he has). The following are his personal thoughts, along with knowledge gained over the past 20 years in various refractive procedures. This chapter should be considered as his opinion based on that experience and nothing more.

## ❧ LASIK PREOPERATIVE COMPLICATIONS

Avoiding complications in LASIK surgery may be impossible but developing a risk avoidance system of green, yellow and red light preferences along with a good history and physical exam may help. Particular attention in history should be paid to a family history of corneal disease such as Fuchs' dystrophy and keratoconus.

### Red Light

Patients with medical diseases such as active autoimmune, uncontrolled diabetes and unstable prescriptions are examples of red lights and should be avoided.[1,2] Large prescriptions are also suspect patients. Large myopes that reduce residual stromal beds (RSB) less than 300 microns are to be avoided. Large hyperopic corrections over 4 diopters risk unusual healing and loss of best-corrected vision. Correcting large amounts of astigmatism can lead to higher

order aberrations and unhappy outcomes.[3] Severe dry eyes preoperatively need aggressive treatment and should be resolved before considering LASIK.

### Yellow Light

There are many items to consider in the yellow light category of possibly good candidates for LASIK. Poor outcomes in family members should require a pristine eye exam and topographical analysis to proceed. Keloids are a relative contraindication in photorefractive keratectomy (PRK) but rarely lead to any problems with LASIK. Controlled autoimmune diseases and diabetes with otherwise good general wound healing should lead to good outcomes with LASIK, but the patient should be informed that the opposite is possible but unlikely.

Patients who have had previous radial keratotomy (RK) present unique challenges. RK incisions need to be well healed without gaping or epithelial ingrowth to survive flap formation in LASIK. Corneal topography should demonstrate a normal posterior float. Those patients that are steep posteriorly in the area of the incisions will show irregular flap healing and unstable prescriptions after LASIK along with the possibility of inducing ectasia in this already weakened eye (Fig. 1). PRK in RK patients is a good option but scarring is possible and mitomycin is required to reduce that occurrence.

Age is a relative contraindication since there is no good history of exactly when keratoconus presents in previously normal patients. Most surgeons believe that a normal topography and leaving a RSB greater than 300 microns ensures strong corneas in these young patients. The possibility of

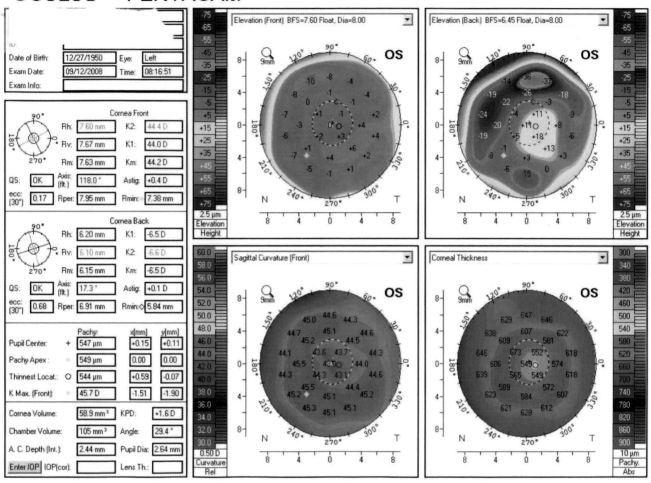

**Fig. 1:** Pentacam posterior elevation Pre-LASIK OS Noncandidate

refractive change should be discussed in young patients. A year of preoperative stability is a requirement but there are numerous examples of young patients exhibiting surprising refractive change over the years.

Amblyopic patients need special consideration, as those with 20/40 or worse visions are essentially one-eyed individuals. As such, an unexpected event could leave them with loss of best-corrected vision in their only useful eye. Special needs and informed consent might make this patient a reasonable LASIK candidate.

Pupil size should lead to a detailed discussion with each patient.[4,5] In reality, there should be a discussion of postoperative glare, halo and aberrations with all patients. Whether or not this is in any way related to pupil size, spherical aberration and coma do occur after LASIK. The simple act of asking patients to assess their preoperative aberrations

leads to fewer postoperative concern since modern software lessens the possibility of induced aberrations.

Presbyopic patients deserve special consideration since the inability to read after a certain age is a relatively foreign concept. Demonstrating eventual reading ability and the eventual need for reading glasses at a future age will avoid postoperative complications of expectations.

LASIK can be problematic in patients whose activities are related to constant physical trauma such as kickboxing or martial arts. There are many patients who do well after physical trauma including vehicular accidents, military service, police and firefighter service. Proper informed consent makes this a yellow light.

Glaucoma is a relative contraindication. PRK might require months of postoperative steroid use so these patients need to be proven as nonsteroid responders if PRK is anticipated. Use of steroids in LASIK is generally limited and makes LASIK a better option here. Timing of pressure induced during flap creation with LASIK should be measured, and visual fields preoperative and 3 months postoperative should demonstrate no loss of visual field from LASIK.

Patients with filtering blebs make poor candidates for LASIK or PRK.

A large percentage of LASIK patients have some symptoms of dry eyes.[6-8] Producing flaps in LASIK seems to temporarily produce dry eye symptoms in many patients, especially those exhibiting preoperative dryness. Aggressive dry eye therapy should occur to reduce postoperative complications. Use of tears, plugs, Restasis and the like are necessary and the relief of symptoms should be documented before surgery is undertaken.

Corneal scars are important to manage in flap formation to avoid problems. Femtosecond lasers that produce flaps need to be able to penetrate the relatively clear corneal surface to the desired depth. An opaque corneal scar should lead to a discussion of microkeratome use or PRK as an alternative.

Providing informed consent to patients is important to highlight issues and avoid one of the most important LASIK complications, unrealized expectations. Surgeons should spend time reviewing with patients one of the many generally published informed consents. Give special emphasis to those findings in the history and eye exam that appear to be outside of the average for the population or that might increase risk, producing a yellow light rather than a green light approach. This includes, but is not limited to, discussions on machine malfunctions, degree of prescription, pupil size, present symptoms of glare and halo, pachymetry and RSB, topographic findings, risk of enhancement, infection, inflammation, and ectasia.

Basement membrane dystrophy or map dot fingerprint corneal dystrophy could be a yellow light for LASIK.[9] In many cases of this dystrophy; epithelial cells are poorly attached to Bowman's membrane. In producing the flap, microkeratome movement across the cornea could disrupt these cells. Femtosecond laser flaps make this disruption much less likely. Doing an adhesion test of the cells preoperatively, helps make an informed decision. PRK is always a reasonable option in these patients. Lifting these flaps for enhancement can be problematic as these cells seemingly have a more difficult time healing the lifted flap edge and epithelial in growth has an increased incidence over the general population (Fig. 2).

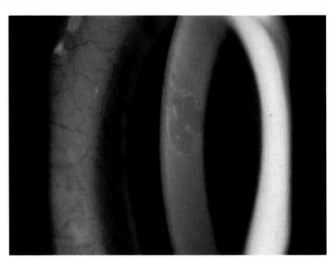

**Fig. 2:** Basement membrane dystrophy

A simple discussion of fainting during medical procedures can help avoid major complications during surgery. Once it is known that fainting has occurred in the past while giving blood or during dental procedures, it allows the surgeon to anticipate this issue and give extra preoperative antianxiety medications and elevate the legs during surgery to allow more blood flow to the head. The surprise of a patient fainting and the many sequelae of the event are enough to make you never forget to ask again.

## Green Light

Once you have decided that you have a green light patient or you have turned the yellow into an acceptable green, it is vital that the eye exam support your decision to avoid complications before they are allowed to happen. Short-cuts never work. Complete cycloplegic refractions avoid surprises and unwanted, complicated results. In having a pre-printed examination form, the surgeon is forced to be complete in the examination of the patient. This form can prompt you to place special emphasis on disorders such as basement membrane dystrophy and scarring. Doing adhesion tests of the corneal epithelium limits postoperative problems. Tests for strabismus, pupil size and unexpected internal eye issues such as cataract, glaucoma or retinal issues, limits unwanted surprises.

Corneal thickness and topography are vital issues. Preoperative determination of postoperative RSB thickness is necessary. Modern topographical analysis is necessary to assess both surface and posterior corneal shapes to determine how each patient relates to the normal population. There are different types of topographers, but viewing of the posterior cornea is a vital predictor of good results.[10] Surgeons have their preferences of various machines but a normal topographic shape avoids unexpected ectasia. Besides the shape and thickness, it is important to note a displaced apex of thinnest cornea and bilaterality of any corneal issues as you combine this knowledge with the age of the patient and the family history, attempting to find a green light patient.

Wavefront analysis in patients complaining of preoperative aberrations can document those symptoms and move the surgeon towards a wavefront guided procedure, if warranted. Routine wavescans can demonstrate patients who already have a higher level of aberrations. They may not be complaining of them but the small amount of induced aberrations from the procedure might be enough to make them notice. A discussion of these findings will avoid unreasonable expectations.

With a green light for LASIK, unwanted results should approach less than 1%. Unexpected complications can occur after the most perfect of LASIK procedures but with proper informed consent, patients can understand risk. Reasonable patients upon being told that the results are excellent in greater than 99%, not 100%, will respond: 'Of course, nothing in life is perfect or guaranteed.' This is when you know that you have done your best to obtain informed consent.

## ⊁ LASIK OPERATIVE COMPLICATIONS

### Use of Machines

Part of avoiding complications involves a basic and sometimes detailed understanding of all machinery used in the LASIK surgery process. Become familiar with how to test femtosecond, excimer and microkeratome technology. By being an active participant with your technicians, you can help avoid unusual machine-based occurrences and help with simple repairs and workarounds when necessary. Be aware of daily energy outputs, line and spot separation, plus x-axis and y-axis offsets. Watch tracking to be certain it is centered.

### Excimer Laser

Know your laser(s).The most common lasers in use are the AMO VISX and the Alcon Wavelight Allegretto. The VISX is generally used as a wavefront-guided excimer laser whereas the Wavelight commonly ablates as a wavefront-optimized laser. Both perform well.

Complications with the excimer laser usually revolve around induced aberrations, errors in tracking, poor refractive results and unrealized expectations. No matter which laser you use, become familiar with the daily testing performed at the beginning of the day. Know your laser is firing optimally and that your tracker is working correctly.

Wavefront-guided versus wavefront-optimized ablations is generally a theoretical, not a clinical issue. All lasers induce aberrations but modern software with extra peripheral shots reduces spherical aberration in both wavefront-guided and optimized lasers. Rarely patients will complain of unusual night vision and, if aberrations are confirmed by wavefront analysis, wavefront guided ablation can reduce the complication of increased glare and halo.[11] Surgeon specific nomograms are vital in improving outcomes, limiting second procedures and reducing postoperative complaints.

### Flap Makers

#### *Microkeratome[12-15]*

Know your device. If it is autoclaved between uses, be certain to inspect before each use. Check that the autoclave is functioning appropriately. If it is a disposable device, continue the habit of inspection before each use. Microkeratomes are well known for issues such as:

- Caps
- Suction loss
- Buttonholes
- Epithelial disruption
- Globe penetration (rare)

Caps occur when the steepness or flatness of a cornea has not been matched correctly to the settings on the microkeratome that stops the unit in time to avoid a full cap rather than a flap with a hinge. Each unit has a unique nomogram and the surgeon, rather than the technician, should be responsible for the correct settings for each patient's corneal topography.

That being said, caps can be easily handled when they occur and not delay the treatment with the excimer laser. Many surgeons mark the corneas before beginning surgery with three lines that are skewed so that alignment is eased and it is impossible to replace the cornea in any way other than epithelial side up. In general, if a cap occurs, it is usually found within the microkeratome. As with any other complication, it is important to slow the process and take the time to view the cap under the microscope as it has come through the microkeratome. This simple act allows you to see the epithelial side of the flap that always faces you. By holding the microkeratome as you did during the procedure, you can tell which way to reorient the flap even if you did not mark the cornea preoperatively.

If excimer ablation occurs quickly, you can remove the flap afterwards. Otherwise, remove the flap and place epithelial side down in the fornix to avoid stromal edema. If no markings occurred preoperatively, use a marking pen to now mark where the hinge should have occurred. After excimer ablation, replace the flap and take extra time to be certain it fits exactly appropriately with marks aligned or the gutters equal surrounding the cap edges (Fig. 3). Use a Weck-Cell sponge to be certain the cap is not movable. Some surgeons place a bandage contact lens over the cap while others tape the lid shut lightly overnight. If it occurs on the first eye, it may be prudent to cancel the second eye until it is certain that this first eye does well (which it usually does). The only thing worse than one cap is two. If the cap is replaced in the incorrect place, induced corneal astigmatism can easily occur. Once stability is reached, PRK with mitomycin is the best choice for treatment.

Suction loss during the procedure is similar in its treatment as a full cap except that excimer treatment might not be possible if the loss happens at any time other than the very end of the run of the microkeratome.[9] Obtaining a good visual outcome in these cases can be problematic due to scarring and epithelial ingrowth, which can occur in the visual axis as a result of the loss of suction as the blade was passing through area of the visual axis. If there is no epithelial ingrowth and a stable preoperative visual acuity

is obtained, PRK with mitomycin is an acceptable answer. Loss of best-corrected visual acuity (BSCVA) will require much more effort. If scarring has occurred leading to loss of BSCVA, an attempt should be made to use Phototherapeutic Keratectomy (PTK) to smooth the scar (with mitomycin). Once BSCVA has been achieved, PRK with mitomycin can achieve an excellent result. Removing epithelial ingrowth can be difficult because of the large incidence of regrowth of cells with a flap edge that was problematic from the beginning. Attempts should be continued until patient/surgeon exhaustion. As a last resort, removing the flap piece with mitomycin, can allow for re-epithelialization and minimal scarring. Obviously, all these procedures should be approached with complete informed consent and in some instances, second opinions.

Buttonholes are a known complication of some microkeratome devices (Fig. 4).[16,17] The single most important act here is not to ever lift the flap. Examining each flap with a wet Weck-Cell after they are produced, will allow the surgeon to spot this complication. By stopping the procedure without lifting, a normal PRK/mitomycin procedure can occur once stable BSCVA is reached. If the flap is lifted, you return to the treatment possibilities outlined above with suction loss (buttonholes are a type of suction loss). Due to the standard deviation of thickness of microkeratome flaps, pachymetry within the bed is appropriate to be certain that RSB will be appropriate.

Epithelial disruption can occur as the microkeratome moves across the epithelial surface. This can be seen as loss of epithelium or piling up epithelial cells without loss. In many instances using a canula or curved typing forceps will

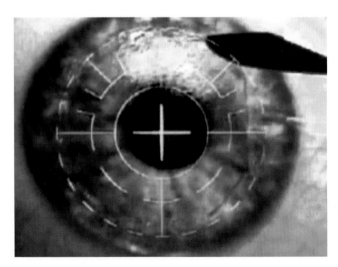

**Fig. 3:** Gutter

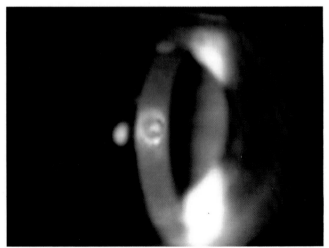

**Fig. 4:** Buttonhole

allow these heaps of cells to fall back into place. In either case, the use of a bandage contact lens at the end of the case will facilitate healing. Whenever the epithelium is insulted in this way, unusual inflammation may occur and should be monitored for extra care and treatment.

## Femtosecond Laser Flaps

Femtosecond lasers are not without their complications. In general, the flap thickness here has a much tighter deviation than the microkeratome, but it is reasonable to prove that occasionally by performing pachymetric measurements. Suction loss is a common problem here. With the IntraLase, it is important to reuse the same cone and redo the ablation at the same depth to affect a good flap. If suction loss occurs before the side cut but the full bed has been ablated, the instrument can be set for side cut only when the same cone is reapplied. It is best to make the side cut slightly deeper and smaller in diameter than originally planned to be certain that all the side cut is within the ablated area (Figs 5A and B).

Breakthrough of the gas producing the flap into the epithelium does not allow the procedure to continue.[18] It is a rare occurrence but should be treated with a bandage contact lens until healing had occurred. Once stable BSCVA has been achieved, PRK/mitomycin with PTK for epithelial removal is perhaps the best choice.

Flaps that are difficult to open could require manufacturer technical review of the laser and spot verification of efficacy. Reducing spot and line separation may help as well as varying of spot energy. Finding the correct balance of energy and spot and line separation for easy lifting versus postoperative inflammation is a tightrope to walk. Too much laser energy might not be apparent for weeks when a seemingly happy patient returns with a painful eye that appears normal. Extra steroid drops here for invisible flap inflammation will cure the problem and a review of your laser settings will be appropriate for the future.

Opaque bubble layer (OBL) occurs commonly as gases produced during the flap making cannot escape through the pocket or canal. These bubbles coalesce and are generally driven deeper within the stroma than the bed. After minutes or hours, these bubbles will dissipate but since these areas usually are not within the visual axis, they can be dispersed with a Weck-Cell sponge if it is necessary to achieve pupil tracking. If pupil tracking cannot be achieved, it is best to replace the flap and have the patient wait for resolution, which generally happens relatively quickly.

In small eyes, the gas bubbles from the femtosecond laser flap can enter the anterior chamber.[19] There are usually multiple bubbles and using the eye tracker on the excimer laser then becomes problematic. It may be necessary to cancel the case and have the patient return the next day when the bubbles have resolved.

Flap lifting seems obvious but there should be a plan. With microkeratomes, once the flap is made, it is free to easily lift. After determining there are no untoward events in the flap production, a spatula may be used, entering beneath the flap opposite the hinge and moving to the hinge lifting and folding the hinge as a taco with the epithelial side up.

Lifting femtosecond flaps is dissimilar to microkeratome flaps in that these flaps are not fully formed until dissected. Using a Sinskey type hook to open the flap edges allows a

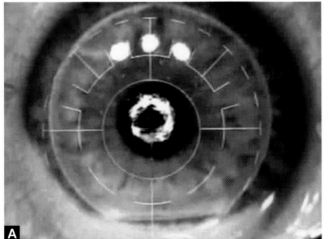 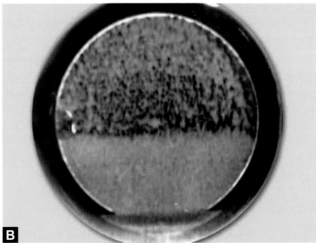

**Figs 5A and B:** Femtosecond flap(s)

spatula to more easily dissect the flap starting at the hinge area and progressing to the opposite edge. Once again 'tacoing' the flap allows the flap to act as a cover to protect the stroma of the flap from laser energy.

Tearing the flap during these maneuvers can be an unforced error. Patient movement could exacerbate this. Limiting this complication comes with positioning the hands on the forehead so that hand movement follows head movement. This gives the surgeon valuable time to remove the instrument with unexpected head movement. Continual downward pressure keeps the spatula on the stromal bed and away from the flap.

Handling the complication of flap tears has everything to do with the position of the tear. If outside the visual axis, it is reasonable to proceed with excimer ablation. If within the visual axis, the case should be aborted, proceeding with PRK/mitomycin with stable and BSCVA obtained.

## ▶ LASIK POSTOPERATIVE COMPLICATIONS

### Overcorrection/Undercorrection[20,21]

It is important to develop an individualized surgeon specific nomogram to achieve better results. If necessary, retreat after stabilization, generally 1–3 months postoperatively. Retreat by either lifting the existing flap or with PRK/mitomycin. In choosing the amount to be corrected, be careful if the original ablation has resulted in an overcorrection. Generally, less treatment than anticipated is required in these cases with much less required when the original prescription was high.

PRK on top of already existing flaps requires mitomycin to reduce the possibility of scarring.[22] In these and most cases, the mitomycin should be left in place for at least 15 seconds before rinsed with copious amounts of BSS solution. Flaps may be lifted at almost anytime postoperatively. However, the longer out from the original procedure, the greater the chance the edges of the flap will not seal as quickly as originally, allowing surface epithelia cells to track beneath the flap. There also seems to be a difference between microkeratome and femtosecond flaps as the occurrence of epithelial ingrowth. Probably due to their more vertical flap edges, femtosecond flaps have less occurrence of epigrowth than microkeratome.

### Epithelial (Epi) Ingrowth[16,9,23]

Almost always seen after lifting a flap for a secondary procedure, epigrowth is generally noted 1–3 weeks post enhancement. If flaps are lifted, a different postoperative

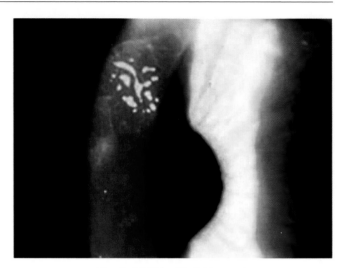

**Fig. 6:** LASIK epithelial ingrowth

appointment schedule should take this fact into account. Epi-ingrowth does not absolutely require removal from beneath the flap (Fig. 6). The decision should be made based on the patient symptoms of pain or photophobia, flap edge melting or reduced visual outcome.

### Epithelial Ingrowth Cell Removal[16,9]

Once the decision is made to remove cells, the flap is lifted with a spatula and a blunt instrument is used to remove all cells visualized from both the stromal bed and flap stroma. It is then important to smooth the flap and spend extra time being certain the flap edges 'stick' down to the stromal bed to attempt to discourage a reappearance of epi-ingrowth. Some surgeons will remove epithelium surrounding the flap edge to allow the flap time to seal down before epithelium challenges the wound edge while others will place a bandage contact lens to force the flap down. These all seem reasonable alternatives without a well-designed study to demonstrate efficacy. Reoccurrence of cells requires suturing the flap down with a running 9-0 or 10-0 nylon suture, leaving it in place for 3–4 weeks. Properly performed, this technique can eliminate cells in the most stubborn of cases (Fig. 7).

### Foreign Bodies Beneath Flaps

Occasionally, a foreign body of some type can become lodged beneath a flap after LASIK and not seen immediately postoperatively.[24] Removing the foreign body is absolutely necessary if it compromises the flap edge, providing a 'wick' for the elements to invade beneath the flap. If the flap edge is sealed well and the foreign body is not eliciting

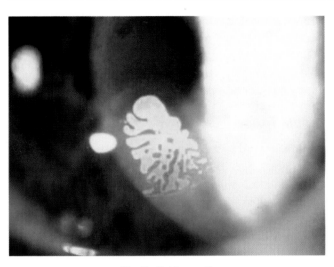

**Fig. 7:** Epi-ingrowth

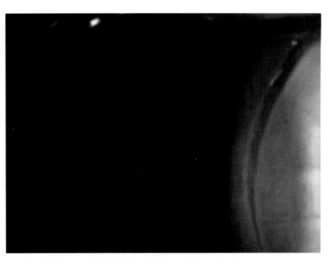

**Fig. 8:** Exposed gutter slipped flap

any symptoms, it may be left in place, unless it is obvious that it harbors bacteria or will become a future visual issue.

## Dislodged Flap[16,9]

Postoperative flaps that have moved enough to expose the gutter and/or demonstrate obvious macrostriae of the flap, need correction. In these cases, the surgeon needs to lift the flap to remove any epi-ingrowth before replacing and smoothing the flap. Depending on the length of time left untreated, it may be difficult to smoothly replace these flaps without much time and effort, constantly smoothing these flaps mainly because these striae may actually be present within the stroma of the flap. In many cases, the surgeon may not see the entire effect of smoothing for 24 hours, but as long as the flap has been replaced, providing the gutter to be closed, a good result can be anticipated (Fig. 8).

## Microstriae[9,25]

Seeing microstriations with the flap challenges the surgeon to determine first whether treatment is even necessary. These are commonly seen after large ablations when the flap attempts to rest back within a stromal bed that has been extensively altered. Visual acuity is the key to the decision making process. If the patient has achieved their uncorrected best visual acuity, these microstriae may be ignored. If the patient realized a difference between the microstriae eye and their other 'normal' eye, then they should be removed. If unanticipated astigmatism in the refraction corrects the visual acuity and coincides with striae, they should be removed. Peripheral striae may cause visual disturbance as much as central flap microstriae (Fig. 9).

### Treatment of Microstriae[9]

One day postoperative, microstriae can be easily handled by smoothing the area of the striae with a Weck-Cell sponge or curved tying forceps without lifting the flap. Leaving the flap down allows the surgeon counter traction to smooth the flap, and since the gutter is not compromised, epi-ingrowth is not a concern. After the first day postoperatively or even the first day, some surgeons prefer to remove the epithelium in the area of the striae and smooth them. Since microstriae are generally present at the level of Bowman's membrane, it makes reasonable sense to break the adhesion between epithelium and Bowman's membrane. This technique allows the surgeon to watch the striae smooth immediately. Breaking the epithelial layer can lead to inflammation and lamellar keratitis that might require intensive steroid treat-

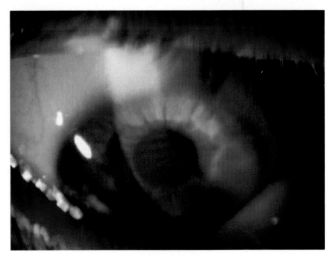

**Fig. 9:** Striae

ment as discussed below. Microstriae left untreated for weeks to months may require flap suturing/stretching. 9-0 or 10-0 nylon should be used as individual or running sutures to stretch the flap continuously, not just in the area of the striae. For those surgeons not used to handling a free flap for suturing, a reasonable technique can employ lifting a few millimeters of the flap before tightening the sutures and observing induced edge striae. A bandage contact lens should be left in place until the epithelium has covered the sutures. The sutures should be left in place approximately a month (Figs 10A and B).

## Postoperative Inflammation[26]

Inflammation is a common complication of LASIK surgery. No one knows with certainty the evolution of this process, but common sense dictates that laser energy or even autoclaved surgical tools can add to an already complicated healing process.

The inflammation can be as simple as a few whitish inflammatory cells seen superiorly beneath the flap. This can respond easily to an increased dosage of steroid drops. Left untreated or in spite of treatment, this inflammatory process can spread throughout the cornea, producing a diffuse lamellar keratitis (DLK) (Fig. 11). This requires a much more intensive steroid regimen including perhaps oral steroids. The timing of this inflammation is within the first week postoperatively and some surgeons believe that if the DLK is particularly intense during this time, with full corneal appearance and loss of visual acuity, rinsing beneath the flap with steroids is warranted. Care should be taken

here, as the stroma is particularly vulnerable and liquefied due to the inflammation. Rinsing could remove the stroma, producing a severe hyperopic shift. If caught early, intense topical/oral steroid therapy should eliminate the need for rinsing beneath the flap.

## Central Toxic Keratopathy[27]

This is a rare and severe form of postoperative inflammation that appears like DLK but doesn't respond appropriately to steroids. After initial use of major steroid therapy for Central toxic keratopathy (CTK), a hyperopic shift occurs and the stroma mysteriously thins. Care should be taken to stop steroid therapy immediately and observe the patient's stromal thickness and refraction. It may take many months for the condition to improve, but steroids do not improve this condition if unknown etiology.

## Pressure-Induced Stromal Keratitis (PISK)[9,28]

Another rare occurrence is a late onset of DLK that is treated with steroids. The DLK responds to steroid treatment but the pressure in the eye increases, as the patient is also a 'steroid responder' with increased pressure in the classic sense. Since a postoperative LASIK patient has a thinner cornea, the surgeon may miss this increased pressure reading with the central tonometer. Off center corneal pressure readings through thicker cornea will demonstrate this increased intraocular pressure. The inflammation in this case increases with increased pressure. Reducing the pressure and removing the steroids will generally clear the cornea of inflammation.

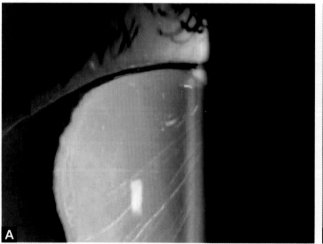 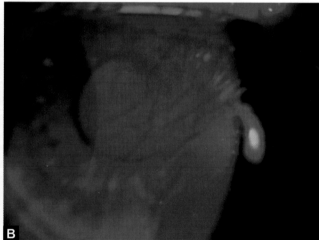

**Figs 10A and B:** Two photos of striae

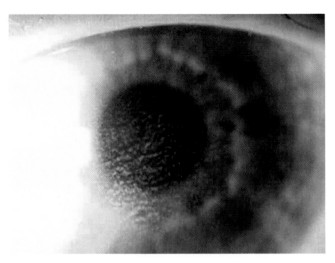

**Fig. 11:** Diffuse lamellar keratitis

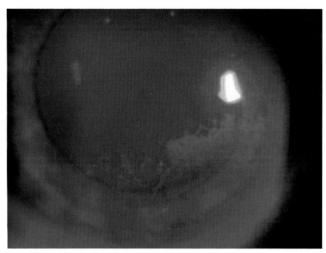

**Fig. 12:** Uncontrolled dry eye

## *Superficial Punctate Keratitis/Dry Eyes*[9]

A common complication of LASIK surgery occurs with increased dryness or poor lid closure. The process of producing a flap severs corneal nerves required in the feedback mechanism, allowing the brain to understand the dryness of the eyes and produce an appropriate amount of tears. Within 3 months, theses nerves have regenerated and normal tear production generally resumes. Producing thinner flaps seems to allow this process to resolve quicker. Managing preoperative dryness reduces this occurrence. Postoperative superficial punctate keratitis (SPK) is treated similarly to preoperatively, with intensive tear replacement drops, including punctual plugs and restasis to improve tear production. Use of steroids can relieve symptoms but corneal stromal loss can occur in dry eye patients with overuse of steroids (Fig. 12).

## Infection[9]

As with any surgical procedure, postoperative infection can occur. Use of preoperative antibiotic drops is commonplace but not proven to reduce the incidence of postoperative infections. Noting a fluffy white infiltrate beneath the flap requires the surgeon to make choices in treatment regimens. Many prefer to stop all antibiotics for a day; lift the flap and culture the exudate before resuming treatment in the hope that knowledge can be gained as to the true nature of the organism and which antibiotics will be most responsive. Depending on growth or no growth of organisms, fortified antibiotics should replace whichever drugs were being used when the infection occurred (Fig. 13).

## Glare/Halo[29,30]

Postoperative aberrations are induced with all LASIK procedures as the cornea is flattened or steepened inducing a small amount of spherical and coma aberrations.[31] Most patients do not notice this due to modern computer programming. In the rare instance of production of enough aberrations to result in permanent symptoms different from preoperative glare, halo or starburst, wave scan measurements should be taken to verify the problem and retreatment with a wavefront-guided ablation may help mitigate the issue.[32] Care must be taken not to overcorrect these patients since the computer program, in its desire to correct the aberration, will smooth the entire cornea to match the ablation needed to solve the problem. This can easily remove too much tissue

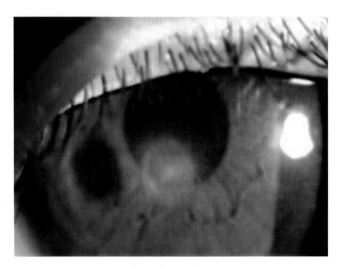

**Fig. 13:** Infection

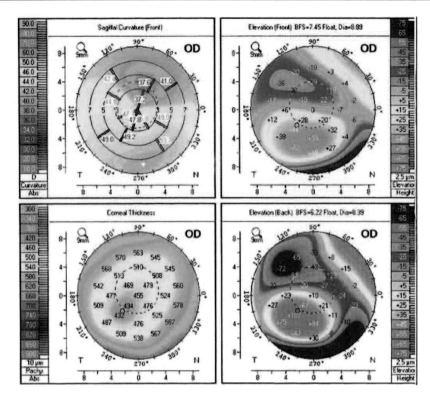

**Fig. 14:** Ectasia

and the surgeon should match the preoperative prescriptive error to the number of microns anticipated for removal.

## Ectasia[33,34]

Ectasia should be defined as an uncontrolled post-LASIK thinning and irregularity of the corneal stroma. Its treatment varies from rigid contact lenses to corneal cross-linking and strengthening to corneal transplantation. The options depend on its severity and patient desires, along with severity and relative stability of the cornea (Fig. 14).

Its etiology can be found in unrealized preoperative corneal disease or thin RSB, producing unstable, continually thinning corneas post-LASIK. Preoperative corneal topography is critical to making the diagnosis of disease. Especially critical is the posterior corneal shape, being certain there is limited deviation from expected normal shapes. Care should be taken in young patients with a family history of keratoconus. Surgeons and the Food and Drug Administration (FDA) have agreed that 250 microns of untouched cornea RSB should remain after LASIK surgery. Many surgeons stretch this number even higher since even the 250 micron number is an estimate of safety based on decades of experience and inadequate prospective analysis.

## ▶ REFERENCES

1. Cobo-Soriano R, Beltrán J, Baviera J. LASIK Outcomes in Patients with Underlying Systemic Contraindications: A Preliminary Study Clínica Baviera, Instituto Oftalmológico Europeo, Madrid, Spain. Ophthalmology. 2006;113(7):1118.
2. Cua IY, Pepose JS. Late corneal scarring after photorefractive keratectomy concurrent with development of systemic lupus erythematosus. J Refract Surg. 2002;18(6):750-2.
3. Urbano AP, Urbano I, Urbano AP. LASIK for compound myopic astigmatism. 18(3suppl):S406.
   Urbano AP, Nogueira MI, Goncalves D, et al. LASIK for hyperopia. 18(3suppl):S406.
   Pozniak S, Pozniak N. LASIK for myopia from −6.00 to−17.00 D with astigmatism. 18(3suppl):S401-2.
4. Schumer DJ. Pupil protocol: A prospective analysis of LASIK using varied treatment sizes based on dark-adapted pupil size. 2002;18(3suppl):S404-5.
5. Chan A, Manche EE. Effect of Preoperative Pupil Size on Quality of Vision after Wavefront-Guided LASIK. Ophthalmology. 2011;118(4):736-41.
6. Issa MK, El-Din S, Abdalla BH, et al. Evaluation of tear secretion after LASIK for myopia. 18(3suppl):S394.
7. Lenton L, Albietz J, McLennan SG. Ocular surface management improves LASIK outcomes. 18(3suppl):S397.
8. Kourenkov VV, Kashnikova OA, Maitchouk DY. Prevention of dry eye complications after photorefractive surgery. 18(3suppl): S396.

9. Rapuano CJ, Belin MW, Boxer-Wachler BS, et al. Refractive surgery. Basic and Clinical Science Course, Section 13. San Francisco CA. AAO. 2009-10.

10. Guarnieri FA, Guarnieri JC. Comparison of placido-based, rasterstereography, and slit-scan corneal topography systems. J Refract Surg. 2002;18(2):169-76.

11. Nagy ZZ, Palágyi-Deák I, Kelemen E, et al. Wavefront-guided photorefractive keratectomy for myopia and myopic astigmatism. J Refract Surg. 2002;18(5):S615-9.

12. Gailitis RP, Lagzdins M. Factors that affect corneal flap thickness with the Hansatome microkeratome. J Refract Surg. 2002; 18(4):439-43.

13. Hagege P. Flap buttonhole in LASIK with the Hansatome microkeratome. 18(3suppl):S393.

14. Shemesh G, Dotan G, Lipshitz I. Predictability of corneal flap thickness in laser in situ keratomileusis using three different microkeratomes. J Refract Surg. 2002;18(3suppl):S347-51.

15. Asano-Kato N, Toda I, Hori-Komai Y, et al. Risk factors for insufficient fixation of microkeratome during laser in situ keratomileusis. J Refract Surg. 2002;18(1):47-50.

16. Azar DT, Koch DD. LASIK: Fundamentals, surgical techniques, and complications. New York. Basel, Marcel Dekker, Inc. 2003.

17. Ambrosio R, Wilson SE. Complications of Laser in situ Keratomileusis: Etiology, Prevention, and Treatment. J Refract Surg. 2001;17:350-79.
Stulting RD, Carr JD, Thompson KP, et al. Complications of laser in situ keratomileusis for the correction of myopia. Ophthalmology. 1999;106:13-20.
Leung ATS, Rao, Cheng ACK, et al. Pathogenesis and management of laser in situ keratomileusis flap buttonhole. J Cataract Refract Surg. 2000;26:358-62.

18. Srinivasan S, Herzig S. Sub-epithelial gas breakthrough during femtosecond laser flap creation for LASIK. Br J Ophthalmol. 2007;91(10):1373.

19. Srinivasan S, Rootman DS. Anterior chamber gas bubble formation during femtosecond laser flap creation for LASIK. J Refract Surg. 2007;23(8):828-30.
Lifshitz T, Levy J, Klemperer I, et al. Anterior chamber gas bubbles after corneal flap creation with a femtosecond laser. J Cataract Refract Surg. 2005;31(11):2227-9.

20. Dedhia N. Outcomes of retreatment after LASIK for myopia and hyperopia. 18(3suppl):S391.

21. Ozdamar A, Sener B, Aras C, et al. Laser in situ keratomileusis after photorefractive keratectomy for myopic regression. J Cataract Refract Surg. 1998;24:1208-11.
Huang D, Stulting RD, Carr JD, et al. Multiple regression and vector analysis of Laser in situ keratomileusis for myopia and astigmatism. J Refract Surg. 1999;15(5):538-49.
Ditzen K, Handzel A, Pieger S. Laser in situ keratomileusis nomogram development. J Refract Surg. 1999;15(suppl): S197-S201.

22. Weisenthal RW, Salz J, Sugar A, et al. Photorefractive keratectomy for treatment of flap complications in laser in situ keratomileusis. Cornea. 2003;22(5):399-404.

23. Asano-Kato N, Toda I, Hori-Komai Y, et al. Epithelial ingrowth after laser in situ keratomileusis: clinical features and possible mechanisms. Am J Ophthalmol. 2002;134(6):801-7.

24. Hirst LW, Vandeleur KW. Laser in situ keratomileusis interface deposits. J Refract Surg. 1998;14(6):653-4.

25. Von Kulajta P, Stark WJ, O'Brien TP. Management of flap striae. Int Ophthalmol Clin. 2000;40(3):87-92.

26. Smith RJ, Maloney RK. Diffuse lamellar keratitis. A new syndrome in lamellar refractive surgery. Ophthalmology. 1998;105 (9):1721-6.
Hadden OB, McGhee CN, Morris AT, et al. Outbreak of diffuse lamellar keratitis caused by marking-pen toxicity. J Cataract Refract Surg. 2008;34(7):1121-4.

27. Moshirfar M, Hazin R, Khalifa YM. Central Toxic Keratopathy after LASIK surgery. Curr Opin Ophthalmol. 2010;21(4):274-9.
Sonmez B, Maloney RK. Central toxic keratopathy: description of a syndrome in laser refractive surgery. Am J Ophthalmol. 2007;143:420-7.
Hazin R, Daoud YJ, Khalifa YM. What is Central Toxic Keratopathy Syndrome if it is not Diffuse lamellar Keratitis Grade IV? Middle East Afr J Ophthalmol. 2010;17(1):60-2.
Moshirfar M, Madsen M, Wolsey D. Re: central toxic keratopathy: description of a syndrome in laser refractive surgery. Am J Ophthalmol. 2007;144(2):332.
Moshirfar M, Kurz C, Ghajarnia M. Contact lens-induced keratitis resembling central toxic keratopathy syndrome. Cornea. 2009;28(9):1077-80.

28. Hamilton DR, Manche EE, Rich LF, et al. Steroid induced glaucoma after laser in situ keratomileusis associated with interface fluid. Ophthalmology. 2002;109:659–65.

29. Kan-xing Z, Yan W, Ying J, et al. Comparison of wavefront aberrations induced by LASIK and PRK. 18(3suppl):S394.

30. Salz JJ. Wavefront-guided treatment for previous laser in situ keratomileusis and photorefractive keratectomy: Case reports. J Refract Surg. 2003;19(6):S697-S702.

31. Sarkisian KA, Petrov AA. Clinical experience with the customized low spherical aberration ablation profile for myopia. J Refract Surg. 2002;18(3suppl):S352-6.

32. McDonald M. Disabling ghosting after laser in situ keratomileusis. J Refract Surg. 2002;18(3):287-8.
Lawless MA. Disabling ghosting after laser in situ keratomileusis. J Refract Surg. 2002;18(3):288-9.
Hardten DR, Lombardo AJ. Disabling ghosting after laser in situ keratomileusis. J Refract Surg. 2002;18(3):289-90.

33. Rao SN, Epstein RJ. Early onset ectasia following laser in situ keratomileusis: Case report and literature review. J Refract Surg. 2002;18(2):177-84.

34. Geggel HS, Talley AR. Delayed onset keratectasia following in situ keratomileusis. J Cataract Refract Surg. 1999;25(4):582-6.
Lifshitz T, Levy J, Klemperer I, et al. Late bilateral keratectasia after LASIK in a low myopic patient. J Refract Surg. 2005;21(5): 494-6.

# CHAPTER 107

# Corneal Applications of Ultrashort Pulse Laser

*Mohamed Abou Shousha, Sonia H Yoo*

## ❧ INTRODUCTION

In 1959, Gordon Gould coined the acronym LASER. He recorded in his laboratory notebook under the heading 'Some rough calculations on the feasibility of a LASER: Light Amplification by Stimulated Emission of Radiation' how to construct a laser and what could be its future applications. He then took his notebook and notarized it in a neighborhood store.[1] He could foresee that his work will change the world and it truly did.[2] Now after five decades, we came to realize that if he had written 'Almost every aspect of our modern life' as the possible applications of laser, he would have been perfectly correct.

Ophthalmologists were one of the pioneers to use this spatially coherent beam of light for the benefit of their patients. Argon, krypton, carbon dioxide, neodymium-doped yttrium aluminum garnet (Nd:YAG), excimer laser and finally neodymium glass femtosecond (FS) laser systems all have been employed in the diagnosis and management of different ocular conditions.

Among all those laser systems, ultrashort pulse laser has proven to be a particularly powerful tool in corneal surgery. Its unique capability to photodisrupt tissue with minimal collateral damage has made it a promising tool to revolutionize corneal surgery, a surgery in which precision has a critical impact on outcomes. Ultrashort pulse laser has been successfully employed in laser *in situ* keratomileusis (LASIK) flap creation, penetrating keratoplasty (PK), anterior lamellar keratoplasty (ALK), endothelial keratoplasty (EK), astigmatic keratectomy (AK), intrastromal corneal ring segment (ICRS) placement and several other corneal surgeries.

## ❧ ULTRASHORT PULSE LASER TECHNOLOGY AND LASER-TISSUE INTERACTION

Laser-tissue interaction varies significantly depending on the properties of the laser as well as the target tissue. Laser parameters such as wavelength, pulse duration and energy, peak power and focusing conditions, determine the nature of the laser-tissue interaction whether being photocoagulation, photoablation or photodisruption (Table 1).

Photodisruption is essentially the use of high power ionizing laser pulses that is concentrated in space and time to create what is known as optical breakdown of tissue.

Photodisruption employs the ionization of the target tissue by dissociating electrons from their atoms creating a rapidly expanding cloud of free electrons and ionized molecules known as plasma. This plasma communicates its energy to the tissue, creating a shockwave and

**Table 1:** The nature of laser-tissue interaction can be roughly determined by laser-tissue exposure time[*,+]

| Laser-tissue Exposure Time | Nature of Laser-tissue Interaction |
|---|---|
| > 100 ms | Photochemical |
| ~ $10^{-5}$–1 s | Photothermal |
| ~ $10^{-9}$–$10^{-7}$ s | Photoablation |
| ~ $10^{-12}$–$10^{-8}$ s | Photomechanical |
| ~ $10^{-13}$–$10^{-10}$ s | Plasma-induced interaction |
| < $10^{-12}$ (ultrashort pulse) | Photodisruption |

*Niemz M. Laser Tissue Interactions. Berlin: Springer; 2007
+Plamann K, Aptel F, Arnold C, et al. Ultrashort pulse laser surgery of the cornea and the sclera. Journal of Optics. 2010;12:1-30

subsequently cavitation bubbles which is quickly resorbed to leave a very localized incision with minimal collateral thermal or mechanical effects.[3,4] Very high power is needed to achieve that kind of laser-tissue interaction. Given the fact that laser power is the energy delivered per unit time, high laser power can be achieved by either increasing the energy or decreasing the period of the laser pulse.[5] After the development of the Q-switching and the mode-locking methods, creation of very brief laser pulses in the subpicosecond range ($< 10^{-12}$ s) became possible and rendered the need to increase the energy unnecessary.[3,6] Those very brief pulses create powers in the tens of megawatts and cause extremely localized temperature rise greater than 10,000°C that photoionize the tissue and bring about photodisruption.

Neodymium-doped yttrium aluminum garnet laser pulses with nanoseconds duration was the first ophthalmic photodisruptor. This laser has become the gold standard in photodisruption of posterior capsule opacification postcataract surgery and iridotomies. However, it was demonstrated that those nanosecond laser pulses produce collateral damage of 100 μm. This rendered the Nd:YAG laser unsuitable for surgeries where more precision is needed such as corneal surgery.[7]

Early 1980s, subpicosecond lasers with pulse durations over the FS range ($10^{-15}$ seconds) were developed. Those new laser pulses were approximately ten thousand times shorter in duration than the nanosecond laser pulses and thus achieved a reduction in collateral tissue damage from 100 μm to only 1 μm.[8-10] They were first used in laboratories to perform microsurgery in cells and did not make it to ophthalmology until the development of diode-pumped solid state lasers in the mid-1990s that were compact enough to make its use outside laboratories feasible.[11,12] Ultrashort pulse laser, namely FS laser, was then ushered into the mainstream of corneal surgery by developing a computer-controlled optical delivery system that had an accuracy of up to 1 μm. This delivery system allowed for placement of FS laser spots with adjustable spot sizes and spacing side to side to create corneal lamellar cuts with unlimited options of geometrical shapes, configurations, depths and diameters.[8]

In 2000, the US Food and Drug Administration (FDA) approved the use of FS laser to perform lamellar corneal surgery and in 2001 the first commercially available FS laser was introduced to the market. It was as if the new millennium had brought with it a revolution in corneal surgery.

Normal human cornea neither absorbs nor scatters visible or near infrared light to any appreciable extent and this is the reason why ultrashort pulse laser systems are so successful in dissecting it with high precision. In opaque corneas, from scars or edema, where the structural arrangement of corneal collagen fibrils is altered, ultrashort pulse laser loses some of its sharpness as it experiences scattering and aberrations while traveling through those distorted lamellae. Similarly but to a lesser extent, when focused at the deep layers of the cornea, ultrashort pulse laser experiences scattering and thus tends to produce relatively inferior interfaces. Plamann et al.[4] have demonstrated that this limitation can be overcome by increasing the laser wavelength as longer wavelengths have the potential to improve penetration of laser and reduce light scattering. Nevertheless, laser machines that can emit those longer wavelengths are relatively complex and still only available in research laboratories. Overcoming this limitation will unlock several applications for ultrashort pulse laser, not only in corneal surgeries but in glaucoma surgeries as well. That is why the market is pushing in that direction and soon laser machines with those capabilities will be released to the market.

## ﹖ FEMTOSECOND LASER LASIK FLAP CREATION

In April 2005, a case of iris lacerations was featured on the cover of Journal of Cataract and Refractive Surgery and it was shocking to know that this was caused by a microkeratome that had cut into the patient's anterior chamber as it was cutting a LASIK flap.[13] Such a catastrophic complication for an elective surgery, regardless of how infrequent it is, was unacceptable. Complications of flap creation using modern microkeratomes are very infrequent, but with more than 1 million surgeries done per year in the United States alone,[14] infrequent complications of such an elective surgery becomes worrisome to patients and surgeons as well as public health authorities. This fact motivated the search for safer technologies that would minimize complications and improve safety and outcomes of LASIK.

A few years before that report, specifically in 2000, the FDA approved the use of FS laser to cut corneal lamellar flaps. This technology was looked at as an overly expensive technology to cut LASIK flaps. Nevertheless, the higher degree of safety and accuracy of FS laser motivated surgeons to adopt it and patients to ask for it and allowed its use to steadily grow to replace microkeratomes in more than one third of the market.[15]

The advantages of FS laser over microkeratomes include better control over flap creation where customization of the diameter, hinge and depth of the flap is more precise and independent of the corneal shape and curvature. This reduced the risk of flap complications such as free caps, buttonhole caps, epithelial abrasions, epithelial ingrowth, blade marks and irregular cuts.[16-18] The controlled fashion of creating LASIK flaps using FS laser have significantly decreased the risk of those complications.

Many of the serious flap complications that have been reported with microkeratomes, such as irregular flap or amputated half flaps have been attributed to loss of suction. With the use of FS laser, consequences were found to be significantly less severe. FS laser machines sense the loss of suction and consequently stop the laser before it cuts in an unintended fashion, unlike microkeratomes that would most probably continue cutting the cornea in a different and irregular plane.

Safety can be improved by improving predictability. The inadvertent creation of thicker LASIK flaps than what was intended and planned has been reported with microkeratomes and has been implicated in the etiology of post-LASIK ectasia. Given that fact, it is clear that creating more precise and predictable LASIK flaps using the FS laser has definitely improved the safety of LASIK; especially in cases with thin corneas or high refractive errors.[19]

Furthermore, the versatility of the FS laser allowed for creating theoretically safer flap configurations such as creating undermined LASIK flap side cuts. Those angulations of the flap edge are thought to improve flap stability and decrease risk of epithelial ingrowth. Moreover, as it has been shown that the FS laser creates stronger adhesion at the flap edge compared to microkeratome flaps, FS laser flaps have shown to be more resilient to trauma.

The shift from microkeratomes to FS laser in cutting LASIK flaps seems to have significantly improved LASIK in terms of safety; but in terms of visual outcomes the improvement was not as significant. Faster visual rehabilitation with less induction of higher order aberrations was reported.[17,20] Nevertheless, it has been shown that long-term visual outcomes of FS laser LASIK flaps were not statistically different from that of microkeratome LASIK flaps.[21]

Disadvantage of FS laser flap creation when compared to microkeratomes include longer operative time, increased cost, more postoperative inflammation in the form of diffuse lamellar keratitis (DLK), harder to lift flaps, granular

stromal bed, opaque bubble layer (OBL) interfering with treatment, vertical gas breakthrough, anterior chamber gas bubbles, transient light-sensitivity syndrome (TLSS) and rainbow glare.[15,22-24] As we have developed more knowledge of the causes of those complications, it became clear that they can be minimized by optimizing the laser technology. Creating a resection plane in the cornea using FS laser entails laying down laser spots side to side, each creating a cavitation bubble that separates the corneal collagen lamellae that results in a resection plane. In an attempt to minimize the operative time of the relatively slow first generation FS lasers, fewer but relatively higher energy laser spots were laid down in the cornea to create larger cavitation bubbles to resect the tissue between relatively distant spots. This high energy was incriminated as the cause of DLK, OBL, TLSS and rainbow glare.[24-26] The widely separated laser spots were obviously the cause of the harder to lift flaps and the granularity of the stromal bed. The advances in laser technology led to newer generation FS lasers with faster firing capabilities. These new fast machines were capable of placing more laser spots with less spacing in between without increasing the operative time and thus allowing delivery of lower energy to the cornea. This resulted in faster and sharper cutting machines that produced smoother interfaces, easier flap lifts and consequently better visual outcomes in addition to minimizing those complications that were attributed to high energy FS laser spots.[27]

Another advancement in the technology was the introduction of FS lasers that employ curved corneal applanators instead of the typically used flat applanators. The corneal lamellar cuts are made parallel to the applanating surface. Thus, applanating the cornea to a flat surface is the simplest optical solution to standardize the anterior surface of the cornea and create a planar flap. However, this employs a relatively high suction pressure and a consequent elevation of the intraocular pressure (IOP). Employing a curved applanator accommodates the anterior curvature of the cornea and causes less distortion to the globe with less induction of IOP elevation, allowing the patient to maintain fixation throughout the surgery and minimizing any theoretical risks on the patient's optic nerve.

In summary, the introduction of FS laser technology to LASIK flap creation has significantly improved the safety of one of the most common elective surgeries in the world. Complications of FS laser flap creation are significantly less serious compared to those reported for microkeratomes and are being addressed by the recent advancements of technology.

## ❖ PENETRATING KERATOPLASTY

In 1905, Eduard Zirm performed the first successful PK and since then PK has remained the gold standard for the management of full thickness corneal pathologies. PK is considered the most successful organ transplantation surgery with more than 100,000 surgeries performed worldwide every year. Nevertheless, this surgery has its complications that advancement in technology did not help to eliminate. Those complications include wound dehiscence, high postoperative regular and irregular astigmatism and delayed visual rehabilitation. PK entails fixing the donor corneal transplant to the graft using sutures and as after more than a century from the first PK we still place sutures, those same complications still exist. The introduction of the surgical microscope and the 10/0 monofilament sutures significantly decreased the severity of those complications but did not eliminate them. In another attempt to limit those complications, multilevel, stepped corneal trephination were suggested to improve tectonic wound stability and consequently decrease the need for high suture tension.[28] Busin et al.[29,30] using suction trephines and microkeratomes have shown that this technique induces less postoperative astigmatism and expedites visual recovery. However, the lacks of reducibility of configuration and depth of corneal

incisions as well as the technical difficulty have prevented this technique from gaining popularity among corneal surgeons.

The introduction of the FS laser to corneal surgery revived that concept. The ability of the FS laser to create highly reproducible accurate incisions was employed to create interlocking multileveled incision. Those incisions allowed for maximizing the surface area of the wound and improving the fit and stability of the graft-host junction.[8,31-33] Laboratory models demonstrated that multileveled FS laser incisions offer PK wounds that are sevenfold more biomechanically stable than the regular PK wound. More stable wounds means that less sutures with less tension are needed to secure them. This is translated to less astigmatism and earlier suture removal and faster visual rehabilitation. The versatility of FS laser incisions unlocked surgeons' imaginations to come up with multiple biomechanically stable wound configurations such as 'top-hat', 'mushroom', 'zig-zag' and 'Christmas tree' shapes[34] (Figs 1A to E).

Top-hat (inverted mushroom) wound configuration (Fig. 1B) was identified as the most mechanically stable wound configuration.[35] It involves transplanting a graft with a larger endothelial diameter and a smaller anterior diameter. The internal tamponade of the peripheral lamellar wound has shown to resist leakage up to seven

**107**
**CHAPTER**

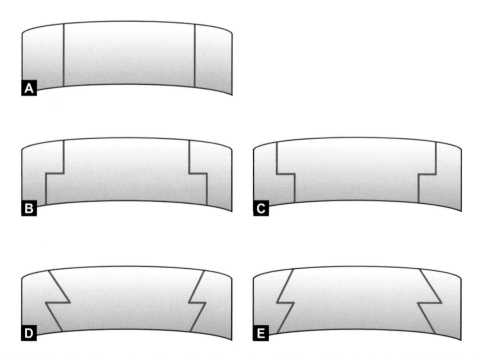

**Figs 1A to E:** Different incision configurations of Femtosecond-assisted penetrating keratoplasty. (A) Traditional incision; (B) Top-hat incision; (C) Mushroom incision; (D) Zig-zag incision; (E) Christmas tree incision

times better than a traditional PK wound thus allowing for early suture removal and visual rehabilitation.[36-38] Price et al.[39] have demonstrated faster healing and earlier suture removal in addition to substantial improvement in best spectacle-corrected visual acuity (BSCVA) when using FS laser top-hat PK. Another advantage of this configuration is that it provides the host with more endothelial cells and this potentially improves graft survival.[40]

Mushroom-shaped wound configuration (Fig. 1C) involves transplanting a graft with a larger anterior diameter and a smaller endothelial diameter. This wound configuration is recommended for cases with anterior corneal pathologies and intact endothelium such as keratoconus and corneal opacities. This configuration allows for placement of the sutures further from the center of the cornea, thus reducing the astigmatism acting on the optical zone without increasing the amount of resected host endothelium. The beveled wound configuration is biomechanically more stable as it takes advantage of the IOP to secure the wound. This allows for using less sutures with less tension as well as earlier removal of sutures that again leads to faster visual rehabilitation and less induced astigmatism.[41,42] However, it is noteworthy that it is technically difficult to include the posterior lip of the wound in sutures and that lip can eventually dehisce in the anterior chamber. This is a known limitation of this wound configuration that limits its use.

Another popular wound configuration that has proven its stability is the zig-zag wound configuration (Fig. 1D). It consists of posterior and anterior angled side cuts connected by a lamellar ring cut in the mid stroma created on the donor cornea with a corresponding interlocking wound configuration on the recipient cornea. This wound configuration has demonstrated more rapid recovery of BSCVA and less induction of surgical astigmatism compared to conventional PK.[43,44]

It is important to note that the significant decrease in the amount of astigmatism in FS laser assisted PK compared to traditional PK is present in the early postoperative period and that this becomes insignificant in the long run. Chamberlain et al. have demonstrated that despite the fact that the FS laser group had significantly less astigmatism initially, after the 6-month postoperative visit—the difference was no longer significant.[45] In other words, FS laser use helps earlier visual rehabilitation but not long-term visual outcomes.

This technology has proven its effectiveness; nevertheless, the high costs, additional operative time and logistic problems are disadvantages seriously affecting its

widespread use. FS laser machines, that lack portability, are usually present in LASIK suites. Consequently, FS laser assisted PK, in most surgical centers, entails cutting the donor and recipient corneas in a laser suite and transferring the patient to the operating room. In addition to being inconvenient and time consuming, it imposes the risk of premature wound rupture during patient transfer to the operating room. Leaving 50–100 μm of uncut gap in the FS posterior aspect of the lamellar cut would decrease the risk of those premature ruptures.[46,47] In conclusion, FS-PK allows for faster visual rehabilitation and improves safety; however, until portable FS machines become available, that technique may be slow to be adopted among surgeons.

## ❧ ANTERIOR LAMELLAR KERATOPLASTY

Anterior lamellar keratoplasty is indicated in cases with anterior corneal pathology and healthy endothelium. Selective transplantation of the diseased anterior layers of the cornea while preserving Descemet's membrane and endothelium will avoid the unnecessary replacement of patient's healthy endothelium with an antigenic and usually older donor endothelium. This dramatically reduces the risk of graft rejection and failure.[48,49] Moreover, ALK, which is essentially an extraocular surgery, preserves the structural integrity of the globe and this allows for earlier suture removal and thus earlier visual rehabilitation compared to PK. Furthermore, it saves the patient the potential devastating intraoperative and postoperative complications of PK.[50-53]

For decades, ALK did not gain popularity despite its potential advantages. Technical difficulties and interface haze with suboptimal visual results inferior to PK has always been the obstacle. The introduction of new technologies namely modern microkeratomes and new microsurgical techniques namely Anwar's big bubble technique revived the interest in ALK.[54-56] Nonetheless, the steep learning curve and lack of reproducibility still hindered ALK widespread use.

The high precision and reproducibility that FS lasers have demonstrated has encouraged corneal surgeons to optimize and standardize ALK.[57,58] In 2008, Yoo et al.[52] reported the first case series of femtosecond laser-assisted anterior lamellar keratoplasty (FALK). They have employed the use of FS laser and anterior segment optical coherence tomography (ASOCT) to selectively cut the diseased corneal lamellae and replace them with identically cut donor tissue. Sparing normal posterior corneal tissue, in addition to Descemet's membrane and endothelium, was enough to maintain the structural integrity of the cornea and allowed for sutureless ALK. This was a new concept in ALK that avoided suture-related complications, most importantly suture-induced astigmatism. Nevertheless, the amount of preserved posterior corneal lamellae enough to conserve the tectonic stability of the globe in sutureless FALK was not identified. Thus, it was advisable to adhere to the 250 μm LASIK residual corneal bed safety margin until FALK safety margins are formulated. In 2011, the long-term results of FALK were reported and have shown that FALK has surpassed all other forms of ALK in terms of the amount of surgically induced astigmatism and the rapidity of visual rehabilitation. That sutureless technique cannot be used in cases with ectasia such as keratoconus and in cases with deeper anterior corneal pathologies where less posterior recipient tissue is left behind after the cut, suturing the graft in such cases would be a better option to guard against induction or exacerbation of ectasia. Several other reports of FALK followed and confirmed the superiority of FALK in providing the patient with superior and faster visual results.[59,60]

Despite that sutureless FALK has proven its efficacy, safety and stability in managing cases with anterior corneal pathologies and healthy posterior stroma and endothelium, this was not the case in FS laser assisted deep ALK. Big bubble technique provided better interfaces than that provided with FS laser. This could be explained by intrinsic limitations in the commercially available FS laser technology as it seemed that as FS laser is employed to deeper corneal lamellae it loses its sharpness and that results in interfaces that are no longer comparable to what could be obtained anteriorly. Scattering of FS laser by corneal lamellae seems to be, at least partially, the reason for those inferior interfaces. Optimization of the FS laser technology seems to have achieved success to reduce the scattering of FS laser by corneal lamellae; however, these new lasers are still in the laboratories and have not made it to clinics yet. In addition to that, it was observed that deep FS laser stromal cuts produce stromal concentric ridges in the interface. Those imperfections in the interfaces were attributed to the fact that laser spots are laid down in reference to the applanation surface, and as a flat applanator will flatten the anterior surface of the cornea but not the posterior surface, as the machine cuts deeper those aberrations will start to become more pronounced.[61] Employment of curved applanators did not seem to resolve that issue as they do not perfectly accommodate the shape

of the anterior surface of the cornea but rather applanate it to a lesser extent than flat applanators. Applanation-free FS laser would probably prevent that distortion from taking place. Prototype applanation-free FS lasers that can apply the laser spots through contact fluid have been reported but have not made it out of laboratories yet for use in lamellar corneal dissections.[62] Finally and most importantly, when the FS laser system cuts corneas with irregular surfaces, as in cases with severely ectatic diseases, irregularities will be imprinted in the stromal bed as the applanator takes the anterior surface of the cornea as its reference plane. Those stromal bed irregularities are transmitted by the uniform planar donor corneal lenticule to the anterior surface of the cornea and result in persistence of the irregular astigmatism. Applanation-free FS laser delivery system will again be the means to overcome such a limitation especially if combined with ASOCT data that could guide and plan uniform lamellar cuts that isolate corneal pathological irregularities.[33]

Femtosecond laser-assisted deep ALK does not match the results of big-bubble deep anterior lamellar keratoplasty (DALK) owing to limitations in current FS laser technology. Nevertheless, both techniques can be combined to get the best of the two worlds. The benefits of 'zig-zag' and 'top-hat' FS laser trephinations were extended to DALK in order to provide faster visual rehabilitations and less surgically induced astigmatism. Moreover, FS laser was used to standardize and simplify several steps in the surgery; such as debulking the anterior lamellae of the cornea and creating the channel from where air can be injected to bare Descemet's membrane. Nevertheless, it is worthy to note that the additional operative time and cost of using FS laser to assist big bubble DALK is a serious disadvantage that might discourage surgeon from adopting that technique.[63-65]

## ENDOTHELIAL KERATOPLASTY

Endothelial keratoplasty has replaced PK for many indications. The selective replacement of the endothelium while preserving the structural integrity of the globe has resulted in earlier visual rehabilitation and less surgically induced astigmatism in cases with endothelium dysfunction. Nevertheless, EK seems to lag behind PK in terms of the final visual outcomes. Less EK patients see 20/20 when compared to PK.[66] This is attributed to the rough corneal lamellar interfaces. Microkeratomes have been the gold standard for preparing those endothelial grafts and they have been the gold standard in cutting LASIK flaps as well. FS laser proved to be superior to microkeratomes as a LASIK flap cutter. That led to enthusiasm that FS laser can also provide a better interface in EK and thus match PK visual results. However, FS laser, with its currently available technology, seemed to have failed to achieve that.[67] The current FS laser technology did not provide superior interfaces than that obtained by manual or microkeratome-assisted techniques.[68,69] Scattering of FS laser by corneal lamellae in addition to the distortion caused by applana-ting the anterior surface of the cornea were incriminated as the causes for the inferior deep lamellar cuts.[70] Prototype FS laser systems with increased laser spot density that will use longer laser wavelengths less prone to scattering have improved the quality of the interfaces in the laboratories.[4] This, in addition to applanation-free delivery systems, is expected to improve the results of FS-DSAEK. However, until this technology becomes available, it is clear that the currently available FS laser technology is unable to provide any advantage over microkeratomes for DSAEK. On the contrary, microkeratome-assisted preparation seems to provide better quality interfaces with better visual results.[71]

## ➤ ASTIGMATIC KERATECTOMY

Astigmatic keratectomy remains the most commonly performed procedure to manage high degrees of regular astigmatism post-PK.[72] Mechanized devices such as the Hanna arcitome have significantly improved the repro-ducibility of the procedure compared to freehand techniques. Nonetheless, decreased efficacy and lack of predictability still question its reliability.[73] Employing FS laser to produce highly reproducible precise lamellar corneal incisions has proved to significantly improve the efficacy, reproducibility and safety of AK.[74-77] FS-AK was used to manage high degrees of post-PK, DALK and DSAEK astigmatism as well as naturally occurring astigmatism with notable success. It allowed for more reduction in postoperative cylinder and less incidence of complications such as microperforation and decentration of incisions.[74,75] Another unique advantage of FS-AK that was brought about by the versatility of the newer FS laser software is the ability to place nonorthogonal incisions that gives the surgeon the ability to manage nonorthogonal astigmatism.[78]

It is worth mentioning that planning FS-AK cuts using ASOCT pachymetry measurements has further improved the safety of the procedure. This is of special importance in post-DSAEK patients, as the DSAEK graft lenticule should not be included while planning the depth of the cut as it does not add to the biomechanical stability of the globe and failure to do so will result in an inadvertent full-thickness recipient corneal incisions and overcorrection.[79]

Despite the favorable results of FS laser AK, nomograms of manual AK are still used and that negatively affects its predictability. Refined nomograms specific to FS laser AK are thus needed to provide a solid base for that technology.[74,75]

## ➤ FEMTOSECOND LASER-ASSISTED PLACEMENT OF INTRASTROMAL CORNEAL RING SEGMENT

Intrastromal corneal ring segment placement is a minimally invasive surgical technique that can delay or prevent corneal transplantation in cases with ectatic corneal conditions such as keratoconus. Those crescent-shaped polymethyl methacrylate implants add thickness to the corneal mid-periphery to anteriorly displace the overlying surface of the cornea and that causes a relative central corneal flattening. This central flattening reduces patients' average keratometry and refractive error and improves their visual acuity.[80] ICRS tunnels can be created mechanically and recently by using FS laser. FS laser creates more reproducible tunnels with more uniform depth and dimensions. This higher degree of precision theoretically reduces the risk of complications reported with mechanical techniques such as anterior or posterior perforation, shallow or uneven placement of ICRS, decentration of rings, epithelial-stromal breakdown and extrusion.

Nevertheless, studies comparing the visual and refractive outcomes as well as safety of ICRS implanted using the mechanical versus FS laser have revealed the absence of statistically significant differences.[81,82]

## ➤ FEMTOSECOND LENTICULE EXTRACTION AND SMALL INCISION LENTICULE EXTRACTION

The term 'all femto LASIK' was recently introduced to corneal refractive surgery. Those relatively new procedures use FS laser to correct myopia and myopic astigmatism without the use of excimer laser or mickrokeratomes. It involves the excision of a corneal lamellar lenticule that is cut by a FS laser and accessed through a FS laser-cut flap that is repositioned back after manually extracting the excised lenticule. This procedure was named femtosecond lenticule extraction (FLEX) and is only offered by the VisuMax femtosecond system (Carl Zeiss Meditec, Jena, Germany). Limited data is available in the literature but all have demonstrated the good predictability and safety of the procedure.[83] However, it seems that it did not offer any advantage over LASIK except that it is logistically more convenient as a refractive suite can run using only a FS laser machine rather than an excimer and FS laser machines. In a modification that could make FLEX a more appealing surgery, a small incision rather than a complete flap is created to allow access to manually extract the lenticule in a procedure named small incision lenticule extraction (SMILE). Performing the surgery through a small incision and avoiding creation of a complete flap mean that less corneal nerve fibers will be cut and thus less dryness would ensue. Additionally, this surgery might have less impact on corneal biomechanical stability and thus can theoretically reduce the risk of ectasia.[84,85] However, those theoretical advantages that have to be yet proven. On the other hand, it is clear that SMILE and to a lesser extent FLEX are technically more challenging than LASIK and both procedures requiring a new learning curve for refractive surgeons familiar with LASIK.

## ➤ OTHER NOVEL FEMTOSECOND LASER APPLICATIONS IN CORNEAL SURGERIES

The high precision and versatility of FS laser technology have allowed for its use in several other corneal surgeries. Obtaining corneal biopsies,[86] corneal tattooing,[87] FLEX,[88] riboflavin FS laser-created pocket for collagen cross-linking,[89] arcuate wedge resection for the correction of high astigmatism[90] and intrastromal correction for presbyopia (INTRACOR procedure)[91] are among those recently introduced FS laser-assisted corneal surgeries.

## ➤ CONCLUSION

The ability of ultrashort pulse laser to photodisrupt corneal tissue with minimal collateral damage and high accuracy and reproducibility has made it a powerful tool capable of improving corneal surgical efficacy, predictability and safety. Nevertheless, ultrashort pulse laser corneal surgeries are not without their limitations and complications. Newer generations with versatile software and optimized laser parameters have successfully addressed some of those limitations and allowed for improved performance, better results and more surgical applications. Better understanding of the laser-tissue interaction will allow for guidance of future ultrashort pulse laser technology to expand its applications even further.

## ➤ REFERENCES

1. Taylor N. LASER: the inventor, the Nobel laureate, and the thirty-year patent war. New York: Simon & Schuster; 2000.
2. Charles H Townes. 'The first laser'. In: Laura Garwin, Tim Lincoln (Eds). A Century of Nature: twenty-one discoveries that changed science and the world. University of Chicago Press; 2003. pp. 107-12.
3. Krauss JM, Puliafito CA. Lasers in ophthalmology. Lasers Surg Med. 1995;17:102-59.
4. Plamann K, Aptel F, Arnold C, et al. Ultrashort pulse laser surgery of the cornea and the sclera. Journal of Optics. 2010;12:1-30.
5. Soong HK, Malta JB. Femtosecond lasers in ophthalmology. Am J Ophthalmol. 2009;147:189-97.
6. McClung FJ, Hellwarth RW. Giant Optical Pulsations from Ruby. Journal of Applied Physics. 1962;33:828-9.
7. Ready JF. Effects of High-Power Laser Radiation. New York: Academic Press; 1971. pp. 133-43.
8. Jonas JB, Vossmerbaeumer U. Femtosecond laser penetrating keratoplasty with conical incisions and positional spikes. J Refract Surg. 2004;20:397.
9. Kurtz RM, Horvath C, Liu HH, et al. Lamellar refractive surgery with scanned intrastromal picosecond and femtosecond laser pulses in animal eyes. J Refract Surg. 1998;14:541-8.
10. Sletten KR, Yen KG, Sayegh S, et al. An in vivo model of femtosecond laser intrastromal refractive surgery. Ophthalmic Surg Lasers. 1999;30:742-9.
11. Berns MW, Aist J, Edwards J, et al. Laser microsurgery in cell and developmental biology. Science. 1981;213:505-13.
12. Vogel A, Hentschel W, Holzfuss J, et al. Cavitation bubble dynamics and acoustic transient generation in ocular surgery with pulsed neodymium: YAG lasers. Ophthalmology. 1986;93:1259-69.
13. Hamill MB, Quayle WH. Iris repair after a catastrophic laser in situ keratomileusis complication. J Cataract Refract Surg. 2005;31:2216-20.
14. Hammond MD, Madigan WP, Bower KS. Refractive surgery in the United States Army, 2000-2003. Ophthalmology. 2005;112:184-90.
15. Slade SG. The use of the femtosecond laser in the customization of corneal flaps in laser in situ keratomileusis. Curr Opin Ophthalmol. 2007;18:314-7.
16. Kezirian GM, Stonecipher KG. Comparison of the IntraLase femtosecond laser and mechanical keratomes for laser in situ keratomileusis. J Cataract Refract Surg. 2004;30:804-11.
17. Durrie DS, Kezirian GM. Femtosecond laser versus mechanical keratome flaps in wavefront-guided laser in situ keratomileusis: prospective contralateral eye study. J Cataract Refract Surg. 2005;31:120-6.
18. Letko E, Price MO, Price FW. Influence of original flap creation method on incidence of epithelial ingrowth after LASIK retreatment. J Refract Surg. 2009;25:1039-41.
19. Zhou Y, Tian L, Wang N, et al. Anterior segment optical coherence tomography measurement of LASIK flaps: femtosecond laser vs microkeratome. J Refract Surg. 2011;27:408-16.

20. Medeiros FW, Stapleton WM, Hammel J, et al. Wavefront analysis comparison of LASIK outcomes with the femtosecond laser and mechanical microkeratomes. J Refract Surg. 2007;23:880-7.

21. Chan A, Ou J, Manche EE. Comparison of the femtosecond laser and mechanical keratome for laser in situ keratomileusis. Arch Ophthalmol. 2008;126:1484-90.

22. Haft P, Yoo SH, Kymionis GD, et al. Complications of LASIK flaps made by the IntraLase 15- and 30-kHz femtosecond lasers. J Refract Surg. 2009;25:979-84.

23. Friedlaender MH. LASIK surgery using the IntraLase femtosecond laser. Int Ophthalmol Clin. 2006;46:145-53.

24. Bamba S, Rocha KM, Ramos-Esteban JC, et al. Incidence of rainbow glare after laser in situ keratomileusis flap creation with a 60 kHz femtosecond laser. J Cataract Refract Surg. 2009;35:1082-6.

25. de Medeiros FW, Kaur H, Agrawal V, et al. Effect of femtosecond laser energy level on corneal stromal cell death and inflammation. J Refract Surg. 2009;25:869-74.

26. Munoz G, Albarran-Diego C, Sakla HF, et al. Transient light-sensitivity syndrome after laser in situ keratomileusis with the femtosecond laser incidence and prevention. J Cataract Refract Surg. 2006;32:2075-9.

27. Sarayba MA, Ignacio TS, Tran DB, et al. A 60 kHz IntraLase femtosecond laser creates a smoother LASIK stromal bed surface compared to a Zyoptix XP mechanical microkeratome in human donor eyes. J Refract Surg. 2007;23:331-7.

28. Franceschetti A. [Combined lamellar and perforant keratoplasty (mushroom graft)]. Bull Schweiz Akad Med Wiss. 1951;7:134-45.

29. Busin M. A new lamellar wound configuration for penetrating keratoplasty surgery. Arch Ophthalmol. 2003;121:260-5.

30. Busin M, Arffa RC. Microkeratome-assisted mushroom keratoplasty with minimal endothelial replacement. Am J Ophthalmol. 2005;140:138-40.

31. Holzer MP, Rabsilber TM, Auffarth GU. Penetrating keratoplasty using femtosecond laser. Am J Ophthalmol. 2007;143:524-6.

32. Seitz B, Brunner H, Viestenz A, et al. Inverse mushroom-shaped nonmechanical penetrating keratoplasty using a femtosecond laser. Am J Ophthalmol. 2005;139:941-4.

33. Yoo SH, Hurmeric V. Femtosecond laser-assisted keratoplasty. Am J Ophthalmol. 2011;151:189-91.

34. Price FW, Price MO, Jordan CS. Safety of incomplete incision patterns in femtosecond laser-assisted penetrating keratoplasty. J Cataract Refract Surg. 2008;34:2099-103.

35. Bahar I, Kaiserman I, McAllum P, et al. Femtosecond laser-assisted penetrating keratoplasty: stability evaluation of different wound configurations. Cornea. 2008;27:209-11.

36. Cheng YY, Tahzib NG, van RG, et al. Femtosecond laser-assisted inverted mushroom keratoplasty. Cornea. 2008;27:679-85.

37. Steinert RF, Ignacio TS, Sarayba MA. 'Top hat'-shaped penetrating keratoplasty using the femtosecond laser. Am J Ophthalmol. 2007;143:689-91.

38. Saelens IE, Bartels MC, van RG. Posterior mushroom keratoplasty in patients with Fuchs endothelial dystrophy and pseudophakic bullous keratopathy: transplant outcome. Cornea. 2008;27:673-8.

39. Price FW, Price MO. Femtosecond laser shaped penetrating keratoplasty: one-year results utilizing a top-hat configuration. Am J Ophthalmol. 2008;145:210-4.

40. Bahar I, Kaiserman I, Lange AP, et al. Femtosecond laser versus manual dissection for top hat penetrating keratoplasty. Br J Ophthalmol. 2009;93:73-8.

41. Saelens IE, Bartels MC, van RG. Manual trephination of mushroom keratoplasty in advanced keratoconus. Cornea. 2008;27:650-5.

42. Busin M, Arffa RC. Microkeratome-assisted mushroom keratoplasty with minimal endothelial replacement. Am J Ophthalmol. 2005;140:138-40.

43. Farid M, Kim M, Steinert RF. Results of penetrating keratoplasty performed with a femtosecond laser zigzag incision initial report. Ophthalmology. 2007;114:2208-12.

44. Farid M, Steinert RF, Gaster RN, et al. Comparison of penetrating keratoplasty performed with a femtosecond laser zig-zag incision versus conventional blade trephination. Ophthalmology. 2009; 116:1638-43.

45. Chamberlain WD, Rush SW, Mathers WD, et al. Comparison of femtosecond laser-assisted keratoplasty versus conventional penetrating keratoplasty. Ophthalmology. 2011;118:486-91.

46. McAllum P, Kaiserman I, Bahar I, et al. Femtosecond laser top hat penetrating keratoplasty: wound burst pressures of incomplete cuts. Arch Ophthalmol. 2008;126:822-5.

47. Price FW, Price MO, Jordan CS. Safety of incomplete incision patterns in femtosecond laser-assisted penetrating keratoplasty. J Cataract Refract Surg. 2008;34:2099-103.

48. Barraquer JI. Lamellar keratoplasty. (Special techniques). Ann Ophthalmol. 1972;4:437-69.

49. Haimovici R, Culbertson WW. Optical lamellar keratoplasty using the barraquer microkeratome. Refract Corneal Surg. 1991;7:42-5.

50. Alio JL, Shah S, Barraquer C, et al. New techniques in lamellar keratoplasty. Curr Opin Ophthalmol. 2002;13:224-9.

51. Bahar I, Kaiserman I, Srinivasan S, et al. Comparison of three different techniques of corneal transplantation for keratoconus. Am J Ophthalmol. 2008;146:905-12.

52. Yoo SH, Kymionis GD, Koreishi A, et al. Femtosecond laser-assisted sutureless anterior lamellar keratoplasty. Ophthalmology. 2008;115:1303-7.

53. Han DC, Mehta JS, Por YM, et al. Comparison of outcomes of lamellar keratoplasty and penetrating keratoplasty in keratoconus. Am J Ophthalmol. 2009;148:744-51.

54. Terry MA. The evolution of lamellar grafting techniques over twenty-five years. Cornea. 2000;19:611-6.

55. Tan DT, Mehta JS. Future directions in lamellar corneal transplantation. Cornea. 2007;26:S21-8.

56. Anwar M, Teichmann KD. Big-bubble technique to bare Descemet's membrane in anterior lamellar keratoplasty. J Cataract Refract Surg. 2002;28:398-403.

57. Mian SI, Soong HK, Patel SV, et al. In vivo femtosecond laser-assisted posterior lamellar keratoplasty in rabbits. Cornea. 2006;25:1205-9.

58. Mian SI, Shtein RM. Femtosecond laser-assisted corneal surgery. Curr Opin Ophthalmol. 2007;18:295-9.

59. Mosca L, Fasciani R, Tamburelli C, et al. Femtosecond laser-assisted lamellar keratoplasty: early results. Cornea. 2008; 27:668-72.

60. Hoffart L, Proust H, Matonti F, et al. [Femtosecond-assisted anterior lamellar keratoplasty]. J Fr Ophtalmol. 2007;30:689-94.

61. Soong HK, Mian S, Abbasi O, et al. Femtosecond laser-assisted posterior lamellar keratoplasty: initial studies of surgical technique in eye bank eyes. Ophthalmology. 2005;112:44-9.

62. Miclea M, Skrzypczak U, Fankhauser F, et al. Applanation-free femtosecond laser processing of the cornea. Biomed Opt Express. 2011;2:534-42.

63. Buzzonetti L, Laborante A, Petrocelli G. Standardized big-bubble technique in deep anterior lamellar keratoplasty assisted by the femtosecond laser. J Cataract Refract Surg. 2010;36:1631-6.

64. Buzzonetti L, Laborante A, Petrocelli G. Refractive outcome of keratoconus treated by combined femtosecond laser and big-bubble deep anterior lamellar keratoplasty. J Refract Surg. 2011;27:189-94.

65. Farid M, Steinert RF. Deep anterior lamellar keratoplasty performed with the femtosecond laser zigzag incision for the treatment of stromal corneal pathology and ectatic disease. J Cataract Refract Surg. 2009;35:809-13.

66. Cheng YY, van Den Berg TJ, Schouten JS, et al. Quality of vision after femtosecond laser-assisted Descemet stripping endothelial keratoplasty and penetrating keratoplasty: a randomized, multicenter clinical trial. Am J Ophthalmol. 2011;152:556-66.

67. Cheng YY, Hendrikse F, Pels E, et al. Preliminary results of femtosecond laser-assisted Descemet stripping endothelial keratoplasty. Arch Ophthalmol. 2008;126:1351-6.

68. Terry MA, Ousley PJ, Will B. A practical femtosecond laser procedure for DLEK endothelial transplantation: cadaver eye histology and topography. Cornea. 2005;24:453-9.

69. Jones YJ, Goins KM, Sutphin JE, et al. Comparison of the femtosecond laser (IntraLase) versus manual microkeratome (Moria ALTK) in dissection of the donor in endothelial keratoplasty: initial study in eye bank eyes. Cornea. 2008;27:88-93.

70. Soong HK, Mian S, Abbasi O, et al. Femtosecond laser-assisted posterior lamellar keratoplasty: initial studies of surgical technique in eye bank eyes. Ophthalmology. 2005;112:44-9.

71. Mootha VV, Heck E, Verity SM, et al. Comparative study of Descemet stripping automated endothelial keratoplasty donor preparation by Moria CBm microkeratome, horizon microkeratome, and Intralase FS60. Cornea. 2011;30:320-4.

72. Poole TR, Ficker LA. Astigmatic keratotomy for post-keratoplasty astigmatism. J Cataract Refract Surg. 2006;32:1175-9.

73. Hoffart L, Touzeau O, Borderie V, et al. Mechanized astigmatic arcuate keratotomy with the Hanna arcitome for astigmatism after keratoplasty. J Cataract Refract Surg. 2007;33:862-8.

74. Hoffart L, Proust H, Matonti F, et al. Correction of postkeratoplasty astigmatism by femtosecond laser compared with mechanized astigmatic keratotomy. Am J Ophthalmol. 2009;147:779-87.

75. Buzzonetti L, Petrocelli G, Laborante A, et al. Arcuate keratotomy for high postoperative keratoplasty astigmatism performed with the intralase femtosecond laser. J Refract Surg. 2009;25:709-14.

76. Kymionis GD, Yoo SH, Ide T, et al. Femtosecond-assisted astigmatic keratotomy for post-keratoplasty irregular astigmatism. J Cataract Refract Surg. 2009;35:11-3.

77. Abbey A, Ide T, Kymionis GD, et al. Femtosecond laser-assisted astigmatic keratotomy in naturally occurring high astigmatism. Br J Ophthalmol. 2009;93:1566-9.

78. Kymionis GD, Yoo SH, Ide T, et al. Femtosecond-assisted astigmatic keratotomy for post-keratoplasty irregular astigmatism. J Cataract Refract Surg. 2009;35:11-3.

79. Yoo SH, Kymionis GD, Ide T, et al. Overcorrection after femtosecond-assisted astigmatic keratotomy in a post-Descemet-stripping automated endothelial keratoplasty patient. J Cataract Refract Surg. 2009;35:1833-4.

80. Kymionis GD, Siganos CS, Tsiklis NS, et al. Long-term follow-up of Intacs in keratoconus. Am J Ophthalmol. 2007;143:236-44.

81. Pinero DP, Alio JL, El KB, et al. Refractive and aberrometric outcomes of intracorneal ring segments for keratoconus: mechanical versus femtosecond-assisted procedures. Ophthalmology. 2009;116:1675-87.

82. Rabinowitz YS, Li X, Ignacio TS, et al. INTACS inserts using the femtosecond laser compared to the mechanical spreader in the treatment of keratoconus. J Refract Surg. 2006;22:764-71.

83. Blum M, Kunert K, Schroder M, et al. Femtosecond lenticule extraction for the correction of myopia: preliminary 6-month results. Graefes Arch Clin Exp Ophthalmol. 2010;248:1019-27.

84. Shah R, Shah S, Sengupta S. Results of small incision lenticule extraction: all-in-one femtosecond laser refractive surgery. J Cataract Refract Surg. 2011;37:127-37.

85. Sekundo W, Kunert KS, Blum M. Small incision corneal refractive surgery using the small incision lenticule extraction (SMILE) procedure for the correction of myopia and myopic astigmatism: results of a 6 month prospective study. Br J Ophthalmol. 2011;95:335-9.

86. Yoo SH, Kymionis GD, O'Brien TP, et al. Femtosecond-assisted diagnostic corneal biopsy (FAB) in l    titis. Graefes Arch Clin Exp Ophthalmol. 2008;246:759-62.

87. Kymionis GD, Ide T, Galor A, et al. Femtosecond-assisted anterior lamellar corneal staining-tattooing in a blind eye with leukocoria. Cornea. 2009;28:211-3.

88. Sekundo W, Kunert K, Russmann C, et al. First efficacy and safety study of femtosecond lenticule extraction for the correction of myopia: six-month results. J Cataract Refract Surg. 2008;34:1513-20.

89. Kanellopoulos AJ. Collagen cross-linking in early keratoconus with riboflavin in a femtosecond laser-created pocket: initial clinical results. J Refract Surg. 2009;25:1034-7.

90. Ghanem RC, Azar DT. Femtosecond-laser arcuate wedge-shaped resection to correct high residual astigmatism after penetrating keratoplasty. J Cataract Refract Surg. 2006;32:1415-9.

91. Ruiz LA, Cepeda LM, Fuentes VC. Intrastromal correction of presbyopia using a femtosecond laser system. J Refract Surg. 2009;25:847-54.

# CHAPTER 108

# Lens Power Calculations in the Postkeratorefractive Eye

*R Duncan Johnson, Uday Devgan*

## ⯈ INTRODUCTION

The advances in modern technology, instrumentation, lens design and surgical technique have allowed us to achieve a safer, more efficient, less invasive and more elegant cataract surgery with minimal recovery time. The eventual postoperative refractive results, however, depend on measurements of the eye taken preoperatively.

Using third generation intraocular lens (IOL) formulas (Hoffer Q, Holladay 1, SRK/T, Haigis) in average eyes with no prior ocular surgery, refractive results are very accurate[1] with excellent reported results[2] of 75% within ±0.5 diopters (D) and 95% within ±1.0 D. A UK benchmark set in 2009 suggested postoperative results in virgin corneas should be within 0.5 D in at least 55% and within 1.0 D in at least 85%.[3]

In eyes with prior keratorefractive surgery, however, reaching such benchmarks is often difficult even with the best techniques.[4] This is primarily due to the difficulty in precisely measuring the corneal refractive power and inaccurate determination of the effective lens position (ELP) of the implant after surgery.

While the cataract surgery itself is generally no more technically challenging in the postkeratorefractive population, calculating the appropriate IOL power is a difficult problem that all anterior segment surgeons must consider. This is a problem that we will inevitably encounter with increasing frequency with nearly 1 million laser refractive procedures being performed in the United States each year (Duffey RJ, Leaming D. US trends in

refractive surgery: ASCRS Survey. ASCRS meeting, San Diego, 2011). As this postrefractive population ages, an ever growing number will eventually develop visually significant cataracts requiring surgical removal. In addition, the population of patients who have already undergone keratorefractive surgery is particularly concerned with achieving a specific refractive outcome. Understanding the limitations of our ability to perform accurate lens power calculations in the postkeratorefractive eye, and advising patients of these limitations is essential for every cataract surgeon.

## ⯈ SOURCES OF ERROR IN CALCULATIONS

The original SRK formula: $P = A - 0.9\,K - 2.5\,L$, highlights the two most important factors in calculating IOL power (P): corneal power (K) and axial length (L). Modern third generation formulas now use these two important factors as well as various other measurements to estimate a third important factor: the Effective Lens Position or 'ELP' (Fig. 1). These variables are altered in various ways in keratorefractive surgery.

### Axial Length

The length of the eye is only minimally,[5] if at all,[6,7] affected by keratorefractive surgery. This is to be expected as photoablative procedures such as photorefractive keratectomy (PRK) or laser *in situ* keratomileusis (LASIK) only remove fractions of a millimeter of corneal tissue and incisional procedures remove no tissue. The biomechanical

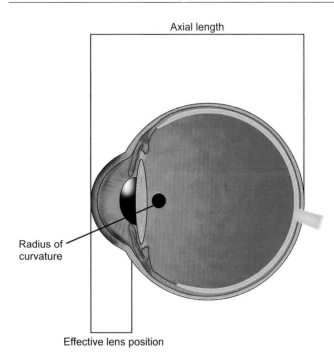

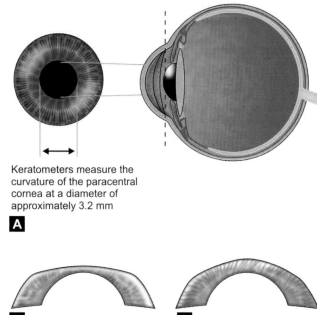

Keratometers measure the curvature of the paracentral cornea at a diameter of approximately 3.2 mm

**A**

**B**        **C**

**Fig. 1:** Diagrammatic eye showing the three most important factors for calculating correct intraocular lens power: axial length, corneal radius of curvature, and effective lens position

**Figs 2A to C:** (A) Most keratometers measure the corneal curvature at a central ring with a diameter of 3.2 mm. This central ring is representative of the central corneal power over a range of curvatures when the central cornea approximates a sphere as shown in A; (B and C) This is inadequate in the postrefractive cornea where the central cornea no longer approximates a sphere. There is central flattening in a postmyopic laser treatment (B) and central steepening in posthyperopic laser treatment (C)

weakening of the cornea due to these procedures may lead to mild anterior bulging of the cornea.[8] However this, too, is of such a low magnitude it is not likely to significantly affect postoperative refractive outcomes.

## Keratometric Power

One of the most important aspects of biometry for lens power calculations is attaining an accurate central corneal power. Most traditional keratometers and topographers used for calculating the corneal power actually measure the curvature at a ring approximately 3.2 mm in diameter surrounding the central cornea. Using various assumptions this paracentral corneal curvature is calculated into the assumed central corneal power using the formula:

$$P = (n' - 1)/r$$

Where P is the keratometric power in diopters, n' is the refractive index of the cornea, and r is the measured radius of curvature in meters.

One of the major assumptions used here is that the central and paracentral cornea approximate a sphere. In a normal, prolate cornea this assumption generally holds true for the central 3 mm (Figs 2A to C). However, after myopic photoablative procedures the central cornea is significantly flatter than the paracentral cornea. In this situation, the measured keratometric power is higher than the true central

corneal power, which leads the observer to overestimate the total power of the eye and choose a weaker IOL power, which leads to a postoperative 'hyperopic surprise'. The opposite holds true in hyperopic procedures where the central cornea is steeper than the paracentral cornea, leading to a postoperative myopic surprise. In radial keratotomy (RK), the central cornea is irregular and variable, especially in treatments where the incisions encroach within the central 3 mm, rendering curvature measurements notoriously inaccurate.

Another major assumption in the above formula is that there is a standard refractive index for all corneas that never changes. The standard Javal-Schiotz keratometer uses a refractive index of 1.3375. This differs from the actual refractive index of the cornea (1.376) in order to take into account the posterior curvature of the cornea, which is significantly steeper than the anterior curvature.[9] This assumed refractive index, however, only works if there is a constant ratio between anterior and posterior curvatures. In incisional refractive surgery such as RK this ratio remains constant, as no tissue has been removed. In corneas that have

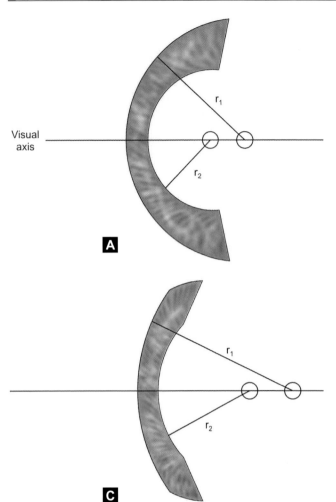

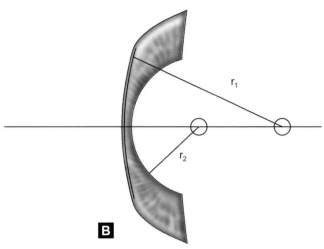

**Figs 3A to C:** (A) In the normal cornea the posterior radius of curvature of the cornea ($r_2$) is steeper than the anterior radius of curvature ($r_1$) at a fairly consistent ratio; (B) In the cornea that has received a myopic laser refractive treatment, the anterior curvature is altered and significantly flattened, while the posterior curvature is mostly unchanged, leading to a large change in the anterior-posterior curvature ratio; (C) In radial keratotomy, the cornea is flattened both anteriorly and posteriorly, thus only minimally affecting the ratio between anterior and posterior curvature

undergone photoablative keratorefractive surgery; however, this relationship is severely altered, rendering the standard corneal refractive index, and thus keratometry readings incorrect (Figs 3A to C). These induced errors become increasingly more significant with higher corrections.[10-14]

### Effective Lens Position

The position of the lens inside the eye varies depending on the depth of the anterior chamber and the length of the eye. In general, eyes that are longer have a steeper cornea and a deeper anterior chamber with a more posterior lens position. In shorter eyes, the cornea is generally flatter with a shallower anterior chamber and thus a more anterior lens position (Figs 4A and B).

The final anterior-posterior position of the lens inside the eye after cataract surgery is the most difficult variable to estimate with our current technology. Most current IOL formulas (except Haigis) rely on the anterior corneal curvature to estimate the final ELP. Corneal refractive surgery alters the anterior corneal curvature, but has no effect on the eventual ELP. This causes the IOL formulas to incorrectly assume a more anterior lens position in the postmyopic keratorefractive patient, leading to an underestimation of the necessary IOL power, and thus resulting in further 'hyperopic surprise'. The opposite is true of posthyperopic corneal treatment.

### ▶ METHODS FOR ESTIMATING EFFECTIVE CENTRAL CORNEAL POWER

The biggest source of error in postrefractive IOL calculations is the effective corneal power used. Various approaches have been used to address this problem, only a

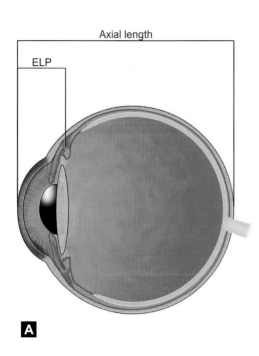

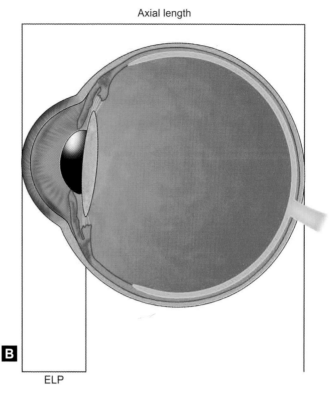

**Figs 4A and B:** Diagrammatic representation of the more anterior effective lens position in the short/hyperopic eye, compared to the more posterior lens position in the longer/myopic eye

portion of which are discussed here. The fact that there are so many different variations and formulas is evidence that none is perfect, or significantly better than the other. Using as many of the methods as possible, and then making an educated guess in choosing the IOL power based on that information is the current standard. It is also important to note that not all methods apply to all types of postrefractive eyes. Table 1 indicates which methods are appropriate with which type of previous surgery.

The various methods basically are divided into two categories: (1) Those that require prerefractive data and (2) Those that do not. Those that require prerefractive data are further divided into those that require preoperative keratometry values and those that only require knowledge of the change in refractive error.

## Preoperative Data Required: Keratometry

### Clinical History Method

The clinical history method was originally introduced by Dr Jack T Holladay in 1989 for IOL calculation in post-RK eyes,[15] but can be used in all types of postrefractive

corneas. Knowledge of preoperative keratometry readings as well as change in refraction (spherical equivalent) is necessary. The corneal power to use in the IOL formula is given by:

$$K_{post} = K_{pre} + (\Delta D)$$

where $K_{post}$ is postrefractive corneal power in diopters, $K_{pre}$ is preoperative keratometric power in diopters and $\Delta D$ is the change in refractive power defined as preoperative spherical equivalent minus the postoperative spherical equivalent.

Originally, refractive change at the corneal plane was used; however, using refraction at the spectacle plane further reduces refractive surprise in the postrefractive cornea.[16]

The clinical history method decreases IOL power error, however, requires preoperative data that is not available for many patients. Its accuracy is limited as well, particularly in corneas that have undergone treatment for larger refractive errors. Mean error is generally ±0.75 D, and errors greater than 2 D are not rare.[4] This increased error is partly due to the incorrect assumption that 1 D of keratometric change is equal to 1 D of refractive change. The history method also lacks any adjustment for true ELP. Therefore, results are

**Table 1:** Appropriate methods with type of previous surgery

| Method | Radial Keratotomy | Myopic Laser Correction | Hyperopic Laser Correction |
|---|---|---|---|
| Clinical history | + | + | + |
| Contact lens | + | + | + |
| Double K method | – | + | + |
| Cornea bypass | – | + | + |
| Modified Maloney | – | + | – |
| Shammas formula | – | + | – |
| Modified Masket | – | + | – |
| Latkany method | – | + | – |
| Haigis L* | – | + | +* |
| Feiz-Mannis nomogram | – | + | + |
| Geggel ratio | – | + | – |
| Aphakic calculations methods | + | + | ± |

*Haigis L for posthyperopic correction available on the IOLMaster 500

augmented when this method is used in conjunction with the double K method (discussed below) to help adjust for the ELP.

### Aramberri Double K Method[17]

The Double K method was originally described in 2003 to adjust for postoperative refractive errors that occurred due to errors in estimated ELP. While the clinical history decreases the magnitude of hyperopic surprise, it does not eliminate it. The reason for this is that while the clinical history method gets a more accurate corneal power, the third generation formulas still use this adjusted postrefractive keratometry value to estimate the postoperative ELP. In postmyopic refractive surgery eyes, using a flatter keratometry value results in an assumed more anterior ELP, which causes an erroneous weak IOL power choice.

To correct this problem, the double K method changed the SRK/T formula to use prekeratorefractive surgery (Kpre) values for the portions of the formula that calculate the ELP, and the postkeratorefractive surgery (Kpost) values for the vergence portions of the formula which give the final IOL power. This same concept may also be applied to other third generation formulas[18] as well with great results.

### Walter Cornea Bypass Method[19]

In this method, the postkeratorefractive corneal measurements can be avoided altogether, as long as the preoperative keratometry readings are known. The pre-LASIK keratometry values are simply plugged into the IOL power

formula and the refractive error (spherical equivalent) corrected for by the previous laser refractive surgery is selected as the postoperative goal refraction. Essentially, using the goal refraction to cancel out the previous refractive change induced on the cornea. This has the drawback of requiring preoperative data, but otherwise is quite simple and makes intuitive sense.

### Feiz-Mannis Method[14]

This method initially uses pre-LASIK keratometry values that are plugged into the SRK/T formula to aim for emmetropia. This IOL power is then adjusted according to the amount of refractive error (spherical equivalent) that had been corrected with LASIK. However, for every diopter of change in the IOL plane, only 0.7 D is changed in the spectacle plane due to the change in vertex distance. The appropriate postrefractive surgery IOL was then calculated using the formula:

$$IOL_{post} = IOL_{pre} - (\Delta D/0.7)$$

where $IOL_{post}$ is the adjusted postrefractive IOL power, $IOL_{pre}$ is the IOL power calculated using the prerefractive surgery keratometry values and $\Delta D$ is the change in spherical equivalent pre- and postrefractive surgery in the spectacle plane.

From this data, a linear relationship between IOL power adjustment and laser corrected spherical equivalent was calculated. This data allows for a simple nomogram to adjust IOL power according to how much refractive error had been corrected.

## Preoperative Data Required: Refractive Error

### Koch-Wang Formula[10,18]

When preoperative keratometry is not available, but an accurate pre- and postrefractive surgery refraction is available, the Koch-Wang formula may be used:

$$Ke = Ccp - (\Delta D \times 0.15)$$

where Ke is the estimated corneal power (diopters), Ccp is the effective central corneal power (EffRP from EyeSys device) and $\Delta D$ is the change in spherical equivalent from prekeratorefractive surgery to postkeratorefractive surgery.

This formula has the advantage of not requiring prerefractive surgery keratometry values, but the refractive change is still needed. The above formula also requires a topographic machine with the ability to give an effective central corneal power such as the EffRP given using the Holladay Diagnostic Summary on the EyeSys device. This formula can be adjusted slightly if only a Sim K of the central cornea is available using the following formula:

$$Ke = TK - (\Delta D \times 0.24)$$

where Ke is the estimated corneal power (diopters), TK is the topographic central corneal power (i.e. Sim K at 3 mm) and $\Delta D$ is the change in spherical equivalent from prekeratorefractive surgery to postkeratorefractive surgery.

### Modified Masket Formula[20,21]

In this method, preoperative keratometry is not needed, however, postrefractive change in refraction is. Intraocular pressure (IOP) power measurements are performed as though the eye was normal; however, the predicted IOL power is adjusted by the formula:

$$IOL_{post} = IOL_{pre} + \Delta D \times 0.4385 + 0.0295$$

where $IOL_{post}$ is the adjusted IOL power, $IOL_{pre}$ is the calculated IOL power and $\Delta D$ is the surgically induced change in manifest refraction (spherical equivalent).

### Latkany Flat K, or Average K Method[22]

In this method, the only prekeratorefractive surgery data needed is the spherical equivalent. The IOL power is then calculated by inserting the average postkeratorefractive surgery keratometry (AvgK) value or flattest postkeratorefractive surgery keratometry (FlatK) value into the SRK/T formula. This IOL power is then adjusted according to a regression formula:

$$\text{Adjustment for } IOL_{flatK} = -(0.47x + 0.85)$$
$$\text{Adjustment for } IOL_{avgK} = -(0.46x + 0.21)$$

where x is the prekeratorefractive surgery spherical equivalent.

## Preoperative Data not Required

### Contact Lens Over-Refraction Method

The contact lens over-refraction method can be used for any postrefractive eye. It also has the advantage of not requiring preoperative data. In this method, the patient is refracted and the spherical equivalent is recorded. A plano contact lens of known curvature is placed on the patient's cornea, and the patient is then refracted again. The corneal power can then be calculated:

$$Ke = BC + Cp + (ORx - SE)$$

where Ke is the effective corneal power (diopters), BC is the base curve of the CTL (diopters), Cp is the CTL power in diopters, ORx is the rigid CTL over-refraction and SE is the spherical equivalent of the manifest refraction sans contact lens.

Disadvantages of this method, however, are many. A full rigid contact lens fitting set with true calibrated lenses is required. The base curve of the contact lens should also nearly approximate that of the cornea, as large differences will lead to errors in refraction. Also, refraction can be difficult in these eyes, and requires sufficient visual acuity to perform an accurate refraction (at least > 20/70).[23] Also, some of the refractive error often is due to nuclear sclerotic changes, and not necessarily only due to changes in corneal curvature.[22]

### Adjusting Postrefractive Keratometry: Regression Formulas

There have been multiple formulas produced that use regression analysis of multiple postrefractive eyes to produce a best-fit regression line equation. This is then used as a formula to correct the measured keratometry. These formulas are often adjusted from time to time as larger numbers of eyes are used, and the regression analysis is updated. The following are representative of these regression formulas:

Modified Maloney[24]

$$Ke = (TK \times 1.1141) - 6.1$$

where Ke is the estimated corneal power (diopters) and TK is the central topographic keratometry (diopters).

Shammas formula[25]

$$Ke = 1.14 \times TK - 6.8$$

where Ke is the estimated corneal power (diopters) and TK is the central topographic keratometry (diopters).

Haigis L for postmyopic laser vision correction[26]

$$r_{corr} = 331.5/(-5.1625 \times r_{meas} + 82.2603 - 0.35)$$

where $r_{corr}$ is the corrected corneal curvature in mm and $r_{meas}$ is the corneal curvature as measured by the IOLMaster (Carl Zeiss, Meditec). This $r_{corr}$ is then inserted into the Haigis formula to derive an adjusted IOL power.

Ferrara formula[27]

In this method, Ferrara et al. use a regression formula to adjust the refractive index of the cornea in postmyopic PRK eyes. They propose a theoretical variable refractive index that is derived from the formula:

$$TRI = -0.0006 \times (AL \times AL) + 0.0213 \times AL + 1.1572$$

where TRI is the theoretical refractive index and AL is the axial length. The corneal power can then be calculated using the formula: $P = (TRI - 1)/r$ (r = corneal curvature in meters).

### Geggel Pachymetric Ratio Method[28]

A novel way of adjusting the postmyopic laser keratorefractive lens power was described by Harry S Geggel in 2009. In this method, it is assumed that there is a constant ratio between superior corneal thickness compared to central corneal thickness, and therefore, any deviations from this constant ratio results from ablation of central corneal tissue. After measuring the superior corneal thickness, the central corneal thickness can then be estimated using the Geggel ratio. The difference between estimated central corneal thickness and measured corneal thickness can then be calculated and taken as the presumed ablation depth as in the formula:

$$A = Geggel\ ratio \times SCP - CP$$

where A is the assumed ablation depth (μm), SCP is the superior corneal pachymetry (μm) and CP is the central corneal pachymetry (μm).

This assumed ablation depth is then applied to the regression formula described by Dr Geggel:

$$-0.399(A/12) - 0.40 = Adjustment\ number$$

where A is the assumed ablation depth (μm).

This adjustment number is then added to the power of the lens power calculated for the eye using the Haigis formula after aiming for slight myopia.

### ⁙ APHAKIC CALCULATION METHODS

Nearly all the calculation methods reviewed above rely on keratometry values in the postkeratorefractive eye, which is highly unreliable. The aphakic calculation method can be used to avoid this confounding factor. In these methods, all corneal measurements are bypassed simply by determining the power of the aphakic eye (i.e. after the cataract is removed), and then inserting the appropriate IOL power to allow emmetropia. This method has the advantage of not needing any pre- or postkeratorefractive surgery measurements. It also can potentially be used after any type of keratorefractive surgery; however, caution should be used particularly in eyes that have had radial keratometry due to changes in refraction secondary to intraoperative corneal hydration. The biggest shortfall of this method is the lack of adjustment for ELP, which likely accounts for a large portion of the variability.

### Mackool Aphakic Refraction Technique[29,30]

In the method described by Richard J Mackool in 2006, cataract surgery is preformed under topical anesthesia and the patient is left aphakic. After 30 minutes of recovery, the eye is refracted with a vertex distance of 12 mm. This refraction is adjusted for the IOL vertex distance using the formula:

$$SE_{aphakic} \times 1.75 = IOL\ power$$

where SE is the spherical equivalent of the aphakic refraction. This also assumes an IOL with A-constant of 118.84.

*Note*: This formula was used only for patients with a history of myopic LASIK.

The patient is then brought back into the operating room (OR) and the appropriate lens is inserted into the capsular bag.

### Intraoperative Aphakic Autorefraction Technique[31]

The obvious drawback of the Mackool technique is the need for a return trip to the OR, within hours to days after the original surgery. This is often neither cost nor time effective. To overcome this problem Ianchulev et al., in 2005, originally described a technique where an autorefractor was used intraoperatively to determine the required IOL power.

The ORange intraoperative wavefront aberrometer (WaveTec vision, Aliso Viejo, CA) operates on similar principles, but uses Talbot-Moiré wavefront technology to more accurately measure eyes with a wider range of axial lengths and estimate the appropriate IOL power intraoperatively. Future intraoperative aberrometers are in development which may provide more accurate results; however, it is important to note that the refraction of the eye intraoperatively will likely change in the postoperative period as the capsular bag contracts and the IOL position shifts.

# ⯈ INTRAOCULAR LENS CHOICE CONSIDERATIONS

In choosing an appropriate lens in the postrefractive patient, lens power is not the only important aspect to consider. The postrefractive cornea has significantly altered spherical aberration compared to the normal cornea. Corneas that have undergone myopic correction have a flatter cornea adding positive spherical aberration. In this situation, implanting an aspheric IOL with negative spherical aberration will result in better visual quality. In eyes that have undergone hyperopic correction, significant corneal negative spherical aberration has been induced, thus placing a lens with negative spherical aberration (i.e. aspheric lens) could actually exacerbate the total spherical aberration in the eye. This is a rare situation where a standard IOL will actually outperform an aspheric lens (Fig. 5).

# ⯈ CONCLUSION

While no one method is truly superior to all others, many investigators have compared many of these techniques head-to-head. Wang et al. evaluated[21] the accuracy of the various methods used on the American Society of Cataract and Refractive Surgery IOL Calculator and found that the methods that used prerefractive surgery keratometry readings and surgically induced refractive change were

actually less accurate than methods using only surgically induced refractive change or used no prekeratorefractive data at all. In fact, all seven of the methods evaluated using only surgi- cally induced refractive change or no prekeratorefractive data actually surpassed the benchmark set by the United Kingdom for cataract surgery refractive results in normal corneas ($\pm 0.5$ D in $\geq 55\%$, and $\pm 1.0$ D in $\geq 85\%$). None of the other methods reached this benchmark. The most accurate method, however, was taking the average IOL power of all methods, which gave an impressive absolute mean error of $0.57$ D $\pm 0.51$ D.

Calculating the appropriate IOL power in the post-keratorefractive surgery eye is a difficult task. The science behind these calculations is improving, and one day soon we may have a single superior method. However, for now, accuracy is still limited compared to IOL calculations in eyes with virgin corneas.

In approaching the postkeratorefractive surgery patient with a visually significant cataract, it is important to understand the limitations of our current technology in estimating a correct IOL power, as well as advising the patient of these limits to set realistic expectations. Gathering as much data as possible and using a variety of power calculation methods will help limit, but still not eliminate, postoperative refractive surprises. Preparing the patient preoperatively for this possibility will help the patient as well as the surgeon.

# ⯈ INTERNET RESOURCES

www.iol.ascrs.org (IOL power calculations in eyes that have undergone LASIK/PRK/RK)
www.hofferprograms.com (Hoffer-Savini LASIK IOL Power Tool)

# ⯈ REFERENCES

1. Hoffer KJ. Clinical results using the Holladay 2 intraocular lens power formula. J Cataract Refract Surg. 2000;26(8):1233-7.
2. Aristodemou P, Knox Cartwright NE, Sparrow JM, et al. Formula choice: Hoffer Q, Holladay 1, or SRK/T and refractive outcomes in 8108 eyes after cataract surgery with biometry by partial coherence interferometry. J Cataract Refract Surg. 2011;37(1):63-71.
3. Gale RP, Saldana M, Johnston RL, et al. Benchmark standards for refractive outcomes after NHS cataract surgery. Eye (Lond). 2009;23(1):149-52.
4. McCarthy M, Gavanski GM, Paton KE, et al. Intraocular lens power calculations after myopic laser refractive surgery: a comparison of methods in 173 eyes. Ophthalmology. 2011; 118(5):940-4.

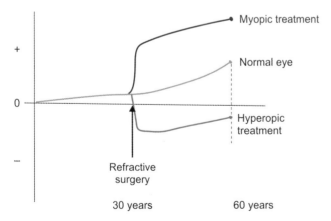

Total eye spherical aberration with age

**Fig. 5:** The cornea naturally has a mild positive spherical aberration which is relatively stable thoughout life. This is canceled out by the negative spherical aberration of the lens in youth giving a total spherical aberration of the eye of near zero in youth. As the lens ages, it gains positive spherical aberration. A myopic laser treatment flattens the cornea, significantly increasing the positive spherical aberration in the eye. A hyperopic treatment steepens the cornea resulting in negative spherical aberration

CHAPTER **108**

5. Rosa N, Capasso L, Lanza M, et al. Axial eye length evaluation before and after myopic photorefractive keratectomy. J Refract Surg. 2005;21(3):281-7.

6. Demirok A, Cinal A, Simsek S, et al. Changes in anterior chamber depth and axial length measurements after radial keratotomy. Eye (Lond). 1999;13:55-8.

7. Winkler von Mohrenfels C, Gabler B, Lohmann CP. Optical bisometry before and after excimer laser epithelial keratomileusis (LASEK) for myopia. Eur J Ophthalmol. 2003;13(3):257-9.

8. Miyata K, Kamiya K, Takahashi T, et al. Time course of changes in corneal forward shift after excimer laser photorefractive keratectomy. Arch Ophthalmol. 2002;120(7):896-900.

9. Lowe RF, Clark BA. Posterior corneal curvature. Correlations in normal eyes and in eyes involved with primary angle-closure glaucoma. Br J Ophthalmol. 1973;57(7):464-70.

10. Hamed AM, Wang L, Misra M, et al. A comparative analysis of five methods of determining corneal refractive power in eyes that have undergone myopic laser in situ keratomileusis. Ophthalmology. 2002;109(4):651-8.

11. Kim JH, Lee DH, Joo CK. Measuring corneal power for intraocular lens power calculation after refractive surgery. Comparison of methods. J Cataract Refract Surg. 2002;28(11):1932-8.

12. Seitz B, Langenbucher A. Intraocular lens calculations status after corneal refractive surgery. Curr Opin Ophthalmol. 2000;11(1):35-46.

13. Seitz B, Langenbucher A, Nguyen NX, et al. Underestimation of intraocular lens power for cataract surgery after myopic photorefractive keratectomy. Ophthalmology. 1999;106(4):693-702.

14. Feiz V, Mannis MJ, Garcia-Ferrer F, et al. Intraocular lens power calculation after laser in situ keratomileusis for myopia and hyperopia: a standardized approach. Cornea. 2001;20(8):792-7.

15. Holladay JT. IOL calculations following radial keratotomy surgery. Refract Corneal Surg. 1989;5(3):36.

16. Hoffer KJ. Calculating intraocular lens power after refractive corneal surgery. Arch Ophthalmol. 2002;120(4):500-1.

17. Aramberri J. Intraocular lens power calculation after corneal refractive surgery: double-K method. J Cataract Refract Surg. 2003;29(11):2063-8.

18. Koch DD, Wang L. Calculating IOL power in eyes that have had refractive surgery. J Cataract Refract Surg. 2003;29(11):2039-42.

19. Walter KA, Gagnon MR, Hoopes PC, et al. Accurate intraocular lens power calculation after myopic laser in situ keratomileusis, bypassing corneal power. J Cataract Refract Surg. 2006;32(3):425-9.

20. Masket S, Masket SE. Simple regression formula for intraocular lens power adjustment in eyes requiring cataract surgery after excimer laser photoablation. J Cataract Refract Surg. 2006;32(3):430-4.

21. Wang L, Hill WE, Koch DD. Evaluation of intraocular lens power prediction methods using the American Society of Cataract and Refractive Surgeons Post-Keratorefractive Intraocular Lens Power Calculator. J Cataract Refract Surg. 2010;36(9):1466-73.

22. Latkany RA, Chokshi AR, Speaker MG, et al. Intraocular lens calculations after refractive surgery. J Cataract Refract Surg. 2005;31(3):562-70.

23. Zeh WG, Koch DD. Comparison of contact lens overrefraction and standard keratometry for measuring corneal curvature in eyes with lenticular opacity. J Cataract Refract Surg. 1999;25(7):898-903.

24. Wang L, Booth MA, Koch DD. Comparison of intraocular lens power calculation methods in eyes that have undergone LASIK. Ophthalmology. 2004;111(10):1825-31.

25. Shammas HJ, Shammas MC, Garabet A, et al. Correcting the corneal power measurements for intraocular lens power calculations after myopic laser in situ keratomileusis. Am J Ophthalmol. 2003;136(3):426-32.

26. Haigis W. Intraocular lens calculation after refractive surgery for myopia: Haigis-L formula. J Cataract Refract Surg. 2008;34(10):1658-63.

27. Ferrara G, Cennamo G, Marotta G, et al. New formula to calculate corneal power after refractive surgery. J Refract Surg. 2004;20(5):465-71.

28. Geggel HS. Pachymetric ratio no-history method for intraocular lens power adjustment after excimer laser refractive surgery. Ophthalmology. 2009;116(6):1057-66.

29. Mackool RJ. The cataract extraction-refraction-implantation technique for IOL power calculation in difficult cases. J Cataract Refract Surg. 1998;24(4):434-5.

30. Mackool RJ, Ko W, Mackool R. Intraocular lens power calculation after laser in situ keratomileusis: aphakic refraction technique. J Cataract Refract Surg. 2006;32(3):435-7.

31. Ianchulev T, Salz J, Hoffer K, et al. Intraoperative optical refractive biometry for intraocular lens power estimation without axial length and keratometry measurements. J Cataract Refract Surg. 2005;31(8):1530-6.

# Light-Adjustable Lenses Postcorneal Refractive Surgery

*Guillermo Rocha, Zale D Mednick*

## ❖ INTRODUCTION

Incisional corneal refractive procedures such as radial and astigmatic keratotomy, developed in the early 1980s, have been followed in increasing popularity by excimer laser refractive procedures. With laser-assisted *in situ* keratomileusis (LASIK) entering its 3rd decade, surgeons are being faced with the reality that many of these patients are now reaching the age of cataract surgery. Refractive surgery has become an increasingly safer and effective proposition since its inception in 1990, with both patients and surgeons expecting excellent predictability in the results.[1] Conversely, when faced with the prospect of inevitable cataract surgery, now patients and surgeons must face a new reality: the fact that our lens power calculations in these circumstances are less than adequate.

In this chapter, we explore a new paradigm in the management of postrefractive surgery patients. We will review basic concepts in intraocular lens (IOL) calculations, the challenges faced in postrefractive surgery lens calculation and discuss the light-adjustable lens technology as a means to raise the bar in the predictability of these cases.

## ❖ BASIC CONCEPTS IN IOL CALCULATION

As cataract surgery has progressed, surgeons have become more concerned with IOL calculations. The advent of microincision cataract surgery technology has afforded the ability to use smaller incisions. This, in turn, has yielded less astigmatic induction following cataract surgery.[2-4] That, coupled with the use of partial coherence interferometry with instruments, such as the Zeiss IOL Master (Carl Zeiss, Germany), has allowed surgeons to increase the predictability of refractive results.[2,5] This has not always been the case. In a review by Apple (2006), the humble beginnings of cataract surgery were explored. The review focused on Harold Ridley, who performed the first IOL implantation in 1949. This first implantation resulted in a postoperative refraction of −20 diopters (D), a result that is almost unthinkable in modern ophthalmology.[6] Even in the 1980s, some surgeons still used the single IOL approach, a model in which surgeons exclusively inserted a +19.0 D lens in all patients, based on Gullstrand's schematic eye. Achieving a postoperative refraction accurate enough to obviate the need for glasses was not even a consideration; it was simply the expectation that glasses would be needed following cataract surgery.

Over the years, many formulas have been used to increase the predictability of IOL calculations following cataract surgery. There are two basic categories of calculations used to determine the IOL power that should be used in cataract surgery: the theoretical formulas and the statistical/regression formulas. The theoretical optical formulas include thin lens formulas, thick lens formulas and exact ray tracing or wavefront technique formulas.[2,7-10] Modern theoretical formulas include the Haigis, Hoffer Q, and Holladay 2 IOL calculation formulas. These formulas take several variables into account: IOL power, keratometric readings, axial length, effective lens position (ELP), postoperative refraction, and vertex distance for postoperative refraction.[11] The ELP is the only one of these variables that cannot be formally measured, and as such, the focus of new theoretical formulas is to most accurately predict the ELP.[11]

The statistical/regression model includes the Sanders Retzlaff Kraff SRK-1 and SRK-2 formulas. These formulas, developed in the 1980s, estimate the power of the IOL implant based on an A-constant provided by the manufacturer and take into account keratometry readings as well as axial length.[2,12] An example is PIOL = A − [(0.9 × K) + (2.5 × AL)], where PIOL = power of the IOL; A = A-constant provided by the manufacturer; K = keratometry readings and AL = axial length. This most basic equation, while fairly simple mathematically, allows a straightforward understanding of some of the factors relevant in lens calculations, and the effect of the error in measuring them. In theory, a 1mm error in AL measurement would result in a 2.50 D lens calculation error. The SRK-2 formula largely replaced the theoretical models due to its easier derivation and use.[5] Binkhorst later modified these earlier SRK formulas to obtain the SRK-T formula, which became more popular in the 1990s.[13]

As technology has improved, so has the ability to measure multiple variables and factors during IOL calculation. Surgeons have enjoyed increasing refractive predictability when moving from A-scan biometry, to A-scan immersion biometry, and furthermore, with different permutations and software changes using partial coherence interferometry. The caveats now include precise measurement of the corneal power, accurate measurement of the axial length, the appropriate predication of postoperative anterior chamber depth (ACD), the refractive effect of the IOL implant itself, and finally optimization and accuracy of the results.

No keratometer measures corneal power directly, but rather the size of the reflected corneal image. This in and of itself represents a caveat in measurement of corneal power. Measurement of the axial length is different when partial coherence interferometry is employed compared to ultrasound biometry.[2] Instruments such as the IOL Master target the retinal pigment epithelium as the end point in axial length measurement, while ultrasonic devices target the internal limiting membrane. Prediction of the postoperative ACD and refractive effect of the IOL are also important variables that must be considered when predicting postoperative refraction. As outlined in the review by Olsen, optimization and accuracy involve several factors, including the role of the capsulorrhexis, as described by Gimbel and Neuhann, and the accuracy of IOL power calculation.[2,14] In Olsen's review, the distribution of the prediction error was analyzed by comparing three types of IOLs.[2] It was evident that although the calculations resulted in high predictability, there was still a spread in outcomes even when considering optical, regression and SRK-1 regression formulas.

In addition to the factors mentioned above, there are other variables, such as corneal radius, axial length, postoperative ACD and IOL power, where errors as little as 1 unit, either in millimeters or diopters depending on the variable, may result in a range of refractive errors from 0.67 to 5.7 D.[2] To further compound the problem, even if all calculations were perfect, there would still be the issue of IOL manufacturing. For example, manufacturers often state that the ACD measurements reported for their lenses are simply estimates. This is because the ACD is dependent on each individual eye, and thus it is not possible for the single ACD measurement provided by the manufacturer to accurately reflect how the lens will behave within the eye.[8] Using this estimated ACD value for a specific lens can result in up to 2.0 D of inaccurate estimation of IOL power.[8] It is possible that a 0.25 D error during the manufacturing process, combined with a 0.25 error in calculation, would result, even before the surgical intervention, in a 0.50 D error from the expected result. The concept of fine-tuning this aspect of the procedure becomes, then, an intriguing proposition.

The increased popularity of the excimer laser in refractive surgery has also strengthened the ability to predict refractive outcomes. Outcome results amongst refractive surgeons revolve around percentages of eyes at or above 20/20, and even 20/16 of uncorrected vision. Refractively, high numbers of eyes are expected to have predictability within the ±0.25 and ±0.50 D ranges. Therefore, the bar has been raised in terms of refractive predictability for both cataract and refractive surgery. In spite of this, Olsen states that with current technology, the IOL refractive predictability would be (reasonably) expected at ±1.0 D in about 90% of eyes and ±2.0 D in 99.9% of eyes.[2]

## ▶ IOL CALCULATION AFTER CORNEAL REFRACTIVE SURGERY

The cornea has two refracting surfaces, and both need to be taken into account in order to calculate corneal power accurately. Eyes that have previously undergone refractive surgery are less amenable to accurate keratometry measurements, due to alterations of these corneal surfaces. Standard keratometry uses four corneal focal points in the paracentral region to obtain its measurement of corneal power. Keratometry, however, becomes inaccurate for corneas that have undergone refractive surgery, because such corneas have experienced a flattening or steepening in the central cornea.[15] Seitz and Langenbucher further outlined that not only does refractive surgery alter the nature of the cornea, but different types of refractive surgery have differing effects on the new corneal measurements.[16] Specifically, excimer laser procedures, such as LASIK and photorefractive keratectomy (PRK) result in different corneal properties when compared to radial keratotomy, in which peripheral relaxing incisions produce a central flattening of the cornea without the removal of central corneal tissue.[16] Based on these findings, it is evident that when using the excimer laser, the relationship between the front and back surfaces of the cornea will be different than that obtained following radial keratotomy.

Many methods have been described to accurately calculate the proper IOL power to be inserted into eyes that have previously undergone refractive surgeries. One group of refractive calculations includes strategies that rely on accessing patient's past optical measurements before they had refractive surgery.[17-19] Some of these methods include the clinical history method, the Feiz-Mannis method, the Hamed method, the Aramberri double-K method, the Latkany method, the Masket method, and the Wake Forest method.[17,20-26] Other methods are more practical, avoiding reliance on past optical history. Among these are the Shammas method, the Maloney/Wang method, the Smith method, the Savini method, and the Ianchulev method.[17,27-31] The inconsistency amongst these various calculations is reflected by the Consensus K technique, which is based on determining a mean of the K values obtained by some of these other formulas.[32]

McCarthy et al. published a study regarding IOL power calculations following myopic laser refractive surgery.[33] The authors compared methods in 173 eyes post myopic laser refractive surgery. They included several of the methods described above, such as the clinical history method, Aramberri Double-K method, Latkany Flat-K, Feiz-Mannis, R Factor, corneal bypass, Masket, Haigis-L, Shammas.cd, and optical version formulas. They compared this against the benchmark of standards for refractive outcomes following cataract surgery that was published by the National Health Services (NHS) in England.[34] Interestingly, the IOL calculation predictability set as a standard by the NHS mentioned that 55% of eyes should be within ± 0.50 D of the targeted outcome, while 85% of eyes should be within 1 D of the desired outcome.[32] McCarthy's study showed that on the high predictability end, 58.8% of eyes were within 0.50 D, and 84.5% were within 1 D of the desired outcome. At the other extreme, low predictability results included 53.8% of eyes within half a diopter, and 80.9% of eyes within 1 D of the desired outcome.[33] This is outlined in Table 1.

**Table 1:** IOL calculation predictability

| Report | ±0.25 D | ±0.50 D | ±1.00 D | ±2.00 D |
|---|---|---|---|---|
| Olsen 2007 | | | 90% | 99.9% |
| NHS Stds | | 55% | 85% | |
| McCarthy(H) | | 58.8% | 84.5% | |
| McCarthy(L) | | 53.8% | 80.9% | |
| Chayet LAL* | 93% | 100% | | |

*FDA Phase I: Sphere Adjustment. Data courtesy of Arturo Chayet, MD. See text for references.
NHS: National Health Services; LAL: Light-adjustable lens

The question then becomes whether surgeons can do better and improve on these refractive aspects. Scheimpflug imaging with instruments such as the Pentacam (Oculus, Germany) provides images of the front and posterior aspects of the cornea (Fig. 1). These are true elevation maps that can be correlated clinically. In particular, by utilizing the Pentacam's Holladay report, which includes equivalent K readings at the 4 mm zone, keratometry values can be combined with axial length and white-to-white measurements from the IOL Master and inputted into the Holladay 2 formula from the Holladay IOL Consultant software.

As an example, we will discuss the case of an individual who underwent successful PRK in 1994, once for the right eye and with two enhancements for the left eye. The preoperative refraction for the right eye was −9.50 − 0.50 × 120 and for the left eye −7.50 D. Our typical patient discussion includes the fact that IOL calculation predictability is quite challenging following laser refractive surgery. Intraocular lens master version 5.4.3 with the postrefractive module was employed. Pentacam with the Holladay equivalent K reading report was used to obtain the K readings, and these were inputted into the Holladay 2 formula. Different printouts were compared, and the discussion explored the options of further vision correction following cataract surgery with the excimer laser, IOL exchange or a piggyback lens.

Postoperatively, uncorrected vision in the right eye for this patient was 20/32, with a refraction of +0.75 + 0.50 x 85 resulting in a corrected vision of 20/16 + 2. The left eye obtained an uncorrected visual acuity of 20/16 and was plano. While the result was better than expected, the patient wanted an enhancement for the right eye, which bares the notion that surgeons could still do better in terms of refractive predictability.

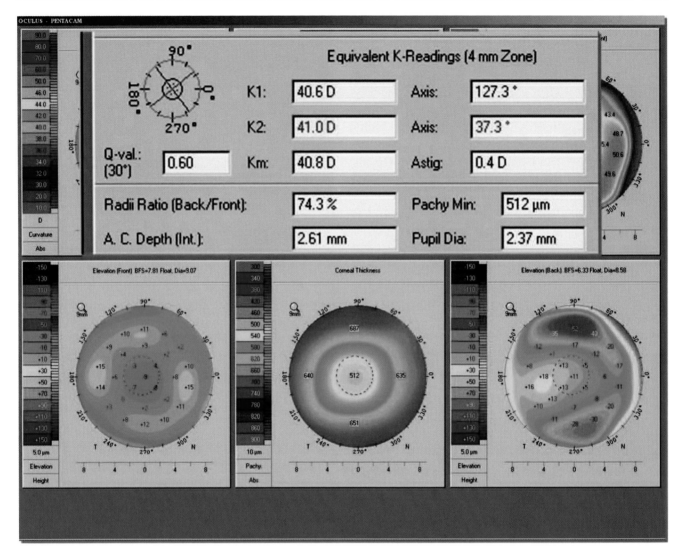

**Fig. 1:** Equivalent K readings from the Holladay display (Pentacam)

## LIGHT-ADJUSTABLE LENS TECHNOLOGY

The light adjustable lens (LAL) is a recent exciting innovation in cataract surgery. Developed by Calhoun Vision Inc (Pasadena, CA), it is the first ever lens to allow for noninvasive power adjustment postimplantation. Essentially, the lens material is amenable to alteration postoperatively, such that the lens power can be changed in order to achieve a more optimal refractive outcome.

The LAL material was originally developed by Dr Robert Grubbs, the 2005 nobel prize winner in Chemistry. The LAL is composed of photosensitive silicone macromers embedded in an ultraviolet (UV) absorbing silicone lens matrix.[35] Upon exposure to UV light, the photoreactive macromers being targeted by the light are photopolymerized. A gradient then develops between the irradiated and nonirradiated macromers of the lens. Adhering to the principle of diffusion, the nonirradiated macromers disperse towards the photopolymerized part of the lens. This causes lens swelling and leads to a change in the shape, and thus, the power of the lens (Figs 2 and 3).[35,36]

The unique features of this lens are exploited during the ensuing weeks following implantation. Once the lens is implanted using standard phacoemulsification techniques, the light delivery device (LDD) is utilized to customize the power of the lens. The LDD has been designed on a standard slit lamp platform, with unlimited flexibility for lens modification (Fig. 4). It consists of a digital mirror

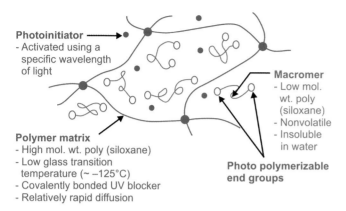

**Photoinitiator**
- Activated using a specific wavelength of light

**Macromer**
- Low mol. wt. poly (siloxane)
- Nonvolatile
- Insoluble in water

**Polymer matrix**
- High mol. wt. poly (siloxane)
- Low glass transition temperature (~ −125°C)
- Covalently bonded UV blocker
- Relatively rapid diffusion

**Photo polymerizable end groups**

Fig. 2: Description of the light-adjustable lens technology
*Source*: Courtesy of Calhoun Vision, Inc

device, which allows customized generation of spatial irradiance profiles. Following surgery, patients are requested to wear UV protecting glasses at all times, both indoors and outdoors, in order to prevent premature unrestricted photopolymerization of the material (Hengerer, 2010). The specific UV treatment parameters, the irradiation dose and spatial irradiation pattern, are altered based on the patient's postoperative refraction in order to achieve the desired change in lens power.[35]

Two weeks after surgery, one or two adjustment treatments are performed on separate occasions, which involve UV light application to alter the lens shape, as explained above. If the desired refraction is achieved following one adjustment treatment, there is no need for a second. Adjustment profiles currently include negative, positive, and toric adjustment (Fig. 5). Twenty-four to forty-eight hours following these adjustments, one or two lock-in treatments are performed, during which UV light is applied to solidify the lens' new shape. Twenty-four hours

following the completion of the second lock-in treatment, patients can stop wearing the UV protecting glasses.

*In vitro* safety studies have shown that in terms of cytotoxicity, sensitization and genotoxicity, this lens meets safety requirements of the industry. *In vivo* animal studies as well as human clinical studies have demonstrated the safety and efficacy of this lens and the implantation material. Studies of the LAL in a rabbit model demonstrated that the UV light exposure does not result in retinal toxicity.[37] The study by Lichtinger et al. diffused concerns that the UV light leads to any more endothelial damage than is incurred in standard cataract surgery.[38]

Typically, patients need to be screened preoperatively for the absence of other conditions aside from cataract, which may compromise the position of the lens, such as pseudoexfoliation syndrome or the ability to deliver the ultraviolet light. For this reason, it is imperative that all patients be screened for the ability to have dilated pupils of 7 mm or more.

Clinically, the results achieved with the LAL have been very encouraging. Up to 2 D of correction for myopia, hyperopia, and astigmatism are possible with this nontoxic and biocompatible material. A pilot study by Chayet et al. showed that 93% of LAL patients achieved a refraction of less than 0.25 D of the intended refraction, and 100% of participants were within 0.5 D of the intended refraction at 9 months postoperatively (Table 1).[35] Salgado et al. conducted a study on 20 eyes, in which all patients were within 0.5 D of the intended refraction at 6 months postoperatively. Furthermore, the spherical equivalent was reduced from + 0.39 D preadjustments, to −0.07 D at 6 months postadjustments.[39] A more recent study of 21 eyes by Hengerer et al. further confirmed these positive results: 96% of eyes were within 0.5 D of the intended

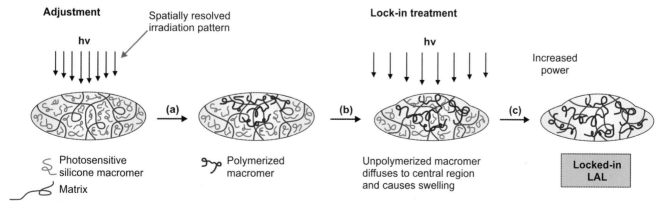

**Adjustment**

Spatially resolved irradiation pattern

hv

**Lock-in treatment**

hv

Increased power

(a)    (b)    (c)

Photosensitive silicone macromer

Matrix

Polymerized macromer

Unpolymerized macromer diffuses to central region and causes swelling

Locked-in LAL

Fig. 3: Mechanism of power adjustment
*Source*: Courtesy of Calhoun Vision, Inc

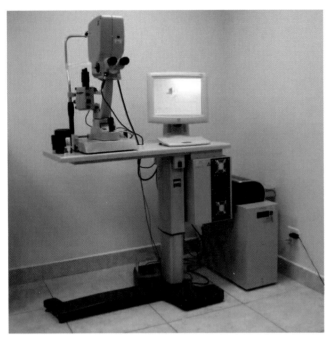

**Fig. 4:** Light delivery device
*Source*: Courtesy of Calhoun Vision, Inc

refraction, and 81% had a predictability of 0.25 D.[40] Such postoperative refractions significantly exceed the predictions set by Olsen in 2007 and the benchmarks established by the NHS Standards.[2,34] The refractive benefits are not limited to myopic correction; Chayet et al. showed that residual hyperopia after cataract surgery, from +0.25 D to +2.0 D, could be significantly improved via UV adjustments.[41]

These optimal refractive results have translated into equally positive visual acuities. In the study by Von Mohrenfels et al. all eyes gained 2 or more lines of corrected visual acuity, while 81% of eyes in the study by Hengerer et al. improved by 2 or more lines.[42,43]

Light-adjustable lens technology provides certain unique features. For example, the LAL offers the option for presbyopic corrections. Multifocality is possible, as well as the creation of central near add or asphericity treatments as a third adjustment protocol. The LAL is also conducive to creating monovision, with the added bonus of being able to eliminate this feature if the patient becomes averse to it. If the patient is not agreeable to the monovision, a further correction can be made within a two-week period to convert the refraction to emmetropia. The LAL may prove particularly valuable in cases of astigmatism. Using the LAL, toric corrections are based directly on the postoperative position of the lens and the manifest refraction (Fig. 6). Thus far, such astigmatic corrections appear to be promising. In the first 13 eyes treated by one of the authors

(GR), mean refractive spherical equivalent (MRSE) of all of the eyes was within 0.25 D of the expected outcome following adjustment and lock-in treatments. The reduction of cylinder was also dramatic, with only one patient having up to 0.5 D of cylinder following the adjustment and no eyes having more than 1.0 D of residual cylinder (Figs 7, 8 and 9).

## ► LIGHT-ADJUSTABLE LENS POSTREFRACTIVE SURGERY

The benefits of using the LAL in patients who have previously undergone refractive surgery are obvious. As already explored in depth, it is difficult to determine the accurate corneal power in an eye that has had prior corneal alterations, such as in refractive surgery. The LAL allows the flexibility of decreased precision of preoperative measurement of corneal power. The ophthalmologist no longer needs to strive for emmetropia right off the bat in these complicated cases; one can simply rely on the properties of the LAL and plan to adjust the corneal power postoperatively.

In the following two cases, we propose a new paradigm for the use of LALs after corneal refractive surgery.

### Case 1–RE

A 55-year-old Caucasian male presented to our office with a diagnosis of a left visually significant posterior subcapsular cataract. He had been a patient at our clinic and had previously received bilateral wavefront LASIK seven years before. His pre-LASIK refraction for the right eye was −7.00 + 2.00 × 130 = 20/20. For the left eye, it was −7.25 + 1.75 × 65 = 20/20.

The LASIK procedure was uneventful and performed using an Amadeus microkeratome as well as a Visx Star S4 CustomVue excimer laser (AMO, California). He presented on January 12, 2011 with a plano correction in the right eye, giving him 20/20 vision, and a refraction of −1.25 − 0.50 × 178 in the left eye, giving him a vision of 20/40. A visually significant cataract was diagnosed, with a component of posterior subcapsular opacity. Due to his job as a truck driver, the decision was made to proceed with surgery.

Several options were discussed, but a LAL implant was used. The calculation involved performing Pentacam and iTrace analysis. From the Pentacam analysis, the Holladay equivalent K readings were obtained, and this, in combination with IOL master biometry, and the use of the Holladay 2 formula, yielded a lens power of +18.0 D. The predicted refractive value was 0.07 D.

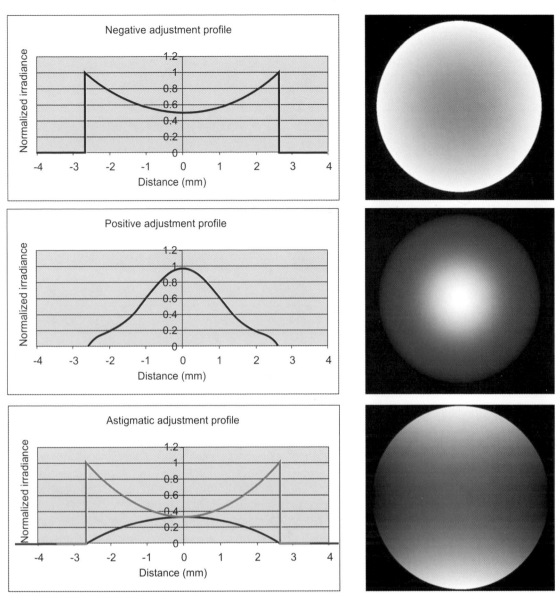

**Fig. 5:** Adjustment profiles
*Source*: Courtesy of Calhoun Vision, Inc

In March 2011, surgery was performed. Two weeks were allowed to elapse before adjustment. Preadjustment measurements included a distance uncorrected visual acuity of 20/40 and a refraction of $+0.75 + 0.50 \times 125 = 20/16$ (Table 2). After the second lock-in treatment, uncorrected visual acuity was 20/20 with a manifest refraction of plano. Near visual acuity was measured at J6.

## Case 2–RS

A 56-year-old Caucasian male underwent successful hyperopic PRK in the left eye in 1997 for a correction of $+3.00 + 2.50 \times 82 = 20/30$. There was documented mild amblyopia in this eye. He was then referred to our clinic in 1999 for a LASIK procedure in the right eye. Preoperative correction in the right eye was $+2.25 + 0.25 \times 113 = 20/20$ and was treated successfully. He presented again to our office on December 9, 2010, now with a cataract in the left eye. Visual acuity was 20/16 in the right eye, with a correction of $+1.50$. Visual acuity was 20/40 in the left eye, with a refraction of $+2.25 + 0.50 \times 35$. He was diagnosed with a nuclear sclerotic cataract, and the option of a LAL was discussed. In addition, it was discussed that the presence of mild amblyopia would limit the final visual acuity result.

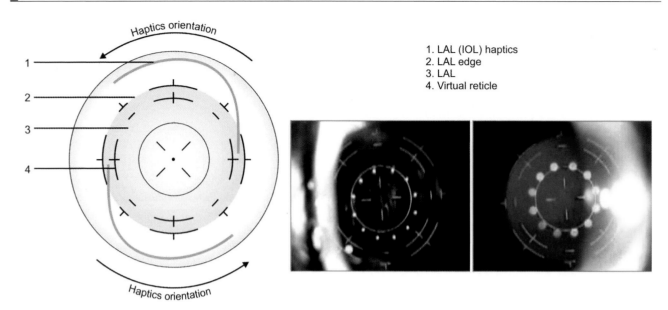

1. LAL (IOL) haptics
2. LAL edge
3. LAL
4. Virtual reticle

**Fig. 6:** Reticle-IOL alignment. This ensures that UV light adjustment for both sphere and cylinder is based in the stabilized lens position
*Source*: Courtesy of Calhoun Vision, Inc

Intraocular lens calculation was performed using a similar approach with the Holladay equivalent K readings from the Pentacam analysis. That, in addition to the IOL Master data, and input into the Holladay IOL consultant and Holladay 2 formula, yielded a proposed lens of +23.0 D with a predicted refraction of +0.24 D (with LAL it is preferable to target for slight hyperopia). Cataract surgery was performed in March of 2011 and was uneventful. Prior to adjustments, uncorrected visual acuity was 20/40 in the left eye, and a refraction of −0.75 resulted in a vision of 20/30 + 2. Following second adjustment and lock-in treatments, his uncorrected visual acuity in the left eye was 20/32 with a near vision of J2. His refraction was −0.75. It was interesting that at one point prior to the second lock-in,

visual acuity improved to an uncorrected and best corrected level of 20/25. This case demonstrates the flexibility of the technology, in that when an adequate result is obtained, lock-in can ensure such outcome is maintained (Table 3).

The authors have since added a third postrefractive surgery case to their database (manuscript in preparation for publication). The end result was once again very precise, with a +0.25 correction, and uncorrected vision of 20/20 following the use of LAL.

Lawrence Brierley has recently reported on the precision of IOL refractive power adjustment of LALs in postrefractive surgery patients which included eyes from Victoria, British Columbia (Brierley); Brandon, Manitoba (Rocha); and Tijuana, Mexico (Chayet) for a total of 16 eyes.

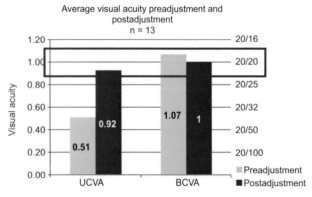

**Fig. 7:** Refractive results in 13 eyes implanted with the Calhoun LAL. Visual acuity after final adjustment

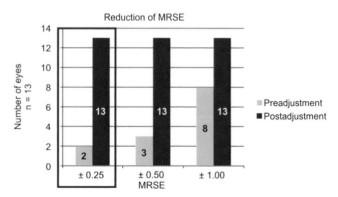

**Fig. 8:** Refractive results in 13 eyes implanted with the Calhoun LAL. Reduction in MRSE

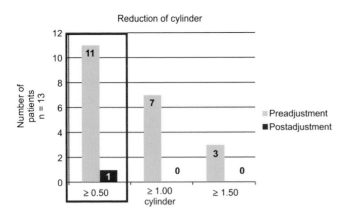

**Fig. 9:** Refractive results in 13 eyes implanted with the Calhoun LAL. Reduction in cylinder

This was presented at the Annual Meeting of the Canadian Ophthalmological Society on Sunday, June 12, 2011. Based on these initial results, the cumulative data of these 16 eyes yielded a predictability of 75% of eyes within 0.25 D, and 94% of eyes within 0.5 D of the desired outcome. These results suggest that LALs result in superior predictability in postrefractive surgery eyes, when compared to the study by Wang et al. which evaluated refractive predictability in postrefractive eyes that did not receive LALs.[44] As such, the approach of the authors is now to include the implantation of LALs in postcorneal refractive surgery patients.

**Table 2:** Case 1

| Visit | UCDVA | M Rx | BCDVA | Near VA |
|---|---|---|---|---|
| Preadjustment 1 | 20/40 | +0.75 + 0.50 x 125 | 20/16 | J10 |
| Preadjustment 2 | 20/16 | −0.25 | 20/16 | J6 |
| Prelock-in 1 | 20/20 | +0.25 | 20/16 | J6 |
| Prelock-in 2 | 20/16 + 1 | +0.25 | 20/16 | J5 |

UCDVA: Uncorrected Distance Visual Acuity; BCDVA: Best Corrected Distance Visual Acuity

**Table 3:** Case 2

| Visit | UCDVA | M Rx | BCDVA | Near VA |
|---|---|---|---|---|
| Preadjustment 1 | 20/40 | −0.75 | 20/32+2 | J2 |
| Preadjustment 2 | 20/40 | −0.75 | 20/40+1 | J2 |
| Prelock-in 1 | 20/25 | −0.50 | 20/25 | J2 |
| Prelock-in 2 | 20/32 | −0.75 | 20/32 | J2 |

UCDVA: Uncorrected Distance Visual Acuity; BCDVA: Best Corrected Distance Visual Acuity

In conclusion, the light-adjustable lens predictability achieves excellent distance visual acuity through accurate correction of defocus and astigmatism, and this translates into clinically successful results in postrefractive surgery eyes. With this, the age of true refractive corneal and cataract surgery has been entered.

## ACKNOWLEDGMENT

We would like to thank Patrick Casey (OD), Calhoun Vision Inc, for all of his help in analyzing and collecting the data presented in this chapter.

*Note*: The authors have no proprietary or financial interests in any aspect of this study.

## REFERENCES

1. Pallikaris IG, Papatzanaki ME, Stathi EZ, et al. Laser in situ keratomileusis. Lasers Surg Med. 1990;10 (5):463-8.
2. Olsen T. Calculation of intraocular lens power: a review. Acta Ophthalmol. Scand. 2007;85:472-85.
3. Olson RJ, Crandall AS. Prospective randomized comparison of phacoemulsification cataract surgery with a 3.2 mm vs a 5.5 mm sutureless incision. Am J Ophthalmol. 1998;125:612-20.
4. Kershner RM. Sutureless one-handed intercapsular phacoemulsification. The key-hole technique. J Cataract Refract Surg. 1991;17:719-25.
5. Drexler W, Findle O, Menapace R, et al. Partial coherence interferometry: a novel approach to biometry in cataract surgery. Am J Ophthalmol. 1998;126:524-34.
6. Apple DJ. Sir Harold Ridley and his fight for sight. Thorofare, NJ: Slack Inc. 2006.
7. Jin H, Rabsilber T, Ehmer A, et al. Comparison of ray-tracing method and thin-lens formula in intraocular lens power calculations. J Cataract Refract Surg. 2009;35:650-62.
8. Preussner PR, Wahl J, Lahdo H, et al. Ray tracing for intraocular lens calculation. J Cataract Refract Surg. 2002;28:1412-9.
9. Norrby S, Lydahl E, Koranyi G, et al. Clinical application of the lens haptic plane concept with transformed axial lengths. J Cataract Refract Surg. 2005;31:1338-44.
10. Norrby S. Using the lens haptic plane concept and thick-lens ray tracing to calculate intraocular lens power. J Cataract Refract Surg. 2004;30:1000-5.
11. Hamilton DR, Hardeten DR. Cataract surgery in patients with prior refractive surgery. Curr Opin Ophthalmol. 2003;14:44-53.
12. Sanders DR, Kraff MC. Improvement of intraocular lens power calculation using empirical data. J Am Intraocul Implant Soc. 1980;6(3):263-7.
13. Binkhorst RD. Intraocular lens power calculation. Int Ophthalmol Clin. 1979;19:237-52.
14. Gimbel HV, Neuhann T. Continuous curvilinear capsulorhexis. J Cataract Refract Surg. 1991;17:110-1.
15. Wang L, Jackson DW, Koch DD. Methods of estimating corneal refractive power after hyperopic laser in situ keratomileusis. J Cataract Refract Surg. 2002;28:954-61.

16. Seitz B, Langenbucher A. Intraocular lens calculations status after corneal refractive surgery. Curr Opin Ophthalmol. 2000;11:35-46.

17. Naseri A, McLeod SD. Cataract surgery after refractive surgery. Curr Opin Ophthalmol. 2010;21:35-8.

18. Sutton GL, Kim P. Laser in situ keratomileusis in 2010—a review. Clin Experiment Ophthalmol. 2010;38:192-210.

19. Diehl JW, Yu F, Olson MD, et al. Intraocular lens power adjustment nomogram after laser in situa keratomileusis. J Cataract Refract Surg. 2009;35:1587-90.

20. Holladay JT. IOL calculations following RK. Refract Corneal Surg. 1989;5:203.

21. Feiz V, Mannis MJ, Garcia-Ferrer F, et al. Intraocular lens power calculation after laser in situ keratomileusis for myopia and hyperopia: a standardized approach. Corneal. 2001;20:792-7.

22. Hamed AM, Wang L, Misra M, et al. A comparative analysis of five methods of determining corneal refractive power in eyes that have undergone myopic laser in situ keratomileusis Ophthalmology. 2002;109:651-8.

23. Aramberri J. Intraocular lens power calculation after corneal refractive surgery: double-K method. J Cataract Refract Surg. 2003;29:792-7.

24. Latkany RA, Chokshi AR, Speaker MG, et al. Intraocular lens calculations after refractive surgery. J Cataract Refract Surg. 2005;31:562-70.

25. Masket S, Masket SE. Simple regression formula for intraocular lens power adjustment in eyes requiring cataract surgery after excimer laser photoablation. J Cataract Refract Surg. 2006;32:430-4.

26. Walter KA, Gagnon MR, Hoopes PC, et al. Accurate intraocular lens power calculation after myopic laser in situ keratomileusis, bypassing corneal power. J Cataract Refract Surg. 2006;32:425-9.

27. Shammas HJ, Shammas MC, Garabet A, et al. Correcting the corneal power measurements for intraocular lens power calculations after myopic laser in situ keratomileusis. Am J Ophthalmol. 2003;136:426-32.

28. Wang L, Booth MA, Koch DD. Comparison of intraocular lens power calculations methods in eyes that have undergone LASIK. Ophthalmology. 2004;11:1825-31.

29. Smith RJ, Chan WK, Maloney RK. The prediction of surgically induced refractive change from corneal topography. Am J Ophthalmol. 1998;125:44-53.

30. Savini G, Barboni P, Zanini M. Intraocular lens power calculation after myopic refractive surgery: theoretical comparison of different methods. Ophthalmology. 2006;113:1271-82.

31. Ianchulev T, Salz J, Hoffer K, et al. Intraoperative optical refractive biometry for intraocular lens power estimation without axial length and keratometry measurments. J Cataract Refract Surg. 2005;31:1530-6.

32. Randleman JB, Foster JB, Loupe DN, et al. Intraocular lens power calculations after refractive surgery: Consensus-K technique. J Cataract Refract Surg. 2007;33:1892-8.

33. McCarthy M, Gavanski GM, Paton KE, et al. Intraocular lens power calculations after myopic laser refractive surgery: a comparison of methods in 173 eyes. Ophthalmology. 2011;118(5):940-4.

34. Gale RP, Saldana M, Johnston RL, et al. Benchmark standards for refractive outcomes after NHS cataract surgery. Eye (Lond). 2009;23:149-52.

35. Chayet A, Sandstedt C, Chang S, et al. Correction of myopia after cataract surgery with a light-adjustable lens. Ophthalmology. 2009;116:1432-5.

36. Hengerer FH, Mellein AC, Buchner SE, et al. The light-adjustable lens: principles and clinical application. Ophthalmologe. 2009;106(3):260-4.

37. Werner L, Chang W, Haymore J, et al. Retinal safety of the irradiation delivered to light-adjustable intraocular lenses evaluated in a rabbit model. J Cataract Refract Surg. 2010;36:1392-7.

38. Lichtinger A, Sandstedt C, Padilla K, et al. Corneal endothelial safety after ultraviolet light treatment of the light-adjustable intraocular lens. J Cataract Refract Surg. 2011;37:324-7.

39. Salgado JP, Khoramnia R, Schweiger B, et al. Six-month clinical results with the light adjustable lens. Klinische Monatsblatter fur Augenheilkunde. 2010;227(12):966-70.

40. Hengerer RH, Hutz WW, Dick HB, et al. Combined correction of sphere and astigmatism using the light-adjustable intraocular lens in eyes with axial myopia. J Cataract Refract Surg. 2011;37(2):317-23.

41. Chayet A, Sandstedt CA, Chang SH, et al. Correction of residual hyperopia after cataract surgery using the light adjustable intraocular lens technology. Am J Ophthalmol. 2009;147:392-7.

42. Von Mohrenfels CW, Salgado J, Khoramnia R, et al. Clinical results with the light adjustable intraocular lens after cataract surgery. J Refract Surg. 2010;26(5):314-20.

43. Hengerer FH, Conrad-Hengerer I, Buchner SE, et al. Evaluation of the Calhoun vision UV light adjustable lens implanted following cataract removal. Journal of Refractive Surgery. 2010;26(10):716-21.

44. Wang L, Hill W, Koch DD. Evaluation of intraocular lens power prediction methods using the American Society of Cataract and Refractive Surgeons Post-Keratorefractive Intraocular Lens Power Calculator. J Cataract Refract Surg. 2010;36:1466-73.

# SECTION 17

# Femtosecond Laser Applications in Anterior Segment Surgery

## CHAPTERS

# Femtosecond Continuous Curvilinear Capsulorhexis

*John P Berdahl*

## ‣ INTRODUCTION

Cataract surgery is the most common ophthalmic surgical procedure worldwide[1] and has helped millions of patients receive better eyesight. The core steps of cataract surgery are: (1) incision, (2) capsulotomy, (3) nuclear fragmentation, (4) cortical removal, and (5) intraocular lens (IOL) insertion.[2] Femtosecond lasers have been approved and are currently in use worldwide for the first three of these steps. Femtosecond lasers have been used extensively in ophthalmology, primarily for creating LASIK (laser-assisted *in situ* keratomileusis) flaps, but to a lesser degree with corneal transplantation. The ability to precisely separate tissue in a very controlled way has led to the rapid adoption of femtosecond technology. As of this writing, femtosecond technology is just starting to be applied to cataract surgery and there are currently four laser platforms that have been approved or are in clinical trials in the United States for use during cataract surgery for the creation of the continuous curvilinear capsulorhexis (CCC) and other steps of the cataract process. We will focus on using a femtosecond laser in the creation of the CCC.

## ‣ HISTORY OF CONTINUOUS CURVILINEAR CAPSULORHEXIS

Thomas Neuhann first developed the original CCC technique, presenting it at the German Society of Ophthalmology meeting in 1985 and publishing a description of the technique in a German medical journal in 1987.[3] Fercho and Shimizu presented similar approaches in 1986 and 1987 respectively.[4] Neuhann coined the term capsulorhexis, deriving its suffix from the Greek 'rhexis' (to tear), to describe the technique.

The CCC is vitally important for cataract surgery because a properly-sized, shaped, symmetrical and centered capsulotomy with an intact posterior capsule prevents vitreous prolapse and determines the centration and effective position of the lens. The CCC is one of the most difficult steps for young cataract surgeons to master.[5] Traditional methods of manual capsulorhexis usually involve a cystotome (or sharp capsulorhexis forceps) to initiate a tear in the anterior capsule under viscoelastic. Once the tear is started, the cystotome (or capsulorhexis forceps) is used to manually tear the anterior capsule in a 5–6 mm circle that is centered on the visual axis. Complications of a traditional capsulorhexis include decentration, asymmetry, anterior capsular tears, improper size, and radialization to the posterior capsule with vitreous prolapse.

## ‣ FEMTOSECOND CONTINUOUS CURVILINEAR CAPSULORHEXIS

One of the most exciting new technologies is the approval of the femtosecond laser for use in cataract surgery. In particular, the creation of the CCC using a femtosecond laser has many potential advantages. Large scale studies are currently being conducted comparing femtosecond continuous curvilinear capsulorhexis (FCCC) to manual CCC methods, but early smaller studies have shown that FCCC are more precise, accurate, reproducible and stronger than those created manually. One year data has shown that there is less IOL shift and decentration with FCCC methods due to symmetric capsulotomy.[6,7] As we await further robust clinical trials, many clinics are still considering the cost-effectiveness of the new technology and other practice-related concerns.

## Femtosecond Capsulotomy Creation

The femtosecond laser is able to focus energy anywhere within transparent tissue. This allows the surgeon to visualize the precise placement of the capsulorhexis prior to creation. The laser creates thousands of individual spots anywhere in a preprogrammed x, y and z axis giving the surgeon the ability to program three-dimensional shapes. Each spot overlaps with the adjacent spot. The spot size, spot separation and energy are calibrated per the manufacturer for each laser.

In order to ensure proper placement along the z-axis (Figs 1A to D), a real-time high-resolution optical coherence tomography (OCT) is used to precisely locate the anterior capsule. After the capsule is identified, virtual calipers are used to determine the capsule displacement in the z-axis. Posterior and anterior buffer zones are used to ensure the programmed cylindrical cut encompasses the entire capsule. The cylindrical pattern starts posteriorly in the anterior cortex of the cataract and proceeds anteriorly through the capsule into the aqueous humor.

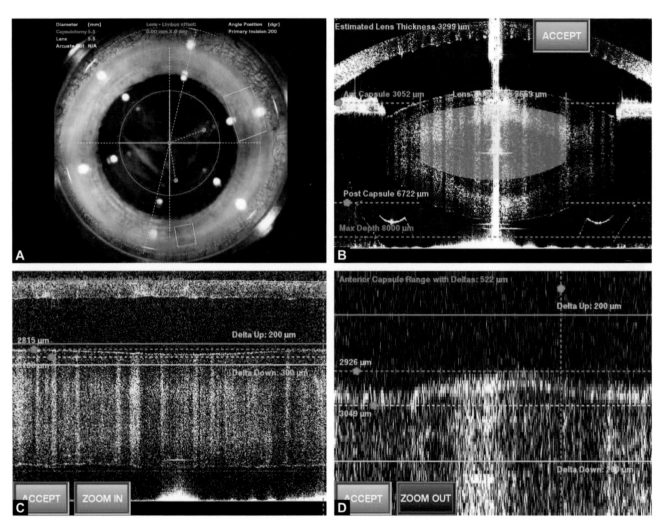

**Figs 1A to D:** (A) The patient interface is docked to the eye and suction is applied. Incision location and capsulotomy location can be changed. The fixation lights help to ensure centration; (B) An anterior/posterior view OCT of the anterior segment allows positioning of the capsulotomy, main incision, paracentesis, lens fragmentation and astigmatic keratotomies; (C) Low magnification OCT of the anterior capsule; (D) High-power magnification of the anterior capsule
*Source*: Courtesy of John Berdahl MD

## Capsule Precision

Femtosecond continuous curvilinear capsulorhexis offers surgeons an unprecedented level of precision in creating incisions, capsulotomies and phacofragmentation. Recent attempts[8,9] have been made to improve the precision of manual CCC techniques through the use of physical or virtual calipers, but FCCC techniques are emerging as the most precise, repeatable CCC technique available to surgeons.[6,7] Additionally, the use of fewer instruments during surgery means less manipulation of the eye and fewer insertion and removal motions, which in sum can be beneficial in terms of precision, postoperative healing, and potentially introducing pathogens.[2]

## Capsule Size

Creating a consistent, repeatable capsule size is important for surgeons to optimize uncorrected visual acuity (UCVA) postoperatively, as a consideration when implanting aspheric and presbyopia correcting and toric IOLs. Capsule size can be planned to 1/100th of a millimeter resulting in average postoperative variation of 29 μm.[6] This precision allows the surgeon to easily customize the capsulotomy size based on the desired IOL. Although most current IOLs benefit from a capsulotomy between 5–6 mm, future lens designs may take advantage of easily customizable capsulotomy size, particularly in combination with emerging accommodating IOLs. The maximum size of the capsulotomy is limited by the pupil size. Patients with particularly small pupils may not be able to receive a FCCC since the femtosecond laser cannot pass through the pigmented iris tissues to reach the capsule. Currently, a pupil size of less than 5.5 mm precludes the creation of an FCCC.

## Capsule Centration

Femtosecond laser platforms allow for an entirely reproducible, centered capsulotomy that cannot be achieved every time using manual methods.[6] One major advantage of an FCCC is the ability to determine the centration of the capsulotomy prior to creating it. The ideal centration is on the visual axis determined by the central corneal light reflex. Often, this does not coincide with the pupil center (the distance between them is known as angle kappa). A perfectly-centered capsulotomy helps to prevent lens tilt, dislocation, and centration, which is critical with the current generation of multifocal IOLs.[2]

## Effective Lens Position

Cataract surgeons have long found value in creating a surgeon-specific A-constant to improve outcomes.[10] The difference in A-constant from one surgeon to another is likely the result of a different effective lens position based on surgical technique. The most important variable in effective lens position (when the IOL is placed in the capsular bag) is the capsulotomy. A larger capsulotomy will lead to a more anterior position of an IOL while a smaller capsulotomy will cause the lens to be more posteriorly positioned.[11] Since a surgeon cannot ensure that a manually created capsulotomy will be identical every time, variability in refractive outcome results since the effective lens position changes. Femtosecond continuous curvilinear capsulorhexis should allow identically reproducible capsulotomies that increase the precision and accuracy of refractive outcomes by ensuring consistency of effective lens position. As the consistency in capsulotomy and effective lens position improves, more accurate IOL power formulas can be developed with tighter outcome tolerances.

## Capsule Tears

Manual CCC results in capsular complications in approximately 1–5% of cases.[12] Capsular tears can cause numerous problems including increased rates of endophthalmitis, retinal detachment, vitreous loss, IOL decentration/dislocation, or the need to place an anterior chamber IOL. Capsular tears with femtosecond capsulorhexis should be less common since the FCCC is performed in a closed eye with no shallowing of the anterior chamber. Additionally, there are no vector forces placed on the zonules with a FCCC, eye movements are limited, and manual surgeon factors should be eliminated. Since the femtosecond capsulotomy is not a 'tear' like the traditional capsulorhexis, studies will determine if the rate of anterior capsular tears is decreased with FCCC (Figs 2A and B).

## Complex Cases

Femtosecond continuous curvilinear capsulorhexis may have important benefits when removing complex cataracts. In situations with loose or weak zonules, such as pseudoexfoliation or traumatic cataracts, a femtosecond laser can create the capsulotomy without putting any additional strain on the zonules (this can be of double benefit if the femtosecond laser is used for nuclear fragmentation). If a natural lens is already partially dislocated (such as in

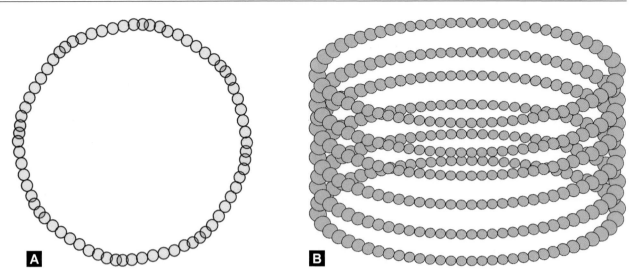

**Figs 2A and B:** (A) The circular capsulotomy created by multiple overlapping small pulses; (B) A cylindrical spiral shape created by multiple overlapping small pulses

Marfan's syndrome), the femtosecond laser can create a capsulotomy and capsular hooks can be used to center the lens in combination with various types of capsular tension rings. Ultra dense and white cataracts can also benefit from FCCC since the capsule can be hard to visualize using traditional methods. White cataracts can also be pressurized inside the capsule leading to rapid radialization when initiating the capsulorhexis with a cystotome. An FCCC may help prevent this radialization. In some cases of mature or traumatic cataracts, an anterior cortical plaque is attached to the overlying capsule. It is extremely difficult to create a capsulotomy in these cases, and the femtosecond laser may allow for a round continuous capsulotomy since it can cause the anterior cortical plaque and the anterior capsule simultaneously.

Pediatric cataracts have more elastic capsules which makes manual capsulotomy more difficult. The elasticity of the capsule is negated during FCCC creation decreasing the likelihood of radialization.

## ADVANCED IOLs

Advanced IOL technology is continuing to improve, and more patients desire the advantages these lenses offer. A key consideration when deciding if and how to implant an advanced IOL is the size, integrity and centration of the CCC. Femtosecond continuous curvilinear capsulorhexis platforms can help maximize capsular performance and minimize complications that lessen the performance of advanced IOLs or, even worse, prevent their use.

Culbertson[2] notes that, using FCCC technology, we can program an exact capsulotomy that matches the design objectives of the preferred IOL with optimal overlap of the lens or an oversized capsulotomy that allows for hinged accommodating IOLs. Additionally, advanced IOLs benefit greatly from the simultaneous astigmatism treatments (typically astigmatic keratotomies) offered by femtosecond platforms.

## ADVANTAGES TO SURGEONS

Many surgeons are proud of their ability to manually create the capsulotomy with a cystotome, and creating a good capsulotomy has been a rite of passage in ophthalmic training. However, FCCC techniques can level the playing field between highly experienced and less experienced surgeons, resulting in less stress for the surgeon and better outcomes for the patient. Both of these are desirable. As FCCC software and clinic practices are streamlined and improved, surgeons should see a more robust and efficient patient throughput, better outcomes, and fewer complications which will increase efficiencies around the femtosecond technology.

## POSTOPERATIVE OUTCOMES

Large studies are currently underway to determine if femtosecond technology in general and FCCC in particular improve outcomes and safety in cataract surgery. Table 1 shows a comparative study between manual CCC methods and FCCC methods in relation to induced aberrations

**SECTION 17**

**Table 1:** Comparison of induced aberrations and tilt between manual CCC and FCCC techniques

Comparison of induced aberrations and tilt[a]

| | Manual (n = 51) | Femtosecond (n = 48) | P |
|---|---|---|---|
| Ocular vertical tilt | 0.09 ± 0.44 | −0.08 ± 0.35 | > 0.05 |
| Ocular horizontal tilt | 0.1 ± 0.49 | 0.16 ± 0.39 | > 0.05 |
| Ocular vertical coma | 0.04 ± 0.19 | −0.02 ± 0.16 | > 0.05 |
| Ocular horizontal coma | −0.01 ± 0.16 | 0.02 ± 0.14 | > 0.05 |
| Internal vertical tilt | 0.27 ± 0.57 | −0.05 ± 0.36 | 0.006 |
| Internal horizontal tilt | 0.15 ± 0.59 | 0.16 ± 0.63 | > 0.05 |
| Internal vertical coma | 0.1 ± 0.15 | 0.003 ± 0.11 | 0.006 |
| Internal horizontal coma | 0.03 ± 0.18 | 0.06 ± 0.11 | > 0.05 |

[a]*Comparison between matched cohorts, with one group's having a manual capsulotomy and the other a femtosecond laser capsulotomy. Source: CRS Today, as noted in text reference list*

and tilt.[2] Given the high success and safety of cataract surgery, the addition of femtosecond technology has a high standard to improve upon. Prohibitively large studies may be necessary to demonstrate a statistically significant improvement.

Like many technologies (such as foldable IOLs and small incisions), simultaneous development of new technologies may provide a synergy that was previously unrealized. Femtosecond technology may provide self-sealing wounds that require less stromal hydration, leaving the eye closer to its physiologic state. Combining self-sealing wounds with interoperative abberometry may allow surgeons to improve refractive outcomes. Combining new generation IOLs with customized FCCCs may allow more predictable treatment of presbyopia.

## FUTURE OF FEMTOSECOND CONTINUOUS CURVILINEAR CAPSULORHEXIS

The accuracy, flexibility, and precision of FCCC are already an improvement over traditional techniques. Future improvements of FCCC will certainly include increased speed. Current generations of femtosecond lasers only allow for circular capsulotomies, however, ovoid or other capsulotomy shapes could be envisioned that may be necessary or complementary to future lens designs.

## SUMMARY

The use of the femtosecond laser in cataract surgery is ushering in an unprecedented level of precision to one of the most commonly performed surgeries worldwide. Although the use of femtosecond technology for cataract surgery is in the earliest stages, one can imagine how the increased precision and accuracy along with customization based on particular IOL technology will lead to improved outcomes and increased functionality for our patients. Robust clinical trials are underway to determine if the increased precision of femtosecond laser applications to cataract surgery result in improved outcomes or safety.

## REFERENCES

1. Nagy Z, Takacs A, Filkorn T, et al. Initial clinical evaluation of an intraocular femtosecond laser in cataract surgery. J Refract Surg. 2009;25:1053-60.
2. Slade SG, Culbertson RR, Krueger RR. Femtosecond lasers for refractive cataract surgery. CRS Today. 2010:67-73.
3. Neuhann T. Theorie und operationstechnik der kapsulorhexis. Klin Monbl Augen- heilkd. 1987;190:542-5.
4. Gimbel HV. The history of the capsulorrhexis technique. CRS Today. 2008:32.
5. Ohmi S. Decentration associated with asymmetrics capsular shrinkage and intraocular lens size. J Cataract Refract Surg. 1993;19:640-3.
6. Kranitz K, Takacs A, Mihaltz K, et al. Femtosecond laser capsulotomy and manual continuous curvilinear campulorrhexis parameters and their effects on intraocular lens centration. J Refract Surg. 2011;27(8):558-63. (Epub ahead of print).
7. Friedman NJ, Palanker DV, Schuele G, et al. Femtosecond laser capsulotomy. J Cataract Refract Surg. 2011;37(7):1189-98.
8. Dick HB, Pena-Aceves A, Manns A, et al. New technology for sizing the continuous curvilinear capsulorrhexis: prospective trial. J Cataract Refract Surg. 2008;34:1136-44.
9. Wallace RB. Capsulotomy diameter mark. J Cataract Refract Surg. 2003;29:1866-8.
10. Kent C. Another Step Closer: Lens Constant Customization. Review of Ophthalmology; 2010.
11. Koeppl C, Findl O, Kriechbaum K, et al. Postoperative change in effective lens position of a 3-piece acrylic intraocular lens. J Cataract Refract Surg. 2003;10:1974-9.
12. Marques FF, Marques DM, Osher RH, et al. Fate of anterior capsule tears during cataract surgery. J Cataract Refract Surg. 2006;32:1638-42.

CHAPTER 110

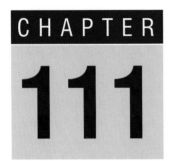

# Femtosecond Laser Lens Fragmentation

*David Smadja, Ronald R Krueger*

## ❧ INTRODUCTION AND CONCEPT OF LENS FRAGMENTATION

### Origin of the Nucleus Fragmentation Concept

The concept of fracturing the nucleus is not new and dates back to 1967, along with the introduction of phaco-emulsification, Kelman used a Ringberg forceps to crack the nucleus (Kelman C, personal communication, 1985). But facing to many complications, this technique was abandoned in favor of the nucleus prolapse method. In 1986, just 1 year after having introduced the continuous curvilinear capsulorhexis (CCC), Gimbel developed a technique to fracture the nuclear rim using the phacoemulsification.[1] This discovery arose from the clinical observation that the rotation of the lens during cataract surgery could result in an inadvertent fracture of the nucleus. Since hard and large nuclei could not be neither safely emulsified *in situ* nor be tipped out through a 5–6 mm CCC, it was therefore necessary to fragment and divide these lenses *in situ* before extraction. This concept of fracturing the nucleus was first termed 'nucleofractis' and has added efficacy and safety to cataract surgery procedure, by easily allowing conquering moderate to hard cataracts. Since its introduction in the 1980s, several methods of nucleofragmentation have been suggested, using different concepts, such as phacoem-ulsification ultrasound, mechanical lens splitting, laser photofragmentation or fluid-based cataract extraction system. However, this fracturing technique makes use of the anatomical features of the lens, since it is based on the anatomic relationship of the lens fibers and the lenticular sutures.

### Lens Anatomic Features

The lens consists of a nucleus and a cortex, and is bordered on its outer surface by the lens capsule, responsible, in part, for the elasticity. During childhood, lens fibers, growing from the lens epithelial cells near the equator, surround the fetal nucleus to become the adult nucleus, whereas subsequent fibers grow to surround the entire nucleus and form the lens cortex. All these fibers join in a Y-shaped suture anteriorly and posteriorly so that the lens is similar to the lamellar organization of an onion. These Y sutures correspond to fault lines in the lens, offering radial cleavage planes through which cracking can be easily made. Under-standings of these anatomical features were essential for the development of the nucleofragmentation technique, improving safety and efficiency in cataract surgery.

## ❧ HISTORY AND TECHNIQUES OF PHACOEMULSIFICATION ULTRASOUND FRAGMENTATION

### Divide and Conquer Sculpting

While the nucleus emulsification was primarily performed in the anterior chamber after having been dislocated, in 1986, Gimbel[2] first introduced the *in situ* nuclear fracturing technique and presented it at the 1987 European Intraocular Implantlens Council (now called 'ESCRS') meeting in Jerusalem. This fracturing maneuver, well-known as the 'divide and conquer technique' was developed to facilitate nuclear fragmentation into small pieces so that they could be removed easily through a small cataract incision and thus, add efficiency and safety during emulsification of moderate to dense cataracts. This technique basically involves four surgical steps as follows: deep sculpting of a groove or trench in the lens nucleus, nucleofractis of the posterior plate and nuclear rim, breaking away a wedge-shaped section of nuclear material for emulsification, and rotation of the remains nucleus for further fracturing and emulsification. Since its introduction, numbers of variations of this technique have been developed to deal with different grade of cataract and challenging situations.[3]

## Choo-choo Chop and Flip Technique

In the early 1990s, along with the desire of cataract surgeon to better achieve phacoemulsification in hard nucleus, Fine[4] developed an alternative technique, taking the maximum advantage of the various new technologies: the choo-choo chop and flip. In this technique, the pulse mode is used to remove nuclear material, thereby decreasing chattering and increasing holding power of the nuclear material. Mechanical forces are substituted to ultrasound energy to further disassembly the nucleus, whereas high vacuum is used as an extractive technique to remove nuclear material rather than the use of ultrasound energy to emulsify the nucleus before extraction. The introduction of this technique has been one more step to optimize safety in cataract surgery. A number of similar techniques have been published in the literature, among which the popular 'crack and flip' technique was developed by Dillman, Maloney and Fine.[5]

## Phaco Chop Technique

In 1993, Kunihiro Nagahara introduced a new technique for nuclear disassembly during phacoemulsification essentially based on mechanical splitting using the natural cleavage planes of the lens. The proposed idea is to split the nucleus by a chopping instrument, taking advantage of these natural cleavage planes, while the nucleus, impaled by the phacoemulsification tip, is maintained stabilized. This popular technique was later slightly modified by some authors to improve its reliability and repeatability (stop and chop technique).[6]

## ❧ CURRENT LIMITATIONS OF ULTRASOUND FRAGMENTATION

Although the use of phacoemulsification for nuclear fragmentation is overall safe and effective, challenging cataracts have a higher risk of intraoperative complications and might particularly benefit from a laser fragmentation that could ease the nuclear disassembly.[7]

Dense nuclei may require excessive ultrasound energy to fragment and remove the cataract, resulting in endothelial damage and thermal incision burns, thereby increasing risk of having leaking incision and induced astigmatism. In addition, fragmentation of hard nuclei may require higher number of intraocular manipulations as well as of generated forces during the nucleus disassembly, increasing risk of capsular tears and zonular dehiscence.[8]

Zonular weakness conditions, commonly seen in patients who have Marfan's disease, pseudoexfoliation, or in eyes with prior trauma or postvitrectomy may compromise the safety of the procedure. Sculpting, cracking and rotation of the nucleus may worsen the situation by breaking additional zonules during surgery. Laser lens fragmentation might be beneficial in those cases by reducing the amount of intraocular maneuvers required, thus lessening the risk of complication such as dropped nuclei.[9]

Poor visualization conditions such as hypermature white cataracts that decrease the visibility of the capsule, or corneal opacities or small pupil size that affect the visibility of lens borders are associated with high risk of accidental damage of the capsule by incorrect assessment of lens width and depth. The safety of the procedure in such eyes might be significantly improved by an adequate visualization of the lens. Therefore, the incorporated imaging system associated with the laser lens fragmentation would be a very useful tool to improve safety by accurately assessing the lens dimensions prior to deliver the treatment.

Corneas with critical endothelium conditions, such as Fuchs' endothelial dystrophy or in a postcorneal transplant eye are predisposed to decompensation from endothelial damage induced by ultrasonic energy. In both, laser lens fragmentation might be beneficial by reducing the amount of ultrasonic energy required to remove the cataract and thus lessen the amount of endothelial cell loss.

## ❧ INTRODUCTION OF LASER LENS FRAGMENTATION

### The Beginning of Lens Photodisruption with the Nd:YAG Laser

In the late 1970s, a young female patient, who underwent a bilateral surgery for congenital cataract was referred to Dr Aron, in Paris, for unilateral endophthalmitis following its secondary cataract treatment with a surgical blade. Having never fully recovered a good visual acuity in this eye, the young girl, despite a 20/400 vision in the contralateral eye, didn't want to further undergo eye surgery procedure. Having at that time no idea how they would accomplish this feat, Dr Aron, in an empathetic impulse, promised the young girl that one day it would be possible to treat her secondary cataract without touching her eye. Few years later, using the physics background of his wife and associate, Dr Aron-Rosa, they reported the first use of the Nd:YAG laser pulse energy for performing posterior capsulotomy.[10] These findings have established the basic framework for the next use of laser in cataract surgery: laser photofragmentation to photodisrupt the lens nucleus, and thus, softening it before phacoemulsification. In the early 1990s, photodisruption with Nd:YAG laser pulses was already a well-established tool for intraocular surgery, such as posterior capsulotomy, iridotomy or pupillary membranectomy. Several studies using Nd:YAG laser pulses to fragment the nucleus have also been published and reported a shorter phaco time and less ultrasound required when using this combination.[11-13] However, by delivering laser pulses with a duration of nanosecond range, and a pulse energy in the millijoule range, the clinical applications of Nd:YAG photodisruption were limited by the large potential for collateral damage in the surrounding tissue. Bille et al.[14] were first, in 1992, to suggest the picosecond Nd:YAG laser as a method to fragment and then aspirate the cataract. In 1994, Vogel et al.[15] confirmed that the use of single picosecond laser pulses and energies in the microjoule range could significantly increase the surgical precision of intraocular Nd:YAG laser surgery and reduce disruptive side effects, thereby further improving the laser photofragmentation technique.

## Nd:YAG Laser Shock Waves Production for Lens Photolysis

The Dodick laser photolysis system has been introduced by Dodick in 1991,[16] and it uses a pulsed Q-switched Nd:YAG laser source to generate shock wave resulting from the impact of the laser radiation on a titanium plate housed within the tip of the probe. In contrast to the other concepts of photofragmentation using an Nd:YAG laser source, no laser beam emerges from the tip, rather, shock waves produced by the interaction with the titanium block, emanate from the mouth of the probe to break-up the lens material. Several studies reporting the results of cataract surgery using the Dodick photolysis system have been published, and two advantages seem to emerge when compared to regular phacoemulsification.[17,18] First, this technique represents a low-energy modality for cataract extraction, with a mean intraocular energy use of 5.65 J

per case, reported in large prospective multicenter study of 1,000 consecutive cases.[19] In addition, this system does not produce significant heat, thus avoiding the risk of corneal burn and subsequent astigmatism and endothelial damage. The second advantage is related to the ability to fragment and extract the cataract through an incision of less than 2 mm. At present, no intraocular lenses (IOLs) are available to be inserted through a 1.4 mm incision, but further improvement in this field are now mandated to achieve a real advantage of this technique.

## Femtosecond Laser Lens Fragmentation

After the surge of interest generated by femtosecond laser in laser-assisted *in situ* keratomileusis (LASIK) surgery, this technology has recently been applied to cataract surgery. Using ultra short laser pulses of low energy (1 µJ/pulse) tightly focus in the lens, the femtosecond laser enables cutting inside the lens to fragment the nucleus without causing damage in the surrounding tissue. Just as for LASIK flap in the early 2000, the introduction of femtosecond laser for the nucleus fragmentation is expected to improve safety in this crucial step of cataract surgery.

## ⋗ TECHNICAL CONSIDERATIONS FOR LASER-ASSISTED FRAGMENTATION

## Technical Requirements

The most challenging technical requirement for a femtosecond laser in cataract surgery is to combine both cutting into the lens and the cornea. The femtosecond laser lens fragmentation targets a volume and thus requires a higher pulse energy to compensate for scattering loss as well as a lower numerical aperture whereas the corneal incisions (primary, secondary and limbal relaxing incisions) target a focal plan and thus requires higher numerical aperture to perform precise cuts (Fig. 1).

In addition, the ability to reliably achieve the threshold energy for a successful fragmentation is highly dependent on the density and dimensions of the treated lens. This feature is one of the critical differentiating factors among the current femtosecond laser platform for cataract surgery. LenSx systems reported an effective nucleofragmentation up to lens opacities classification system (LOCS) II Grade 3.0 cataracts.[20] Optimedica claimed a successful fragmentation up to LOCS II Grade 4.0 cataracts,[21] whereas with the LensAR laser system, effective fragmentation of LOCS II Grade 5.0 cataracts have been reported.[22]

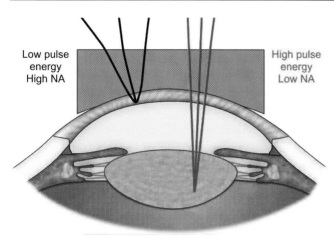

**Fig. 1:** Scheme to represent the differences of laser technical requirements to perform femtosecond laser lens surgery versus corneal surgery
*Source*: Holger Lubatschowski

**Fig. 2:** Safety zones preoperatively programmed using a high-resolution OCT with the LenSx laser. The yellow area corresponds to the volume of fragmentation. The safety zone below to protect the posterior capsule from inadvertent laser pulses from the fragmentation was programmed to be about 800–1,000 µm. The edges of the iris are clearly seen, and the treatment was delivered within a 5 mm diameter, away from the pupil edge

## Imaging System

Another critical differentiating factor between laser platforms is the associated imaging system. Since proper alignment of the cutting pattern inside the lens is essential to avoid inadvertent laser pulses delivery in the capsular bag or on the iris, the capacity to readily identify lens structures as well as adjacent intraocular tissue become one of the most critical part of the image-guided femtosecond laser surgery. A treatment pattern that does not fit within the capsular bag because of tilted lens is likely to encroach the capsule and might lead to complication, such as capsular rupture and vitreous loss. To prevent such complications, all the current laser systems are equipped with different imaging system that can help in defining precise safety zones to avoid laser pulses delivery to occur in critical zones, such as the posterior capsule or iris (Fig. 2).

The LenSx and Optimedica laser are equipped with a real time high-resolution optical coherence tomography (OCT), whereas the LensAR laser uses a high-resolution 3D confocal structured illumination (3D CSI). This imaging system is an infrared-based imaging with a resolution of approximately 12 µm. The 3D CSI has the particularity of using ray tracing to precisely determine boundaries of the different intraocular structures.[23] In addition, it allows to obtain high contrast images of the lens by enhancing detail and imaging through denser cataracts by varying scanning beam intensity (Fig. 3).

## Treatment Algorithms

Currently, three commercial systems are developing treatment algorithm for nuclear disassembly using the femtosecond laser technology: LensAR (LensAR Inc,

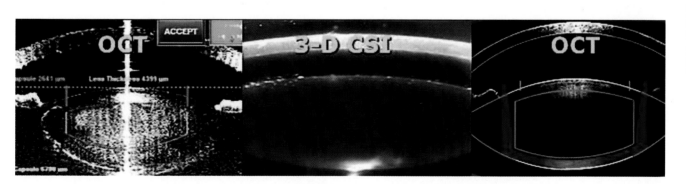

**Fig. 3:** Difference in quality of images obtained with high-resolution OCT used respectively by LenSx (left) and Optimedica (right) versus 3D CSI used by LensAR (center)

Winter Park, FL); LenSx (LenSx Lasers Inc., Aliso Viejo, CA); Optimedica (OptiMedica Corporation, Santa Clara, CA). Depending on nuclear density and surgeon preferences, different treatment profiles to successfully achieve lens fragmentation may be programmed with the FS laser system software. The wide choice of treatment algorithm available varies between laser platforms but aims to facilitate and reduce the amount of ultrasonic energy needed for nuclear disassembly. With the LensAR system, an integrated software uses the high contrast images generated by the 3D CSI imaging system to suggest a plan of necessary laser pulse energy and pattern needed for that specific nucleus density. For Dr Harvey Uy, who is working with LensAR, the 'pie shape' fragmentation pattern that first divides the nucleus into 20 slices before further subdividing these wedges into inner, middle and outer segments seems to be the most successful in reducing ultrasonic energy.

As prechopping surgeons, Dr Slade and Dr Donnenfeld, working with LenSx are mostly using the four-chop radial pattern with circular cuts and say that it appears to work best to facilitate nuclear disassembly[24] (Figs 4A and B). Surgeons using the Optimedica Catalys FS laser reported similar results to those reported by LensAR when using the four-quadrants pattern. Although different in shape and setting parameters (energy, spot separation and volume), all current commercial lasers are delivering the treatment in a posterior to anterior direction, starting posteriorly and leaving a safety zone between the lens tissue targeted for photodisruption and the posterior capsule of about 800–1,000 μm. Thus, it reduces the risk that femtosecond pulses delivery during fragmentation interferes with the cavitation bubbles generated in a more superficial plane. The surgical duration for this specific step varies with laser platform and the algorithm chosen, but usually ranges between 30 and 60 seconds.

A wide choice of pattern has been developed (cubes, cylinder, cross-shape, ellipsoidal, pie, circles and many other shapes) to perform nuclear disassembly but studies are still underway to optimize the available treatment patterns for each commercial system.

## Advantages of Laser Lens Fragmentation

The laser-assisted lens fragmentation can facilitate removal of nearly all types of cataract and may be of particular interest in complicated cases. Sculpting, cracking and rotation are critical steps during the attempt to fragment such challenging cataracts as brunescent cataracts or zonular weakness. Because additional forces generated to achieve nuclear disassembly are transmitted to the capsule and zonules, the risk of capsular tears and zonular dehiscence significantly increase in these cases. Therefore, any maneuver that can reduce the amount of sculpting and

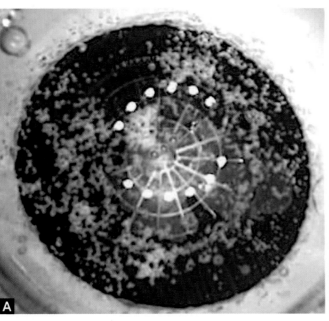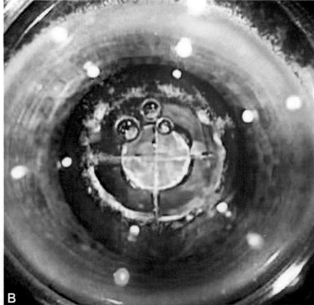

**Figs 4A and B:** Photos of different laser lens fragmentation treatment profiles. (A) In the left side, is represented the subdivided pies shape used by the LensAR system; (B) In the right side, the four-chop radial pattern with circular cuts used by the LenSx system

cracking motions to remove the cataract, such as laser lens fragmentation to pretreat and liquefy the lens will significantly lessen the risk of associated complications.

Another major safety advantage of preliminary using femtosecond laser to fragment the lens is the possibility to create an epinuclear safety plate between the posterior capsule and the targeted lens volume. This plate, easily removable by using aspiration at the end of the nucleus removal, can serve as an armor to reduce the risk of accidental posterior capsular rupture or puncture by surgical instruments. In addition, preliminary femtosecond nucleus fragmentation allows reducing the subsequent amount of ultrasound energy required with phacoemulsification and thus, diminishes the complications related to excessive use of energy such as damage in the corneal endothelium, thermal burn incision and risk of posterior capsular tears. This particularity of laser lens fragmentation to allow for less ultrasonic dissipated energy to emulsify is of great advantage for patients who have preoperative critical endothelium conditions.

## ꙮ EARLY CLINICAL RESULTS

The three main measurable benefits directly related to the preliminary use of femtosecond laser to fragment the lens before its extraction are the reduction of ultrasonic energy needed as the surgical impact, the reduction of endothelial cells as the safety impact and the postoperative visual recovery delay as the clinical impact.

All of the three companies have studied, as an efficacy parameter, the amount of ultrasound energy still needed for the nuclear disassembly after femtosecond laser lens fragmentation, and depending on the grade of cataract. In overall, the percentage of ultrasound energy reduction after photofragmentation varied from 33% to 100%, depending on the company and the cataract grade.[25-27]

Edwards and colleagues, using the LensAR system, compared preliminary fragmented lenses with the pie shape pattern to traditional phacoemulsification surgery and reported a reduction of cumulative dissipated energy by 100%, 64%, 39% and 42% for Grades 1, 2, 3 and 4 cataracts respectively.[25] Nagy et al., using the LenSx system to fragment Grade 1 to Grade 2 cataracts with a cross-pattern treatment, reported a reduction of 43% of phacoemulsification power and a 51% decrease in phacoemulsification time.[28]

Regarding the safety impact of preliminary using laser lens fragmentation for nucleus disassembly, Dr Slade reported a statistically significant decrease in endothelial cell loss when comparing eyes treated with the LenSx laser to conventionally treated eyes. The average cell loss 3 months after surgery in the manual group was 6.3% compared to 2.5% in the LenSx group, meaning a reduction of 60% in endothelial cell loss.[24] This lower cell loss with the laser pretreatment might result in fewer complications such as postoperative cloudy corneas leading to penetrating or endothelial keratoplasty.

Reduction in phacoemulsification time and power might also directly influence the postoperative inflammatory reaction as well as the visual recovery often delayed by temporary corneal edema. Although not yet scientifically demonstrated in peer review publication, many surgeons that recently started using the LenSx system (only system currently available for clinical purpose) in their practice observed exceptionally clear cornea the day after surgery. The reason is believed to be due to less intraocular manipulations required, less dissipated ultrasonic energy and less fluid flow used during phacoemulsification as well as phacoemulsification time.[24] Nagy et al., in their first series of eyes treated with laser, reported a visual acuity superior or equal to 20/40 in 100% of eyes after 1 week and 20/20 in 100% of eyes after 1 month.[28]

## ꙮ CONCLUSION

The first reported results of femtosecond laser lens fragmentation showed its capacity to significantly facilitate removal of nearly all kinds of cataract (except white cataracts) while improving the safety of the procedure. The added safety of reducing sculpting and cracking motion for nucleus disassembly may be particularly beneficial in challenging cases such as compromised zonules, traumatic cataract or brunescent cataracts.

## ꙮ REFERENCES

1. Gimbel HV. Principle of nuclear phacoemulsification. Cataract surgery, techniques, complications and management, 2nd edition. 2004:153-81.
2. Gimbel HV. Divide and conquer. Presented at the European intraocular implant lens council meeting. Jerusalem, Israel. 1987.
3. Gimbel HV. Divide and conquer nucleofractis phacoemulsification: development and variations. J Cataract Refract Surg. 1991;17(3):281-91.
4. Fine I. The chip and flip phacoemulsification technique. J Cataract Refract Surg. 1991;17(3):267.
5. Fine I, Maloney W, Dillman D. Crack and flip phacoemulsification technique. J Cataract Refract Surg. 1993;19(6):797-802.
6. Koch P, Katzen L. Stop and chop phacoemulsification. J Cataract Refract Surg. 1994;20(5):566-70.

7. Naranjo-Tackman R. How a femtosecond laser increases safety and precision in cataract surgery? Curr Opin Ophthalmol. 2011;22(1):53-7.

8. Agarwal A. Mature cataracts and dyes. In: Agarwal (Ed). Phaco nightmares: conquering cataract catastrophes. 2006; Section II: Chapter 8.

9. Felipe Vejarano L, Tello A. Complications in phacoemulsification. In: Agarwal (Ed). Phaco nightmares: conquering cataract catastrophes. 2006; Section II: Chapter 19.

10. Aron-Rosa D, Aron J, Griesemann M, et al. Use of the neodymium-YAG laser to open the posterior capsule after lens implant surgery: a preliminary report. J Am Intraocul Implant Soc. 1980;6(4):352-4.

11. Ryan E, Logani S. Nd:YAG laser photodisruption of the lens nucleus before phacoemulsification. Am J Ophthalmol. 1987;104:382-6.

12. Zelman J. Photophaco fragmentation. J Cataract Refract Surg. 1987;13:287-9.

13. Chambless WS. Nd:YAG laser photofracture: an aid to phacoemulsification. J Cataract Refract Surg. 1988;14(2):180-1.

14. Bille J, Klancnik E, Niemz M. Principles of operation and first clinical results using the picosecond IR laser. Parel JM (Ed). Ophtalmic Technologies II. SPIE Proc. 1992:88-95.

15. Vogel A, Capon M, Asiyo-Vogel M, et al. Intraocular photodisruption with picosecond and nanosecond laser pulses: tissue effects in cornea, lens, and retina. Invest Ophthalmol Vis Sci. 1994;35(7):3032-44.

16. Dodick J. Laser phacolysis of the human cataractous lens. Dev Ophthalmol. 1991;22:58-64.

17. Kanellopoulos AJ, Dodick J. Dodick photolysis for cataract surgery: early experience with the Q-switched neodymium:YAG laser in 100 consecutive patients. Ophthalmology. 1999;106(11):2197-202.

18. Huetz W, Eckhardt H. Photolysis using the Dodick-ARC laser system for cataract surgery. J Cataract Refract Surg. 2001;27(2):208-12.

19. Kanellopoulos AJ, Group PI. Laser cataract surgery: A prospective clinical evaluation of 1000 consecutive laser cataract procedures using the Dodick photolysis Nd:YAG system. Ophthalmology. 2001;108(4):649-54.

20. Nagy ZZ. Femtosecond laser lens fragmentation, personal communication. ASCRS congress, San Diego, CA. 2011.

21. Battle J. Prospective study of size and shape accuracy of optimedica femtosecond laser capsulotomy vs manual capsulorohexis. Personal communication, XXVIII Congress of the ESCRS, Paris, France. 2010.

22. Krueger RR. Personal experience with the LensAR system. Personal communcation, XXIX Congress of the ESCRS, Vienna. 2011.

23. Klyce S. Evolution of imaging technology for laser refractive cataract surgery. Personal communication, ICFLO 4th, Dana Point, CA. 2011.

24. Slade SG. First U.S. clinical experience with laser cataract surgery. In: Krueger RR, Talamo J, Lindstrom R (Eds). Femtosecond laser refractive cataract surgery. 2011: Chapter 13.

25. Edwards K, Uy H, Scheinder S. The effect of laser lens fragmentation on the use of ultrasound energy in cataract surgery. Poster, ARVO meeting, Ft. Lauderdale, FL; 2011.

26. Fishkind W, Uy H, Tackman R, et al. Alternative fragmentation patterns in femtosecond laser cataract surgery (abstract). In: Program and Abstracts of American Society of Cataract and Refractive Surgeons Symposium on Cataract, IOL and Refractive Surgery, Boston, Massachusetts. 2010.

27. Koch D, Batlle J, Feliz R. The use of OCT-guided femtosecond laser to facilitate cataract nuclear disassembly and aspiration (abstract). In: Program and Abstracts of XXVIII Congress of the ESCRS, Paris, France. 2010.

28. Nagy Z, Takacs A, Filkorn T, et al. Initial clinical evaluation of an intraocular femtosecond laser in cataract surgery. J Refract Surg. 2009;25(12):1053-60.

# Femtosecond Laser Presbyopia Correction

*Mike P Holzer*

## ✛ INTRODUCTION

The use of the femtosecond laser in corneal refractive surgery first came to the forefront in 1990s, and it has become a well-established technique for precise and predictable laser-assisted *in situ* keratomileusis (LASIK) flap creation since 2000.[1,2] Subsequently, the femtosecond laser started to be used in therapeutic applications, such as lamellar keratoplasty, tunnels for intracorneal ring segments and astigmatic keratoplasty owing to the ability of the femtosecond laser technology to accurately cut corneal tissue, and considered in the application for intracorneal refractive correction.[3-8]

Following feasibility studies into the application of the femtosecond laser for intracorneal correction, the use of the femtosecond laser to treat presbyopia using a technique known as the INTRACOR® procedure (Technolas Perfect Vision GmbH, Munich, Germany) was first performed in patients by Dr Luis Ruiz from Bogotá, Colombia in 2007.[9] Dr Ruiz is the co-inventor of the procedure and a leading pioneer in the field of refractive surgery.

In 2008, a prospective, multicenter CE study was conducted to further evaluate this new procedure.[10] CE mark approval was obtained in April 2009. The procedure does not currently have Food and Drug Administration (FDA) approval.

## ✛ THE INTRACOR® PROCEDURE

The INTRACOR® procedure is performed using the VICTUS™ Femtosecond Laser Platform (Bausch + Lomb/ Technolas Perfect Vision) (Fig. 1). The VICTUS Platform

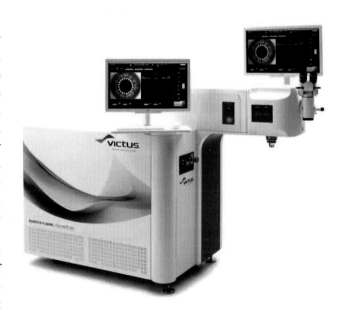

**Fig. 1:** VICTUS Femtosecond Laser Platform

uses a proprietary curved patient interface which adapts to the natural shape of the cornea and does not applanate it (Figs 2 and 3). INTRACOR® is a minimally-invasive procedure, performed only within the stroma, so no incisions to the cornea or Bowman's membrane occur. The technique involves making a series of five concentric rings within the stroma, starting in the center with a diameter of 1.8 mm and moving to the periphery, where using the company's proprietary nomogram, the cut design depends upon the refractive error. These ring cuts result in a localized biomechanical change which causes a central steepening of the cornea (Fig. 4). The duration of the procedure is between 15 and 20 seconds.

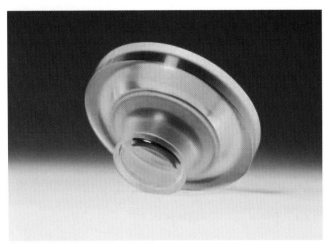

**Fig. 2:** TECHNOLAS curved patient interface

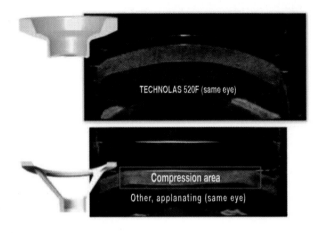

**Fig. 3:** Nonapplanating vs applanating

## ► EVALUATION OF THE INTRACOR® PROCEDURE—2-YEAR FOLLOW-UP DATA

Following ethics committee approval from the University of Heidelberg, 63 patients were recruited to undergo the intrastromal treatment of presbyopia with the femtosecond laser at the four study sites of Heidelberg, Mannheim, Duisburg and Munich. Treatments took place between July and October of 2008. The results of the Heidelberg subgroup of 25 patients are presented in this chapter.

Within the study group at Heidelberg University, 25 patients of mean age $56.2 \pm 5.79$ years (range 47–67 years) underwent an INTRACOR® treatment in the nondominant eye only between July and September of 2008. Patients required a minimum addition of +2.0 D and all were

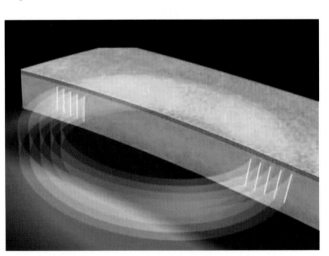

**Fig. 4:** Schematic of INTRACOR® concentric, intrastromal ring pattern

slightly hyperopic with a preoperative spherical equivalent of $0.6 \pm 0.26$ D, sphere of $0.75 \pm 0.23$ D and cylinder of $-0.33 \pm 0.17$ D. Uncorrected distance visual acuity (UDVA) was $0.11 \pm 0.11$ logMAR and uncorrected near visual acuity (UNVA) was $0.70 \pm 0.16$ logMAR. Postoperative follow-up was at 1 day, 1 week, 1, 3, 6, 12, 18 and 24 months. In addition, patients were checked immediately after the procedure to check the quality of the cuts with a slit-lamp examination.

## ► STEPS FOR PERFORMING THE INTRACOR® PROCEDURE

### Preoperative Measurements

Preoperatively, the patient should undergo a complete ocular examination and complete an ocular and medical history. Furthermore, a slit-lamp examination should be performed to exclude any previous ocular surgeries as well as corneal or ocular diseases. Careful patient selection is imperative, and the patient's visual needs should be discussed in detail and expectations carefully managed (see section on patient selection and managing expectation below). Monocular and binocular uncorrected and best corrected near and distance visual acuities should be measured, along with the refraction which should be stable for the year previously. It is also important to obtain K readings and corneal thickness readings using corneal topography, where the thinnest pachymetry values at 2, 4, 6 and 8 mm diameter are registered. Since a slight myopic shift is induced by the procedure, this should be tested and simulated for the patient.

The VICTUS system operates at a pulse frequency of 40 kHz when performing the INTRACOR® procedure. After selecting the INTRACOR® module on the main menu, the patient's details should be entered, along with subjective refraction and K readings. Next, the pachymetry values from the IntraCalc software should be entered. A summary of the selected treatment and the pachymetry values will be displayed on the screen.

## INTRACOR® Procedure

Anesthetic drops should be applied when the patient is lying on the laser bed. It is then very important to optimize centration. The author's preferred technique is to center on the visual axis, whereby the patient is instructed to focus on the red fixation light to allow the visual axis to be marked with a small instrument. The suction ring should then be positioned on the patient's eye, centering on the mark with the aid of an ASICO ring. Vacuum is commenced with the foot pedal or by pressing the 'Suction Status'

button of the computer software, and the patient interface vacuum is managed via the computer software, clicking the 'PI Fixation' button. The patient's eye is docked into the curved patient interface by raising the patient bed and maneuvering with the joysticks until optimal contact, i.e. suction and centration is achieved.

The green light on the docking control indicates when ideal contact between the eye and patient interface has been achieved. Any final adjustments of the centration can be performed using the INTRACOR® centration software (Fig. 5). Redocking should be performed in the cases of poor centration. When centration is optimal, the suction ring clip should be closed in order to proceed with the procedure.

The procedure can then be started by pressing the procedure pedal. The five concentric intrastromal ring cuts take approximately 15–20 seconds. Once completed, the vacuum is released and the patient is undocked from the patient interface and the laser. A slit-lamp examination should be performed immediately after the procedure to

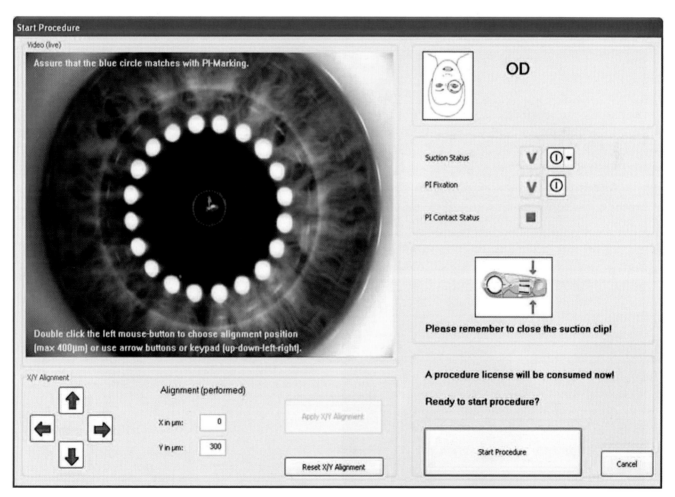

**Fig. 5:** INTRACOR® centration software

check the quality of the cuts. Patients should then return for follow-up examinations at 1 day and 2–4 weeks or as needed. Patients are provided with steroid-containing eye drops and artificial tear drops to administer if needed.

## ⁖ RESULTS

One hour after the procedure, the slit-lamp examination shows the expanded intrastromal rings which are clearly visible owing to the cavitation gas from the photodisruption. However, these gas bubbles typically disappear after a few hours postoperatively and within a day the cuts are barely visible (Figs 6A to C).

At 24 months postoperative, the mean UNVA was 0.20 logMAR (20/30) compared with 0.70 logMAR (20/100) preoperative. This improvement was statistically significant (p < 0.05, Wilcoxon test) and there was no change between 12 and 24 months which demonstrates the results are stable over time. Similar results were found with the distance corrected near visual acuity (Fig. 7). Patients typically gain 4–5 lines of near vision on the ETDRS chart used measured at 40 cm distance. The achieved mean near acuity of 0.2 logMAR is equivalent with reading newspaper print. Cumulative results on UNVA also show a marked increase in near visual acuity with less than 5% achieving 0.4 logMAR (20/50) preoperatively, and 84% achieving 0.3 logMAR (20/40) at 24 months postoperatively (Fig. 8).

Intermediate vision was also evaluated using a Sloan reading chart and showed a statistically significant difference between pre-and postoperative UNVA (p < 0.05, Wilcoxon test). Defocus curves performed on a selected number of patients also demonstrate the patients achieve good intermediate vision.

In terms of safety, there is in some cases some impact on the best-corrected distance visual acuity (BCDVA), with all patients achieving 20/32, following an initial myopic shift of −0.5 D. A few patients lost one or two lines of BCDVA.[11] No differences between the pre- and the postoperative straylight measurements or endothelial cell counts were observed. Further studies have also indicated that normal intraocular lens (IOL) power calculations can be used if the patient subsequently develops a cataract.[12]

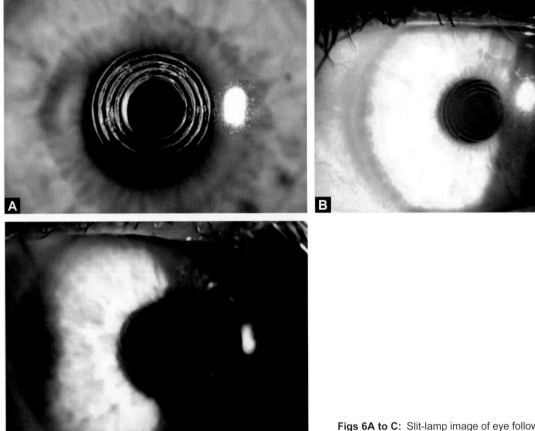

**Figs 6A to C:** Slit-lamp image of eye following INTRACOR® treatment at (A) 1 hour; (B) 1 week; (C) 2 years

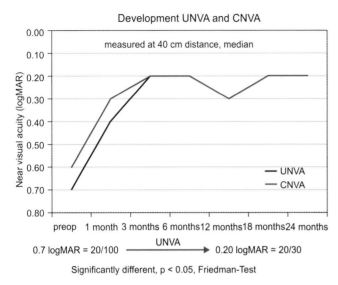

**Fig. 7:** Development of UNVA and CNVA over 24 months
*Source*: Mike P Holzer

## WORKING PRINCIPLE

The five-ring pattern of the INTRACOR® procedure induces some changes of the cornea with a typical outcome of the central corneal steepening of around 2 D. Corneal topography also shows no change between 1 month, 12 and 24 months postoperatively. Changes in the spherical aberrations as well as the corneal asphericity are also observed.

## PATIENT SELECTION AND MANAGING EXPECTATIONS

Based upon the author's experience at Heidelberg, where he has now performed over 300 cases, he has adopted the following patient selection criteria. Patients should require a near addition of greater than or equal to +1.50 D and have a stable refraction. The procedure should be performed in the nondominant, virgin eye. Patients should have hyperopia of +0.5 to +1.25 D (SEQ), although surgeon's first starting with INTRACOR® should consider a more conservative approach of +0.5 to +1.0 D of hyperopia in order to assess the myopic shift, which in the author's experience is around −0.5 D. Slightly hyperopic patients are more suitable to this procedure owing to this myopic shift. All candidates should be advised of the possible slight loss of distance vision. Patients should have a subjective astigmatism not exceeding 0.5 D, pachymetry should be > 500 μm; angle κ < 10° and K max < 48 D; K min > 39 D. A full ocular examination including mydriasis and cycloplegic refraction should be performed to ensure the cornea is healthy with no retinal diseases, such as age-related macular degeneration (AMD) or diabetic retinopathy.

Patients should also be advised of what to expect in terms of the improvement of near vision of 4–5 lines, and the author uses the ETDRS chart to demonstrate this

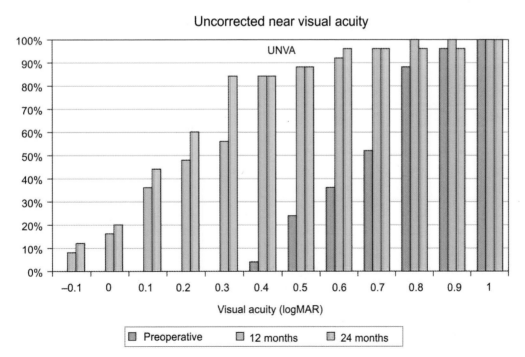

**Fig. 8:** Cumulative UNVA
*Source*: Mike P Holzer

improvement beforehand. The author also informs patients that they might typically see rings around light sources in the first few weeks, or in some cases for longer, but these rings aren't really disturbing in night driving conditions.

## SUMMARY

In summary, at 24 months postoperative, the outcomes following INTRACOR® treatment remain stable. Patients normally gain between 4 and 5 lines of near vision, and over 80% of the author's patients read without glasses. No regression has been observed to date and no severe side effects have occurred. However, some compromise might be a slight loss in distance visual acuity. One further issue is the current lack of retreatment possibilities. INTRACOR® is a minimally-invasive procedure, and hence has a low risk of infection. As it is a very fast procedure and painless postoperatively, with a quick recovery time, patients can quickly resume their normal activities. As with all presbyopic procedures, it is very important to carefully manage patient selection and managing patient expectations.

*Acknowledgment*: Lindsay Brooks, PhD helped in preparing the manuscript.

## REFERENCES

1. Heisterkamp A, Mamom T, Kermani O, et al. Intrastromal refractive surgery with ultrashort laser pulses: in vivo study on the rabbit eye. Graefes Arch Clin Exp Ophthalmol. 2003;241:511-7.

2. Holzer MP, Rabsilber TM, Auffarth GU. Femtosecond laser assisted corneal flap cuts: Morphology, accuracy and histopathology. Invest Ophthalmol Vis Sci. 2006;47:2828-31.

3. Lubatschowski H, Maatz G, Heisterkamp A, et al. Application of ultrashort laser pulses for intrastromal refractive surgery. Graefes Arch Clin Exp Ophthalmol. 2000;238:33-9.

4. Lubatschowski H. Overview of commercially available femtosecond lasers in refractive surgery. J Refract Surg. 2008;24:S102-7.

5. Meltendorf C, Schroeter J, Bug R, et al. Corneal trephination with the femtosecond laser. Cornea. 2006;25:1090-2.

6. Nordan LT, Slade SG, Baker RN, et al. Femtosecond laser flap creation for laser in situ keratomileusis: six-month follow-up of initial U.S. clinical series. J Refract Surg. 2003;19:8-14.

7. Ratkay-Traub I, Ferincz IE, Juhasz T, et al. First clinical results with the femtosecond neodynium-glass laser in refractive surgery. J Refract Surg. 2003;19:94-103.

8. Sletten KR, Yen KG, Sayegh S, et al. An in vivo model of femtosecond laser intrastromal refractive surgery. Ophthalmic Surg Lasers. 1999;30:742-9.

9. Ruiz LA, Cepeda LM, Fuentes VC. Intrastromal correction of presbyopia using a femtosecond laser system. J Refract Surg. 2009;25:847-54.

10. Holzer MP, Mannsfeld A, Ehmer A, et al. Early outcomes of INTRACOR femtosecond laser treatment for presbyopia. J Refract Surg. 2009;25:855-61.

11. Fitting A, Ehmer A, Rabsilber TM, et al. Agreement of subjective and objective refraction measurements following INTRACOR femtosecond laser treatment. Ophthalmologe. 2011;108(9):852-8.

12. Rabsilber TM, Haigis W, Auffarth GU, et al. Intraocular lens power calculation after intrastromal femtosecond laser treatment for presbyopia: Theoretic approach. J Cataract Refract Surg. 2011;37(3):532-7.

# CHAPTER 113

# Wound Creation

*Brett P Bielory, Terrence J Doherty, James C Loden, George O Waring IV, Richard M Awdeh*

## ✦ THE SCIENCE OF THE FEMTOSECOND LASER

Ever since the creation of the Ruby laser by Maimon[1] nearly one-half a century ago, the application of laser technology has made considerable strides in the field of medicine and dentistry. Maimon discovered that laser pulses excite unattached electrons within organic or inorganic matter causing them to collide with nearby atoms creating heat and vibration. This, in turn, causes chemical bonds to break and reform more stable compounds. The end result is the creation of water and carbon dioxide gas molecules (cavitation bubbles), which ultimately dissipate as the tissue is literally vaporized into plasma. This process is called laser induced optical breakdown (LIOB).

The optically transparent tissues of the eye, such as the cornea and lens, do not absorb electromagnetic radiation in the visible or near-infrared spectrum at low-power density. However, at higher power densities, these tissues will absorb energy leading to plasma generation. Laser power can be understood as energy delivery per unit time, as demonstrated by the following simple equation:

$$P = e/t$$

Where $P$ equals the power threshold needed to produce tissue breakdown, $e$ equals the energy delivery of the laser and $t$ equals the pulse duration. Increasing the energy of the laser will deliver the adequate power, but will lead to a larger amount of collateral damage to surrounding tissue and would therefore be impractical for precise incisions needed with corneal wound creation. The YAG laser, for instance, operates at the energy level of several millijoules in the nanosecond ($10^{-9}$ seconds) range and has a collateral tissue damage zone of about 100 μm. The goal of each successive generation of laser technology has been to reduce the pulse duration, which in effect decreases the threshold energy for LIOB. Femtosecond (FS) laser technology uses near-infrared ultrashort wavelengths, which when directed at tissue structures results in the maximal absorption of light energy. By shortening the pulse duration and energy of the near-infrared laser (femto; $10^{-15}$ seconds), the zone of collateral tissue disruption and damage is significantly reduced to about 1 μm, thus making the femtosecond laser an ideal laser for use in the eye.[2]

## ✦ APPLICATION OF FEMTOSECOND TECHNOLOGY IN OPHTHALMOLOGY

Maimon's technology spurred the development of the argon, krypton, carbon dioxide, neodymium-doped yttrium aluminum garnet (ND: YAG), excimer and femtosecond laser systems to treat a vast array of ophthalmic disorders. FS is the latest and most recent technology pioneered by ophthalmologists to dramatically revolutionize the management of ocular conditions, particularly for anterior segment surgery. The strongly localized interaction process of ultrashort laser pulses with tissue makes FS lasers a powerful tool for ophthalmic surgery.

Femtosecond laser technology allows for precise, reproducible, placement of laser spots with adjustable spot size, spot separation, pulse energy and pulse patterns. The modern FS lasers allow for laser incisions in both the horizontal and vertical planes, creating corneal lamellar cuts of various geometrical patterns, configuration depths, and diameters.[3] Additionally, there are numerous technical features that vary between FS laser devices (Table 1). These include: (1) Differences in the applanation interfaces, which can be a flat (as in the Intralase IFS—Abbott Medical Optics, Santa Ana CA; Alcon FS 200—Alcon Laboratories, Fort Worth, TX; Ziemer LDV—Germany) or a curved interface (Visumax—Carl Zeiss Meditech—Germany, Technolas Perfect Vision—Bausch & Lomb, Rochester, NY); (2) Differences in where the interface docks (for example, the corneal limbus as in the Visumax vs the conjunctiva for other systems); (3) Differences in the amount of intraocular pressure elevation induced by applanation (high as in the Intralase and low in the Visumax); (4) Loss of vision during treatment (which is secondary to IOP rise). The available pulse duration and pulse rate ranges from as low as 200–300 kHz (Ziemer LV) to greater than 500 kHz (Intralase IFS and Technolas) and greater than 1 MHz (Zemer LDV) to 500 kHz (Carl Zeiss Visumax) respectively. These differences lead to a different side-effect profile with the various FS lasers on the market. For instance, Carl Zeiss Visumax has a curved docking system, similar to the Technolas laser uses a limbal suction mechanism compared to the standard conjunctival suction. As such, limbal docking of the applanation interface leads to a decreased risk of postoperative subconjunctival hemorrhage. In summary, the ideal device would include a high-repetition rate, small spot size and low-energy pulse.

## Laser *in situ* Keratomileusis (LASIK)

The versatility of FS technology allows the surgeon to precisely plan all parameters of the lamellar LASIK flap, including the hinge position, hinge angle, flap diameter, flap thickness, flap shape and side-cut angle.[4] It has been suggested that these advantages, as well as the theoretical

biomechanics have allowed patients with higher refractive errors and/or thinner corneas to become appropriate candidates for LASIK.[5,6] Gil-Carzola et al. reported 3-month refractive outcomes in hyperopic LASIK patients comparing the IntraLase FS 60-kHz laser to the Moria M2 microkeratome and found improved outcomes with the femtosecond laser.[7] Ideal lamellar flap characteristics include, but are not limited to: planarity, minimal residual microadhesions, complete side cut, smooth lamellar bed, minimal opaque bubble layer (OBL) and minimal but adequate energy. The ease of flap lift is directly related to the number of pulses, distance between pulse shots, orientation of pulses in the x-y and z dimensions, overlap of pulses, and bed energy. However, there is a balance that is necessary, as more pulses with closer pulse shots and higher energy will allow for the easiest flap lift, but can cause an increase in procedure time, incidence of DLK and inflammation.[8] Alternatively, wide spot and line settings, without multidimensional overlapped pulses may result in a more difficult flap lift and increased forward light scatter, particularly with deeper cuts with less compact stroma (data on file Waring IV GO). It has been reported that FS lasers create reproducible planar flaps, resulting in a less-meniscus shape, theoretically improving the biomechanical and neuronal properties of a flap.[9,10] Others have reported that reverse bevel side cuts and elliptical flaps may enhance the aforementioned benefits with less chance of flap dislocation.[11-13]

## Penetrating Keratoplasty (PKP)

Historically, penetrating keratoplasty (PKP) has been the primary means of visual restoration for severe damage of any and all corneal layers. There has been little evolution

| **Table 1:** Comparison of commercially available FS lasers | | | | |
|---|---|---|---|---|
| Femtosecond Laser* | Intralase (AMO) | Zeimer LDV | Technolas (Femtec) | Zeiss VisuMax |
| Pulse duration fs | 600-800 | 200-350 | 500-700 | 220-580 |
| Laser engine | 150 kHz | 20.8 mHz | 80 kHz | 200-500 kHz |
| Pulse energy max | 0.6-1 µJ | 10-20 ηJ | 4.6 µJ | 50-420 ηJ |
| Side cut angles | 30-150 | 28(fixed) | 30-90 | 45-135 |
| Mobile | No | Yes | No | No |
| Keratoplasty | Yes | No | Yes | Yes |
| No. of cases | 4,000,000 | 100,000 | 20,000 | 7500 |
| IOP increase | 30-60 mm Hg | >25 mm Hg | >26 mm Hg | >26 mm Hg |
| Thickness (µm) | 90-400 | 90-200 (foils) | 100-200 | 80-220 |

*Information adapted from AAO subspecialty day presentation 2010. Binder PS and Juhasz T

in technique or postoperative visual rehabilitation in the past 25 years and healing has been plagued by delayed visual recovery, high astigmatism, and life-long risk of wound dehiscence. For both full thickness and partial thickness transplantation, the FS laser has revolutionized the trephination process by enabling surgeons to create a wide variety of shaped or geometric corneal incisions with much better precision and reproducibility than previously attempted by manual means.[14,15] The FS laser can be programmed to precisely cut the exact dimensions in both the recipient and donor tissues, allowing an ideal fit during transplantation. This, in turn, allows the transplanted grafts to have a larger contact area at the donor-host junction for better wound sealing and less suture tension.

Femtosecond laser technology has revolutionized the penetration keratoplasty (PKP) procedure by allowing for laser trephination in lieu of the conventional blade punch trephine during corneal transplantation. Femtosecond laser technology assisted corneal transplantation helps to achieve a better and quicker visual recovery with less total astigmatism and fewer aberrations, in addition to strong architectural wound construction, allowing for earlier suture removal.[16] The three most-popular FS-PKP incisions profiles are: mushroom, top-hat, and zig-zag, each being customizable based on the surgeon's preference. The mushroom-shaped incision preserves more host endothelium than the traditional trephine. The top-hat-shaped incision allows for the transplantation of large endothelial surfaces. The zigzag-shaped incision provides a smooth transition between host and donor tissue and allows for a hermetic wound seal, thereby minimizing the risk for postoperative wound leak.

## ⋗ LASER SETTINGS AND TECHNIQUES

Modern FS lasers allow a high amount of versatility for the diameter, depth, and angle of both the lamellar and side-cut laser incisions. Because of this, a virtually unlimited number of graft sizes and shapes are possible (Fig. 1).

The IntraLase FS™ Laser (Abbot Medical Optics, Santa Ana, CA) is currently the most widely used FS laser for both LASIK and keratoplasty in the United States. The suction rings, applanation cones and docking process are all the same for both procedures. This laser creates the keratoplasty incisions by programming two side-cut incisions (anterior and posterior) and one lamellar incision, each of which can also be turned off or on, depending on the desired shape. Small radial alignment marks can also be created along the circumference of the anterior side

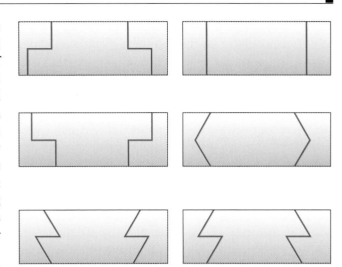

**Fig.1:** Schematic cross-sections of the various laser incision patterns that can be created with the femtosecond laser

cut at evenly spaced intervals within the 9.5 mm surgical field. The settings for these alignment marks are fixed, and have a length of 500 μm. The cuts begin posteriorly and move toward the epithelium starting with the posterior side cut, followed by the lamellar cut and anterior side cut respectively. The side cut angles can range from 30–150° referenced from the central anterior surface of the cornea. Therefore, larger angles bevel out toward the limbus, while acute angles bevel centrally. Diameters of the side cuts are also reference from the anterior perspective. This means that an anterior cut that is programmed to be 8.0 mm, but has an angle of greater than 90°, will actually have a larger posterior diameter, the size of which will be determined by the side-cut angle and the depth of the cut. The maximum diameter allowed with this laser is 9.5 mm, with a minimum diameter of 3 mm. The depth of the cuts can reach as far as 1,200 μm from the anterior surface (Fig. 2).

It is important when creating the various patterns of corneal incisions with the FS laser, that adequate overlap of the incisions be instituted to allow continuity and ease of dissection. Typically the vertical overlap of the side-cut incisions should be 20–30 μm past the lamellar incision

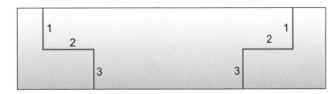

**Fig. 2:** A schematic cross-section of a 'mushroom' shaped corneal graft demonstrating the types of cuts programmed into the Intralase™ FS laser. 1: anterior side cut; 2: lamellar cut; 3: posterior side cut

and the horizontal overlap of the lamellar incision should be 0.1 mm relative to the side cuts. Therefore, if the lamellar cut is set at a depth of 300 μm, the anterior side-cut depth should be set for 330 μm, while the posterior side cut should end at an anterior depth of 270 μm. Horizontally, a 90° anterior side-cut diameter of 9.0 mm and a posterior side cut of 7.0 mm should be paired with a lamellar incision that is set for an inner diameter of 6.9 mm and an outer diameter 9.1 mm.

These calculations are very simple when using vertical or 90° side-cut incisions, but can become a bit trickier when the side cuts are angled to any degree. This is because the posterior diameter will be determined by the angle and depth of the cut as described by the trigonometric equation:

$$W = d/\tan\theta$$

where, $W$ equals the deviation from the set anterior diameter, $d$ equals the depth of the cut, and $\theta$ equals the side-cut angle. For example, an anterior side cut set at an 8.0 mm diameter with a 30° angle and 300 μm depth will have a posterior diameter of about 7.0 mm. If the paired lamellar cut was mistakenly set to range from 9.5 mm to 7.9 mm to overlap an 8.0 mm setting by 0.1 mm, it actually would leave a gap of uncut tissue approximately 0.9 mm in width, which may require manual dissection. The angled side cuts may also cause difficulty if the posterior diameter goes past the maximum 9.5 mm surgical field allowed by the laser. This will usually result in an error message on the laser, which will not allow the surgeon to proceed with the desired settings.

The laser can be programmed to perform full thickness corneal incisions by having the posterior side-cut depth set deeper than the peripheral corneal thickness. This is how donor tissues for keratoplasty are prepared using an artificial anterior chamber. However, for the recipient cornea, leaving approximately 60 μm of uncut tissue posteriorly will allow for more stability and a safer patient transfer to the operating room. For the IntraLase FS Laser, this needs to be calculated by performing either peripheral corneal ultrasound pachymetry at the 7–8 mm zone or using imaging modalities such as an anterior segment OCT to determine the thinnest region of the cornea. The posterior side-cut depth is then programmed to be 60 μm above this depth. This remaining bridge of tissue can then be easily dissected with standard instruments in the operating room. Using other nonintersecting patterns is also possible. A tissue gap can be left between either the anterior side cut and the lamellar cut, or the posterior side cut and the lamellar cut. This potentially negates the need to have to measure and calculate the thinnest area of the cornea to

ensure a posterior tissue bridge, but may result in a more difficult surgical dissection that could cause irregularity in the interface.

In our experience, we have encountered no difficulties with patient transfer, retrobulbar blocks, or placement of the Honan pressure balloon after the incisions have been made by the FS laser. One patient had a small area of unidentified full-thickness penetration, but still encountered no issues with this regimen. It is our usual practice to administer the 5% betadine on the conjunctiva before the laser incisions are created and to perform only the betadine skin preparation once the Honan balloon has been removed.

With the increasing use of the FS lasers for keratoplasty, precut donor tissue from eye banks has become readily available. Eye banks will often have a list of parameter settings to choose from when ordering the tissue, but the surgeon is also able to specify any number of custom cuts and sizes to fit individual needs. The precut tissue arrives with the FS laser printout to verify the settings for the donor incision. This printout is very useful to double check against the settings planned for the recipient corneal incisions.

The three most popular or well-reported corneal-shaped grafts for FS laser keratoplasty are the top hat, the zig-zag, and the mushroom (Fig. 1). Each shape has theoretical advantages depending upon the need of the recipient, and all significantly increase the overall area of the graft-host interface.

## ❧ TOP-HAT-SHAPED GRAFTS

Top-hat configurations provide a larger posterior diameter which acts as a shelf of tissue that has been shown in laboratory studies by Steinert and others to increase the amount of intraocular pressure needed for wound leakage to occur.[16] This was confirmed by a 2008 study by Bahar et al. in which the burst pressure of top-hat grafts (102 mm Hg) was far greater than traditional (49 mm Hg), zig-zag (48 mm Hg), 'Christmas tree' (52.3 mm Hg), and mushroom (65.8 mm Hg) grafts after 16 radial sutures were placed.[17] A larger posterior diameter also replaces more of the recipients endothelium and posterior stroma and would perhaps be theoretically advantageous for diseases such as Fuch's corneal dystrophy or posterior polymorphous dystrophy (PPMD) that may not be appropriate candidates for Descemet's stripping endothelial keratoplasty (DSEK). Top-hat grafts can also potentially re-establish thinned peripheral corneal tissue as the larger posterior section is placed under the thinned periphery. This is possible because the lamellar ring cut is always uniform relative to the anterior surface. Dr Francis Price beautifully demonstrated this advantage at the 2007 meeting of the American Academy of Ophthalmology (AAO). Price also reported 1-year results for the top-hat configuration of 6 eyes with BSCVA ranging from 20/25 to 20/400. Two patients had underlying retinal conditions. Mean time to complete suture removal was 7 months.[18]

## ZIGZAG-SHAPED GRAFTS

Zig-zag shapes have the advantages of providing excellent corneal tissue alignment, tapered anterior edge, and a posterior shelf that provides a potentially self-sealing wound similar to the top-hat shape. This shelf also promotes the even and stable alignment of the anterior surface. Results of this shape in full-thickness keratoplasty have been well established, particularly by Farid et al. who published a relatively large comparative study.[19] Zig-zag shapes and other configurations that use angled side cuts are potentially more difficult to program given the need to calculate the difference in the posterior diameters based on the tangent of the side-cut angle. However, templates are well established for the zig-zag shape and are readily available from eye banks that provide precut donor tissue.

Farid's (2009) comparative study between the zig-zag incision grafts and traditional PK concluded that the zig-zag shaped resulted in a more rapid visual recovery of BSCVA and induced less astigmatism compared with blade trephination.[19] However, these results were somewhat disputed in a subsequent larger comparative study by Chamberlin et al. who found the difference in the astigmatism results was no longer present after 6 months and he found no improvement in BSCVA at any time point for the zig-zag shape.[20] This study did however note faster suture removal in the zig-zag grafts and identified the limitations of multiple suturing techniques, multiple surgeons, and retrospective design.

## MUSHROOM-SHAPED GRAFTS

Mushroom-shaped grafts are the inverse of the top-hat, with a larger anterior diameter and 90° side cuts. This shape does not provide a posterior shelf and may be tectonically less stable compared to the top-hat and zig-zag configurations. However, the mushroom shape actually had higher burst pressures than the zig-zag grafts in Bahar's comparative study.[17] It also does not naturally promote the even alignment of the anterior surface. However, it does offer the advantages of creating a larger diameter on the anterior surface with potentially less central astigmatism

and higher visual quality. The posterior margin is also farther away from the limbus which may decrease the incidence of graft rejection, although this has not been established by any review studies. Dissection of the tissue bridges and placement of the donor graft may also be a technically easier with the mushroom shape. We have found that the larger anterior diameter sits very nicely on the host tissue during suture placement, perhaps protecting the endothelium from possible intraoperative damage (See Video Clip).

In our practice, the surgeon (TJD) has had great success using predominately the mushroom-shaped graft. The decision to choose this shape was influenced by the reports presented by Dr William Culbertson at the 2007 American Academy of Ophthalmology (AAO) meeting (Course 596) in which his first 13 cases of mushroom-shaped keratoplasty for keratoconus all had UCVA 20/50 or better and BCVA of 20/25 or better in 2–15 months of follow up. Our unpublished results also reflect a high-success rate, especially for young patients with no other ocular comorbidities. Our average amount of postoperative astigmatism for all patients who followed up for 12 months (n = 18) was 2.88 D. All patients with no comorbidities (n = 10) had the best spectacle corrected vision (BSCVA) 20/25 or better at 12 months, with 50% being 20/20. Eighty percent had BSCVA of 20/25 or better at 6 months, with one patient at 20/30 and another 20/100. Both of these patients eventually obtained a BSCVA of 20/20.

Blunt dissection of the laser incisions is very easily performed using a Sinsky hook or other blunt instrument. The anterior chamber is entered with a 15° blade to instill a viscoelastic material and the dissection is completed using standard corneal-scleral scissors angled parallel to the angle of the posterior side cut. The graft is then sewn into place in the standard fashion with bites taken as far posteriorly as possible. We use an interrupted suturing technique to allow earlier selective suture removal postoperatively, but using a continuous suture is also possible. We have found that the tighter sealing graft shape allows for better anterior chamber stability during suturing. After each needle pass, the chamber can be gently refilled with balanced salt solution to maintain a good physiologic intraocular pressure and promote a more even suture tension. This is another potential advantage of interrupted suturing technique. It is also possible to slightly oversize either all or part of the graft to allow a potentially tighter fit. It is our standard practice to oversize only the posterior side cut by 0.1 mm to promote a better seal while maintaining an exact fit anteriorly for a smoother surface contour (Fig. 3).

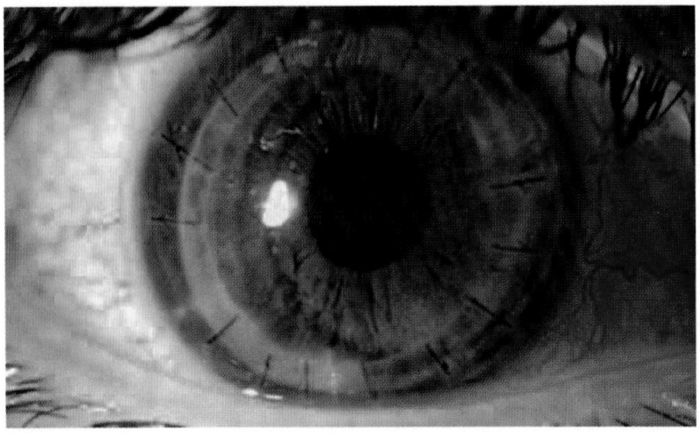

**Fig. 3:** Photo of a mushroom shaped PK one month postoperative. Three sutures have already been removed due to loosening with no evidence of leakage. Fibrotic scarring of the lamellar shelf is readily visible. Uncorrected visual acuity was 20/25

Case reports and series of other various laser trephine cuts have been published, including noncircular decagonal shapes that are designed to prevent torqueing of the graft and provide ideal alignment during transplantation.[21,22] FS lasers are also being applied to facilitate and improve partial thickness anterior lamellar grafts, including deep anterior lamellar keratoplasty (DALK), sutureless anterior grafts and corneal biopsies.[23-27]

Potential problems or complications of FS laser keratoplasty include inability to apply or applanate the suction ring, loss of suction during the procedure, poor centration, inadvertent full-thickness incisions, incomplete laser dissection through densely scarred tissue, problems related to patient transport to the operating room table, as well as the more devastating complications of choroidal hemorrhage and endophthalmitis that can occur with standard PK. To our knowledge, none of these complications have been reported to any large degree.[28] Adjusting laser setting to higher powers and smaller spot size separation can also aid in dissecting through scarred tissue, although we have found no issue with incomplete dissection in any of our cases with our standard settings.

Femtosecond laser keratoplasty has had a remarkable early history for safety and results. This precise surgical instrument has finally provided the answer to a surgical theory that has existed for many years but has heretofore been unobtainable by manual means. As the results continue to accumulate and the technology continues to be refined, there is little doubt that the femtosecond laser will grow as an integral and standard device for the corneal surgeon.

## Additional Corneal Procedures

Aside from LASIK and PKP, the clinical application of FS laser has been successfully used in endothelial keratoplasty (EK), astigmatic keratotomy (AK), intrastromal corneal ring segment (ICRS) placement for keratoconus and corneal ectasias, intrastromal pockets for presbyopic corneal inlays and other corneal surgeries. More recently, FS laser technology has extended itself to anterior lens capsulorrhexes surgery, diagnostic corneal biopsies for infectious ulcers, and intrastromal correction of presbyopia.[29,30] For the remainder of this chapter, we will focus on corneal wound creation for cataract surgery using FS laser technology as compared to traditional blade-based wound creation.

## ❧ HISTORICAL CORNEAL INCISIONS FOR CATARACT SURGERY

As cataract surgery techniques have improved over the years, corneal incision size has decreased. Smaller corneal incisions with more sophisticated architecture decrease the opportunity for postoperative wound leaks thereby decreasing the chance of postoperative infectious endophthalmitis. In addition, smaller corneal incisions may result in a more stable anterior chamber during surgery as well as provide more rapid visual recovery and greater refractive stability following surgery. The evolution of surgical incisions in phacoemulsification began in the late 1960s with large extracapsular scleral tunnel incisions. Smaller extracapsular incisions followed in the early 1970s and clear corneal incisions (CCI) were developed a decade later. McFarland reported the first series of patients undergoing phacoemulsification with a sutureless CCI in 1990. He theorized that a CCI behaved like a flutter-valve, and could allow a sutureless technique that would prevent astigmatic instability associated with uneven suture tension, as long as the intrastromal incision depth and width were equally maintained.[31] With the advent of improved foldable intraocular lens (IOL) delivery systems in the mid-1990s, it became possible to perform an entire cataract procedure through an incision of 3 mm or less. With the widespread use of topical anesthesia, sutureless CCI gained more popularity with ophthalmic surgeons who wanted their patients to have the most rapid postoperative recovery possible. These sutureless CCI were refined during the 1990s when Pfleger and Skorpik et al. reported topographic data suggesting a novel square clear corneal incision which provided short-term and long-term astigmatic stability.[32] Square limbal incisions also helped to decrease wound leak, a major risk factor for endophthalmitis, in the early postoperative period.[33] Researchers and clinicians continued to develop and refine incision architecture in an effort to decrease the risk of endophthalmitis which led to the introduction of multiplanar CCI. Biplanar and triplaner incisions both involve the combination of partial-thickness perpendicular grooves and beveled entry into the anterior chamber with the goal of creating incisions that function as a one-way valve and produce a self-sealing, water-tight wounds, thereby decreasing the risk of wound leak and infectious endophthalmitis. McDonnell et al. have studied the closure of 'near clear' corneal or incisions intentionally placed juxtalimbally, through limbal vessels to create an additional seal, in cadaveric human and rabbit eyes. Using an artificial anterior chamber, India ink was applied to the surface of cadaveric human corneas with near clear corneal incisions in order to detect whether any ink would reflux into the anterior chamber through a clear corneal incision (essentially as a proxy to detect the potential reflux of conjunctival bacteria, lipids and other toxins into the anterior chamber) when the IOP decreases postoperatively, giving an explanation for the increased frequency of acute bacterial endophthalmitis. Although some intentional hemorrhage seemed to increase wound integrity, it is important to note that an inherent shortcoming with the cadaveric data was the lack of an active endothelial pump, which certainly plays a role in wound closure. With the advent of the FS laser technology, and the ability to create incisions with greater accuracy, and potential tongue-and-groove or valve incision, we hypothesize that the risk of postoperative complication secondary to poor-wound creation should decrease.

## ➤ BENEFIT OF USING THE FS LASER FOR WOUND CREATION

Though the development of CCIs have improved refractive outcomes, precise construction of wound architecture is dependent on surgical skill, keratometry, limbal anatomy, intraocular pressure, tissue variation and keratome design. The FS laser may allow for optimized wound construction despite these variables. FS enabled CCIs provides flexibility with surgical planning, including primary incision and paracentesis shape, size and placement. Like FS enabled lamellar flaps, surgeons can custom-design preferred wound architecture and preprogram all parameters to their preference. Although further studies are needed, the precise cutting mechanisms of a FS laser should theoretically allow for minimal induction of operative astigmatism, minimal

risk of postoperative wound leak, and minimal disruption to the adjacent Descemet's membrane, surrounding stroma and epithelium.

Currently in the United States, both LenSX (Alcon, Fort Worth, TX) and LensAR (LensAR Corp., Winter Park, FL), FS lasers are FDA approved for anterior capsulotomy and to create CCI for cataract surgery, and Optimedica (Optimedica Corp., Santa Clara, CA) is in the FDA regulatory process pursuing FDA approval.[34] All three lasers have onboard high-resolution imaging where wound architecture can be planned specifically for the patients' anatomy.

Surgeons are exploring ways to customize and optimize CCIs with FS lasers approved for corneal refractive surgery, though this is currently an off label application. The most widely used FS laser for LASIK in the United States is the IntraLase FS™ Laser (Abbot Medical Optics, Santa Ana, CA). The keratoplasty software for the IntraLase allows surgeons to create a very wide range of full-thickness incisions of various shapes, dimensions and degrees that have the potential to be used for cataract surgery. We are currently undertaking pioneering work with this laser in Nashville (JCL) to potentially make a widely distributed laser beneficial to the cataract surgeon.

The keratoplasty software for the IntraLase FS™ 60 kHz and iFS™ 150 kHz laser has three separate programmable cuts to make various incisions: anterior side cut; lamellar cut; and posterior side cut (Fig. 2). Each of these settings can be enabled or disabled with any planned incision. The anterior side cut has the most versatility because it can be set to create a full 360° incision or 1–2 arcuate incisions centered at any position and spanning any angle degree. The lamellar and posterior side-cut incisions can only currently be programmed to create a 360° circular incision. The anterior side-cut incision has been used to create paired arcuate incisions for the reduction of astigmatism in both healthy corneas and patients with cornea transplants (See Section on Limbal Relaxing Incisions).

By angling the anterior side to an angle of less than 90° (typically 30–45°) and setting it to span the full thickness of the cornea, the two arcuate incisions can be used to create a paracentesis and main corneal incision for cataract surgery. However, while there may be the potential for the laser incisions to heal with a tighter seal compared to blade incisions as has been shown for LASIK flaps,[12] creating a single-plane incision could potentially negate any advantage this may have and perhaps increase the risk of endophthalmitis.

In order to create a triplanar incision with the IntraLase laser, it is necessary to utilize the lamellar and posterior side cuts, but somehow prevent them from creating a 360° incision. To solve this issue, we have designed a disk-shaped mask called the iCatnavigator™ (Fig. 4) that fits inside the standard suction ring after the gantry has been docked onto the patient's cornea. The mask is an opaque black disk made of semi-pliable plastic that has two precise cut-outs along the circumference representing the location of the CCI and paracentesis. The mask blocks the passage of laser energy to the cornea except in the areas that are cut out. The location of the cut-outs can be varied depending on surgeon preference. We currently use a diameter of 2.3 mm on the mask for the CCI and a 1.2 mm diameter for the paracentesis set 60° apart.

We have been successful in creating very well-defined triplanar incisions verified by OCT (Fig. 5). Comparatively, our biplanar blade incisions demonstrate almost an entirely linear shape (Fig. 6). In addition, the three plane incision seems to promote much better alignment of the anterior surface and epithelium compared to the more linear-shaped blade incision that can demonstrate an uneven surface contour. Accurate and reproducible triplanar incisions at this high of quality may potentially be self-sealing at 3–4 mm in diameter, and may facilitate the design and insertion of more complex IOL designs without the need to suture a larger wound.

As previously mentioned, one of the most powerful aspects of a FS laser is the ability to customize wound architecture. Three-dimensional, multiplanar self-sealing incisions can be customized to allow for precise, self-sealing CCIs. A longer tunnel and small internal wound opening, can be easily programmed with a FS and may provide a more stable wound for cases of intraoperative floppy iris syndrome cases. Though, wounds like this can be constructed with a manual keratome, FS lasers may allow for enhanced precision and reproducibility. Furthermore, various external opening configurations can be programmed with FS lasers such as bevel, reverse bevel or ellipses (such as those used in small incision extracapsular surgery). Square incisions have been shown to be most stable with a keratome,[33] and exact dimensions can be programmed with a FS laser. Further studies are needed to establish the safety and efficacy of these FS enabled wound configurations relative to current keratome microincisions.

Additionally, FS lasers may be programmed to simultaneously place limbal relaxing incisions (LRI) or arcuate incisions for the intraoperative management of astigmatism. The same precision and customization previously described for CCIs can be applied to the creation of these arcuate incisions. The FS laser will allow for unique customization of these incisions, even allowing for sub-Bowman's incisions, which would leave the corneal epithelium intact and lead to a faster postoperative recovery and decreased postoperative dry eye and foreign body sensation.[35]

The way the incisions are made with the IntraLase FS laser is once again using the anterior side cut setting of the keratoplasty software. The lamellar and posterior side cuts are turned off. Determining the steep axes and marking the limbus is done in the usual fashion as with any LRI utilizing a Mendez ring or other calibrated limbal marking system. We find it easiest to use the oculars of our excimer laser for this step because of the better optics and close

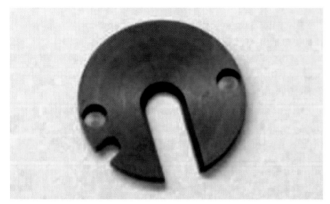

**Fig. 4:** iCatnavigator™: This device is used to facilitate cornea cataract incisions with the intraLase laser. The cut-outs represent the location of the CCI and paracentesis.
*Note*: iCatnavigator™ is a trademarked and a patent pending design by author (JCL)

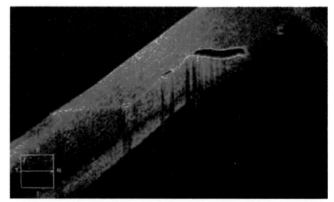

**Fig. 5:** A stepped triplanar incision made by the FS laser 5 minutes postoperatively. Note the smooth anterior contour

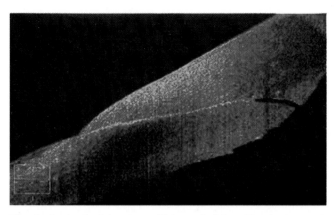

**Fig. 6:** A standard keratome biplanar incision 30 minutes postoperatively. The incision line appears linear and there is poor alignment of the anterior surface

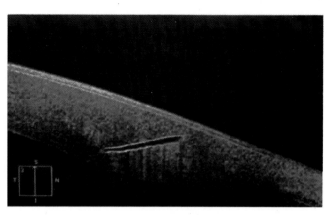

**Fig. 7:** OCT image of a sub-Bowman's intrastromal accurate incision for the correction of corneal astigmatism

proximity to the FS laser. It is also a good idea to mark the limbus at the 180° axis so that better alignment with the reticle can be achieved.

The anterior side cut settings include: entries for 'Cut Position 1', 'Cut Angle 1', 'Cut Position 2' and 'Cut Angle 2'. The position entries determine the axes where the arc positions will be centered. Position 1 can range from 0–180° and position 2 can range from 180–360°. The angle entries determine the amount of arc in degrees for each corresponding cut position. If a full-thickness incision is desired, the 'Depth in Glass' entry is set to 50 µm. This means that the laser will not stop proceeding anteriorly until it has cut 50 µm into the applanation cone. If a completely stromal or sub-Bowman's incision is desired, the 'Depth in Glass' is set to about −100 µm to keep the epithelium intact (Fig. 7). The depth of the incision can be set according to surgeon preference. The maximum depth allowed by the laser is 1,200 µm. The diameter of the incisions can range from 3 mm to 9.5 mm.

Performing LRIs and cataract surgery incisions for the same person in one procedure with the IntraLase laser at this point requires a double-docking technique, as developed by author (JCL) (See Video Clip). The gantry needs to be reapplied for each step and the laser settings changed appropriately. The use of the FS laser for the treatment of astigmatism is described in a separate chapter in this book.

In closing, FS laser technology has contributed to ophthalmic surgery by giving the surgeon the confidence of safety, predictability and reproducibility of surgical incisions.

More than ever, the subspecialties of refractive surgery and lens surgery are colliding. FS laser applications in intraocular surgery represent another step in the marriage

of these disciplines. FS laser enabled CCIs should allow for improved wound healing and rapid visual rehabilitation. FS technology is constantly evolving and advanced refinements in wound creation are currently being developed in the newer generation femtosecond laser devices.

## ⧁ REFERENCES

1. Maiman TH. Stimulated optical radiation in ruby. Nature. 1960;187:493-4.
2. Reggiani-Mello G, Krueger RR. Comparison of commercially available femtosecond lasers in refractive surgery. Expert Rev Ophthalmol. 2011;6:55-65.
3. Jonas JB, Vossmerbaeumer U. Femtosecond laser penetrating keratoplasty with conical incisions and positional spikes. J Refract Surg. 2004;20:397.
4. Salomao MQ, Wilson SE. Femtosecond laser in laser in situ keratomileusis. J Cataract Refract Surg. 2010;36:1024-32.
5. Slade SG, Durrie DS, Binder PS. A prospective, contralateral eye study comparing thin-flap LASIK (sub-Bowman keratomileusis) with photorefractive keratectomy. Ophthalmology. 2009;116:1075-82.
6. Durrie DS, Kezirian GM. Femtosecond laser versus mechanical keratome flaps in wavefront-guided laser in situ keratomileusis: prospective contralateral eye study. J Cataract Refract Surg. 2005;31:120-6.
7. Gil-Cazorla R, Teus MA, de Benito-Llopis L, et al. Femtosecond Laser vs Mechanical Microkeratome for Hyperopic Laser In Situ Keratomileusis. Am J Ophthalmol. 2011.
8. Gil-Cazorla R, Teus MA, de Benito-Llopis L, et al. Incidence of diffuse lamellar keratitis after laser in situ keratomileusis associated with the IntraLase 15 kHz femtosecond laser and Moria M2 microkeratome. J Cataract Refract Surg. 2008;34:28-31.
9. Stahl JE, Durrie DS, Schwendeman FJ, et al. Anterior segment OCT analysis of thin IntraLase femtosecond flaps. J Refract Surg. 2007;23:555-8.

10. Jaycock PD, Lobo L, Ibrahim J, et al. Interferometric technique to measure biomechanical changes in the cornea induced by refractive surgery. J Cataract Refract Surg. 2005;31:175-84.

11. Vaddavalli PK, Yoo SH. Femtosecond laser in-situ keratomileusis flap configurations. Curr Opin Ophthalmol. 2011;22:245-50.

12. Knorz MC, Vossmerbaeumer U. Comparison of flap adhesion strength using the Amadeus microkeratome and the IntraLase iFS femtosecond laser in rabbits. J Refract Surg. 2008;24:875-8.

13. Lohmann CP, von Mohrenfels CW, Herrmann W, et al. Elliptical ELSA (LASEK) instruments for the treatment of astigmatism. J Cataract Refract Surg. 2003;29:2174-80.

14. Busin M. A new lamellar wound configuration for penetrating keratoplasty surgery. Arch Ophthalmol. 2003;121:260-5.

15. Barraqueri J. Special Methods in corneal surgery. In: King H, McTigue JW (Eds). The Cornea World Congress. Washington, DC, USA: Butterworths; 1965. pp. 586-604.

16. Steinert RF, Ignacio TS, Sarayba MA. 'Top hat'-shaped penetrating keratoplasty using the femtosecond laser. Am J Ophthalmol. 2007;143:689-91.

17. Bahar I, Kaiserman I, McAllum P, et al. Femtosecond laser-assisted penetrating keratoplasty: stability evaluation of different wound configurations. Cornea. 2008;27:209-11.

18. Price FW, Price MO. Femtosecond laser shaped penetrating keratoplasty: one-year results utilizing a top-hat configuration. Am J Ophthalmol. 2008;145:210-4.

19. Farid M, Steinert RF, Gaster RN, et al. Comparison of penetrating keratoplasty performed with a femtosecond laser zig-zag incision versus conventional blade trephination. Ophthalmology. 2009;116:1638-43.

20. Chamberlain WD, Rush SW, Mathers WD, et al. Comparison of femtosecond laser-assisted keratoplasty versus conventional penetrating keratoplasty. Ophthalmology. 2011;118:486-91.

21. Proust H, Baeteman C, Matonti F, et al. Femtosecond laser-assisted decagonal penetrating keratoplasty. Am J Ophthalmol. 2011;151:29-34.

22. Lee J, Winokur J, Hallak J, et al. Femtosecond dovetail penetrating keratoplasty: surgical technique and case report. Br J Ophthalmol. 2009;93:861-3.

23. Shousha MA, Yoo SH, Kymionis GD, et al. Long-term results of femtosecond laser-assisted sutureless anterior lamellar keratoplasty. Ophthalmology. 2011;118:315-23.

24. Chan CC, Ritenour RJ, Kumar NL, et al. Femtosecond laser-assisted mushroom configuration deep anterior lamellar keratoplasty. Cornea. 2010;29:290-5.

25. Buzzonetti L, Laborante A, Petrocelli G. Standardized big-bubble technique in deep anterior lamellar keratoplasty assisted by the femtosecond laser. J Cataract Refract Surg. 2010;36:1631-6.

26. Farid M, Steinert RF. Deep anterior lamellar keratoplasty performed with the femtosecond laser zigzag incision for the treatment of stromal corneal pathology and ectatic disease. J Cataract Refract Surg. 2009;35:809-13.

27. Yoo SH, Kymionis GD, O'Brien TP, et al. Femtosecond-assisted diagnostic corneal biopsy (FAB) in keratitis. Graefes Arch Clin Exp Ophthalmol. 2008;246:759-62.

28. Price FW, Price MO, Jordan CS. Safety of incomplete incision patterns in femtosecond laser-assisted penetrating keratoplasty. J Cataract Refract Surg. 2008;34:2099-103.

29. Buzzonetti L, Laborante A, Petrocelli G. Refractive outcome of keratoconus treated by combined femtosecond laser and big-bubble deep anterior lamellar keratoplasty. J Refract Surg. 2011;27:189-94.

30. Ruiz LA, Cepeda LM, Fuentes VC. Intrastromal correction of presbyopia using a femtosecond laser system. J Refract Surg. 2009;25:847-54.

31. Ernest PH, Lavery KT, Kiessling LA. Relative strength of scleral corneal and clear corneal incisions constructed in cadaver eyes. J Cataract Refract Surg. 1994;20:626-9.

32. Pfleger T, Skorpik C, Menapace R, et al. Long-term course of induced astigmatism after clear corneal incision cataract surgery. J Cataract Refract Surg. 1996;22:72-7.

33. Masket S, Belani S. Proper wound construction to prevent short-term ocular hypotony after clear corneal incision cataract surgery. J Cataract Refract Surg. 2007;33:383-6.

34. He L, Sheehy K, Culbertson W. Femtosecond laser-assisted cataract surgery. Curr Opin Ophthalmol. 2010.

35. Donnenfeld E. Multicenter prospective evaluation of effects of cataract extraction and limbal relaxing incisions on corneal sensation and dry eye. In: American Society of Cataract and Refractive Surgery Annual Meeting. San Diego, CA; 2011.

# CHAPTER 114

# Femtosecond Refractive Lenticule Extraction and Small Incision Lenticule Extraction

*Karim Mohamed-Noriega, Jodhbir S Mehta*

## ❖ INTRODUCTION

Refractive lenticule extraction (ReLEx) is a new and promising cornea refractive procedure and that is an alternative to laser *in situ* keratomileusis (LASIK). ReLEx is the first all-in-one femtosecond (FS) laser refractive procedure that does not require an excimer or mechanical microkeratome. It corrects the refractive error by creating a refractive intrastromal lenticule that is manually extracted out of the cornea. Refractive lenticule extraction consists of two surgical procedures: (1) femtosecond lenticule extraction (FLEx) and (2) small incision lenticule extraction (SMILE).[1] FLEx requires the creation of a flap, akin to

LASIK, to remove the lenticule. SMILE is a flapless and minimally invasive procedure that extracts the lenticule from a small cornea incision (Fig. 1).[2,3]

## ❖ FEMTOSECOND LASER

The FS laser is a near-infrared, photodisruptive neodymium-doped yttrium aluminum garnet (Nd:YAG) laser.[4] It works at a wavelength of 1053 nm, and the laser beam has a diameter of 1 micron, that can be focused to a 3-$\mu$m spot and is accurate to within 5 $\mu$m.[4] It can produce ultrashort pulses of light ($10^{-15}$ of a second or femtosecond) at high repetition rates.[4] These pulses elicit a cleavage

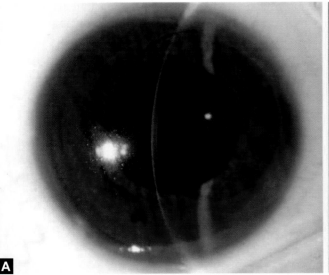
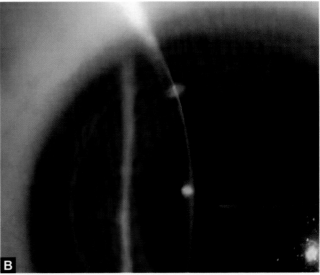

**Figs 1A and B:** SMILE 1 month after surgery. (A) A clear cornea is observed after SMILE. Only a fine superficial scar, corresponding to the small arcuate incision, is observed in the superotemporal cornea. No haze is observed; (B) Higher magnification of "A" at the area of the incision

of tissue planes by creating small bubbles, thus making highly accurate incisions with minimal tissue damage and exothermic reaction.[4-7]

Currently, the only FS laser that has the software to do ReLEx is the VisuMax® FS laser (Carl Zeiss Meditec, Jena, Germany).[2,3] The new version of the VisuMax® produces ultrashort pulses of light at a repetition rate of 500 kHz (older machines were 200 kHz).[7,8] The typical pulse energy used for ReLEx is between 130–200 nJ and a spot distance of 2–6 μm.[3,8,9] The laser disrupts the cornea by delivering the laser pulses in a spiral scanning pattern, either in a centripetal direction from the periphery to the center of the cornea (scanning pattern spiral-in) or in a centrifugal direction from the center to the periphery of the cornea (scanning pattern spiral-out).[10,1] Hence, there are four possible scanning pattern combinations that can be used to cut the stromal lenticule: (1) spiral in/out: spiral-in for the posterior lenticule surface and spiral-out for the anterior lenticule surface; (2) spiral out/in: Spiral out for the posterior lenticule and spiral in for the anterior lenticule; (3) spiral in/in: Spiral in for the posterior and the anterior lenticule surface; (4) spiral out/out: spiral out for the posterior and the anterior lenticule surface. The posterior surface must always be disrupted first since the laser cannot focus through previous cavitation bubbles. The scanning pattern spiral in/out is the one that yields the best clinical outcomes with respect to visual acuity.[10] Even though other patterns produced equivalent ultrastructural results, spiral in/out is the recommended scanning pattern since it maintains fixation for the longest duration during the lenticule formation.[10,1,11] The VisuMax® FS laser has a unique curved suction contact glass (so-called treatment pack or cone) that allows minimal distortion of the cornea and minimal elevation of intraocular pressure (IOP) during suction and placement of laser pulses.[4,10-12] The curved suction contact glass comes in three sizes (S, M, L) depending on the white-to-white diameter of the cornea on which it is to be applied and to the size of the desired flap/cap. For a minimum white-to-white diameter of 11.2 mm, it is advised to use an S cone, for a minimum of 11.7, a M cone and for a minimum of 12.4 mm, a L cone.[13] The smallest possible treatment pack should be selected. For Asian eyes, we use in most of the cases the S-cone. If the suction ring of the cone is too large for the cornea, it may cause loss of suction due to inadvertent sucking in of the loose conjunctiva hence disrupting the suction ring.[13] Current company recommendation for ReLEx is to always use an S cone (unpublished data). The S cone allows for a lenticule diameter of 6.5 mm and a cap diameter of up to 7.9 mm.

## ⊁ INDICATIONS

At the moment of writing this chapter, ReLEx is indicated to correct myopia with or without astigmatism. The maximum spherical equivalent (SE) refraction that can be corrected is −10.0 diopters (D), the maximum myopia is −10.0 D and the maximum cylinder is −5.00 D.[3] However, the treatment range may be increased in the near future. Nomogram adjustment for hyperopic treatment is also under study.

## ⊁ PREOPERATIVE ASSESSMENT AND FOLLOW-UP

Preoperative evaluation is the same as for LASIK,[14] and the same precautions should be made to avoid iatrogenic cornea ectasia.[14] In the future, deeper ablations may be possible if superior biomechanical stability is shown but further research is required in this area. In the authors' center,[11] the patients should be at least 21 years old, should have stable manifest cycloplegic refraction for at least 12 months, a stable and regular topography and pachymetry maps, and normal anterior segment and fundal examination. The estimated residual stromal bed (RSB) should not be less than 250 μm, avoid thin corneas (< 500 μm), steep corneas (> 47.00 D), irregular topographic images, asymmetric thinning and inferior steepening. Keratoconus and fruste-keratoconus remain a contraindication. If patients use contact lens, they should be off them for at least 1 week if wearing soft contact lenses and 3 weeks if wearing rigid gas permeable lenses before the assessment examination to avoid irregular topography maps compatible with contact lens wearpage. If irregular maps are found, the patient must refrain from contact lens wear until the anterior topographic maps return to normal.

A slit-lamp evaluation is important to confirm that the eye is normal and to rule out severe dry eye, meibomian gland dysfunction, cataract, atopy, eyelid disorders that prevent correct eyelid closure and conditions that may compromise a healthy ocular surface. Patient with diseases of the cornea should be excluded. Attention should be made to look for cornea scars, because the FS laser may not be able to cut through the scar. Dry eye patients may be better candidates for SMILE because there is less risk of having neurotrophic dry eye after the surgery due to less damage to the cornea nerves (unpublished data, presented in APACRS 2012, Karim Mohamed). Dilated posterior fundus evaluation to verify that the optic nerve is normal and to rule out peripheral retinal disorders as retinal tears, retinal holes or lattice with holes that may increase the probability of retinal detachment related to the suction of the FS-laser machine. However, in these eyes, a prophylactic treatment with laser photocoagulation of the peripheral retina should allow the patient to have surgery. Rule out manifest or subclinical strabismus. Consider not operating on patients with glaucoma, history of ocular trauma or previous ocular surgery. Active ocular or systemic disease likely to affect corneal wound healing should also be excluded. Ideally, the patient eyes should be healthy without any eye disease and the only problem should be the refractive error. Although amblyopic patients may have surgery, the ideal candidate should have a best spectacle-corrected visual acuity (BSCVA) of 20/20 or better. Pregnancy and breastfeeding are a contraindication.[11]

Follow-up is the same as for LASIK, i.e. 1 day, 1 week, 1 month then 3 months.[11,14] Postoperative treatment is topical corticosteroids eyedrops four times a day for 1 or 2 weeks, 3rd or 4th generation fluoroquinolones four times a day for 1 week and preservative free artificial tears four times a day for 1 month. Artificial tears can be used more often and longer time if needed.[2,3,11]

## ▶ SURGICAL PROCEDURE

All ReLEx procedures share similar surgical steps at the beginning of the procedure (first half, shared steps). After these common steps, there are specific steps for FLEx or SMILE (second half, specific steps).

Before starting the surgery, it is important to verify that the correct patient and eye is undergoing the correct refractive correction. The authors preprogram the laser before the patient enters the laser room to ensure the laser settings and parameters are correct (see the laser settings in Table 1), verify that the correct refractive treatment is programmed in the machine, confirm the correct eye is selected and the correct cone size has been chosen. The shape and thickness of the lenticule depends on the refractive correction. However, there is no transition zone as seen in LASIK and lenticule sizes of between 6 and 7 mm in diameter may be chosen.[2,3,9,11,12] The reason there is no transition zone is due to the fact the lenticule shape is designed to preserve the normal prolate curvature of the cornea and to allow a smooth transition to the untreated cornea. The lenticule edge thickness is approximately 15 μm to facilitate its removal from the eye when grasping it with the forceps especially in low power treatments.[12] The flap/cap diameter compared to the lenticule diameter can be altered depending on surgeon preference but is normally at least 0.5 mm. Hence if a 6.5 mm lenticule size

is chosen then a flap/cap of 7 mm is selected.[11] Currently, no nomogram is used for programming the laser and normally the full manifest refraction is entered. However, a nomogram adjustment may be required in the future as more clinical data is acquired. In the authors' experience, they have found that for myopic correction greater than or equal to −5 D the postoperative outcome has been very accurate but in lower myopic corrections, they have aimed for an overcorrection of 0.25 D. Accurate centration is very important. Only when appropriate centration on the visual axis is achieved, is the suction applied. A low IOP rise and low suction pressure ensures that there are no blackouts and enables continuous visualization of the fixation target by the patient. Following creation of the posterior lenticule surface, the fixation target becomes more blurred than at the beginning of the procedure. It is recommended to continuously talk to the patient, to reassure him/her that everything is going fine and to keep him/her calm. That is to prevent excessive eye squeezing and eye movements what may cause a loss of suction. Excessive tearing may also cause suction loss but this can be prevented by meticulous drying of the ocular surface prior to the start of the procedure.

## Common ReLEx, FLEx and SMILE Steps (First Half Shared Steps)

After the application of topical anesthesia and povidone-iodine (betadine) scrub of the skin and eyelids, a standard sterile drape and the speculum are inserted. The patient is directed to stare at the fixation target and the laser is centered on the target eye. After correct alignment, the eye is docked under the curved interface cone (the standard cone size that the authors use in their Asian eyes in S due to the small white-to-white diameter in their patient population) attached to the optical aperture and application of suction is applied. After full suction is acquired and pupil centration confirmed (an infrared light on the laser can be used to confirm centration), the laser treatment is started. As previously mentioned, a spiral in/out scanning pattern is chosen (see laser settings in Table 1) (Figs 2A to C and 3A to C). First, the posterior surface of the refractive lenticule is cut (spiral in), followed by the lenticule side cut. Second, the anterior surface of the lenticule is cut (spiral out), and then the flap/cap is created by extension of 0.5 mm beyond the edge of the anterior surface of lenticule. The next surgery steps are specific for either FLEx or for SMILE. Either a complete rim cut is made with a hinge similar to LASIK for FLEx, or a small circumferential incision is made for SMILE.

**Table 1:** The authors' laser parameters in refractive lenticule extraction

|  | FLEx | SMILE |
| --- | --- | --- |
| Pulse frequency | 500 kHz | 500 kHz |
| Pulse energy | 145 nJ | ≤ 145 nJ |
| *Lenticule* | | |
| Posterior surface scanning pattern | Spiral in | Spiral in |
| Diameter (mm) | 6.5 | 6.5 |
| Edge thickness (µm) | ≥ 15 | ≥ 15 |
| Spot distance/tracking space (µm) | 3/3 | 3/3 |
| Side cut angle | 90º | 90º |
| Side cut spot distance/tracking space (µm) | 2.5/2.5 | 2.5/2.5 |
| *Flap/Cap* | | |
| Lenticule anterior surface and flap/cap scanning pattern | Spiral out | Spiral out |
| Diameter (mm) (≥ 0.5 mm than lenticule) | 7.5 | 7.5 |
| Flap/cap thickness (µm) | 120 | 120 |
| Flap/SMILE access incision, side cut angle | 90º | 90º |
| Flap/SMILE access incision, spot distance/tracking space (µm) | 3/3 | 3/3 |
| Flap/SMILE access incision side cut, spot distance/tracking space (µm) | 2/2 | 2/2 |
| Flap hinge/SMILE incision, location and length | Superior, 50º cord length | Superior, 3–4 mm |

FLEx: Femtosecond lenticule extraction; SMILE: Small incision lenticule extraction

## Femtosecond Lenticule Extraction Specific Steps (Second Half Steps)

After the flap is created by extension of the anterior lenticule surface, the flap side cut is created leaving a superior hinge (similar to LASIK). After the laser firing is completed, the suction is automatically released. A superior located hinge is set for default, however, the surgeon can change its location. Before lifting the flap is important to mark the cornea with asymmetrical ink markings to allow an adequate and aligned flap repositioning at the end of the procedure. A Seibel spatula (Rhein Medical, Heidelberg, Germany) is inserted under the flap near the hinge to find the dissection plane, the flap is separated and reflected, similar to LASIK. The lenticule edge is identified with a Sinsky hook and is separated from the residual stromal. A Seibel spatula is introduced in the plane of the posterior lenticule surface and the posterior surface of the lenticule is partially separated from the residual stromal bed to the point that part of the lenticule is free. By gently grasping the free end of the lenticule with non-toothed serrated forceps the lenticule is peeled off from the residual formal bed. The flap is repositioned, the interface is flushed with BSS, and the flap is placed in correct position and dried with sponges, as in LASIK. Topical steroid and antibiotic eye drops are applied (Figs 4A to F).

## Pseudo-SMILE

The laser is performed exactly the same as FLEx, but the flap is not lifted, only a small incision is opened and the lenticule is extracted akin to SMILE. Since it is easier to

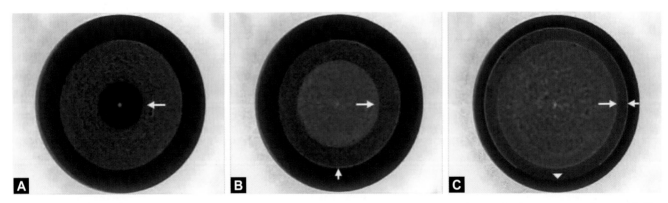

**Figs 2A to C:** FLEx laser firing sequence. After full suction is acquired and pupil centration confirmed, the laser treatment is started. The patient must always look at the fixation target (green light). (A-C) Representative and consecutive images of FLEx laser firing sequence; (A) First the posterior lenticule surface is cut in a spiral-in scanning pattern (arrow); (B) The lenticule side-cut is created (small arrow) and followed by the anterior lenticule surface in a spiral-out scanning pattern (long arrow); (C) A peripheral extension of anterior lenticule surface creates the flap. Following, the flap side-cut (small arrow) is created leaving a superior hinge (arrowhead). The laser firing sequence is concluded and the lenticule edge can easily be observed (long arrow).

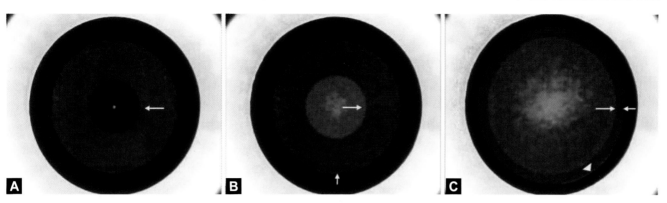

**Figs 3A to C:** SMILE laser firing sequence. After full suction is acquired and pupil centration confirmed, the laser treatment is started. The patient must always look at the fixation target (green light). (A-C) Representative and consecutive images of SMILE laser firing sequence; (A) First the posterior lenticule surface is first cut in a spiral-in scanning pattern (arrow); (B) The lenticule side-cut is created (small arrow) and followed by the anterior lenticule surface in a spiral-out scanning pattern (long arrow); (C) A peripheral extension of anterior lenticule surface creates the cap (small arrow). Finally an arcuate incision is created at the edge of the cap (arrowhead) and the laser firing sequence is concluded. The lenticule edge can easily be observed (long arrow).

remove the lenticule from the superior location, the laser is programmed so that the hinge position is rotated to the upper temporal quadrant. A 5–6 mm superior opening is created in order to remove the lenticule, care is taken during the lenticule dissection not to inadvertently open the complete side cut hence converting to a standard FLEx procedure. It is a procedure that is generally performed during the learning curve and transition from FLEx to SMILE.

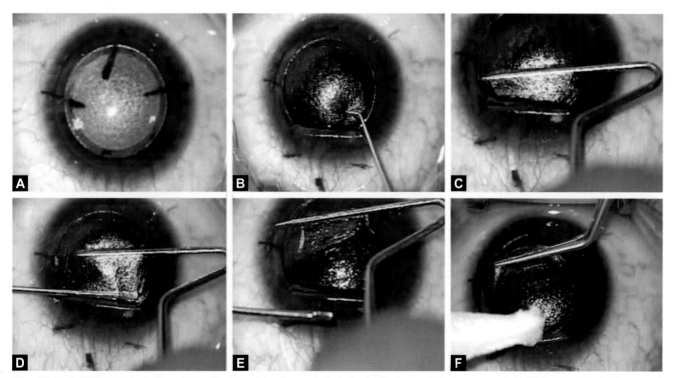

**Figs 4A to F:** FLEx surgical steps. Once the laser firing is concluded, the lenticule needs to be removed. (A-F) Representative images of sequential surgical steps in FLEx; (A) Before lifting the flap is important to mark the cornea with asymmetrical marking; (B) After the flap has been lifted with a Seibel spatula, the lenticule edge is identified and the posterior surface of the lenticule is located with aid of a Sinsky hook; (C) A Seibel spatula is introduced in the plane of the posterior surface of the lenticule; (D-E) The posterior surface of the lenticule is partially separated from the residual stromal bed with the Seibel spatula to the point that part of the lenticule is free; (F) The free segment of the lenticule is grasped with Kelman forceps and the lenticule is completely peeled off from the residual stromal bed. Finally the flap is repositioned (image not shown).

## Small Incision Lenticule Extraction Specific Steps (Second Half Steps)

After the cap is created by extension of the anterior lenticule surface, the laser creates a small 2.5–4 mm arcuate opening in the superior/superior temporal part of the cornea. In the first published series of SMILE surgeries, a superior and an inferior incision were performed to aid removal of the lenticule. Currently, only one incision 2.5–4 mm long is required. The incision is opened with a Sinskey hook and the anterior and posterior surface of the lenticule are localized. The anterior surface of the lenticule is first dissected and separated from the cap with a femtolamellar dissector (Asico®) in a smooth rotational movement similar to a cornea lamellar dissection. Following which the posterior surface of the lenticule is dissected and separated from the RSB using the same dissector in a similar motion. The rotational movement is important to achieve a smooth lamellar dissection. The lenticule edge is then grasped and extracted from the cornea with forceps. The authors use the Tan DSAEK Forceps AE-4226 to remove the lenticule since the grip is reliable (Asico®). The interface is flushed with BSS and topical steroid and antibiotic eye drops are applied. The time for the laser procedure is 28–55 seconds depending on the size of lenticule and speed of laser (Figs 5A to F).[9-11]

## ⯈ BASIC SCIENCE

### Surface Regularity of Stromal Bed and Lenticule

The surface of the corneal stromal bed and the extracted lenticules in FLEx is regular and smooth.[11,15,16] The surface quality of the lenticule anterior surface has been qualitatively comparable to the RSB after FS-LASIK with the same FS laser system, but smoother than the RSB after removal of the lenticule in FLEx. The smoothness of the RSB has not been found to be related to the degree of myopic correction or depth of laser cutting;[11] however, it is related to the scanning pattern of the laser delivery.[1] Riau et al. analyzed

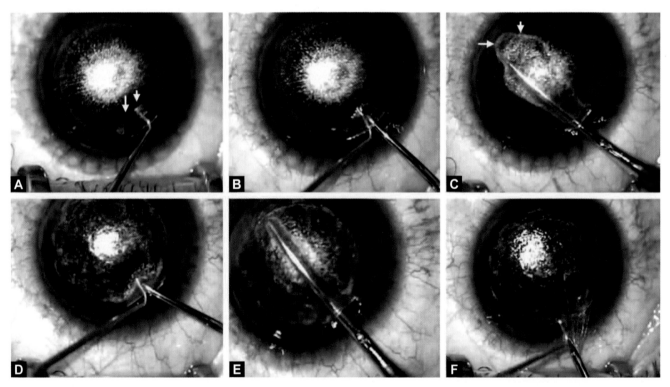

**Figs 5A to F:** SMILE surgical steps. Once the laser firing is concluded, the lenticule needs to be dissected and extracted. (A-F) Representative images of sequential surgical steps in SMILE; (A) The anterior (long arrow) and posterior (small arrow) surface of the lenticule are identified with a Sinskey hook; (B) The femto-lamellar dissector is introduced, with aid of a Sinskey hook, in the plane of the lenticule anterior surface; (C) The anterior surface of the lenticule is dissected with the femtolamellar dissector. It is essential to dissect (long arrow) beyond the margins of the lenticule (small arrow) in order to release the lenticule from the stroma; (D) After complete dissection of the lenticule anterior surface and with aid of a Sinskey hook, the femtolamellar dissector is introduced in the previously located plane of the lenticule posterior surface; (E) A complete dissection of the posterior surface of the lenticule is performed beyond the edge of the lenticule; (F) Finally the lenticule is extracted from the cornea with forceps.

the cornea collagen surface of rabbit eyes after four different laser scanning patterns and found that the corneal collagen arrangement is more disrupted with a scanning pattern spiral out/out. On the contrary, the scanning pattern spiral in/spiral out produced less collagen fibrillar disruption. Hence, a scanning pattern spiral in/spiral out and careful manual dissection, peeling and extraction of the lenticule are related to an earlier VA recovery during the first week after surgery.[1,11] Most surface irregularities are caused by tissue bridges and cavitation bubbles, although not both types of irregularities are present in every lenticule.[15,16] Tissue bridges produce a serrated surface. Cavitation bubbles produce ring-like slot irregularities of different sizes called cavitation marks. Third surface irregularities are the grooves that run crisscross over the cutting surface of some of the lenticules. They may be surgically induced at the moment of removing tissue bridges; however, they do not affect the surface quality as much as the other two irregularities.[15] Cavitation bubbles and tissue bridges reduce the surface regularity more than the grooves. The surface quality of the refractive lenticule has been shown to decrease as pulse energy is increased.[15,16] Cavitation bubbles and tissue bridges are reduced with lower pulse energies, higher frequencies and smaller spot sizes; thus making it easier to dissect and lift the flap and lenticule.[15,16]

## Early Inflammation, Cell Proliferation and Wound Healing

Refractive lenticule extraction (FLEX) has been shown to result in less inflammation and early extracellular matrix deposition than LASIK, especially at higher corrections.[12] An early inflammation marker (antibody anti-CD11b, expressed in monocytes) and an extracellular matrix marker (fibronectin) were expressed 1 day after FLEx, located in the interface and the flap margin (side cut).[1,12] The expression of CD11b in ReLEx was significantly less when compared to LASIK in higher myopic corrections (−6.00 D and −9.00 D). At lower corrections (−3D), the expression was less than LASIK but not statistically significant. The reason for this difference is because in ReLEx the amount of inflammation induced by the laser and lenticule extraction remains constant regardless of the myopic correction. Whereas in LASIK, the amount of inflammation increases with increasing levels of excimer ablation. Hence, a −9D ablation causes more inflammation than a −3D ablation.[12] However, there was minimal CD11b expression in eyes that did not have the lenticules removed compared to those that had the full ReLEx procedure.[12] This suggested that

the laser itself induced minimal inflammation and that the inflammatory response following ReLEx was related to the lenticule extraction and the flap lift.

Fibronectin expression was similar in eyes that had a complete ReLEx procedure (i.e. had lenticules extracted) and in eyes where the flap was not lifted and the lenticule removed. This indicated there was no excessive extracellular matrix formation from the lenticule removal. Cell proliferation after ReLEx (FLEx) was detected 1 day after surgery with the proliferation marker Ki-67.[12] However, most of the proliferation was restricted to the epithelial cells of the flap margin and was not significantly different to changes following LASIK.[12] The cell proliferation at the flap margin in FLEx and LASIK is likely due to the flap itself, hence with SMILE this will be less. In the same rabbit model, in vivo confocal microscopy (CM) showed significantly less light-scattering particles at the flap interface after FLEx compared with LASIK at higher corrections (−6 D and −9 D). A similar trend but not significant was observed at −3D.[12] This suggests more damage to the stromal bed in LASIK than in ReLEx at higher corrections and this damage is related to the increased levels of laser ablation, supporting the previous findings of greater inflammation and extracellular matrix deposition after LASIK particularly at higher corrections. Also in ReLEx, the light scattering was similar in all eyes independent of the level of myopic correction.[12]

## Cell Death, Keratocyte Viability after Refractive Lenticule Extraction

In a rabbit model comparing FLEx and LASIK, there was no significant difference in the number of apoptotic keratocytes in the cornea following surgery in the two groups[12] as detected with deoxynucleotidyl transferase-mediated nick end labeling (TUNEL) assay. TUNEL assay detects fragmented DNA and allows the observation of apoptotic cells, but is not completely specific.[7] After FLEx more TUNEL positive cells were detected in the periphery than in the center of the flap area after removal of the lenticule.[12] Interestingly, eyes that underwent FLEx but in which the flap was not lifted and hence the lenticule were not extracted only showed apoptotic cells at the margins of the lenticule.[12] This result showed that the apoptotic cells of the lenticule were caused by the laser formation of the lenticule and not related to the tissue manipulation by the surgeon during the lenticule extraction. It also showed that the laser was very precise with respect to lenticule formation. After ReLEx, live and dead keratocytes were observed in the lenticule as shown in both animal[12] and in human cadaveric corneas;[7] however, the majority of cells were alive. The lenticules also show significantly more dead cells in the anterior and posterior surface than in the center.[7] Transmission electron microscopy analysis of the extracted lenticules found a mixture of normal and dead keratocytes. The mechanism of cell death was found to be mixed, apoptosis or necrosis, and mainly located on surface of the lenticule.[7] However, the majority of the cells identified in the lenticule stained with DAPI and were not detected by TUNEL. This implied that the majority of cells were alive. This was proved following collagenase digestion of the lenticules and cell culture. The isolated cells from the lenticule were able to be grown in a serum containing medium and express keratocyte specific markers, human aldehyde dehydrogenase 3A1 (ALDH3A1) and keratocan (KERA).[7]

## Topographic and Keratometric Changes

Refractive lenticule extraction may result in less topographic changes than LASIK at higher corrections (e.g. −9 D), however, no significant differences were observed after −3 D and −6 D corrections as showed in a rabbit model.[12] After a −9.00 D correction, the average K was 34.9 ± 2.9 D after LASIK and 37.3 ± 1.2 D after FLEx (P = 0.097).[12] However, more work needs to be done in this area in both animal studies and human clinical trials to confirm this initial observation.

## ▸ CLINICAL OUTCOMES

The first published paper on the safety of ReLEx (FLEx) was published in 2008 by Sekundo and Blum.[8] At the time of writing this chapter, the majority of published series used the 200 kHz VisuMax® laser. Newer hardware improvements with the 500 kHz laser may yield even better outcomes. Visual outcomes after refractive surgery in general include the following evaluations: (1) predictability [postoperative mean manifest refraction spherical equivalent (MRSE), attempted versus achieved refraction, and mean induced astigmatism]; (2) stability (SE regression); (3) efficacy (uncorrected visual acuity, UCVA); (4) safety (loss and gain lines of BSCVA); (5) contrast sensitivity; (6) higher order aberrations (HOA); (7) side effects.

## Femtosecond Lenticule Extraction

A summary on the visual outcomes and safety of FLEx is in Table 2. Results with FLEx have been very encouraging, but since this is a new refractive procedure, the longest published follow-up time is 12 months (range: 3–12 months) and the number of eyes, in each series are small (< 108 eyes). The following outcomes are expressed up to the latest follow-up for each paper (please see detailed data in Table 2). These studies show that FLEx has good predictability, with 75–84% of eyes being within ± 0.50 D of target refraction and 96–100% within ± 1.00 D of target refraction.[2,11,17-19] The exception of these results was in the first reported series of 10 eyes where only 40% of eyes were within ± 0.50 D and 90% was within ± 1.00 D of target refraction.[8] The fact that this first report showed inferior outcomes in predictability than all of the published data is to be expected since this was a more proof of concept paper and as more experience has been obtained, the outcomes have improved. Future refinement of the nomogram might be helpful to improve results further. Postoperative results with FLEx have shown to be predictable achieving a mean MRSE that was between −0.06 ± 0.35 D and −0.23 ± 0.35 D.[2,11,17-19] Once again, excluding the first reported series, that showed inferior levels of predictability with a mean MRSE of −0.33 ± 0.61 D.[8]

Femtosecond lenticule extraction has been shown to be a very stable procedure with a mean SE regression ranging from 0.09 to 0.19 D.[2,11,17-19] The papers with longer follow-up (12 months) show a similar SE regression of 0.15 D[17] and 0.14 D[19] respectively.

The efficacy of FLEx has been good with a cumulative UCVA of 20/25 or better achieved in 87–90% of the eyes.[2,11,18,19] The safety of FLEx has also been demonstrated. The majority of eyes maintain or improve their preoperative BSCVA after FLEx.[2,8,9,11,17-19] It is surprising to see that the percentage of eyes that gain one or more lines of BSCVA ranges from 21% to 60%.[2,8,11,17-19] However, in a few series, there is reported loss of BSCVA.[2,17,18] Overall, the percentage of eyes that experience loss of one line of BSCVA range from 3% to 12.5%.[2,8,11,17-19] Two series reported loss of two lines of BSCVA in two eyes (5%) at 3 months[18] and in one eye (0.9%) at 6 months[2] respectively. Best spectacle corrected visual acuity seems to improve over time; no eyes have been reported loss of two or more lines of BSCVA after 12 months in the series with longer follow-up.[17,19] Blum et al. mention that those eyes with loss of BSCVA may benefit from prolonged steroid eye drops therapy and improve their BSCVA to preoperative values.[2] However, one eye in their series lost two lines of BSCVA, due to the cessation of prolonged steroid therapy due to pregnancy.[2] Vestergaard et al. mentioned that the two eyes

**Table 2:** Review of published papers on FLEx outcomes

| Outcomes/Author | Sekundo, Blum, et al. 2008[8] | Blum, Sekundo, et al. 2010[2] | Blum, Sekundo, et al. 2010[17] | Ang M, Jodhbir S Mehta, et al. 2012[11] | Vestergaard A, Ivarsen A, et al. 2012[18] | Gertnere J, Sekundo W, et al. 2012[19] |
|---|---|---|---|---|---|---|
| Follow-up (months) | 6 | 6 | 12 | 3 | 3 | 12 |
| Eyes (number) | 10 | 108 | 62 | 66 | 80 | 44 |
| Preoperative refractive error | Myopia | Myopia and myopic astigmatism | Myopia and myopic astigmatism | Myopia and myopic astigmatism | Myopia and myopic astigmatism | Myopia and myopic astigmatism |
| Preoperative mean MRSE (D) | −4.73 ± 1.48 D | −4.59 ± 1.30 D | −4.81 ± 1.16 D | −5.77 ± 2.04 D | −7.50 ± 1.16 D | −5.13 D ± 1.41 D |
| *Predictability* | | | | | | |
| Postoperative mean MRSE (D) | −0.33 ± 0.61 D | −0.19 ± 0.47 D | −0.15 ± 0.46 D | 0.14 ± 0.53 D (1.75 to −1.63) | −0.06 ± 0.35 D | 0.23 ± 0.35 D |
| Attempted vs achieved refraction within ± 0.50 D | 40% | 74.8% | — | 81.8% | 83% | 84% |
| Attempted vs achieved refraction within ± 1.00 D | 90% | 98.1% | 100% | 95.5% | 100% | 100% |
| Induced astigmatism: Mean ± SD (range) | −0.12 | −0.40 ± 0.38 D (−1.75 to 0.0) | −0.02 ± 0.03 D (−0.87 to +0.75) | −0.38 ± 0.43 D | — | — |
| *Stability* | | | | | | |
| SE regression (D) | 0.19 | 0.16 | 0.15 | 0.14 | 0.09 | 0.14 |
| *Safety* | | | | | | |
| Lost > 2 lines of BSCVA | 0% | 0% | 0% | 0% | 0% | 0% |
| Lost 2 lines of BSCVA | 0(0%) | 1 (0.9%) | 0 (0%) | 0 (0%) | 2 (5%) | 0% |
| Lost 1 line of BSCVA | 1 (10%) | 8 (7.4%) | 7 (11.3%) | 3% | 5 (12.5%) | 5% |
| Unchanged BSCVA | 3 (30%) | 42 (39.3%) | 21 (33.9%) | 76% | 21 (52.5%) | 49% |
| Gained 1 line of BSCVA | 4 (40%) | 46 (43%) | 28 (45.2%) | 9% | 12 (30%) | 46% |
| Gained 2 lines of BSCVA | 2 (20%) | 10 (9.3%) | 5 (8.1%) | 12% | 0 (0%) | 0% |
| Gained > 2 lines of BSCVA | 0 (0%) | 0 (0%) | 0 (0%) | 0% | 0 (0%) | 0% |
| *Efficacy* | | | | | | |
| Cumulative UCVA ≥ 20/20 (%) | — | 73% | — | 65% | 56% | 68% |
| Cumulative UCVA ≥ 20/25 (%) | — | 87% | — | 88% | 88% | 90% |
| Cumulative UCVA ≥ 20/32 (%) | — | 96% | — | — | 100% | 95% |
| Cumulative UCVA ≥ 20/40 (%) | 90% | 97% | — | — | 100% | 100% |

*Contd...*

| Outcomes\ Author | Sekundo, Blum, et al. 2008[8] | Blum, Sekundo, et al. 2010[2] | Blum, Sekundo, et al. 2010[17] | Ang M, Jodhbir S Mehta, et al. 2012[11] | Vestergaard A, Ivarsen A, et al. 2012[18] | Gertnere J, Sekundo W, et al. 2012[19] |
|---|---|---|---|---|---|---|
| *Higher order aberrations* | | | | | | |
| Total induction of RMS HOA | 0.03 ± 0.08 | — | — | 0.12 ± 0.02 Significant | — | 0.08 |
| Induction of spherical aberration Z4, 0 | −0.02 ± 0.08 | — | — | +0.11 Significant | Increase but significantly less than LASIK | −0.087 |
| Induction of Coma Z3, +1 | 0.05 ± 0.07 | — | — | +0.07 Significant | Increase but not significantly more than LASIK | — |

FLEx: Femtosecond lenticule extraction; D: Diopter; MRSE: Manifest refraction spherical equivalent; SE: Spherical equivalent; UCVA: Uncorrected visual acuity; BSCVA: Best spectacle-corrected visual acuity; RMS: Root mean square; HOA: Higher order aberrations

that lost two lines of BSCVA in their series were related to difficulties during the surgical procedure that led to the development of corneal haze (i.e. difficult to remove the lenticule from the stromal bed and a central corneal abrasion during surgery).[18] Therefore, we speculate that with longer steroid eyedrops (2 weeks), it can be possible to reduce this early loss of BSCVA. There have been few reported side effects following FLEx, these have been documented in detail, later in this chapter. The most common is transient dry eye that resolves with lubricant eyedrops.[2,8,11,17-19] There are a couple of studies that have retrospectively compared FLEx and LASIK and are documented later in this chapter. However, there is a need for more prospective and comparative studies of FLEx and LASIK.

### Small Incision Lenticule Extraction

A detailed description on the visual outcomes and safety of SMILE is displayed in Table 3. In published studies, SMILE has shown satisfactory results, but again since this is a relatively new surgical procedure, there are only a few published papers on visual outcomes at the moment of writing this chapter.[3,9] The maximum published follow-up time is 6 months and sample sizes vary between 51 and 91 eyes. The following outcomes are documented with the latest follow-up available for each paper (see data in Table 2). These studies show that SMILE has good predictability, with 80–91% of eyes being within ± 0.50 D of target refraction, 95–100% within ± 1.00 D of target refraction and with no significant induction of astigmatism.[3,9] Also, postoperatively, the residual refractive error achieved had a mean MRSE of between −0.01 ± 0.49 D and 0.03 ± 0.30 D after 6 months in the two published papers respectively.[3,9] Small incision lenticule extraction has proved to be a very stable procedure with a mean SE regression ranging from −0.06 to 0.10 D at 6 months.[2,17] It has been shown to be efficacious, 79–91% of eyes have UCVA of 20/25 or better and 95–98% have an UCVA of 20/32 or better.[3,9] SMILE is a safe procedure and the majority of the eyes maintain or even improve their preoperative BSCVA after SMILE.[3,9] It is interesting to note that the percentage of eyes that gain one or more lines of BSCVA ranges from 25% to 35%.[3,9] However, 4–8% of eyes lost one line of BSCVA and in one series two eyes (2.2%) were reported to have lost two or more lines of BSCVA at 6 months.[3]

There are few side effects, which are commented later in this chapter, and the most common is transient dry eye that resolves with lubricant eyedrops.[3,9] There is a need for more studies with longer follow-up and greater sample sizes; as well as prospective and comparative studies of SMILE and LASIK.

### ❧ REFRACTIVE LENTICULE EXTRACTION (FLEx AND SMILE)

### Early Visual Acuity, Stability of Refraction and Regression of Refractive Error

Early visual recovery, UCVA greater than or equal to 20/25 1 day after FLEx was achieved only in 41% of the eyes.[7] However, this is temporal and visual acuity and refractive error seems to be stabilized after 1 month from ReLEx.[2,3,9,17] After 3 months, the percentage of eyes with

**Table 3:** Review of published papers on SMILE outcomes

| Outcomes | Sekundo, Blum, et al. 2011[3] | R Shah, MS, S Shah, et al. 2011[9] |
|---|---|---|
| Follow-up (months) | 6 | 6 |
| Eyes (number) | 91 | 51 |
| Preoperative refractive error | Myopia and myopic astigmatism | Myopia and myopic astigmatism |
| Preoperative mean MRSE (D) | −4.75 ± 1.56 D | −4.87 ± 2.16 D |
| *Predictability* | | |
| Postoperative mean MRSE (D) | −0.01 ± 0.49 D | +0.03 ± 0.30 D (0.75 to −0.75) |
| Attempted vs achieved refraction within ± 0.50 D | 80.2% | 91% |
| Attempted vs achieved refraction within ± 1.00 D | 95.6% | 100% |
| Induced astigmatism: Mean ± SD (range) | No topographic induction of | −0.07 D |
| *Stability* | | |
| SE regression at 6 or 12 months (D) | 0.10 | −0.06 |
| *Safety* | | |
| Lost > 2 lines of BSCVA | 1 (1.1%) | 0% |
| Lost 2 lines of BSCVA | 1 (1.1%) | 0% |
| Lost 1 line of BSCVA | 8 (8.8%) | 4% |
| Unchanged BSCVA | 49 (53.8%) | 70% |
| Gained 1 line of BSCVA | 29 (31.8%) | 21% |
| Gained 2 lines of BSCVA | 3 (3.3%) | 4% |
| Gained > 2 lines of BSCVA | 0 (0%) | 0% |
| *Efficacy* | | |
| Cumulative UCVA ≥ 20/20 (%) | 83.5 | 62 |
| Cumulative UCVA ≥ 20/25 (%) | 91 | 79 |
| Cumulative UCVA ≥ 20/32 (%) | 97.6 | 95 |
| Cumulative UCVA ≥ 20/40 (%) | 98.9 | 95 |
| *Higher order aberrations* | | |
| Total induction of RMS HOA | 0.04 ± 0.07 | +0.13 Significant |
| Induction of spherical aberration Z4, 0 | 0.008 ± 0.07 | +0.11 Significant |
| Induction of Coma Z3, +1 | 0.04 ± 0.12 | +0.07 Significant |
| Induction of Coma Z3, −1 | −0.09 ± 0.13 | |
| Induction of 4th order astigmatism | | +0.03 Significant |
| Induction of trefoil | | +0.01 No significant |

SMILE: Small incision lenticule extraction; D: Diopter; MRSE: Manifest refraction spherical equivalent; SE: Spherical equivalent; UCVA: Uncorrected visual acuity; BSCVA: Best spectacle-corrected visual acuity; RMS: Root mean square; HOA: Higher order aberrations

UCVA greater than or equal to 20/25 was 88%.[18] There is no significant regression in mean manifest refraction spherical equivalent (MRSE) after 1 month and over all there is a slight trend towards slight over correction in low myopia and undercorrection in high myopia.[2,3,9,11,17-19]

## Topographic Changes

The treatment zone is observed as a slightly prolated and well-centered area delineated by a small step corresponding to the edge of the lenticule after FLEx[8] and SMILE.[3] Scanning pattern in/out has shown to produce more regular topographic mires than scanning pattern out/in in the early postoperative period.[10]

## Higher Order Aberrations

There is a small induction of total root mean square (RMS) HOA, mainly coma and spherical aberration; and in some series also high order astigmatism and trefoil after FLEx (see Table 2)[8,11,18,19] and SMILE (see Table 3).[3,9] However, ReLEx has been shown to induce less HOA than LASIK at 4 and 6 mm pupil.[18] This difference is mainly attributed to the significantly less induced spherical aberration with 6 mm pupil after ReLEx than after standard FS-LASIK[18] or even wavefront-optimized FS-LASIK.[19]

## Contrast Sensitivity

Photopic and mesopic contrast sensitivity is improved after FLEx, particularly in highest frequencies.[19] Photopic contrast sensitivity is similarly increased after ReLEx and LASIK.[19] Mesopic contrast sensitivity was significantly improved after ReLEx but not after FS-LASIK.[19]

## Quality of Life Questionnaires

A standardized questionnaire has been performed to evaluate the quality of life following FLEx procedure. Patients were satisfied or very satisfied with the procedure [(the mean score was 90.4–96.7, (100 being the highest)][2,3,8,9,] no patient reported a worsening of vision, and most of FLEx patients (97.1–100%) never wore glasses for distance at 6 month follow-up.[2,3,8] All SMILE patients reported full independence from spectacle correction.[3] The presence of glare or halos was reported in between 0 and 17% of patients who underwent FLEx,[2,8] but has not been reported after SMILE.[3] The more common subjective symptom was occasional mild dryness that required the use of lubricant eyedrops.[2,3,8,9] Between 0 and 6% of patients reported some deterioration of night-driving vision in FLEx[2,8] and SMILE.[3]

## Different Laser Scanning Patterns and Visual Outcomes

Shah et al. showed that the spiral in/out pattern provides better early visual recovery, refractive outcomes and is safer and more effective than the spiral out/in pattern.[10] They analyzed the visual outcomes 6 months after ReLEx using two different scanning patterns in 329 eyes with myopia or myopic astigmatism.[10]

The benefits of the spiral in/out scanning pattern has being previously mentioned earlier in this chapter from animal studies by Riau et al.[1] The benefits of this firing sequence is due to the shorter time between the cutting of the posterior and anterior lenticule surface in the central cornea.[10] On the contrary, in the spiral out/in pattern, there is a significant time delay between the posterior lenticule cut in the central cornea and the anterior lenticule cut in the central cornea. This allows time for the accumulation of gas bubbles above the posterior surface of the lenticule in the central cornea. As the cavitation bubble expand, they can exert a compressive force and distort the area where the anterior lenticule surface is going to be cut in the center of the cornea.[10] These eyes had irregular topographic mires in the early postoperative period and visual recovery tended to be delayed.[10] UCVA at 1 week was the same or better than preoperative BSCVA in 48% of scanning pattern out/in eyes and 66% of scanning pattern in/out eyes (P = 0.02). At 1 month, however, the results were 65% for the scanning pattern out/in and 85% for scanning pattern in/out (P < 0.01) and after 6 months 82% for the former and 91% for the latter, these results were not statistically significant anymore.[10] The percentage of eyes that achieved a SE of ± 0.50 D after 1 week was 90% with scanning pattern in/out and 84% with scanning pattern out/in (P = 0.03).[10] After 6 months, the percentage increased to 95% for pattern in/out and 92% for pattern out/in and that difference was not significant anymore.[10] Scanning pattern in/out is significantly safer than out/in (P < 0.01) mainly because after 1 week of ReLEx (FLEx and SMILE), the BSCVA was the same or better than preoperative BSCVA in a higher percentage of eyes with scanning pattern in/out (94%) than with scanning pattern out/in (65%).[10] After 6 months, the percentage of eyes that achieved the same or better preoperative BSCVA were still higher in the scanning pattern in/out (99%) than out/in (83%), but this was not significant anymore.[10]

## Intraocular Pressure

In ReLEx as in LASIK or in any other procedure involving FS laser or microkeratome, there is a transient rise in IOP that occurs while the suction is active. The safety of IOP rise in ReLEx was evaluated with real time trans-surgical IOP measurements in rabbit eyes and the IOP during FLEx was found to be 34–39 mm Hg.[11] A considerable lower value than reported with other FS-laser systems and this was not significantly different from the measured IOP during FS-LASIK flap creation with VisuMax® in the same experiment.[11] Due to the small increase in IOP, patients do not experience blackout during the procedure with the VisuMax®. Although ReLEx patients are exposed to longer period of time than with LASIK (45–55 vs 25 sec respectively), this small increase in IOP should not represent a greater risk for optic nerve damage than with LASIK done with the same FS laser.[11] The ReLEx procedure is not associated with high IOP after the surgery, however, the use of postoperative steroids for a short period may induce high IOP in steroid responder patients similar to the risk in LASIK patients.

## ▸ SIDE EFFECTS

The most common side effect reported after ReLEx was transient dry eye that is resolved in most cases by 3 months.[2,3,8,9,17] Dry eye symptoms are resolved with the use of lubricants and only few patients developed punctate epithelial erosions during the first week. Transient corneal haze grade 1 during the first week that later resolved may be observed in some eyes (0–60%),[2,8] but no cases of permanent haze have been reported. Stationary epithelial ingrowth, at the edge of the flap in FLEx, has been reported in two series in only one eye (0–1%).[3,10] Occasional presence of debris in the interface can be observed in 0–8.5% of eyes.[2,8] Subconjunctival hemorrhage in 0–2.8% of eyes has also been reported. Diffuse lamellar stromal keratitis (DLK) grade 0.5 that later resolved with topical steroids has been reported in 0.0–0.9% in 2 series, all other series reported no cases.[2,10] Transient optically insignificant microstriae in the periphery can be observed in 10–20% of eyes. There are no reported cases of transient light-sensitivity syndrome (TLSS) reported after ReLEx. There is one reported case of cornea ectasia after FLEx, all other series reported no cases neither in FLEx or SMILE.[17] This patient developed unilateral ectasia 12 months from FLEx. His cylinder progressed from $-1.75 \times 80°$ 9 months after surgery to a cylinder of $-5.0 \times 90°$ 12 months after surgery. The patient was treated with collagen cross-linking and his cylinder improved to $-3.25 \times 82°$. In FLEx as in LASIK, a corneal flap is created and the strength and biomechanics of the cornea may be similarly altered. Hence, the risk of ectasia after FLEx may be similar to LASIK. On the other hand, SMILE does not require a flap, but instead only a small incision is required. Therefore, the cornea biomechanics should be less altered and the risk of cornea ectasia should be lower than in LASIK and FLEx. However, there is the need for more research on cornea biomechanics following these procedures.

Suction loss is one of the most important complications during the surgery and occurs in 0.9–2% of eyes. The management of suction loss depends on the surgical step at which it occurs. Current recommendations during each stage are now as follows: Stage 1 (lenticule cut < 10%): restart; Stage 2 (lenticule cut > 10%): abort and repeat ReLEx 1 month later or switch to LASIK or PRK; Stage 3 (lenticule side cut): repeat lenticule side cut with decreased size (0.02 mm diameter smaller than original); Stage 4 (flap/incision cut): repeat flap/incision cut; and Stage 5 (flap side cut): repeat flap/incision side cut with decreased size (0.02 mm diameter smaller than original).[11,20] Shah et al. reported in her series that one eye had suction loss and was successfully managed with a second pass with the laser without added side effects, i.e. induced astigmatism, loss of BSCVA or poor UCVA.[9] We reported one case of suction loss during the procedure where less than 10% of the lenticule cut was completed. The laser pass was restarted and 1 month after surgery had a UCVA of 20/60 and BCVA of 20/25 with $-2.0$ D of induced astigmatism.[11] The patient underwent a excimer ablation to correct the induced astigmatism. At the time of the procedure, no guidelines (as documented above) were available.

Specific complications related to SMILE are uncommon but have been reported. Perforation of the anterior flap with the dissecting spatula, tears at the incision edge and incomplete laser incision have been reported.[3] However, all flap-related complications are avoided in SMILE (Fig. 6).

## ▸ ADVANTAGES AND DISADVANTAGES OF ReLEx OVER LASIK

Refractive lenticule extraction still a new surgical procedure and visual outcomes are at least comparable or even better to LASIK.[18,19] Stability of refraction, predictability, efficacy, safety, contrast sensitivity and induction of HOAs have been reported to be similar or better than FS-LASIK.[18,19] Photopic contrast sensitivity is similarly increased after ReLEx and LASIK.[19] Mesopic contrast sensitivity was significantly improved after ReLEx and only maintained at preoperatively levels after wavefront-optimized FS-LASIK.[19]

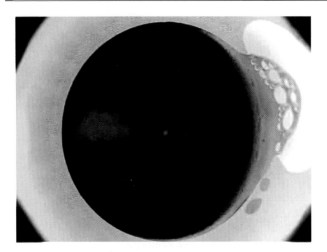

**Fig. 6:** Suction loss. Representative image of suction loss. Suction loss is preceded by the formation of air bubbles with the tear at the edge of the cone

The fact that the corneal lenticule is cut independently to any changes in cornea hydration has many advantages, especially with high myopic treatments. The predictability of excimer ablation is dependent on the amount of cornea hydration.[18] Early visual recovery after ReLEx may not be as good as with LASIK, UCVA greater than or equal to 20/25 was achieved only in 41% of the eyes 1 day after FLEx, contrary to an achievement in 61% of eyes after FS-LASIK (P = 0.033).[18] However, this is temporal and refraction seems to be stabilized after 1 month from ReLEx. Three months after surgery, ReLEx seems to have comparable or better visual outcomes than LASIK, as shown in the percentage of eyes that achieved UCVA greater than or equal to 20/25, 88% for FLEx and 69% for FS-LASIK (P = 0.030).[18] The predictability after ReLEx is comparable or even better than LASIK as observed in one study that showed a statistically significant less difference in attempted versus achieved SE after FLEx than after LASIK and the percentage of eyes with a target refraction within 0.5 and 1.0 D of attempted refraction was higher after FLEx.[18] Another study found similar predictability after LASIK and ReLEx with a mean SE in ReLEx of −0.23 ± 0.35 D and in FS-LASIK of −0.15 ± 0.27 D.[19] The safety after ReLEx is comparable and may be better than LASIK as it is observed that 1 year after surgery, the incidence of one line loss of BSCVA was 5% in ReLEx as compared to 8% in LASIK.[19] Furthermore, in the same study 46% of ReLEx eyes gained one line of BSCVA as compared to 22% in LASIK eyes.[19]

The ReLEx procedure may result in less topographic changes (cornea flattening), inflammation (CD11b), less light scattering in corneal CM and early extracellular matrix (fibronectin) deposition than LASIK, especially at high refractive correction as previously commented above.[12] Energy levels as well as the inflammation and early wound healing is constant in ReLEx whereas in LASIK increases with higher corrections because this requires more energy.[12] These may impact favorably on visual results and outcomes.[12] These disparities were only significant at moderate refractive corrections (−6 D >). In SMILE, with a much smaller incision, all these parameters may be further reduced with the added benefits of a non-neutrophic cornea.[12]

A substantial number of LASIK complications, which are believed to be linked to the creation of the flap (regardless of the method of flap formation) have the potential to be avoided after SMILE. Therefore, significant potential advantages of SMILE surgery lie in the flapless nature of the procedure because the lenticule is extracted through a small pocket incision, causing less postoperative discomfort, better corneal strength, better biomechanical stability, reduced risk of flap dislocation and less dry eye (neurotrophic status). However, this needs to be confirmed with more prospective studies in human and animal models. Dry eye patients may be better candidates because there is less damage to the cornea anterior stromal nerves and sub-basal nerve plexus, therefore less risk for developing neurotrophic cornea state after surgery (unpublished data, presented in APACRS 2012, Karim Mohamed). A reduced risk of cornea ectasia is expected because of better preservation of anterior layers of the cornea. Another advantage of ReLEx is that it could potentially be a reversible refractive procedure, because the removal of the refractive intrastromal lenticule *in situ* allows the possibility of reimplantation at a future date.[7] In ReLEx, only one laser is used, therefore, there is less surgical time than standard FS-LASIK where two different laser machines are needed. The new generation VisuMax® 500 kHz should produce better outcomes and faster surgical procedure reducing the risk of suction loss. However, further studies are required to prove its superiority.

## FUTURE PROSPECTS AND DEVELOPMENTS

### Lenticule Long-Term Storage

The lenticule can safely be stored long-term in cryopreservation.[7] The extracted refractive lenticule is still viable after cryopreservation, with live keratocytes that express keratocyte specific markers (ALDH3A1 and KERA) on RT-PCR and able to proliferate in serum-containing culture.[7] The lenticule collagen fibril architecture after cryopreservation is comparable to that of freshly extracted lenticules with a well-preserved and aligned structure, without fragmented fibrils or areas of collagen disruption as evidenced by TEM.[7] Because of the expected tissue hydration after cryopreservation, the lenticule collagen fibril density is lower than after cryopreservation (from $15.75 \pm 1.56$ to $12.05 \pm 0.62$, P = 0.02).[7] More live than dead keratocytes are observed in the lenticule before than after cryopreservation and a mixed pattern of apoptosis and necrosis has been observed. Cells located in the center of the lenticule are more susceptible to damage during cryopreservation and thawing process. After cryopreservation, there are significantly more TUNEL positive cells in the center of the lenticule. Similarly, the surface of the lenticule showed an increase in the number of TUNEL positive cells after cryopreservation.[7]

### Lenticule Reimplantation

Regular collagen architecture is one of the key factors to maintain corneal transparency. Following cryopreservation, the authors were able to show that the extracted lenticule can safely be stored following cryopreservation with maintenance of regular collagen structure and organization after thawing.[7] It has been proposed that the lenticule can be reimplanted if needed at a future date, making the ReLEx procedure a reversible refractive technique.[7] The lenticule can be reimplanted as means of correcting iatrogenic corneal ectasia, reversing presbyopia or to allow a monovision correction after reshaping the lenticule before reimplantation. The proof of concept of this idea has been demonstrated in rabbit[21] and in a long-term monkey model (unpublished data).

### Enhancement Procedures for Small Incision Lenticule Extraction

If a regression or under/overcorrection occurs, at the moment the only possibility is to do an enhancement with an excimer laser. For FLEx and pseudo-SMILE, the procedure is like a LASIK enhancement, i.e. lifting the complete flap and performing an excimer ablation on the RSB. For SMILE, the options are to do surface ablation over the cap or to form a flap and do excimer ablation on the RSB like a LASIK enhancement; unfortunately, this will eliminate any extra advantage that SMILE may have over LASIK. There is a need to develop software profiles

that enable the performance of FS laser enhancements without the need of cutting the cap, thus maintaining the advantages of SMILE. However, enhancement rates are likely to be lower after SMILE compared to LASIK. In the authors' center, LASIK enhancement rate is 4–5% per annum and ReLEx enhancement rate is 1%.

### Hyperopic Correction

Clinical studies are in progress for hyperopic correction, no published results yet.

## CONCLUSION

Refractive lenticule extraction, especially SMILE, is a promising new refractive procedure with excellent early results. By July 2012, there will be 80 sites worldwide doing ReLEx and more than 13,000 procedures performed to date. We are waiting to see more prospective studies with longer follow-up to validate this procedure as a true alternative for LASIK with comparable or even better outcomes.

## ACKNOWLEDGMENTS

We would like to express our thanks to Lions Eye Bank, Miami, FL for providing human corneas. Ms Livia Yong, Ms Jessica Yu, Mr Tarak Pujara and Carl Zeiss Meditec, for their assistance in the operation of VisuMax® Femtosecond Laser System.

## REFERENCES

1. Riau A, Angunawela RI, Chaurasia SS, et al. Effect of differential femtosecond laser firing patterns on collagen disruption during Refractive Lenticule Extraction (ReLEx) procedure. J Cataract Refract Surg. 2012 Aug;38(8):1467-75.
2. Blum M, Kunert K, Schröder M, et al. Femtosecond lenticule extraction for the correction of myopia: preliminary 6-month results. Graefes Arch Clin Exp Ophthalmol. 2010;248:1019-27.
3. Sekundo W, Kunert KS, Blum M. Small incision corneal refractive surgery using the small incision lenticule extraction (SMILE) procedure for the correction of myopia and myopic astigmatism: results of a 6 months prospective study. Br J Ophthalmol. 2011;95:335-9.
4. Kullman G, Pineda R. Alternative applications of the femtosecond laser in ophthalmology. Semin Ophthalmol. 2010; 25:256-64.
5. Vaddavalli PK, Yoo SH. Femtosecond laser in-situ keratomileusis flap configurations. Curr Opin Ophthalmol. 2011; 22:245-50.
6. Tran DB, Binder PS, Brame CL. LASIK flap revision using the IntraLase femtosecond laser. Int Ophthalmol Clin. 2008;48: 51-63.

CHAPTER 114

SECTION 17

7. Mohamed-Noriega K, Toh K-P, Poh R, et al. Cornea lenticule viability and structural integrity after refractive lenticule extraction (ReLEx) and cryopreservation. Mol Vis. 2011; 17:3437-49.

8. Sekundo W, Kunert K, Russmann C, et al. First efficacy and safety study of femtosecond lenticule extraction for the correction of myopia: six-month results. J Cataract Refract Surg. 2008;34:1513-20.

9. Shah R, Shah S, Sengupta S. Results of small incision lenticule extraction: All-in-one femtosecond laser refractive surgery. J Cataract Refract Surg. 2011;37:127-37.

10. Shah R, Shah S. Effect of scanning patterns on the results of femtosecond laser lenticule extraction refractive surgery. J Cataract Refract Surg. 2011;37:1636-47.

11. Ang M, Chaurasia SS, Angunawela RI, et al. Femtosecond lenticule extraction (FLEx): clinical results, interface evaluation, and intraocular pressure variation. Invest Ophthalmol Vis Sci. 2012;53:1414-21.

12. Riau AK, Angunawela RI, Chaurasia SS, et al. Early corneal wound healing and inflammatory responses after refractive lenticule extraction (ReLEx). Invest Ophthalmol Vis Sci. 2011; 52:6213-21.

13. Flap Option. Visumax Laser Keratome. Documentation set. Jena, Germany: Carl Zeiss Meditec AG; 2011. pp. 12.

14. Yuen LH, Chan WK, Koh J, et al. A 10-year prospective audit of LASIK outcomes for myopia in 37932 eyes at a single institution in Asia. Ophthalmology. 2010;117:1236-44.

15. Kunert KS, Blum M, Duncker GIW, et al. Surface quality of human corneal lenticules after femtosecond laser surgery for myopia comparing different laser parameters. Graefes Arch Clin Exp Ophthalmol. 2011;249:1417-24.

16. Heichel J, Blum M, Duncker GIW, et al. Surface quality of porcine corneal lenticules after femtosecond lenticule extraction. Ophthalmic Res. 2011;46:107-12.

17. Blum M, Kunert KS, Engelbrecht C, et al. [Femtosecond lenticule extraction (FLEx) - Results after 12 months in myopic astigmatism]. Klin Monbl Augenheilkd. 2010;227:961-5.

18. Vestergaard A, Ivarsen A, Asp S, et al. Femtosecond (FS) laser vision correction procedure for moderate to high myopia: a prospective study of ReLEx(*) flex and comparison with a retrospective study of FS-laser in situ keratomileusis. Acta Ophthalmol. 2012; doi: 10.1111/j.1755-3768.2012.02406.

19. Gertnere J, Solomatins I, Sekundo W. Refractive Lenticule Extraction (Relex) and Wavefront Optimized Femto-Lasik: comparison of contrast sensitivity and high order aberrations at one year. Graefes Arch Clin Exp Ophthalmol. (in Press).

20. FLEx Option. Visumax Operation Manual. Jena, Germany: Carl Zeiss Meditec AG; 2011. pp. 24-5.

21. Angunawela RI, Riau A, Chaurasia SS, et al. Refractive lenticule re-implantation after myopic ReLEx: a feasibility study of stromal restoration after refractive surgery in a rabbit model. Invest Ophthalmol Vis Sci. 2012. Jul 26;53(8):4975-85.

# CHAPTER 115

# Femtosecond Laser Keratoplasty

*M Farid, S Garg, Roger F Steinert*

## ❖ INTRODUCTION

In the 1930s, Dr Castroviejo experimented with a variety of customized hand trephination patterns to increase wound surface area and improve outcomes in penetrating keratoplasty (PKP).[1,2] Multi level stepped corneal incisions for improving donor to host alignment and wound stability were also ideas that were introduced initially by Franceschetti and Doret in the 1950s and expanded on by Dr Barraquer.[3-5] Technical difficulty kept these methods from becoming widely adopted at that time. Penetrating keratoplasty using a standard straight edge blade trephination creating a 'butt' joint wound became the standard. The advent of the femtosecond laser technology has now added a new array of options for the transplant surgeon. Using near-infrared light to cut corneal tissue via photodisruption, the laser can create nonplanar cuts at a precise depth and pattern with limited damage to surrounding tissue. The femtosecond laser cuts are consistent and reproducible, allowing for the creation of a variety of incision types using combinations of lamellar and vertical cuts. The femtosecond laser has also been used to create straight cuts in shapes too complex for standard trephines, such as decagonal, and circular with a series of orientation teeth and notches.[6,7]

The first customized trephination pattern using the femtosecond laser was the 'top-hat' shape. Studies demonstrated that the 'top-hat' shape led to increased biomechanical wound stability with a sevenfold increase in resistance to leakage and possibly less astigmatism than traditional trephination PKP wounds.[8,9] Subsequently, a variety of other biomechanically stable wound configurations were identified. Corneal surgeons now have a variety of

trephination patterns to choose from, including 'top-hat', 'mushroom', 'zig-zag', and 'Christmas tree' shapes (Figs 1A to D). All of these wound configurations create more surface area for healing and have superior biomechanical strength as compared to the traditional 'butt' joint (Fig. 1E).

Optical perfection in PKP is limited by multiple factors. These include donor-host misalignment of the anterior surface, rotational misalignment and poor tissue distribution, excess and uneven suture tension, and postoperative slow and uneven wound healing. The femtosecond laser incision for PKP has allowed for certain improvements in these variable factors and improved optical and mechanical outcomes.

Early surgical outcomes with the femtosecond laser assisted PKP show better natural alignment of the donor and host anterior surface, reducing one source of distortion. Improved sealing of the incision permits the surgeon to use only enough suture tension to keep the incision apposed, reducing distortion from the suture itself. In addition, the increased surface area of these incisions leads to improved tensile strength of the wound, improving both patient safety and allowing earlier suture removal when indicated. Furthermore, early studies of femtosecond laser assisted PKP have shown rapid visual recovery and astigmatism comparable to or slightly better than traditional blade trephination PKP.[10-14]

The first femtosecond laser platform to accomplish the full thickness corneal cuts for PKP was the Intralase (IntraLase Femtosecond Laser, AMO, Irvine, California). A second femtosecond laser platform, FEMTEC (Bausch & Lomb and 20/10 Perfect Vision, Heidelberg, Germany) has also subsequently created stable full thickness PKP wounds

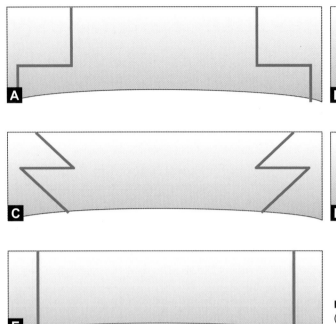

**Figs 1A to E:** (A) Top-hat configuration; (B) Mushroom configuration; (C) Zig-zag configuration; (D) Christmas tree configuration; (E) Traditional (straight) configuration

and demonstrates short-term visual results analogous to other femtosecond laser-assisted PKP studies.[15-18] Additional refractive femtosecond lasers in use include VisuMax (Carl Zeiss Meditec AG, Jena, Germany) and Femto LDV (Ziemer Ophthalmic Systems AG, Port, Switzerland).

## PATIENT SELECTION AND PREOPERATIVE EVALUATION

Proper patient selection is crucial to successful femtosecond laser assisted PKP. Any conditions preventing proper laser applanation and suction, such as severe ocular surface irregularity, active or elevated bleb, or glaucoma implant are a contraindication to the procedure. Although the femtosecond laser has shown excellent cut penetration through even dense scars, severe peripheral corneal neovascularization may be a relative contraindication in certain cases. Small orbits or narrow palpebral fissures may not be able to accommodate the limbal suction ring required for laser use.

Graft size selection depends on a combination of factors, including host corneal diameter (especially vertical), location of thinning or active corneal infection, and presence of prior graft. Large or eccentric grafts may be necessary in cases of ectasia, especially pellucid marginal degeneration.

A posterior bridge of uncut tissue will maintain a closed eye and formed anterior chamber between laser cut and tissue removal. Therefore, accurate preoperative pachymetry can be crucial in cases where deep anterior lamellar keratoplasty (DALK) is to be attempted, or, as is usually the case, the femtosecond laser is not located in the operating suite and corneal stability is required in the time between laser cut and corneal removal. A preoperative pachymetry map either by anterior segment optical coherence tomography (Visante OCT, Carl Zeiss Meditec, Inc., Dublin, California), Pentacam (Oculus USA, Lynwood, Washington), or ultrasound is performed to adequately assess and program depth settings for the femtosecond laser incision.

## GRAFT CUTTING AND SURGERY

By mounting the tissue on an anterior artificial chamber (Fig. 2), donor corneas can be cut by the femtosecond laser using preprogrammed parameters set by the surgeon. Alternatively, the tissue can be ordered "pre-cut" with the same laser parameters as those to be used on the patient, a service now provided by numerous eye bank facilities. The donor tissue diameter should be set to the same size as the host. Using the zig-zag incision where donor and host diameters were set to the same size, Farid et al. report an average keratometry value of 44.4 diopters.[19]

Host laser cut can be done under topical or retrobulbar anesthesia. Although newer model femtosecond lasers work faster than older models, more complex cutting patterns and alignment marks can increase the amount of time the suction ring remains on the eye, prompting more surgeons

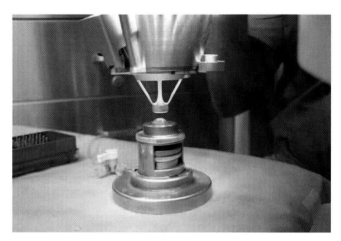

**Fig. 2:** Graft mounted on artificial anterior chamber

to opt for preoperative retrobulbar block to ensure patient comfort. Proper centration of the suction ring on the patient is crucial to ensure centration of the graft. A customized trephination pattern per surgeon's preference is selected and programmed into the laser computer. The laser pattern always starts from the deepest portion of the cornea and works its way anteriorly. The software of the Intralase laser allows for a maximum diameter of 9 mm, with the ability to vary the side cut angle from 30° to 150°. In the example of the zig-zag incision, the laser parameters are a posterior side cut from deep stroma to anterior stroma at 30° to the periphery. The second cut is a lamellar cut at a depth of 320 μm from the anterior surface, which is intersected by the third incision, the anterior side cut that advances toward the anterior corneal surface at 30°. Anterior diameter of the zig-zag cut can be set at 8, 8.5, or 9 mm, based on the patient's corneal diameter and surgeon preference. The femtosecond laser also allows for the placement of radial alignment marks on the host and donor that facilitate ease of precise suture placement and improved tissue distribution.

If small bubbles are seen at the initiation of the laser, then the laser energy is in the anterior chamber fluid and a full thickness incision is being performed. If a full thickness incision was not the intended action, then a quick cessation of the laser should be done by lifting off of the foot pedal. As long as the laser has not reached Descemet's membrane, then resetting of the posterior depth can be done and the laser restarted within the posterior corneal stroma to maintain a bridge of uncut tissue. If transporting a patient to the operating room after the laser corneal cut is necessary, a posterior bridge of uncut corneal tissue is essential to ensure globe stability. Studies have demonstrated that side cut bridges are stronger than lamellar bridges, with median burst pressures in the top-hat configuration exceeding approximately 735 mm Hg compared to lamellar bridges at approximately 350 mm Hg, in artificial anterior chambers. Both types of tissue bridges were stronger than full-thickness cuts which had a median burst pressure of approximately 140 mm Hg.[20,21] Posterior side-cut bridge is preferred over anterior side-cut to minimize irregularities in anterior contour and poor anterior graft-host fit. Furthermore, a posterior side-cut bridge is easily extended with a blade into the anterior chamber without compromising the laser cut shape. In one study, a 70–75 μm posterior lamellar bridge provided ample wound stability.[21]

After completion of the femtosecond laser incision, the eye is treated with antibiotic drops and shielded prior to transport to the operating suite. The host corneal button is separated with a blunt lamellar dissector to reveal lamellar and side-cut incisions made by the laser. Although laser incisions usually separate cleanly, limited sharp dissection with a surgical blade or scissors may be needed in areas of dense corneal scarring. After completion of the blunt dissection, the anterior chamber is entered with a blade and the corneal bridging tissue (if any) is cut with corneal scissors. The donor cornea is then sutured into place using the surgeon's suturing pattern of choice. Care should be taken to match the depth of the suture in the donor and host to achieve a true 'lock and key' configuration.[22] Postoperative results show excellent donor-host apposition and the zig-zag incision pattern can be seen on narrow beam slit lamp microscopy (Figs 3A and B).

## ▶ REVIEW OF RECENT OUTCOMES

Results of multiple studies using femtosecond laser assisted PKP have shown endothelial cell loss, postoperative astigmatism and best spectacle corrected visual acuity (BSCVA) better than or equal to conventional PKP. In a small study using the top-hat configuration, Price et al. showed endothelial cell loss comparable to conventional PKP at 1-year postoperative exams. Complete suture removal was accomplished at an average of 7 months and there was a substantial improvement in BSCVA post-transplant.[12] In a series of five patients undergoing inverted mushroom type configuration, Cheng et al. reported an average best corrected visual acuity of 20/32, with average refractive and topographical cylinder of 3.20 and 3.26 respectively. Mean endothelial cell density at 1 year was similar to prior studies.[13] In a nonrandomized study comparing top-hat configuration femtosecond laser

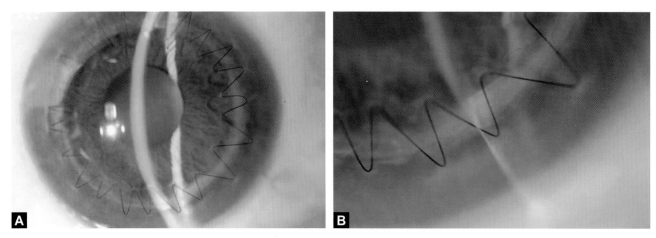

**Figs 3A and B:** (A) Slit-lamp photo of postoperative zig-zag femtosecond keratoplasty; (B) High-magnification slit-lamp photo of postoperative zig-zag femtosecond keratoplasty. Note smooth anterior contour

keratoplasty with manual trephinated top-hat PKP, Bahar et al. showed higher endothelial cell counts and faster suture removal compared to manual top hat trephination.[14] Burrato and Bohm similarly showed faster visual recovery and low amounts of astigmatism in top-hat cuts.[11]

In an initial report and follow-up study, Farid et al. demonstrated that the femtosecond laser-generated zig-zag incision induces less astigmatism and results in a more rapid recovery of BSCVA compared to conventional blade trephination PKP in patients with 24 bite running sutures. Eighty-one percent of the zig-zag group versus 45% of the conventional group achieved BSCVA of greater than or equal to 20/40 by postoperative month 3.[10,19] In a study of 50 patients undergoing zig-zag PKP compared to 50 patients who underwent conventional PKP, Chamberlain et al. showed significantly less astigmatism prior to postoperative month 6, as well as earlier suture removal. The results in the two groups showed no significant difference in the long-term, however.[23] The angled edge of the zig-zag cut, provides a smooth anterior transition between donor and host that allows for a smooth donor to host transition and a hermetic wound seal. This improved natural alignment intrinsically produces less optical distortion, and combined with a watertight seal and less suture tension, results in lower amounts of induced astigmatism.

The two most popular patterns remain the top-hat and zig-zag incisions. Part of the advantage of femtosecond laser assisted keratoplasty to conventional PKP is the accuracy to which the donor and host fit. It is for this reason that the zig-zag incision may prove to be the most biomechanically sound incision pattern. The zig-zag pattern allows for consistent suture placement at approximately 50% depth, where the posterior side cut and lamellar incision intersect

(Fig. 4). With the top-hat incision, suture placement can vary leading to the possibility of posterior wound gape that may negatively impact refractive outcomes (Figs 5A and B). With suture placement at the inner point of the Z, the biomechanics of the zig-zag incision results in good wound apposition at the deeper layers and anterior cornea.

At the Gavin Herbert Eye Institute (University of California, Irvine), the most updated review of 173 eyes having undergone femtosecond laser keratoplasty at an academic center, shows average manifest astigmatism of less than or equal to 3 diopters and average topographic astigmatism less than or equal to 4 diopters as early as 3 months postoperatively and remaining so throughout the 2-year follow-up period (unpublished data). The rapid wound healing from increased surface area and excellent donor-host apposition are achieving corneal transplantation results that are unprecedented in conventional keratoplasty.

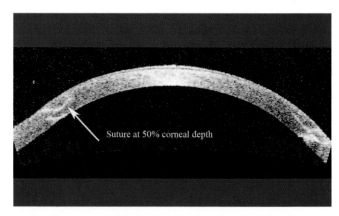

**Fig. 4:** Anterior segment OCT of zig-zag femtosecond keratoplasty. Note smooth anterior and posterior corneal curvatures and placement of suture at 50% corneal depth

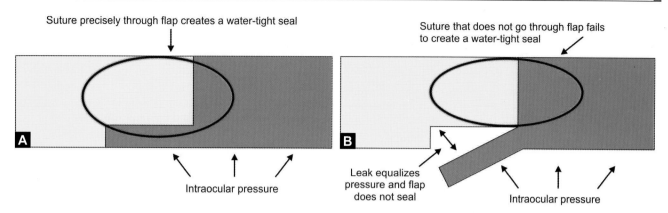

**Figs 5A and B:** (A) Schematic of top-hat femtosecond keratoplasty with well-placed suture; (B) Schematic of top-hat femtosecond keratoplasty with improperly placed suture. Note resultant posterior lip which does not oppose the host cornea

## ❧ FEMTOSECOND LASER ASSISTED LAMELLAR KERATOPLASTY

Along with full thickness keratoplasty, the femtosecond laser technology can be applied to numerous other forms of corneal transplantation. Femtosecond assisted techniques have been used in deep anterior lamellar keratoplasty (DALK), anterior lamellar keratoplasty (ALK), Descemet's stripping endothelial keratoplasty (DSEK), and deep lamellar endothelial keratoplasty (DLEK).

Deep anterior lamellar keratoplasty via the 'big-bubble' technique has been employed successfully for multiple cases of stromal pathology with healthy endothelium, including infections, anterior stromal dystrophies, keratoconus, and postrefractive ectasia.[24-30] Customized femtosecond trephinations, such as zig-zag or mushroom patterns, have assisted the DALK technique by creating a posterior cut whose posterior depth lies within 50–100 microns of the endothelium, providing a guide for needle insertion and big-bubble dissection. If the dissection of Descemet's membrane fails, easy conversion to a full thickness transplant can be done while maintaining the benefits of the femtosecond laser incision.[31,32] Buzzonetti et al. describe a technique whereby a channel in the posterior stroma, 50 microns above the endothelium, is created using the femtosecond laser. A blunt cannula, minimizing risk of Descemet's perforation, can be passed through the tunnel to facilitate big-bubble dissection at the proper corneal plane.[33] There are multiple benefits to the femtosecond DALK technique for stromal corneal pathology and ectatic corneal disease which make it a more preferable treatment than traditional PKP. Some of these include the safety of extraocular surgery, no risk of endothelial rejection due to preservation of the host endothelium, and shorter postoperative course of topical corticosteroid use. Care to monitor for epithelial and stromal rejection, although rare, is still required.[34] A successful case of femtosecond assisted DALK in a cornea with previous radial keratotomy (RK) incisions has also been reported.[35]

Anterior lamellar keratoplasty is a treatment option for patients with relatively anterior pathology, including scars and anterior dystrophies. Using the femtosecond to create smooth lamellar dissections just inferior to the corneal pathology, a sutureless technique has been described by Yoo et al. which resulted in a mean gain of 3.8 lines of BCVA.[36] In a study showing long term results, Shousha et al. showed no significant difference in astigmatism or spherical equivalent compared to preoperative values at 1-year follow-up.[37]

Descemet's stripping endothelial keratoplasty (DSEK) allows for replacement of diseased host endothelium with retention of normal stroma and epithelium, decreased healing time, decreased astigmatism and a predictable change in corneal power.[38] While investigators were quick to make use of the femtosecond laser's ability to create lamellar cuts to prepare the donor button, outcomes yield mixed results.[39,40] Cheng et al. randomized a group of 80 eyes with endothelial disease to femtosecond laser endothelial keratoplasty (FLEK) versus conventional PKP. The FLEK group had significantly less postoperative astigmatism. However, the postoperative BSCVA was significantly lower in the FLEK group. This may be a result of interface haze resulting from the roughened collagen fibrils produced by the femtosecond laser.[39] A recent study also showed a smoother stromal bed in corneas cut with either of two tested microkeratomes as compared to those cut with the femtosecond laser.[41]

Further studies looking at various energy and spot size patterns of the femtosecond laser as well as multiple passes to create a smoother donor bed are in progress and may lead to improved outcomes.

CHAPTER **115**

## ❧ REFERENCES

1. Castroviejo R. Keratoplasty: a historical and experimental study, including a new method: Part I. Am J Ophthalmol. 1931;15:905-16.
2. Castroviejo R. Keratoplasty: a historical and experimental study, including a new method: Part II. Am J Ophthalmol. 1932;15:825-37.
3. Franceschetti A, Doret M. Lamellar and perforating keratoplasty. Concilium Ophthalmologicum. 1950.
4. Barraquer J. Queratoplastia: problemas que plantea la fijacion del injerto. Proceedings of the XVI Concilium Ophtalmologicum 1950. Acta 1950; II 999-1004.
5. Barraquer J. Two level keratoplasty: keratoplasty and the eye and diabetes. Int Ophtalmol Clin. 1963;3:515-39.
6. Proust H, Baeteman C, Matonti F, et al. Femtosecond laser-assisted decagonal penetrating keratoplasty. Am J Ophthalmol. 2011;151(1):29-34.
7. Mastropasqua L, Nubile M, Lanzini M, et al. Orientation teeth in nonmechanical femtosecond laser corneal trephination for penetrating keratoplasty. Am J Ophthalmol. 2008;146(1):46-9.
8. Ignacio TS, Nguyen TB, Chuck RS, et al. Top-hat wound configuration for penetrating keratoplasty using the femtosecond laser: a laboratory model. Cornea. 2006;25:336-40.
9. Steinert RF, Ignacio TS, Sarayba MA. Top-hat shaped penetrating keratoplasty using the femtosecond laser. Am J Ophthalmol. 2007;143(4):689-91.
10. Farid M, Kim M, Steinert RF. Results of penetrating keratoplasty performed with a femtosecond laser zigzag incision: initial report. Ophthalmology. 2007;114(12):2208-12.
11. Buratto L, Böhm E. The use of the femtosecond laser in penetrating keratoplasty. Am J Ophthalmol. 2007;143(5):737-42.
12. Price FW, Price MO. Femtosecond laser shaped penetrating keratoplasty: one-year results utilizing a top-hat configuration. Am J Ophthalmol. 2008;145(2):210-4.
13. Cheng YY, Tahzib NG, van Rij G, et al. Femtosecond-laser-assisted inverted mushroom keratoplasty. Cornea. 2008;27(6):679-85.
14. Bahar I, Kaiserman I, Lange AP, et al. Femtosecond laser versus manual dissection for top-hat penetrating keratoplasty. Br J Ophthalmol. 2009;93(1):73-8.
15. Seitz B, Brunner H, Viestenz A, et al. Inverse mushroom-shaped nonmechanical penetrating keratoplasty using a femtosecond laser. Am J Ophthalmol. 2005;139(5):941-4.
16. Meltendorf C, Schroeter J, Reinhold B, et al. Corneal trephination with the femtosecond laser. Cornea. 2006;25(9):1090-2.
17. Holzer MP, Rabsilber TM, Auffarth GU. Penetrating keratoplasty using femtosecond laser. Am J Ophthalmol. 2007;143(3):524-6.
18. Hoffart L, Proust H, Matonti F, et al. Short-term results of penetrating keratoplasty performed with the femtec femtosecond laser. Am J Ophthalmol. 2008;146(1):50-5.
19. Farid M, Steinert RF, Gaster RN, et al. Comparison of penetrating keratoplasty performed with a femtosecond laser zig-zag incision versus conventional blade trephination. Ophthalmology. 2009;116(9):1638-43.
20. McAllum P, Kaiserman I, Bahar I, et al. Femtosecond laser top hat penetrating keratoplasty: wound burst pressures of incomplete cuts. Arch Ophthalmol. 2008;126(6):822-5.
21. Price FW, Price MO, Jordan CS. Safety of incomplete incision patterns in femtosecond laser-assisted penetrating keratoplasty. J Cataract Refract Surg. 2008;34(12):2099-103.

22. Heur M, Tang M, Yiu S, et al. Investigation of femtosecond laser-enabled keratoplasty wound geometry using optical coherence tomography. Cornea. 2011. [Epub ahead of print]
23. Chamberlain WD, Rush SW, Mathers WD, et al. Comparison of femtosecond laser-assisted keratoplasty versus conventional penetrating keratoplasty. Ophthalmology. 2011;118(3):486-91.
24. Anwar M, Teichmann KD. Deep lamellar keratoplasty: surgical techniques for anterior lamellar keratoplasty with and without baring of Descemet's membrane. Cornea. 2002;21(4):374-83.
25. Tan DT, Parthasarathy A. Deep anterior lamellar keratoplasty for keratoconus. Cornea. 2007;26(8):1025-6.
26. Park KA, Ki CS, Chung ES, et al. Deep anterior lamellar keratoplasty in Korean patients with Avellino dystrophy. Cornea. 2007;26(9):1132-5.
27. Parthasarathy A, Tan DT. Deep lamellar keratoplasty for acanthamoeba keratitis. Cornea. 2007;26(8):1021-3.
28. Susiyanti M, Mehta JS, Tan DT. Bilateral deep anterior lamellar keratoplasty for the management of bilateral post-LASIK mycobacterial keratitis. J Cataract Refract Surg. 2007;33(9):1641-3.
29. Villarrubia A, Pérez-Santonja JJ, Palacín E, et al. Deep anterior lamellar keratoplasty in post-laser in situ keratomileusis keratectasia. J Cataract Refract Surg. 2007;33(5):773-8.
30. Colin J, Velou S. Current surgical options for keratoconus. J Cataract Refract Surg. 2003;29:379-86.
31. Farid M, Steinert RF. Deep anterior lamellar keratoplasty performed with the femtosecond laser zig-zag incision for the treatment of stromal corneal pathology and ectatic disease. J Cataract Refract Surg. 2009;35(5):809-13.
32. Price FW, Price MO, Grandin JC, et al. Deep anterior lamellar keratoplasty with femtosecond-laser zigzag incisions. J Cataract Refract Surg. 2009;35(5):804-8.
33. Buzzonetti L, Laborante A, Petrocelli G. Standardized big-bubble technique in deep anterior lamellar keratoplasty assisted by the femtosecond laser. J Cataract Refract Surg. 2010;36(10):1631-6.
34. Mosca L, Fasciani R, Mosca L, et al. Graft Rejection After Femtosecond Laser-Assisted Deep Anterior Lamellar Keratoplasty: Report of 3 Cases. Cornea. 2011. [Epub ahead of print]
35. Chamberlain W, Cabezas M. Femtosecond-assisted deep anterior lamellar keratoplasty using big-bubble technique in a cornea with 16 radial keratotomy incisions. Cornea. 2011;30(2):233-6.
36. Yoo SH, Kymionis GD, Koreishi A, et al. Femtosecond laser-assisted sutureless anterior lamellar keratoplasty. Ophthalmology. 2008;115(8):1303-7.
37. Shousha MA, Yoo SH, Kymionis GD, et al. Long-term results of femtosecond laser-assisted sutureless anterior lamellar keratoplasty. Ophthalmology. 2011;118(2):315-23.
38. Gorovoy MS. Descemet-stripping automated endothelial keratoplasty. Cornea. 2006;25(8):886-9.
39. Cheng YY, Schouten JS, Tahzib NG, et al. Efficacy and safety of femtosecond laser-assisted corneal endothelial keratoplasty: a randomized multicenter clinical trial. Transplantation. 2009;88(11):1294-302.
40. Cheng YY, Hendrikse F, Pels E, et al. Preliminary results of femtosecond laser-assisted descemet stripping endothelial keratoplasty. Arch Ophthalmol. 2008;126(10):1351-6.
41. Mootha VV, Heck E, Verity SM, et al. Comparative study of descemet stripping automated endothelial keratoplasty donor preparation by Moria CB microkeratome, horizon microkeratome, and Intralase FS60. Cornea. 2011;30(3):320-4.

# CHAPTER 116

# Femtosecond Laser Enabled Correction of Postkeratoplasty Astigmatism

*Nikhil L Kumar, David S Rootman*

## ⋗ INTRODUCTION

Visual rehabilitation after penetrating keratoplasty (PKP) is frequently limited by significant astigmatism and aniso-metropia. Once all sutures have been removed, greater than five diopters of astigmatism is common.[1-3] Conservative options for treatment includes spectacles and contact lenses. Spectacle use can lead to intolerable aniseikonia and distortion, due to the distance of the correction from the nodal point of the eye. Contact lenses may be challenging to fit over an irregular corneal topography.[4] Consequently conservative therapy may not achieve the desired visual outcome.[5]

Within a year postkeratoplasty, selective intermittent suture removal and continuous suture adjustment are possible, but may not exert a permanent effect. Once all sutures are removed, surgical options include manual astigmatic keratotomy with and without compression sutures, astigmatic keratotomy using mechanical devices, manual wedge resections and keratorefractive surgery (surface ablation and LASIK).[6-15] Despite their potential to reduce high amounts of astigmatism, manual relaxing procedures are difficult to produce in a reliable and uniform pattern. They are known to suffer from poor predictability, higher order aberrations, wound gape, and perforation. In the literature, mechanical astigmatic keratotomy reports show low reliability.[12-14] Although laser keratorefractive surgery is an excellent option for stable and predictable astigmatic reduction, it is limited to lower amounts of correction and may offer complications in terms of haze in PRK and flap problems with LASIK.[15]

There are encouraging preliminary data supporting the use of femtosecond laser technology to improve patient outcomes and decrease complications in penetrating keratoplasty, and particularly for the correction of high astigmatism.[16-20] Currently, femtosecond laser technology may facilitate reduction of postkeratoplasty astigmatism in two ways: by enabling flap creation for LASIK, and by creating incisions for astigmatic keratotomy or wedge resection within the graft. Femtosecond enabled astigmatic keratotomy has the capacity to reduce large amounts of astigmatism by producing extraordinarily even astigmatic arcuate cuts, such that wedge resections may not be necessary. This chapter will focus principally on femtosecond enabled astigmatic keratotomy.

## ⋗ THE PRINCIPLES OF ASTIGMATIC KERATOTOMY POSTKERATOPLASTY

Astigmatic keratotomy postkeratoplasty is a quick, safe, and minimally invasive technique to reduce high astig-matism.[2,3,21] The aim of the procedure is to reduce high astigmatism to facilitate spectacle or contact lens wear, or once stabilized, to render the astigmatism amenable to excimer laser ablation. The aim should not be to eliminate the astigmatism completely, as overzealous large inci-sions may produce overcorrections necessitating incision resuturing.

Astigmatic keratotomy postkeratoplasty involves placement of paired arcuate incisions on the steep axis, within the corneal stroma and inside the graft-host inter-face to reduce high astigmatism. The graft-host interface is thought to act as a new functional limbus. Astigmatic keratotomy postkeratoplasty is thought to induce an exaggerated response due to the greater tension within the graft.[22]

There is usually no change in spherical equivalent, because the flattening produced by the incisions in the steep axis is countered by the steepening of the unincised meridian. This is known as the 'coupling effect'. When there is little or no change in spherical equivalent, the corneal steepening-flattening coupling ratio is close to one.[23] This has been reported in several other studies analyzing the effect of relaxing incisions.[22-28] A coupling ratio greater than one will lead to hyperopic shift, whereas a coupling ratio less than one will lead to myopic shift. Shorter incisions are associated with greater flattening, and longer incisions with greater steepening.

Parameters associated with increased magnitude of effect include longer incision length, deeper incisions, incisions closer to the central corneal optical zone, and incisions in an older patient's cornea. Because the graft-host interface is thought to act as a new limbus, incisions are usually placed 0.5 mm within the interface. Incision placement must be at an adequate distance from the interface to prevent wound destabilization, and at an adequate distance from the central cornea to prevent glare and higher order aberrations.

## ▶ FEMTOSECOND ENABLED ASTIGMATIC KERATOTOMY (FEAK) POST KERATOPLASTY

### Surgical Assessment

To ensure appropriate candidacy, all sutures should have been removed at least 6 months prior to intervention. The surgical wound is inspected for wound slippage, a separate issue best addressed by wound revision.

Preoperative planning includes assessment of the axis, amount and regularity of corneal astigmatism, and graft thickness and size. Patients undergo imaging with a placido disk topographer (NIDEK, OPD Scan III, Gamagori, Japan), and with the Pentacam rotating Scheimpflug camera (Oculus, Wetzlar, Germany). Pre- and postoperative topographic monitoring is essential in assessing the effect of incisions. Pachymetry is best performed with a handheld ultrasonic pachymeter at the time of surgery in the area where the incision will be placed. Anterior chamber OCT is an alternative method using the caliper tool to determine depth at the suitable location.

If there is disagreement between the axis of the manifest refraction and the topography, we favor the topography axis. The amount of topographic cylinder rather than the manifest cylinder is used to determine the length (degrees) of the keratotomy.[29]

We recommend femtosecond enabled astigmatic keratotomy for high degrees (greater than 5–6 diopters) of regular astigmatism. At lower levels of astigmatism, PRK, Microkeratome LASIK, intraocular lens exchange with a toric IOL, or piggyback secondary toric IOL implantation may be considered due to their greater accuracy and ability to alter the spherical equivalent and astigmatism. In a phakic patient, toric intraocular lenses may be considered as well.

Treatment parameters are based upon the topographic location and radial extent of the steep meridian. Our initial experience of early overcorrections prompted us to alter the treatment nomogram. Currently, up to 6 diopters of cylinder are treated with 45–50 degree arc length, 6–10 diopters with 50–60 degree arc length, and greater than 10 diopters with 60–70 degree arc length.

### Surgical Technique

Our technique has been outlined previously.[29] Treatments are paired symmetric (same length) incisions, centered on the steep axis. The depth of the incisions is set at approximately 90% depth, based on either the Pentacam or ultrasound pachymetry at the incision location. Each incision is made 0.5 mm within the graft-host junction, such that the diameter is 1 mm less than the graft diameter measured by calipers at the time of surgery.

The surgery may be performed using the 60 kHz (with the IEK software upgrade) or 150 kHz IntraLase FS (IFS) system in keratoplasty mode (IntraLase Corp, Irvine, California, USA). Using the 30 kHz IntraLase FS system, treatment depth is limited to 400 microns and does not have the proper software for astigmatic cuts. The Femto LDV (Ziemer Group, Port, Switzerland) is an alternative system with software for astigmatic keratotomy. Other commercially available systems include the Technolas Perfect Vision 520 FS (Technolas Perfect Vision, Munich Germany) and the VisuMax Femtosecond System (Carl Zeiss Meditec, Jena, Germany). These other systems are not discussed, as we have no experience with their use.

On the IntraLase system, the laser is adapted by using the Anterior Side Cut Planning Window. The side cut is set at 90°. The position of the center of the steep axis is entered. Variable parameters include posterior depth (incision depth in microns), diameter (optical zone diameter in millimeters), and cut angle (angular length of incision in degrees). Irregular astigmatism can be treated with unpaired incisions requiring resetting of the planning window.

Surgery is commenced under topical anesthesia (proparacaine 0.5%). The eyelids are prepared with betadine sponges. Using a sterile marking pen, the graft host junction is marked in the steep and flat axis, as this helps to center the incisions on the graft, which is often not obvious once applanation is achieved. The diameter of the graft is measured. This, minus one millimeter is used to determine the diameter of the arcuate cuts. Pachymetry is performed in the proposed area of the cuts with an ultrasound device. Cuts are made at a depth equal to 90% of the thinnest measurement taken in the area of the proposed cuts. The IntraLase limbal suction ring is then applied and the cone is positioned. Applanation is judged as adequate if the fluid meniscus is at least beyond the graft host junction. The X–Y position of the cuts are then adjusted using the software program on the IntraLase. Cuts are made with the laser and usually take less than 10 seconds. Once complete, suction is released and the ring is removed. We do not routinely open incisions though they can be expanded with the forceps if the expected effect is minimal. Topography is repeated immediately after the procedure.

After surgery, patients are treated with topical tobramycin and dexamethasone (TobraDex; Alcon, Mississauga, Ontario, Canada) four times daily for 1 week. Thereafter they are placed on a maintenance dose of topical steroid according to their individual requirements. The patients are seen 24 hours later and effect is observed. Often the effect is less than desired immediately after the procedure and at 24 hours. There is usually an increased effect up to 1 week postoperative. Thus undercorrection is desirable immediately after the procedure.

## ❯ RESULTS

For postkeratoplasty astigmatism, femtosecond enabled astigmatic keratotomy results are encouraging. There are now several reports verifying the effectiveness of the technique. Kiraly et al.[19] reported their experience of FEAK in 10 patients with postkeratoplasty astigmatism,

showing a reduction in astigmatism of three diopters with improvement of best-corrected visual acuity in 8 patients. Nubile et al.[30] investigated the feasibility and initial outcomes of FEAK for high postkeratoplasty astigmatism using the Femtec (20/10 Perfect Vision, GmbH, Heidelberg, Germany) femtosecond laser. Incision sites were 1.0 mm within the graft-host interface. In 12 patients, mean preoperative astigmatism of 7.16 ± 3.07 diopters (D) reduced to 2.23 ± 1.55 D at 1 month after surgery ($P = 0.002$) and remained stable thereafter. Kymionis et al.[31] have reported their experience with FEAK for irregular nonorthogonal astigmatism postkeratoplasty. They observed a significant reduction in irregular astigmatism from 4.0 diopters to 0.5 diopters, with an improvement in best-corrected visual acuity from 20/50 to 20/32. Levinger et al.[32] have reported a case of FEAK after endothelial keratoplasty. A reduction of absolute cylinder from 5.75 diopters to 2.75 diopters was observed, with improvement of best-corrected visual acuity from 20/100 to 20/40. It is recommended that calculation of incision depth should exclude the donor lenticule.

Comparison studies between FEAK and manual and mechanized astigmatic keratotomy have been performed. Our group, Bahar et al.[20] have compared manual astigmatic keratotomy with IntraLase enabled astigmatic keratotomy (IEAK). Twenty eyes were allocated to each treatment group. Mean cylinder reduction was 3.23 +/− 4.69 diopters in the manual AK group and 4.26 +/− 1.72 diopters in the IEAK group ($P = 0.36$). Treatment with IEAK was found to be safe and effective, with a significant improvement in uncorrected and best-corrected visual acuity when compared to manual astigmatic keratotomy. Hoffart et al.[14] compared mechanized astigmatic keratotomy produced with the Hanna keratome (Moria, Anthony, France) with FEAK. Using the Alpins method of arithmetic and vector analysis, the mean arithmetic change was significantly higher after FEAK with a decrease of −55.4 +/− 20.7% ($P = 0.011$). A larger misalignment of treatment using mechanized astigmatic keratotomy was suggested.

We reported our results of FEAK for high postkeratoplasty astigmatism in 37 eyes with a minimum of 3 months and a mean of 7 months follow-up.[29] Incision depth was 90% and cuts were placed 0.5 mm within the graft-host interface. UCVA (logMAR) improved significantly from 1.08 ± 0.34 preoperatively to 0.80 ± 0.42 postoperatively (p = 0.0016, paired t-test). BCVA (logMAR) improved significantly from 0.45 ± 0.27 preoperatively to 0.37 ± 0.27 postoperatively (p = 0.018). Both absolute orthogonal and oblique astigmatism were significantly reduced (p = 0.005 and p = 0.04, respectively). For orthogonal and lower degrees of oblique astigmatism, a precise relationship between achieved and intended correction was established. For higher degrees of oblique astigmatism, a slight overcorrection was achieved for high minus cylinder and a slight undercorrection was achieved for high plus cylinder. There was a significant increase in total higher order aberrations. The effect of the astigmatic keratotomy was maximal after 6 weeks, with stabilization after 3 months. The defocus equivalent, proportional to the diameter of the blur circle on the retina for a given pupil size, was significantly reduced by more than one diopter (from 8.5 ± 3.5 to 7.2 ± 4.59, p = 0.025). The mean astigmatism vector reduced from 2.52 × 122° ± 5.4 to 0.41 × 126° ± 4.0 (p = 0.07). A larger sample size would have been required to produce a treatment nomogram.

## ▶ COMPLICATIONS

Potential complications of FEAK include overcorrection requiring resuturing, infective keratitis, graft rejection, and graft perforation. In our series, 8% experienced an episode of graft rejection and each case resolved on topical steroid therapy. A high initial overcorrection rate (24%) prompted a change in the surgical nomogram to shorter arcuate cuts, with a corresponding fall in the rate of overcorrection from 24% to 11%. Overcorrection tended to occur more in keratoconic eyes. There were no cases of perforation or infective keratitis, though we later had one after the study was concluded. Nubile et al.[30] reported two cases of microperforation of a total of 12 eyes. This may have been related to mechanical stress induced by opening incisions.

### Discussion

The femtosecond laser facilitates a precise astigmatic keratotomy incision length, depth, curvature and symmetry.

Results of FEAK for high astigmatism postkeratoplasty (greater than five diopters) compare favorably with astigmatic keratotomy performed with other techniques. FEAK also has an encouraging refractive predictability.

Two factors limit the application of FEAK in lesser degrees of astigmatism postkeratoplasty (less than five diopters). First, astigmatic reduction after FEAK is subject to unpredictable corneal wound healing. Keratotomy healing begins with an epithelial plug that is eventually replaced by hypercellular scar tissue, explaining delayed changes in corneal curvature.[33] Second, due to the coupling effect, FEAK should induce little or no change in spherical equivalent. At lower degrees of astigmatism postkeratoplasty, a better alternative may be excimer surface ablation or nonfemtosecond assisted LASIK. This is due to higher predictability of refractive effect and significant reduction in the spherical equivalent. Our experience with IntraLase LASIK post PKP has been variable, with poor flap formation due to gas breakthrough old suture tracts. We thus prefer PRK in these cases with mitomycin C as haze is more likely in these cases. For presbyopic phakic patients, an alternative is lens exchange with a toric intraocular lens (IOL) or toric implantable collamer lenses (ICL). For pseudophakic patients, an alternative is a toric sulcus lens. However, these approaches are more invasive, damaging to the graft endothelium, and necessitate a potentially traumatic IOL removal should the keratoplasty fail.

FEAK represents a significant advance in the treatment of high astigmatism postkeratoplasty. Perfectly centered, arc shaped incisions of a prescribed depth are greatly facilitated and it is possible to achieve improved best-corrected acuity with greater reliability and power. Where a reduction in spherical equivalent and better unaided visual acuity is desired, a staged procedure may be considered: primary FEAK, observation for wound stabilization, followed by secondary excimer laser treatment. A new treatment nomogram is required to further refine refractive outcomes. This should be possible with greater use of femtosecond technology for this application.

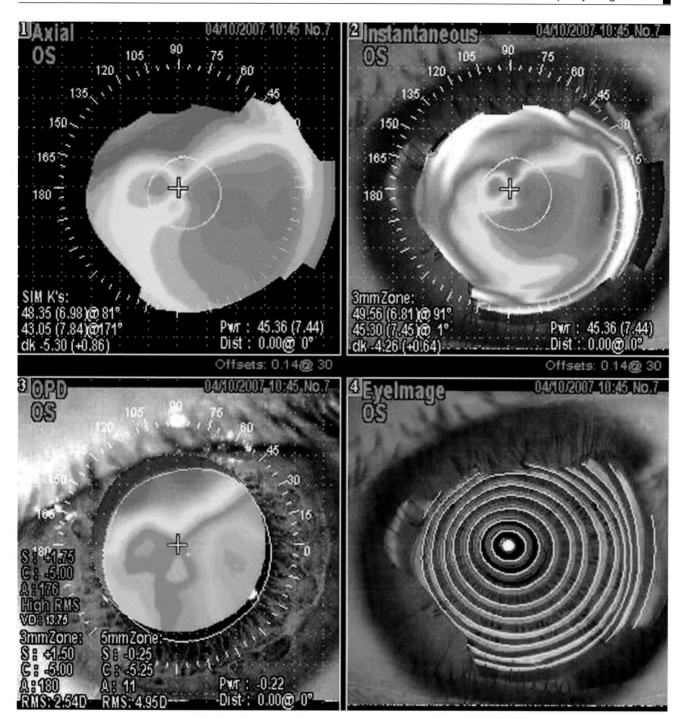

**Fig. 1:** A 37-year-old female underwent penetrating keratoplasty for keratoconus 8 years prior to the featured topography. Preoperatively, her uncorrected visual acuity was 20/200. With a subjective manifest refraction of +1.75–5.00×178, her best-corrected visual acuity was 20/60. Topography reveals 5.30 diopters of astigmatism with the steep axis at 81°

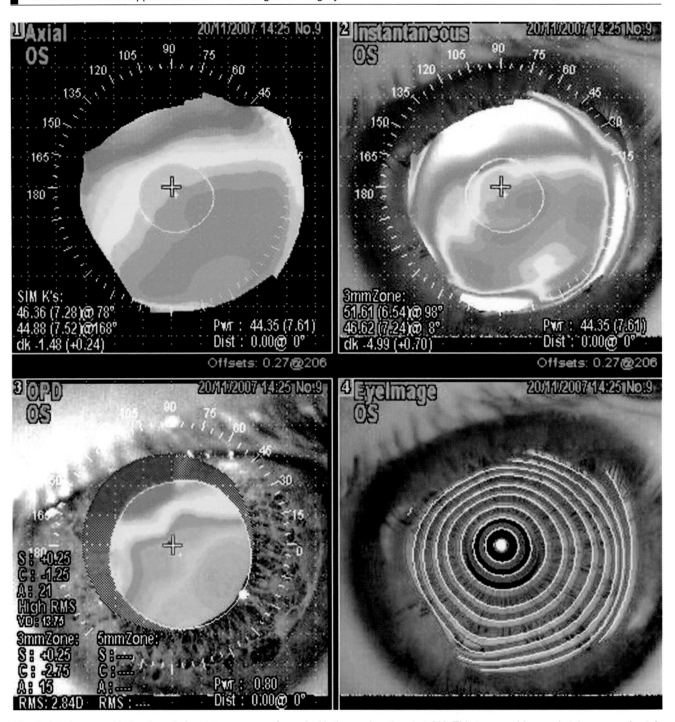

**Fig. 2:** IntraLase enabled astigmatic keratotomy was performed with the arc length set at 60°. This topographic map is taken approximately 1 month after surgery. Topography confirms approximately 1.50 diopters of residual astigmatism. Uncorrected visual acuity improved to 20/40, and with a subjective manifest refraction of +1.00–1.75×85 her best-corrected visual acuity improved to 20/30

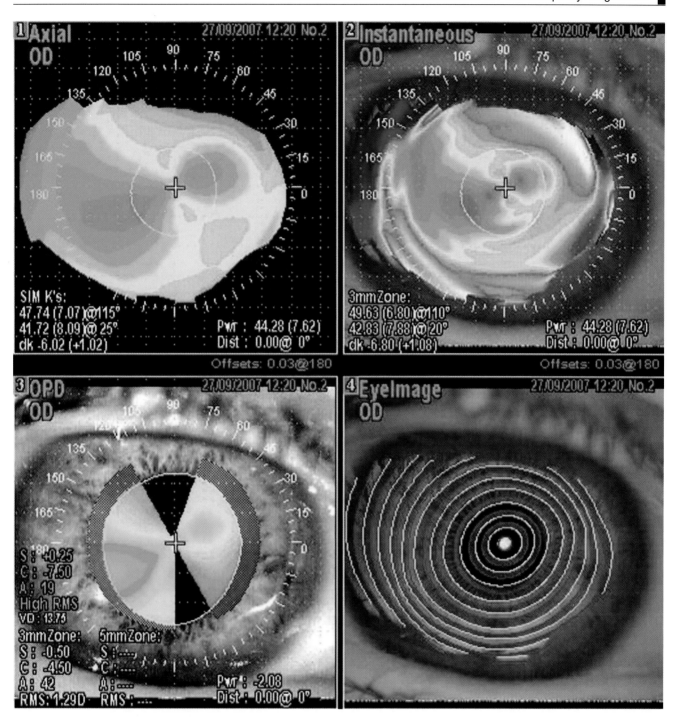

**Fig. 3:** A 44-year-old female underwent penetrating keratoplasty for keratoconus 4 years prior to the featured topography. Preoperatively, her uncorrected visual acuity was 20/70. With a subjective manifest refraction of 0.25–6.00×31, her best-corrected visual acuity was 20/30. Topography reveals 6.02 diopters of astigmatism with the steep axis at 115°

116
CHAPTER

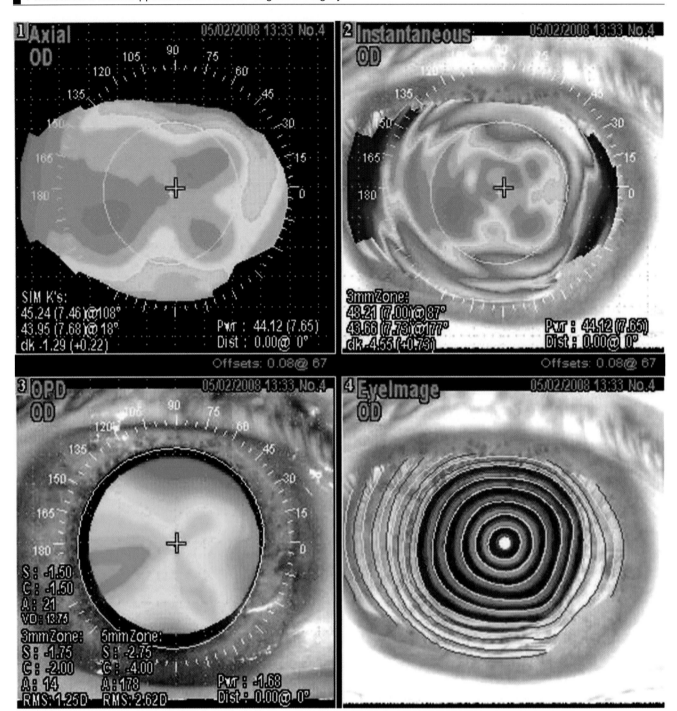

**Fig. 4:** IntraLase enabled astigmatic keratotomy was performed with the arc length set at 55°. This topographic map is taken approximately 3 months after surgery. Topography confirms approximately 1.30 diopters of residual astigmatism. Uncorrected visual acuity improved to 20/40, and with a subjective manifest refraction of −1.00−1.00×15 her best-corrected visual acuity improved to 20/25

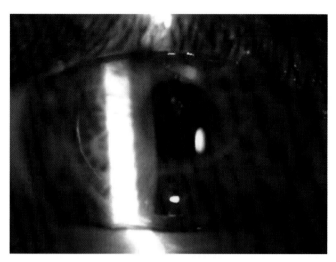

**Fig. 5:** This clinical photo displays a curvilinear femtosecond astigmatic keratotomy approximately 0.5 mm within the graft-host junction. The meticulous architecture of the incision length, depth and curvature are difficult to replicate using manual techniques

## ❧ REFERENCES

1. Williams KA, Roder D, Esterman A, et al. Factors predictive of corneal graft survival: report from the Australian Corneal Graft Registry. Ophthalmology. 1992;99:403-14.
2. Poole TR, Ficker LA. Astigmatic keratotomy for post-keratoplasty astigmatism. J Cataract Refract Surg. 2006;32:1175-9.
3. Bochmann F, Schipper I. Correction of post-keratoplasty astigmatism with keratotomies in the host cornea. J Cataract Refract Surg. 2006;32:923-8.
4. Genvert GI, Cohen EJ, Arentsen JJ, et al. Fitting gas permeable contact lenses after penetrating keratoplasty. Am J Ophthalmol. 1989;99:511-4.
5. Forseto AS, Francesconi CM, Nose RA, et al. Laser in situ keratomileusis to correct refractive errors after keratoplasty. J Cataract Refract Surg. 1999;25:479-85.
6. Hardten DR, Lindstrom RL. Surgical correction of refractive errors after penetrating keratoplasty. Int Ophthalmol Clin. 1997;37(1):1-35.
7. Troutman RC. Corneal wedge resections and relaxing incisions for postkeratoplasty astigmatism. Int Ophthalmol Clin. 1983;23(4):161-8.
8. Arffa RC. Results of a graded relaxing incision technique for postkeratoplasty astigmatism. Ophthalmic Surg. 1988;19:624-8.
9. Lugo M, Donnenfeld ED, Arentson JJ. Corneal wedge resection for high astigmatism following penetrating keratoplasty. Ophthalmic Surg. 1987;18:650-3.
10. Gothard TW, Agapitos PJ, Bowers RA, et al. Four incision radial keratotomy for high myopia after penetrating keratoplasty. J Refract Corneal Surg. 1993;9:51-7.
11. John ME, Martines E, Cvintal T, et al. Photorefractive keratectomy following penetrating keratoplasty. J Refract Corneal Surg. 1994;10(suppl):S206-10.
12. Borderie VM, Touzeau O, Chastang PJ, et al. Surgical correction of post-keratoplasty astigmatism with the Hanna arcitome. J Cataract Refract Surg. 1999;25:205-11.
13. Hanna KD, Hayward JM, Hagen KB, et al. Keratotomy for astigmatism using an arcuate keratome. Arch Ophthalmol. 1993;111:998-1004.
14. Hoffart L, Touzeau O, Borderie V, et al. Mechanized astigmatic arcuate keratotomy with the Hanna arcitome for astigmatism after keratoplasty. J Cataract Refract Surg. 2007;33:862-8.
15. Vajpayee RB, Sharma N, Sinha R, et al. Laser in-situ keratomileusis after penetrating keratoplasty. Surv Ophthalmol. 2003;48:503-14.
16. Slade SG. Applications of the femtosecond laser in corneal surgery. Curr Opin Ophthalmol. 2007;18:338-41.
17. Buratto L, Bohm E. The use of the femtosecond laser in penetrating keratoplasty. Am J Ophthalmol. 2007;143:737-42.
18. Harissi-Dagher M, Azar DT. Femtosecond laser astigmatic keratotomy for postkeratoplasty astigmatism. Can J Ophthalmol. 2008;43:367-9.
19. Kiraly L, Herrmann C, Amm M, et al. Reduction of astigmatism by arcuate incisions using the femtosecond laser after corneal transplantation [in German]. Klin Monatsbl Augenheilkd. 2008;225:70-4.
20. Bahar I, Levinger E, Kaiserman I, et al. Intralase-enabled astigmatic keratotomy for postkeratoplasty astigmatism. Am J Ophthalmol. 2008;146:897-904.
21. Wilkins MR, Mehta JS, Larkin FP. Standardized arcuate keratotomy for postkeratoplasty astigmatism. J Cataract Refract Surg. 2005;31:297-301.
22. Wu E. Femtosecond-assisted astigmatic keratotomy. International Ophthalmology Clinics. 2011;51:77-85.
23. Krachmer JH, Fenzl RE. Surgical correction of high postkeratoplasty astigmatism: relaxing incisions vs wedge resection. Arch Ophthalmol. 1980;98:1400-2.
24. Hjortdal JO, Ehlers N. Paired arcuate keratotomy for congenital and postkeratoplasty astigmatism. Acta Ophthalmol Scand. 1998;76:138-41.
25. Cohen KL, Tripoli NK, Noecker RJ. Prospective analysis of photokeratoscopy for arcuate keratotomy to reduce postkeratoplasty astigmatism. J Refract Corneal Surg. 1989;5:388-93.
26. Koay YP, McGhee CN, Crawford GJ. Effect of a standard paired arcuate incision and augmentation sutures on postkeratoplasty astigmatism. J Cataract Refract Surg. 2000;26:553-61.
27. Akura J, Matsuura K, Hatta S, et al. A new concept for the correction of astigmatism: full-arc, depth-dependent astigmatic keratotomy. Ophthalmology. 2000;107:95-104.
28. Price FW, Grene RB, Marks RG, et al. Astigmatism reduction clinical trial: a multicenter prospective evaluation of the predictability of arcuate keratotomy; evaluation of surgical nomogram predictability. Arch Ophthalmol. 1995;113:277-82.

CHAPTER **116**

29. Kumar NL, Kaiserman I, Shehadeh-Mashor R, et al. IntraLase enabled astigmatic keratotomy for post-keratoplasty astigmatism: on-axis vector analysis. Ophthalmol. 2010;117:1228-35.

30. Nubile M, Carpineto P, Lanzini M, et al. Femtosecond laser arcuate keratotomy for the correction of high astigmatism after keratoplasty. Ophthalmol. 2009;116:1083-92.

31. Kymionis GD, Yoo SH, Ide T, et al. Femtosecond-assisted astigmatic keratotomy for post-keratoplasty astigmatism. J Cataract Refract Surg. 2009;35:11-3.

32. Levinger E, Bahar I, Rootman DS. IntraLase-enabled astigmatic keratotomy for correction of astigmatism after descemet stripping automated endothelial keratoplasty: a case report. Cornea. 2009;28:1074-6.

33. Eiferman RA, Schultz GS, Nordquist RE, et al. Corneal wound healing and its pharmacologic modification after refractive keratotomy. In: Waring GO III (Ed). Refractive Keratotomy for Myopia and Astigmatism. St Louis, MO: Mosby; 1992. pp. 749-79.

# Complications of Femtosecond Laser Procedures

*George D Kymionis, Vardhaman P Kankariya*

## ⋗ INTRODUCTION

Femtosecond (FS) lasers are solid state Nd:Glass lasers similar to a Nd:YAG lasers, which work on the principle of photoionization (also known as laser induced optical breakdown). FS lasers produce photodisruption at its focal point, resulting in a rapidly expanding cloud of free electrons and ionized molecules (plasma), in turn creating an acoustic shock wave that disrupts the surrounding tissue. In this event, small volumes of tissue are vaporized with the formation of cavitation gas bubbles consisting of carbon dioxide and water, which eventually dissipate into the surrounding tissues.[1] Additionally collateral damage seen with FS laser is $10^6$ times less than Nd:YAG laser, thus demonstrating its precision and safety when used in corneal surgeries.[2] It is important to understand the principles of operation to appreciate mechanism of FS lasers related complications and to plan preventive strategy.

Femtosecond laser enabled common procedures include hinged flap creation in LASIK,[3-10] keratoplasty (penetrating,[11-15] anterior lamellar[16] and deep anterior lamellar[17,18]); and channel creation for INTACS (intracorneal segments) implantation.[19-21] Other procedures utilizing FS lasers include astigmatic keratotomy,[22-24] lamellar pocket creation (corneal inlays), corneal biopsy[25] and cataract surgery[26] (capsulorhexis, lenticular fragmentation and corneal incisions) amongst others.

Most frequent FS laser enabled procedure currently is flap creation LASIK. More than 55% of the all LASIK surgeries in the United States were performed with FS lasers in 2009.[27] Proportion is even more in high volume practices and FS lasers are gaining more acceptance worldwide. Several studies have shown FS lasers to be superior to microkeratome in terms of predictability of flap thickness and diameter; planar architecture of flap, better predictability of hinge position and size; and astigmatic neutrality.[28-31] FS enabled flaps also demonstrate less incidence of complications like induced dry eye, epithelial ingrowth, optical abberations, flap slippage, free cap and buttonholes.[32-39]

Femtosecond lasers promise excellent reproducibility and versatility in applications, at the same time they demonstrate 'unique' set of complications. Lately, there has been a great interest in complications related to use of FS lasers namely formation of opaque bubble layer, vertical gas break through, air in anterior chamber, transient light-sensitivity syndrome (TLSS), rainbow glare and lamellar keratitis. Currently most relevent complications unique to FS lasers are as flap maker in LASIK surgeries. All complications are herein described in terms of mechanisms, risk factors, management and preventive measures.

## ⋗ COMPLICATIONS

### Cavitation Bubble Related Complications

Femtosecond lasers work on the principle of photoionization by creation of series of cavitation bubbles, which ultimately join to create a cleavage plane in the corneal tissue. Expansion of these bubbles outside cleavage plane produces opaque bubble layer (OBL). Furthermore, if expansion occurs anteriorly or in posterior stroma, it results in vertical gas breakthrough (VGB) resulting in buttonhole formation and presence of air bubble in anterior chamber respectively.

## Opaque Bubble Layer

High energy used in the previous generation FS lasers (6 kHz, 15 kHz) was related to uncontrolled expansion of these high-pressure bubbles into a path of least resistance resulting in OBL. Two mechanisms for formation of OBL have been described; first states that OBL is a microplasma of corneal byproducts that results from laser vaporization of corneal tissue.[40] Alternatively, OBL simply may be the gas bubbles formed between collagen lamellae in the cleavage plane. The collagen lamellae are forced apart by the shock wave generated because of the laser induced optical breakdown of corneal tissue if energy used is too high.[41,42] These cavitation bubbles (by producing carbon dioxide and water) ultimately disappear by diffusion and corneal endothelial pump.[43]

Kaiserman et al. described two types of OBL depending upon location of cavitation bubbles.[44] An early (or hard) opaque bubble layer appears when gas bubbles spread into the tissue anterior or posterior to the plane. Hard type of OBL is formed in the stroma and does not disappear quickly after lifting the flap. A late (diffuse) opaque bubble layer occurs when gas travels into the intralamellar spaces after the laser pulses have passed through a particular portion of the resection. Diffuse OBL is formed in the cleavage plane of the cornea, as it's usually the path of least resistance. Late OBL gets absorbed quickly, though it may interfere with pupillary tracking (Figs 1A to C).

Risk factors for excessive OBL include higher raster energy (more common with 15 Hz Intralase laser than present generation FS lasers), thicker corneas, smaller flap diameter and harder applanation of cornea while docking.[44] Once developed, excessive OBL demands wait for at least few minutes for the bubbles to disappear. Some surgeons prefer to swipe the stroma with Weck cell sponge after lifting the flap to hasten absorption. OBL may interfere with optimal outcome of LASIK procedure. Studies have reported worse visual acuity and increased higher order aberrations postoperatively (not statistically significant) in eyes with OBL, especially the hard type.[44] They associate this outcome with possibility of irregular flap interface generated due to attenuation and scatter of laser beam. Moreover, it may also be required to postpone the excimer ablation, if excessive OBL interferes with papillary tracking. In addition, OBL can give erroneous reading on intraoperative pachymetry as gas bubbles are reflective to acoustic signals.

Considering potential delay and other risks involved, prevention is crucial to avoid these complications and surgeons would want to reduce the incidence of this complication. There are inbuilt features in the FS laser systems to reduce risk of formation of OBL. For instance, Intralase creates a peripheral pocket at depth of approximately 300 μ located just behind the hinge, thus allowing gas bubbles to be released outside the flap.[45] Wavelight FS200 creates a similar channel behind the hinge, which has a posterior vent to the surface for the bubbles to escape.[46] Femto LDV creates the side cuts at the same time with flap creation, thus side cuts provide access in close proximity for the bubbles to get away. In addition, optimizing laser settings in the form of reducing raster energy, changing pocket/channel specifications will reduce incidence of OBL.[47] 'Soft' docking and a well-centered applanation distributes applanation pressure evenly over the cornea and provide thin sliver of applanated tissue posterior to the pocket. Furthermore, for the pocket to serve its function, it has to be anterior to the low-resistance tissue. Hence, it is important to position pocket away from limbus otherwise cavitation bubbles encounter great resistance at perilimbal area and form OBL.

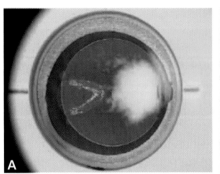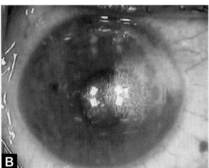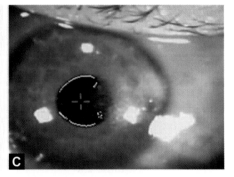

**Figs 1A to C:** (A) Opaque bubble layer as seen on monitor seen at the time of flap creation with femtosecond laser; (B) Diffuse opaque bubble layer as seen under the microscope before lifting the flap; (C) Opaque bubble layer interfering with pupillary tracking. Note, though pupil is tracked incompletely due to opaque bubble layer on temporal side

## Vertical Gas Breakthrough

Photodisruption creates multiple cavitation bubbles, which coalesce together forming the cleavage plane in the corneal stroma. However, they can occasionally coalesce and travel within the cornea to undesired locations. Vertical gas breakthrough is the escape of bubbles from the stroma to the corneal surface during the keratectomy.[48] Vertical gas breakthrough can be subepithelial or could produce full thickness defect creating (more visual threatening) buttonhole formation.[48,49] Mechanism of formation of VGB is microbubbles, which are under significant pressure due to suction ring and glass applanation, breaks vertically through areas of corneal weakness. The predisposing factors have been largely unknown. Some of the suspected factors are focal defects in the Bowman's membrane,[48] previous incisional surgery like radial keratotomy, corneal scars and ocular rosasea.[49] In ocular rosasea, focal area of altered epithelium and thinned stroma provides a low-resistance pathway for early gas-bubble escape to the surface instead of advancing in lamellar plane.[49] In incisional surgeries and corneal scars, there is an obvious low-resistance pathway leading gas-bubbles to the superficial surface. VGB is also associated with thin flap thickness e.g. in sub-Bowman keratomileusis (SBK).

Epithelial breakthrough may result in obstruction of subsequent laser spots to the area and even risk of epithelial ingrowth if the flap is lifted. To prevent VGB, flap creation should be done with caution and close observation in patients with risk factors like corneal scars or postradial keratotomy. Lowering the raster energy has been seen to be successful in avoiding this complication. Buttonhole formation because of epithelial breakthrough can be prevented in high-risk corneas by use of microkeratome instead.

Management of the VGB depends on the stage at which it is noticed and location of epithelial breakthrough. If intraoperative epithelial breakthrough is noticed before the side cuts are made, then a second 40 μ deeper flap is suggested. One should keep in mind that in such attempt, there is a possibility of recurrence of VGB. On the other hand, if the vertical side cut has been completed before VGB is noticed, then it is advisable not to lift the flap. Chang et al.[50] have reported use of microkeratome in such situations. The FS-enabled flap is not lifted; instead a microkeratome is used to recut the flap in the same sitting. The FS laser cut and microkeratome cut creation have to be kept in the same direction e.g. if it is superior hinge flap with laser, then an inferior hinge flap is created with microkeratome because that is the direction of raster energy. A cut from any other side would result in flap movement and possible flap shredding.[50]

## Air Bubble in the Anterior Chamber

Gas bubbles can occasionally coalesce and travel within the cornea to undesired locations through posterior stroma and endothelium producing air bubbles in anterior chamber. There are several mechanisms proposed for this phenomenon.[51-55] Lifshitz et al. proposed that multiple bubbles coalesce to form larger bubble which migrates to posterior stroma and endothelim without being absorbed by the endothelial pump.[40] Srinivasan et al. suggested that the positive pressure from suction device and docking forced expanding airbubble in anterior chamber though peripheral stroma and trabecular meshwork.[52] In addition, Utine et al. proposed that FS lasers produce direct photo dissociation of aqueous humor, or direct cavitation effect in aqueous humor due to rapid pressure changes in corneal lamellar interface.[55]

Once formed, the anterior chamber bubbles generally get absorbed within 30 minutes, thus causing no harm. Although they may interfere with fixation, iris registration and eye tracking during procedure. If persistent, they may even necessitate postponement of excimer ablation on next day. In case of persistent air bubbles, if cylindrical error or customized treatment is not planned, then the procedure can be done on the same day with manual centration.[55] Otherwise, it is advisable to wait until the air bubble is totally absorbed for facilitating iris registration and pupillary tracking.

## Transient Light Sensitivity Syndrome

Transient light sensitivity syndrome (TLSS) is characterized by severe photophobia starting from 2 to 6 weeks after uneventful LASIK surgery and normal visual acuity with unremarkable slitlamp examination.[56,57] There are other terms used for TLSS like delayed acute photophobia and good acuity plus photophobia. Slit lamp examination shows no signs of inflammation like hyperemia, anterior chamber reaction or inflammation in the interface. The differential diagnosis of TLSS should include dry eye syndrome and diffuse lamellar keratitis (DLK). Presence of disproportionate photophobia in relation to corneal findings, lack of staining, absence of interface cells and normal visual acuity suggest diagnosis of TLSS.

Proposed mechanisms consist of inflammation caused by subproducts of gas bubbles, cytokines from flap interface, activated keratocytes and necrotic cell debris. Laser energy has been strongly implicated in pathogenesis of TLSS, lowering energy by 20% has been reported to have resulted in decreased incidence by fivefolds.[56] There has been a reported association of DLK with TLSS, suggesting that inflammation in early postoperative period can be a predisposing factor.[57] Treatment of TLSS essentially consists of anti-inflammatory agents like steroids and cyclosporion. It is suggested that steroids decrease activated keratocytes in the corneal stroma, thus controlling inflammation.[56]

## Rainbow Glare Phenomenon

Rainbow glare is an optical phenomenon experienced as colored bands of light radiating from a white light source, when viewed in dark environment. Micro-irregularities on the back surface of the FS laser enabled LASIK flap are implicated. It is also related to poor optical beam quality due to lack of maintenance of optics. This phenomenon was described with previous generations of lasers.[58,59] The incidence of rainbow glare decreased from 19.07% to 2.32% with 60 kHz laser (instead of 15 kHz) and small numeric aperture, thus supporting the role of energy and optics. Present FS lasers with frequency of 150 kHz, 200 kHz and above will reduce the incidence further or make it obsolete. On slit lamp examination, all the findings are essentially normal. Patients notice reduction in the symptoms as the time goes by. There is no specific treatment required. Although rainbow glare is not debilitating, its association with higher raster energy and improper or insufficient machine maintenance shows the importance of quality control in the flap-creation process.[58,59]

## Lamellar Keratitis

Diffuse lamellar keratitis (DLK), also known as sands of Sahara syndrome or interface keratitis, is a noninfectious condition in which white blood cells infiltrate the space between the flap and the stromal bed shortly after LASIK with microkeratome.[60] It is a vision threatening complication which may be associated with redness, tearing, pain, photophobia, and decline in vision. In contract to DLK related to microkeratomes, FS laser related lamellar keratitis (LK) is more focal i.e. dusting of cells more in periphery in doughnut shape. Lamellar keratitis is seen predominantly in periphery as more energy is used for side-cut creation. Studies have shown that incidence of LK is much higher in Intralase enabled LASIK compared to microkeratome.[61] Confocal and histological studies of human and rabbit corneas reveal that femtosecond LASIK flap creation resulted in a higher wound-healing index, greater stromal

cell apoptosis and influx of inflammatory cells than microkeratome flap creation.[62] Furthermore, studies have shown that higher frequency FS lasers caused less corneal inflammation and that a 60 kHz FS laser induced a similar amount of inflammation as a microkeratome.[63] Thus as expected, higher frequency lasers of today (Intralase 150, Wavelight FS200) demonstrate infrequent incidence of LK. Change in laser raster energy, side-cut energy will reduce incidence further. Treatment of LK is same as DLK seen with microkeratome use. Intensive topical steroids are the mainstay to reduce inflammation.

## Other Complications

### Decentered Flap

While docking, if the applanation is not achieved keeping the applanation glass plate centered on pupil, decentered flap can occur. It is an outcome of improper patient positioning and off centered docking, more than a true complication of FS lasers. A decentered flap itself doesn't result in visual threatening complication unless it is accompanied by decentered ablation. It can occur in inaccurate suction ring placement, pupil centroid shift due to dilation and an abnormal papillary center. Occurence of decentered cap can be avoided by putting reference markings at the limbus before starting of the procedure and orienting suction ring accordingly.[64]

### Suction Loss and Partial Flap

During the creation of the flap, the FS suction ring may lose suction, and the applanation plate may become separated from the cornea. Suction loss can be attributed to number of factors, such as the patient squeezing the eyelid, conjunctival chemosis and epithelial breakthrough.[49] Consequences and management of suction loss depends on the stage at which it was encountered. If it occurs before starting of laser lamellar cut, then suction ring is reapplied and procedure is done as routine. On the contrary, if suction is lost after partial propagation of laser, then an incomplete/partial flap is encountered (Fig. 2). Some surgeons make a second pass after achieving sufficient suction, using conjunctival markings as the reference mark.[65] Study on porcine eyes have shown that, in case of double pass after partial flap, there can be an irregular surface, multiple flaps, a free sliver of the corneal stroma, and crossing of the two cut planes because of differences in applanation pressure, hydration conditions and chemosis. This can result in long-lasting, sight-threatening complications such as mismatch of the flap and the bed, larger aberrations, glare and halos.[66]

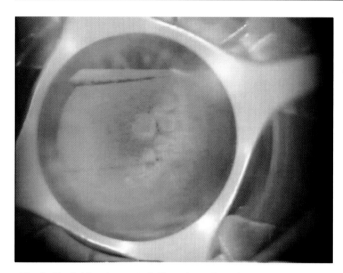

**Fig. 2:** Partial flap is created due to loss of suction towards the end of complete propagation of laser pulse

Furthermore, if suction is lost during the side cut, then the diameter of the side cut is decreased by 1 mm, the suction ring is reapplied, and the side cut is performed just inside the outside diameter of the lamellar cut.

### Interface Haze

Roch et al. reported occurrence of interface haze formation after thin flap IntraLASIK (FS60, AMO, Irvine, CA).[67] Mild haze was observed in 15% of eyes treated for moderate to high myopia at 3 months postoperatively. Ultrathin IntraLASIK flaps (= 90 μm) and younger age were strongly associated with an increased risk for postoperative interface haze. Haze formation is presumed as an effect of TGF-B cytokine release from the epithelial basement membrane in response to energy of FS laser. Epithelial injuries are associated with increased inflammation and diffuse lamellar keratitis. Occasionally, epithelial defects occur adjacent to the side cut after IntraLASIK. In these cases, corticosteroids should be used more often during the first 24–48 hours.

### Unintended Epithelial Flap

Despite the high predictability and safety of the FS laser in terms of flap thickness, complications may occur. Kymionis et al.[68] reported occurrence of unintended epithelial flap with femto-enabled flap (Intralase FS150) when attempted flap thickness was 100 μ. A possible explanation for this incidence could be the inadequate corneal applanation by the glass cone. A similar case of thin flap creation including stroma by Choi et al.[69] suggests that FS laser flap

thickness creation is correlated to cone glass thickness, and thicker glass cones may produce thinner than usual flaps. Epithelial flap is assumed to have resulted from variation in the glass applanation plate thickness. Case was successfully converted into photorefractive keratectomy (PRK) with anti- metabolite (mitomycin C) with good outcome.

### Interface Stromal Irregularities

Kymionis et al.[70] reported a case of interface corneal stromal irregularities after flap creation with the IntraLase FS (150 Hz) laser system. As irregular stromal interface did not interfere with the final refractive results. The presence of this complication is not a contraindication to continue with the LASIK procedure.

### Air Under Conjunctiva

Ide et al.[71] reported a case of subconjunctival airbubbles during IntraLase flap creation. A possible explanation for this finding could be the migration of the created bubbles to the peripheral corneal, perilimbal area and subconjuctival space. It did not interfere with the procedure or the visual results.

### Macular Hemorrhage

Macular hemorrhage after LASIK has been reported more commonly with microkeratome enabled flap with the associated sudden increase in intraocular pressure (IOP) to 60–70 mm Hg, followed by a rapid IOP decrease upon suction release. This results in a mechanical stress that may rupture Bruch membrane in susceptible eyes, leading to macular hemorrhage. Predisposing factors include high myopia, lacquer cracks, choroidal neovascularization. There is also a reported case of macular hemorrhage after intralase enabled LASIK in a patient with no predisposing factors. The rare occurrence of this entity should be kept in mind and patients 'at risk' should be counseled accordingly.[72]

### ▶ CONCLUSION

To conclude, complications related to use of FS laser are rare and fortunately, not vision threatening. Understanding the mechanisms of these complications have enabled us to decrease incidence and severity of these unique entities. Many of these complications were more common with previous generations of FS lasers, which used more raster energy and low frequency; thus contributing to lamellar keratitis, TLSS and corneal edema. Present generation FS lasers use less energy resulting in decrease in the incidence and severity of

**CHAPTER 117**

**17 SECTION**

these complications. New FS technology possesses better algorithm to reduce possibility of cavitation bubble related complications (OBL, vertical gas breakthrough and bubbles in AC); modified planar applanation and automated suction mechanisms. FS technology holds great promise and will continue to provide more applications in ophthalmic surgery, ultimately contributing to our goal of emmetropia.

## Financial Support: None

The authors have no proprietary or commercial interest in any material discussed.

## ❧ REFERENCES

1. Chung SH, Mazur E. Surgical applications of femtosecond laser. J Biophotonics. 2009; 2(10):557-72.
2. Stern D, Schoenlein RW, Puliafito CA, et al. Corneal ablation by nanosecond, picosecond, and femtosecond lasers at 532 and 625 nm. Arch Ophthalmol 1989;107:587-92.
3. Ratkay-Traub I, Ferincz IE, Juhasz T, et al. First clinical results with the femtosecond neodymium-glass laser in refractive surgery. J Refract Surg. 2003;19:94-103.
4. Kezirian GM, Stonecipher KG. Comparison of the IntraLase femtosecond laser and mechanical keratomes for laser in situ keratomileusis. J Cataract Refract Surg. 2004;30:804-11.
5. Durrie DS, Kezirian GM. Femtosecond laser versus mechanical microkeratome flaps in wavefront-guided laser in situ keratomileusis: prospective contralateral eye study. J Cataract Refract Surg. 2005;31:120-6.
6. Binder PS. One thousand consecutive IntraLase laser in situ keratomileusis flaps. J Cataract Refract Surg. 2006;32:962-9.
7. Kim JY, Kim MJ, Kim T-I, et al. A femtosecond laser creates a stronger flap than a mechanical microkeratome. Invest Ophthalmol Vis Sci. 2006;47:599-604.
8. Netto MV, Mohan RR, Medeiros FW, et al. Femtosecond laser and microkeratome corneal flaps: comparison of stromal wound healing and inflammation. J Refract Surg. 2007;23:667-76.
9. Slade SG. The use of the femtosecond laser in the customization of corneal flaps in laser in situ keratomileusis. Curr Opin Ophthalmol. 2007;18:314-7.
10. Montés-Micó R, Rodríguez-Galietero A, Alió JL. Femtosecond laser versus mechanical keratome LASIK for myopia. Ophthalmology. 2007;114:62-8.
11. Farid M, Kim M, Steinert RF. Results of penetrating keratoplasty performed with a femtosecond laser zig-zag incision: Initial report. Ophthalmology. 2007;114:2208-12.
12. Por YM, Cheng JY, Parthasarathy A, et al. Outcomes of femtosecond laser-assisted penetrating keratoplasty. Am J Ophthalmol. 2008;145:772-4.
13. Price FW, Price MO. Femtosecond laser shaped penetrating keratoplasty: One-year results utilizing a top-hat configuration. Am J Ophthalmol. 2008;145:210-4.
14. Steinert RF, Ignacio TS, Sarayba MA. 'Top-hat'-shaped penetrating keratoplasty using the femtosecond laser. Am J Ophthalmol. 2007;143:689-91.
15. Bahar I, Kaiserman I, McAllum P, et al. Femtosecond laser-assisted penetrating keratoplasty: stability evaluation of different wound configurations. Cornea. 2008;27(2):209-11.
16. Yoo S, Kymionis G, Koreishi A, et al. Femtosecond laser assisted sutureless anterior lamellar keratoplasty. Ophthalmology. 2008;115:1303-7.
17. Chan CC, Ritenour RJ, Kumar NL, et al. Femtosecond laser-assisted mushroom configuration deep anterior lamellar keratoplasty. Cornea 2010;29(3):290-5.
18. Price FW, Price MO, Grandin JC, et al. Deep anterior lamellar keratoplasty with femtosecond-laser zig-zag incisions. J Cataract Refract Surg. 2009;35(5):804-8.
19. Ertan A, Kamburoglu G, Bahadir M. Intacs insertion with the femtosecond laser for the management of keratoconus: One year results. J Cataract Refract Surg. 2006;32:2039-42.
20. Rabinowitz YS, Li X, Ignacio TS, et al. Intacs inserts using the femtosecond laser compared to the mechanical spreader in the treatment of keratoconus. J Refract Surg. 2006;22:764-71.
21. Coskunseven E, Kymionis GD, Tsiklis NS, et al. One-year results of intrastromal corneal ring segment implantation (KeraRing) using femtosecond laser in patients with keratoconus. Am J Ophthalmol. 2008;145(5):775-9.
22. Ghanem RC, Azar DT. Femtosecond-laser arcuate wedge-shaped resection to correct high residual astigmatism after penetrating keratoplasty. J Cataract Refract Surg. 2006;32:1415-9.
23. Harissi-Dagher M, Azar DT. Femtosecond laser astigmatic keratotomy for postkeratoplasty astigmatism. Can J Ophthalmol. 2008;43:367-9.
24. Abbey A, Ide T, Kymionis GD, et al. Femtosecond laser-assisted astigmatic keratotomy in naturally occurring high astigmatism. Br J Ophthalmol. 2009;93(12):1566-9.
25. Yoo SH, Kymionis GD, O'Brien TP, et al. Femtosecond-assisted diagnostic corneal biopsy (FAB) in keratitis. Graefes Arch Clin Exp Ophthalmol. 2008;246(5):759-62.
26. Kullman G, Pineda R. Alternative applications of the femtosecond laser in ophthalmology. Semin Ophthalmol. 2010;25 (5-6):256-64.
27. Binder PS. Femtosecond applications for anterior segment surgery. Eye Contact Lens. 2010;36(5):282-5.
28. Shemesh G, Dotan G, Lipshitz I. Predictability of corneal flap thickness in laser in situ keratomileusis using three different microkeratomes. J Refract Surg. 2002;18:S347-51.
29. Kim J-H, Lee D, Rhee K-I. Flap thickness reproducibility in laser in situ keratomileusis with a femtosecond laser: optical coherence tomography measurement. J Cataract Refract Surg. 2008;34:132-6.
30. Sutton G, Hodge C. Accuracy and precision of LASIK flap thickness using the IntraLase femtosecond laser in 1000 consecutive cases. J Refract Surg. 2008;24:802-6.
31. Stahl JE, Durrie DS, Schwendeman FJ, et al. Anterior segment OCT analysis of thin IntraLase femtosecond flaps. J Refract Surg. 2007;23:555-8.

32. Salomão MQ, Ambrósio R, Wilson SE. Dry eye associated with laser in situ keratomileusis: mechanical microkeratome versus femtosecond laser. J Cataract Refract Surg. 2009;35:1756-60.

33. Soong HK, Malta JB. Femtosecond lasers in ophthalmology. Am J Ophthalmol. 2009;147:189-97.

34. Sarayba MA, Ignacio TS, Binder PS, et al. Comparative study of stromal bed quality by using mechanical, IntraLase femtosecond laser 15- and 30-kHz microkeratomes. Cornea. 2007;26:446-51.

35. Medeiros FW, Stapleton WM, Hammel J, et al. Wavefront analysis comparison of LASIK outcomes with the femtosecond laser and mechanical microkeratomes. J Refract Surg. 2007;23:880-7.

36. Buzzonetti L, Petrocelli G, Valente P, et al. Comparison of corneal aberration changes after laser in situ keratomileusis performed with mechanical microkeratome and IntraLase femtosecond laser: One-year follow-up. Cornea. 2008;27:174-9.

37. Durrie DS, Kezirian GM. Femtosecond laser versus mechanical keratome flaps in wavefront-guided laser in situ keratomileusis; prospective contralateral eye study. J Cataract Refract Surg. 2005;31:120-6.

38. Tran DB, Sarayba MA, Bor Z, et al. Randomized prospective clinical study comparing induced aberrations with IntraLase and Hansatome flap creation in fellow eyes: potential impact on wavefrontguided laser in situ keratomileusis. J Cataract Refract Surg. 2005;31:97-105.

39. Stonecipher K, Ignacio TS, Stonecipher M. Advances in refractive surgery: microkeratome and femtosecond laser flap creation in relation to safety, efficacy, predictability, and biomechanical stability. Curr Opin Ophthalmol. 2006;17:368-72.

40. Lifshitz T, Levy J, Klemperer I, et al. Anterior chamber gas bubbles after corneal flap creation with a femtosecond laser. J Cataract Refract Surg. 2005;31:2227-9.

41. Juhasz T, Hu Xh, Turi L, et al. Dynamics of shock waves and cavitation bubbles generated by picosecond laser pulses in corneal tissue and water. Lasers Surg Med. 1994;15:91-8.

42. Juhasz T, Kastis GA, Suarez C, et al. Time-resolved observations of shock waves and cavitation bubbles generated by femtosecond laser pulses in corneal tissue and water. Lasers Surg Med. 1996;19:23-31.

43. Kurtz RM, Liu X, Elner VM, et al. Photodisruption in the human cornea as a function of laser pulse width. J Refract Surg. 1997;13:653-8.

44. Kaiserman I, Maresky HS, Bahar I, et al. Incidence, possible risk factors, and potential effects of an opaque bubble layer created by a femtosecond laser. J Cataract Refract Surg. 2008;34:417-23.

45. IntraLase Corporation/Advanced Medical Optics. The IntraLase FS Laser: Training Manual. Santa Ana: IntraLase Corp; 2006.

46. Mrochen M, Wüllner C, Krause J, et al. Technical aspects of the WaveLight FS200 femtosecond laser. J Refract Surg. 2010;26(10):S833-40.

47. Faktorovich EG. Femtodynamics: optimizing femtosecond laser settings and procedure techniques to optimize outcomes. Int Ophthalmol Clin. 2008;48(1):41-50.

48. Srinivasan S, Herzig S. Sub-epithelial gas breakthrough during femtosecond laser flap creation for LASIK. Br J Ophthalmol. 2007;91:1373.

49. Seider MI, Ide T, Kymionis GD, et al. Epithelial breakthrough during IntraLase flap creation for laser in situ keratomileusis. J Cataract Refract Surg. 2008;34:859-63.

50. Chang JS, Lau S. Intraoperative flap re-cut after vertical gas breakthrough during femtosecond laser keratectomy. J Cataract Refract Surg. 2010;36(1):173-7.

51. Kuo AN, Kim T. Persistent anterior chamber gas bubbles during IntraLASIK. J Cataract Refract Surg. 2007;33:1134-5.

52. Srinivasan S, Rootman DS. Anterior chamber gas bubble formation during femtosecond laser flap creation for LASIK. J Refract Surg. 2007;23:828-30.

53. Srinivasan S, Herzig S. Management of Anterior Chamber Gas Bubbles During IntraLASIK. Ophthalmic Surg Lasers Imaging. 2010;41(4):482-4.

54. Tomita M, Watabe M, Waring Iv GO, et al. Corneal endothelial cell density after myopic intra-LASIK and the effect of AC gas bubbles on the corneal endothelium. Eur J Ophthalmol. 2010.

55. Utine CA, Altunsoy M, Basar D. Visante anterior segment OCT in a patient with gas bubbles in the anterior chamber after femtosecond laser corneal flap formation. Int Ophthalmol. 2010;30(1):81-4.

56. Stonecipher KG, Dishler JG, Ignacio TS, et al. Transient light sensitivity after femtosecond laser flap creation: clinical findings and management. J Cataract Refract Surg. 2006;32(1):91-4.

57. Munoz G, Albarran-Diego C, Sakla HF, et al. Transient light-sensitivity syndrome after laser in situ keratomileusis with the femtosecond laser Incidence and prevention. J Cataract Refract Surg. 2006;32(12):2075-9.

58. Krueger RR, Thornton IL, Xu M, et al. Rainbow glare as an optical side effect of IntraLASIK. Ophthalmology. 2008;115:1187-95.

59. Bamba S, Rocha KM, Ramos-Esteban JC, et al. Incidence of rainbow glare after laser in situ keratomileusis flap creation with a 60 kHz femtosecond laser. J Cataract Refract Surg. 2009;35:1082-6.

60. Smith RJ, Maloney RK. Diffuse lamellar keratitis; a new syndrome in lamellar refractive surgery. Ophthalmology. 1998;105:1721-6.

61. Gil-Cazorla R, Teus MA, de Benito-Llopis L, et al. Incidence of diffuse lamellar keratitis after laser in situ keratomileusis associated with the IntraLase 15 kHz femtosecond laser and Moria M2 microkeratome. J Cataract Refract Surg. 2008;34(1):28-31.

62. Javaloy J, Vidal MT, Abdelrahman AM, et al. Confocal microscopy comparison of IntraLase femtosecond laser and Moria M2 microkeratome in LASIK. J Refract Surg. 2007;23:178-87.

63. Netto MV, Mohan RR, Medeiros FW, et al. Femtosecond laser and microkeratome corneal flaps: comparison of stromal wound healing and inflammation. J Refract Surg. 2007;23:667-76.

64. Christopher Kent. Femtosecond Laser Flaps: Managing Complications. Rev Ophthalmology. 2011.

65. Lim T, Yang S, Kim MJ, et al. Comparison of the IntraLase femtosecond laser and mechanical microkeratome for laser in situ keratomileusis. Am J Ophthalmol. 2006;141:833-9.

66. Ide T, Yoo SH, Kymionis GD, et al. Second femtosecond laser pass for incomplete laser in situ keratomileusis flaps caused by suction loss. J Cataract Refract Surg. 2009;35(1):153-7.

67. Rocha KM, Kagan R, Smith SD, et al. Thresholds for interface haze formation after thin-flap femtosecond laser in situ keratomileusis for myopia. Am J Ophthalmol. 2009;147:966-72.

68. Kymionis GD, Portaliou DM, Krasia MS, et al. Unintended epithelium-only flap creation using a femtosecond laser during LASIK. J Refract Surg. 2011;27(1):74-6.

69. Choi SK, Kim JH, Lee D, et al. Creation of an extremely thin flap using IntraLase femtosecond laser. J Cataract Refract Surg. 2008;34(5):864-7.

70. Kymionis GD, Kounis GA, Grentzelos MA, et al. Interface corneal stromal irregularities after flap creation using femtosecond laser. Eur J Ophthalmol. 2011;21(2):207-9.

71. Ide T, Kymionis GD, Goldman DA, et al. Subconjunctival gas bubble Formation during LASIK flap creation using femtosecond laser. J Refract Surg. 2008;24(8):850-1.

72. Principe AH, Lin DY, Small KW, et al. Macular hemorrhage after laser in situ keratomileusis (LASIK) with femtosecond laser flap creation. Am J Ophthalmol. 2004;138(4):657-9.

# Corneal Instrumentation

CHAPTER

**Corneal Instrumentation**
*Ying Qian, Bennie H Jeng*

# CHAPTER 118

# Corneal Instrumentation

*Ying Qian, Bennie H Jeng*

## ❧ INTRODUCTION

Coincident with the recent explosion of new corneal surgical techniques, there has been a huge increase in the number of different corneal surgical instruments that are available for the corneal surgeon's use. As the new corneal surgical procedures continue to be refined, more and more instruments will continue to be developed and modified to meet newly found needs. This chapter will outline the basic corneal surgical instruments that are currently used for both traditional penetrating keratoplasty, as well as the newer lamellar and laser procedures.

## ❧ PENETRATING KERATOPLASTY

Since Dr Ramon Castroviejo pioneered the use of fine and delicate instruments for modern corneal transplantation in the mid-20th century,[1] penetrating keratoplasty (PK) has been the mainstay of surgery to replace diseased corneas. While innovations such as the operating microscope, antibiotics, corticosteroids and improvements in surgical instrumentation have dramatically improved clinical outcomes, the basic principles of removing full thickness host cornea, punching donor cornea and suturing in the graft largely remain the same.

The basic PK set includes instruments that grasp, cut and tie. The 0.12 mm toothed Castroviejo forceps remains the most versatile grasping instrument for the corneal surgeon (Fig. 1). The caliber of the teeth is strong enough to hold tissue, yet fine enough to manipulate the graft without causing undue damage to the tissue. With a flat tying platform, suturing efficiency can be maximized by eliminating the need to hand off and exchange the instrument for separate tying forceps. Care should be taken to avoid

grabbing larger objects, such as the globe support rings, or to overcompress the forceps, as the tips can deform. Other forceps available include the 0.3 mm and 0.5 mm toothed Castroviejo forceps, which generally have a lesser role in corneal transplantation.

Tying forceps have smooth and fine jaws that allow for manipulation and tying of the fine sutures used in corneal transplantation surgery (Fig. 2). The needle holder used for the fine sutures ideally has delicate curved jaws with a nonlocking round handle. A round handle is useful for fine rotation and torque action required for corneal suturing (Fig. 3). The standard straight needle holder can be used for passing sutures in conjunctival or episcleral tissue (Fig. 4). Typical suture used in PK is the 3/8 circle 10–0 monofilament nylon suture on a spatulated needle with cutting sides.

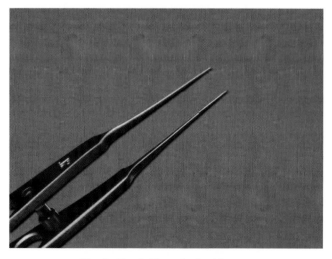

**Fig. 1:** Fine 0.12 mm toothed forceps

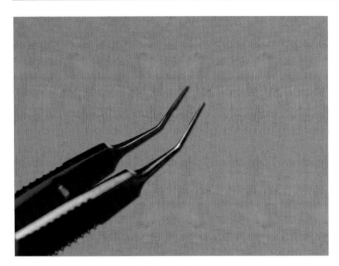

**Fig. 2:** Tying forceps

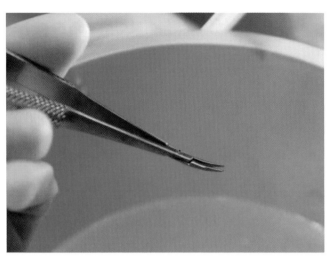

**Fig. 3:** Barraquer curved delicate needle holder with round handle

Specialized curved corneal scissors are essential to the corneal surgeon for excising the remaining host cornea after a partial trephination has been made. These scissors are made with various degrees of curvature to accommodate a range of graft diameters, as well as different surgeon preferences (Fig. 5). Other scissors are also useful, such as straight and curved Westcott scissors and the smaller Vannas scissors, and these are standard instrumentation for most any anterior segment surgery (Fig. 6). The small curved Vannas are especially useful for trimming the wall of the host bed after trephination.

A globe support ring such as the Flieringa ring or the blepharostat is critical to preventing globe collapse during the open sky portion of PK, especially in aphakic or vitrectomized eyes or any eye without adequate scleral rigidity, such as in children. The Flieringa ring is a metal ring of varying sizes (Fig. 7) which is secured onto the episclera with four to eight 5-0 or 6-0 vicryl or merselene sutures. Some surgeons leave the ends of the sutures long so as to tether them to the speculum or drape to provide further support. The McNeill-Goldmann blepharostat incorporates a support ring to a lid retractor.

Ophthalmic viscoelastic devices, more commonly known as viscoelastic agents, are gel-like substances that have dramatically improved the safety of ophthalmic surgery. They coat and protect the corneal endothelium, maintain the anterior chamber, and protect intraocular structures such as the iris and lens during corneal trephination.

Calipers are frequently used to measure the horizontal and vertical diameters of the host cornea to help select

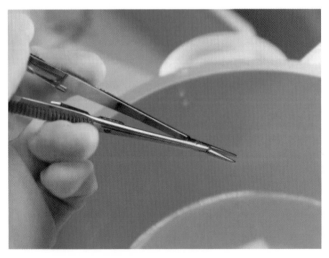

**Fig. 4:** Castroviejo standard straight needle holder

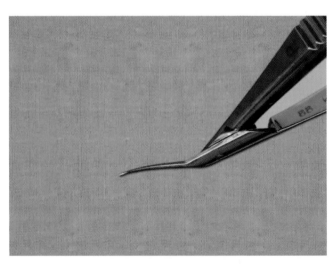

**Fig. 5:** Corneal scissors

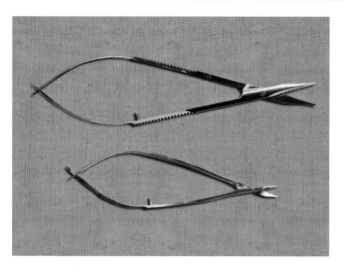

**Fig. 6:** Large and small Westcott scissors

**Fig. 7:** Flieringa ring sewn on with vicryl sutures intentionally left long. These long ends can be fixated to the speculum or drape to suspend the ring and therefore help prevent collapse of the globe

the appropriate size trephine to use to trephinate the host cornea. Trephines are disposable circular metal blades used to cut corneal tissue. Trial trephines with blunt edges in various sizes can be used to mark the cornea. Trephine punches typically range from 6.0 mm to 9.5 mm in 0.25 mm increments. One half mm increments are available for the smallest and largest sizes. Dermal skin biopsy punches 5 mm or less may be used for smaller grafts intended for tectonic support. Larger 12.0–13.0 mm trephines are also commercially available and can be used in combination to cut crescentic tectonic grafts, for example, in cases of peripheral corneal thinning and perforation. Preparation of

the donor cornea is typically done on a separate back table with a sterile field. The donor corneoscleral rim is centered endothelial side up on a cutting block, which has a well to accommodate the curvature of the cornea (Figs 8A and B). Cutting blocks typically have either a red target or rings of vents to guide centration. Examples of donor punches include the Barron disposable trephine, the Hanna trephine and the Iowa punch (Fig. 9). The Hanna and Barron trephines can be connected to suction to prevent movement of the donor cornea during trephination. After the donor cornea is punched, it is immersed in storage media, protected by a lid cover (Fig. 10) and set aside until it is needed.

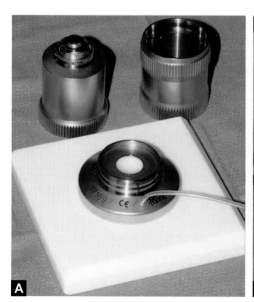

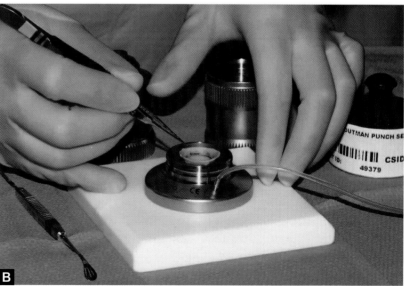

**Figs 8A and B:** (A) The cutting block with the Hanna donor punch; (B) The corneoscleral rim oriented endothelial side up on the cutting block

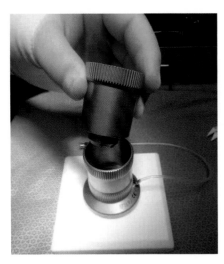

**Fig. 9:** The Hanna donor punch, assembled

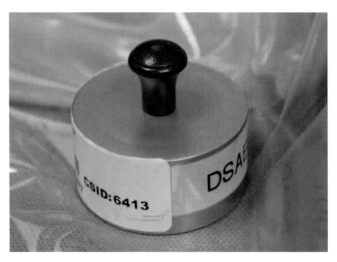

**Fig. 10:** Lid cover to provide moisture chamber to store punched corneal button until ready for use

Host corneal trephination is typically performed with either vacuum-assisted trephines, or hand-held trephines. Vacuum-assisted host trephines include the Hessburg-Barron disposable vacuum trephine and the Hanna corneal trephine. When using vacuum-assisted trephines with a globe support ring in place, care must be taken to size the ring big enough to allow the suction chamber to contact the conjunctiva for a complete seal (Fig. 11). The advantages of suction trephines include globe stabilization and minimization of trephine tilt that can result in undercutting or overcutting. They can also allow for relatively precise depth of cuts: the Hessburg-Barron trephine has an outer vacuum barrel and an inner rotating blade manually driven by four

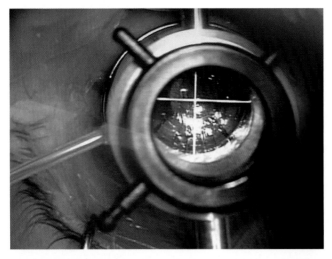

**Fig. 11:** Hessburg-Barron disposable vacuum trephine positioned on the host. Note the Flieringa ring outside of the trephine. The trephine is tilted to demonstrate the view of the host cornea visible down the core of the trephine

spokes with a complete revolution cutting 250 microns of tissue. The Hanna trephine is about the size and shape of the Goldmann 3-mirror goniolens. The disposable blade is turned by an obliquely inserted knob. Unlike the Hessburg-Barron system, the Hanna can be preset to cut to a specified depth, which makes it useful for lamellar keratoplasty such as the deep anterior lamellar keratoplasty (DALK). Both trephines allow the surgeon to visualize and center the host cornea prior to trephination. Trephine blades can also be used free hand or with a handle. These blades are necessary when performing keratoplasty procedures in the setting of an open eye such as a perforation, a situation whereby a suction trephine would be contraindicated.

Once cut, the corneal button can be transferred to the recipient bed with the Paton spatula, which has slits so that excess fluid on the donor epithelial surface can be dried with surgical spears without any manipulation of the graft (Fig. 12). It is then inverted so that the endothelial side faces down and onto the host which is coated with viscoelastic agents. Grasping of the donor button for placement of the first cardinal suture is greatly facilitated by the Pollock forceps, which has parallel toothed prongs through which a suture can be passed without torquing of the tissue (Fig. 13). The spatulated needle on 10-0 nylon suture with the cutting surface on the leading edge and on the sides is ideal for passing through cornea.

In the case of combined PK with pars plana vitrectomy, to maximize the surgical view afforded to the retina surgeon and to minimize surgical trauma to the donor graft, the diseased cornea can first be replaced with a temporary intraoperative keratoprosthesis such as the Eckhardt keratoprosthesis (Figs 14A to C) for use during

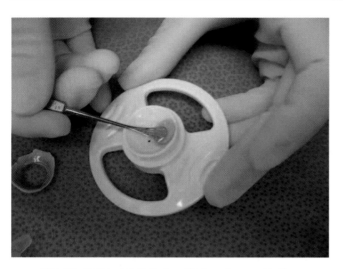

**Fig. 12:** Paton spatula for transferring of corneal button

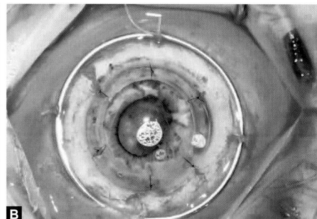

**Fig. 13:** Pollock forceps for placement of the first cardinal suture

the vitrectomy. This silicone device is sewn in place with 9-0 nylon suture, and it provides the retina surgeon with a closed chamber and clear view to the posterior segment. Once the posterior procedures are completed, the temporary keratoprosthesis is removed and replaced with the donor cornea. The Cobo temporary keratoprosthesis is a tapered plug mounted on a handle that can hook to suction (Fig. 15). It can be used in case of expulsive choroidal hemorrhage to quickly tamponade the corneal defect and to insufflate the globe with saline or air.

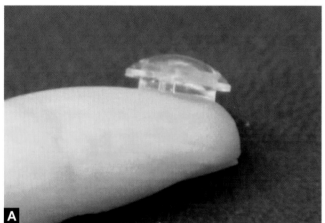

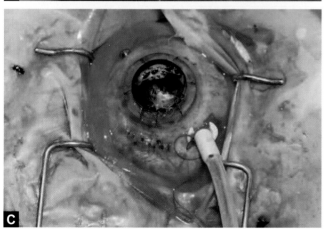

**Figs 14A to C:** (A) Eckhardt temporary keratoprosthesis; (B) The Eckhardt temporary keratoprosthesis placed on an eye in preparation for vitrectomy; (C) The same case at the completion of the vitrectomy. Note the scleral plug and the pars plana infusion port used during retina surgery

118
CHAPTER

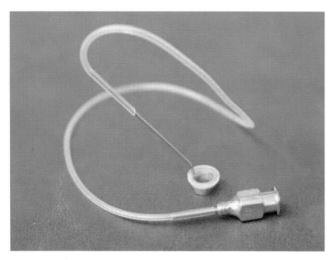

**Fig. 15:** Cobo temporary keratoprosthesis

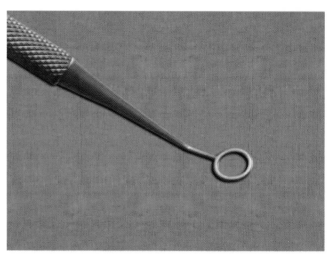

**Fig. 16:** Mandel intraoperative keratometer

After all the sutures have been placed, it can be helpful to perform intraoperative keratometry to guide in assessment of corneal toricity. An oval mire implicates a steeper meridian in the short axis of the oval. Suture tension can then be adjusted accordingly. Different types of intraoperative keratometers include a ring of lights mounted on the operating microscope or a hand held ring keratometer such as the Mandel keratometer (Fig. 16).

## ▶ DEEP ANTERIOR LAMELLAR KERATOPLASTY

In corneas with isolated stromal pathology and healthy endothelium, as in keratoconus or corneal stromal scarring or dystrophy, host Descemet can be preserved by performing DALK. Despite the technical difficulty in performing this procedure compared to PK, there has been a renewed interest in this procedure as it holds many potential advantages for the patient. Compared to PK, DALK achieves the same level of postoperative visual acuity but has no advantage in refractive error outcomes.[2] However, there is a significant advantage of DALK over PK in that the integrity of the eye is stronger, there is virtually no risk of endothelial rejection, and visual rehabilitation occurs faster due to more surface area for healing.

Most of the instruments used for PK are also used for DALK. However, partial thickness trephination of the host can be performed with more reliability of depth with a vacuum trephine such as the Hanna trephine to debulk stroma in preparation for manual dissection down to Descemet's membrane. The Hanna trephine has an internal

dial, which can be set to the desired cut depth with a key (Fig. 17). An angled knob is turned to start the trephination. Tactile resistance in the knob is met when the blade has cut down to the specified depth. Turning the knob further at this point simply spins the blade and does not advance it further into stroma. Typical trephination depth is 350–400 μm, but it can vary depending on the host cornea. The anterior stromal lamella is removed with a crescent blade or a blunt long dissector (Fig. 18).

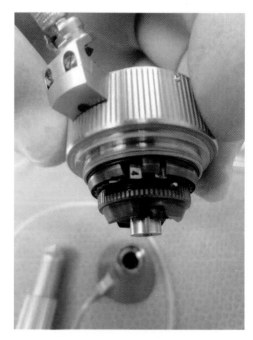

**Fig. 17:** Internal dial of Hanna trephine. The key and housing are visible in the background

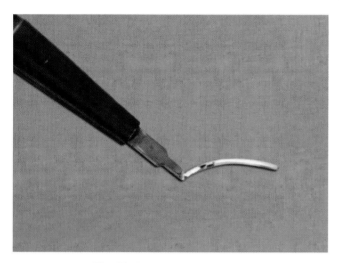

**Fig. 18:** DALK lamellar dissector

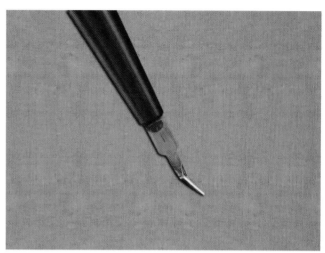

**Fig. 19:** DALK pointed dissector

Lamellar dissection down to Descemet's membrane is commonly performed using the 'big bubble' technique[3] which begins with inserting a blunt tapered instrument such as the pointed dissector into the stroma (Fig. 19). This instrument is inserted from the periphery towards the center and downward towards Descemet's membrane to create a track. Early reports of DALK utilized a bent 30G or 27G needle for air injection to accomplish Descemetic dissection with the big bubble.[4] However, the use of a flat and blunt 27G cannula with the exit port facing down (Fig. 20) enables a safer approach to creating the big bubble with lower risk of perforation.[5] Viscoelastic agents can be injected to fill the space between stroma and Descemet's membrane, and the space can then be entered using a super sharp blade with the blade facing up. The Fogla trifacet spatula can be inserted to divide the lamellar dissection into quadrants. The superior edge of this trifacet spatula is sharp which allows the overlying stroma to be incised. The dissected lamella is then excised with DALK scissors (Fig. 21) which resemble cornea scissors but has a thinner, longer and flatter lower blade that protects Descemet's membrane from inadvertent cuts. The donor preparation proceeds in the same way as for PK. Most surgeons either mechanically remove Descemet's membrane by stripping with toothed forceps, or they remove donor endothelium by wiping with a surgical spear before sewing on the full thickness graft onto the host Descemet's membrane bed.

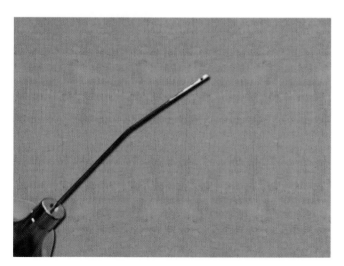

**Fig. 20:** DALK air injection cannula

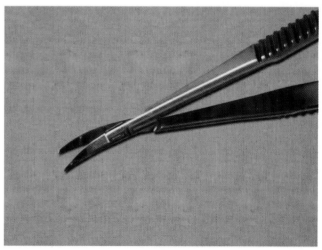

**Fig. 21:** DALK scissors

# ▶ DESCEMET'S STRIPPING ENDOTHELIAL KERATOPLASTY

Few surgical procedures have gained such widespread acceptance as Descemet's stripping endothelial keratoplasty (DSEK), and in less than 10 years after its initial introduction in 2004, it has replaced PK as the standard of care for surgical management of endothelial disease.[6-8] Advantages of DSEK over PK include faster recovery time, more refractive neutrality and predictability, and more tectonically stable globe. While the learning curve for even experienced corneal surgeons is steep for DSEK, innovations in surgical instrumentation and techniques have allowed this form of corneal transplantation to supplant PK as the most commonly performed procedure for isolated corneal endothelial disease.[8] When donor dissection is performed by the surgeon with a microkeratome on an artificial anterior chamber at the time of surgery (Figs 22A and B), the technique is referred to as Descemet's stripping automated endothelial keratoplasty (DSAEK).[9] Different thickness of the donor lenticule can be achieved using different microkeratome heads, and sometimes by performing multiple passes. Most surgeons will ensure an accurate microkeratome cut before bringing the patient into the operating room in the event of an errant cut requiring cancellation of the case. Once the donor tissue is cut, it is immersed in storage media and set aside in a humid chamber until it is needed. The increasing availability of eye bank prepared precut donor tissue has decreased operative time and contributed to DSEK's

appeal. The precut cornea typically is supplied with its 10–11 mm free cap of anterior stroma, marked with surgical ink at the edge, and it is punched during surgery in the same manner as for PK (Fig. 23). A randomized prospective double-masked clinical trial comparing 20 precut (at the eye bank) donor corneas to 20 surgeon-dissected grafts did not find significant differences in endothelial cell loss, visual and refractive outcomes, and dislocation rates at 1 year postoperatively.[10] Another comparative study of 225 DSAEK procedures found no higher risk of complications in the precut tissue group and possibly less early endothelial cell loss with precut tissue.[11]

In DSEK, the pupil is dilated at the start of the case to maximize the red reflex for descemetorhexis. Trial trephines can be used to mark the placement of the host cornea and to guide the descemetorhexis. The donor cornea is prepared and punched to the desired size on the back table and set aside in storage media for later use. A paracentesis is created using an angled super sharp blade or diamond blade. Viscoelastic agent is injected into the anterior chamber. Alternatively, an anterior chamber maintainer can be used to continuously irrigate balanced salt solution into the eye to maintain the stability of the anterior chamber (Fig. 24). A scleral tunnel or clear corneal incision is created with standard instrumentation. Descemet's membrane is scored with an angled reverse Sinskey hook (Fig. 25), and a stripper instrument with its wider surface and angled blunt tip is used to rake Descemet's membrane centrally. The 90° bend is most widely used, but a 45° is also available

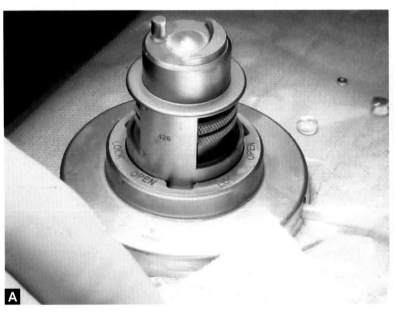
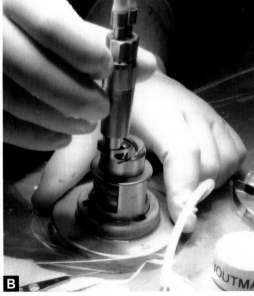

**Figs 22A and B:** (A) Donor cornea mounted on the Moria artificial chamber; (B) Cutting the donor with the microkeratome

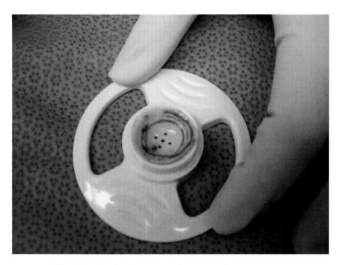

**Fig. 23:** Eye bank prepared pre-cut donor cornea.
Edge of the free cap is inked and is faintly visible

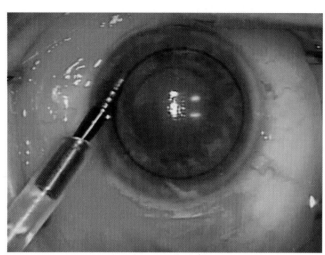

**Fig. 24:** Anterior chamber maintainer

(Fig. 26). The reverse Utrata forceps are useful for removing Descemet's membrane in an inverted capsulorrhexis motion (Fig. 27). Roughening of the peripheral host stroma can be accomplished with the blunt-tipped stripper or with the sharp-tipped Terry scraper (Fig. 28).

Many surgeons prefer making small venting incisions to decompress fluid from the graft-host interface. If venting incisions are to be made, the epithelium is often first debrided in the areas of the proposed vents with a #69 beaver blade to prevent epithelial downgrowth. A diamond blade or metal blade can be used to perform the venting. The Triamond blade is a diamond blade used to create such vertical stab incisions, which is typically placed tangentially in the corneal mid-periphery (Fig. 29). However, incisions at 4 mm and 6 mm optical zone have been shown to induce

irregular astigmatism compared to the 7 mm zone in one *in vitro* and *in vivo* study.[12] If viscoelastic agents were used, it is now, after the venting incisions are made, removed with an automated irrigation/aspiration hand piece attached to a phacoemulsification unit.

There are many techniques and instruments for insertion of the donor lenticule. Folding the graft into a 'taco' shape and inserting it with forceps was one of the original techniques described.[7] The single point fixation forceps (Fig. 30) minimize compression of the graft but still requires folding of the lenticule. Other techniques include suture pull-through[13] and cartridge injector with or without suture pull-through[14,15] which both aim to minimize crush injury. Various inserters such as the Busin glide[16] (Moria USA, Doylestown, Pennsylvania, USA) and EndoGlide[17]

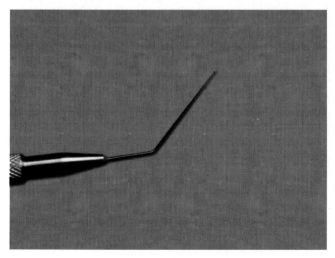

**Fig. 25:** Reverse Sinsky hook

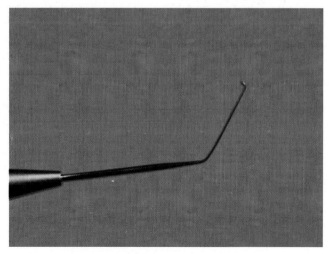

**Fig. 26:** A 90° Descemet membrane stripper

**118**
CHAPTER

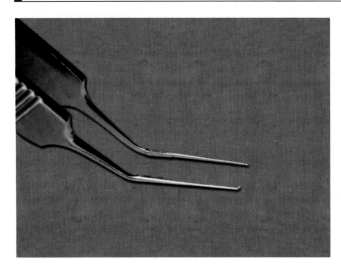

**Fig. 27:** Reverse Utrata forceps

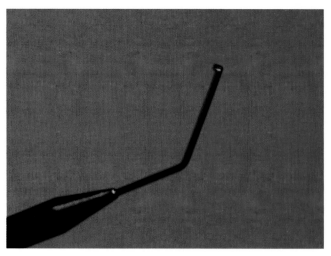

**Fig. 28:** Terry peripheral scraper

(Angiotech, Reading, Pennsylvania, USA/Network Medical Products, North Yorkshire, UK) have also been developed to minimize donor manipulation and endothelial cell loss.

A retrospective study of 179 cases comparing forceps and cartridge injector suture pull-through insertion technique[18] reported endothelial cell loss rates of 42.5% versus 51.4%, respectively, at 12 months with no significant differences in postoperative complications, endothelial cell loss, visual acuity or graft survival. One of the longest follow-up studies to date for DSEK was reported by Price et al.[19] One hundred and sixty-five eyes received DSEK with the forceps delivery technique. The median 5-year endothelial cell loss was 53% (range 7.5–89%) which compares favorably with 5-year loss of 70% found after penetrating keratoplasty in the multicenter Cornea Donor Study.[19,20]

The Busin glide is a metal instrument with an open plate upon which the donor lenticule is placed endothelial side up and forceps are then used to pull the graft through the funnel portion of the glide which curls the sides of the lenticule up without touching each other. The device is inverted and placed at the main wound. Forceps from an opposite paracentesis are used to pull the graft through the incision and into the anterior chamber where it unfolds spontaneously (Figs 31A and B). A prospective series of 10 consecutive patients undergoing DSAEK with the Busin glide reported mean endothelial cell loss of 20.0% at 6 months, 23.5% at 12 months and 26.4% at 18–24 months.[16]

The EndoGlide is a medical device that was approved for DSEK by the United States Food and Drug Administration (FDA) in 2009 (Figs 32A to C). It is comprised of three

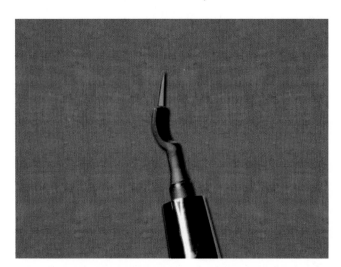

**Fig. 29:** Triamond blade for venting incisions

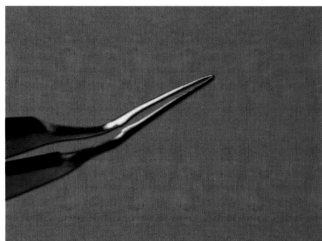

**Fig. 30:** Single-point fixation forceps for inserting donor tissue in Descemet's stripping endothelial keratoplasty

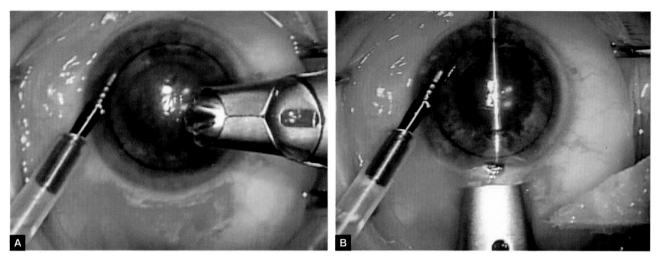

**Figs 31A and B:** (A) The Busin glide with a graft curled up inside; (B) The Busin glide inserted at the main incision with forceps from an opposite paracentesis pulling the donor into the anterior chamber. The anterior chamber maintainer is present.

pieces: the glide capsule, the glide introducer and the preparation base. This instrument folds the donor lenticule into a 'double-coil' configuration in the glide capsule without touching the endothelium. The capsule fits snugly into the corneal wound much like the lens cartridge for intraocular lens implants during cataract surgery. The glide introducer

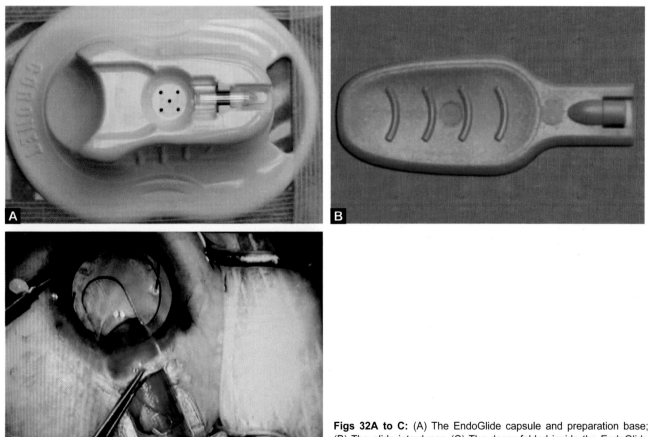

**Figs 32A to C:** (A) The EndoGlide capsule and preparation base; (B) The glide introducer; (C) The donor folded inside the EndoGlide capsule being inserted into the anterior chamber, before forceps are used to pull the graft into the anterior chamber.

locks into the posterior opening of the capsule and forms a closed system, analogous to an intraocular lens inserter. The capsule is inserted into the anterior chamber, and the graft is pulled out of the capsule by forceps coming from an opposite paracentesis. The graft uncoils spontaneously without collapse of the anterior chamber. In a prospective series of 25 eyes undergoing DSAEK,[17] the mean endothelial cell loss was 13.1% at 6 months and 15.6% at 12 months.

Gangwani and coworkers prospectively compared graft insertion with Busin glide versus with EndoGlide in 52 consecutive eyes undergoing DSEK. At 6 months follow-up, there was lower endothelial cell loss in the EndoGlide group (cell count 1919 cells/mm$^2$ or 25.76% loss) compared to the Busin group (cell count 1374 cells/mm$^2$ or 47.46% loss), p < 0.0001.[21] There was no difference in logMAR visual acuity, spherical equivalent or cylinder. The authors attributed the difference in endothelial cell loss to maintaining a closed system with a more stable anterior chamber with the EndoGlide technique.

## ‣ DESCEMET'S MEMBRANE ENDOTHELIAL KERATOPLASTY

In 2006, Melles reported a technique for transplanting only Descemet's membrane and endothelium into a recipient eye, and this procedure is referred to as Descemet's membrane endothelial keratoplasty (DMEK).[22] In theory, it is the purest form of endothelial keratoplasty, eliminating the graft-host stromal interface in DSEK that may possibly limit visual recovery and adding the thinnest amount of tissue that can minimize postoperative refractive shift. In practice, it is technically very challenging and has not yet been widely adopted. The donor tissue is prepared by scoring Descemet's membrane of the donor cornea, staining with trypan blue, and then carefully stripping with nontoothed forceps. Descemet's membrane has a natural tendency to coil and can be inserted into the anterior chamber with forceps or fit inside a cartridge injector through a 3.0–3.5 mm scleral incision or clear corneal incision. Dislocation rates have been reported at 20–30% early in the learning curve.[23,24] However, excellent clinical outcomes can be achieved, with 77–80% of eyes reaching 20/25 or better at 6–12 months.[25,26] DMEK is currently still in the refining stage, much like DSEK was in its beginning. Much of the challenge lies in harvesting the thin and delicate Descemet's membrane and unfurling it in the anterior chamber without damaging the endothelium. Some eyebanks are now pre-harvesting Descemet's membrane to help streamline DMEK for the surgeon. However, until the definite advantages of this procedure outweigh the technical challenges, DMEK may be slow to become a mainstream alternative for endothelial transplantation.

## ‣ FEMTOSECOND LASER ASSISTED CORNEAL SURGERY

The femtosecond laser was initially used to create flaps in laser *in situ* keratomileusis (LASIK). Initial programming allowed tissue cuts in only a raster pattern in one plane, which was the LASIK flap. Modifications in software and hardware allowed circular cuts, at different levels which have expanded its role in corneal surgery. The cornea is applanated with a single use glass applanator, and depth of the tissue is referenced with respect to the applanator. The femtosecond laser is in the near-infrared frequency and relies on photodisruption of tissue to create a nonthermal cut in tissue without collateral damage to surrounding tissue.[27] It is able to deliver precision and reproducibility and can produce near perfect tissue match between the host and donor in keratoplasty. The laser cuts from the posterior edge to anterior to avoid obscuration of the laser path by the gas produced. Even though the femtosecond laser can and has been applied to almost any type of corneal surgery traditionally performed manually or by microkeratome, its use is still limited by the expense of the laser, the increased operating time, and the disruption to workflow, as most laser suites are not adjacent to the operating room.

Currently, there are several commercially available lasers: the Intralase (Irvine, California), the Femtec (Heidelberg, Germany), the Femto LDV (Port, Switzerland) and the VisuMax (Jena, Germany). The Intralase provided the first capability to produce expanded cuts, and thus the first femtosecond laser assisted penetrating keratoplasties were dubbed Intralase-Enabled Keratoplasty (IEK).[28] The concept was to create identically shaped cuts for both donor and host so that the wound can fit together like a jigsaw puzzle. The increased wound surface area allows for faster healing times and a stronger wound that requires fewer sutures and allows for earlier suture removal. The most commonly used cut patterns are mushroom, top hat and zigzag. The mushroom shaped graft has a wider diameter anteriorly and smaller diameter posteriorly, making it more suitable for patients with keratoconus in which more anterior diseased tissue is replaced and less endothelium is transplanted. The top hat configuration has the opposite properties and is suitable in cases of endothelial dysfunction in which a wider posterior diameter allows transplantation of more endothelial tissue while the anterior wound is smaller so as to avoid a wound too close to the limbus.

Femtosecond laser assisted lamellar procedures include the femtosecond laser assisted anterior lamellar keratoplasty (FALK), the femtosecond laser assisted deep anterior lamellar keratoplasty (FDALK), and femtosecond laser assisted endothelial keratoplasty (FLEK). A randomized clinical trial of 80 eyes undergoing either FLEK or PK showed less astigmatism in the FLEK group, but lower best correct visual acuity of 20/70 ± 2 compared to 20/44 + 2 in the PK group and higher endothelial cell loss of 65% compared to 23% in the PK group at 12 months.[29] Differences were attributed to interface opacification and lenticule insertion, respectively.

Because of near perfect fit between the host and donor from identical cuts by the laser, FALK can be performed without sutures, thus eliminating postoperative suture-related complications. However, optically dense corneal scarring obscuring iris detail attenuates the penetration of the laser, and laser use in this setting is not advised. A retrospective series of 13 patients undergoing sutureless FALK showed rapid visual rehabilitation and minimal induced astigmatism at an average follow-up of 31 months.[30]

Astigmatic keratotomy and instrastromal ring segments can also be created with the femtosecond laser. More recently, the technology has been applied toward creating cataract surgery incisions and capsulorrhexis.

## ❧ SUMMARY

The past 10 years have seen a revolution in corneal transplantation which has spurred tremendous innovations in corneal surgical instrumentation. From PK to DALK to DSEK to DMEK, the field continues to evolve. With continued advances in surgical techniques, newer instruments are constantly being designed to keep up with our needs and to provide for the most efficient performance of surgical procedures, which ultimately provides for the best outcomes for our patients.

## ❧ REFERENCES

1. Moffatt SL, Cartwright VA, Stumpf TH. Centennial review of corneal transplantation. Clin Experiment Ophthalmol. 2005;33(6):642-57.
2. Reinhart WJ, Musch DC, Jacobs DS, et al. Deep anterior lamellar keratoplasty as an alternative to penetrating keratoplasty: a report by the American Academy of Ophthalmology. Ophthalmology. 2011;118(1):209-18.
3. Anwar M, Teichmann KD. Big-bubble technique to bare Descemet's membrane in anterior lamellar keratoplasty. J Cataract Refract Surg. 2002;28(3):398-403.
4. Anwar M, Teichmann KD. Deep lamellar keratoplasty: surgical techniques for anterior lamellar keratoplasty with and without baring of Descemet's membrane. Cornea. 2002;21(4):374-83.
5. Sarnicola V, Toro P. Blunt cannula for descemetic deep anterior lamellar keratoplasty. Cornea. 2011;30(8):895-8.
6. Melles GR, Wijdh RH, Nieuwendaal CP. A technique to excise the Descemet membrane from a recipient cornea (descemetorhexis). Cornea. 2004;23(3):286-8.
7. Price FW, Price MO. Descemet's stripping with endothelial keratoplasty in 50 eyes: a refractive neutral corneal transplant. J Refract Surg. 2005;21(4):339-45.
8. Ghaznawi N, Chen ES. Descemet's stripping automated endothelial keratoplasty: innovations in surgical technique. Curr Opin Ophthalmol. 2010;21(4):283-7.
9. Gorovoy MS. Descemet-stripping automated endothelial keratoplasty. Cornea. 2006;25(8):886-9.
10. Price MO, Baig KM, Brubaker JW, et al. Randomized, prospective comparison of precut vs surgeon-dissected grafts for Descemet stripping automated endothelial keratoplasty. Am J Ophthalmol. 2008;146(1):36-41.
11. Terry MA. Endothelial keratoplasty: a comparison of complication rates and endothelial survival between precut tissue and surgeon-cut tissue by a single DSAEK surgeon. Trans Am Ophthalmol Soc. 2009;107:184-91.
12. Moshirfar M, Lependu MT, Church D, et al. In vivo and in vitro analysis of topographic changes secondary to DSAEK venting incisions. Clin Ophthalmol. 2011;5:1195-9.
13. Macsai MS, Kara-Jose AC. Suture technique for Descemet stripping and endothelial keratoplasty. Cornea. 2007;26(9):1123-6.
14. Harvey TM. Small incision insertion of posterior lamellar button. J Refract Surg. 2006;22(5):429.
15. Kuo AN, Harvey TM, Afshari NA. Novel delivery method to reduce endothelial injury in Descemet stripping automated endothelial keratoplasty. Am J Ophthalmol. 2008;145(1):91-6.
16. Busin M, Bhatt PR, Scorcia V. A modified technique for Descemet membrane stripping automated endothelial keratoplasty to minimize endothelial cell loss. Arch Ophthalmol. 2008;126(8):1133-7.
17. Khor WB, Mehta JS, Tan DT. Descemet stripping automated endothelial keratoplasty with a graft insertion device: surgical technique and early clinical results. Am J Ophthalmol. 2011; 151(2):223-32.
18. Wendel LJ, Goins KM, Sutphin JE, et al. Comparison of bifold forceps and cartridge injector suture pull-through insertion techniques for Descemet stripping automated endothelial keratoplasty. Cornea. 2011;30(3):273-6.
19. Price MO, Fairchild KM, Price DA, et al. Descemet's stripping endothelial keratoplasty five-year graft survival and endothelial cell loss. Ophthalmology. 2011;118(4):725-9.
20. Lass JH, Gal RL, Dontchev M, et al. Donor age and corneal endothelial cell loss 5 years after successful corneal transplantation. Specular microscopy ancillary study results. Ophthalmology. 2008;115(4):627-32.

21. Gangwani V, Obi A, Hollick EJ. A Prospective Study Comparing EndoGlide and Busin Glide Insertion Techniques in Descemet Stripping Endothelial Keratoplasty. Am J Ophthalmol. 2012;153 (1):38-43.

22. Melles GR, Ong TS, Ververs B, et al. Descemet membrane endothelial keratoplasty (DMEK). Cornea. 2006;25(8):987-90.

23. Dapena I, Ham L, Droutsas K, et al. Learning curve in Descemet's membrane endothelial keratoplasty: first series of 135 consecutive cases. Ophthalmology. 2011;118(11):2147-54.

24. Melles GR, Ong TS, Ververs B, et al. Preliminary clinical results of Descemet membrane endothelial keratoplasty. Am J Ophthalmol. 2008;145(2):222-7.

25. Dirisamer M, Ham L, Dapena I, et al. Efficacy of Descemet membrane endothelial keratoplasty: clinical outcome of 200 consecutive cases after a learning curve of 25 cases. Arch Ophthalmol. 2011;129(11):1435-43.

26. Guerra FP, Anshu A, Price MO, et al. Descemet's membrane endothelial keratoplasty: prospective study of 1-year visual outcomes, graft survival, and endothelial cell loss. Ophthalmology. 2011;118(12):2368-73.

27. Soong HK, Malta JB. Femtosecond lasers in ophthalmology. Am J Ophthalmol. 2009;147(2):189-97.

28. Buratto L, Bohm E. The use of the femtosecond laser in penetrating keratoplasty. Am J Ophthalmol. 2007;143(5):737-42.

29. Cheng YY, Schouten JS, Tahzib NG, et al. Efficacy and safety of femtosecond laser-assisted corneal endothelial keratoplasty: a randomized multicenter clinical trial. Transplantation. 2009;88 (11):1294-1302.

30. Shousha MA, Yoo SH, Kymionis GD, et al. Long-term results of femtosecond laser-assisted sutureless anterior lamellar keratoplasty. Ophthalmology. 2011;118(2):315-23.

# Appendices

## CHAPTER: SURGICAL PROCEDURE GUIDELINES

# Physical Trauma of the Cornea

*Mikelson MomPremier, Robert A Copeland Jr*

## ➤ PROCEDURAL STEPS FOR THE REPAIR OF CORNEAL LACERATIONS

Once the decision has been made to operate on a patient with corneal laceration, the eye should certainly be protected with a shield. The patient should be placed *nil per os* (NPO) and broad-spectrum systemic antibiotic(s) instituted. Please note that succinylcholine should be avoided if possible as neuromuscular depolarizing agents can cause co-contraction of the extraocular muscles thereby increasing intraocular pressure (IOP) leading to intraocular content extrusion. After obtaining the proper informed consent, the patient is prepped and draped in standard sterile fashion avoiding undue pressure on the globe.

Identify ocular structures and findings such as corneal pieces, sclera or flat anterior chamber. Iris prolapse can be addressed with gently repositioned with blunt instruments. In the event that this cannot be accomplished, anterior chamber fluid (aqueous or viscoelastic material) should be removed in order to decrease the IOP facilitating prolapse structure repositioning. Nonviable iris structure can be cut at the wound interface preserving as much tissue as possible (Fig. 5 of the chapter 'Physical Trauma of the Cornea'). Vitreous should be cut and removed at the laceration interface with dry Weck-cel sponge and Wescott scissors. In the setting of lens subluxation, a lensectomy may be required.

Perform a 360° peritomy whenever a corneal laceration extends to the limbus (Fig. 6 of the chapter 'Physical Trauma of the Cornea'). Start by making a conjunctival incision at the superior limbus. Proceed with blunt dissection (closed scissors slowly opened when in position) 180° at a time. Avoid including Tenon's in your conjunctival dissection. Repeat the process at the inferior limbus. Of note, peritomy may also be performed starting four to six millimeters from the limbus as a surgeon's preference.

The repair of corneal lacerations can be accomplished using 10-0 nylon sutures in the cornea, 9-0 nylon sutures at the limbus and 8-0 nylon sutures on the sclera; this can be remembered by the mnemonic 10, 9, 8. The first suture is placed at the limbus. Using interrupted sutures, start with long sutures peripherally. Maintain a 90% depth with each bite, but the suture total length should be gradually decreased as you approach the central cornea. Perform equal bites on each side of the corneal wound for each suture. A slipknot tying method should be employed in order to maintain the ability to adjust the suture's tightness and prevent air-knots. Finally, sutures should be buried away from the visual axis.

Flat or otherwise shallow anterior chamber should then be reformed with balanced salt solution (BSS), viscoelastic material or sterile air in the absence of the former two. A Seidel test should be performed to detect leaks which may be sealed with cyanoacrylate tissue adhesive.

The peritomy is closed using interrupted 8-0 vicryl sutures. It is important to remember that surgery does not end once the last suture is secured. Great coordination is required with your anesthesiology colleague to assure that bucking does not occur during the case and when bringing the patient out of anesthesia again to decrease the risks of intraocular content extrusion.

# Conjunctival Flaps

*Anne S Steiner, Ira J Udell*

1. A retrobulbar injection is performed.
2. The eye is prepped and draped in the usual sterile ophthalmic fashion.
3. A lid speculum is placed into the surgical eye.
4. The corneal epithelium is removed in its entirety either with a dry Weck-cel sponge or #59, #15 or #57 blade.
5. A 6-0 spatulated double-armed nylon or similar traction suture is placed in the superior cornea or perilimbal sclera at approximately 12 o'clock position, depending on the status of the superior limbal tissue.
6. A 360° peritomy is performed. Others perform the superior dissection described below first and then proceed to complete the peritomy 360°.
7. The eye is infraducted to expose the entire superior bulbar conjunctiva. Ideally, one would like to obtain access 16–18 mm posterior to the limbus as the free flap tends to retract especially if partially scarred. It is helpful to use a marking pen to mark the distance from the limbus prior to the dissection.
8. Two percent lidocaine with 2.5% epinephrine is injected in the subconjunctival space posterior to the intended incision taking care not to penetrate the conjunctiva in the area which will be used to create the flap.
9. A 2 cm incision 16–18 mm posterior to the limbus, concentric with the limbus is made with the aid of a blunt tip scissors and nontoothed anatomical forceps.
10. The dissection of the conjunctiva from tenon's capsule is continued anteriorly to the limbus, taking great care not to create a buttonhole in the conjunctiva.
11. The traction suture is removed and the bipedicle flap is slid over the surface of the cornea. It may be necessary to create relaxing incisions at 4 and 8 o'clock positions for this purpose.
12. The flap is secured to the inferior conjunctiva and to the superior limbus with interrupted nylon or vicryl sutures.
13. The superior tenon's is left bare to re-epithelialize.

# Scleral Transplantation: Supportive and Protective

*Frank W Bowden III*

## ❧ SUTURELESS REPAIR OF CONJUNCTIVAL EROSION ASSOCIATED WITH SCLERAL RESORPTION FOLLOWING TUBE SHUNT SURGERY

Following placement of a glaucoma drainage tube device with a scleral reinforcement graft, the overlying conjunctiva may breakdown due to scleral resorption and tube erosion. The eye becomes exposed to the risk of bleb failure and endophthalmitis. When the conjunctival erosion is clinically detected early in the process, an operative repair may be accomplished with a scleral reinforcement graft and direct conjunctival closure with advancement flaps. The procedure may involve a suture fixation of the sclera with a suture repair of the conjunctiva. Alternatively, a bio-adhesive material may be used to secure the scleral graft and close the conjunctival wound.

The operative repair of an exposed tube illustrated in the video begins with the usual ophthalmic surgical prep and drape technique. Topical anesthetic drops were administered. A 6-0 vicryl bridle suture was placed inside the limbus superiorly to facilitate inferior rotation of the globe with fixation to the drape. With adequate exposure of the tube present, lidocaine 2% was infiltrated into the adjacent subtenons space on either side of the tube. Sharp dissection with Vannas scissors was used to meticulously create a subtenons pocket space surrounding the conjunctival opening over the tube. The conjunctival opening was enlarged over the tube to 4 mm. The subtenons dissection extended 3–4 mm on either side of the tube. Hemostasis was achieved with direct pressure using Weck spears.

The scleral graft was cut to the dimensions of 4 × 6 mm, then placed in the operative field. The graft was tucked into the subtenons pocket over the tube to assess the fit, and then removed. Tisseel glue components were instilled via cannula into the subtenons space. The scleral graft was replaced into the subtenons pocket with care to ensure tube coverage without kinking or retraction. Additional Tisseel glue was instilled over the scleral graft. Forceps were used to advance the edges of conjunctival wound for direct coaptation. The glue effectively sealed the wound in a watertight fashion. The excess dried glue on the surface was excised with Vannas scissors. A collagen shield sealed with a fluoroquinolone antibiotics and steroid solutions was placed over the eye along with an occlusive patch.

# Superficial Keratectomy and Epithelial Debridement

*Julian A Procope*

## ⃗ INSTRUMENTATION

- Topical proparacaine
- Povidone-iodine 5%
- Balanced salt solution
- Eyelid speculum
- #57 Beaver blade(with or without a handle)
- Tooke knife
- Diluted (20%) alcohol
- Cellulose sponges
- Bandage soft contact lens (BSCL)
- 0.12 or Clibri forceps if dissecting lesion off cornea
- Diamond burr (optional)
- Postoperative drops to include an antibiotic, a topical NSAID, a topical steroid and artificial tears.

## ⃗ PROCEDURE TECHNIQUE

For the author's typical superficial keratectomy procedure on a patient with recurrent epithelial erosions, the lids and lashes are first sterilized with povidone-iodine 5% on a cotton-tip applicator. A drop of topical proparacaine is placed on the eye followed by a drop of povidone-iodine 5% diluted by 50% with balanced salt solution into the conjunctival fornix. The patient is then positioned at the slit lamp, and with the aid of a surgical assistant, a wire lid speculum is inserted into the palpebral fissure to retract the eyelids. An 8.0 mm optical zone marker is then used to delineate the area of the cornea to be treated. Twenty percent ethanol on a cotton-tip applicator is then applied to the area of pathology to loosen the epithelium. Then, using a #57 Beaver blade without a handle, the keratectomy is performed with swift, sure strokes. Care is taken to ensure

that the blade remains perpendicular to the dome of the cornea at all times, so as to avoid sharp dissection into and damage of subepithelial and Bowman's layers.

Following epithelial removal, it is paramount that the corneal bed be left as smooth as possible to facilitate re-epithelialization. To this end, the author utilizes a Tooke corneal knife to smooth Bowman's layer (a diamond burr may alternatively be used), again employing swift, sure strokes while maintaining perpendicularity of the blade to the corneal dome. This ensures that no linear defects are induced in Bowman's layer. The author is also careful to avoid injuring the limbal epithelium, as the limbal stem cells are vital for subsequent re-epithelialization.

Upon completion of the superficial keratectomy, the lid speculum is removed, and the patient is allowed to recline in the exam chair. The bandage soft contact lens (BSCL) is placed onto the cornea and one drop each of nepafenac (nevanac), moxifloxacin (vigamox) and prednisolone acetate 1% is administered. The patient is discharged home with a pair of postmydriatic sunglasses and instructed to keep the above drops chilled for enhanced analgesic effect. Aggressive topical ocular lubrication with chilled artificial tears is also encouraged.

The author's postoperative regimen calls for QID dosing of all prescription drops and hourly dosing of artificial tears until re-epithelialization is complete—usually around postoperative day three or four. At that time, the BSCL is removed and the topical steroid and NSAID are discontinued. The topical antibiotic is continued for a total of 1 week of therapy. Aggressive topical lubrication is continued for a few weeks, and may sometimes be augmented with topical sodium chloride 5% ointment for additional nocturnal lubrication.

# Evaluation and Management of Eyelid and Eyelash Malposition for the Anterior Segment Surgeon

*Salman J Yousuf, Earl D Kidwell*

Anderson RL, Gordy DD. The tarsal strip procedure. Arch Ophthalmol. 1979;97(11):2192-6.

In summary:

- Administration of local anesthesia
- Performing a lateral canthotomy
- Incision of the inferior crus of lateral canthal tendon
- Spliting the eyelid into anterior and posterior lamellae
- Formation of the tarsal strip
- Shaving off the palpebral conjunctiva of the tarsal strip
- Excision of excess anterior lamella
- Suturing the lateral tarsal strip into the periosteum of the inner lateral orbital rim
- Closure of the lateral canthotomy wound.

See Figures 3A to F of the chapter 'Evaluation and Management of Eyelid and Eyelash Malposition for the Anterior Segment Surgeon'.

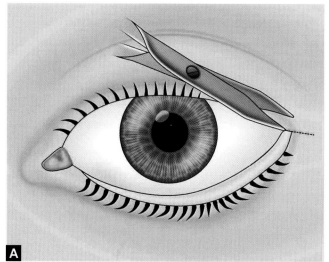 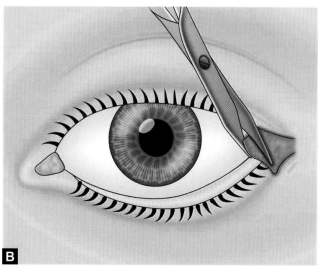

**Figs 3A and B**

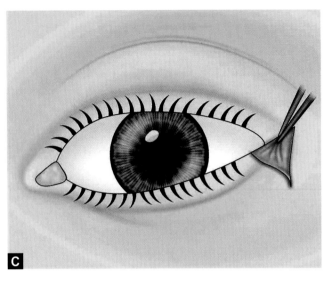

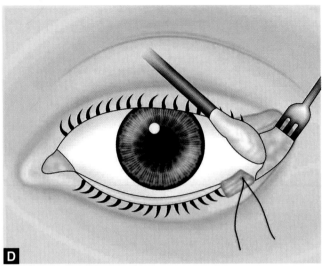

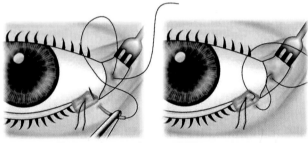

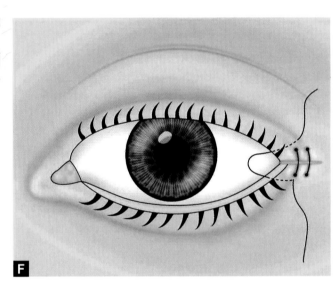

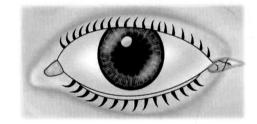

**Figs 3A to F:** Lateral tarsal strip

# Pterygium Surgery

*Alfred L Anduze*

## ꞏ CONJUNCTIVAL FLAPS PROCEDURE FOR PTERYGIUM SURGERY

### Preoperative

Topical NSAIDs and decongestants for 3–5 days

*Instruments*: Wire lid speculum, small Westcott scissors, 0.12 forceps with teeth, 2 tying forceps, no. 64 Beaver blade, needle holder, 9-0 nylon suture, gauze sponges, cotton-tipped swabs, disposable cautery (low temp), 2.5% phenylephrine drops for hemostasis, 0.1 cc of 0.4 mg/ml mitomycin-C in tuberculoin syringe fitted with 27 gauge cannula.

### Conjunctival Flaps Procedure: Five Steps

1. *Initial incision*: Made into the body (2–4 mm from the limbus). This isolates the head for better visibility, easier access and safer excision along a distinct cleavage plane. Apply light cautery to minimize sclera injury, and 2.5% phenylephrine drops for hemostasis. Do only minimal to moderate tenonectomy and avoid the muscle sheath. Less trauma to the tissues results in less postoperative inflammation.
2. *Excision of the head*: Excise the head with the no. 64 Beaver blade from the limbal side. Use a superficial plane and carefully shave it from the cornea to minimize the damage and prevent dellen.
3. *Conjunctival flaps*: Make vertical superior and inferior relaxing incisions along the limbus (5–6 mm in each direction) to create easily opposable flaps to cover the sclera defect entirely. The limbus should be covered or no more than 1 mm exposed.
4. *Initial closure*: Use 9-0 nonabsorbable suture to minimize the inflammatory reaction. Use three or four short bite sutures to achieve apposition and three to four long bite sutures to minimize tension and ensure that the flaps remain in place and the sclera remains covered for the healing period (2 weeks). Knots should be moved to the midline or inferior and not buried.
5. *Completed closure*: Conjunctival flaps should be oriented so that the blood vessels are directed vertically away from the limbus. Closure should be neat and flat.

### Postoperative

Apply topical antibiotic ointment and cover with a patch for 24 hours. Oral analgesics are optional. No steroids should be used in the initial phase to enhance early corneal healing. Upon removal of the patch, use topical tears and decongestants, three to four times daily. NSAIDs may be used if needed. Use of sunglasses, avoidance of irritants and abstention from rubbing should be emphasized. Irritating tips of suture can be trimmed at any time.

# Amniotic Membrane Transplantation

*Soosan Jacob, Amar Agarwal*

The amniotic membrane, first used by De Rotth in 1940 and popularized by Kim and Tseng in 1995, consists of a single layer of cells on a thick basement membrane. It has anti-inflammatory, antiangiogenic, antibacterial, wound protecting, pain reducing and antifibrotic properties as well as the ability to promote epithelial differentiation, adhesion and migration. It also has the advantage of being nonimmunogenic.

It can be used as a graft where it fills defects and promotes epithelialization or it can be used as a patch where it is used for its anti-inflammatory and antiangiogenic properties.It may also be used as a patch-graft simultaneously according to the underlying condition being treated. During surgery, the stromal side is differentiated from the basement membrane by touching with a sponge. The stromal side is sticky whereas the basement membrane side is nonsticky.

Amniotic membrane can be used as a graft for conditions, such as persistent epithelial defects, bullous keratopathy, etc. by spreading out the membrane under tension and suturing onto the cornea with the stromal side facing down after denuding the unhealthy epithelium. A Patch-graft or an inlay-onlay graft is performed by using multilayered amniotic membrane. The amniotic membrane is repeatedly folded on itself using fibrin glue to stick the multiple layers together. The base and edges of the defect are scraped and all necrotic tissue as well as loose epithelium is removed. The inlay is used to fill the defect and is stuck into place using glue and/or anchoring sutures. An amniotic membrane patch or an onlay graft is then used to cover the inlay graft in such a manner as to extend beyond the denuded epithelium. It is also used to protect donor tissue in limbal stem cell transplants and for lining part of or the entire ocular surface in situations, such as after excision of pterygia; acute corneal or conjunctival injuries such as chemical burns, Steven-Johnson syndrome, etc.; as well as for procedures such as fornix reconstruction, repair of leaking blebs, etc. In all these conditions, it is anchored in place using sutures and if available, fibrin glue.

# Autologous Ex Vivo Cultivated Limbal Epithelial Transplantation

*Sayan Basu, Virender S Sangwan*

## ☞ TECHNIQUE OF LIMBAL BIOPSY

A biopsy was taken from a healthy part of the limbus; a 2 × 2 mm piece of conjunctival epithelium with 1 mm into clear corneal stromal tissue at the limbus was dissected; conjunctiva was excised just behind the pigmented line (palisades of Vogt), and the limbal tissue that contained epithelial cells and a part of the corneal stroma was obtained.

## ☞ TECHNIQUE OF LIMBAL CULTURE

The tissue was transported to the laboratory in human corneal epithelium (HCE) medium. HCE is composed of modified Eagle's medium/F12 medium (1:1) solution containing 10% (vol/vol) autologous serum (AS), 2 mM l-glutamine, 100 U/ml penicillin, 100 µg/ml streptomycin, 2.5 µg/ml amphotericin B, 10 ng/ml human recombinant epidermal growth factor and 5 µg/ml human recombinant insulin. Under strict aseptic conditions, the donor limbal tissue was shredded into small pieces. Human amniotic membrane (HAM), prepared and preserved by the authors' eye bank, was used as a carrier. A 3 × 4 cm HAM sheet was de-epithelized using 0.25% recombinant trypsin and EDTA solution for 15 minutes. The shredded bits of limbal tissue were explanted over the center of de-epithelized HAM with the basement membrane side up. A similar parallel culture was also prepared as a backup. A submerged explant culture system without a feeder-cell layer was used. The authors used the HCE medium to nurture the culture. The culture was incubated at 37°C with 5% $CO_2$ and 95% air. The growth was monitored daily under an inverted phase contrast microscope and the medium was changed every other day. The culture was completed when a monolayer of the cells growing from the explants became confluent, typically in 10–14 days.

## ☞ TECHNIQUE OF LIMBAL TRANSPLANTATION

Any symblepharon which prevented adequate separation of the lids was released to permit the insertion of a wire speculum (no additional surgery to treat the symblepharon was performed). A peritomy was performed and the corneal fibrovascular pannus was excised. If excessive corneal thinning or perforation was noted at this stage, a lamellar or penetrating keratoplasty was performed. The human amniotic membrane and monolayer of cultivated limbal epithelial cells were spread over the cornea with epithelial side up. The graft was then secured to the peripheral cornea by interrupted, circumferential 10-0 nylon sutures and to the surrounding conjunctival edge by interrupted 8-0 polyglactin sutures. Alternately, using a sutureless technique, the graft was secured to underlying ocular surface with fibrin glue (TISSEEL™ Kit from Baxter AG, Austria) and the margins of the graft were tucked under the surrounding conjunctival edge. Bandage contact lenses were not applied at the end of surgery.

## ☞ POSTOPERATIVE MANAGEMENT

All patients were treated with 1% prednisolone acetate eye drops eight times a day tapered to once a day in 35–42 days and 0.3% ciprofloxacin hydrochloride eye drops four times a day for 1 week. The latter were continued, as needed, if an epithelial defect was present. No systemic antibiotics or steroids were administered to any patients. Patients were examined on postoperative days 1, 7, 42 and at an interval of 90–180 days thereafter, as customized by the clinical appearance of the transplant. Each examination included a complete history, visual acuity assessment with Snellen's charts, intraocular pressure measurement and detailed ocular examination with slit-lamp biomicroscopy.

# Penetrating Keratoplasty: Surgical Techniques and Pre- and Postoperative Care

*John W Cowden*

## ✈ PENETRATING KERATOPLASTY: SUMMARY OF OPERATION

The lids are separated with a wire lid speculum, and superior and inferior rectus traction sutures are placed in phakic eyes to stabilize the globe during trephination. In pseudophakic or aphakic eyes and in infant eyes, a double Flieringa ring or the McNeill-Goldmann ring is sewn to the episclera or sclera in four to six locations in order to support the cornea. This technique is particularly important in cases of decreased scleral rigidity or in which a vitrectomy might be utilized. The diameter of the trephine to be utilized can be determined by using calipers or sizer trephine blades, in 0.25-mm increments. The marking or sizer trephine blade is selected to surround the central pathology adequately and to be large enough to supply adequate endothelial cells but not extend to the limbus.

A partial-thickness trephination is done to two thirds to three fourths of the depth of the cornea. The cornea is then marked with a four- or an eight-bladed radial keratotomy marker in order to facilitate suture placement. At this point, attention is directed to trephination of the donor button. The donor corneal scleral tissue is placed on a concave Teflon cutting block, endothelial side up, centered and punched by hand using the Castroviejo-type disposable trephine blade with the obturator retracted. A guillotine-type corneal donor punch, such as a Hessburg-Barron disposable donor trephine or one of several other corneal trephine punches, may also be used. The proper size of the donor corneal button and the trephine diameter in the recipient is determined by selecting a donor button size that is 0.25–0.50 mm larger than the diameter of the recipient trephine. The cornea must be punched so as to be centered entirely within the limbus. To minimize astigmatism, the trephine blade is positioned to cut the cornea perpendicularly to the table. Once cut, the cornea is immersed with several drops of preservation media, covered and set aside until it will be sutured into the patient's eye.

Once the donor cornea is trephined and stored, attention is redirected to the patient's cornea. A #75 blade is used to enter the anterior chamber at the 9 o'clock position (for a right-handed surgeon). Using a sweeping motion in the previous groove, the incision is extended for about 2 o'clock hours to permit the insertion of the Katzin corneal transplant scissors. The right cutting scissors are used to complete the corneal incision inferiorly, from the 9 o'clock position and around to the 2 o'clock position. The left corneal scissors are used to complete the incision superiorly. Some surgeons prefer to leave a small inner lip by tilting the scissors slightly.

Care is taken not to injure the iris or lens during entrance with the knife or while extending the incision with the scissors. A viscoelastic material may be injected into the anterior chamber to protect the iris and lens. Any necessary trimming of the recipient incision is done at this time. A small amount of viscoelastic material is placed in the pupillary area, especially if an intraocular lens is in place, following which the donor cornea is brought into position using a Paton spatula.

The Pierce Colibri forceps are used to hold the donor cornea at the 12 o'clock position. Using forceps, the assistant stabilizes the cornea at the 6 o'clock position. The double-pronged Pollack corneal forceps can be used at 12 o'clock in lieu of an assistant holding the cornea at the 6 o'clock position. A 10-0 nylon suture on a spatula needle is placed at the 12 o'clock position by the surgeon. Hold ing the donor cornea at exactly the 6 o'clock position, the needle is passed under the forceps and through the donor and recipient corneas, utilizing the previously placed markings as a guide. The 3 and 9 o'clock sutures are placed similarly, forming in the cornea a square crease with equal sides. The four interrupted cardinal sutures are placed perpendicular to the corneal surface in order to obtain a deep, 80–90% depth of the corneal thickness, with approximately a 0.75- to 1.0-mm bite on each side of the corneal incision. A triple throw followed by two single throws is used to tie the knot. The 6 o'clock suture is the most important for determining the degree of astigmatism and must equally bisect the cornea.

The final decision on the type of suture technique—which includes interrupted, interrupted running, running and double running techniques—is determined after the cardinal sutures are placed. The suture technique utilized depends on both the surgeon's preferences and the circumstances. For infants and patients with vascularized corneas, 16 interrupted sutures are used. All knots are buried. For relatively clear corneas, which are not vascularized, a single or double running suture may be appropriate, which could allow quicker visual rehabilitation. A combination of 8 or 12 interrupted sutures and a running 10-0 or 11-0 nylon suture is used by some surgeons so that astigmatism can be adjusted by early selective suture removal.

A single running nylon suture is often used in cases of keratoconus, since healing usually occurs sooner in the younger individual. A double running 10-0 and 11-0 nylon suture may be utilized in older individuals, with the 11-0 sutures remaining in place indefinitely after removal of the 10-0 suture 3–6 months postoperatively, after which spectacles are prescribed. When a running suture is used, the cardinal sutures are typically removed before the running suture has been tied and adjusted. The running suture is tightened slightly, to remove any slack and to prevent any leakage of aqueous, and then tied. The knot is buried in the incision, if it was not buried when tied in the incision. Intraoperative keratoscopy is utilized to determine if significant astigmatism exists by projecting a ring of light or reflections onto the corneal surface. If any ovality of the circle is noted, the sutures are adjusted to make the circle round, tightening the area of the suture that is the longest dimension of the oval ring.

# Glaucoma Surgery in Penetrating and Nonpenetrating Keratoplasty Patients

*Oluwatosin Smith, Davinder Grover*

## ⮞ TRABECULECTOMY (FORNIX-BASED APPROACH)

- After local anesthesia is administered—retrobulbar block or subconjunctival anesthesia, a traction suture is placed; this could be a superior rectus bridle suture or a corneal traction suture depending on surgeon preference.
- A fornix-based conjunctival opening is then created at the limbus with subsequent dissection posteriorly creating a pocket in subtenon space using blunt forceps. Careful manipulation of the conjunctiva is important to avoid formation of conjunctival buttonholes.
- Hemostasis is maintained, avoiding excessive cauterization.
- Antimetabolite can then be applied to the sclera/subtenon space at this point making sure to apply over a wide area and not just in the area of planned scleral flap.
- A half-thickness scleral flap is then created in the preferred shape (rectangular, triangular, square, or trapezoid) depending on surgeon preference. This is dissected anteriorly all the way to clear cornea.
- A paracentesis is then created, preferably temporally for easy access if needed postoperatively.
- The anterior chamber is then entered under the flap with a 15° blade and a block of tissue is then excised using the blade and a Vannes scissors. An alternative way of creating the sclerostomy is to use a Kelly Descemet's punch.
- A surgical peripheral iridectomy is then done and hemostasis is maintained under the flap.
- 10-0 nylon interrupted sutures are then used to suture down the flap titrating for flow at different intraocular pressure (IOP) levels while reforming the anterior chamber. Releasable sutures could be used especially if lasers are not readily available for suturelysis in the postoperative period. Preplacement of the initial sutures is an option that is performed by some surgeons prior to creating the sclerostomy.
- After adequate titration of flow from under the flap with more flow at higher IOP, the conjunctival wound is then pulled up to the limbus and closed in the surgeon's preferred method. Conjunctival closure at the limbus varies from interrupted closure to more complex closure to attain water tightness.
- Anterior chamber is reformed to create a bleb and to check for the presence of any leaks.
- Prophylactic antibiotics and steroids are used as indicated.

## ⮞ TRABECULECTOMY (LIMBUS-BASED APPROACH)

- After local anesthesia is administered—retrobulbar block or blitz anesthesia, a traction suture is placed; this could be a superior rectus bridle suture or a corneal traction suture depending on surgeon preference.
- A limbus-based conjunctival opening is then created about 5 mm posterior to the limbus with subsequent dissection anteriorly in the subtenon space using blunt forceps. Careful manipulation of the conjunctiva is important to avoid formation of conjunctival buttonholes.
- Hemostasis is maintained, avoiding excessive cauterization.
- Antimetabolite can then be applied to the sclera/subtenon space at this point making sure to apply over a wide area and not just in the area of planned scleral flap.

- A half-thickness scleral flap is then created in the preferred shape (rectangular, triangular, square and trapezoid) depending on surgeon preference. This is dissected anteriorly all the way to clear cornea.
- A paracentesis is then created, preferably temporally for easy access if needed postoperatively.
- The anterior chamber is then entered under the flap with a 15° blade and a block of tissue is then excised using the blade and a Vannes scissors. An alternative way of creating the sclerostomy is to use a Kelly Descemet's punch.
- A surgical peripheral iridectomy is then done and hemostasis is maintained under the flap.
- 10-0 nylon interrupted sutures are then used to suture down the flap titrating for flow at different IOP levels while reforming the anterior chamber. Releasable sutures could be used especially if lasers are not readily available for suturelysis in the postoperative period. Preplacement of the initial sutures is an option that is performed by some surgeons prior to creating the sclerostomy.
- After adequate titration of flow from under the flap with more flow at higher IOP, the conjunctival wound is then sutured closed in the surgeon's preferred method. This can be done in two separate layers closing Tenon's capsule in running locking fashion and the conjunctiva in a running nonlocking fashion. Care must be taken to use a tapered needle to avoid large holes in the conjunctiva.
- Anterior chamber is reformed to create a bleb and to check for the presence of any leaks.
- Prophylactic antibiotics and steroids are used as indicated.

## GLAUCOMA DRAINAGE DEVICES

- After local anesthesia is administered—retrobulbar block or blitz anesthesia, a traction suture is placed; this could be a superior rectus bridle suture or a corneal traction suture depending on surgeon preference.
- A conjunctival peritomy with relaxing incisions at either end is created over 3–4 clock hours in the quadrant of tube placement (usually superotemporal for the first device if there is no contraindication) with subsequent dissection posteriorly in the subtenon space using blunt forceps between the recti muscles bordering that quadrant. Careful manipulation of the conjunctiva is important to avoid formation of conjunctival buttonholes.
- The recti muscles are identified or isolated depending on the type of device.
- Nonvalved devices like Baerveldt (AMO) and Molteno (Molteno Ophthalmic Limited) devices may require

manipulation prior to placement during surgery to prevent immediate postoperative hypotony. The options include ligating the tube with an absorbable suture like a 6-0 vicryl close to the plate or a prolene suture in which case the tube will need to be opened at a later date with a laser. Stenting the tube with a 4-0 nylon suture ,'ripcord suture', prior to ligature makes allowance for opening the tube at the slit lamp by pulling out the ripcord suture in either of the prior scenarios.

- Valved glaucoma drainage devices like the Ahmed Glaucoma valve (New World Medical, Inc.) may require priming with balanced salt solution prior to placement.
- Hemostasis can be maintained with wet field cautery as there may be some amount of bleeding.
- After device is prepared, the device is placed in the quadrant either between the muscles or under the muscles depending on the type and size of the glaucoma drainage device.
- The plate is then secured to the sclera using nonabsorbable suture like a 9-0 prolene or nylon about 8 mm posterior to the limbus.
- The tube is then cut to the approximate length required for good placement in the anterior chamber.
- A paracentesis is then created, preferably temporally for easy access if needed postoperatively.
- A 23-gauge needle is then used to enter the anterior chamber and the tube is inserted into the opening. Slight tunneling in the sclera prior to entering the anterior chamber parallel to the iris will help prevent erosion. The tube position should preferably be away from the cornea and the iris.
- The tube is secured to the sclera with sutures and covered with a donor scleral or corneal patch graft is preferred. There are some alternative bioengineered patch grafts available in the market.
- Slits could be made in the tube at this point to vent the anterior chamber while waiting for the ligature sutures to dissolve in the case of nonvalved devices. The anterior chamber can also be filled with a small amount of viscoelastic material at the end of the case if a valved device is used to prevent early postoperative hypotony.
- The ripcord suture is buried in the subconjunctival space adjacent to the tube in an area where it could be accessed easily usually the inferotemporal subconjunctival space.
- The conjunctiva is then closed at the limbus as water as possible in the surgeon's preferred manner.
- Prophylactic antibiotics and steroids are used as indicated.

# Pediatric Corneal Transplant Surgery

*Gerald W Zaidman*

## ➤ SURGICAL TECHNIQUE

All transplants are done under general anesthesia with corneal donor tissue preferably between the ages of 4 and 19. At the beginning of the case, intravenous mannitol is given. Children are then hyperventilated by the anesthesiologist. A scleral support ring is sutured to the sclera. The donor tissue is usually 0.5 mm larger than the recipient tissue. After the initial trephination, the anterior chamber is entered with a #75 blade. The anterior chamber is then reformed with a dispersive viscoelastic. A specially designed pediatric cyclodialysis spatula is then used to lyse any synechiae between the iris and the cornea (manufactured by Storz). The patient's corneal button is then excised with pediatric corneal transplant scissors also designed by Storz (E 3320 RL). Because of the likelihood that infants and children will develop significant amounts of positive pressure during excision of the cornea, the surgeon will often begin by placing the donor cornea on top of the recipient corner before it is fully excised. For example, the patient's cornea is excised for approximately 270°. While it is being excised, one suture, usually 7'o silk, is placed at the 9 o'clock position to temporarily close the wound. Viscoelastic is then placed on the surface of the patient's cornea and the donor cornea is then sutured in position with two 9-0 nylon sutures, one at 6 o'clock and one at 12 o'clock. The surgeon then continues excision of the donor cornea using corneal scissors and eventually slides the patient's cornea out from underneath the donor cornea. This way one never has a completely open eye and this avoids loss of lens or vitreous as a result of the high positive pressure typically seen in these children's eyes. The corneal wound is then closed with between 12 to 16 interrupted 10-0 sutures. All the sutures knots are trimmed and buried and the scleral support ring is excised.

Any other indicated surgical procedures such as cataract extraction, pupilloplasty, vitrectomy, etc. are typically performed after the donor cornea is partially sutured into position, but the timing of these additional procedures will vary depending on the patient's underlying pathology and the surgeon's preference.

In children and infants with anterior stromal corneal scarring typically due to an infectious etiology such as herpes simplex keratitis, a lamellar keratoplasty is often the procedure of choice. Finally, in cases of endothelial decompensation, such as congenital hereditary endothelial dystrophy (CHED), if the surgeon is experienced with endothelial keratoplasty, Descemet's stripping automated endothelial keratoplasty (DSAEK) can be attempted instead of a penetrating keratoplasty. Finally, a keratoprosthesis may be indicated in a small number of patients. It is rarely indicated as a primary procedure, but may be useful in children who had multiple failed corneal transplants.

# DLEK, DSAEK, DSEK, DMEK

*Marianne O Price, Francis W Price, Arundhati Anshu*

## Recipient Preparation (Note: Donor tissue should be prepared before entering the recipient eye)

1. Make a paracentesis with 75 super-sharp blade marked with Gentian violet. Place it slightly to the right of where the temporal incision will be placed (for right handed surgeons).
2. Inject 1% lidocaine in eye.
3. Fill eye with air bubble; if unstable chamber, may use anterior chamber (AC) maintainer or viscoelastic.
4. With reverse Price/Sinskey hook (Moria), score 6–7 mm diameter without engaging stroma.
5. Strip Descemet's membrane (DM) from within scored area without tearing stromal fibers.
6. Inject Trypan blue into anterior chamber to show up any residual DM tags.
7. Create another paracentesis with 75 super-sharp blade for left hand.
8. Create temporal incision (5 mm scleral tunnel for DSEK or 2.8 mm corneal for DMEK).
9. Irrigate AC with balanced salt solution (BSS), remove residual Trypan blue.
10. Remove any residual tags of DM with intraocular forceps or irrigation/aspiration (IA) handpiece.
11. For DMEK only: create inferior peripheral iridectomy with intraocular scissors or vitrector in IA/PI cut mode, and use bimanual IA to aspirate posterior pigment layer to ensure a patent PI.

## Donor Preparation and Insertion

### Descemet's Stripping Endothelial Keratoplasty (DSEK)

1. Obtain precut tissue from eye bank or dissect tissue using a microkeratome.
2. Trephine the donor to the desired diameter.
3. Insert the graft using taco fold, suture pull-through, funnel glide or insertor technique.
4. Watch graft closely to make sure endothelial side faces downwards.
5. Inject air beneath the graft to lift and press it against the host stroma.
6. Fill AC with air—ensure patient can still see light.
7. Using a LASIK roller, massage the host cornea to position the graft and drain residual fluid from the graft/host interface.
8. After 8 minutes remove most of the air from the AC and replace with BSS.
9. Patient lays face up in recovery room and is instructed to lay face up as much as possible until returning for examination the next day.

### Descemet's Membrane Endothelial Keratoplasty (DMEK)

1. Step-by-step donor preparation—Submerged Cornea Using Backgrounds Away Technique (SCUBA) technique.

a. Score DM with blunt-tipped instrument or small tying forceps.

b. Stain with Trypan blue and rinse with corneal storage medium.

c. Using microfinger instrument, strip DM inward from trabecular meshwork about 1–2 mm, 360°, and remove any tears in edge.

d. Lightly pull DM off about halfway to center, 360°.

e. Lightly punch tissue with 8.0–9.0 trephine.

f. Finish stripping DM while watching closely for any tearing.

g. Lay tissue scroll on donor corneal-scleral rim and cover with storage solution until ready to insert.

2. Stain donor tissue with Trypan blue and insert using a glass pipette or intraocular lens (IOL) injector.

3. Suture the temporal incision with 10-0 nylon.

4. Rotate the scrolled donor tissue, so, endothelial side faces downward and it begins to unfold by injecting bursts of BSS through any paracentesis.

5. Once the graft starts to unfold, place a small air bubble under it and tap on cornea to allow bubble to unroll scrolled side; as more unfolds, inject larger air bubble.

6. Position graft by making 'golf swings' on corneal surface with irrigating cannula.

7. Once the graft is fully unfolded, fill AC with air—ensure patient can still see light.

8. In recovery room, patient lays face up for 60 minutes.

9. Check to make sure intraocular pressure (IOP) is okay and PI not blocked by air.

10. Instruct patient to lay face up as much as possible until examination next day and give pupillary block warning signs.

*Surgical technique videos can be viewed at:* http://www.youtube.com/user/DSEKdoc/feed

## Direct Links to Specific Technique Videos

### DSEK

*Donor dissection with the microkeratome*: http://youtu.be/XczfGXp0uCc

*Donor insertion through a funnel glide*: http://youtu.be/ZyxnDB_KtSg

*DSEK surgery*: http://youtu.be/yOh_4hG8gJw

### DMEK

*Donor preparation (SCUBA technique)*: http://youtu.be/_RUvYAG1VWg

*DMEK surgery*: http://youtu.be/ECn43kLK2EE

# Descemet's Membrane Endothelial Keratoplasty

*Isabel Dapena, Vasilios S Liarakos, Martin Dirisamer, Miguel Naveiras, Ru-Yin Yeh, Ruth Quilendrino*
*Konstantinos Droutsas, Kyros Moutsouris, Marieke Bruinsma, Gerrit RJ Melles*

## ⮞ DESCEMET'S MEMBRANE ENDOTHELIAL KERATOPLASTY SURGICAL STEPS

### Obtaining a Soft Eye

- Surgical bed in anti-Trendelenburg position
- Manual ocular massage after retrobulbar injection
- Ten minutes oculopressure with Honan balloon
- Eye speculum tightness control during surgery.

### Incisions and Descemetorhexis

- Mark a 3.0 mm incision at 12 o'clock.
- Make three side ports (10:30, 01:30 and 07:30 (right eye)/04:30 (left eye)).
- Fill the anterior chamber (AC) with air.
- Score and strip Descemet's membrane (DM) with reversed Sinskey hook and/or scraper.
- Complete main incision creating a clear corneal tunnel.
- Remove recipient DM from the AC through corneal incision.
- Keep the AC filled with air.

### Intraoperative Preparation of the Descemet's Membrane Endothelial Keratoplasty (DMEK) Graft

- Rinse the roll with balanced salt solution (BSS) 2–3 times making sure that the roll opens a few times.
- Stain the DMEK roll with vision blue 0.06% twice (for about 1–2 minutes each).
- Remove the excess of stain and rinse on top of the membrane with BSS to obtain a double roll.
- Aspirate the stained DMEK-double roll into the injector.

## Donor Implantation and Unfolding

- Remove air from AC and pressurize the eye with BSS.
- Turn the injector so that the double-roll is facing upwards (i.e. hinge down).
- Carefully inject the DMEK-roll into the AC.
- Check the orientation of the graft in the AC with *Moutsouris sign* (i.e. position a cannula inside one of the rolls and observe the tip turning blue).
- Unfold and center the graft by careful indirect maneuvers with air and BSS, and by gently tapping onto the recipient outer corneal surface with a cannula.
- Position the DMEK graft against recipient posterior stroma by lifting the donor with an air bubble under its surface.
- Completely fill the AC with air pressurizing the eye during 60 minutes.
- After this time, remove half of the air and pressurize with BSS.
- After surgery, keep patient in a supine position for 24–48 hours.

## ⮞ BIBLIOGRAPHY

1. Dapena I, Moutsouris K, Droutsas K, et al. Standardized "no-touch" technique for Descemet membrane endothelial keratoplasty. Arch Ophthalmol. 2011;129:88-94.
2. Liarakos V, Dapena I, Ham L, et al. Intraocular graft unfolding techniques in Descemet membrane endothelial keratoplasty (DMEK). Arch Ophthalmol. (In press).
3. http://www.niios.com.

# Deep Anterior Lamellar Keratoplasty

*David D Verdier*

1. Determine size and centration of lamellar bed and graft. Lamellar bed diameter is usually 8.0–8.25 mm. Donor diameter is typically 0.25 mm larger than lamellar bed, or matched in keratoconus or high axial myopia eyes.
2. Trephine recipient cornea 60–80% stromal depth with a Hessburg-Barron vacuum trephine.
3. Big-bubble technique: Place a 27-guage 5/8 inch needle bevel down in the trephine groove at 4/5 stromal depth, advance 3–4 mm into the stroma to a paracentral location, and inject 0.5 cc of air to form the big bubble.
4. To confirm the presence of the big bubble, a small air bubble can be placed in the anterior chamber through a self-sealing limbal paracentesis incision either before or after the big-bubble air injection is performed. The small anterior chamber air bubble will be displaced peripheral by a successful big bubble.
5. Debulk the anterior 2/3 corneal stroma with an angled crescent blade.
6. Lower intraocular pressure by releasing a small amount of fluid from a self-sealing limbal paracentesis site.
7. Make a quick nick incision ('brave slash') with a 15° blade into the central cornea stroma just deep enough to enter the big bubble, and quickly withdraw the blade to avoid the anteriorly displaced Descemet's membrane.
8. Dissect posterior stroma from Descemet's membrane. First enter the nick incision with a blunt-tip cyclodialysis spatula and advance to form tunnel dissections extending to the 3, 6, 9 and 12 o'clock lamellar bed edge. Unroof each tunnel with blunt-tip curved Vannas scissors to form four quadrants. Complete dissection with a blunt-tip instrument such as the Tan marginal dissector and remove stromal wedges by severing the peripheral edge with blunt-tip DALK scissors.
9. Donor preparation: Stain donor tissue endothelium with trypan blue, then score peripheral endothelium with a Sinskey hook and remove endothelium by gently grasping edges with tie forceps. Trephine donor tissue to desired diameter.
10. Place donor tissue in lamellar bed epithelial side up, and secure with 16 interrupted 10-0 nylon sutures. Bury suture knots.
11. Place antibiotic and corticosteroid drops of choice, followed by placement of a pressure patch and shield.

# UVA-light and Riboflavin Mediated Corneal Collagen Crosslinking

*Erik Letko, William B Trattler, Roy S Rubinfeld*

The procedure consists only of eye drops and a UV light. The procedure would be:

1. The patients are administered riboflavin eye drops.
2. The patient is examined in the slit lamp to ensure sufficient riboflavin saturation of the cornea.
3. The patient receives X # of minutes of UV treatment (based on the UV device used).
4. The patient is sent home.

With epithelial on CXL—it is not surgery—just eye drops followed by a UV light.

However, some doctors remove the epithelium. But the future is epithelial on CXL, which is actually performed by the technician.

# Phototherapeutic Keratectomy

*John W Josephson, Jay M Lustbader*

## ▶ PHOTOTHERAPEUTIC KERATECTOMY PROCEDURE

1. Program the excimer laser. Usually a circular treatment, with a diameter a bit larger than the area of corneal pathology. The number of pulses varies with the underlying corneal pathology. Usually 30 pulses for recurrent erosions and several hundred for other disorders.
2. Position the patient under the laser.
3. Apply topical anesthetic.
4. Remove the epithelium over the area of corneal pathology. For recurrent erosions, the epithelium can be removed with a cellulose sponge. For other conditions, an instrument such as a surgical blade should be used.
5. Apply a moistened cellulose sponge over the debrided area, followed by a dry cellulose sponge.
6. Adjust the excimer beam to center the treatment over the de-epithelialized area of the cornea.
7. Apply the laser treatment.
8. For recurrent erosion, apply 20–30 laser pulses and stop. For treatment of other conditions, apply enough pulses to remove the majority of the corneal pathology (approximately 4 pulses of laser remove 1 micron of tissue).
9. Bring the patient to the slit lamp to examine the cornea and see if sufficient tissue has been removed to treat the underlying disease.
10. If necessary, apply additional laser treatment and re-examine.
11. At the conclusion of the procedure, apply topical antibiotic, steroid, nonsteroidal drops, and a bandage contact lens.
12. Examine the patient at the slit lamp before discharge.

# Boston Keratoprosthesis in the Management of Limbal Stem Cell Failure

*Kenneth M Goins*

## ▶ BOSTON KERATOPROSTHESIS TYPE I SURGERY: STEP BY STEP SURGICAL PREPARATION

1. Indication: high-risk keratoplasty candidate; in this case, chemical burn with a previous failed keratoplasty approximately 50 years ago.
2. B-scan ultrasound needed for opaque media; in this case, no excavation of the optic disc or retinal detachment is present. Dense lens cataract is noted. Axial eye length is calculated in the event that a keratoprosthesis model for aphakia is planned.
3. Anesthesia type depends upon the patient and clinical situation; monitored anesthesia care with a retrobulbar block using 2% lidocaine and 0.75% bupivacaine is most common, followed by general endotracheal anesthesia.
4. Flieringa scleral support ring is secured into position with 6-0 vicryl suture.
5. Trephination may be done using either manual or vacuum trephines; to accommodate the 8.5 mm posterior plate, an 8.5 mm recipient and 9.0 mm donor trephination is preferred.
6. Keratoprosthesis assembly:
   - Place the adhesive strip to surgical drape.
   - Place the anterior surface of the optic portion of the keratoprosthesis to the adhesive strip.
   - Cut the donor cornea centrally using a 3 mm trephine or skin punch.
   - Center the cut donor cornea onto either a 9.0 mm manual or vacuum trephine, and perform trephination.
   - After trephination, place the donor onto the optic portion of the keratoprosthesis.
   - Apply viscoelastic to the posterior surface of the corneal donor.
   - Place the 8.5 mm posterior plate onto the stem of the optic portion of the keratoprosthesis, posterior to the donor cornea.
   - Fixate the optic, corneal donor and posterior plate into position using a titanium ring using a plastic hand wrench.
7. Trephine the recipient cornea at 8.5 mm.
8. Iris hook placement is used to facilitate extracapsular cataract surgery in cases with poor dilation as shown.
9. Open sky can-opener capsulotomy or capsulorhexis is used to gain access to the lens nucleus.
10. Delivery of the lens nucleus
11. Cortex removal with either manual or automated irrigation/aspiration handpiece.
12. Contrary to the video shown, the posterior capsule should be left intact, and a posterior chamber lens implant should be inserted into either the sulcus or capsular bag to help reduce the risk of retinal detachment; in the case shown, it was chosen to leave the patient aphakic, perform a posterior capsulotomy and anterior vitrectomy intraoperatively.
13. The keratoprosthesis is secured into position using 16–24 9-0 nylon interrupted sutures. In this case, a kertaoprosthesis model for aphakia is used, which provides optical correction, based on the preoperative axial length. In cases with an intraocular lens in place, a keratoprosthesis model for pseudophakia, which has no additional optical correction, would be preferred.

14. Seton placement is recommended afterward to help reduce the risk of vision loss from glaucoma; the Ahmed FP-7 model is most commonly used.

15. Following seton placement, subconjunctival injections of cephazolin 50–100 mg, dexamethasone 5 mg, and triamcinolone 40 mg are given at the end of the case.

16. The following day, a bandage contact lens, Kontur model (base curve 9.8, power plano, diameter 16.0 mm) is placed onto the ocular surface for protection.

17. Standard medications: prednisolone 1%, medroxyprogesterone 1%, levofloxacin 0.5%, and vancomycin 16 mg/ml are given QID for 1 month, TID for 1 month, BID for 1 month, and continued daily thereafter.

# Radial Keratotomy

*John B Cason, Kerry K Assil*

When performing radial keratotomy (RK) for the correction of myopia, there are several key steps to keep in mind. First and foremost, an appropriate nomogram needs to be consulted, which takes patient's age and degree of myopia into account, thereby recommending an appropriate diameter optical zone and number of incisions, for desired correction.

Following the instillation of topical antibiotics and anesthetic, a lid speculum is placed. With the patient fixating upon the operating microscope light, the corneal light reflex is used as a landmark to identify the corneal apex (closest anatomical neighbor to 'the line of sight') and a Sinskey hook is used to indent the epithelium at this location (compensating for any operating microscope associated parallax).

An optical zone marker is then used to indent the corneal epithelium, concentric to this centration mark. Next, the appropriate number (4, 6 or 8) winged, preinked RK marker is centered around the optical zone and compressed against the cornea, thus leaving an inked epithelial imprint. Following confirmatory pachymetry (coinciding with the thinnest corneal point by OrbScan imaging), the Diamond keratome tip is extended to 90% of the pachymetric site measurement.

Next, a guarded bidirectional diamond blade (such as the Genesis blade) is used to make sequential radial incisions beginning with the thinnest corneal site first and sequentially proceeding to progressively thicker quadrants. Forceps globe stabilization should be carried out during this portion of the procedure. The guarded diamond incisions should be initiated at the optical zone margin, with the diamond blade tracing centrifugally (down-hill) along the inked markings, towards the limbus and then retracing centrally back to the optical zone. Care should be taken to terminate each incision one millimeter shy of the corneal-scleral limbus.

Postoperative steroid and antibiotic drops should be administered for 2 weeks.

# Incisional Surgery for Natural and Surgically-Induced Astigmatism

*Matthew D Council*

- Determine the amount and location of the patient's corneal astigmatism. This should be verified with multiple modalities, including corneal topography and manual keratometry.
- Use a nomogram or online calculator to prepare a surgical plan documenting the location and extent (clock hours) of the incisions.
- Preoperatively, place reference marks on the patient's eye with the patient in the upright position prior to any sedation.
- Intraoperatively, align an axis marker with the previously placed reference marks.
- Use the axis marker to identify the beginning and end point for each incision.
- Place viscoelastic over the cornea in the area of the planned incision.
- Prepare the blade for use: if the DONO nomogram is used, the blade is set to 600 microns. If the NAPA nomogram is used, the blade is set to 90% of the thinnest pachymetry reading.
- Fully insert the blade in the peripheral cornea just inside the limbus at the starting point of the incision. The blade should enter perpendicular to the corneal surface.
- Draw the blade back toward the surgeon in a curvilinear fashion, completing the incision.
- If the limbal relaxing incision (LRI) overlaps a planned clear corneal phacoemulsification incision, first create a partial LRI corresponding to the width of your planned incision. Enter the eye with the keratome through the partial LRI. After cataract removal and before the removal of viscoelastic, extend the LRI to its full length on either side.
- Perform the second incision as indicated by the nomogram.
- Use balanced salt solution on a blunt tip cannula to irrigate the incisions. This will ensure they are of the proper length and are not full thickness.
- Proceed with the remainder of the cataract surgery if indicated.
- Postoperatively, treat with antibiotic and anti-inflammatory drops as per usual care. Continue the antibiotic drops until the epithelium is healed.

# Excimer Laser Surface Ablation: Photorefractive Keratectomy and Laser Subepithelial Keratomileusis

*Noel Rosado-Adames*

Laser surface treatment procedures, including photorefractive keratectomy (PRK) and laser subepithelial keratomileusis (LASEK), use the excimer laser to ablate corneal tissue without the need of a partial-thickness incision in the corneal stroma.

The initial step of these procedures consists of removal of the corneal epithelium, and leaving a smooth, undamaged Bowman's membrane. Removal of the corneal epithelium can be achieved by mechanical, chemical or laser techniques. Mechanical removal of corneal epithelium can be performed with the use of a spatula, blunt blade or with the use of a motorized brush. Chemical removal of the corneal epithelium involves the use of 20% ethanol solution applied to the corneal epithelium for 20–40 seconds in a well or on a corneal light shield and thoroughly irrigated with balanced salt solution (BSS). After application of alcohol, the corneal epithelium is easily debrided with a spatula or microsponge. LASEK is a modification of this technique in which the corneal epithelium is partially trephined with the use of a corneal marker and 20% alcohol solution is applied for 20–40 seconds to loosen the epithelium. A flap of corneal epithelium is then raised, hinged usually at the 12 o'clock meridian, and protected for postoperative repositioning. The excimer laser in phototherapeutic keratectomy (PTK) mode has also been used to completely remove the corneal epithelium before stromal ablation.

After epithelial removal/flap formation, PRK and LASEK techniques are identical. Before beginning the procedure, a reference mark may be placed on the eye at 180°. The patient is then laid flat under the laser. A small dose of anxiolytic such as diazepam may be given preoperatively for patient comfort. A topical anesthetic, such as tetracaine or proparacaine should be used. The head should be positioned such that the alignment marks placed at the limbus preoperatively coincide with the laser reticule to minimize cyclotorsion. The reticule is centered on the pupil. Iris registration may be used to reduce error from cyclotorsion, while pupil tracking may help to account for eye movement. It is still important, however, to encourage the patient to stare at the fixation target during the procedure. The foot pedal is depressed to engage the laser treatment. In eyes with high myopia or after previous corneal surgery, mitomycin C (MMC) 0.02% may be applied topically to help prevent the potential complication of corneal haze. At the conclusion of the treatment, the cornea is irrigated with cool BSS solution to lower the corneal temperature and remove any debris from the ocular surface. In LASEK, the epithelial flap is repositioned. A drop of a topical steroid, nonsteroidal anti-inflammatory drug (NSAID), and antibiotic are usually given. A bandage contact lens is then placed, and a clear eye shield is positioned over the eye. If bilateral treatment is planned, this is normally performed concurrently.

# LASIK Technique with the Mechanical Microkeratome Hansatome

*Roberto Pineda, Andrea Cruzat*

1. *Sterile surgery*: Hat, facemask, sterile gown, sterile field, sterile equipment and sterile powder-free surgical gloves.

2. *Laser calibration and input*: Before surgery, perform a laser fluence test. Check the refractive correction, diameter of the ablation, calculation of the tissue to be removed and personal settings of the patient.

3. *Microkeratome preparation prior to surgery*:
   - Check the blade under high magnification of a microscope.
   - Assemble the microkeratome (MK) and check that each component has been inserted correctly.
   - Check the gears for any debris and that they can be moved manually without friction.
   - Visually check the blade movement and that the suction ring is free of debris and the suction ring orifice is clean.
   - Check the electrical and suction connections with the console, that the suction is working correctly and that the manometer for the vacuum reading is on the desired setting.
   - Place the MK on the suction ring and check the complete movement (backward and forward) before placing it on the eye and check the reading on the voltmeter to make sure that the blade is moving correctly.

4. *Preoperative medication and pachymetry*: Instill a topical antibiotic and a topical anti-inflammatory drop. Also, apply one to two drops of topical anesthetic (0.5% proparacaine) to anesthetize the ocular surface once the patient is lying on the operating bed. Obtain two to three measurements of central pachymetry and record the lowest of these.

5. *Positioning and preparing the field*: Check chin and forehead positioned on the same plane, cover the fellow eye, clean the skin of the eyelids with a solution of povidone iodine and dry, apply disposable sterile self-adhesive drape excluding the eyelashes from the operating field.

6. *Speculum and corneal preplaced marks*: Check that the opening after the gentle position of the speculum is enough for the application of the suction ring and MK pass. Mark with corneal markers stained with methylene blue the peripheral cornea previously dried to allow the exact repositioning of the flap. Irrigate the cornea and conjunctiva with balanced salt solution (BSS) and clean with Merocel sponges to remove the excess of dye, any secretions, eyelashes or other debris.

7. *Suction ring application and tonometry*: Reassure the patient and tell them what to anticipate. With the handle positioned nasally, place the ring on the center of the cornea and center it on the pupil. Apply certain degree of pressure for good adhesion and activate the suction until vacuum is achieved and it emits a signal, the pupil diameter has increased and corneal pressure can be checked with a surgical tonometer (Barraquer) to indicate that the intraocular pressure (IOP) is sufficiently high (approximately 65 mm Hg if the applanation by the tonometer on the cornea lies inside the circle inscribed on the inferior surface of the tonometer).

8. *Microkeratome advancement*: Apply some drops of liquid (proparacaine is recommended by several MK manufacturers) to wet the corneal surface and the suction ring pivot to facilitate insertion and reduce friction. Insert the microkeratome on the suction ring pivot until it locks

into the teeth. Press the foot pedal to pass the MK forward along the suction ring grooves until it is interrupted by a stop, change to the other pedal to reverse and return to its original position. Release the suction by pushing its foot pedal and remove the ring together with the MK.

9. *Lifting the flap*: Check head position of the patient and fixation on the target light. Dry the fornices after removal of the MK and suction ring to minimize tear debris into the flap interface. A spatula, hook or irrigating cannula is used to lift the flap and reflect it superiorly. It might be necessary to use a dry Merocel sponge to wipe any fluid or blood pooling the flap edge and at the hinge.

10. *Ablation depth and pachymetry*: The flap thickness performed with the MK may vary from the manufacturer's flap thickness setting. The calculated ablation depth can be reconfirmed prior to the laser ablation and pachymetry can be obtained intraoperatively when treating corneas where the residual stromal bed could approach the limit.

11. *Refractive ablation*: Use dim oblique illumination to allow physiologic dilation of the pupil, decreased light sensitivity and improve patient's cooperation and ability to fixate on the blinking target. Check focus and pupil centration of laser and connect the eye tracker. Push the laser foot pedal and perform the laser ablation monitoring centration and protecting the hinge if it is necessary (i.e. against-the-rule astigmatism, big ablation zone).

12. *Flap reposition*: Apply some BSS to the stromal surface to clean of any debris and to allow the flap to distend easily to its original position. Reposition the flap with the cannula towards the center of the cornea starting from the hinge. Reirrigate interface to loosen adherent debris in a centrifugal direction.

13. *Flap realignment*: The aim is to obtain a symmetrical gutter, realignment of the preplaced corneal marks and a clean interface with the observation of a round placido reflex in the case of ring illumination as in the case with the VISX laser. Gently sweep the epithelial surface of the flap with a wet Merocel sponge from the hinge to the inferior margin to distend the flap and multiple centrifugal pararadial sweeps. Dry the remaining liquid with a dry Merocel sponge and check flap position increasing magnification and using direct light (using the placido single-ring light source), checking the preoperative marks and performing the gutter test (margins of the flap are symmetrical). Push gently the cornea about 1 mm outside the margin of the flap to check adequate adhesion (slade striae test).

14. *Speculum removal and double-check*: Gently remove the speculum taking care to avoid any contact with the cornea and displacing the flap. Ask the patient to blink softly and check the flap is in position. Instill one drop of antibiotic and anti-inflammatory and put a transparent eye shield to protect. Thirty minutes after surgery, examine the patient at the slit lamp to insure correct flap alignment and absence of significant interface debris and give postoperative instructions to the patient and follow 1 day after surgery.

# Light Adjustable Lenses Post Corneal Refractive Surgery

*Guillermo Rocha, Zale D Mednick*

## ❧ LIGHT ADJUSTABLE LENS TECHNOLOGY

### Device Description

#### Light Adjustable Intraocular Lens

The Calhoun Vision light adjustable lens (LAL) (Figs 1A and B) is a foldable posterior chamber, ultraviolet (UV) absorbing, three-piece photoreactive silicone lens with blue polymethyl- methacrylate (PMMA) modified-C haptics, a 6.0 mm biconvex optic with squared posterior edge, and an overall length of 13.0 mm. The LAL optic design incorporates a silicone posterior surface layer of 100 μm or less with a higher concentration of UV absorber than the photoreactive bulk lens material to further enhance the UV absorbing properties of the LAL lens and provide additional retinal safety during the lens power adjustment procedures.

Implanted LALs can be treated for spherical power adjustments in the range of –2.0 to +2.0 diopters (D) and cylindrical power adjustments in the range of 0.75 to 2.0 D in 0.25 D increments with controlled application of UV light (365 nm) using the light delivery device (LDD). Lenses are manufactured in a range from 10 to 30 D.

A summary of the LAL design characteristics is presented below:

*Lens Optic*
- Material: Photoreactive, UV absorbing silicone
- Light transmission: UV cutoff at 10% T = 390 ± 2 nm

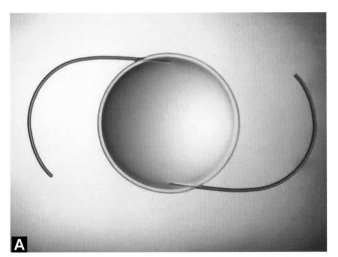
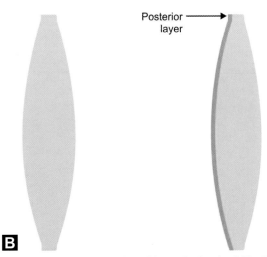

**Figs 1A and B:** Calhoun Vision light adjustable intraocular lens (IOL). (A) Top view; (B) Cross-section view of the optic showing LAL with and without a posterior layer. The posterior layer of up to 100 microns of a higher UV absorber concentration further enhances the UV absorbing properties of the lens and safety of the retina during irradiation procedures

for a +20 D lens
- Index of refraction: 1.43
- Diopter power: +10 to +15.0 D and +25.0 to +30 D in 1.0 D increments; and +16.0 to +24.0 D in 0.5 D increments
- Optic type: Biconvex with posterior layer of 100 μm or less with a higher concentration of UV absorber than optic bulk
- Optic edge: Square on posterior surface and round on anterior surface
- Overall diameter: 13.0 mm
- Optic diameter: 6.0 mm

*Haptics*
- Configuration: Modified C
- Material: Blue PMMA
- Haptic angle: 10°

### Light Delivery Device

The light delivery device (LDD) is used to deliver UV light of a selected wavelength [365 nm ± 5 nm full width half maximum (FWHM)], spatial irradiance profile and diameter to produce a predictable change in the power of the Calhoun Vision LAL.

The LDD (Fig. 2) consists of a UV light source, projection optics and control interface installed on a standard slit lamp. The light source employed is a mercury (Hg) arc lamp delivered to the projection optics through a liquid filled light guide. The light source includes a narrow band-pass interference filter producing a beam with a center wavelength of 365 nm.

The LDD is designed to guarantee alignment of the adjustment and photolocking beam with the LAL. The LDD projects an alignment reticle image to the surgeon's eye through a common optical path shared with the UV light projection optics. The reticle image and UV light profile are both parfocal and parcentral to within 50 microns. The reticle image is visualized through the microscope of a standard slit lamp, which serves as the mechanical support for the LDD. The line width of each reticle feature is 35 ± 5 microns, giving good visualization of the alignment target.

The subject participates in alignment by attending a fixation target, parcentral to the delivery beam. The fixation target appears at infinity to the subject, and subtends 0.20° of arc from the subject point of view. The fixation target has an adjustable intensity and is modulated to flash at a frequency of 5 Hz to maintain the subject's attention. The fixated subject is perfectly aligned and treatment will occur on the visual axis of the subject.

The LDD is operated through a computer interface, which controls the characteristics and initiation of the light beam delivery. A joystick or foot switch is used to activate light beam delivery, and a touchscreen is used to control

System Overview
Light Delivery Device

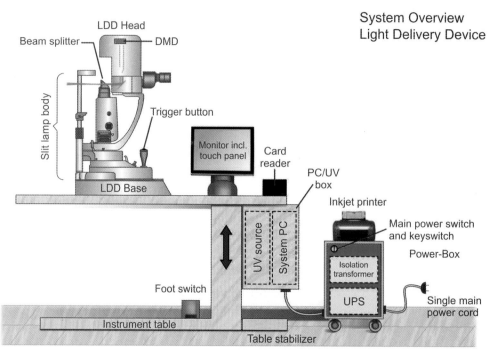

**Fig. 2:** Slit lamp based light delivery device

the user interface.

The LDD uses two different methods for the generation of the light beam irradiance profile or pattern required for the refractive adjustment treatment and the lock-in treatment. The profiles for the refractive power adjustments are digitally created while the lock-in profiles are generated using a static apodizing filter.

## Indications for Use

The light adjustable lens is an IOL intended for the treatment of aphakia in patients in whom the cataractous natural lens has been removed by phacoemulsification and who wish to minimize their postoperative refractive error. Following implantation, UV light is used to adjust the LAL power using the LDD to correct residual postoperative hyperopia or myopia up to 2 D with up to 2 D postoperative cylinder with a maximum defocus equivalent of 2.0 D.

## Patients

The preoperative examination will be performed no more than 60 days prior to surgery and consists of a complete ophthalmic examination. Only subjects meeting all inclusion/exclusion criteria will be implanted with the LAL. The implant lens power required for the refractive target will be calculated based upon the ocular biometry data and a standard IOL power calculation formula for the surgeon.

## Light Adjustable Lens Implantation and Refractive Adjustment

### Surgical Procedure

The LAL will be implanted using standard microsurgical techniques. All instruments and procedures used will be identical to those routinely used for phacoemulsification-type cataract extraction. The surgical procedure will be performed as follows:

- The eye will be prepared for surgery and draped according to the surgeon's standard procedure.
- A clear corneal or scleral incision of approximately 3.0–3.8 mm will be made using the surgeon's standard instrumentation and techniques.
- Viscoelastic will be used to fill the anterior chamber through the incision opening. A hyaluronic based viscoelastic (e.g. Viscoat, Amvisc, Healon or similar) is

recommended.

- The surgeon will perform an anterior circular capsulorhexis of a maximum of 5.5 mm using his standard technique.
- The surgeon will extract the cataract by phacoemulsification.
- The LAL will be introduced into the eye using the Naviject 2.9-3P injector. Only this validated instrument may be used to introduce the LAL into the eye.
- Residual viscoelastic will be aspirated from the eye using the surgeon's preferred technique.
- Routinely, the wound will be closed without a suture. If the unsutured wound is not watertight, it will be closed with a suture by the surgeon using his/her standard technique.
- Immediately after completion of the surgery, a non-steroidal anti-inflammatory such as nepafenac (nevanac), bromfenac (xibrom), acular LS and a 4th generation fluoroquinolone antibiotic such as gatifloxacin or moxifloxacin will be applied to the eye. Additional medications as deemed necessary will be used at the surgeon's discretion.
- The subject will be instructed to use the UV protective eyewear provided at all times indoors and outdoors, until the lock-in treatments are completed. If an optional patch is used postoperatively according to the surgeon's preference, the subject will be instructed not to remove the patch and keep it in place until the surgeon removes it at the 1 day postoperative visit. The UV protective eyewear will be provided once the patch is removed at the 1 day postoperative visit.

The UV protective spectacles (UVEX Bandit™ #S1600 with clear lens and #S1603 with Espresso tinted lens) are supplied to the patient as a two-pair set, with one having clear lenses for indoor use and the other pair with tinted lenses for outdoor use. The patient will be instructed to wear the spectacles at all times, keeping the eyes closed when changing spectacles.

For subjects requiring spectacle correction for refractive errors in the fellow eye, 'fitover' UV protective spectacles (Cocoons Models C202, C302, C422, C402 or C412 with clear lens or gray lens; manufactured by Live Eyewear) are supplied to the patients as a two-pair set, with one pair having clear lenses for indoor use and the other pair with tinted lenses for outdoor use. The patient will be instructed to wear the 'fitover' UV protective eyewear over their existing corrective spectacles at all times, keeping the eyes closed when changing spectacles.

CHAPTER 119

## Power Adjustment Procedure

Seventeen to twenty-one days after surgery, the subject will return for examination and adjustment treatment.

Any eye with evidence of premature photopolymerization as detected by slit lamp examination will be scheduled for a power neutral adjustment in 0–2 days after detection. The lock-in treatments will be scheduled for 3 days post previous LDD treatment. The patient is cautioned to be vigilant in wearing the UV protective eyewear at all times until 1 day after the second lock-in treatment.

The refractive adjustment is based on the difference between the measured manifest refraction and emmetropia [manifest refraction spherical equivalent (MRSE) = 0.0 D]. For eyes not requiring an adjustment (where MRSE is within ±0.125 D of emmetropia), a power neutral dose will be given.

- The eye will undergo study examination prior to the adjustment treatment. The manifest refraction measured prior to adjustment will be performed results will be recorded. The surgeon then takes the MRSE of the final refraction to enter into the LDD for spherical adjustments and the sphere, cylinder and axis of the final refraction for spherocylindrical adjustments.

- The eye will be dilated using tropicamide 1.0% and phenylepherine 2.5% and positioned in front of the LDD. The subject will be comfortably situated with chin in the chinrest and forehead against the support bar.

- The eye will be examined using the LDD slit lamp to determine if the complete LAL edge around the circular periphery is visualized without any obstruction by the pupil. If some part of the LAL is obscured by the pupil, additional dilation drops will be administered.

- To adjust the lens power, the surgeon will follow the touchscreen prompts to enter the subject identification, eye to be treated, i.e. OD or OS, and manifest refraction (sphere, cylinder and axis), target refraction, LAL ID, LAL base power, and K values on the LDD.

- For LALs not requiring a refractive adjustment (MRSE within ±0.125 D of emmetropia), the investigator will treat the lens with a power neutral dose and will follow the touchscreen prompts to enter the subject identification, eye to be treated, i.e. OD or OS, LAL ID, LAL base power, and K values on the LDD. Values of '0' are entered for manifest refraction (sphere, cylinder and axis) and target refraction.

- The surgeon will confirm all information by pressing the 'Confirm' button.

- A topical anesthetic such as proparacaine HCL or tetracaine HCL (alcaine, ophthaine, ophthetic or equivalent) will be applied to the cornea in order to facilitate insertion of a contact lens required for focusing of the LDD and stabilizing the eye.

- The Calhoun Vision supplied contact lens (0.835X) will be positioned on the cornea using hydroxypropyl methylcellulose as the coupling media. The contact lens supplied will be similar to those used in other ophthalmic procedures in which customized magnification is required. To assure correct magnification for treatment, only the Calhoun Vision designated contact lens will be used.

- Using the slit lamp, the surgeon will focus on the LAL with the contact lens in place on the cornea.

- The LDD alignment reticle image and fixation light will be activated. The surgeon will instruct the subject to focus on the LDD fixation light with the study eye and align the irradiation reticle with the periphery of the LAL.

- The surgeon will initiate the irradiation delivery as prompted by the LDD display using the joystick to keep the LAL centered in the alignment reticle. In the case of subject movement, loss of alignment or loss of focus, the surgeon will pause the irradiation, quickly refocus and realign the lens with respect to the irradiation beam, and immediately resume irradiation to limit the duration of any pauses once the irradiation delivery has been initiated.

- Following the light adjustment, the patient will be instructed to continue to wear the UV protective eyewear provided at all times.

- For spherocylindrical adjustments only, the patient will return 3–5 days following the power adjustment treatment and will be refracted following the procedures described above. The manifest refraction will be entered into the LDD and an additional adjustment or lock-in #1 will be performed. The same procedures followed for the first adjustment will be repeated.

## Lock-in Irradiation Procedure

All subjects will return at 3–5 days following the final power adjustment treatment for lock-in treatments using the LDD. The lock-in procedure is comprised of two lock-in treatments delivered 3–5 days apart.

The patient is cautioned to be vigilant in wearing the UV protective eyewear at all times until 1 day after the second lock-in treatment.

- The first lock-in treatment will be administered 3–5 days postadjustment treatment.
- The subject will be refracted and examined prior to each lock-in treatment.
- The subject will be dilated using tropicamide 1.0% and phenylepherine 2.5% and positioned in front of the LDD. The subject should be comfortably situated with chin in the chinrest and forehead against the support bar.
- The subject will be examined using the LDD slit lamp to ensure that the complete LAL edge around the circular periphery is visualized without any obstruction by the pupil. If some part of the LAL is obscured by the pupil, additional dilation drops will be administered.
- If adequate pupil dilation is not achieved with additional drops, it is recommended that the treatment be rescheduled and that the dilation is attempted at another visit.
- The surgeon will enter the subject ID, eye to be treated, i.e. OD or OS, and manifest refraction (sphere and cylinder), LAL ID and base power as directed on the touchscreen of the LDD.
- The surgeon will confirm all information by pressing the 'Confirm' or 'OK' button.
- The surgeon will select 'LOCK IN' on the screen.
- The surgeon will confirm the selection by pressing the 'Confirm' or 'OK' button.
- A topical anesthetic such as proparacaine HCL or tetracaine HCL (alcaine, ophthaine, ophthetic or equivalent) will be applied to the cornea, to facilitate insertion of the contact lens required for focusing of the LDD and to stabilize the eye.
- The contact lens (0.835X) supplied by Calhoun Vision will be positioned on the subject's cornea using hydro-xypropyl methylcellulose as the coupling media. The contact lens supplied will be similar to those used in other ophthalmic procedures in which a customized magnification is required. To assure correct magnification for treatment, only the Calhoun Vision designated contact lens will be used.
- Using the slit lamp, the surgeon will focus on the LAL with the contact lens in place on the cornea.
- The alignment reticle image and fixation light will be activated. The surgeon will instruct the subject to focus on the fixation light and align the irradiation reticle with the periphery of the LAL.
- The surgeon will perform the irradiation delivery as prompted by the LDD display using the joystick to keep the LAL centered in the alignment reticle. In the case of subject movement, loss of alignment or loss of focus, the investigator will pause the irradiation, quickly refocus and realign the lens with respect to the irradiation beam, and immediately resume irradiation to limit the duration of any pauses once the irradiation delivery has been initiated.
- The subject will be instructed to continue to wear the UV protective eyewear provided at all times.
- The subject will return for the second lock-in treatment at 3–5 days after the first lock-in treatment.
- The subject will be permitted to discontinue wear of the UV protective eyewear the next day after the second lock-in treatment.

Typically, a follow-up examination will be performed 1 week after the last lock-in treatment.

*Note*: The authors have no proprietary or financial interests in any aspect of this study.

# Femtosecond Refractive Lenticule Extraction and Small Incision Lenticule Extraction

*Karim Mohamed-Noriega, Jodhbir S Mehta*

All ReLEx procedures share similar surgical steps at the beginning of the procedure (first-half, shared steps). After these common steps, there are specific steps for FLEx or SMILE (second-half, specific steps).

## ☞ COMMON ReLEx, FLEx AND SMILE STEPS (FIRST-HALF SHARED STEPS)

- Verify that patient is candidate for the surgery.
- Selection of laser settings (The authors' current standard setting parameters for the Visumax 500 are shown in Table 1 of chapter Femtosecond Refractive Lenticule Extraction and Small Incision Lenticule Extraction).
- Confirm that correct refractive treatment is programmed in the computer.
- Confirm correct eye.
- Confirm small cone size.
- Application of topical anesthesia.
- Povidone-iodine (betadine), scrub of the skin and eyelids.
- Standard sterile draping and insertion of the speculum.
- Eye is docked under the curved cone.
- Patient must fixate on the green target light.
- Eye is centered on the visual axis.
- Suction is applied, only when appropriate centration on the visual axis is achieved.
- Confirm pupil centration with infrared scan and wait for full suction to be achieved.
- Laser treatment can be started in a scanning pattern spiral in/out.

## ☞ FLEx SPECIFIC STEPS (SECOND-HALF STEPS)

- After the laser firing is completed, mark the cornea with asymmetric ink marker.
- Lift the flap with a Seibel spatula.

- The lenticule edge is identified with a Sinsky hook. Then it is partially separated from the residual stromal bed (RSB) with a Seibel spatula and gently grasped with nontoothed serrated forceps to fully separate the lenticule from the RSB.
- Flush the RSB with balanced salt solution (BSS).
- Reposition the flap.
- Flush the RSB with BSS.
- Make sure the flap is placed in correct position according to markings.
- Dry the flap and flap edge with sponges.
- A bandage contact lens may be applied if needed if epithelium disrupted.
- Topical steroid and antibiotic eyedrops are applied.

## ☞ SMILE SPECIFIC STEPS (SECOND-HALF STEPS)

- After the laser firing is completed, the superior incision is opened with a Sinskey hook.
- The anterior and posterior surfaces of the lenticule are identified by using the Sinskey hook.
- The anterior surface of the lenticule is first dissected and separated from the cap with a femtolamellar dissector (Asico®) in a smooth rotational movement similar to a cornea lamellar dissection. Make sure the dissection goes beyond the lenticule margins.
- The posterior surface of the lenticule is dissected as previously described for the anterior surface of the lenticule.
- The lenticule is grasped from the edge with forceps (Tan DSAEK Forceps AE-4226, ASICO) and is extracted from the cornea.
- The interface is flushed with BSS.
- Topical steroid and antibiotic eyedrops are applied.

# Femtosecond Laser Keratoplasty

*M Farid, S Garg, Roger F Steinert*

## ✢ GRAFT CUTTING AND SURGERY

The donor tissue is mounted on an anterior artificial chamber and cut by the femtosecond laser using preprogrammed parameters set by the surgeon. Alternatively, the tissue can be ordered 'precut' with the same laser parameters as those to be used on the patient, a service now provided by numerous eyebank facilities. The donor tissue diameter should be set to the same size as the host.

The laser cut for the recipient can be done under topical or retrobulbar anesthesia. Although new model femtosecond lasers work faster than the older models, more complex cutting patterns and alignment marks can increase the amount of time the suction ring remains on the eye, prompting more surgeons to opt for preoperative retrobulbar block to ensure patient comfort. Proper centration of the suction ring on the patient is crucial to ensure centration of the graft. A customized trephination pattern per surgeon's preference is selected and programmed into the laser computer. The laser pattern always starts from the deepest portion of the cornea and works its way anteriorly. The software of the Intralase laser allows for a maximum diameter of 9 mm, with the ability to vary the side-cut angle from 30° to 150°. In the example of the zigzag incision, the laser parameters are a posterior side-cut from deep stroma to anterior stroma at 30° to the periphery. The second cut is a lamellar cut at a depth of 320 μm from the anterior surface, which is intersected by the third incision, the anterior side-cut that advances toward the anterior corneal surface at 30°. Anterior diameter of the zigzag cut can be set at 8, 8.5, or 9 mm, based on the

patient's corneal diameter and the surgeon's preference. The femtosecond laser also allows for the placement of radial alignment marks on the host and donor that facilitate ease of precise suture placement and improved tissue distribution.

If small bubbles are seen at the initiation of the laser, then the laser energy is in the anterior chamber fluid and a full thickness incision is being performed. If a full thickness incision was not the intended action, then a quick cessation of the laser should be done by lifting off of the foot pedal. As long as the laser has not reached Descemet's membrane, then resetting of the posterior depth can be done and the laser restarted within the posterior corneal stroma to maintain a bridge of uncut tissue. If transporting a patient to the operating room after the laser corneal cut is necessary, a posterior bridge of uncut corneal tissue is essential to ensure globe stability.

After completion of the femtosecond laser incision, the eye is treated with antibiotic drops and shielded prior to transport of the patient to the operating suite. The host corneal button is separated with a blunt lamellar dissector to reveal lamellar and side-cut incisions made by the laser. Although laser incisions usually separate cleanly, limited sharp dissection with a surgical blade or scissors may be needed in areas of dense corneal scarring. After completion of the blunt dissection, the anterior chamber is entered with a blade and the corneal bridging tissue is cut with corneal scissors. The donor cornea is then sutured into place using the surgeon's suturing pattern of choice. Care should be taken to match the depth of the suture in the donor and host to achieve a true 'lock and key' configuration.

# Femtosecond Laser Enabled Correction of Postkeratoplasty Astigmatism

*Nikhil L Kumar, David S Rootman*

## Femtosecond Enabled Astigmatic Keratotomy: Surgical Procedure

Preoperative planning includes the assessment of the amount and axis of corneal astigmatism, corneal thickness and graft size. When there is a disagreement between the axis of the manifest refraction and the topography, the topography axis is favored. The amount of topographic cylinder rather than the manifest cylinder is used to determine the length (degrees) of the keratotomy.

All treatments are paired symmetric incisions of the same length, centered on the steep axis. The depth of the incisions is set at approximately 90%, based on either the Pentacam or ultrasound pachymetry at the incision location. Each incision is made 0.5 mm within the graft-host junction, such that the diameter is set at 1 mm less than the graft diameter measured by calipers at the time of surgery.

The surgery is performed using the 150 kHz IntraLase FS system (IntraLase Corp, Irvine, California, USA) under topical anesthesia (proparacaine 0.5%), with the laser adapted to make therapeutic cuts. The eyelids are prepared with Betadine sponges. Using a sterile marking pen, the graft host junction is marked in the steep and flat axis, as this helps to center the incisions on the graft. The IntraLase limbal suction ring is then applied and the cone is positioned. The cone is centered on the graft host junction. Applanation is judged as adequate if the fluid meniscus is at least beyond the graft host junction. The position of the programmable arcuate cuts are checked and repositioned as necessary. Once satisfied with incision location, the foot pedal is depressed and the cuts completed. Suction is released and the ring removed.

Treatment parameters are based upon the topographic location and radial extent of the steep meridian. Up to 6 diopters of cylinder was treated with 45–50 degree arc length, 6–10 diopters with 50–60 degree arc length, and greater than 10 diopters with 60–70 degree arc length.

After surgery, patients are treated with topical tobramycin and dexamethasone (TobraDex; Alcon, Mississauga, Ontario, Canada) four times daily for 1 week. Thereafter, they are placed on a maintenance dose of topical steroid according to their individual requirements.

# Corneal Instrumentation for Femtosecond Laser Enabled Penetrating Keratoplasty

*Ying Qian, Bennie H Jeng*

## ‣ DONOR CORNEA LASER RESECTION WITH FEMTOSECOND LASER*

1. A flat lockable table should be placed under the gantry and leveled so that the edge of the table does not go past the joystick toward the surgeon.
2. A sterile drape is placed on the lockable table.
3. Balance salt solution and intravenous tubing should be connected to the artificial anterior chamber making sure that tight connection is established and all air has been vented.
4. The donor cornea is centered and mounted carefully on the artificial anterior chamber. Viscoelastic may be placed on the artificial anterior chamber before mounting the donor cornea
5. Donor epithelium is removed at the discretion of the surgeon.
6. The central mark is made with the marking pen.
7. Central and peripheral (7 mm) pachymetry should be performed with ultrasound sterile pachymeter on the cornea. In most cases donor tissue will be de-epithelialized generally requiring differences to the programmed depths for the donor and recipient.
8. A sterile cone is placed in the cone holder and the gantry is lowered carefully to obtain full applanation of the donor cornea.
   a. Make sure the IV line from the IV bottle to the artificial anterior chamber is open to allow back-flow during the applanation.
   b. Make sure the cone applanates the cornea evenly. The laser objective may have to be pushed up manually to obtain green light during docking.
   c. If there is movement of the corneal central mark, elevate the gantry so the cornea is not applanated and reposition in the X-Y direction. Using the X-Y movement when the cornea is applanated can produce an elliptical cut.
9. Do not overapplanate the cornea. However, some wrinkles can be seen when full applanation is achieved.
10. Depressed the foot pedal and perform the laser cut.
11. Reduce the fluid pressure in the artificial anterior chamber prior to removing applanation.
12. When the laser treatment is complete, lift the gantry and mark the cornea with an eight-cut RK marker across the cut.
13. Perform blunt dissection of the graft with a Sinskey hook. Vannas scissors can be used if significant attachments are found.
14. Place the graft endothelial side up in a storage media and stored until ready for transplantation as per normal protocol.

## ‣ RECIPIENT CORNEA LASER RESECTION WITH FEMTOSECOND LASER

1. Determine patient appropriateness for FS laser keratoplasty:
   a. Corneas which have areas that are too thin to make lamellar cuts or who have a high risk of graft dehiscence in the laser suite due to large areas of thinning are not good candidates for the procedure. Corneas that are very scarred or vascular may also need special consideration.

---

*Adapted from IntraLase FS™ Laser Training Manual: Section 7 IntraLase Enabled Keratoplasty

b. Patients should have relatively normal conjunctival and limbal architecture to ensure ability to place suction ring and applanate. Cystic glaucoma blebs, tight interpalpebral fissures, or shortened fornices can create difficulty. Placing a ring on the patient's anesthetized eye in the clinic as a trial may be beneficial.

c. Ensure patient's ability to cooperate and remain still during the procedure. Depending upon the location of the femtosecond laser, monitored anesthesia care may be limited. It is possible to perform a retrobulbar block before the FS laser incisions are placed.

d. Evaluate ability of the patient to be safely transported from the laser to the OR. An obese patient or one with limited mobility may require more effort upon transferring to the bed, which could pose a risk for graft dehiscence, especially if a full thickness incision has been inadvertently made.

2. Obtain ultrasound pachymetry at the 7–8 mm zone at 45° intervals for 360° around the cornea, noting the thinnest area measured. Alternatively, anterior segment OCT can be used to obtain serial measurement in the same fashion.

3. Measure white-to-white diameter horizontally and vertically with calipers while patient is reclined in the examination room.

4. Determine the particular shape of the graft based upon the patient's pathology. Most shapes will work equally well, but special considerations can be made for thin cornea periphery, or patients who may pose a higher risk of graft dehiscence in which case a top-hat configuration may be most appropriate.

5. Determine the diameter of the graft to be transplanted. Note the diameter in the chart and surgical planning to refer to if the donor tissue is to be cut in house by the surgeon on the day of the transplantation. It is also necessary to determine an appropriate diameter preoperatively for those ordering precut tissues from the eye bank.

6. Request the cornea tissue as usual. If using a precut order, determine whether a standard template from the eye bank is appropriate for the patient, or if custom sizes and shapes are needed.

a. If custom cuts are being requested, all side cut and lamellar-cut parameters need to be entered in the ordering sheet clearly, specifying all depths and diameters. If side-cut angles are angled greater or less than 90°, it is very important to check that the cuts will be intersecting and overlapping, remembering that only the anterior diameters of the side cuts are entered as settings into the IntraLase FS laser, while the posterior diameters are determined based upon the trigonometric equation $w = d/\tan\theta$. This is mainly a concern for the anterior side cut because it is important to ensure overlap with the lamellar cut. The posterior side cut will intersect the lamellar cut at its anterior depth which is set into the laser.

b. Example (Fig. 1): Anterior side-cut diameter = 8.0 mm (set into laser), Lamellar depth = 300 μm; Anterior side-cut angle = 30°. What is the posterior diameter of the anterior side cut? ($w = d/\tan\theta$; where, $w$ = deviation from anterior diameter, $d$ = lamellar depth, $\theta$ = side-cut angle)

    i. Tan 30° = 0.577

    ii. 300 μm/0.577 = 520 μm

    iii. 520 μm × 2 = 1,040 μm (multiplied × 2 because the deviation occurs at both ends of the diameter)

    iv. 8.0 mm − 1,040 μm = 6.96 mm or roughly 7.0 mm

7. On the day of surgery, patient is brought to the laser suite and placed supine on the femtosecond bed. If necessary, an IV can be started and mild sedation can be administered by anesthesia preoperatively for patient comfort.

8. Topical anesthetic drops (proparacaine) are placed on the operative eye.

9. A drop of dilute 5% betadine solution is placed on the conjunctiva.

10. Peripheral pachymetry can be performed once again if desired.

11. Ensure the posterior side cut depth is about 60 μm less than the thinnest measurement made preoperatively.

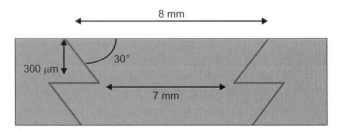

**Fig. 1:** A schematic cross section of a 'zig-zag' shaped corneal graft demonstrating the types of cuts (anterior angle; lamellar; posterior angle) and suggested cut profile measurements

12. A centration mark is placed on the epithelium over the center of the pupil with a Genetian Violet marker. This can be done with or without the aid of the laser microscope.

13. If precut tissue has been ordered, confirm the settings from the eye bank against the settings that are to be used for the patient. Diameter and depths can be matched exactly or slightly oversized depending upon surgeon preference.

14. Decide if energy levels of the cuts need to be increased above the average setting due to dense scarring or other factors. (Our typical settings are below)

15. Decide if the radial alignment marks are to be used. If the diameter of the graft causes the 500 μm marks to go outside the 9.5 mm surgical zone, the laser will not let the surgeon proceed.

16. Place the applanation cone onto the laser.

17. Place the suction ring on the patient's eye. This should be placed as centrally as possible. This again can be done with or without the aid of the surgical microscope.

18. Place the patient under the laser and lower the gantry onto the center of the suction ring with the joystick until adequate depression of the gantry is reached and the green light indicator has lit.

19. Begin applanating the cone onto the cornea by squeezing the suction ring handles and applying gentle pressure upwards onto the cone. The gantry can also be lowered a bit further during this process. Some prefer to lock to suction ring handles during this step and applanate by lowering the gantry until the adequate applanation is achieved.

20. Observe the meniscus ring through the oculars or viewing screen to ensure that it reaches as far peripherally as possible to avoid the possibility of incomplete cuts.

21. Once adequate applanation has been reached, release the handles of the suction ring to lock it onto the cone.

22. Using the centration mark (or pupil if visible) center the cornea in the reticle of the laser.

23. After good centration, have the laser technician confirm and lock the laser to proceed with the treatment.

24. If no error messages have occurred, depress the food pedal. Closely observe the cornea while the incisions are being made to ensure no suction loss, shrinking of the meniscus inside the incision diameter, or evidence of full-thickness penetration.

25. Once the incisions are complete, release suction on the ring.

26. Observe the patients eye for any evidence of fluid leak or flattening of the anterior chamber.

27. Close the patient's eyelid and place a gentle patch and shield over the eye.

28. Assist the patient off the table and into a wheel chair for immediate transport into the operating room.

29. Place patient supine and administer a retrobulbar block as usual. Place Honan pressure balloon on the eye for 20–30 minutes.

30. Remove the Honan and thoroughly prepare the lashes and skin with betadine as per usual protocol with no additional drop on the conjunctiva to avoid the possibility of betadine into the wound or anterior chamber.

31. Place radial alignment marks onto the epithelium if desired or highlight the laser alignment marks with a Genetian Violet marker.

32. Bluntly dissect the laser incisions with a Sinsky hook. Enter the anterior chamber with 15° blade and instill a viscoelastic device.

33. Finish the posterior dissection with corneal-scleral scissors along the plane of the posterior side cut.

34. Bring the donor tissue into the surgical field and proceed with the transplant as per usual fashion using an interrupted or continuous suturing technique.

35. Postoperative management is the same for standard penetrating keratoplasty.

119 CHAPTER

# INDEX

*Page numbers followed by f refer to figure and t refer to table*